PHYSICAL REHABILITATION OF THE INJURED ATHLETE

PHYSICAL REHABILITATION OF THE INJURED ATHLETE

4th EDITION

James R. Andrews, MD

Orthopaedic Surgeon, Andrews Sports Medicine and Orthopaedic Center
Medical Director, The Andrews Institute, Gulf Breeze, Florida;
Medical Director, The American Sports Medicine Institute
Clinical Professor, Department of Orthopaedic Surgery
The University of Alabama Birmingham Medical School, Birmingham, Alabama;
Clinical Professor, Department of Orthopaedic Surgery
University of South Carolina School of Medicine, Columbia, South Carolina;
Clinical Professor of Orthopaedics and Sports Medicine
University of Virginia Medical School, Charlottesville, Virginia

Gary L. Harrelson, EdD, ATC

Director, Organizational Development and Education, DCH Health System
Tuscaloosa, Alabama

Kevin E. Wilk, PT, DPT

Adjunct Assistant Professor, Programs in Physical Therapy
Marquette University, Milwaukee, Wisconsin;
Associate Clinical Director, Champion Sports Medicine, Physiotherapy Associates
Director of Rehabilitative Research, American Sports Medicine Institute
Birmingham, Alabma;
Rehabilitation Consultant, Tampa Bay Rays Baseball Club, Tampa Bay, Florida

ELSEVIER
SAUNDERS

1600 John F. Kennedy Blvd.
Ste 1800
Philadelphia, PA 19103-2899

PHYSICAL REHABILITATION OF THE INJURED ATHLETE   ISBN: 978-1-4377-2411-0

Library of Congress Cataloging-in-Publication Data
Physical rehabilitation of the injured athlete/[edited by] James R. Andrews, Gary L. Harrelson, Kevin E. Wilk. – 4th ed.
    p. ; cm.
    Includes bibliographical references and index.
    ISBN 978-1-4377-2411-0 (hardcover : alk. paper)
    I. Andrews, James R. (James Rheuben), 1942- II. Harrelson, Gary L. III. Wilk, Kevin E.
    [DNLM: 1. Athletic Injuries–rehabilitation. 2. Physical Therapy Modalities. QT 261]

617.1'027–dc23   2011043782

Content Strategist: Don Scholz
Content Specialist: Julia Bartz
Publishing Services Manager: Anne Altepeter
Senior Project Manager: Doug Turner
Designer: Ellen Zanolle

Printed in the People's Republic of China

Last digit is the print number: 9   8   7   6   5   4   3   2   1

To my wife, Lisa, and my son, Noah,

who did not write a word of this text or edit a single paragraph

but rather sacrificed much more…our time together.

I'm grateful for your abounding love and blessed that you are both in my life.

Love, Gary

Contributors

James R. Andrews, MD
Orthopaedic Surgeon
Andrews Sports Medicine and Orthopaedic Center;
Medical Director
The Andrews Institute
Gulf Breeze, Florida;
Medical Director
The American Sports Medicine Institute;
Clinical Professor
Department of Orthopaedic Surgery
The University of Alabama Birmingham Medical School
Birmingham, Alabama;
Clinical Professor
Department of Orthopaedic Surgery
University of South Carolina School of Medicine
Columbia, South Carolina;
Clinical Professor of Orthopaedics and Sports
Medicine
University of Virginia Medical School
Charlottesville, Virginia
Chapter 13: Rehabilitation of Elbow Injuries

Christopher Arrigo, PT, MS, ATC
Owner
Advanced Rehabilitation
Tampa, Florida
Chapter 12: Shoulder Rehabilitation
Chapter 13: Rehabilitation of Elbow Injuries

Michael J. Axe, MD
Clinical Professor
Department of Physical Therapy
University of Delaware
Newark, Delaware
Chapter 3: Developing Treatment Pathways

Victoria L. Bacon, EdD
Professor of Counselor Education
Licensed Psychologist
Licensed School Counselor
Certified Group Psychotherapist
Bridgewater State University
Bridgewater, Massachusetts
Chapter 1: Psychologic Factors of Rehabilitation

Jake Bleacher, PT, MS, CSCS
Board Certified Specialist in Orthopaedic Physical Therapy
Staff Physical Therapist
The Ohio State University Sports Medicine Center and
    Rehabilitation Services at Care Point
Gahanna, Ohio
Chapter 24: Proprioception and Neuromuscular Control

Jason Brumitt, PT, PhD, SCS, ATC, CSCS
Assistant Professor
School of Physical Therapy
Pacific University
Hillsboro, Oregon
Chapter 18: Rehabilitation of Thigh Injuries

Gray Cook, PT, MS, OCS, CSCS
Adjunct Professor, Athletic Training
Averitt University
Danville, Virginia
Chapter 22: Functional Movement Assessment
Chapter 23: Functional Training and Advanced Rehabilitation

Bradley Cummings, PT, CHT
Center Manager
Director of Physical Therapy
Kentucky Hand and Physical Therapy
Richmond, Kentucky
Chapter 14: Rehabilitation of Wrist and Hand Injuries

Anthony Cuoco, DPT, MS, CSCS
President
Aeon Physical Therapy, PC
Monroe, Connecticut;
Adjunct Faculty
Department of Exercise Science
College of Health Professions
Sacred Heart University
Fairfield, Connecticut
Chapter 26: Plyometric Training and Drills

R. Barry Dale, PT, PhD, DPT, ATC, OCS, SCS, CSCS
UC Foundation Associate Professor
University of Tennessee at Chattanooga
Chattanooga, Tennessee
Chapter 4: Principles of Rehabilitation
Chapter 21: Clinical Gait Assessment

George J. Davies, DPT, MEd, SCS, ATC, CSCS
Professor
Armstrong Atlantic State University
Savannah, Georgia;
Professor Emeritus
University of Wisconsin-LaCrosse;
Consultant, Clinician, and Co-Director
Sports Physical Therapy Residency Program
Gundersen Lutheran Sports Medicine
LaCrosse, Wisconsin
Chapter 24: Proprioception and Neuromuscular Control
Chapter 25: Application of Isokinetics in Testing and
*   Rehabilitation*

Todd S. Ellenbecker, DPT, MS, OCS, SCS, CSCS
Clinical Director
Physiotherapy Associates Scottsdale Sports Clinic;
National Director of Clinical Research
Physiotherapy Associates;
Director
Sports Medicine ATP Work Tour
Scottsdale, Arizona
Chapter 24: Proprioception and Neuromuscular Control
Chapter 25: Application of Isokinetics in Testing and
*   Rehabilitation*

Matthew J. Failla, DPT
Sports Physical Therapy Resident
Department of Physical Therapy
University of Delaware
Newark, Delaware
Chapter 3: Developing Treatment Pathways

Julie Fritz, PT, PhD, ATC
Associate Professor
Department of Physical Therapy
University of Utah
Salt Lake City, Utah
Chapter 17: Low Back Rehabilitation

Kurt A. Gengenbacher, DPT
Sports Physical Therapy Resident
Department of Physical Therapy
University of Delaware
Newark, Delaware
Chapter 3: Developing Treatment Pathways

Gary L. Harrelson, EdD, PCC, ATC
Director
Organizational Development and Education
DCH Health System
Tuscaloosa, Alabama
Chapter 5: Measurement in Rehabilitation

Timothy E. Hewett, PhD, FACSM
Professor and Director of Research
Sports Medicine and The Sports Health and Performance
   Institute
Departments of Physiology and Cell Biology, Orthopaedic
   Surgery, Family Medicine, and Biomedical Engineering
The Ohio State University, Columbus, Ohio;
Professor and Director
Cincinnati Children's Hospital Medical Center
Cincinnati, Ohio
Chapter 9: Rehabilitation Considerations for the Female Athlete

Barb Hoogenboom, PT, EdD, SCS, ATC
Associate Professor
Department of Physical Therapy
Grand Valley State University
Grand Rapids Michigan;
Senior Associate Editor
International Journal of Sports Physical Therapy
Indianapolis, Indiana
Chapter 22: Functional Movement Assessment
Chapter 23: Functional Training and Advanced Rehabilitation

**Todd R. Hooks, PT, SCS, ATC, MOMT, MTC,
   CSCS, FAAOMPT**
Coordinator of Rehabilitation Research and Education
Beacon Orthopaedics and Sports Medicine;
Co-Director of Physical Therapy Services
Cincinnati Reds Baseball Organization
Cincinnati, Ohio
Chapter 15: Temporomandibular Joint
Chapter 16: Cervical Spine Rehabilitation

Brittany Jessee, PT, DPT
Rehabilitation Hospital of Southwest Virginia
Bristol, Virginia;
Alumnus of the University of St. Augustine
St. Augustine, Florida
Chapter 6: Range of Motion and Flexibility

Jeff G. Konin, PT, PhD, ATC, FACSM, FNATA
Associate Professor and Vice Chair
Department of Orthopaedics and Sports Medicine;
Associate Professor
College of Public Health;
Executive Director
Sports Medicine and Athletic Related Trauma (SMART)
   Institute
University of South Florida
Tampa, Florida
Chapter 6: Range of Motion and Flexibility

Leonard C. Macrina, MSPT, SCS, CSCS
Physical Therapist
Board Certified Sports Specialist
Certified Strength and Conditioning Specialist
Champion Sports Medicine
Birmingham, Alabama
Chapter 12: Shoulder Rehabilitation

Terry Malone, PT, EdD, ATC, FAPTA
Professor
Department of Rehabilitation Sciences
University of Kentucky
Lexington, Kentucky
Chapter 7: Principles of Rehabilitation for Muscle and Tendon Injuries

Bob Mangine, PT, MEd, ATC
Associate Director of Sports Medicine
University of Cincinnati;
National Director of Sports Physical Therapy Residency Program
NovaCare Rehabilitation
Cincinnati, Ohio
Chapter 2: Physiologic Factors in Rehabilitation

Mark A. Merrick, PhD, ATC
Associate Professor and Director
Division of Athletic Training
The Ohio State University
Columbus, Ohio
Chapter 8: Therapeutic Modalities As an Adjunct to Rehabilitation

W. Andrew Middendorf, PT, ATC
Center Manager
NovaCare Rehabilitation at the University of Cincinnati;
Clinical Instructor
NovaCare Sports Physical Therapy Residency Program
Cincinnati, Ohio
Chapter 2: Physiologic Factors in Rehabilitation

Edward P. Mulligan, PT, DPT, OCS, SCS, ATC
Assistant Professor and Residency Director
UT Southwestern Medical Center
School of Health Professions
Department of Physical Therapy
Dallas, Texas
Chapter 20: Lower Leg, Ankle, and Foot Rehabilitation

Brian Noehren, PT, PhD
Assistant Professor
Division of Physical Therapy
University of Kentucky
Lexington, Kentucky
Chapter 7: Principles of Rehabilitation for Muscle and Tendon Injuries

Stacey Pagorek, PT, DPT, SCS, ATC, CSCS
Physical Therapist
Board Certified Clinical Specialist in Sports Physical Therapy
Department of Sports Physical Therapy
University of Kentucky
Lexington, Kentucky
Chapter 7: Principles of Rehabilitation for Muscle and Tendon Injuries

Greg Pitts, MS, OTR/L, CHT
Clinical Director
Kentucky Hand and Physical Therapy, LLC
Lexington, Kentucky
Chapter 14: Rehabilitation of Wrist and Hand Injuries

Joseph T. Rauch, PT, ATC
Director of Rehabilitation
University of Cincinnati Football;
Head Athletic Trainer
University of Cincinnati Baseball
Cincinnati, Ohio
Chapter 2: Physiologic Factors in Rehabilitation

Michael M. Reinold, PT, DPT, SCS, ATC, CSCS
Head Athletic Trainer
Assistant Director of Medical Services
Boston Red Sox Baseball Club
Boston, Massachusetts
Chapter 10: Biomechanical Implications in Shoulder and Knee Rehabilitation

Charles D. Simpson II, DPT, CSCS
Minor League Physical Therapist
Boston Red Sox Baseball Club
Boston, Massachusetts
Chapter 10: Biomechanical Implications in Shoulder and Knee Rehabilitation

Lynn Snyder-Mackler, PT, ScD, FAPTA
Alumni Distinguished Professor
Department of Physical Therapy
University of Delaware
Newark, Delaware
Chapter 3: Developing Treatment Pathways

Elizabeth Swann, PhD, ATC
Program Director
Athletic Training and Exercise Science;
Associate Professor
Farquhar College of Arts and Science
Nova Southeastern University
Fort Lauderdale, Florida
Chapter 5: Measurement in Rehabilitation

Jill M. Thein-Nissenbaum, PT, DSc, SCS, ATC
Assistant Professor
Doctor of Physical Therapy Program
University of Wisconsin-Madison;
Staff Physical Therapist
University of Wisconsin Athletics
Badger Sportsmedicine
Madison, Wisconsin
Chapter 11: Aquatic Rehabilitation

Timothy F. Tyler, PT, MS, ATC
Clinical Research Associate
The Nicholas Institute of Sports Medicine and Athletic Trauma
Lenox Hill Hospital
New York, New York
Chapter 26: Plyometric Training and Drills

Tim L. Uhl, PT, PhD, ATC, FNATA
Associate Professor
Co-Director of Musculoskeletal Laboratory
Department of Rehabilitation Sciences
Division of Athletic Training
University of Kentucky
Lexington, Kentucky
Chapter 14: Rehabilitation of Wrist and Hand Injuries

Michael L. Voight, PT, DHSc, OCS, SCS, ATC, CSCS, FAPTA
School of Physical Therapy
Belmont University
Nashville, Tennessee
Chapter 22: Functional Movement Assessment
Chapter 23: Functional Training and Advanced Rehabilitation

Mark Weber, PT, PhD, ATC, SCS
Professor
Department of Physical Therapy
School of Health Related Professions
University of Mississippi Medical Center
Jackson, Mississippi
Chapter 19: Knee Rehabilitation

Kevin E. Wilk, PT, DPT
Adjunct Assistant Professor
Programs in Physical Therapy
Marquette University
Milwaukee, Wisconsin;
Associate Clinical Director
Champion Sports Medicine
Physiotherapy Associates;
Director of Rehabilitative Research
American Sports Medicine Institute
Birmingham, Alabama;
Rehabilitation Consultant
Tampa Bay Rays Baseball Club
Tampa Bay, Florida
Chapter 12: Shoulder Rehabilitation
Chapter 13: Rehabilitation of Elbow Injuries
Appendix A: Throwers' Ten Exercise Program
Appendix B: Interval Rehabilitation Program
Appendix C: Upper Extremity Plyometrics
Appendix D: Advanced Throwers' Ten Program

Jason Willoughby, MS, OTR/L, CHT
Manager
Kentucky Hand and Physical Therapy, LLC
Lexington, Kentucky
Chapter 14: Rehabilitation of Wrist and Hand Injuries

William R. Woodall, PT, EdD, ATC, SCS
Professor
Department of Physical Therapy
School of Health Related Professions
University of Mississippi Medical Center
Jackson, Mississippi
Chapter 19: Knee Rehabilitation

A.J. Yenchak, PT, DPT, CSCS
Director of Physical Therapy
Associate Clinical Instructor for Orthopaedic Surgery
Strength and Conditioning Specialist
Columbia University Orthopaedics—New York
Presbyterian Hospital
New York, New York;
Physical Therapy Fellow
Champion Sports Medicine
Birmingham, Alabama
Chapter 13: Rehabilitation of Elbow Injuries

Bohdanna T. Zazulak, DPT, MS, OCS
Staff Physical Therapist
Department of Sports Physical Therapy
Yale New Haven Hospital
New Haven, Connecticut
Chapter 9: Rehabilitation Considerations for the Female Athlete

Preface

Therapeutic rehabilitation used to be a product of philosophies based on traditions handed down through the years from clinician to clinician. These concepts were usually based on the premise, "Well, it has always worked for me," with the subsequent blending of these philosophies and exercises into therapeutic rehabilitation programs without an underlying scientific rationale for their implementation. Many early rehabilitation concepts and exercises were extrapolated from scientific models using biomechanical principles without empirical research data to support the theories. Today, 20 years since this book's initial publication, the plethora of research to support the scientific underpinnings for rehabilitation principles and concepts for the physically active is astounding. As orthopedic surgical techniques have advanced to help injured athletes regain their abilities to compete at their former levels, so have the scientific (evidence-based) bases for implementing and sequencing therapeutic exercises along a continuum of care. The fourth edition of *Physical Rehabilitation of the Injured Athlete* incorporates these ever-expanding scientific bases for rehabilitation of the physically active.

So, why a fourth edition? What has changed? What is new? What is now considered cutting edge? As in the previous editions, we have brought together contributors who are experts in the field of sports rehabilitation, and many have the monumental task of both practicing clinically and feeling the desire or responsibility to share their research, knowledge, and experience with others through their writings. We have also added some new contributors to provide different perspectives on the content. Furthermore, as with the previous editions, the primary audience for this text is the practicing clinician. Yet we realize that this book is used as a textbook in many educational settings, thus we also took that into consideration when reworking the content and format.

Aside from the obvious fact that this text is in color, what specific content changes and additions will you find in the fourth edition?

- The rehabilitation protocols, or progressions, have been updated to reflect the current research and state of practice. We have found that the rehabilitation protocols are an important feature in this book. Our purpose for inclusion of the protocols is to provide a set of parameters for rehabilitation and

are by no means the only way to do it. Rather, advancement through a rehabilitation program should be based on clinical findings such as the athlete's level of pain tolerance, joint effusion, known tissue-healing parameters, and achievement of specific criteria before the rehabilitation program is advanced. Additionally, surgeons vary their surgical techniques for specific lesions, and this must be considered when developing a rehabilitation regimen. Rehabilitation can by no means be "cookbooked," with a program developed for every injury for every athlete. Each athlete brings a unique set of personal qualities that must be addressed by the clinician to facilitate the athlete's rehabilitation.

- Five new chapters have been added. These include "Developing Treatment Pathways," "Principles of Rehabilitating Muscle and Tendon Injuries," "Temporomandibular Rehabiliation," "Gait Assessment," and "Functional Movement Assessment."
- Chapters have been updated to reflect the latest surgical techniques and subsequent evidence-based rehabilitation rationales. Surgical techniques that are no longer as prevalent as they once were have been deleted. This editon contains an entire section on resortration of athletic performance (Section IV), with an emphasis on functional exercise and testing.
- Not only is this book in color but also has an Expert Consult website that contains content from some chapters that we could not include in the printed text due to space limitations. This allowed us to present the full content that in the past would have been edited out.

It is our hope that this edition of *Physical Rehabilitation of the Injured Athlete* will serve as both a reference for clinicians and a text for students interested in the area of sports rehabilitation. We further hope that this book will serve as a clinician's reference source to improve their clinical practice and will also provide students with the basic knowledge for the development and implementation of rehabilitation programs for the injured athlete.

James R. Andrews, MD
Gary L. Harrelson, EdD, ATC
Kevin E. Wilk, PT, DPT

Contents

Online-Only Material

The appendixes in this section can be found on the Expert Consult website accompanying this text. You can access this site by activating the PIN code on the inside front cover of this book.

Foundational Concepts in Rehabilitation

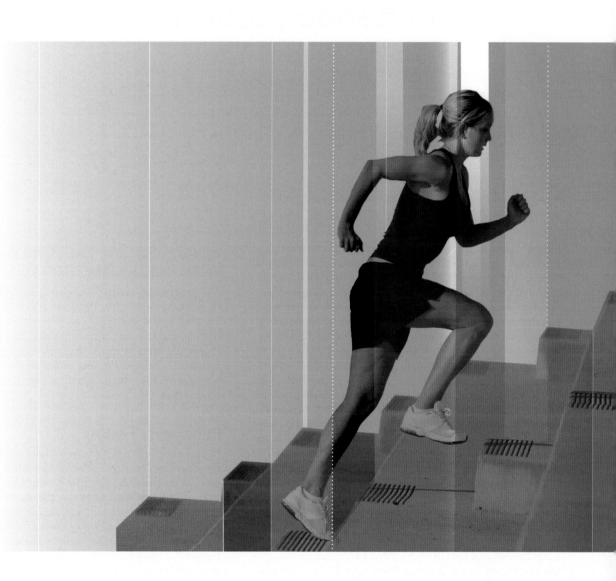

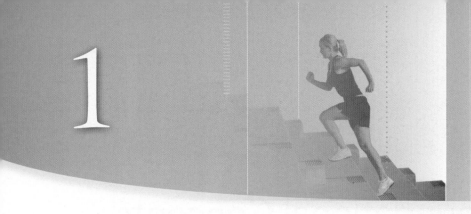

Psychologic Factors in Rehabilitation

Victoria L. Bacon, EdD

CHAPTER OBJECTIVES

- Explain the relationship between psychosocial factors and the potential for sports-related injury.
- Identify signs of psychologic distress in the injured athlete.
- Describe the psychologic response to athletic injury.

- Explain psychologic coping strategies.
- List psychosocial interventions for enhancing rehabilitation.

Sports-related injury is a major concern for athletes, coaches, and teammates. The incidence of sports injuries continues to increase at every level of participation. A great deal of information is available about injury prevention, improved athletic equipment and facilities, and increased safety precautions in most sports. Much less attention has been devoted to understanding the psychologic factors associated with sports-related injuries and rehabilitation, yet the role of psychologic factors has been considered a critical variable.

Sports psychology began as a discipline in the 1960s with the goal of expanding research related to psychologic factors as they relate to athletes and the sports context.[1] Advances in applied psychology in sports did not flourish until years later. MacIntoch et al[2] conducted research in the early 1970s on sports injuries at the University of Toronto over a 17-year time frame that led him to postulate that psychologic factors were critical for understanding sports injuries. A few years later, Taerk[3] continued this line of thinking and offered a multifaceted perspective in which psychosocial factors were proposed as 1 of 10 key elements associated with sports injuries. The 1980s was fertile ground for both evidence-based research and theoretic conceptualizations that served to further advance our understanding of the psychologic factors associated with sports injury and rehabilitation. Figure 1-1 depicts the predominant model of stress and athletic injury in the field today. The purpose of this chapter is to provide an overview of the psychologic factors associated with rehabilitation.

PSYCHOSOCIAL FACTORS ASSOCIATED WITH INJURY AND REHABILITATION

The stress-injury model developed by Anderson and Williams[4,5] in 1988 and updated in 1998 (see Fig. 1-1) is the most widely accepted model and depicts an interrelationship between three psychosocial factors: personality traits, history of stressors, and coping resources as risk factors associated with preinjury vulnerability. These risks factors are believed to influence the stress response of the athlete, which in turn increases the risk for sports injury.

Personality Factors

In the stress-injury model, the authors assert that certain personality characteristics influence the stress response. Various personality characteristics have been studied over the years, yet only a few are believed to temper the effects of stress, including hardiness, locus of control, trait anxiety, motivation, and sensation seeking.[4,6] More recently, Johnson[7] conducted a review of the literature for empiric findings from studies investigating personality variables in the stress-injury model and determined that personality characteristics may serve to moderate the effects of stress for some athletes and, for others, predispose them for risk for injury. This review of the literature revealed evidence in support of the following personality variables as antecedents of sports injury: locus of control, competitive trait anxiety,

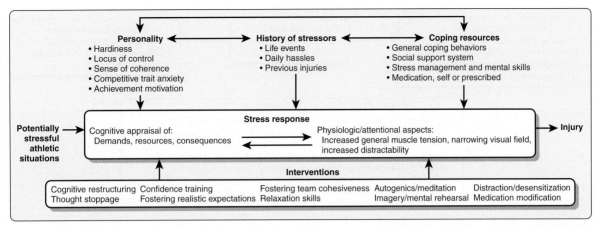

FIGURE 1-1 A model of stress and athletic injury. *(Modified from Anderson, M.B., and Williams, J.M. [1988]: A model of stress and athletic injury: Prediction and prevention. J. Sport Exerc. Psychol., 10:297. Copyright 1988 by Human Kinetics Publishers, Inc. Reprinted by permission.)*

perfectionism, mood states, and self-confidence/self-esteem. Competitive anxiety has received the most attention, with athletes having high trait anxiety being more prone to injury.[8]

Stressors

A large body of knowledge supports the relationship between life stress and risk for injury.[7,8] Although terminology such as *stress* and *stressors* is widely used, it is always helpful to convey clarity with reminders of their meanings. Selye[9] defined stress as "the nonspecific response of the body to any demand." The stimulus that evokes a stress response in individuals is what is referred to as a stressor.[10] There are two types of stressors, acute and chronic. Acute stressors are associated with stressful life events, such as the death of a loved one, natural disasters, or terrorist-related activity. Chronic stressors are longer lasting, with the stressor lasting for months or years. Examples of chronic stress include homelessness, loss of job, or living in a neighborhood with high crime. Athletes experiencing increased stress levels may turn to alcohol, substance use/abuse, disordered eating, high-risk behavior, or other injurious stress-relieving activity.

Assessment of an athlete's history of stressors provides crucial information about key variables related to life events, daily stressors, and previous history of stress.[4] Holmes and Rahe[11] developed the well-known Social and Readjustment Rating Scale in 1967, and it has been widely used to assess an individual's level of stress. This early work laid the groundwork for the development of instruments to assess stress in athletes, such as the Social and Athletic Readjustment Rating Scale[12] and the Athletic Life Experience Survey,[13] as well as the Life Events Survey for Collegiate Athletes, to measure an athlete's history of stressors.[14] See Box 1-1 for examples of positive and negative stress factors.

To further understand the relationship between stress and injury, Nideffer[15] developed a model to describe two potential scenarios, the first being the injured athlete and subsequent considerations regarding the rehabilitation process and the second concerning the athlete with anticipatory anxiety around the possibility of injury. This model (Fig. 1-2) attempts to depict the impact of situational stressors, physiologically and psychologically, as well as potential performance problems. Nideffer contends that athletes' performance will

Box 1-1
Sources of Life Stress*

Examples of negative life stress:

- Death of a significant other
- Illness of a significant other
- Breakup of a relationship
- Loss of job/team position
- Illness or injury to self
- Previous injury
- Academic failure or threat of failure
- Daily hassles

Examples of positive life stress:

- Made captain of the team or a starter
- Moved up a competitive level (e.g., junior varsity to varsity)
- Received media recognition for previous performance
- Experienced changes in what others expect because of success of a sibling
- Made all-star team
- Had a new significant other (boyfriend/ girlfriend)

*Remember that it may not be the event itself, such as those listed, but how the athlete perceives the demands of the event and his or her ability to cope with it.

be hindered if they are worried about the possibility of sustaining an injury or getting reinjured. These situational stressors are thought to have a direct impact on physiologic and psychologic flexibility, which in turn has a negative impact on concentration. This cycle can become a chronic condition resulting in an increase in frustration and anxiety and lower performance for the athlete.

Coping Resources

Cohen and Lazarus[16] define coping as "efforts, both action-oriented and intrapsychic, to manage (that is, master, tolerate, reduce, minimize) environmental and internal demands, and

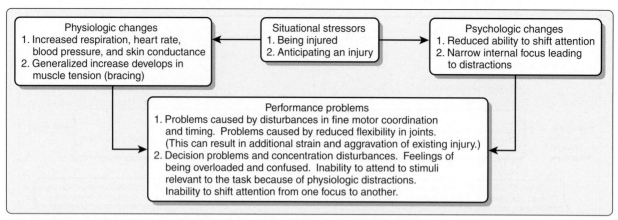

FIGURE 1-2 Physical and psychologic changes accompany increases in pressure as a result of injury or the fear of injury. Problems in performance resulting from stress and reduced physiologic and psychologic flexibility can become chronic. Disturbances in physical flexibility affect concentration, and as the athlete becomes upset at his or her own failure (frustration or anxiety increases), the attentional and physiologic disturbances become stronger and more intractable. *(Modified from Nideffer, R.M. [1983]: The injured athlete: Psychological factors in treatment. Orthop. Clin. North Am., 14:373–385.)*

conflicts among them, which tax or exceed a person's resources." Individuals have two ways of coping. The first, problem-focused coping, is coping by managing the stressor—that is, reducing the demands being made on the athlete. The second, emotion-focused coping, is managing the feelings related to the stressor, which requires the acquisition of additional skills for working with stress.[16] Coping resources refer to coping behavior, social support, and psychologic skills and are believed to moderate the effects of stress and therefore reduce the risk for injury; they can be used for both problem-focused and emotion-focused coping. Box 1-2 lists some of the commons signs and symptoms associated with stress.[17]

Coping behavior encompasses a wide range of behavior and can serve to potentiate the stress response when the athlete lacks good coping behavior. For others, it appears to enhance their ability to cope with stress as a result of using effective ways of coping. An assessment is initiated with an intake interview conducted by a mental health professional. The use of assessment instruments may assist in this process. An appraisal of coping behaviors often includes behaviors associated with health-related factors, such as nutrition and sleep; personal attributes that have an impact on academic success, such as study skills and time management; and overall self-esteem.[4]

A wealth of evidence-based research supports the significance of social support as it relates to health and well-being. In addition, numerous studies have explored social support and risk for injury. Study findings have shown that athletes with high social support have fewer injuries than athletes with little or no social support.[8,18] Social support is defined as "an exchange of resources between at least two or more individuals perceived by the provider or the recipient to be intended to enhance the well-being of the recipient."[19] The Social Support Survey (SSS)[20] assesses an individual's perception of social support on eight scales. Key support factors measured on the SSS include listening support, emotional support, assistance, and reality confirmation. Social support typically comes from key persons in the athlete's family, circle of friends, teammates, coaches, and medical staff. Begel and Baum[21] contend that the potential for increased social support may be jeopardized because athletes spend numerous hours each week on their sport, which in turn places them at risk for social isolation.

Box 1-2

Common Signs and Symptoms Associated with Stress

COGNITIVE
Confusion in thinking
Difficulty making decisions
Decrease in concentration
Memory dysfunction
Poor judgment
Lowered academic performance

EMOTIONAL
Emotional shock
Feelings of anger, grief, loss, or depression
Feeling overwhelmed
Presents with flattened affect
Displays inappropriate and/or excessive affect

PHYSICAL
Excessive sweating
Feeling dizzy
Increased heart rate
Elevated blood pressure
Rapid breathing
Increased symptoms of anxiety

BEHAVIORAL
Changes in behavior patterns
Changes in eating
Decreased personal hygiene
Withdrawal or isolative behavior
Less attention to presentation

From Bacon, V., and Anderson, M. (2007): The Athletic Trainer's Role in Facilitating Healthy Behavior Change: the Psychosocial Domain. Unpublished study. (Reprinted by permission.)

Coping resources also include psychologic coping skills. Examples of psychologic skills that may reduce the risk for sports injury are having the ability to concentrate, remain positive, and regulate arousal states.[5] Social support has been shown to have a positive influence on rehabilitation and recovery.[5,22] Given the significance of social support, it is essential that key players on the rehabilitation team provide the injured athlete with ample support and connection to additional support resources to ensure better health outcomes.

Clinical Pearl #1

It appears that a positive relationship exists between stressful life events, especially those with high negative stress, and the occurrence of injury and disease.

Clinical Pearl #2

Although life stress is most often thought to result from negative events, positive events can also produce stress that can influence life experiences.

PSYCHOLOGIC SEQUELAE OF INJURY

When an athlete is injured, the immediate response of the coach, medical staff, teammates, and family is to assess the severity of the injury and medical needs. Although the physical concerns and welfare of the athlete take precedent, it is essential to remember that psychologic reactions accompany the sports injury. It is important to note that the athlete will experience a range of emotions (e.g., sadness, anger, frustration, fear), which will then be perceived by the athlete as a major stressor.[23] The more serious the injury, the more likely that the athlete will experience intense emotions, as well as the potential loss of primary coping mechanism—that is, exercise, physical activity, and sport involvement—which in turn, creates even more emotional stress for the injured athlete.[24]

Feltz[25] contends that a sports injury has three psychologic effects on an athlete: (1) emotional trauma of the injury, (2) psychologic factors associated with rehabilitation and recovery, and (3) the psychologic impact of the injury on the athlete's future. Box 1-3 lists some of the possible consequences of emotional trauma. Of particular importance are young athletes because adolescents are more likely to experience psychologic distress after injury.[26]

Various stage or phase theories have been offered about sports injury and the grief response (Table 1-1). Evans and Hardy[27] conducted an extensive literature review of grief response models that have been offered to account for the psychologic responses to sports injury. After a careful review of the literature, the authors concluded that no one model addressed the atypical grief reaction experienced by injured athletes. The most well-supported grief model in sports is Kubler-Ross's stages—(1) disbelief, denial, and isolation; (2) anger; (3) bargaining; (4) depression; and (5) acceptance—because these stages may be at play in the grief process experienced by the injured athlete (see Table 1-1).[28-30]

Box 1-3
Possible Consequences of Emotional Trauma

Loss of confidence
Fear
Difficulty concentrating
Changes in appetite
Sleep disturbances
Feeling sad, angry, and/or frustrated
Lack of motivation
Substance use
Engaging in high-risk behavior
Decrease in self-esteem
Negativity

Table 1-1 Summary of Three Injury/Grief Response Models

Model	Stage	Characteristics
Kubler-Ross's Grief Model	Denial	Experiences state of disbelief that something happened
	Anger	Asks "why did this happen and what did I do to deserve it?"
	Bargaining	Negotiates with God: "If you only allow this injury to not be as bad as they think, then I will _____."
	Depression	Comes to terms with what has happened and is able to be sad about the situation
	Acceptance	Accepts what has happened
Affective Cycle of Injury	Distress	Exhibits anxiety and depression, fear, guilt, bargaining
	Denial	Does not acknowledge distress, such as pain, feeling of loss, separation from teammates
	Determined coping	Looks for possibilities, seeks out resources, sets goals, manifests commitment
Cognitive-Appraisal Theory		Process of how people perceive a situation and assign an emotion to it, such as anger, fear, guilt, joy

---

Box 1-4

Signs of Adjustment Problems

Emotional displays of anger, depression, confusion, or apathy

Obsession with the question, "When will I be able to play again?"

Denial—athlete leads you to believe that the injury is no big deal

History of coming back too fast from an injury

Exaggerated storytelling or bragging about accomplishments

Dwelling on minor somatic complaints

Remarks about letting the team down or feeling guilty

Dependence on the therapist—hanging around the athletic training room

Withdrawal from teammates, coaches, or friends

Rapid mood swings or changes in behavior

Statements indicating feeling of helplessness to have an impact on recovery

---

Adopted from Petitpas, A., and Danish, S. (1995): Caring for the injured athlete. In: Murphy, S.M. (ed.), Sport Psychology Interventions. Champaign, IL, Human Kinetics, pp. 255–281.

Additionally, the cognitive-appraisal model further explains why athletes' response to being injured cannot be explained by using a grief model. The cognitive-appraisal model asserts that both emotional and behavioral responses are shaped by the athlete's appraisal of the incident, as well as throughout rehabilitation.[30] It is therefore postulated that the injured athlete's experience is a complex interrelationship of thoughts, feelings, and behaviors.[23,25,30] It would be helpful for health care practitioners to be mindful that each individual's experience is unique; consequently, no single theory or model can be applied indiscriminately.

Heil[31] proposed an alternative stage theory, the Affective Cycle of Injury. He contends that the stresses of injury affect four components in the injured athlete: physical well-being, emotional well-being, social well-being, and self-concept. The three elements of the affective cycle are distress, denial, and determined coping (see Table 1-1). In this model, Heil views distress as emotional disequilibrium and denial as disbelief or lack of acceptance of the injury by the athlete. Determined coping, in contrast, implies acceptance and the use of effective coping skills by the athlete. Specifically, determined coping involves setting new goals, seeking out resources, learning new skills, and demonstrating resolve and commitment to a new perspective of the future.[32] Key factors in assisting an athlete move from distress and denial to determined coping are education, goal setting, and social support.

Each athlete will exhibit a range of emotions and varying levels of intensity in response to being injured. Learning to identify the typical signs displayed is paramount in ensuring overall health and well-being of the athlete and success in the rehabilitation process. Poor adjustment after injury will be manifested as psychologic distress. Box 1-4 provides some common signs associated with adjustment problems for the injured athlete.[33]

Petitpas and Danish[33] recommend ongoing assessment of psychologic signs and symptoms and paying close attention to any changes, particularly when the athlete exhibits several warning signs signifying psychologic distress and poor adjustment (see Box 1-4). Henderson[34] contends that high school, college, and professional athletes are considered to be at risk for suicide if they share several high-risk factors:

- Age
- Fluctuations in diet, weight, and training regimen
- Having sustained a head injury
- Having experienced a personal loss
- Personality characteristics
- Alcohol or substance abuse
- Issues related to sexual identity

Coaches, parents, and medical staff should be aware of the warning signs of suicidal behavior (e.g., changes in behavior, anxiety, depression, substance abuse, hopelessness, loss of interest in activities, isolation, preoccupation with death)[34,35] because they are in key positions to monitor changes in affect and behavior. Any change in behavior or concern about the psychologic safety and well-being of an injured athlete warrants an immediate risk assessment by a licensed mental health professional.

Clinical Pearl #3

Acceptance by the athlete of the athletic trainer's and physician's appraisal of the injury is important. If an athlete lacks confidence in the ability of medical personnel to appraise and treat the injury properly, the athlete can reject and ignore the medical advice, thereby resulting in a stronger negative rehabilitation outcome.

REHABILITATION CONSIDERATIONS

Adherence to the Rehabilitation Regimen

Adherence to the rehabilitation program is regarded as being necessary to achieve positive postinjury outcomes. Athletes who adhere to their rehabilitation regimen, use mental skills for managing pain, have a strong social support system, and limit risk-taking behavior that has a negative impact on rehabilitation often have better postinjury outcomes.[36] Unfortunately, studies report adherence to rehabilitation to be rather low, with estimates of as little as one third to one half of patients following their treatment plan.[37] Granquist et al[38] reported rates of adherence to rehabilitation after sports injury to be 47% in division II college athletes, whereas in community-based sports medicine settings, adherence rates ranged from 40% to 91%.

Research investigating psychosocial factors and adherence to rehabilitation in athletes is limited. One study examined psychologic factors in athletes that affect adherence to sports rehabilitation programs and found that adherence rates were highest in those who reported high motivation, higher tolerance of pain, and greater effort in their rehabilitation program.[35] A review of studies that investigated psychosocial factors and adherence outcomes of athletes with anterior cruciate ligament injuries showed that motivation, self-efficacy, and the athlete's perception of control were associated with good adherence and better outcomes after recovery from the injury.[39]

Heil[31] identified psychologic factors demonstrated by injured athletes that were associated with positive rehabilitation outcomes. These factors include motivation, tolerance of pain, goal orientation, and good physical training habits. Factors associated with negative or poor rehabilitation outcomes were found to be a sense of loss, threat to self-esteem, heavy demands of their sport, and an unrealistic recovery time.

Psychosocial Interventions for Successful Rehabilitation

Researchers have identified postinjury psychosocial intervention strategies that have been shown to be effective in assisting athletes in rehabilitation and recovery. These intervention strategies include education, goal setting, social support, and the use of mental skills.[30,31,40] More recently, studies have identified another key factor associated with postinjury rehabilitation outcomes: positive relationships with key health care professionals (i.e., athletic trainer or physical therapist). Athletic trainers and physical therapists who exhibited a positive attitude about the rehabilitation process, particularly regarding the use of mental skills, appear to have a significant positive impact on athletes' recovery rates and adherence to rehabilitation.[41,42]

Education

Education is important because it provides information to athletes to assist them in achieving a sense of understanding, fostering a sense of control, and encouraging commitment to the recovery process. Early education helps injured athletes learn about the nature of their injury, the process of rehabilitation, and realistic postinjury outcomes. Ongoing education is needed about the rehabilitation plan, the athlete's progress, and addressing challenges as they arise. Information allows the athlete to make informed decisions about various treatment options and decreases risky postinjury behavior.

Goal Setting

Goal setting is well established as a significant psychologic skill in sports for enhancement of performance and rehabilitation of injuries.[24,31,33] Goal setting serves to provide motivation for taking action.[40] It is important to help athletes set clear goals so that they can monitor progress and maintain a sense of control during the treatment process. Although goal setting has been shown to be effective, research indicates that it is not widely used and that when used, goals are often vague and not measurable.[31,43] The following guidelines for setting goals offered by Gould[43] will help ensure greater success for athletes:

- Set measurable goals.
- Make the goals moderately difficult yet realistic.
- Set both short-term and long-term goals.
- Have both process and performance goals.
- Set goals for a specific program.
- Make the goals positive.

All goals should have a target date and be monitored and evaluated. A longitudinal study of 70 patients conducted by Levy et al[44] found that to improve patient motivation and result in favorable postinjury outcomes, health care professionals need to set the stage early in treatment by increasing patient awareness about the severity of the injury, creating a learning environment, and encouraging a positive attitude toward the rehabilitation process.

Box 1-5

Reminders for the Sports Medicine Team When Working with Injured Athletes

Important rehabilitation concerns:

- Athlete must feel understood
- Athlete must accept the reality of the injury
- Athlete must understand the rehabilitation plan
- Athlete must adhere to the rehabilitation plan

To be successful in achieving these rehabilitation concerns, you must

- Build rapport with the injured athlete
- Educate the athlete about the rehabilitation process
- Teach the athlete coping skills
- Identify and help develop the athlete's social support system

---

Social Support

The role of social support, as discussed earlier, has been extensively researched and is well documented as playing a significant role in the recovery process for injured athletes.[8,18,31] Granito[45] conducted a qualitative study of injured athletes' personal experiences and found that athletes benefited by having a connection to other athletes with similar injuries.

The SSS[20] measures the athlete's perception of support experienced with respect to a variety of factors—listening, emotional, assistance, and reality confirmation—yet athletes report insufficient support from health care professionals[46] and the least support from coaches.[47] Box 1-5 provides reminders for sports medicine professionals working with injured athletes.

Clinical Pearl #4

Of prime importance in providing medical services to an athlete during recovery is identifying and developing a strong social support system.

Mental Skills

The same mental skills used to enhance performance can be used to assist in recovery and rehabilitation. Research evidence suggests that the use of mental skills during rehabilitation will facilitate the recovery process of injured athletes.[36,40,43] These skills will need to be included in the rehabilitation plan and taught to the injured athlete. After the athlete has learned how to set realistic goals, athletic trainers and physical therapists will need to educate athletes about the value of mental skills in the healing process. Several skills and techniques have been found to be effective during the rehabilitation process: relaxation techniques, imagery, enhancement of concentration skills, and positive self-talk.[23,31,40] It is important for professionals to receive training to become proficient in the use of mental skills before using these skills in treatment. The following is an overview of such skills.

RELAXATION

Learning how to relax will benefit athletes over the course of their career and life. Relaxation reduces the negative effects of stress (e.g., tension, anxiety, pain) by decreasing the heart rate, slowing breathing, and increasing blood flow.[40] Two types of relaxation techniques are used: muscle-to-mind and mind-to-muscle techniques. The muscle-to-mind technique seems to be preferred by athletes. Breathing exercises and progressive relaxation (e.g., the Jacobsonian method) are examples. These methods of relaxation teach athletes to release tension in their muscles. Mind-to-muscle techniques involve training the mind to relax. Meditation and visualization are good examples of mind-to-muscle techniques. As with any skill, practice is essential for these skills to be effective.

IMAGERY

Imagery has been shown to be an effective tool in sports. Vealey and Greenleaf[48] define imagery as "using one's senses to re-create or create an experience in the mind" (p. 268). Athletes use imagery for a number of applications[48]:

- Learning and practicing sports skills and performance enhancement techniques
- Correcting mistakes
- Getting focused
- Automating routines
- Helping in recovery and rehabilitation after injury

Athletes have effectively used imagery for healing, coping with pain, and reducing stress. Use of imagery in rehabilitation can assist athletes in managing pain following surgery and when engaging in exercise during the rehabilitation process.

CONCENTRATION SKILLS

Enhancement of concentration skills is essential in sports. In 1978, Nideffer and Sharpe[49] introduced attention control training (ACT) to enhance and control concentration. ACT involves a number of strategies to improve performance. One ACT strategy, focus training, is also effective for pain management. Focus training techniques involve either association or dissociation. Dissociation techniques are easy to learn and widely used by injured athletes because they appear to reduce tension and therefore reduce pain.[31]

SELF-TALK

Positive self-talk is a powerful cognitive reframing tool that can reduce or eliminate negative thoughts. Preoccupation with negative thinking has an impact on the affective domain and often results in low self-esteem and interferes with performance in sports. Negative self-talk is associated with depression. Fostering positive self-talk serves to enhance recovery and increases the athlete's motivation for rehabilitation.

Heil[31] identified 10 keys for achieving a "remarkable recovery" (p. 205): (1) acquisition of knowledge, (2) goal-directed behavior, (3) focused attention, (4) controlled affect, (5) precise skill execution, (6) exercising without overloading, (7) mastering mind-body control (pain), (8) calculated risk taking, (9) mental toughness, and (10) self-actualization. These 10 keys summarize the various components for athletic trainers and physical therapists to keep in mind when considering how to foster the use of mental skills for rehabilitation in injured athletes.

Psychosocial Interventions to Enhance Coping and Facilitate Adherence to Rehabilitation

Adherence to the rehabilitation program may well be the most significant challenge that athletic trainers and physical therapists face when working with injured athletes. Various models have been proposed over the years that identify factors associated with athletes' compliance with medical regimens and the rehabilitation program. Considerable effort in recent years has been devoted to understanding change in behavior and finding ways to facilitate patient adherence rates. Two of the more prominent models, the Health Belief Model (HBM) and the Transtheoretical Model, most often referred to as Change Theory, are helpful in understanding injured athletes' compliance with the medical regimen and rehabilitation program.

The HBM was developed in the 1950s by psychologists working in the U.S. Public Health Service and has been enhanced over the years. The HBM is based on value expectancy theory and is built on the belief that individuals will take action on their health if they believe that they are susceptible to the health condition, that the planned course of action would make them less susceptible to this condition, and that the benefits outweigh the costs.[50] Heil[31] suggests that when applying this model to injured athletes, health care professionals should investigate issues related to the treatment schedule, financial burden, and poor understanding of the injury and rehabilitation plan by the athlete.

The Transtheoretical Model, or Change Theory, has received considerable attention in recent years. Prochaska et al[51] introduced Change Theory in their book *Changing for Good* in 1994. Change Theory is based on five stages of change: precontemplation, contemplation, preparation, action, and maintenance (Table 1-2). This theory provides a framework for assessing an athlete's readiness for change, in this case rehabilitation. Change Theory offers health care practitioners strategies to facilitate patient readiness for the various stages of change. Assessing the athlete's readiness to engage in rehabilitation is crucial because such assessment provides invaluable information about the athlete's level of readiness and potential adherence to the rehabilitation plan. It also helps the health care practitioner identify and use effective strategies aimed at facilitating readiness to move forward through the rehabilitation process toward a satisfactory outcome.[25,52]

Motivational Interviewing (MI) is a method for enhancing a patient's motivation to change. It was developed by Miller in 1983 for counseling problem drinkers and is now an effective strategy used by practitioners for patients in many, if not all, health care matters.[53] MI is an evidenced-based strategy that has been demonstrated to increase change talk and decrease resistance to change.[54] Change talk refers to identification of

Table 1-2 Stages of the Transtheoretical Model, or Change Theory

Stage	Description
Precontemplation	Individual does not intend to change behavior in the next 6 months.
Contemplation	Individual is strongly inclined to change behavior in the next 6 months.
Preparation	Individual intends to act in the near future.
Action	Behavior has already been incorporated for at least 6 months.
Maintenance	Action has already taken place for more than 6 months and changes to return to old behavior are few.

language used by a patient that shows a readiness for change. The elements of MI for heath care practitioners to learn are as follows[53]:

- Work in collaboration with the athlete.
- Listen for change talk used or not used by the athlete.
- Listen for language from the athlete about wanting to maintain the status quo.
- Think about resistance from athletes as being related to one or more of the following factors:
  - Lack of agreement between the practitioner and athlete
  - Little to no collaboration
  - Low empathy from the practitioner
  - Little athlete autonomy

Four basic principles should guide the health care practitioner when conversing with athletes: (1) express empathy, (2) develop discrepancy, (3) manage resistance (avoid arguing), and (4) support self-efficacy.[53] MI is often used in conjunction with Change Theory. MI has been shown to be effective in facilitating motivation for the different stages of change.[55,56]

It is important for professionals to receive education and training so that they can become proficient in the use of various psychosocial intervention strategies before applying these skills to treatment.

CONCLUSION

- Certain psychosocial factors such as personality traits, history of stressors, and coping resources are believed to influence the stress response.
- Sports injury has a psychologic effect on athletes.
- Effective postinjury psychosocial intervention strategies include education, goal setting, social support, and the use of mental skills.
- Health care practitioners can enhance coping and facilitate adherence to rehabilitation by assessing patient readiness and fostering change.
- Athletes who adhere to their rehabilitation program use mental skills for managing pain, have a strong social support system, limit risk-taking behavior that has a negative impact on rehabilitation, and often have better postinjury outcomes.
- Each athlete will exhibit a range of emotions and varying levels of intensity in response to being injured. Learning to identify the typical signs displayed is paramount for ensuring overall health and well-being of the athlete and adherence to the rehabilitation process.

REFERENCES

1. Pargman, D. (ed.). (2007): Psychological Bases of Sport Injuries. 3rd ed. Morgantown, WV, Fitness Information Technology.
2. MacIntoch, D.L., Skrien, T., and Shepard, R. (1972): Physical activity and injury: A study of sports injuries at the University of Toronto. J. Sports Med. Phys. Fitness, 12:224–237.
3. Taerk, G.S. (1977): The injury-prone athlete: A psychosocial approach. J. Sports Med. Phys. Fitness, 17:186–194.
4. Anderson, M.B., and Williams, J.M. (1988): A model of stress and athletic injury: Prediction and prevention. J. Sport Exerc. Psychol., 10:294–306.
5. Anderson, M.B., and Williams, J.M. (1999): Athletic injury, psychosocial factors, and perceptual changes during stress. J. Sport Sci., 17:735–741.
6. Hanson, S.J., McCullagh, P., and Tonymon, P. (1992): The relationship of personality characteristics, life stress, and coping resources to athletic injury. J. Sport Exerc. Psychol., 14:262–272.
7. Johnson, U. (2007): Psychosocial antecedents of sport injury, prevention, and intervention: An overview of theoretical approaches and empirical findings. Int. J. Sport Exerc. Psychol., 5:352–369.
8. Maddison, R., and Prapavessis, H. (2005): A psychological approach to the prediction and prevention of athletic injury. J. Sport Exerc. Psychol., 27:289–310.
9. Selye, H. (1974): Stress Without Distress. Philadelphia, Lippincott, p. 14.
10. Everly, G.S. (1989): A Clinical Guide to the Treatment of the Human Stress Response. New York, Plenum.
11. Holmes, T.H., and Rahe, R.H. (1967): The Social Readjustment Scale. J. Psychosom. Res., 11:213–218.
12. Bramwell, S.T., Masuda, M., Wagner, N.N., and Homes, T.H. (1975): Psychosocial factors in athletic injuries: Development and application of the Social Athletic Readjustment Rating Scale (SARRS). J. Hum. Stress, 1(2):6–20.
13. Passer, M.W., and Seese, M.D. (1983): Life stress and athletic injury: Examination of positive versus negative events and three moderating variables. J. Hum. Stress, 9:11–16.
14. Petrie, T.A. (1992): Psychosocial antecedents of athletic injury: The effects of life stress and social support on female collegiate gymnasts. Behav. Med., 18:127–138.
15. Nideffer, R.M. (1983): The injured athlete: Psychological factors in treatment. Orthop. Clin. North Am., 14:373–385.
16. Cohen, F., and Lazurus, R.S. (1979): Coping with the stresses of illness. In: Stone, G., Cohen, F., and Adler, N. (eds.). Health Psychology. San Francisco, Jossey-Bass, pp. 217–254.
17. Bacon, V.L., and Anderson, M.K. (2007): The Athletic Trainer's Role in Facilitating Healthy Behavior Change: The Psychosocial Domain. Center for Research and Teaching Grant Workshop, Bridgewater State University.
18. Williams, R.A., and Newcomer Appaneal, R. (2010): Social support and sport injury. Athl. Ther. Today, 15:(4)46–49.
19. Shumaker, S.A., and Brownell, A. (1984): Toward a theory of social support: Closing conceptual gaps. J. Social Issues, 40:11–36.
20. Richman, J.M., Rosenfeld, L.B., and Hardy, C.J. (1993): The Social Support Survey: A validation of a clinical measure of the social support process. Res. Social Work Pract., 3:288–311.
21. Begel, D., and Baum, A. (2000): The athlete's role. In: Begel, D., and Burton, R. W. (eds.). Sports Psychiatry. New York, Norton, pp. 55–56.
22. Bone, J.B., and Fry, M.D. (2006): The influence of injured athletes' perceptions of social support from ATCs on their beliefs about rehabilitation. J. Sport Rehabil., 15:156–167.
23. Weiss, M.R., and Troxel, R.K. (1986): Psychology of the injured athlete. Athl. Train., 21:104–109.
24. Team Physician Consensus Statement (2006): Psychological issues related to injury in athletes and the team physician. Med. Sci. Sports Exerc., 38:2030–2034.
25. Feltz, D.L. (1986): The psychology of sport injuries. In: Vinger P.F., and Hoerner E.F. (eds). Sports Injuries: The Unthwarted Epidemic. 2nd ed. Littleton, MA, PSG Publishing, pp. 336–344.
26. Newcomer, R.R., and Perna, F.M. (2003): Features of posttraumatic distress among adolescent athletes. J. Athl. Train., 38:163–166.
27. Evans, L., and Hardy, L. (1995): Sport injury and grief responses: A review. J. Sport Exerc. Psychol., 17:227–245.
28. Kubler-Ross, E. (1969): On Death and Dying. New York, MacMillan.
29. Rotella, R.J. (1982): Psychological care of the injured athlete. In: Kulund, D.N. (ed.). The Injured Athlete. Philadelphia, Lippincott, pp. 213–224.
30. Brown, C. (2005): Injuries: The psychology of recovery and rehab. In: Murphy, S. (ed.). The Sport Psychology Handbook. Champaign, IL, Human Kinetics.
31. Heil, J. (1993): Psychology of Sport Injury. Champaign, IL, Human Kinetics.
32. Hanin, Y.L. (ed.) (2000): Emotions in Sport. Champaign, IL, Human Kinetics.
33. Petitpas, A., and Danish, S. (1995): Caring for the injured athlete. In: Murphy, S.M. (ed.). Sport Psychology Interventions. Champaign, IL, Human Kinetics, pp. 255–281.
34. Henderson, J.C. (2007): Suicide in sport: Athletes at risk. In: Parman, D. (ed.). Psychological Basis of Sport Injuries. 3rd ed. Morgantown, WV, Fitness Information Technology, pp. 267–285.
35. MedicineNet.com. Suicide warning signs, symptoms, and causes. Retrieved on 11/24/10 from http://www.medicinenet.com/suicide/article.htm.
36. Wiese-Bjornstal, D.M., Smith, A.M., and LaMott, E.E. (1995): A model of psychologic response to athletic injury and rehabilitation. Athl. Train. Sports Health Care Perspect., 1:17–30.
37. Danish, S.J. (1986): Psychological aspects in the care and treatment of athletic injuries. In: Vinger, P.F., and Hoerner, E.F. (eds). Sports Injuries: The Unthwarted Epidemic. 2nd ed. Littleton, MA, PSG Publishing, pp. 345–353.
38. Granquist, M.D., Gill, D.L., and Appaneal, R.N. (2010): Development of a measure of rehabilitation adherence for athletic training. J. Sport Rehabil., 19:249–267.
39. Mendonza, M., Patel, H., Bassett, S., and Phty, D. (2007): Influences of psychological factors and rehabilitation adherence on the outcome of post anterior cruciate ligament injury/surgical reconstruction. N. Z. J. Physiother., 35:62–71.
40. O'Connor, E., Heil, J., Harmer, P., and Zimmerman, I. (2005): Injury. In: Taylor, J., and Wilson, G. (eds). Applying Sport Psychology: Four Perspectives. Champaign, IL, Human Kinetics, pp. 187–206.
41. Tracey, J. (2008): Inside the clinic: Health professionals' role in their clients' psychological rehabilitation. J. Sport Rehabil., 17:413–431.
42. Hamson-Utley, J.J., Martin, S., and Walters, J. (2008): Athletic trainers' and physical therapists' perceptions of the effectiveness of psychological skills within sport injury rehabilitation programs. J. Athl. Train., 43:258–264.

43. Gould, D. (2010): Goal setting for peak performance. In: William, J. M. (ed.). Applied Sport Psychology: Personal Growth to Peak Performance. 6th ed. Boston, McGraw-Hill, pp. 201–220.

44. Levy, A.R., Polman, R.C.J., and Clough, P.J. (2008): Adherence to sport injury rehabilitation programs: An integrated psycho-social approach. Scand. J. Med. Sci. Sports, 18:798–809.

45. Granito, V.J. (2001): Athletic injury experience: A qualitative focus group approach. Sport Psychologist, 24:63–82.

46. Mainwaring, L.M. (1999): Restoration of self: A model for the psychological response of athletes to severe knee injuries. Can. J. Rehabil., 12:143–154.

47. Robbins, J.E., and Rosenfels, L.B. (2001): Athletes' perceptions of social support provided by their head coach, assistant coach, and athletic trainer, pre-injury and during rehabilitation. J. Sport Behav., 24:277–297.

48. Vealey, R.S., and Greenleaf, C.A. (2010): Seeing is believing: Understanding and using imagery in sport. In: William J.M. (ed.). Applied Sport Psychology: Personal Growth to Peak Performance. 6th ed. Boston, McGraw-Hill, pp. 267–299.

49. Nideffer, R.M., and Sharpe, R. (1978): A.C.T.: Attention Control Training. New York: Wyden.

50. Janz, N.K., Champion, V.L., Strecher, V.J. (2002): The health belief model. In: Glanz K., Rimer, B.K., and Lewis, F.M. (eds). Health Behavior and Health Education: Theory, Research and Practice, 3rd ed, San Franciso, John-Wiley & Sons, pp. 45–66.

51. Prochaska, J.O., Norcross, J.C., and DiClemente, C.C. (1994): Changing for Good. New York, Harper-Collins.

52. Singer, E.A. (2007): The transtheoretical model and primary care: "The Times They Are A Changing." J. Am. Acad. Nurse Pract., 19:11–14.

53. Rollnick, S., Miller, W.R., and Butler, C.C. (2008): Motivational Interviewing in Health Care: Helping Patients Change Behavior. New York, Guilford.

54. Motivational Interviewing Bibliography. Retrieved on 12/02/10 from http://motivationalinterview.org/library/biblio.html.

55. Kittles, M., and Atkinson, C. (2009): The usefulness of motivation interviewing as a consultation and assessment tool for working with young people. Pastoral Care Educ., 27:241–254.

56. Lundahl, B.W., Kunz, C., Tollerfson, D., and Burke, B.L. (2010): A meta-analysis of motivational interviewing: Twenty-five years of empirical studies. Res. Social Work Pract., 20:137–160.

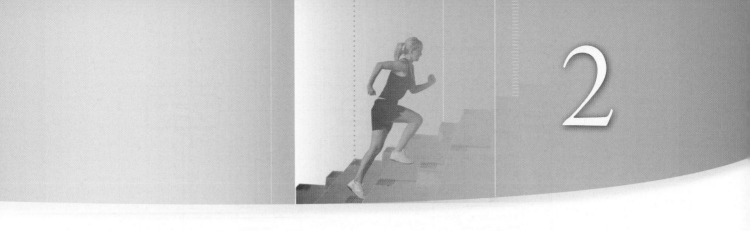

Physiologic Factors in Rehabilitation

Bob Mangine, PT, MEd, ATC, Joseph T. Rauch, PT, ATC, and W. Andrew Middendorf, PT, ATC

CHAPTER OBJECTIVES

- Explain the body's chemical, metabolic, permeability, and vascular changes that occur as a result of trauma.
- Explain how different joint structures respond to the inflammatory process.
- Summarize the effect that immobilization has on muscle, periarticular connective tissue, articular cartilage, ligaments, and bone.
- Describe the sequelae of events that result in synovitis.
- Describe the process that can result in arthrofibrosis.

- Summarize how muscle, periarticular connective tissue, articular cartilage, ligaments, and bone respond to exercise following a period of immobilization.
- Explain the therapeutic benefits of the use of continuous passive motion.
- List several ways to help deter the deleterious effects of immobilization on specific body structures.
- Describe the mechanism and appropriate use of plasma-rich platelet therapy.
- Explain the physiology and rationale for appropriate pre-participation warm-up techniques.

The effects of immobilization on bone and connective tissue have been widely reported in the literature. The evolution from immobilization to implementation of early motion programs has become accepted practice in the orthopedic community. Proper use of specific exercises can accelerate the healing process, whereas lack of exercise during the early stages of rehabilitation can result in long-term functional impairment. Caution must be observed, however, because exercise that is too vigorous can also result in undesired effects on healing tissues. Immobilization initially results in loss of tissue substrate, with subsequent loss of basic tissue components. The reversibility of these changes appears to depend on the length of immobilization.

To understand the body's response to immobilization and remobilization, its normal reaction to injury must be addressed. The sequence of events that transpire after trauma to a joint can cause cartilage degradation, chronic joint synovitis, and stretching of the joint capsule as a result of increased effusion.

REACTION TO INJURY

Inflammation is the body's response to injury, and optimally, it results in healing of tissues by replacement of damaged and destroyed tissue, along with associated restoration of function.[1]

Repeated injury or microtrauma to a specific region can cause a cumulative effect that results in adverse effects on the joint and its surrounding structures. The inflammatory response is the same, regardless of the location and nature of the injurious agent, and consists of chemical, metabolic, permeability, and vascular changes, followed by some form of repair.[2]

Figure 2-1 illustrates the primary and secondary injuries affiliated with trauma and the associated inflammation and repair processes. Primary injury is the result of trauma that directly injures the cells themselves. Secondary injury (sometimes referred to as secondary hypoxia) is precipitated by the body's response to trauma. This response includes decreased blood flow to the traumatized region as a result of vasoconstriction, which decreases the amount of oxygen to the injured area. Thus, additional cells die because of secondary hypoxia; these dead cells organize and ultimately develop into a hematoma.

Cell degeneration or cell death perpetuates the release of potent substances that can induce vascular changes. The most common of these substances is histamine, which increases capillary permeability and allows fluid and blood cells to escape into the interstitial spaces. In the noninjured state, plasma and blood proteins escape from capillaries by osmosis

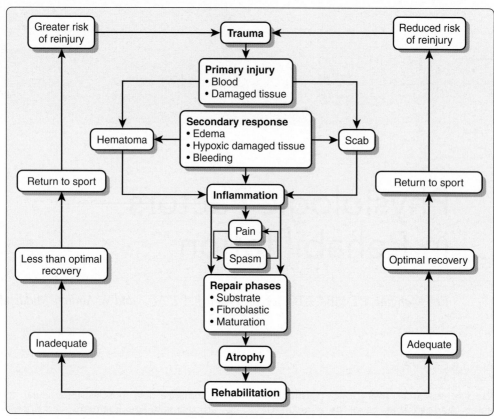

FIGURE 2-1 Cycle of athletic injury. *(From Booher, J.M., and Thibodeau, G.A. [1989]: Athletic Injury Assessment. St. Louis, Times Mirror/Mosby.)*

and diffusion into the interstitial spaces but are reabsorbed. This homeostasis is maintained by colloids present within the blood system. However, trauma leads to increased capillary permeability as a result of the release of cell enzymes, which allows blood plasma and proteins to escape into surrounding tissues. Concurrently, the concentration of colloids greatly increases in the surrounding tissues, thus reversing the colloidal effect. Rather than the colloids pulling fluid back into the capillaries, the presence of colloids outside the vessels causes additional fluid to be pulled into the interstitial tissues with resultant swelling and edema.

The body's reaction after injury is to mobilize and transport the defense components of the blood to the injured area. Initially, blood flow is reduced, which allows white blood cells to migrate to the margins of the blood vessels. These cells adhere to the vessel walls and eventually travel into the interstitial tissues. When in the surrounding tissues, the white cells remove irritating material by the process of phagocytosis. Neutrophils are the first white blood cells to arrive, and they normally destroy bacteria. However, because bacteria are not usually associated with athletic injuries, these neutrophils die.[2] Macrophages then appear and phagocytize the dead neutrophils, cellular debris, fibrin, red cells, and other debris that may impede the repair process.[2] Unfortunately, destruction of the neutrophils results in the release of active proteolytic enzymes (i.e., enzymes that hasten the hydrolysis of proteins into simpler substances), which can attack joint tissues, into the surrounding inflammatory fluid.[3] Although this is the natural response of ridding the body of toxic or foreign material, prolongation of this process can damage surrounding joint structures.

After the inflammatory debris has been removed, repair can begin. Cleanup by macrophages and repair often occur simultaneously. However, for repair to occur, enough of the hematoma must be removed to permit ingrowth of new tissue. Thus, the size of the hematoma or the amount of the exudate is directly related to the total healing time. If the size of the hematoma can be minimized, healing can begin earlier and total healing time is reduced.[2]

Clinical Pearl #1

The primary role of the rehabilitation specialist during the acute phase of injury is to decrease inflammation and prevent damaging secondary effects, such as decreased range of motion (ROM), decreased muscle strength, and prolonged edema. The presence of inflammation must be regarded with caution because too much activity can prolong the inflammation and increase pain. Inflammation is controlled with ice, rest, and electrical stimulation, such as electrical galvanic stimulation or transcutaneous electrical stimulation. Secondary effects are prevented with gentle ROM exercises, isometrics, and avoidance of maladaptive postures or gait patterns.

Response of Joint Structures to Injury

As a result of the inflammatory process, each joint structure responds differently to injury (Fig. 2-2). The reaction of the synovial membrane to injury involves the proliferation of

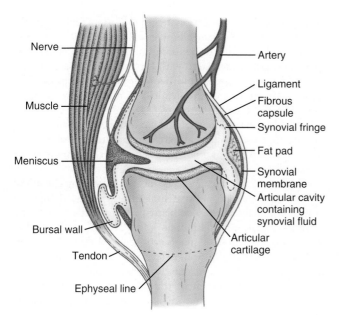

FIGURE 2-2 Synovial joint structures. *(From Wright, V., Dowson, D., and Kerry, J. [1973]: The structure of joints. Int. Rev. Connect. Tissue Res., 6:105–125.)*

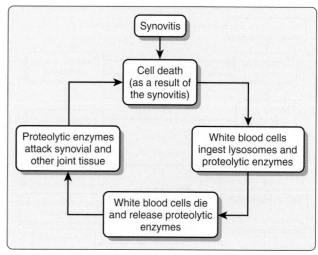

FIGURE 2-3 Continued mechanical irritation of a joint can result in perpetuation of chronic synovitis in a vicious inflammatory cycle. This keeps the reactive synovitis alive even without further trauma.

surface cells, an increase in vascularity, and gradual fibrosis of subsynovial tissue. Posttraumatic synovitis is not uncommon after most injuries. Continued mechanical irritation can produce chronic synovitis, which results in the reversal of normal synovial cell ratios.[3,4] Changes in synovial fluid occur as a result of alterations in the synovial membrane. Cells are destroyed as a consequence of the synovitis; white blood cells ingest the lysosomes and proteolytic enzymes. This ingestion and the subsequent death of white blood cells in the transudate result in the further release of proteolytic enzymes. The overall consequence is spawning of a vicious inflammatory cycle, which can keep reactive synovitis active for some time, even without further trauma (Fig. 2-3).[5] As chronic posttraumatic effusions occur, changes in the synovial membrane can continue, with progressing sclerotic alterations as a sequela.[6] If conservative treatment consisting of antiinflammatory medications, rest, aspiration, and application of cold does not relieve the symptoms, synovectomy may be necessary.

Articular cartilage lesions within a synovial joint or meniscal lesions within the knee, whether acute or chronic, are invariably accompanied by increased synovial effusion. Surgical correction is often required to prevent secondary damage to other joint structures as a result of prolonged inflammation. After the problem has been corrected, the synovial irritation usually subsides. If, however, the problem is left uncorrected, tissues not injured by the original trauma can be damaged from the prolonged inflammation, thus resulting in progressive degradation of the synovial membrane.

Fortunately, when the inflammation begins to abate, synovial tissue can regenerate remarkably well, an ability that possibly stems from its excellent blood supply and origin. Synovium regenerates completely within several months into tissue that is indistinguishable from normal tissue.[3] Acute and chronic synovitis directly affects the amount and content of synovial fluid produced. Synovitis can result in an increased protein level within the synovial fluid. In addition, chronic synovitis can cause a reduction in the viscosity of synovial fluid and a decrease in the concentration of hyaluronic acid.[7] The concentration of hyaluronic acid is directly related to synovial fluid viscosity. Minor joint trauma results in no change in either the concentration or molecular weight of hyaluronic acid.[7] As the severity of trauma increases, however, the concentration of hyaluronic acid decreases to levels below normal, and when the inflammatory process becomes sufficiently disruptive, joint-lining cells fail not only to maintain the hyaluronic acid concentration but also to maintain normal polymer weight.[7]

Hemarthrosis, or bleeding into a joint, can have an effect on joint structures. When a vascular joint structure is damaged, the synovial fluid has a lower sugar concentration, blood clots can be found in the synovial fluid, and fibrinogen can be detected as a result of bleeding into the joint. Although the average time for natural evacuation of a hemarthrosis is approximately 4 days,[8] it depends on individual factors, such as the magnitude of injury, the nature of the structures injured, and the individual's activity level after injury. The presence of blood in a joint has a damaging effect on articular cartilage, with a potentially irreversible decrease in proteoglycan synthesis.[9] In addition, younger individuals with hemarthrosis have been shown to have a greater decrease in proteoglycan synthesis and a slower return to normal rates of synthesis.[10]

The absorption rate of solutions from the joint space is inversely proportional to the size of the solutes: the larger the molecules, the slower the clearance. Clinically, absorption from a joint is increased by active or passive ROM, massage, intraarticular injection of hydrocortisone, or acute inflammation, whereas the effect of external compression is variable.[11]

The reaction of the joint capsule to injury is similar to that of the synovial membrane. If the inflammatory process continues, the joint capsule eventually becomes a more fibrous tissue, and effusion into the joint cavity can lead to stretching of the capsule and its associated ligaments. The higher the hydrostatic pressure and volume of effusion, the faster the fluid reaccumulates after aspiration.[3,12] Conversely, a significant rise in intraarticular hydrostatic pressure contributes to the joint damage by stretching the capsule and associated ligaments.

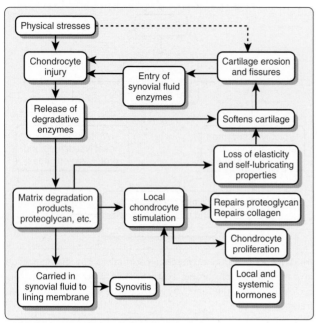

FIGURE 2-4 Postulated final pathway of cartilage degeneration. *(From Howell, D.S. [1976]: Osteoarthritis—Etiology and pathogenesis. In: American Academy of Orthopaedic Surgeons: Symposium on Osteoarthritis. St. Louis, Mosby.)*

The load-carrying surfaces of the synovial joint are covered with a thin layer of specialized connective tissue referred to as articular cartilage. The response of articular cartilage to trauma is not unlike that of the other structures within the joint. The mechanical properties of articular cartilage are readily affected by enzymatic degradation of the components of cartilage. This can occur after acute inflammation, synovectomy, immobilization, or other seemingly minor insults.[13] When articular cartilage loses its content of proteoglycan (a protein aggregate that helps establish the resiliency and resistance of articular cartilage to deformation), the physical properties of the cartilage are changed; this renders the collagen fibers susceptible to mechanical damage.[13] The opposite is also true: if a joint loses collagen in the outer layer of the articular surface, the proteoglycans beneath are subject to damage. As a result of either of these two types of degradation, articular cartilage can erode and leave denuded bone, which results in early, irreversible osteoarthritis or degenerative joint disease (Fig. 2-4).

Reduction of posttraumatic joint effusion is paramount in the early rehabilitation process and is important for restoration of joint kinematics. Prolonged effusion, if left unchecked, can result in reactive synovitis, damage to the joint capsule, and degradation of articular cartilage. Early use of mobilization techniques, such as continuous passive motion (CPM) and modalities such as cryotherapy and vasopneumatic compression, can aid in reducing joint effusion.

EFFECTS OF IMMOBILIZATION

Muscle

One of the first and most obvious changes that occur as a result of immobilization is loss of muscle strength. This correlates with a reduction in muscle size and a decrease in tension per unit of muscle cross-sectional area.[14-16] MacDougall et al[16] reported that 6 weeks of elbow cast immobilization results in greater than a 40% decrease in muscle strength. This deficit in strength is correlated with loss of fiber cross-sectional area and with an associated decrease in muscle mass. The cross-sectional area of the quadriceps muscle may decrease from 21% to 26% with 4 to 6 weeks of immobilization in an individual without a pathologic condition.[17] It is important to note that immobilization atrophy is due to loss of fiber cross-sectional area and not to loss of fibers, as seen in older persons.[18]

The rate of loss appears to be most rapid during the initial days of immobilization. Structural and metabolic changes in muscle cells have been documented after as little as 2 hours of immobilization.[19,20] Lindboe and Platou[20] reported that in humans, muscle fiber size is reduced by 14% to 17% after 72 hours of immobilization. After 5 to 7 days of immobilization, the absolute loss in muscle mass appears to slow considerably.[21,22] The amount of training before immobilization may dramatically decrease the amount of atrophy during immobilization.[21]

Both type I (slow-twitch) and type II (fast-twitch) muscle fibers atrophy. It is generally accepted that a selective decrease in type I (redundant) fibers occurs.[23,24] However, conflicting evidence is found in the literature.[25] After immobilization, the contractile ability of type I fibers is more adversely affected than that of type II fibers.[24,26-28] The decreased contractile ability of type I fibers, rather than decreased fiber proportion, may be more clinically relevant, which implies that exercises involving decreased intensity and increased frequency should be performed after immobilization. This is particularly relevant in an athlete who is specifically conditioned to aerobic activity because of the more dramatic decrease in the percent area of type I fibers. These studies evaluated the effect of immobilization only on muscle fiber composition, not the combined effect of injury and immobilization. Muscle fiber atrophy after injury or surgery may be different from that occurring when a healthy muscle is immobilized.

The mechanical properties of the myotendinous junction are changed as a result of immobilization. The contact area between the muscle cells and the collagen fibers of the tendon is decreased by 50%[29]; the glycosaminoglycan (GAG) content of the myotendinous junction is also decreased.[29] These changes can predispose the myotendinous junction to injury after immobilization. A dramatic increase in activity after immobilization may lead to secondary tendinopathy.

In addition to causing changes in muscle size and volume, immobilization also results in histochemical changes. Such changes include a reduction in levels of adenosine triphosphate (ATP), adenosine diphosphate, creatine, creatine phosphate, and glycogen and a greater increase in lactate concentration with work. Furthermore, the rate of protein synthesis decreases within 6 hours of immobilization.[16,30-33]

Immobilization also causes an increase in muscle fatigability as a result of decreased oxidative capacity. Reductions occur in maximum oxygen consumption, glycogen levels, and high-energy phosphate levels.[14,16,30,34,35] Rifenberick and Max[36] reported fewer mitochondria in atrophic muscle and a significant decrease in mitochondrial activity by day 7 after immobilization, which causes a reduction in cell respiration and contributes to decreased muscle endurance (Box 2-1).

Box 2-1

Summary of the Effects of Immobilization on Muscle

Decrease in muscle fiber size

Change in muscle resting length

Decrease in size and number of mitochondria

Decrease in total muscle weight

Increase in muscle contraction time

Decrease in muscle tension produced

Decrease in resting levels of glycogen and adenosine triphosphate (ATP)

More rapid decrease in ATP levels with exercise

Increase in lactate concentration with exercise

Decrease in protein synthesis

It appears that the muscle atrophy that occurs after immobilization is selective. For example, immobilization of the thigh is often associated with selective atrophy of the quadriceps femoris muscle.[37] Although the knee is the area traditionally noted for selective atrophy, this phenomenon can also be observed in the triceps brachii of an immobilized elbow. Clinically, one can observe that atrophy of the quadriceps is greater than that of the hamstrings. This finding is supported by evidence on computed tomography that despite significant loss of quadriceps cross-sectional area, no significant difference in hamstring or adductor muscle cross-sectional area is seen after 5 weeks of immobilization.[37]

The selective atrophy that occurs in the quadriceps femoris and the triceps brachii with immobilization of the knee and elbow, respectively, may be due to their roles as primarily one-joint muscles. Three of the four heads of the quadriceps cross only the knee joint, and two of the three triceps heads cross only the elbow joint. In contrast, all heads of the biceps and the hamstrings cross two joints. The biceps and hamstrings are therefore less immobilized by having all portions contract across one of the two joints that they cross (the hip or the shoulder), which may be the reason that cross-sectional area is preserved in these muscles.[28]

Clinical Pearl #2

The volume of muscle in the thigh decreases after immobilization, but the volume of subcutaneous adipose tissue does not change. This can mask the amount of quadriceps atrophy and invalidate girth measurements as a tool for measuring atrophy.[38] Girth measurements also do not distinguish between muscle groups and can therefore underestimate the amount of quadriceps atrophy. Girth measurements do not correlate with deficits in strength.

Reflexive inhibition, or arthrogenous muscle wasting, can contribute to selective muscle atrophy, particularly of the quadriceps, after trauma to or surgery on a joint. Pain has traditionally been regarded as the general cause of reflex inhibition. The perception and fear of pain can greatly affect muscular strength. Athletes who fear that muscle contraction will result in pain may be very apprehensive about contracting these particular muscles, but severe inhibition of muscle strength is seen even after the pain subsides.[39] At 1 to 2 hours after arthrotomy and meniscectomy, a 62% decrease in quadriceps electromyographic (EMG) activity occurs.[40] This decrease is due to reflexive inhibition. A significant amount of anesthetic injected into the knee may decrease (but not eliminate) the inhibition temporarily, but the effects are lost after 4 to 5 hours.[40] Ten to 15 days after surgery, quadriceps EMG activity decreases by 35%.[40] Whether this reduced activity is due to reflexive inhibition or disuse atrophy is unclear. Pain has been shown to inhibit strength in patients with preoperative pathologic changes in the shoulder, but postoperative reflex inhibition has not been investigated.[41-43] In studies investigating arthrogenous muscle wasting, the level of quadriceps activation is typically determined by EMG testing. The degree of unilateral quadriceps inhibition is then judged by the difference in maximum voluntary activation between the two limbs. Because no method is available to directly measure inhibition, it is indirectly quantified by EMG testing. This may not be a valid measure of true reflex inhibition during the first few hours after injury or surgery. After injury, reflex inhibition leads to muscle atrophy. When the inhibition has ceased, muscle weakness from disuse or immobilization atrophy will continue. Caution must be used when one generalizes the findings of studies pertaining to arthrogenous muscle weakness.

The nature of the surgical procedure performed may have an effect on the amount of arthrogenous muscle wasting after surgery. Advances in technology have led to the use of a less invasive arthroscope for many procedures that previously required an arthrotomy. A significant decrease in quadriceps muscle EMG activity is seen after arthrotomy of the knee. Although this decrease in EMG activity is still present after arthroscopy of the knee, the magnitude of the change is much decreased.[44] Two-portal arthroscopy produces a lesser decrease in quadriceps strength after surgery than three-portal arthroscopy does.[45] Clinically, patients undergoing an arthroscopic procedure would be expected to recover at a more rapid rate, but consideration must be given to the specific surgical procedure. In general, patients who have undergone less invasive procedures (arthroscopy) will initially recover faster than those who have undergone more invasive procedures (arthrotomy), but the long-term outcome is usually the same. This has been demonstrated in the knee[46] and shoulder.[47]

Tourniquet-related ischemia has also been thought to contribute to quadriceps shutdown. When a tourniquet is used to provide a relatively bloodless field during surgery, the pressure required to staunch blood flow is also enough to damage the tissues being compressed. Use of a tourniquet, although necessary, leads to postoperative EMG changes[48,49] and increased quadriceps atrophy.[48] Nonroutine complications from tourniquet use include compression neurapraxia, wound hematoma, tissue necrosis, vascular injury, and compartment syndrome.[50]

Research has shown that distension of a knee with plasma can lead to quadriceps shutdown and subsequent quadriceps weakening in normal individuals, even in the absence of pain.[51-55] Young et al[56] and others[53] reported that injection of small volumes of fluid (20 to 30 mL) into normal knees results in 60% quadriceps inhibition, with the inhibition increasing as the infusion increases. Spencer et al[54] found the threshold amount of effusion for reflexive shutdown to be between 20 and 30 mL for the vastus medialis and between 50 and 60 mL for the vastus lateralis and rectus femoris. The decreased threshold for the vastus medialis can contribute to patellar tracking problems when the knee is even slightly effused. Inhibition is directly related to the degree of effusion and increases as the amount of effusion increases.[57] With a chronically effused joint, aspiration of the effusion does not result in any difference in quadriceps inhibition.[58] This may be attributed to concomitant disuse atrophy.

Joint angle has also been shown to have an effect on quadriceps inhibition. In normal knees, the highest quadriceps EMG activity is obtained with the knee in the shortened position, or full extension.[59] Stratford[60] reported that effusion inhibits quadriceps contraction less when the knee is in 30° of flexion than when it is fully extended. Similar results have been found even after arthrotomy with meniscectomy, with isometric quadriceps contraction being inhibited less in flexion than in extension.[18,39,59] This has been postulated to occur because intraarticular pressure is less when the knee is in 30° of flexion than when in full extension.[39,52,61-63] Despite higher EMG activity being obtained with the knee in flexion, it is not desirable to perform all exercises in the clinic with a flexed knee position. On the contrary, this information emphasizes to the clinician the importance of training the quadriceps in a fully extended position to overcome the biomechanical disadvantage.

The length at which the muscle is immobilized also affects selective atrophy. Tardieu et al[64] suggested that muscle fibers under stretch lengthen by adding sarcomeres in series whereas those immobilized in a shortened position lose sarcomeres. Thus, when a muscle is immobilized in a lengthened position, the length of the muscle fibers increases to accommodate the muscle's new length, along with other connective tissue changes. A similar adjustment in sarcomere number occurs in muscle that is immobilized in a shortened position; the length of the fibers decreases, and the number of sarcomeres is reduced to achieve the physiologic change.[65] Immobilization of a muscle in a shortened position leads to increased connective tissue and reduced muscle extensibility.[64] Muscle immobilization in a lengthened position maintains muscle weight and fiber cross-sectional area better than does immobilization in a shortened position.[66,67] This theoretically explains the selective atrophy of the quadriceps when the knee is immobilized in full extension. Because the knee is usually immobilized in an extended or slightly flexed position, the hamstrings are placed in a lengthened position and the quadriceps in a shortened position. These positions help preserve muscle cross-sectional area and strength, but the sarcomeres will no longer be able to shorten enough to achieve maximal extension. Clinically, the position of the joint cannot be the only factor that influences muscle atrophy; for example, in a shoulder that is immobilized in internal rotation, the external rotators (the rotator cuff muscles) still demonstrate marked atrophy.

Despite the fact that the knee is typically immobilized in extension, patients tend to hold the knee in a slightly flexed position, either sitting with the hips flexed or supine with the pelvis tilted posteriorly, which shortens the hamstrings. Hamstring stretches to increase the resting length of the spindle are an important part of a knee rehabilitation program after immobilization. Increasing the length of the hamstrings will decrease the amount of resistance that the quadriceps must contract against to achieve full knee extension. Stretching of the posterior capsule may also be required if the knee is held in a flexed position.

Clinical Pearl #3

One of the factors that may also influence reflex inhibition is the muscle spindle. When a muscle is immobilized in a shortened or lengthened position, the spindle will assume a new resting length.[68] A muscle in the shortened position will then have greater resistance to stretch, and a muscle immobilized in the lengthened position will have decreased contractile ability. This is especially true at the shoulder, which is typically immobilized in internal rotation, and at the elbow, which is typically immobilized in flexion. The shortened position facilitates the shortened muscles (elbow flexors and shoulder internal rotators) and may account for the decreased strength of the shoulder external rotators and elbow extensors. Treatment of these joints should include facilitatory techniques for the lengthened muscles and inhibitory techniques for the shortened muscles. The shortened muscles should be stretched often but gently because quick or aggressive stretching can cause a facilitatory response. Isometric contractions can also preserve tension in the muscle spindle while allowing healing of damaged tissues.

Clinical Pearl #4

Despite the increased preservation of quadriceps muscle cross-sectional area and increased EMG activity in flexion, this is not the preferential position for immobilization of the knee after injury or surgery. If the knee is immobilized in flexion, full passive extension must be maintained by passively extending the knee to 0° several times per day (barring medical or surgical precautions.) This ensures that the quadriceps will maintain proper length to allow shortening of the muscle to full knee extension.

Active quadriceps exercises should be done in full extension for several reasons. Full active knee extension is needed for a proper gait pattern during initial contact (heel strike). A quadriceps contraction in full extension allows maximal superior glide of the patella in the trochlear groove, thereby preventing patella infera. If patients do not have full active extension, they must be taught to glide the patella superiorly to preserve length of the patellar tendon. If patients do not have full passive knee extension after immobilization, a motion complication program should be initiated.

Periarticular Connective Tissue

The periarticular connective tissue consists of ligaments, tendons, synovial membrane, fascia, and joint capsule. As a consequence of immobilization, injury, or surgery, biochemical and histologic changes occur in the periarticular tissue around synovial joints and may result in arthrofibrosis. Arthrofibrosis has been referred to as ankylosis, joint stiffness, or joint contracture.[69] It is a term that describes excessive formation of scar tissue around a joint

on an adequate blood supply, and immobilization may therefore delay healing of the meniscus. Knee joint immobilization decreases the proteoglycan and water content of the meniscus,[127] which changes its ability to distribute compressive force. In the absence of weight bearing, active joint motion has been shown to decrease the loss of ligament and meniscal mass.[128]

Bone

The effects of immobilization on bone are similar to those on other connective tissues. A consistent finding in response to diminished weight bearing and muscle contraction is bone loss. Changes in bone can be detected as early as 2 weeks after immobilization.[87,96,134] Although the pathogenesis of immobilization-associated osteoporosis is unclear, animal studies have shown decreased bone formation and increased bone resorption.[135-138]

Bone hardness decreases steadily with the duration of immobilization, with hardness dropping to 55% to 60% of normal by 12 weeks.[139] A decline in elastic resistance also occurs—the bone becomes more brittle and thus more susceptible to fracture.

It appears that mechanical strain influences osteoblastic and osteoclastic activity on the bone surface.[140] Bone loss from disuse atrophy occurs at a rate 5 to 20 times greater than that resulting from metabolic disorders affecting bone.[141] The primary cause of this immobilization osteoporosis appears to be mechanical unloading, which may be responsible for the inhibition of bone formation during immobilization.[142] Therefore, non–weight-bearing immobilization of an extremity should be limited to as short a period as possible.

CONTINUOUS PASSIVE MOTION

In 1970, Salter[143] originated the biologic concept of CPM of synovial joints to stimulate healing, regenerate articular tissue, and avoid the harmful effects of immobilization.[144] In 1978, Salter and Saringer (who was an engineer) collaborated to develop the first CPM device for humans.[143] A CPM machine is an electrical, motor-driven device that helps support the injured limb. It is used to move a joint at variable rates through progressively increasing ROM; no muscular exertion is required of the patient.

Salter et al[102,143] provided the first histologic evidence in support of CPM. They reported[143,145] that CPM significantly stimulates healing of articular tissues, including cartilage, tendons, and ligaments; prevents adhesions and joint stiffness; does not interfere with healing of incisions over the moving joint; and influences the regeneration of articular cartilage through neochondrogenesis.

When compared with immobilization of tendons, CPM has proved effective in increasing linear and maximum stress, linear load, and ultimate strength in tendons.[144] Salter and Minster[146] reported the preliminary results of semitendinous tenodesis for MCL reconstruction in experimental animals, in which increased strength was reported after the use of CPM. The application of early tensile force appears to facilitate proper alignment of collagen fibers during the initial healing process. In addition, decreases in medication requests and in wound edema and effusion in operative knees were reported in patients undergoing CPM.[147] The greatest benefit of CPM appears to be the prevention of articular cartilage degradation. Salter[143] reported that healing of cartilage defects in rabbits appears to be more

---

> ### Box 2-5
> #### Benefits of the Early Use of Passive Motion
>
> No deleterious effects on stability of the ligament
> Decrease in joint swelling and effusion
> Decrease in pain medication taken
> Faster regaining of range of motion
> Reduced muscle atrophy

---

rapid and complete when CPM is used. More recently, a 2007 study reported that the use of CPM stimulates chondrocyte PRG4 metabolism, which benefits cartilage and joint health.[148]

CPM has received widespread attention for use in treating pathologic conditions of the knee. However, CPM machines have been developed for the shoulder as well. Raab et al[149] found increased ROM and decreased pain with the use of CPM after rotator cuff repair, although no difference in combined outcome measures was seen 3 months postoperatively. Lastayo et al[150] found no difference in outcomes between subjects who used a CPM machine and those who had a friend or relative perform manual ROM exercises, thus indicating that the presence of passive motion is more important than the mode of delivery.

It is well established in the literature that the use of CPM is not associated with a significant difference in outcome measures at approximately 4 weeks postoperatively.[151-153] However, when the short-term effects of CPM are examined, subjects undergoing CPM regain their motion faster and with less pain than do those who are not undergoing CPM.[154,155] Although there may be no long-term difference, CPM appears to be beneficial to patients in the short term (Box 2-5).[115,154,156-158]

Use of CPM units is considered an acceptable practice after most orthopedic procedures. Although initially designed for the lower extremities, CPM units are available for the upper extremities as well. CPM has helped counteract the deleterious effects of immobilization by allowing early protected ROM. Some indications for the use of CPM include ligament reconstruction or repair, total joint replacement, release of joint contractures, tendon repair, open reduction of fractures, and articular cartilage defects.

EFFECTS OF REMOBILIZATION

Physical forces provide important stimuli to tissues for the development and maintenance of homeostasis.[116] Lack or denial of mobilization results in deleterious effects on bone, muscle, connective tissue, and articular cartilage. The advent of CPM in the late 1970s and early 1980s provided an impetus for the initiation of early motion to repair tissues and for using early electrical stimulation of muscle to decrease atrophy and promote early muscle reeducation. In addition, the emergence of hinged braces, which allow early protected motion, has helped foster early mobilization.

Early motion and loading and unloading of joints through partial weight bearing promote the diffusion of synovial fluid to nourish articular cartilage, menisci, and ligaments. Moreover, research has shown that motion enhances transsynovial flow of nutrients.[63,97,159] Regardless of the cell-stimulating mechanism, it is clear that fibroblasts and chondrocytes respond to physical forces by increasing their rate of synthesis, and the extracellular degradation of matrix components is similarly controlled.[79]

Immobilization is still used, however, in the treatment of many ligamentous reconstructions and fractures. It is not known whether the deleterious effects of prolonged immobilization can be reversed with remobilization techniques. These structural changes generally appear to depend on the duration and angle of immobilization and on weight-bearing status.

Clinical Pearl #8

Rehabilitation protocols for specific injuries and surgical procedures are popular and commonly used. These protocols must be viewed as guidelines and not as rules. Each patient's condition must be taken into account when determining appropriate progression of activities. Objective and subjective findings are used to determine the patient's tolerance of a new activity. Signs of intolerance include increased effusion, pain, erythema, or an inability to perform a task correctly. These are signs that the activity should be modified or delayed.

Muscle

Many researchers have investigated the process of remobilization after immobilization. Extrapolation of the results of these studies to an injured or postoperative patient population must be done with caution, however, because injury may compound the effects of immobilization. It is critical to consider how the specific injury or surgical procedure and the length of immobilization will affect the rate of return of muscle strength.

To achieve gains in muscle strength, the principle of overload must be used.[160] Overload involves the application of a stimulus that is greater than the stimulus to which the muscle is accustomed. This principle must be used with caution in an injured population, however, because excessive overload can be detrimental to healing tissues.

Return of quadriceps strength after knee surgery has been widely investigated. With ACL reconstruction, loss of quadriceps strength appears to be greater with bone–patellar tendon–bone autografts than with semitendinosus-gracilis autografts.[161,162] Despite quadriceps weakness being associated with patellar tendon–bone autografts, only a slight amount of hamstring weakness is associated with semitendinosus-gracilis autografts.[163] This may be due to the previously discussed reasons for predisposition of the quadriceps to atrophy. After ACL reconstruction with patellar tendon–bone autografts, quadriceps strength has been found to be less than 50% of that on the contralateral side 3 months postoperatively[156] and 72% to 78% of that on the contralateral side from 6 to 12 months postoperatively.[156,161] Six months after ACL reconstruction with a semitendinosus-gracilis autograft, quadriceps strength has been found to be 88% of that on the contralateral side, and hamstring strength has been found to be 90% of that on the contralateral side.[163] In both a human[164] and an animal model,[55] performance of this type of reconstruction in a female patient[156,165] and older age are factors associated with increased risk for prolonged muscle weakness after surgery.

Shoulder strength after rotator cuff injury has been studied. In shoulders with a rotator cuff tear, strength is decreased by one third to two thirds with respect to abduction, flexion, and external rotation.[42,43] Strength is decreased by one third 6 months after repair and becomes comparable to that on the contralateral side at 1 year after repair.[166] Shoulder strength is positively correlated with the size of the rotator cuff tear.[166]

It has been theorized that electrical muscle stimulation (EMS) can provide enough muscle activity to deter atrophy and the deleterious effects of immobilization on muscle. EMS has been investigated primarily as a tool to preserve muscle strength and cross-sectional area after knee surgery, particularly with ACL reconstruction. EMS has been shown to preserve quadriceps cross-sectional area and protein synthesis in an immobilized injured knee[167,168] when combined with traditional rehabilitation exercises.[162,169,170] EMS has also been shown to be associated with a more normalized gait pattern postoperatively.[171] It may be particularly effective in women.[165]

Some reports in the literature do not support the effectiveness of EMS in preserving muscle strength after injury or surgery.[172] This lack of support may be due to the type and individual parameters of the electrical stimulation used. EMS is comparable to voluntary exercise only when the exercises are required to be performed at the same intensity as the EMS.[173] In addition, EMS is effective only when used at a level strong enough to produce a contraction in a shortened position that is greater than what the patient can produce voluntarily. Biofeedback training has been shown to be as effective as EMS in recovery of quadriceps strength.[174]

Clinical Pearl #9

EMS can provide clinical benefit when a patient does not have active full knee extension. It can be especially helpful if the patient is immobilized in a flexed position. The patient must apply EMS on a regular basis (three to five times a day at home) with the knee in full extension during each use to preserve full ROM.

Many clinicians use EMS for the quadriceps after knee surgery or injury. However, EMS can help preserve motion and allow early neuromuscular reeducation at other joints. Functional electrical stimulation is used on the rotator cuff of patients who have a subluxated shoulder after a cerebral injury.

Articular Cartilage

The effects of remobilization on articular cartilage seem to depend on time. Many studies have examined the effects of remobilization on articular cartilage after a period of immobilization. The period of remobilization required to restore articular cartilage structure and function is significantly longer than the immobilization period required to cause those changes.[175-177] Kiviranta et al[111,175] found that 50 weeks of remobilization after 11 weeks of immobilization is not sufficient to restore GAG content. Haapala et al[178] used a similar protocol to demonstrate the inability of 50 weeks of remobilization to reverse cartilage softening in the cartilage of immature beagles. This indicates that younger individuals may sustain long-term damage to their articular surfaces as a result of immobilization. Evans et al[179] reported alterations in cartilage, such as matrix fibrillation, cleft formation, and ulceration, that are not reversible in rats after immobilization for up to 90 days. They noted, however, that the soft tissue changes are reversible if the period of immobilization does not exceed 30 days. Clinically, it is rare that an extremity would be immobilized for longer than the 30 days that is required to cause irreversible damage.

The remobilization process after immobilization must consist of controlled stress. Although moderate activity after a period of immobilization causes increases in cartilage thickness and proteoglycan content, strenuous activity can cause damage to the articular structures.[111] It is important to watch for signs of intolerance of a new activity. Signs of intolerance include increased effusion or edema, erythema, pain, or inability to complete a task correctly.

Bone

Immobilization results in disuse osteoporosis, which may not be reversible on remobilization of the limb. Reversibility is related to the severity of changes and to the length of immobilization. Permanent osseous changes appear to occur with an immobilization period exceeding 12 weeks.[55] Even though bone lost in the first 12 weeks is regained, the period of recovery is at least as long as and may be many times longer than the immobilization period.[76] The most effective means of modifying osteoporosis caused by reduced skeletal loads appears to be through exercise. Isotonic and isometric exercises decreased bone loss in subjects who were exposed to prolonged periods of weightlessness and bed rest.[180,181] Activity increases bone formation in these situations and can hasten recovery after return to a normal loading environment. If an appropriate environment can be maintained during immobilization of a limb, the deleterious effects of disuse on bone can be partially prevented, and rehabilitation can be accelerated.[76]

Ligaments

Remobilization after immobilization of ligaments occurs in an asynchronous fashion. It appears that the bone-ligament junction recovers at a much slower rate than do the mechanical or midsubstance properties of the ligament.[182,183] Cabaud et al[112] reported that ligament strength and stiffness in rat ACLs can increase with endurance-type exercises. Others have noted similar results.[99,184] Moreover, not only does the ligament injury result in weaker mechanical properties at midsubstance and at the bone-ligament complex, but nontraumatized ligaments also become weaker as a result of immobilization. These weakened mechanical properties of ligaments must be considered when a rehabilitation program is being planned.

Recovery from immobilization depends on the duration of immobilization. Woo et al[182] noted that 1 year of remobilization is required before the architectural components of the MCL-tibia junction return to normal after 12 weeks of immobilization. Noyes[117] reported that after 5 months of remobilization following total body immobilization in primates, ligament strength recovers only partially, although ligament stiffness and compliance parameters return to control values. It was reported that 12 months is required for complete recovery of ligament strength parameters.[117] Tipton et al[185] observed recovery of 50% of normal strength in a healing ligament by 6 months, 80% after 1 year, and 100% after 1 to 3 years, depending on the type of stress placed on the ligament and on prevention of repeated injury.

It appears that the properties of ligaments return to normal with remobilization, but this depends on the duration of the immobilization, with the bone-ligament junction taking longer to return to normal after immobilization.

Connective Tissue

Few studies have documented the effects of remobilization after immobilization on the formation of cross-links.[75] Movement maintains lubrication and critical fiber distance within the matrix and ensures an orderly deposition of collagen fibrils, thereby preventing abnormal cross-link formation.[75] Frequently, for ROM to be restored, forceful manipulation to break the intracapsular fibrofatty adhesions may need to be performed.[75] Although ROM is restored, it has been speculated that fibrofatty tissue is peeled from the ends of bones, with ragged edges of adhesions remaining in the joint.[106,179] Increased joint inflammation also occurs as a result of the manipulation and enhances the potential for chronic synovitis.

TISSUE HEALING WITH PLATELET-RICH PLASMA THERAPY

As sports medicine has developed, clinicians have searched for ways to create a competitive advantage for their athletes. Musculoskeletal injury has often resulted in loss of playing time and continues to increase in active populations.[186,187] Returning these athletes to sports participation can be the difference between winning and losing. New science involving tissue regeneration techniques along with other ways of speeding the recovery process has been developed, including the use of platelet-rich plasma (PRP) therapy. An understanding of the physiology of injury leads to a better understanding of the healing process and effective use of PRP. Originally, PRP was shown to enhance bone formation and antiinflammatory function after oral and maxillofacial applications.[188,189] Today, more information is being presented on the various beneficial ways in which autologous platelet therapy can benefit a broader patient population, specifically athletes for the purposes of this book.

Blood is made up of many different components. Plasma, the liquid form of blood, is made mostly of water and transports all other components of blood. Red blood cells transport oxygen to the body, and white blood cells fight off infection and act as a defense for the body. Platelets are responsible for homeostasis, revascularization, and construction of new connective tissue. Human blood is composed of 93% red blood cells, 6% platelets, and 1% white blood cells. For many years, platelets were believed to have an effect only on clotting. However, new evidence has shown that they release multiple growth factors that may enhance tissue regeneration and healing.[190] Injection of whole blood has been shown to decrease subjective pain scores in humans with tendon injury, but it lacks the healing properties of other injection treatment options.[191] PRP is useful as an activator of circulation-derived cells for enhancement of the initial healing process.[192] The rationale for the use of PRP is to reverse the blood ratio by decreasing red blood cells, which are less useful in healing, to 5% and increase the platelet ratio to 94%.[193] This will stimulate a supraphysiologic release of growth factors in an attempt to jump-start healing.[190]

The normal human concentration of platelets is 200,000 platelets/μL. Injection of concentrated autologous PRP can increase the platelet concentration by four to eight times the normal value.[193,194] The PRP injection procedure is relatively quick and can be done in the doctor's office, athletic training room, or outpatient clinic. It begins by drawing 30 to 60 mL of blood from the patient, usually the arm. The blood is then placed in a microwave-size centrifuge and spun down to extract the platelets from the other components of blood. Depending on the unit, this process can take 5 to 30 minutes. After separation, 3 to 6 mL of isolated PRP is removed and secured in a separate sterile syringe. After the injury site has been prepared, the injection can be completed. The use of diagnostic ultrasound or magnetic resonance imaging is recommended for accurate injection into the specific damaged tissue. At rest, platelets require a trigger to become active in healing and homeostasis.[195] Thrombin will trigger release of the pool of growth factors over the injured tissue. Peerbooms et al[196] described a peppering technique for the injection of platelets that naturally causes release of thrombin. A normal platelet's life span is 7 to 10 days. During this time it is recommended that the use of antiinflammatory drugs, which can kill the injected platelets, be avoided. After injection, rest, ice, compression, and elevation (RICE), as well as acetaminophen or prescription pain medication in extreme cases, have been used to negate pain. Depending on the sensitivity of the injection site, an immediate, short-term increase in pain may be expected by the patient as a normal biologic response to the injection. An important benefit of this procedure is the very low risk for immunogenic reactions or transfer of disease secondary to the autologous nature of the procedure. When compared with injection of isolated growth factors, PRP offers multiple healing components in one treatment. Growth factors act solely on cell membranes with no effect on the cell nucleus, thereby decreasing the chance of hyperplasia, carcinogenesis, or tumor growth.[190,197] Sampson et al[190] found minimal contraindications, including the presence of tumor, metastasis, active infection, and low platelet or hemoglobin count.

The value of concentrated platelets lies in their ability to release numerous growth factors that promote specific components of the healing process.[198,199] Neutrophils and macrophages naturally respond to injury by releasing growth factors, including platelet-derived growth factor, transforming growth factor, vascular endothelial growth factor, and epithelial growth factor. Following injury, administration of concentrated platelets will accelerate the process of releasing growth factors. In tendon injury, this leads to an earlier increase in tendon breaking strength, arguably the most important tendon-healing parameter.[200,201] Table 2-1 summarizes the various growth factors that are released as a result of injury.[195,202-205] Many other growth factors are also found that will aid in stimulating angiogenesis, regulating cell migration and proliferation, activating satellite cells, and supporting other growth factors.[202,206]

To date, much of the literature on PRP is anecdotal and derived from small sample case studies. However, many have attributed decreased pain and decreased loss of function to the use of PRP injection. Early research has shown PRP injection to be effective in treating Achilles tendinopathy after failed physical therapy, with patients reporting significantly reduced or eliminated clinical symptoms.[207] A study by Peerbooms et al[196] is one of a limited number of randomized controlled studies that compared PRP and corticosteroid injections for the

Table 2-1 Various Growth Factors Released as a Result of Injury

Growth Factor	Purpose
PDGF	Helps promote tissue remodeling and stimulates the production of other growth factors. It is hypothesized that PDGF is the first growth factor found in injured tissue and initiates healing.[195]
TGF	Promotes the extracellular matrix and regulation of cell replication.[202]
VEGF	Stimulates angiogenesis, which is instrumental in accelerating tendon cell proliferation and stimulating type I collagen synthesis.[203]
IGF-I	Stimulates the proliferation of myoblasts and improves skeletal muscle regeneration.[204]
FGF-2	Enhances the number and diameter of regenerating muscle fibers.[205]

FGF-2, Fibroblast growth factor-2; *IGF-I,* insulin-like growth factor I; *PDGF,* platelet-derived growth factor; *TGF,* transforming growth factor; *VEGF,* vascular endothelial growth factor.

treatment of lateral epicondylitis. Corticosteroid injection has long been considered the "gold standard" treatment, but it has been shown to have limited long-term effects and requires multiple treatments.[208] The results demonstrated initial improvement in the corticosteroid group, but a rapid decline and return to preinjection complaints. PRP-injected subjects showed gradual improvement with decreased subjective pain reports and improved function without relapse at 26-week and 1-year followup. Using the DASH (Disabilities of the Arm, Shoulder, and Hand) Outcome Measure, 73% of patients injected with PRP demonstrated improvement versus only a 51% success rate in steroid-injected patients.[196] In this case it can be hypothesized that PRP administration will decrease the need for multiple injections. Barrett and Erredge[209] reported almost 78% complete resolution of symptoms and return to previous levels of function in patients with plantar fasciitis at 1-year followup after a single PRP injection. Even though this was a small sample pilot study, the conclusions were intriguing, but it should be kept in mind that treatment of plantar fasciitis with multiple injections has been shown to be a factor contributing to eventual rupture of the tendon.[210-213] Research is also favorable for surgical patients. Berghoff et al[214] compared 137 patients undergoing total knee arthroscopy, 71 treated with PRP and 66 controls, and found increased hemoglobin, fewer transfusions, shorter hospital stay, and quicker return of ROM in those treated with PRP. Similar results were found in the same population by Gardner et al.[215] and Everts et al.[197] Studies involving animal models have shown increased mechanical properties after cartilage defects,[216] as well as support for chondrogenesis and healing of meniscal defects with use of PRP.[217,218]

More specific uses of PRP have been reported in other studies. Hammond et al[206] studied the use of PRP for muscle injuries in rats. Using the anterior tibialis muscles, the authors created two different protocols. One involved inducing a single, large strain injury and compared it with an injury caused by multiple small strain stretching contractions. Interestingly, the specimens with a large, single injury showed improvement only on day 3 with a significant increase in generation of muscle force. Conversely, the multiple small strain–injured specimens improved at several different time points and showed greater overall healing and return to function. This was attributed to the need for myogenesis to take place for complete healing in the multiple-injury group. The authors concluded that PRP was useful for muscle injuries only when myogenesis is required for recovery.[206]

More examples of the use of PRP are being presented, with increasing use in the field of sports medicine.[219] The efficacy of this treatment continues to improve with continued positive results. Combining PRP therapy with appropriate mechanical loading properties can lead to speedier recovery and faster return to sport.[220] When treating elite, high-level athletes, clinicians should be aware of concerns expressed by the World Anti-Doping Agency about the use of PRP to create an unfair advantage against competition rules. Care should be taken before treatment to receive an exemption for therapeutic reasons, if necessary.

In the future, PRP treatments can be improved with a standardized method of application, including the optimal time frame after injury for injection. Little is known about tendon healing time after injection or any deleterious effects with rapid return to sport. The literature also lacks a postinjection rehabilitation protocol, neither standard nor injection site specific. No concrete evidence has been presented for the appropriate time to resume antiinflammatory or oral steroid use. Other possible indications for the use of PRP have yet to be studied, including limiting inflammation, which could speed return to sport. Further information must be presented by clinicians with specific results for the increasingly wide use of PRP injection. Injuries, including osteoarthritis, bursitis, acute ligament injuries versus overuse injury, and postoperative joint reconstruction, can be experimented with to create possible future uses of this increasingly popular tool.

DYNAMIC FLEXIBILITY

Preexercise routines have long been practiced as a way to prepare for activity. Historically, various stretches and movements to "loosen" or "warm up" the body have been implemented despite limited evidence of effectiveness. Warm-up should be designed to increase muscle/tendon suppleness, stimulate blood flow to the periphery, increase body temperature, and enhance coordinated movement.[221] The objectives of a warm-up routine developed at West Point also include increasing body temperature, as well as promoting the responsiveness of nerves and muscles, in preparation for activity.[222] Traditionally, the main component of these routines has been static stretching. Many different stretching options and methods of coaching an athlete can be used to properly prepare for sports activity (Table 2-2).

Over time, each has fallen in and out of popularity, and health care professionals and strength and conditioning coaches still debate the most effective way to put together a warm-up routine. For years the gold standard included numerous static stretches that isolate specific muscle groups, such as the hamstrings, quadriceps, triceps, and pectorals, among others. Current research has proposed that a static stretching program may no longer be the most appropriate. Movement toward dynamic flexibility warm-up has gained recognition as a more effective method of preparation. Others note that a specific combination of stretching options in a controlled order will create a well-prepared athlete.

A 2010 literature review by McHugh and Cosgrave[223] examined the results of studies reporting the effects of static and dynamic stretching. Nineteen papers were reviewed that used a strength measurement after static stretching. All 19 reported a loss in strength after using static stretch to warm up. Losses ranged from 2% to 28% of function. Eighteen studies chose power as their outcome measure, with 14 of these studies showing that athletes have an average decreased power output of 4.5% after the implementation of preexercise static

Table 2-2 **Summary of Common Stretching Methods**

Type of Stretch	Definition
Static stretching	Involves the inhibition of tension receptors in muscles. When done properly, static stretching slightly lessens the sensitivity of tension receptors, which allows the muscle to relax and be stretched to greater length. Often referred to as the "reach and hold" technique, an athlete will stretch an isolated muscle to end ROM in an elongated position and typically hold it for 10-30 seconds at a time. Note the difference between static stretching and passive stretching.
Passive stretching	Involves no active movement by the athlete. Passive stretching usually requires an outside force to stretch the muscle, for example, another person or a stretch band.
Dynamic flexibility	Active motion of a body part through full ROM in a functional movement to increase tissue temperature, improve neuromuscular control and speed, and prepare for physically demanding activity. Properly done, it involves slow, controlled movements with a slow increase in speed and ROM.
Ballistic stretching	Sometimes known as the "bouncing technique," ballistic stretching uses body momentum to passively or dynamically move into an extended ROM unable to be reached with a static approach.
Proprioceptive neuromuscular facilitation	Normally found in rehabilitation protocols but can also be used in preparation for exercise. Proprioceptive neuromuscular techniques include agonist contraction, hold-relax, or rhythmic stabilization. Perceived benefits include enhanced neuromuscular control, greater increased ROM than with other techniques, and improved joint stability.
Myofascial release	Creates breaking of adhesions between muscle, fascia, skin, and bone to decrease pain and increase tissue extensibility. Manually disturbing the fascia promotes reorganization of connective tissue in a pattern of greater functional extensibility.
Eccentric training	Eccentric training begins with the muscle to be stretched in a shortened position, followed by active elongation to end ROM to create an eccentric contraction.

ROM, Range of motion.

stretching.[222] Other authors have compared static versus dynamic flexibility. In a study measuring knee flexor strength after a 6-minute stretch time, athletes who used static stretching demonstrated a 14% loss of isometric strength as compared with just a 4% drop in the dynamic group.[224] Manoel et al[225] performed a similar study in 2008 on the knee extensors, but isokinetic tests were used as an outcome measure. Again, the static group had a 4% decrease in power. Comparatively, the dynamic group was shown to have gained 9% in power. In 2009, Sekir et al[226] statically stretched the knee extensors and dynamically stretched the knee flexors via an isokinetic test to measure outcomes. Interestingly, the statically stretched knee extensors lost 14% of their strength, whereas the dynamically stretched knee flexors gained 15% in strength. In a 2006 study, Yamaguchi et al[227] concluded that a quadriceps statically stretched to the point of discomfort decreased in power by 12%. A year later this group measured quadriceps power after dynamic stretching and reported a 9% increase in power output.[118] Although both groups have been shown to exhibit some deleterious effect on strength, statically stretched tissue consistently exhibited greater loss. In terms of power, many times the dynamically stretched athlete shows an increase in output.

With continuing laboratory evidence that static stretching can inhibit performance, Nelson et al[228] examined carryover to sport-specific trials. In measuring 20-m dash times, statically stretched athletes were consistently slower on average by 0.04 second. The dynamic groups had better results than the static groups in high-speed performance activity,[229] agility testing, upper extremity power, and lower extremity power.[222]

Dynamic warm-up leads to a lesser increase in ROM than static stretching does.[230] This provides a possible explanation for better performance in high-speed activity. Conversely, the inhibited function after static stretch has been attributed to muscle having less resistance to passive stretch. This has been referred to as "stress relaxation," or loss of tension after stretch at a constant length.[231] The increased muscle compliance resulting from stretching is suggested as a possible explanation for the decreased muscle performance after static stretching. Improved tolerance of stretching, not mechanical change, causes inhibition of muscle, tendon, or joint receptors (nociceptors) and decreases the body's natural protection of commonly injured structures. A period of delayed neuromuscular response is also reported following stretching exercise. It is possible that these results combined with overwhelming evidence of decreased contracture strength can lead to an increased rate of injury.

To rationalize the loss of strength performance after static stretching it was hypothesized that an alteration in viscoelastic properties has an effect on the length-tendon relationship of the muscle. However, there is no evidence of permanent modification of muscle length at 90 minutes after acute stretching, nor at 24 hours after a 3-week stretch program.[232] Strains as little as 20% beyond resting fiber length can cause muscle damage and subsequent decreased force.[233] Walking alone can cause a 20% strain in sarcomeres.[234] It is a relative certainty that greater than 20% strain occurs with normal stretching routines.

Although most recent research has swung in the direction of dynamic warm-up, this does not mean complete avoidance of static stretching. Static stretching is recommended only after appropriate warm-up and facilitation of the tissue at all times.

Recommended use of static stretching includes equalizing any bilateral differences in ROM that can lead to pathology. A popular static stretch is the "sleeper" stretch for the rotator cuff and capsule stretching in overhead athletes.[235] Such stretching has been shown to be effective in increasing ROM in individuals exhibiting posterior shoulder tightness. As with any static stretch, the sleeper stretch should never be implemented on cold tissue.

It is important to understand the difference between preexercise training and flexibility training. Preexercise dynamic warm-up specifically prepares the athlete for optimal performance in competition. Flexibility training is aimed at changing the resting state of available ROM with little regard for immediate high-level functional performance in competition. Flexibility training is specific to individual needs, whereas dynamic warm-up is specific to the activity. A large, randomized controlled trial in 2005 concluded that dynamic, functional warm-up also reduced rates of injury.[236] Athletes should be sweating after warm-up. If the athlete complains of being tired, the level of activity may be too high. Too large an energy consumption before activity could cause decreased performance secondary to early fatigue. Despite this possibility, dynamic warm-up appears to be the best option to acutely prepare for sports activity.

CONCLUSION

Effects of Immobilization

- Motion problems should be detected early, joint end-feel assessed by palpation, and the reason for the motion problem determined.
- If manipulation is the treatment of choice, it should be performed early in the recovery process to decrease the amount of joint damage resulting from manipulation and to prevent changes in connective tissue from becoming morphologic changes.

Connective Tissue

- The deleterious effects of immobilization on bone and connective tissue have been widely reported. The efficacy of early, controlled mobilization to allow orderly organization of collagen along lines of stress and to promote healthy joint arthrokinematics is supported by many studies.
- Acute injury that is not treated adequately by early concentration on decreasing joint effusion and pain and restoration of normal joint arthrokinematics can result in a vicious inflammatory cycle in which articular cartilage degradation is perpetuated by the enzymes released after cell death. This articular cartilage damage is a secondary injury induced by inadequate attention to decreasing the severity of the early inflammatory process.

Muscle

- The harmful effects of immobilization on muscle are the most obvious changes. Muscle atrophy can be detected as early as 24 hours after immobilization.
- Muscle responds to immobilization by decreases in muscle fiber size, total muscle weight, mitochondrial size and number, muscle tension produced, resting levels of glycogen and ATP, and protein synthesis. Exercise increases muscle contraction time and the lactate level.

- Muscle shutdown is a phenomenon generally seen after immobilization, but it can also be readily detected after most surgical procedures. It is observed in the quadriceps muscle after knee surgery. Although many reasons for muscle shutdown have been postulated, it appears to be affected by one or more of the following factors: joint effusion, angle of joint immobilization, and periarticular tissue damage from surgery or trauma.

Periarticular Tissue

- Immobilization leads to the biochemical and histochemical changes in periarticular tissue that ultimately contribute to arthrofibrosis. Immobilization-induced arthrofibrosis has been widely documented, although the exact mechanism is still speculative.
- Connective tissue usually responds to immobilization by a reduction in water and GAG content; a decrease in the extracellular matrix, which leads to a reduction in the lubrication between fiber cross-links; a decrease in collagen mass; an increase in collagen turnover, degradation, and synthesis rates; and an increase in abnormal collagen fiber cross-links.

Ligaments

- Ligaments are similarly affected by immobilization. It appears that the bone-ligament junction undergoes an increase in osteoclastic activity, which results in a weaker junction. Ligament atrophy also occurs along with a corresponding decrease in linear stress, maximum stress, and stiffness.

Articular Cartilage

- The greatest effect of immobilization appears to be on articular cartilage. Intermittent loading and unloading of synovial joints promotes the metabolic exchange necessary for the proper structure and function of articular cartilage.
- Joint immobilization, in which articular cartilage is in constant contact with opposing bone ends, can cause pressure necrosis. Conversely, noncontact between joint surfaces can promote the ingrowth of connective tissue into the joint.
- Diminished weight bearing and loading and unloading of an extremity also cause an increase in bone resorption in that area.

Continuous Passive Motion

- CPM devices allow early joint motion with no detrimental side effects. CPM has a significantly stimulating effect on healing articular tissues, including cartilage, tendons, and ligaments, and prevents joint adhesions and stiffness. Patients using CPM devices have shown decreases in joint hemarthrosis and in requests for pain medication.

Effects of Remobilization

- Tissues appear to recover at different rates with remobilization after immobilization, with muscle recovering the fastest.
- Although few studies on the effects of remobilization on immobilized connective tissue have been conducted, it has been proved that early mobilization maintains lubrication and a critical fiber distance between collagen fibrils in the matrix, thereby preventing abnormal cross-link formation.

- After immobilization, articular cartilage and bone respond the least favorably to remobilization. Changes in articular cartilage depend on the length and angle of immobilization. Prolonged immobilization can result in irreversible changes in articular cartilage.
- Early protected motion and weight bearing, as healing restraints allow, are therefore advocated to avoid the deleterious effects of immobilization and to deter the secondary problems perpetuated by immobilization.

Tissue Healing with Platelet-Rich Plasma Therapy

- PRP has recently become a popular treatment option for orthopedic injuries. Currently, proper uses and dosages are being developed.
- Continued research is needed to establish appropriate injection methods and follow-up treatment to optimize effectiveness. Recommendations at this time include 48- to 72-hour rest of the injection site, as well as cessation of antiinflammatory medication to increase the total number of platelets reaching the injury site.

Dynamic Flexibility

- Incorporating dynamic flexibility into the warm-up routine is best suited for preparing athletes to participate in sports. Use of static stretching only will result in a decrease in muscle strength and power and can lead to an increased incidence of injury.
- By using progressive, active movement to increase tissue temperature, muscle will respond with increased extensibility in a functional capacity. A properly constructed active warm-up will cause the athlete to perspire, but not fatigue, before participating in practice or games.

REFERENCES

1. Golden, A. (1980): Reaction to injury in the musculoskeletal system. In: Rosse C., and Clawson DK. (ed.). The Musculoskeletal System in Health and Disease. New York, Harper & Row, pp. 89–93.
2. Knight, K. (1976): The effects of hypothermia on inflammation and swelling. Athl. Train., 11:7–10.
3. Hettinga, D.L. (1979): I. Normal joint structures and their reaction to injury. J. Orthop. Sports Phys. Ther., 1:16–22.
4. Roy, S., Ghadially, F.N., and Crane, W.A.J. (1966): Synovial membrane and traumatic effusion: Ultrastructure and autoradiography with tritiated leucine. Ann. Rheumatol. Dis., 25:259–271.
5. Bozdech, Z. (1976): Posttraumatic synovitis. Acta Chir. Orthop. Traumatol. Cech., 43:244–247.
6. Soren, A., Rosenbauer, K.A., Klein, W., and Hugh, F. (1973): Morphological examinations of so-called posttraumatic synovitis. Beitr. Pathol. 1950:11–30.
7. Castor, C.W., Prince, R.K., and Hazelton, M.J. (1966): Hyaluronic acid in human synovial effusions: A sensitive indicator of altered connective tissue cell function during inflammation. Arthritis Rheum., 9:783–794.
8. Roosendaal, G., Vianen, M.E., and Marx, J.J. (1999): Blood-induced joint damage: A human in vitro study. Arthritis Rheum., 42:1025–1032.
9. Roosendaal, G., Vianen, M.E., and van der Berg, H.M. (1997): Cartilage damage as a result of hemarthrosis in a human in vitro model. J. Rheumatol., 24:1350–1354.
10. Roosendaal, G., Tekoppele, J.M., and Vianen, M.E. (2000): Articular cartilage is more susceptible to blood induced damage at young than at old age. J. Rheumatol., 27:1740–1744.
11. Stravino, V.D. (1972): The synovial system. Am. J. Phys. Med., 51:312–320.
12. Hettinga, D.L. (1979): II. Normal joint structures and their reaction to injury. J. Orthop. Sports Phys. Ther., 1:83–88.
13. Sledge, C.B. (1975): Structure, development, and function of joints. Orthop. Clin. North Am., 6:619–628.

14. Booth, F.W., and Kelso, J.R. (1973): Effect of hindlimb immobilization on contractile and histochemical properties of skeletal muscle. Pflugers Arch., 342:231–238.
15. MacDougall, J.D., Elder, G.C.B., and Sale, D.G. (1980): Effects of strength training and immobilization on human muscle fibers. Eur. J. Appl. Physiol., 43:25–34.
16. MacDougall, J.D., Ward, G.R., Sale, D.G., and Sutton, J.R. (1977): Biochemical adaptation of human skeletal muscle to heavy resistance training and immobilization. J. Appl. Physiol., 43:700–703.
17. Venn, M.F. (1979): Chemical composition of human femoral and head cartilage: Influence of topographical position and fibrillation. Ann. Rheum. Dis., 38:57–62.
18. Stokes, M., and Young, A. (1984): The contribution of reflex inhibition to arthrogenous muscle weakness. Clin. Sci., 67:7–14.
19. Leivo, I., Kauhanen, S., and Michelsson, J.E. (1998): Abnormal mitochondria and sarcoplasmic changes in rabbit skeletal muscle induced by immobilization. APMIS, 106:1113–1123.
20. Lindboe, C.F., and Platou, C.S. (1984): Effects of immobilization of short duration on muscle fiber size. Clin. Physiol., 4:183–188.
21. Appell, H.J. (1986): Morphology of immobilized skeletal muscle and the effects of a pre- and postimmobilization training program. Int. J. Sports Med., 7:6–12.
22. Binkley, J.M., and Peat, M. (1986): The effects of immobilization on the ultrastructure and mechanical properties of the medial collateral ligament of rats. Clin. Orthop. Relat. Res., 203:301–308.
23. Haggmark, T., Eriksson, E., and Jansson, E. (1986): Muscle fiber type changes in human skeletal muscle after injuries and immobilization. Orthopedics, 9:181–185.
24. Haggmark, T., Jansson, E., and Eriksson, E. (1981): Fiber type area and metabolic potential of the thigh muscle in man after knee surgery and immobilization. Int. J. Sports Med., 2:12–17.
25. Labarque, V.L., Op't Eijnde, B., and Van Leemputte, M. (2002): Effect of immobilization and retraining on torque-velocity relationship of human knee flexor and extensor muscles. Eur. J. Appl. Physiol., 86:251–257.
26. Hayashi, K. (1996): Biomechanical studies of the remodeling of knee joint tendons and ligaments. J. Biomech., 29:707–716.
27. Wolf, J. (1982): Das Gesetz der Transformation der Knochen. Berlin, A. Hirschwald.
28. Young, D.R., Niklowitz, W.J., and Steele, C.R. (1983): Tibial changes in experimental disuse osteoporosis in the monkey. Calcif. Tissue Int., 35:304–308.
29. Kannus, P., Jozsa, L., and Kvist, M. (1992): The effect of immobilization on myotendinous junction: An ultrastructural, histochemical and immunohistochemical study. Acta Physiol. Scand., 144:387–394.
30. Booth, F.W. (1987): Physiological and biochemical effects of immobilization on muscle. Clin. Orthop. Relat. Res., 219:15–20.
31. Booth, F.W., and Seider, M.J. (1979): Recovery of skeletal muscle after 3 months of hindlimb immobilization in rats. J. Appl. Physiol., 47:435–439.
32. Maier, A., Crockett, J.L., and Simpson, D.R. (1976): Properties of immobilized guinea pig hindlimb muscles. Am. J. Physiol., 231:1520–1526.
33. Trias, A. (1961): Effects of persistent pressure on articular cartilage. J. Bone Joint Surg. Am., 43:376–386.
34. Cooper, R.R. (1972): Alternatives during immobilization and regeneration of skeletal muscle in cats. J. Bone Joint Surg. Am., 54:919–953.
35. Max, S.R. (1972): Disuse atrophy of skeletal muscle: Loss of functional activity of mitochondria. Biochem. Biophys. Res. Commun., 46:1394–1398.
36. Rifenberick, D.H., and Max, S.R. (1974): Substrate utilization by disused rat skeletal muscles. Am. J. Physiol., 226:295–297.
37. Ingemann-Hansen, T., and Halkjaer-Kristensen, J. (1980): Computerized tomographic determination of human thigh components. The effects of immobilization in plaster and subsequent physical training. Scand. J. Rehabil. Med., 12:27–31.
38. Ingemann-Hansen, T., and Halkjaer-Kristensen, J. (1977): Lean and fat composition of the human thigh. The effects of immobilization in plaster and subsequent physical training. J. Rehabil. Med., 9:67–72.
39. Shakespeare, D.T., Stokes, M., Sherman, K.P., and Young, A. (1983): The effect of knee flexion on quadriceps inhibition after meniscectomy. Clin. Sci., 65:64P–65P.
40. Shakespeare, D.T., Stokes, M., Sherman, K.P., and Young, A. (1985): Reflex inhibition of the quadriceps after meniscectomy: Lack of association with pain. Clin. Physiol., 5:137–144.
41. Ben-Yishay, A., Zuckerman, J.D., Gallagher, M., and Cuomo, F. (1994): Pain inhibition of shoulder strength in patients with impingement syndrome. Orthopedics, 17:685–688.
42. Itoi, E., Minagawa, H., and Solo, T. (1997): Isokinetic strength after tears of the supraspinatus tendon. J. Bone Joint Surg. Br., 79:77–82.
43. Kirschenbaum, D., Coyle, M.P., and Leddy, L.P. (1993): Shoulder strength with rotator cuff tears: Pre- and postoperative analysis. Clin. Orthop. Relat. Res., 288:174–178.
44. Hess, T., Gleitz, M., and Hopf, T. (1995): Changes in muscular activity after knee arthrotomy and arthroscopy. Int. Orthop., 19:94–97.
45. Stetson, W.B., and Templin, K. (2002): Two versus three portal technique for routine knee arthroscopy. Am. J. Sports Med., 30:108–111.
46. Rabb, D.J., Fischer, D.A., and Smith, J.P. (1993): Comparison of arthroscopic and open reconstruction of the anterior cruciate ligament. Early results. Am. J. Sports Med., 21:680–683.
47. T'Jonck, L., Lysens, R., and De Smet, L. (1997): Open versus arthroscopic subacromial decompression: Analysis of one-year results. Physiother. Res. Int., 2:46–61.
48. Arciero, R.A., Scoville, C.R., Hayda, R.A., and Snyder, R.J. (1996): The effect of tourniquet use in anterior cruciate ligament reconstruction. A prospective, randomized study. Am. J. Sports Med., 24:758–764.
49. Saunders, K.C., Louis, D.L., Weingarden, S.I., and Waylonis, G.W. (1979): Effect of tourniquet time on postoperative quadriceps function. Clin. Orthop. Relat. Res., 143:194–199.

50. Walsh, S., Frank, C., Shrive, N., and Hart, D. (1993): Knee immobilization inhibits biomechanical maturation of the rabbit medial collateral ligament. Clin. Orthop. Relat. Res., 297:253–261.
51. DeAndrade, J.R., Grant, C., and Dixon, A. (1965): Joint distension and reflex inhibition in the knee. J. Bone Joint Surg. Am., 47:313–322.
52. Jayson, M.I.V., and Dixon, A. (1970): Intra-articular pressure in rheumatoid arthritis of the knee. III. Pressure changes during joint use. Ann. Rheum. Dis., 29:401–408.
53. Kennedy, J.C., Alexander, I.J., and Hayes, K.C. (1982): Nerve supply of the human knee and its functional importance. Am. J. Sports Med., 10:329–335.
54. Spencer, J.D., Hayes, K.C., and Alexander, I.J. (1984): Knee joint effusion and quadriceps inhibition in man. Arch. Phys. Med. Rehabil., 65:171–177.
55. Ziechen, J., van Griensven, M., and Albers, I. (1999): Immunohistochemical localization of collagen VI in arthrofibrosis. Arch. Orthop. Trauma Surg., 119:315–318.
56. Young, A., Stokes, M., and Iles, J.F. (1987): Effects of joint pathology on muscle. Clin. Orthop. Relat. Res., 219:21–27.
57. Geborek, P., Moritz, U., and Wollheim, F.A. (1989): Joint capsular stiffness in knee arthritis. Relationship to intraarticular volume, hydrostatic pressures, and extensor muscle function. J. Rheumatol., 16:1351–1358.
58. Jones, D.W., Jones, D.A., and Newham, D.J. (1987): Chronic knee effusion and aspiration: The effect on quadriceps inhibition. Br. J. Rheumatol., 26:370–374.
59. Krebs, D.E., Staples, W.H., Cuttita, D., and Zickel, R.E. (1983): Knee joint angle: Its relationship to quadriceps femoris activity in normal and post-arthrotomy limbs. Arch. Phys. Med. Rehabil., 64:441–447.
60. Stratford, P. (1981): Electromyography of the quadriceps femoris muscles in subjects with normal knees and acutely effused knees. Phys. Ther., 62:279–289.
61. Eyring, E.J., and Murray, W.R. (1964): The effect of joint position on the pressure of intra-articular effusion. J. Bone Joint Surg. Am., 46:1235–1241.
62. Levick, R.J. (1983): Joint pressure-volume studies: Their importance, design and interpretation. J. Rheumatol., 10:353–357.
63. Levick, R.J. (1983): Synovial fluid dynamics: The regulation of volume and pressure. In: Holborrow E.J., and Maroudas V. (eds). Studies in Joint Disease. London, Pitman Medical, pp. 153–240.
64. Tardieu, C., Tabary, J.C., Tabary, C., and Tardieu, G. (1982): Adaptation of connective tissue length in immobilization in the lengthened and shortened positions in cat soleus muscle. J. Physiol., 78:214–217.
65. Witzmann, F.A., Kim, D.H., and Fitts, R.H. (1982): Hindlimb immobilization: Length-tension and contractile properties of skeletal muscle. J. Appl. Physiol., 53:335–345.
66. Jarvinen, M.J., Einola, S.A., and Virtanen, E.O. (1992): Effect of the position of immobilization upon tensile properties of rat gastrocnemius muscle. Arch. Phys. Med. Rehabil., 73:253–257.
67. Jokl, P., and Konstadt, S. (1983): The effect of limb immobilization on muscle function and protein composition. Clin. Orthop. Relat. Res., 174:222–229.
68. Edin, B.B., and Vallbo, A.B. (1988): Stretch sensitization of human muscle spindles. J. Physiol., 400:101–111.
69. Hugheston, J.C. (1985): Complications of anterior cruciate ligament surgery. Orthop. Clin. North Am., 16:237–240.
70. Paulos, L., Rosenberg, T., and Drawbert, J. (1987): Infrapatellar contracture syndrome: An unrecognized cause of knee stiffness with patella entrapment and patella infera. Am. J. Sports Med., 15:331–342.
71. Sprangue, N.F., O'Conner, R.L., and Fox, J.M. (1982): Arthroscopic treatment of postoperative knee fibroarthrosis. Clin. Orthop. Relat. Res., 166:165–172.
72. Jackson, D.W., and Shafer, R.K. (1987): Cyclops syndrome: Loss of extension following intra-articular anterior cruciate ligament reconstruction. Arthroscopy, 6:171–178.
73. Fujimoto, D., Moriquichi, T., Ishida, T., and Hayashi, H. (1978): The structure of pyridinoline, a collagen cross link. Biochem. Biophys. Res. Commun., 84:52–57.
74. Ham, A.C., and Cormack, D. (1979): Histology, Vol. 8. Philadelphia, Lippincott.
75. Donatelli, R., and Owens-Burkhart, A. (1981): Effects of immobilization on the extensibility of periarticular connective tissue. J. Orthop. Sports Phys. Ther., 3:67–72.
76. Burr, D.B., Frederickson, R.G., and Pavlinch, C. (1984): Intracast muscle stimulation prevents bone and cartilage deterioration in cast-immobilized rabbits. Clin. Orthop. Relat. Res., 189:264–278.
77. Akeson, W.H., Amiel, D., and Woo, S. (1980): Immobility effects of synovial joints: The pathomechanics of joint contracture. Biorheology, 17:95–110.
78. Swann, D., Radin, E., and Nazimiec, M. (1976): Role of hyaluronic acid on joint lubrication. Ann. Rheum. Dis., 33:318–326.
79. Akeson, W.H., Amiel, D., and Abel, M.F. (1987): Effects of immobilization on joints. Clin. Orthop. Relat. Res., 219:28–37.
80. Akeson, W.H., Amiel, D., and LaViolette, D. (1967): The connective tissue response to immobility: A study of the chondroitin-4- and 6-sulfate and dermatan sulfate changes in periarticular connective tissue of control and immobilized knee of dogs. Clin. Orthop. Relat. Res., 51:183–197.
81. Akeson, W.H., Woo, S.L.Y., and Amiel, D. (1984): The chemical basis of tissue repair. In Hunter, L.Y., and Funk, F. J. (eds): Rehabilitation of the Injured Knee. St. Louis, Mosby, pp. 93–148.
82. Bosch, U., Ziechen, J., and Skutek, M. (2001): Arthrofibrosis in the result of a T-cell mediated immune response. Knee Surg. Sports Trauma Arthrosc., 9:282–289.
83. Akeson, W.H., Woo, S.L.Y., and Amiel, D. (1973): The connective tissue response to immobility: Biochemical changes in periarticular connective tissue of the immobilized rabbit knee. Clin. Orthop. Relat. Res., 93:356–362.
84. Hunter, R.E., Mastrangelo, J., and Freeman, J.R. (1996): The impact of surgical timing on postoperative motion and stability following anterior cruciate ligament reconstruction. Arthroscopy, 12:667–674.

85. Shelborne, K.D., Wilchkens, J.H., Mollabashy, A., and DeCarlo, M. (1991): Arthrofibrosis in acute anterior cruciate ligament reconstruction: The effect of timing on reconstruction and rehabilitation. Am. J. Sports Med., 19:332–336.

86. Wakai, A., Winter, D.C., Street, J.T., and Redmond, P.H. (2001): Pneumatic tourniquets in extremity surgery. J. Am. Acad. Orthop. Surg., 9:345–351.

87. Mariani, P.P., Santori, N., and Rovere, P. (1997): Histological and structural study of the adhesive tissue in knee fibroarthrosis: A clinical-pathological correlation. Arthroscopy, 13:13–18.

88. Tamberello, M., Mangine, R.E., and Personius, W. (1982): Patella hypomobility as a cause of extensor lag. Presented at Total Care of the Knee: Before and After Injury (Cybex Conference),Overland Park, KS, May 17-19, 1985.

89. Arem, A.J., and Madden, J.W. (1976): Effects of stress on healing wounds: Intermittent noncyclical tension. J. Surg. Res., 20:93–102.

90. Wright, V., Dowson, D., and Kerr, J. (1973): The structure of joints. Int. Rev. Connect. Tissue Res., 6:105–125.

91. Williams, P.E., and Goldspink, G. (1978): Changes in sarcomere length and physiological properties in immobilized muscle. J. Anat., 127:459–468.

92. Wronski, T., and Morey, E.R. (1982): Skeletal abnormalities in rats induced by simulated weightlessness. Metab. Bone Dis., 4:69–74.

93. Videman, T. (1981): Changes of compression and distances between tibial and femoral condyles during immobilization of rabbit knee. Arch. Orthop. Trauma Surg., 98:289–294.

94. Elliot, R.J., and Gardner, D.L. (1979): Changes with age of the glycosaminoglycans of human cartilage. Ann. Rheum. Dis., 38:371–377.

95. Westers, B.M. (1982): Review of the repair of defects in articular cartilage: Part I. J. Orthop. Sports Phys. Ther., 3:186–192.

96. Uhthoff, H.K., and Jaworski, Z.F.G. (1978): Bone loss in response to long-term immobilization. J. Bone Joint Surg. Br., 60:420–429.

97. Maroudes, A., Bullough, P., Swanson, S., and Freemna, M. (1968): The permeability of articular cartilage. J. Bone Joint Surg. Br., 50:166–177.

98. Jozsa, L., Jarvinen, M., Kannus, P., and Reffy, A. (1987): Fine structural changes in the articular cartilage of the rat's knee following short-term immobilization in various positions: A scanning electron microscopical study. Int. Orthop., 11:129–133.

99. Jurvelin, J., Kiviranta, I., Tammi, M., and Helminen, J.H. (1986): Softening of canine articular cartilage after immobilization of the knee joint. Clin. Orthop. Relat. Res., 207:246–252.

100. Radin, E.L., Paul, I.L., and Pollock, D. (1970): Animal joint behavior under excessive loading. Nature, 266:554–555.

101. Virchenko, O., and Aspenberg, P. (2006): How can one platelet injection after tendon injury lead to a stronger tendon after 4 weeks? Interplay between early regeneration and mechanical stimulation. Acta Orthop. 77:806–812.

102. Salter, R.B., and Field, P. (1960): The effects of continuous compression on living articular cartilage. J. Bone Joint Surg. Am., 42:31–49.

103. Hall, M.C. (1963): Cartilage changes after experimental relief of contact in the knee of the mature rat. J. Bone Joint Surg. Am., 45:36–44.

104. Broom, N.D., and Myers, D.B. (1980): A study of the structural response of wet hyaline cartilage to various loading situations. Connect. Tissue Res., 7:227–237.

105. Ekholm, R. (1955): Nutrition of articular cartilage: A radioautographic study. Acta Anat., 24:329–338.

106. Enneking, W.F., and Horowitz, M. (1972): The intra-articular effects of immobilization on the human knee. J. Bone Joint Surg. Am., 54:973–985.

107. Eronin, I., Videman, T., Friman, C., and Michelsson, J.E. (1978): Glycosaminoglycan metabolism in experimental osteoarthritis caused by immobilization. Acta Orthop. Scand., 49:329–334.

108. Langenskiold, A., Michelsson, J.E., and Videman, T. (1979): Osteoarthritis of the knee in the rabbit produced by immobilization: Attempts to achieve a reproducible model for studies on pathogenesis and therapy. Acta Orthop. Scand., 50:1–14.

109. Sherman, K.P., Young, A., Stokes, M., and Shakespeare, D.T. (1984): Joint injury and muscle weakness. Lancet, 2:646–651.

110. Roth, J.H., Mendenhall, H.V., and McPherson, G.K. (1988): The effect of immobilization on goat knees following reconstruction of the anterior cruciate ligament. Clin. Orthop. Relat. Res., 229:278–282.

111. Kiviranta, I., Tammi, M., and Jurvelin, J. (1992): Articular cartilage thickness and glycosaminoglycan distribution in the canine knee joint after strenuous running exercise. Clin. Orthop. Relat. Res., 283:302–308.

112. Cabaud, H.E., Chatty, A., and Gildengorin, V. (1980): Exercise effects on the strength of the rat anterior cruciate ligament. Am. J. Sports Med., 8:79–86.

113. Amiel, D., Woo, S.L.Y., Harwood, F.L., and Akeson, W.H. (1982): The effect of immobilization on collagen turnover in connective tissue: A biochemical-biochemical correlation. Acta Orthop. Scand., 53:325–332.

114. Noyes, F.R., Mangine, R.E., and Barber, S. (1974): Biomechanics of ligament failure. II. An analysis of immobilization, exercise, and reconditioning effects in primates. J. Bone Joint Surg. Am., 56:1406–1418.

115. Noyes, F.R., Mangine, R.E., and Barber, S. (1987): Early knee motion after open and arthroscopic anterior cruciate ligament reconstruction. Am. J. Sports Med., 15:149–160.

116. Woo, S., Gomez, M.A., and Sites, T.J. (1987): The biomechanical and morphological changes in the medial collateral ligament of the rabbit after immobilization and remobilization. J. Bone Joint Surg. Am., 69:1200–1211.

117. Noyes, F.R. (1977): Functional properties of knee ligaments and alterations induced by immobilization. Clin. Orthop. Relat. Res., 123:210–242.

118. Yamaguchi, T., Ishii, K., Yamanaka, M., et al. (2006): Acute effects of static stretching on power output during concentric dynamic constant external resistance leg extension. J. Strength Cond. Res., 20:804–810.

119. Gamble, J.G., Edwards, C.C., and Max, S.R. (1984): Enzymatic adaptation in ligaments during immobilization. Am. J. Sports Med., 12:221–228.

120. Newton, P.O., Woo, S.L., and Kitabayashi, L.R. (1990): Ultrastructural changes in knee ligaments following immobilization. Matrix, 10:314–319.

121. Yasuda, K., Ohkoshi, Y., Tanabe, Y., and Kaneda, K. (1992): Quantitative evaluation of knee instability and muscle strength after anterior cruciate ligament reconstruction using patellar tendon and quadriceps tendon. Am. J. Sports Med., 20:471–475.

122. Boorman, R.S., Shrive, N.G., and Frank, C.B. (1998): Immobilization increases the vulnerability of rabbit medial collateral ligament autografts to creep. J. Orthop. Res., 16:682–689.

123. Thornton, G.M., Boorman, R.S., Shrive, N.G., and Frank, C.B. (2002): Medial collateral ligament autografts have increased creep response for at least two years and early immobilization makes this worse. J. Orthop. Res., 20:346–352.

124. Weiss, C. (1979): Normal and osteoarthritic articular cartilage. Orthop. Clin. North Am., 10:175–189.

125. Ochi, M., Kanda, T., Sumen, Y., and Ikuta, Y. (1997): Changes in the permeability and histologic findings of rabbit menisci after immobilization. Clin. Orthop. Relat. Res., 334:305–315.

126. Bray, R.C., Smith, J.A., and Eng, M.K. (2001): Vascular response of the meniscus to injury: Effects of immobilization. J. Orthop. Res., 19:384–390.

127. Djurasovic, M., Aldridge, J.W., and Grumbles, R. (1998): Knee joint immobilization decreases aggrecan gene expression in the meniscus. Am. J. Sports Med., 26:460–466.

128. Klein, L., Heiple, K.G., and Torzilli, P.A. (1989): Prevention of ligament and meniscus atrophy by active joint motion in a non–weight-bearing model. J. Orthop. Res., 7:80–85.

129. Butler, D.L., Grood, E.S., and Noyes, F.R. (1989): Mechanical properties of primate vascularized versus nonvascularized patellar tendon grafts, changes over time. J. Orthop. Res., 7:68–79.

130. Falconiero, R.P., DiStefano, V.J., and Cook, T.M. (1998): Revascularization and ligamentization of autogenous anterior cruciate ligament grafts in humans. Arthroscopy, 14:197–205.

131. Rougraff, B.T., and Shelbourne, K.D. (1999): Early histologic appearance of human patellar tendon autografts used for anterior cruciate ligament reconstruction. Knee Surg. Sports Trauma Arthrosc., 7:9–14.

132. Papageorgiou, C.D., Benjamin, C., and Abramowitch, S.D. (2001): Multidisciplinary study of the healing of an intraarticular anterior cruciate ligament in a goat model. Am. J. Sports Med., 29:620–626.

133. Scranton, P.E., Lanzer, W.L., and Ferguson, M.S. (1998): Mechanism of anterior cruciate neovascularization and ligamentization. Arthroscopy, 14:702–716.

134. Hardt, A.B. (1972): Early metabolic responses of bone to immobilization. J. Bone Joint Surg. Am., 54:119–124.

135. Burdeaux, B.D., and Hutchinson, W.J. (1953): Etiology of traumatic osteoporosis. J. Bone Joint Surg. Am., 35:479–488.

136. Fleisch, H., Russell, R.G., Simpson, B., and Muhlbauer, R.C. (1969): Prevention by a diphosphonate of immobilization osteoporosis in rats. Nature, 223:211–212.

137. Geiser, M., and Trueta, J. (1985): Muscle action, bone rarefaction, and bone formation. J. Bone Joint Surg. Br., 40:282–311.

138. Landry, M., and Fleisch, H. (1964): The influence of immobilization on bone formation as evaluated by osseous incorporation of tetracyclines. J. Bone Joint Surg. Br., 46:764–771.

139. Steinberg, F.U. (1980): The Immobilized Patient: Functional Pathology and Management. New York, Plenum Press.

140. Epker, B.N., and Frost, H.M. (1965): Correlation of bone resorption and formation behavior of loaded bone. J. Dent. Res., 44:33–41.

141. Mazess, R.B., and Whedon, G.D. (1983): Immobilization and bone. Calcif. Tissue Int., 35:265–267.

142. Wrotniak, M., Bielecki, T., and Gazdzik, T. (2007): Current opinion about using the platelet-rich gel in orthopaedics and trauma surgery. Orthop. Traumatol. Rehabil., 9:227–238.

143. Salter, R.B. (1989): The biologic concept of continuous passive motion of synovial joints. Clin. Orthop. Relat. Res., 242:12–25.

144. Loitz, B.J., Zernicke, R.F., and Vailas, A.C. (1989): Effects of short-term immobilization versus continuous passive motion on the biomechanical and biochemical properties of the rabbit tendon. Clin. Orthop. Relat. Res., 244:265–271.

145. Salter, R.B., Simmonds, D.F., and Malcolm, B.W. (1975): The effect of continuous passive motion on the healing of articular cartilage defects: An experimental investigation in rabbits [Abstract]. J. Bone Joint Surg. Am., 57:570.

146. Salter, R.B., and Minster, R.R. (1982): The effect of continuous passive motion on a semitendinous tenodesis in the rabbit knee [Abstract]. Orthop. Trans., 6:292.

147. McCarthy, M.R., Buxton, B.P., and Yates, C.K. (1993): Effects of continuous passive motion on anterior laxity following ACL reconstruction with autogenous patellar tendon grafts. J. Sport Rehabil., 2:171–178.

148. Nugent-Derfus, G., Takara, T., O'Neill, J.K., et al. (2007): Continuous passive motion applied to whole joints stimulates chondrocyte biosynthesis of PRG4. Osteoarthritis Cartilage, 15:566–574.

149. Raab, M.G., Rzeszutko, D., O'Conner, W., and Greatting, M.D. (1996): Early results of continuous passive motion after rotator cuff repair: A prospective, randomized, blinded, controlled study. Am. J. Orthop., 25:214–220.

150. Lastayo, P.C., Wright, T., Jaffe, R., and Hartzel, J. (1998): Continuous passive motion after repair of the rotator cuff: A prospective outcome study. J. Bone Joint Surg. Am., 80:1002–1111.

151. Engstrom, B., Sperber, A., and Wredmark, T. (1995): Continuous passive motion in rehabilitation after anterior cruciate ligament reconstruction. Knee Surg. Sports Trauma Arthrosc., 3:18–20.

152. Gasper, L., Farkas, C., Szepesi, K., and Csernatony, Z. (1997): Therapeutic value of continuous passive motion after anterior cruciate replacement. Acta Chir. Hung., 36:104–105.

153. Rosen, M.A., Jackson, D.W., and Artwell, E.A. (1992): The efficacy of continuous passive motion in the rehabilitation of anterior cruciate ligament reconstruction. Am. J. Sports Med., 20:122–127.

154. McCarthy, M.R., Yates, C.K., Anderson, M.A., and Yates-McCarthy, J.L. (1993): The effects of immediate continuous passive motion on pain during the inflammatory phase of soft tissue healing following anterior cruciate reconstruction. J. Orthop. Sports Phys. Ther., 17:96–101.

155. Lenssen, T., van Steyn, M.J., Crijns, Y.H., et al. (2008): Effectiveness of prolonged use of continuous passive motion (CPM) as an adjunct to physiotherapy, after total knee arthroplasty. BMC Musculoskel. Disord., 9:1–11.

156. Yates, C.K., McCarthy, M.R., Hirsch, H.S., and Pascale, M.S. (1992): Effects of continuous passive motion following ACL reconstruction with autogenous patellar tendon grafts. J. Sport Rehabil., 1:121–131.

157. Dehert, W.J., O'Driscoll, S.W., van Royen, B.J., and Salter, R.B. (1988): Effects of immobilization and continuous passive motion on postoperative muscle atrophy in mature rabbits. Can. J. Surg., 31:185–188.

158. Gebhard, J.S., Kabo, J.M., and Meals, R.A. (1993): Passive motion: The dose effects on joint stiffness, muscle mass, bone density, and regional swelling. A study in an experimental model following intra-articular injury. J. Bone Joint Surg. Am., 75:1636–1647.

159. Renzoni, S.A., Amiel, D., Harwood, F.L., and Akeson, W.H. (1984): Synovial nutrition of knee ligaments. Trans. Orthop. Res. Soc., 9:277–283.

160. Kannus, P., Jozsa, L., and Jarvinen, T.L. (1998): Free mobilization and low- to high-intensity exercise in immobilization-induced muscle atrophy. J. Appl. Physiol., 84:1418–1424.

161. Keays, S.L., Bullock-Saxton, J., and Keays, A.C. (2000): Strength and function before and after anterior cruciate ligament reconstruction. Clin. Orthop. Relat. Res., 373:174–183.

162. Snyder-Mackler, L., Delitto, A., Bailey, S.L., and Stralka, S.W. (1995): Strength of the quadriceps femoris muscles and functional recovery after reconstruction of the anterior cruciate ligament: A prospective, randomized clinical trial of electrical stimulation. J. Bone Joint Surg. Am., 77:1166–1173.

163. Keays, S.L., Bullock-Saxton, J., Keays, A.C., and Newcombe, P. (2001): Muscle strength and function before and after anterior cruciate ligament reconstruction using semitendinosis and gracilis. Knee, 8:229–234.

164. Osteras, H., Augestad, L.B., and Tondel, S. (1998): Isokinetic muscle strength after anterior cruciate ligament reconstruction. Scand. J. Med. Sci. Sports, 8:279–282.

165. Arvidsson, I., Arvidsson, H., Eriksson, E., and Jansson, E. (1986): Prevention of quadriceps wasting after immobilization: An evaluation of the effect of electrical muscle stimulation. Orthopedics, 9:1519–1528.

166. Rokito, A.S., Zuckerman, J.D., Gallagher, M.A., and Cuomo, F. (1996): Strength after surgical repair of the rotator cuff. J. Shoulder Elbow Surg., 5:12–17.

167. Gibson, J.N., Smith, K., and Rennie, M.J. (1988): Prevention of disuse muscle atrophy by means of electrical muscle stimulation: Maintenance of protein synthesis. Lancet, 7:767–770.

168. Morrissey, M.C., Brewster, C.E., Shields, C.L., and Brown, M. (1985): The effects of electrical stimulation on the quadriceps during postoperative knee immobilization. Am. J. Sports Med., 13:40–45.

169. Delitto, A., Rose, S.J., and McKowen, J.M. (1988): Electrical stimulation versus voluntary exercise in strengthening thigh musculature after anterior cruciate ligament surgery. Phys. Ther., 68:660–663.

170. Eriksson, E., and Haggmark, T. (1979): Comparison of isometric muscle training and electrical stimulation supplementing isometric muscle training in the recovery after major knee ligament surgery. Am. J. Sports Med., 7:169–171.

171. Snyder-Mackler, L., Ladin, Z., Schepsis, A.A., and Young, J.C. (1991): Electrical stimulation of the thigh muscles after reconstruction of the anterior cruciate ligament: Effects of electrically elicited contraction of the quadriceps femoris and hamstring muscles on gait and on strength of the thigh muscles. J. Bone Joint Surg. Am., 73:1025–1036.

172. Paternostro-Sluga, T., Fialka, C., and Alacamlioglu, Y. (1999): Neuromuscular electrical stimulation after anterior cruciate ligament surgery. Clin. Orthop. Relat. Res., 368:166–175.

173. Lieber, R.L., Silva, P.D., and Daniel, D.M. (1996): Equal effectiveness of electrical and volitional strength training for the quadriceps femoris muscles after anterior cruciate ligament surgery. J. Orthop. Res., 14:131–138.

174. Draper, V., and Ballard, L. (1991): Electrical stimulation versus electromyographic biofeedback in the recovery of quadriceps femoris muscle function following anterior cruciate ligament surgery. Phys. Ther., 71:455–461.

175. Kiviranta, I., Tammi, M., and Jurvelin, J. (1994): Articular cartilage thickness and glycosaminoglycan distribution in the young canine knee joint after remobilization of the immobilized limb. J. Orthop. Res., 12:161–167.

176. Van, H., Lillich, J.D., and Kawcak, C.E. (2002): Clinical evaluation of the effects of immobilization followed by remobilization and exercise on the metacarpophalangeal joint in horses. Am. J. Vet. Res., 63:282–288.

177. Veldhuizen, J.W., Verstappen, F.T., and Vroemen, J.P. (1993): Functional and morphological adaptations following four weeks of knee immobilization. Int. J. Sports Med., 14:283–287.

178. Haapala, J., Arokoski, J., and Pirttimaki, J. (2000): Incomplete restoration of immobilization induced softening of young beagle knee articular cartilage after 50-week remobilization. Int. J. Sports Med., 21:76–81.

179. Evans, E.B., Egger, G.W.N., Butler, M., and Blumel, J. (1960): Experimental immobilization and remobilization of rat knee joints. J. Bone Joint Surg. Am., 42:737–758.

180. Lynch, T.N., Jensen, R.L., and Stevens, D.M. (1967): Metabolic effects of prolonged bed rest: Their modification by simulated altitude. Aerosp. Med., 38:10–20.

181. Wahl, S., and Renstrom, R. (1991): Fibrosis in soft-tissue injuries. In: Leadbetter, W., Buckwalter, J., and Gordon, S. (eds). Sports-Induced Inflammation: Clinical and Basic Science Concepts. Park Ridge, IL, American Academy of Orthopaedic Surgeons, pp. 63–82.

182. Woo, S., Inoue, D.M., McGurk-Burleson, E., and Gomez, M.A. (1987): Treatment of the medial collateral ligament injury. II: Structure and function of canine knees in response to differing treatment regimes. Am. J. Sports Med., 15:22–29.

183. Woo, S., Matthew, J.V., and Akeson, W.H. (1975): Connective tissue response to immobility. Arthritis Rheum., 18:257–264.

184. Jurvelin, J., Helminen, H.J., and Laurisalo, S. (1985): Influences of joint immobilization and running exercise on articular cartilage surfaces of young rabbits. Acta Anat., 122:62–68.

185. Tipton, C.M., James, S.L., and Mergner, W. (1970): Influence of exercise on strength of medial collateral knee ligament of dogs. Am. J. Physiol., 218:894–902.

186. Cassel, E.P., Finch, C.F., and Stathakis, V.Z. (2003): Epidemiology of medically treated sport and active recreation injuries in the Latrobe Valley, Victoria. Australia. Br. J. Sports Med., 37:405–409.

187. Timpka, T., Ekstrand, J., and Svanstrom, L. (2006): From sports injury prevention to safety promotion in sports. Sports Med., 36:733–745.

188. Anitiua, E. (1999): Plasma-rich in growth factors: preliminary results of the use in the preparation of future sites for implants. Int. J. Oral Maxillofac. Implants, 14:529–535.

189. Marx, R.E., Carlson, E.R., Eichstaedt, R.N., et al. (1998): Platelet-rich plasma: growth factor enhancement for bone grafts. Oral Surg. Oral Med. Oral Pathol. Oral Radiol. Endod., 85:638–646.

190. Sampson, S., Gerhardt, M., and Mandelbaum, B. (2008): Platelet rich plasma injection grafts for musculoskeletal injuries: A review. Curr. Rev. Musculoskel. Med., 1:165–174.

191. Edwards, S.G., and Calandruccio, J.H. (2003): Autologous blood injections for refractory lateral epicondylitis. Am. J. Hand Surg., 28:272–278.

192. Kajikawa, Y., Morihara, T., Sakamoto, H., et al. (2007): Platelet-rich plasma enhances the initial mobilization of circulation-derived cells for tendon healing. J. Cell. Physiol., 215:837–845.

193. Marx, R., and Garg, A. (2005): Dental and Craniofacial Applications of Platelet-Rich Plasma. Hanover Park, IL, Quintessence Publishing.

194. Creaney, L., and Hamilton, B. (2008): Growth factor delivery methods in the management of sports injury: The state of play. Br. J. Sports Med., 42:314–320.

195. Everts, P., Knape, J., Weirich, G., et al. (2006): Platelet-rich plasma and platelet gel: a review. J. ECT, 38:174–187.

196. Peerbooms, J.C., Sluimer, J., Bruijn, D.J., and Gosens, T. (2010): Positive effect of an autologous platelet concentrate in lateral epicondylitis in a double blind randomized controlled trial; platelet-rich plasma versus corticosteroid injection with a 1-year follow up. Am. J. Sports Med., 38:255–262.

197. Everts, P., Deville, R., Mahoney, C., et al. (2006): Platelet gel and fibrin sealant reduce allogenic blood transfusions in total knee arthroplasty. Acta Anaesthesiol. Scand., 50:593–599.

198. Yamaguchi, T., Ishii, K., Yamanaka, M., and Yasuda, K. (2006): Acute effects of static stretching on power output during concentric dynamic constant external resistance leg extension. J. Strength Cond. Res., 20:804–810.

199. Everts, P.A., Overdevest, E.P., Jakimowicz, J.J., et al. (2007): The use of autologous platelet-leukocyte gels in enhancing the healing process in surgery: A review. Surg. Endosc., 21:2063–2068.

200. Aspenberg, P., and Virchenko, O. (2004): Platelet concentrate injection improves Achilles tendon repair in rats. Acta Orthop. Scand., 75:93–99.

201. Vogt, F.B., Mack, P.B., and Beasley, W.G. (1965): The effect of bed rest on various parameters of physiological function. Part XII. The effect of bed rest on bone mass and calcium balance. Washington, DC, National Aeronautics and Space Administration.

202. Molloy, T., Wang, Y., and Murrell, G. (2003): The roles of growth factors in tendon and ligament healing. Sports Med., 33:381–394.

203. Anitiua, E., Andia, I., Sanchez, M., et al. (2005): Autologous preparations rich in growth factors promote proliferation and induce VEGF and HGF productions by human tendon cells in culture. J. Orthop. Res., 23:281–286.

204. Mentry, J., Kasemkijwattana, C., Day, C.S., et al. (2000): Growth factors improve muscle healing in vivo. J. Bone Joint Surg. Br., 82:131–137.

205. Lefaucheur, J.P., and Sebille, A. (1995): Muscle regeneration following injury can be modified in vivo by immune neutralization of basic fibroblast growth factor, transforming growth factor beta 1 or insulin-like growth factor 1. J. Neuroimmunol., 57:85–91.

206. Hammond, J.W., Hinton, R.Y., Curl, L.A., et al. (2009): Use of autologous platelet-rich plasma to treat muscle strain injuries. Am. J. Sports Med., 37:1135–1142.

207. Gaweda, K., Tarczynska, M., and Krzyzanowski, W. (2010): Treatment of Achilles tendonopathy with platelet-rich plasma. Int. J. Sports Med., 31:577–583.

208. Smidt, N., van der Windt, D.A., Assendelft, W.J., et al. (2002): Corticosteroid injections, physiotherapy or a wait-and-see policy for lateral epicondylitis: A randomized controlled trial. Lancet, 359:657–662.

209. Barrett, S., and Erredge, S. (2004): Growth factors for chronic plantar fasciitis. Podiatry Today, 17:37–42.

210. Cole, C., Seto, C., and Gazewood, J. (2005): Plantar fasciitis: Evidence-based review of diagnosis and therapy. Am. Fam. Physician, 72:2237–2242.

211. Acevedo, J., and Beskin, J. (1998): Complications of plantar fascia rupture associated with corticosteroid injection. Foot Ankle Int., 19:91–97.

212. Sellman, J. (1994): Plantar fascia rupture associated with corticosteroid injection. Foot Ankle Int., 15:376–381.
213. Leach, R., Jones, R., and Silva, T. (1978): Rupture of the plantar fascia in athletes. J. Bone Joint Surg. Am., 60:537–539.
214. Berghoff, W., Pietzak, W., and Rhodes, R. (2006): Platelet-rich plasma application during closure following total knee arthroscopy. Orthopedics, 29:590–598.
215. Gardner, M.J., Demetrakopoulos, D., Klepchick, P., and Mooar, P. (2006): The efficacy of autologous platelet gel in pain control and blood loss in total knee arthroplasty: An analysis of the hemoglobin, narcotic requirement and range of motion. Int. Orthop., 31:309–313.
216. Sanchez, M., Azofra, J., Aizpurua, B., et al. (2003): Plasma rich in growth factors to treat articular cartilage avulsion: A case report. Med. Sci. Sports Exerc., 35:1648–1652.
217. Akeda, K., An, H.S., Okuma, M., et al. (2007): Platelet-rich plasma stimulates porcine articular chondrocyte proliferation and matrix biosynthesis. Osteoarthritis Cartilage, 14:1272–1280.
218. Ishida, K., Kuroda, R., Miwa, M., et al. (2007): The regenerative effects of platelet-rich plasma on meniscal cells in vitro and its in vivo application with biodegradable gelatin hydrogel. Tissue Eng., 13:1103–1112.
219. Sanchez, M., Anitua, E., Orive, G., et al. (2009): Platelet-rich therapies in the treatment of orthopaedic sports injuries. Sports Med., 39:345–354.
220. Aspenberg, P. (2007): Stimulation of tendon repair: mechanical loading. GDFs and platelets. A mini-review. Acta Orthop. Scand., 31:783–789.
221. Smith, C.A. (1994): The warm-up procedure: to stretch or not to stretch. A brief review. J. Orthop. Sports Phys. Ther. 19:12–17.
222. McMillian, D.J., Moore, J.H., Hatler, B.S., and Taylor, D.C. (2006): Dynamic vs. static-stretching warm up: The effect on power and agility performance. Strength Cond. Res, 20:492–499.
223. McHugh, M.P., and Cosgrave, C.H. (2010): To stretch or not to stretch: the role of stretching in injury prevention and performance. Scand. J. Med. Sci. Sports, 20:169–181.
224. Herda, T.J., Cramer, J.T., Ryan, E.D., et al. (2008): Acute effects of static versus dynamic stretching on isometric peak torque, electromyography, and mechanomyography of the biceps femoris muscle. J. Strength Cond. Res., 22:809–817.
225. Manoel, M.E., Harris-Love, M.O., Danoff, J.V., and Miller, T.A. (2008): Acute effects of static, dynamic, and proprioceptive neuromuscular facilitation stretching on muscle power in women. J. Strength Cond. Res., 22:1528–1534.
226. Sekir, U., Arabaci, R., Akova, B., and Kadagan, S.M. (2009): Acute effects of static and dynamic stretching on leg flexor and extensor isokinetic strength in elite women athletes. Scand. J. Med. Sci. Sports, 20:268–281.
227. Yamaguchi, T., Ishii, K., Yamanaka, M., and Yasuda, K. (2007): Acute effects of dynamic stretching exercise on power output during concentric dynamic constant external resistance leg extension. J Strength Cond. Res., 21:1238–1244.
228. Nelson, A.G., Driscoll, N.M., Landin, D.K., et al. (2005): Acute effects of passive muscle stretching on spring performance. J. Sports Sci., 23:449–454.
229. Little, T., and Williams, A.J. (2006): Effects of differential stretching protocols during warm-ups on high speed motor capacities in professional footballers. J. Strength Cond. Res., 20:203–207.
230. Bandy, W.D., Irion, J.M., and Briggler, M. (1998): The effect of static stretch and dynamic range of motion training on the flexibility of the hamstring muscles. J. Orthop. Sports Phys. Ther., 27:295–300.
231. McHugh, M.P., Magnusson, S.P., Gleim, G.W., et al. (1992): Viscoelastic stress relaxation in human skeletal muscle. Med. Sci. Sports Exerc., 24:1375–1382.
232. Toft, E., Sinkjaer, T., Kalund, S., et al. (1989): Biomechanical properties of the human ankle in relation to passive stretch. J. Biomech., 22:1129–1132.
233. Shrier, I. (2004): Does stretching improve muscle performance? A systematic and critical review of the literature. Clin. J. Sports Med., 14:267–273.
234. Macpherson, P.C.D., Schork, M.A., and Faulkner, J.A. (1996): Contraction-induced injury to single fiber segments from fast to slow twitch muscles of rats by single stretches. Am. J. Physiol., 271:C1438–C1446.
235. Laudner, K.G., Sipes, R.C., and Wilson, J.T. (2008): The acute effects of sleeper stretch on shoulder range of motion. J. Athl. Train., 43:359–363.
236. Olsen, O.E., Myklebust, G., Engebretsen, L., et al. (2005): Exercises to prevent lower limb injuries in youth sports: Cluster randomized control trial. BMJ, 330:449.

3

Developing Treatment Pathways

Lynn Snyder-Mackler, PT, ScD, FAPTA, Michael J. Axe, MD, Matthew J. Failla, DPT, and Kurt A. Gengenbacher, DPT

CHAPTER OBJECTIVES

- Explain the impact that biologic healing rates have on postoperative or postinjury rehabilitation programs.
- Explain how various biologic variables and functional parameters affect the progression of rehabilitation for knee injuries.
- Discuss how surgical techniques that are directed at repairing or reconstructing injured tissues affect the progression of rehabilitation.

- Apply the principles gleaned from review of two knee injury treatment pathways to develop other treatment pathways for various pathologies.

Treatment guidelines or pathways based on the best available evidence provide several advantages. First, they help us choose the right care for most patients. Second, they allow us to distinguish those who need more hands-on care and those who can manage their condition themselves. Finally, they allow acceleration of the transition from novice to expert clinician. The aim of this chapter is to describe the development of treatment pathways that ensure the highest probability of success in advancing an athlete from injury back to sport. The knee will be used as an example in this chapter.

Rehabilitation specialists strive to resolve impairments (range of motion, weakness, inflammation) as quickly as possible. We coined the term *procedure-*(e.g., surgery) *modified rehabilitation* to underscore the concept that the speed, volume, and intensity of rehabilitation are dependent on the surgical procedure. Not all tissue is of good quality, and not all fixation is rigid. Therefore, adjustments in protocol are necessary to protect the surgical site until biologic healing has progressed to permit the demands of a rehabilitation program. We coined the term *rehabilitation-modified surgery* to describe the mindset of a surgeon who is willing to spend the extra time to better fix a pathologic structure and thereby allow more timely advancement to return to functional activities. This chapter concentrates on the process of developing postoperative treatment guidelines. First, common knee diagnoses that require surgical intervention are described. For each diagnosis, the primary and associated pathologies are discussed. The indications for

surgery, the primary surgical procedure, and the associated surgeries are explained. Critical surgical decisions, extra intraoperative measures taken to allow accelerated rehabilitation (i.e., rehabilitation-modified surgery), and intraoperative and postoperative surgical concerns are discussed. All is presented in the context of what the clinician needs to create and modify in regard to the rehabilitation pathways.

BASIC PRINCIPLES

Ultimately, success is a race between biologic healing and failure of fixation. In the knee, pathology involves healing of soft tissue, bone, and articular cartilage. All soft tissue healing is not created equal. Both the quality of the injured tissue and its intrinsic healing potential determine the timing and magnitude of the stress applied to the healing structures (e.g., functional activities, exercises, mobilization). Surgical repair is restricted to structures with healing potential. Repair restores normal anatomy (e.g., suturing an injured structure back together). When healing potential is limited, either because of the inherent properties of the tissues involved (e.g., anterior cruciate ligament [ACL]) or because the extent of the injury is too great (e.g., complex tear of the meniscus), repair is unlikely to be successful even with significantly modified rehabilitation. Repair in this instance would be a failure for the surgeon, the rehabilitation specialist, and most importantly, the patient; therefore, the structure must be resected (removed) or reconstructed (replaced). Resection of pathology is rarely without consequence, and thus reconstruction is preferred whenever possible.

Soft tissue healing potential varies from tissue to tissue—meniscus versus ligament/tendon, intraarticular versus extraarticular, allograft versus autograft.[1-4] Menisci have good healing potential limited to the periphery, they hold sutures well, but repairs are technically difficult. Tendons (e.g., patellar tendon) have excellent healing potential but tear in a nonuniform manner that demands the use of special suturing techniques to allow the ends to be approximated without pulling through the tissue until biologic healing takes place. Extraarticular ligaments (e.g., medial collateral ligament [MCL]) have excellent healing potential and a good environment for healing but present the same dilemmas and require the same protection as tendons.[5,6] Surgical repair makes a grade III ligament sprain only a grade II sprain. Surgeons constantly struggle to achieve appropriate tightness without constraining the joint and resulting in loss of motion or increased articular stress. Intraarticular ligaments have a poor blood supply and a hostile environment for healing; consequently, successful repair is rarely possible and reconstruction is the norm. Allograft tissue poses special problems. Although rejection and infection are exceedingly rare, incorporation can be slower than occurs with analogous autograft tissue (i.e., allograft bone heals more slowly than autogenous bone graft).

Healing of bone in the knee is generally good and nonunion is rare. Therefore, surgical procedures in the knee that depend on bone healing for success have predictably good results (e.g., bone–patellar tendon–bone ACL reconstruction), although healing of bone does require a healthy bone base.

Articular (hyaline) cartilage does not have a blood supply and its healing potential is limited. Normally, articular cartilage defects heal with the formation of fibrocartilage, but new techniques for cartilage repair boast of healing with hyaline cartilage (e.g., autologous chondrocyte implantation).[7-9]

With repair and reconstruction, the concepts of fixation become critical to the timing of progression of the rehabilitation program. Rigid fixation is optimal but unusual. It implies that the fixed structure can withstand normal forces without protection. Other than fractures and bone–patellar tendon–bone autografts, rigid fixation is most times an unrealizable ideal. Most knee surgeons seek to achieve semirigid fixation. Soft tissue screws have enhanced surgical procedures that require ingrowth of bone into soft tissue. Techniques to hold the graft firmly in place (though not strictly providing rigid fixation) are being advanced by surgeons and orthopedic implant manufacturers around the world. Soft tissue fixation always depends on the inherent biologic healing potential of the injured tissue and the individual patient variables (e.g., age, diabetes, peripheral vascular disease). When fixation is possible only with sutures, both the surgery and the rehabilitation are at major risk of losing the race between biologic healing and failure of fixation.

The addition of *tension bands* to protect the primary quadriceps or patellar tendon repair is the classic rehabilitation-modified surgery. Band sutures are used to pull the tissues closer to the patella as the knee flexes, thereby protecting the repair sutures while allowing flexion to 120°. Like most rehabilitation-modified surgery, it is more time-consuming, with an additional 10 minutes being needed.

In addition to the inherent healing potential of each tissue, the injury itself has an impact on healing. Many studies of healing in animals models (see Chapter 2), on which our estimates of healing have traditionally been based, involved cutting of structures (e.g., clean cuts) in otherwise healthy, young animals. This represents the ideal situation but is seldom found in the operating room. The tissue encountered is often degenerated, stretched, macerated, or torn at different levels (e.g., "mop end"). In addition, concomitant illness or injury and age affect healing. Healing rates of tissues are typically described as ranges (Fig. 3-1). The development and implementation of contemporary evidence-based rehabilitation protocols are predicated on the rehabilitation specialist's knowledge of these time frames and moderators.

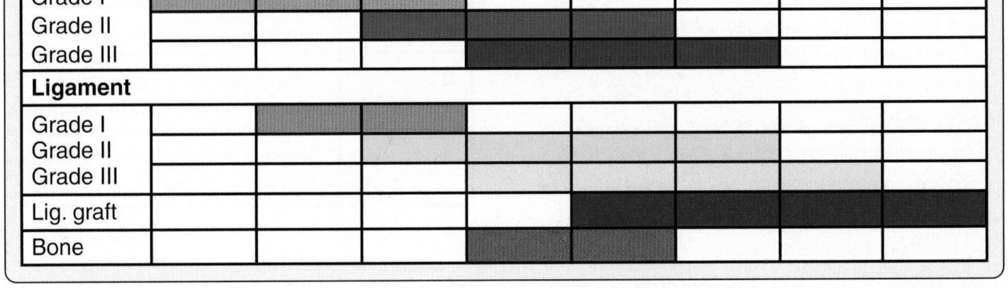

	0–3 days	4–14 days	3–4 wk	5–7 wk	2–3 mo	3–6 mo	6 mo–1 yr	2 yr
Tendon								
Tendinitis			░					
Rupture				▓	▓	▓		
Muscle								
Exercise induced	░							
Grade I	▓	▓						
Grade II			▓	▓				
Grade III				▓	▓			
Ligament								
Grade I		▓	▓					
Grade II			░	░				
Grade III				░	░			
Lig. graft					▓	▓	▓	▓
Bone			▓	▓				

FIGURE 3-1 Tissue-healing time line.

REHABILITATION PROGRESSION

All rehabilitation practice guidelines included in this chapter are criterion based. The criteria for progression are similar for each. Pain and swelling are the main indicators that the rehabilitation is progressing too quickly. In addition, quadriceps strength and inhibition and the results of performance on functional tests and self-report questionnaires are used to gauge progress and readiness (Box 3-1).

Soreness Rules

We have developed and previously reported the use of soreness rules for functional progression in individuals with a variety of pathologic conditions.[10-12] Soreness is defined as soreness of the involved structure (e.g., knee joint, not the quadriceps muscle). These guidelines are presented in Box 3-2.

Effusion

Knee effusion is an indicator of healing and response to treatment progression. Careful assessment of effusion is necessary for effective implementation of progressive rehabilitation. Girth measurements do not adequately quantify effusion, particularly if the effusion is small. Instead, the stroke test can give more meaningful information about the presence and amount of effusion.[13] The stroke test is performed with the patient supine and the knee relaxed in full extension. The test starts with the examiner performing several strokes upward from the medial joint line toward the suprapatellar pouch in an attempt to move the effusion from the medial aspect of the knee. The examiner then strokes downward on the lateral side of the knee from the suprapatellar pouch toward the lateral joint line and observes the medial aspect of the knee in an effort to appreciate a fluid wave emanating from the suprapatellar pouch[13] (Fig. 3-2). Four different grades are used to describe the amount of effusion. If no wave is produced with the downward stroke, no effusion is present. If the downward stroke produces a small wave on the medial side of the knee, the effusion is given a "trace" grade; a larger bulge is given a "1+" grade. If the effusion returns to the medial side of the knee without a downward stroke, the effusion is given a "2+" grade. Inability to move

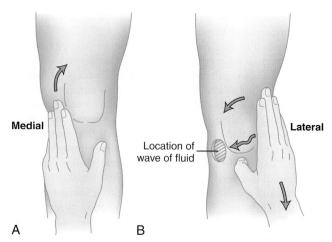

FIGURE 3-2 Diagram depicting the stroke test. **A,** The examiner strokes upward from the medial joint line toward the suprapatellar pouch. **B,** A downward stroke on the distal lateral aspect of the thigh from the suprapatellar pouch toward the lateral joint line is performed; a wave of fluid is observed at the medial aspect of the knee. *(From Sturgill, L.P., Snyder-Mackler, L., Manal, T.J., Axe, M.J. (2009): Interrater reliability of a clinical scale to assess knee joint effusion. J. Orthop. Sports Phys. Ther., 39:845–849. Doi:10.2519/jospt.2009.3143, with permission of JOSPT and the Orthopaedic and Sports Physical Therapy Sections of the American Physical Therapy Association.)*

the effusion out of the medial aspect of the knee equates to a "3+" grade (Table 3-1). The reliability of this test is excellent.[13]

Quadriceps Strength Testing

Quadriceps weakness is common after a knee injury; therefore, measurement of quadriceps strength is important to ensure full resolution of this impairment before return to sport. Biomechanical studies have demonstrated that a deficit in quadriceps strength is correlated with altered gait.[14]

A variety of methods can be used to test quadriceps strength. The two most common methods used in the clinical setting are manual muscle testing and isokinetic testing (see Chapter 25). Manual muscle testing is one of the easiest to use; however, the results are less accurate when a patient is able to generate high force or when the difference in strength between limbs is minimal. Isokinetic testing offers the benefit of objective

---

Box 3-1

Clinical Pearls for Progression of Treatment

Use validated performance measures.
Monitor pain, swelling, and fatigue.
Know tissue-healing time frames.
Follow the soreness rules.

Box 3-2

Exercise Progression Guidelines Based on Soreness

If no soreness is present from the previous day's exercise, advance the level of exercise by modifying one variable.
If soreness is present from the previous day's exercise but recedes with warm-up, stay at the same level.
If soreness is present from the previous day's exercise but does not recede with warm-up, decrease exercise to the level before progression. Consider taking the day off if soreness is still present with the reduced level of exercise. When exercise is resumed, it should be at the reduced level.

Table 3-1 Effusion Grading Scale for the Knee Joint Based on the Stroke Test

Grade	Test Result
Zero	No wave produced with a downstroke
Trace	Small wave on the medial side with a downstroke
1+	Larger bulge on the medial side with a downstroke
2+	Effusion spontaneously returns to the medial side after an upstroke (no downstroke necessary)
3+	So much fluid that it is not possible to move the effusion out of the medial aspect of the knee

From Sturgill, L.P., Snyder-Mackler, L., Manal, T.J., Axe, M.J. (2009): Interrater reliability of a clinical scale to assess knee joint effusion. J. Orthop. Sports Phys. Ther., 39:845–849. Doi:10.2519/jospt.2009.3143, with permission of JOSPT and the Orthopaedic and Sports Physical Therapy Sections of the American Physical Therapy Association.

measurement through a force transducer, but the most clinically significant testing speed has not been established. Faster speeds better approximate the speed of joint motion during function; however, they underestimate deficits in strength.[15,16]

Neither manual muscle testing nor isokinetic testing measures a patient's effort or offers a method to quantify quadriceps inhibition (inability to fully activate the quadriceps voluntarily). The quadriceps can be inhibited following a knee injury.[17,18] The burst superimposition method of testing quadriceps strength is not used as commonly in the clinical setting as in research studies, but this method offers the ability to measure inhibition.[18] For this type of testing, an electrical stimulus is applied (superimposed) while the patient produces a maximum voluntary isometric contraction. If the patient has fully activated the quadriceps, no force augmentation will occur when the electrical stimulus is delivered. Up to 5% inhibition is considered normal. If the burst superimposition method of testing is not available to the clinician, targets should be set and verbal encouragement given during testing to improve the quality of the effort.

Hop Testing

In sports rehabilitation, hop testing is a commonly used clinical test of function. Many clinics use one or all of the hop tests described by Noyes et al,[19] which include the single-hop test, triple-hop test, crossover triple-hop test, and timed hop test. Testing in an uninjured population showed that 92% to 93% had a symmetry index (side-to-side comparison) of at least 85% for the single-hop and timed hop tests[20]; thus, a score of less than 85% on the hop tests can be indicative of disability. Hop testing has good reliability, particularly when patients are given more than one practice trial.[21] See Chapter 22 for more on functional testing.

Other Functional Measures

In patients who are older and not athletes, other functional tests can provide insight into functional progression. Tests such as the Timed-Up-and-Go (TUG), Functional Stair Test (FST), and 6-minute walk have been used for the evaluation of patients recovering from knee surgery, typically for those with osteoarthritis. The first two are timed tests and the last is a walking distance measure. The TUG test is a measure of the ability to rise from a chair, walk 3 m, and return to sit in the chair.[22] The FST is a timed measure of the ability to ascend and descend a flight of stairs. The 6-minute walk measures the distance that an individual can walk in 6 minutes with unrestricted rest times.

Self-Report Questionnaires

The use of self-report questionnaires to measure health-related quality of life and self-assessment of function is helpful in assessing the progress of rehabilitation after knee surgery. In our clinic a generic health status index is typically used, the Medical Outcomes Trust SF-36, as well as a regional (knee-specific) health status index, the Knee Outcome Survey (KOS). The KOS has two forms, the Activities of Daily Living Scale and the Sports Activity Scale.[23]

Running Progression

Progression of aerobic conditioning often includes a running program that is usually initiated in this phase of rehabilitation. To start running, quadriceps strength on the athlete's injured side must be restored to at least 80% of that on the uninvolved side, and sufficient healing of the injured structure must have occurred (e.g., ACL reconstruction at approximately 8 weeks, grade I MCL injury at 1 to 2 weeks).[3-6] Soft tissue healing is generally sufficient at 4 to 6 weeks. Running progression starts on a treadmill and then moves to running on a track. Track workouts are initiated by running the straightaways and walking the corners. The intensity is gradually increased until the athlete can run the full length of the track. Road running and finally off-road running represent the least controlled training situations and are instituted as a final stage in running progression. Jogging duration may start with as much as 2 miles and may be progressed on a weekly basis if no pain or swelling occurs. Completion of a full running progression can take as long as 2 to 3 months.

ORGANIZATION

The remainder of this chapter follows a precise format. First, two specific knee pathologies that require operative management (meniscus tear and posterior cruciate ligament [PCL] rupture) are described. The primary pathology and common associated pathologies will be detailed, and surgical indications will be described. The description of the surgery includes a brief account of each primary procedure and common associated procedures, followed by critical surgical decisions that may have an impact on rehabilitation. Efforts that the surgeon can make during the surgical procedure to allow a more progressive rehabilitation program to take place (i.e., rehabilitation-modified surgery) are then described. Intraoperative and postoperative surgical concerns are also included along with information about how they might be manifested in the postoperative period. Finally, procedure-modified, criterion-based, rehabilitation practice guidelines are presented for each scenario and the rehabilitation pathway presented.

Meniscus Repair

The primary pathology amenable to meniscal repair is a tear in the red (vascular) zone (the outer third of the meniscus) in a young person, although certain red-white zone tears are also repairable.[2,24] Common associated pathology includes chondral defects and ACL injury. Indications for meniscal repair are mechanical signs (e.g., locked knee) and good tissue for repair. The primary surgery involves a multiple-fixation repair of the tear, with less than 5 mm per fixation. If the ACL is also torn, it is usually reconstructed at the same time. Concomitant ACL reconstruction is associated with a higher percentage of healing of repaired menisci.

The critical surgical decision is determination of the healing potential of the tear when it is actually visualized and probed. Here, the surgeon assesses the location and type of tear, and makes the ultimate decision about whether the potential is good for successful repair. Another critical surgical decision is whether the repair be done "all inside" or whether a posterior incision is necessary to tie the sutures in an "inside-out" technique. To "rehabilitation-proof" the surgery, the surgeon uses multiple nonabsorbable sutures or other fixation devices, performs the surgery through an arthrotomy if necessary, and ties the sutures with the knee fully extended. If a posterior incision is made either laterally or medially, this poses a special problem in preventing adherence of the scar to the underlying structures. Intraoperative surgical concerns include using one suture every

5 mm or less and taking care to avoid neurovascular structures. With medial meniscal repair, the concern is capture of the saphenous nerve medially by a suture and rarely the popliteal artery and tibial nerve posteriorly. In addition, the surgeon is concerned about capturing the posterior capsule and inducing a flexion contracture. Therefore, the sutures are tied in extension to prevent this capsular problem.

Lateral meniscal repair poses a somewhat more difficult problem in two respects. First, the popliteal hiatus has to be maintained and many times created with sutures both anteriorly and posteriorly to the popliteus tendon. Structures at risk from repair of the lateral meniscus are the peroneal nerve laterally and the popliteal artery and tibial nerve centrally.

Postoperative concerns include nerve entrapment–related flexion contracture and failed repair. If the sutures are tied in extension, the repair is stressed only in deep knee flexion in non–weight-bearing situations or in loaded (weight-bearing) knee flexion in greater than 45° of flexion. Typically, a knee immobilizer is worn for 4 to 6 weeks. A postoperative surgical concern is full range of motion and the potential for retearing in loaded flexion before healing is completed. The rehabilitation specialist must be concerned about achieving full range of motion while preventing undue stress on the fixation. Recovery from both medial and lateral meniscal repair takes a minimum of 12 weeks, with a knee immobilizer being used for at least 4 weeks and frequently for 8 weeks. Passive range of motion is strongly encouraged, with full flexion being achieved by 8 weeks. Electrical stimulation is used to maintain quadriceps strength so that when the meniscus has healed, quadriceps atrophy has been minimized. The rehabilitation pathway is presented in Table 3-2.

Table 3-2 Rehabilitation Practice Guidelines for Meniscal Repair

Assumptions	Isolated meniscal repair
Primary surgery	Meniscal repair; arthroscopically assisted open repair or all-inside repair
Secondary surgery (possible)	ACL reconstruction, PCL reconstruction, chondroplasty
Precautions	No loaded knee flexion beyond 45° for 4 weeks No loaded knee flexion beyond 90° for 8 weeks
Expected number of visits	12 to 24

	Treatment	Milestones
Weeks 1-2 (total visits, 1-3)	Immobilizer for ambulation or a brace locked at 0° extension Crutches as needed (WB per surgeon) OKC AROM and PROM exercises Scar mobilization Patellar mobilization NMES for the quadriceps Modalities as needed No resisted hamstring exercise	Full knee extension AROM knee flexion to 90° Superior patellar glide with QS AROM of the hip/ankle WNL SLR without quadriceps lag
Weeks 3-4: 1-3 visits/wk (total visits, 6-12)	Immobilizer for ambulation or a brace locked at 0° extension Crutches with WB per surgeon OKC PREs of the hip, knee, ankle Multiangle isometric knee extension NMES for the quadriceps at 60° Gait training (WB per surgeon) on week 4 CKC to 45° knee flexion on week 4	Full scar mobility AROM knee flexion within 10° of the uninvolved knee Full patellar mobility Zero to trace effusion
Weeks 5-7: 0-2 visits/wk (total visits, 6-16)	Immobilizer d/c per surgeon Increase PREs for the hip, knee, ankle Begin to advance WB flexion 45° to 90° Endurance training via bike/StairMaster	Full AROM Normal gait MVIC >60% No effusion
Weeks 8-11: 0-2 visits/wk (total visits, 6-20)	Increase PREs Begin loaded flexion beyond 90° at 8 weeks	MVIC >80%
Weeks 12-14: visits as needed (total visits, 2-10)	Functional hop test if MVIC >80% When MVIC >80%, initiate running progression, sports-specific drills, and agility drills PREs at fitness facility Follow-up functional testing at 6 months and 1 year postoperatively Progression of strengthening in gym Emphasize plyometrics, jumping, and cutting	Maintaining or gaining quadriceps strength MVIC, KOS, and hop test >90% for return to sport (per surgeon)

Used with permission from the University of Delaware.

ACL, Anterior cruciate ligament; *AROM*, active range of motion; *CKC*, closed kinetic chain; *d/c*, discontinued; *KOS*, Knee Outcome Survey; *MVIC*, maximum voluntary isometric contraction; *NMES*, neuromuscular electrical stimulation; *OKC*, open kinetic chain; *PCL*, posterior cruciate ligament; *PRE*, progressive resistive exercise; *PROM*, passive range of motion; *QS*, quadriceps sets; *SLR*, straight leg raises; *WB*, weight bearing; *WNL*, within normal limits.

Posterior Cruciate Ligament Rupture

A torn PCL without other ligamentous compromise rarely requires surgery. A PCL-deficient knee is at risk for early degenerative arthritis in the medial compartment, particularly if the medial meniscus is not reparable. Even in the busiest centers, it is rare that a knee service will perform more than 25 isolated PCL repairs per year. Identification of appropriate tunnels in both the femur and tibia, use of multiple grafts, and better fixation have led to improved results. The largest intraoperative surgical concern is the neurovascular bundle posteriorly on the tibia. Techniques have evolved just to protect these vital structures.

Postoperatively, the surgeon is often concerned about recurrent laxity, and generally discourages any accelerated rehabilitation beyond patellar mobilization and maintenance of quadriceps strength. Graft site morbidity is less common because allograft tissue is frequently the graft of choice. The rehabilitation protocol for the PCL reflects the surgeon's concern that early activity will lead to increased residual laxity. When the PCL and the posterolateral corner are involved, the patient has both symptomatic instability and an increased likelihood of degenerative arthritis in the medial compartment. In addition to the PCL being compromised, the main stabilizer of the posterolateral corner, the popliteal fibular ligament, has also been injured. Other associated pathology includes the fibular collateral ligament, the arcuate complex, the ACL, and too often, the peroneal nerve.[25,26] If the ACL is also injured, knee dislocation has to be suspected. The amount of tourniquet time becomes critical, and reconstruction of the PCL and posterolateral corner demands special expertise. Reconstruction of the posterolateral corner, even in the largest regional centers, seldom exceeds 25 cases per year, and most centers rarely see patients who have undergone this surgery. In reconstructing the posterolateral corner, full range of motion must be achieved with the graft under appropriate tension throughout the entire range. Intraarticular ligamentous procedures must be performed in such a way that they too do not capture the knee. If the surgeon is successful, full range of motion is achieved and the constructs do not stretch out. As with isolated PCL repair, the rehabilitation process is much slower than for ACL reconstruction alone. The rehabilitation pathway is presented in Table 3-3.

Table 3-3 Rehabilitation Practice Guidelines for Reconstruction of the Posterior Cruciate Ligament

Assumptions	Isolated PCL injury or PCL/PL
Primary surgery	PCL reconstruction with or without PL repair/reconstruction
Secondary surgery (possible)	Meniscal injury, chondroplasty
Precautions	See later
Expected number of visits	30 to 40

Electrode Placement and Stimulation Parameters

1	Electrodes placed over the proximal lateral and distal medial aspects of the quadriceps (modify distal electrode placement by not covering the superior median [VMO] arthroscopy portal or incision until the stitches are removed)
2	Stimulation parameters: 2500 Hz, 75 bursts, 2 sec ramp, 2 sec on, 50 sec rest, intensity to maximum tolerable (at least 50% MVIC [see Maximum Volitional Isometric Contraction section on next page]), 10 contractions per session, 3 sessions per week until quadriceps strength MVIC is 80% of the uninvolved side
3	Stimulation performed **isometrically** at **30°**

Electrodes
Dynamometer motor
0°

	Treatment	Milestones
Week 1: 1 visit	NMES (see guidelines) QS SLR Patellar mobilization HEP: patellar mobilization 30-50×, QS and SLR 3 × 10 (3× per day)	Good quadriceps contraction Superior patellar glide Ambulating PWB with crutches and postoperative orthosis locked

Continued

Table 3-3 Rehabilitation Practice Guidelines for Reconstruction of the Posterior Cruciate Ligament—cont'd

	Treatment	Milestones
Week 2: 2-3 visits (total visits, 3-4)	Portal/incision mobilization as needed SAQ 30°-0°	Full extension Flexion to 60° SLR without lag (full quadriceps contraction)
Weeks 3-5: 2-3 visits/wk (total visits, 9-13)	Prone knee flexion of 0°-60°, therapist assisted Supine knee flexion while holding tibia forward OKC 60°-0° Stationary bike for ROM—easy Gait-training PWB with crutches, no orthosis	Flexion to 110° Quad strength >60% of the uninvolved side Wean from orthosis, normalize gait crutches
Weeks 6-10: 2-3 visits/wk (total visits, 19-28)	Stationary bike—easy Begin closed chain if good quadriceps control: wall sits, wall squats at 0°-45°	Normal gait without crutches Quadriceps strength >80% of the uninvolved side
Week 12: twice per week to rechecks	Advance exercise intensity and duration 0°-90° hamstring exercises against gravity	Pain-free AROM to within 10° of the uninvolved side Maintaining or increasing quadriceps strength (≥90%)
Week 16: twice per week to rechecks	Begin running progression with functional brace (see Running Progressing section below) PRE hamstring curls at 0°-90° Transfer to fitness facility (if all milestones are met)	Full ROM (compared with uninvolved side) Maintaining quadriceps strength ≥95%

Week 20: rechecks (total visits, 25-44)	Return-to-sport transition
	Proprioceptive, static balance, dynamic balance, functional activities:
	  Slow to fast speed
	  Low to high force
	  Controlled to uncontrolled
		Global report >70%
		KOS ADLS > 90%

Precautions	
1. Partial meniscectomy	No modifications required, progress per patient tolerance and protocol
2. Meniscal repair	No modifications required, progress per patient tolerance and protocol Weight bearing in full extension OK
3. Chondroplasty	Restricted weight bearing for 4 weeks No weight-bearing exercises for 4 weeks Consider tibiofemoral unloading brace to help facilitate earlier participation in functional rehabilitation activities if limited by pain
4. MCL injury	Restrict motion to the sagittal plane until week 4-6 to allow healing of the MCL Perform PREs with the tibia in internal rotation during the early postoperative period to decrease MCL stress Consider a brace for exercise and periods of activity if severe sprain and/or pain is present
5. ACL injury	Follow PCL guidelines

Maximum Volitional Isometric Contraction	
Guideline	Patient is asked to volitionally extend the involved leg as hard as possible while the knee is maintained isometrically at 30° of knee flexion. Side-to-side comparison: involved/uninvolved × 100 = % MVC

Running Progression	
1	Treadmill walking
2	Treadmill walk/run intervals
3	Treadmill running
4	Track: run straights, walk turns
5	Run on road
	Progress to the next level when the patient is able to perform activity for 2 miles without increased effusion or pain. Perform no more than 4 times in 1 week and no more frequently than every other day. Do not progress more than 2 levels in a 7-day period.

Used with permission from the University of Delaware.

ACL, Anterior cruciate ligament; *ADLS,* Activities of Daily Living Scale; *AROM,* active range of motion; *HEP,* Home Exercise Program; *KOS,* Knee Outcome Survey; *MCL,* medial collateral ligament; *MVC,* maximum voluntary contraction; *MVIC,* maximum voluntary isometric contraction; *NMES,* neuromuscular electrical stimulation; *OKC,* open kinetic chain; *PCL,* posterior cruciate ligament; *PL,* posterolateral corner; *PRE,* progressive resistive exercise; *PWB,* partial weight bearing; *QS,* quadriceps sets; *ROM,* range of motion; *SLR,* straight leg raises; *SAQ,* short arc quadriceps; *VMO,* vastus medialis obliquus.

RETURN TO SPORT

When the athlete has achieved all the milestones necessary (Box 3-3), return-to-sport progression may begin. The basic return-to-sport lower extremity progression incorporates the following: straight-plane movements, lateral movements, cutting at progressive angles, sport-specific agility, mirroring practice, return to practice, and return to sport[27] (Box 3-4). When to advance athletes along this continuum is based on clinical decision making that involves all the aforementioned aspects mentioned in this chapter. The basis behind this is to slowly introduce these complex movements in a controlled environment before returning to play. The intensity and difficulty can be altered as progression continues. The athlete must be able to complete each progression at 100% intensity before moving to the next level. An often forgotten aspect of the return-to-sport progression is psychologic readiness to return to sport (see Chapter 1). One way to objectively assess this factor is through the use of outcome measures, such as the Tampa Scale of Kinesiophobia.[28] These short forms are filled out by the athlete to give the clinician an idea of how kinesiophobic the athlete is with activities and how much change has occurred with treatment. They need to be filled out starting at the initial evaluation to monitor the change in score. When the time comes for return to sport, the athlete may be permitted either full return or a graded return. A graded return to sport occurs when the athlete is limited to a certain amount of playing time, which is then progressed until unlimited play occurs.

The last step in formulating treatment pathways is to develop a way to help prevent the athlete from becoming reinjured.[29] One of the biggest predictors of risk for injury is previous injury. The athlete must have a plan in place to minimize this risk. This may be a set of home exercises, bracing, technique modification, or a combination of these factors.

Box 3-3

General Return-to-Sport Guidelines After Rehabilitation

>90% Strength
>90% Functional testing score
>90% Global Rating Scale score
Absence of effusion
Absence of pain
Full active range of motion
The results of strength and functional testing are relative
  to the uninvolved limb

Box 3-4

Clinical Pearls for Return to Sport

Return to play is a progression.
Start with general agility and move toward sport- and position-
  specific exercises.
Pain, swelling, fatigue, and soreness rules still apply.

CONCLUSION

- *Procedure-modified rehabilitation* refers to the concept that the speed, volume, and intensity of rehabilitation are dependent on the surgical procedure. *Rehabilitation-modified surgery* describes the practice of a surgeon who is willing to spend the extra time to better fix a pathologic structure and thereby allow more timely advancement to return to functional activities.
- All soft tissue healing is not created equal. Both the quality of the injured tissue and its intrinsic healing potential determine the timing and magnitude of the stress applied to the healing structures.
- When healing potential is limited either because of its inherent properties or because the extent of the injury is too great, repair is unlikely to be successful even with significantly modified rehabilitation.
- Soft tissue healing potential varies from tissue to tissue.
- With repair and reconstruction techniques, the concepts of fixation become critical to the timing of progression of rehabilitation.
- The development and implementation of contemporary evidence-based rehabilitation protocols are predicated on the rehabilitation specialist's knowledge of tissue healing time frames and other variables, such as age and other health issues.
- Pain and swelling are the main indicators that the rehabilitation is progressing too quickly.
- The two most common methods used in the clinical setting to assess muscle strength are manual muscle testing and isokinetic testing.
- A surgeon's choice of how to repair or reconstruct damaged tissues has a direct impact on the rehabilitation process.
- Basic return-to-sport lower extremity progression includes straight-plane movements, lateral movements, cutting at progressive angles, sport-specific agility, mirroring practice, return to practice, and return to sport. Advancing athletes along this return-to-sport continuum involves clinical decision making that must take into account many variables.

REFERENCES

1. Gross, M.T. (1992): Chronic tendinitis: Pathomechanics of injury factors affecting the healing response and treatment. J. Orthop. Sports Phys. Ther., 16:248–261.
2. Cooper, D.E., Arnoczky, S.P., and Warren, R.F. (1991): Meniscal repair. Clin. Sports Med., 10:529–548.
3. Rodeo, S.A., Arnoczky, S.P., Torzilli, P.A., et al. (1993): Tendon-healing in a bone tunnel. A biomechanical and histological study in the dog. J. Bone Joint Surg. Am., 75:1795–1803.
4. Bosch, U., Kasperczyk, W., Marx, M., et al. (1989): Healing at graft fixation site under functional conditions in posterior cruciate ligament reconstruction. A morphological study in sheep. Arch. Orthop. Trauma Surg., 108:154–158.
5. Woo, S.L., Inoue, M., McGurk-Burleson, E., and Gomez, M.A. (1987): Treatment of the medial collateral ligament injury. II: Structure and function of canine knees in response to differing treatment regimens. Am. J. Sports Med., 15:22-29.
6. Woo, S.L., Buckwalter, J.A. (1988): AAOS/NIH/ORS workshop. Injury and repair of the musculoskeletal soft tissues. Savannah, Georgia, June 18–20, 1987. J. Orthop. Res., 6:907–931.
7. Brittberg, M., Peterson, L., Sjogren-Jansson, E., et al. (2003): Articular cartilage engineering with autologous chondrocyte transplantation. A review of recent developments. J. Bone Joint Surg. Am., 85(Suppl 3):109–115.
8. Brittberg, M., Lindahl, A. Nilsson, A., et al. (1994): Treatment of deep cartilage defects in the knee with autologous chondrocyte transplantation. N. Engl. J. Med., 331:889–895.
9. Steadman, J.R., Miller, B.S., Karas, S.G., et al. (2003): The microfracture technique in the treatment of full-thickness chondral lesions of the knee in National Football League players. J. Knee Surg., 16:83–86.
10. Fees, M., Decker, T., Snyder-Mackler, L., and Axe, M.J. (1998): Upper extremity weight-training modifications for the injured athlete. A clinical perspective. Am. J. Sports Med., 26:732–742.

11. Axe, M.J., Windley, T.C., and Snyder-Mackler, L. (2002): Data-based interval throwing programs for collegiate softball players. J. Athl. Train., 37:194–203.

12. Axe, M.J., Snyder-Mackler, L., Konin, J.G., and Strube, M.J. (1996): Development of a distance-based interval throwing program for Little League–aged athletes. Am. J. Sports Med., 24:594–602.

13. Sturgill, L.P., Snyder-Mackler, L., Manal, T.J., and Axe, M.J. (2009): Interrater reliability of a clinical scale to assess knee joint effusion. J. Orthop. Sports Phys. Ther., 39:845–849.

14. Snyder-Mackler, L., Delitto, A., Bailey, S.L., and Stralka, S.W. (1995): Strength of the quadriceps femoris muscle and functional recovery after reconstruction of the anterior cruciate ligament. A prospective, randomized clinical trial of electrical stimulation. J. Bone Joint Surg. Am., 77:1166–1173.

15. Gapeyeva, H., Paasuke, M., Erreline, J., et al. (2000): Isokinetic torque deficit of the knee extensor muscles after arthroscopic partial meniscectomy. Knee Surg. Sports Traumatol. Arthrosc., 8:301–304.

16. Keays, S.L., Bullock-Saxton, J., and Keays, A.C. (2000): Strength and function before and after anterior cruciate ligament reconstruction. Clin. Orthop. Relat. Res., 373:174–183.

17. Chmielewski, T.L., Stackhouse, S., Axe, M.J., and Snyder-Mackler, L. (2004): A prospective analysis of incidence and severity of quadriceps inhibition in a consecutive sample of 100 patients with complete acute anterior cruciate ligament rupture. J. Orthop. Res., 22:925–930.

18. Snyder-Mackler, L., De Luca, P.F., Williams, P.R., et al. (1994): Reflex inhibition of the quadriceps femoris muscle after injury or reconstruction of the anterior cruciate ligament. J. Bone Joint Surg. Am., 76:555–560.

19. Noyes, F.R., Barber, S.D., and Mangine, R.E. (1991): Abnormal lower limb symmetry determined by function hop tests after anterior cruciate ligament rupture. Am. J. Sports Med., 19:513–518.

20. Barber, S.D., Noyes, F.R., Mangine, R.E., et al. (1990): Quantitative assessment of functional limitations in normal and anterior cruciate ligament–deficient knees. Clin. Orthop. Relat. Res., 255:204–214.

21. Bolgla, L.A., and Keskula, D.R. (1997): Reliability of lower extremity functional performance tests. J. Orthop. Sports Phys. Ther., 26:138–142.

22. Podsiadlo, D., and Richardson, S. (1991): The timed "Up and Go": a test of basic functional mobility for frail elderly persons. J. Am. Geriatr. Soc., 39:142–148.

23. Irrgang, J.J., Snyder-Mackler, L., Wainner, R.S., et al. (1998): Development of a patient-reported measure of function of the knee. J. Bone Joint Surg. Am., 80:1132–1145.

24. McAndrews, P.T., and Arnoczky, S.P. (1996): Meniscal repair enhancement techniques. Clin. Sports Med., 15:499–510.

25. Lunden, J.B., Bzdusek, P.J., Monson, J.K., et al. (2010): Current concepts in the recognition and treatment of posterolateral corner injuries of the knee. J. Orthop. Sports Phys. Ther., 40:502–516.

26. McCarthy, M., Camarda, L., Wijdicks, C.A., et al. (2010): Anatomic posterolateral knee reconstructions require a popliteofibular ligament reconstruction through a tibial tunnel. Am. J. Sports Med., 38:1674–1681.

27. Myer, G.D., Paterno, M.V., Ford, K.R., et al. (2006): Rehabilitation after anterior cruciate ligament reconstruction: criteria-based progression through the return-to-sport phase. J. Orthop. Sports Phys. Ther., 36:385–402.

28. Chmielewski, T.L., Jones, D., Day, T., et al. (2008): The association of pain and fear of movement/reinjury with function during anterior cruciate ligament reconstruction rehabilitation. J. Orthop. Sports Phys. Ther., 38:746–753.

29. Paterno, M.V., Schmitt, L.C., Ford, K.R., et al. (2010): Biomechanical measures during landing and postural stability predict second anterior cruciate ligament injury after anterior cruciate ligament reconstruction and return to sport. Am. J. Sports Med., 38:1968–1978.

Principles of Rehabilitation

R. Barry Dale, PT, PhD, DPT, ATC, SCS, OCS, CSCS

CHAPTER OBJECTIVES

- Differentiate between rehabilitation and physical conditioning.
- List the general goals of rehabilitation.
- Define and explain the general phases of rehabilitation and the objectives for each phase.
- Explain the influence and importance of the neurologic system in rehabilitation.
- List and describe the types of therapeutic exercise.

- List and summarize the methods of progressive resistive exercise.
- Discuss the differences between and implications for using open versus closed chain exercises.
- Discuss strategies of physical conditioning during rehabilitation.
- Explain the parameters of conditioning and rehabilitation.
- Explain the importance of function-based rehabilitation.

This chapter provides an overview of the rehabilitation process and reviews key concepts that need attention during the development of athletic rehabilitation programs. The first part of the chapter begins with a broad definition of rehabilitation and a discussion of the various stages of rehabilitation. Next, key concepts pertaining to the neuromuscular system and motor learning are reviewed. This is followed by an account of the different types of exercise used in the rehabilitation process and considerations for their incorporation into rehabilitation programs. Finally, physical conditioning during rehabilitation and the various parameters pertinent to program progression are discussed. Many of the concepts are explained briefly, and the reader is referred to other specified sources, some located within this text.

Rehabilitation, from the Medieval Latin root word *rehabilitare*, literally means "to restore to a rank."[1] From the aforementioned definition, *rehabilitation* is a broad conceptual term used to describe restoration of physical function. Physical rehabilitation reverses various physical conditions associated with injury or dysfunction.

Rehabilitation is similar to other types of physical conditioning. Essentially, body systems respond to physical stress by undergoing adaptations that ultimately improve their functioning (see the section on conditioning later in this chapter). Rehabilitation is the process of applying stress to healing tissue in accordance with specific stresses that the

tissue will face on return to a particular activity. Thus, rehabilitation involves reconditioning injured tissue. When the healing tissue is mature, the emphasis moves to more aggressive conditioning in preparation for the athlete returning to his or her sport.

The physical rehabilitation process often involves many health care professionals, each with their specific role to help the athlete progress through recovery (Box 4-1). Sometimes professional responsibilities overlap, but each plays an active role in the rehabilitation process while working together to meet the many needs of an athlete undergoing physical rehabilitation.

Before implementing a rehabilitation program, the rehabilitation specialist should perform and be familiar with the findings of a thorough physical examination.[2,3] The physical examination should rule out other pathologic conditions and reveal problems inherent in the athlete's current physical condition. Clinical decisions regarding the course of rehabilitation depend on adequate information derived from a comprehensive clinical examination.[4] The physical examination should address joint range of motion, muscle flexibility, muscle strength, proprioception, posture, and ambulation and gait patterning, in addition to other specific criteria.[2,3] Thus, depending on the findings, the rehabilitation program may address multiple problem areas. Box 4-2 lists the key components of a physical examination.

Clinical Pearl #1

Effective rehabilitation occurs when health professionals coordinate their efforts based on written and verbal communication and documentation. As appropriate, research the medical records to obtain the most accurate picture of an athlete's condition. Next, make sure to document the athlete's condition on your examination and frequently record changes in status. This helps other health care providers who may need information at a point later in the rehabilitation process.

Rehabilitation programs, whether conservative or occurring after invasive procedures, are specifically tailored to an injury or surgical intervention. No matter how specific the rehabilitation is to a particular condition, general physiologic events that occur in response to trauma must be considered (see Chapters 2 and 7). Remember that the effectiveness of rehabilitation during the recovery period usually determines the degree and success of future athletic competition.[5] Thus, it is the clinician's role to optimize the healing environment of the injured tissue and return the athlete to competition as soon as possible without compromising the healing process. At least two foundational goals are applicable to any rehabilitation program: (1) reverse or deter the adverse sequelae resulting from immobility or disuse and (2) facilitate tissue healing and avoid excessive stress on immature tissue. The generic goals of any rehabilitation program are listed in Box 4-3.

Incomplete rehabilitation and premature sports re-entry predispose the athlete to reinjury. Figure 4-1 illustrates the body's response to injury and the result of inadequate rehabilitation.[6]

Clinical Pearl #2

The cardinal rule of rehabilitation is to avoid exacerbating the athlete's present condition. The athlete's pain and tissue responses dictate progression through the various stages of rehabilitation.

Box 4-1

Examples of Professions Potentially Influencing Athletic Rehabilitation

Physician
Athletic trainer
Physical therapist
Nutritionist
Registered nurse
Strength and conditioning specialist
Coach
Clergy
Psychologist

Box 4-3

Generic Goals of Rehabilitation

Decrease pain
Decrease the inflammatory response to trauma
Return to full active and pain-free range of motion
Decrease effusion
Return to full muscular strength, power, and endurance
Return to full asymptomatic functional activities at the
    preinjury level

Box 4-2

Foundation of Any Rehabilitation Program: Key Components of Physical Examination

1. History (subjective)
2. Examination of specific systems (objective)
   a. Neurologic: sensation via dermatome assessment, gross strength via myotome assessment, and reflexes
   b. Musculoskeletal: range of motion/flexibility, strength, coordination, agility, special tests, and functional performance tests
   c. Cardiopulmonary: respiratory rate, heart rate, and blood pressure
   d. Integumentary: skin condition, color, and temperature
3. Assessment
   a. Problem list, short-term goals (1 to 2 weeks), long-term goals (functional goals), and rehabilitation potential
   b. Summarizing the evaluation
4. Plan
   a. Specifying interventions and the frequency and duration of treatment

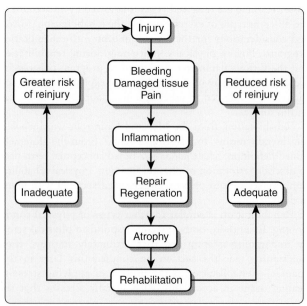

FIGURE 4-1 The body's response to injury and the role of rehabilitation. *(From Welch, B. [1986]: The injury cycle. Sports Med. Update, 1:1.)*

GENERAL REHABILITATION CONSIDERATIONS

Specific problems associated with injury include swelling, pain, and muscle spasm. On a positive note, pain and swelling serve to alert the rehabilitation specialist and athlete that tissue damage is present, which facilitates clinical decision making and proper determination of exercise progression. However, the presence of these injury by-products may hinder early therapeutic exercise because of pain and muscle inhibition.[6-13]

Peripheral Receptor Afferent Activity

Pain is something directly unseen by clinicians, yet we must rely on the patient's subjective complaint and interpret it according to the nature and time frame of the injury.[14] Pain may be acute, chronic, or persistent.[14,15] Acute pain occurs soon after the injury and is typically of short duration (matter of days). Acute pain is often a protective response that alerts us that something is wrong. Chronic pain is present for at least 6 months, frequently recurs, and resists alleviation with intervention.[15] It may continue long after the original injury has healed as a result of factors such as altered biomechanics or learned habits of guarding. In a person with chronic pain, the pain may become a dysfunction in itself.[16] Persistent pain, unlike chronic pain, generally occurs with a condition that responds to treatment over a period of time, which is variable according to the condition and the individual's interpretation of pain (pain threshold).[14] The latter type of pain may have a cognitive-behavioral component that may require counseling or other psychologic intervention.[17]

Controlling existing edema (present in soft tissue outside a joint) and prevention of further effusion (excess fluid inside a joint) are critical in the rehabilitation process for several reasons. Edema increases localized pressure, which compresses sensory nerve endings and contributes to the sensation of pain. Joint effusion increases intraarticular pressure and afferent activity, which contributes to muscle inhibition.[18] In fact, even small increases in fluid in a joint (as little as 10 mL) can produce a 50% to 60% decrease in maximal voluntary contractions of the quadriceps.[7-10,19] (See the section on arthrogenic inhibition later in this chapter and in Chapter 2.)

Rehabilitation adjuncts, such as electrophysical modalities (see Chapter 8), are instrumental in controlling and reducing these responses and allowing the athlete to begin early range-of-motion and strengthening exercises.[20-25] The modality itself, however, is almost never considered the only course of treatment of most athletic injuries. Therapeutic modalities assist the body's response to inflammation, but most do little to stress healing tissue. An exception is low-intensity ultrasound, which can facilitate the healing process when applied during the granulation phase of healing.[26] Only with therapeutic exercise can the injured body part or parts be restored to their preinjury level through the adaptation process associated with physical activity when prescribed in the correct dosage.[27-31] Therefore, the injury cycle may continue if therapeutic exercise is not included—or if improperly instituted—within a rehabilitation program.

Furthermore, exercise in the early rehabilitation phases diminishes the adverse effects of disuse or immobility. Athletes can improve their physical condition by training, yet those training responses readily reverse when activity ceases or diminishes, with ill effects becoming evident in as short a time as a few days.[32] Unfortunately, the rate of reversal is much

---

Box 4-4

Adverse Effects of Immobility (Unilateral Limb Suspension or Absolute Bed Rest)

1. Muscle
   a. Cross-sectional area: atrophy rates of 0.5% to 1% per day of inactivity for the quadriceps
   b. Strength: decreases 0.5% to 2% per day of inactivity for the plantar flexors and quadriceps
2. General deconditioning (reduced strength production and endurance capacity)
3. Structural changes in articular capsule connective tissue causing decreased range of motion
4. Degeneration of articular cartilage
5. Cardiovascular deconditioning
6. Reduced stimulus for bone mineral deposition, possibly contributing to diminished bone density

Data from Adams, G.R., Hather, B.M., and Dudley, G.A. (1994): Effect of short-term unweighting on human skeletal muscle strength and size. Aviat. Space Environ. Med., 65:1116–1121; Bamman, M.M., Clarke, M.S.F., Feeback, D.L., et al. (1998): Impact of resistance exercise during bed rest on skeletal muscle sarcopenia and myosin isoform distribution. J. Appl. Physiol., 84:157–163; Bamman, M.M., Hunter, G.R., Stevens, B.R., et al. (1997): Resistance exercise prevents plantar flexor deconditioning during bed rest. Med. Sci. Sports Exerc., 29:1462–1468; Bortz, W. (1984): The disuse syndrome. West. J. Med., 141:169; Cooper, D.L., and Fair, J. (1976): Reconditioning following athletic injuries. Phys. Sports Med., 4:125–128; Houglum, P. (1977): The modality of therapeutic exercise: Objectives and principles. Athl. Train., 12:42–45; and Noyes, F.R. (1977): Functional properties of knee ligaments and alterations induced by immobilization. Clin. Orthop. Relat. Res., 123:210–242.

---

faster than the rate of improvement. For example, untrained individuals can improve their cardiovascular conditioning by 1% per day of training, but the rate of reversal can be as high as 3% to 7% if they suddenly become totally inactive (Box 4-4).[32] Therefore, the longer an athlete is inactive, the longer it takes to return to preinjury fitness levels.[32-37]

Clinical Pearl #3

Remove or diminish the presence of pain, edema, and joint effusion as soon as possible. These sources of afferent activity result in reflex inhibition of associated musculature, which delays the rehabilitation process.

REHABILITATION CONCEPTS

Healing Constraints

The most important factors to consider when designing a rehabilitation program are the physiologic constraints to healing. Generally, across different tissue types, tissue strength decreases after injury, but as time elapses and healing occurs, tissue strength increases (Table 4-1).[38-40] The athlete's age, health, and nutritional status and the magnitude of injury are the primary factors influencing the rate of physiologic healing, and the rehabilitation program must be structured around these constraints (see Chapters 2, 3, and 7). New medicinal advances, however, may facilitate the healing process, such as autologous platelet-rich plasma technologies (see Chapter 2) and matrix metallo-proteinase inhibitors.[41,42]

Connective tissue, present in some form or another in almost all tissue, accommodates force—or stress—in a manner described by Hooke's law and the stress-strain curve (see Box 4-5 for definitions of force terms).[39,40,43] The specific composition and fiber arrangement of connective tissue determine the tissue's relative reaction to stress. For example, ligaments stretch relatively farther than tendons with the same magnitude of tensile force.[43] Ligaments stretch farther because of the more irregular or multidirectional arrangement of their collagen fibers in comparison to those of tendons, which are more specialized to resist tensile force.[43]

The aforementioned stress-strain curve graphically depicts how stress affects connective tissue.[39,43] It is described as a sinusoidal curve with specific areas that include the toe, elastic region, plastic region, and point of failure (Fig. 4-2).[39] The toe area is the elongation of connective tissue up to its point of stretch (e.g., taking up the slack in the tissue).[39] The elastic point begins when the tissue stretches beyond approximately 2% of its resting length. Within the elastic region, tissue returns to

its prestretch length. Permanent elongation occurs to a degree when the tissue surpasses its resting length by approximately 4%, known as the plastic region. Permanent elongation results from actual disruption of a few but not all collagen fibers present within the connective tissue. Finally, the failure point of connective tissue results from stretch beyond 6% to 10% of the tissue's resting length.[39] Thus, excessive stress applied to tissue may result in failure of that tissue. Rehabilitation must accommodate the fragility of healing tissue because its ability to withstand tensile stress is compromised early in rehabilitation.[38]

Stages of Rehabilitation

"Time waits for no one" and "timing is everything" are clichés that describe how dependent we are on time. Just as in everything else, timing is crucial during recovery from injury and rehabilitation. It has already been mentioned that proper intervention by the rehabilitation expert may include the use of therapeutic modalities or therapeutic exercises. However, certain intensities of therapeutic exercise and certain forms of therapeutic modalities may damage immature tissue in the early phases of rehabilitation. Damage to immature tissue incites further inflammation and prolongs the recovery process.

Rehabilitation phases are time frames that consider general healing constraints and assist the rehabilitation specialist in planning rehabilitative interventions.[44] However, it is important to recognize that there is no absolute transition from one rehabilitation phase to the next. In fact, the phases may overlap.[44] Furthermore, there is interindividual variability within these time constraints. Therefore, these stages or phases should not dictate progression of rehabilitation but should serve as a guide for the clinician because the experience of the rehabilitation specialist is important in maneuvering through the sometimes murky waters of rehabilitation and recovery.[5,39,45]

Overall, the phases are progressive in nature; that is, they should build on one another like building blocks.[45] When tasks that are relatively basic are accomplished, such as range of motion, the athlete may progress to strengthening within the

Table 4-1 Healing Rates for Various Tissue Types

Tissue	Time to Return to Approximately Normal Strength
Bone	12 weeks
Ligament	40-50 weeks
Muscle	6 weeks up to 6 months
Tendon	40-50 weeks

Data from Houglum, P. (1992): Soft tissue healing and its impact on rehabilitation. J. Sports Rehabil., 1:19–39; and Houglum, P. (2001): Muscle strength and endurance. In: Houglum, P. (ed.). Therapeutic Exercise for Athletic Injuries. Champaign, IL, Human Kinetics, pp. 203–265.

Box 4-5

Definitions of Key Terms Specific to Physical Stress

Force: something that causes or tends to cause a change in the motion or shape of tissue

Stress: generally synonymous with force; types include compression, tension, torsion, and shear

Compression: pushing or squeezing tissue together

Tension: pulling tissue apart

Torsion: twisting tissue

Shear: tearing across tissue

Strain: deformation of tissue

Elasticity: ability of tissue to accommodate strain and return to its original length

Plasticity: permanent change in tissue structure resulting from strain beyond the elastic region

Failure: tissue disruption resulting from strain beyond the plastic region

Data from Kreighbaum, E., and Barthels, K.M. (1996): Biomechanics: A Qualitative Approach for Studying Human Movement, 4th ed. Boston, Allyn & Bacon.

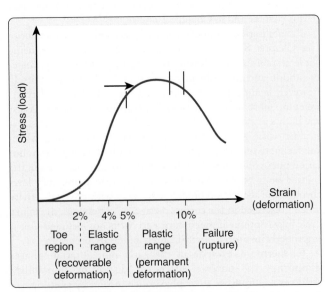

FIGURE 4-2 The stress-strain curve. *(Modified from Houglum, P. [2001]: Muscle strength and endurance. In: Houglum, P. (ed.). Therapeutic Exercise for Athletic Injuries. Champaign, IL, Human Kinetics, pp. 203–265.)*

newly acquired range of motion. As healing occurs and newly formed connective tissue matures, tolerance of increased exercise intensity improves.

Phases of rehabilitation include the acute, subacute (intermediate), and chronic or return-to-sport phases.[44] Other authors describe a fourth phase, the advanced strengthening phase, that follows the subacute (intermediate) phase and precedes the return-to-sport phase.[46]

Acute Phase

The acute phase occurs from the moment that tissue sustains injury until the time that inflammation becomes controlled. Generally, the acute phase of soft tissue healing lasts 4 to 6 days after injury.[44] The goals of the acute phase of rehabilitation are to diminish pain, control inflammation, and begin the restoration of joint range of motion, muscle flexibility and strength, and proprioception in a pain-free fashion.[46]

Rest, ice, compression, and elevation are necessary to combat pain and swelling in the acute injury state. Rest is paramount to manage inflammation during the first 24 hours after injury.[44] Therapeutic modalities, especially cryotherapy and electrophysical agents, play a crucial role in controlling the inflammation process and the athlete's pain early in rehabilitation. Cryotherapy helps prevent secondary hypoxic injury and aids in controlling hemorrhage and edema.[20] Application of external pressure to the injury site assists in limiting the amount of soft tissue edema. Compression wraps are applied from a distal to proximal direction, with a decreasing pressure gradient as the wrap moves proximally. Stockinettes are excellent for compression and can be applied and removed easily by the athlete. Elevation assists the lymphatic system in moving any extracellular tissue fluid away from the injury site. Passive and active assisted movements, when indicated, are beneficial in assisting proper healing of soft tissue.[44,47,48] Motion stresses immature collagen, which assists in alignment of its fiber along lines of stress while preventing excessive development of adhesions. Table 4-2 summarizes treatment considerations during the acute stage of soft tissue healing.

Advancement from the acute stage to the intermediate phase begins when the effects of cryotherapy have plateaued, as

Table 4-2 Rehabilitation During the Acute Phase of Soft Tissue Healing

Goals	Treatment
Control inflammation	Rest and protection of the injured area, cryotherapy, compression, elevation, gentle (grade I) pain-free mobilization of the affected joint
Minimize deleterious effects of immobilization	Passive motion within limits of pain, isometric muscle setting, electrical stimulation, axial loading for early proprioception
Reduce joint effusion	Pain-free active range of motion as tolerated, medical intervention (joint aspiration) if necessary
Maintain condition of noninjured areas	Activity of nonaffected extremities as tolerated

Data from Kisner, C., and Colby, L.A. (2002): Therapeutic Exercise: Foundations and Techniques, 4th ed. Philadelphia, Davis.

manifested by the stabilization of edema, relative restoration of pain-free range of motion, and removal of hyperemia.[49] Another way to view the criteria for progression to the subacute or intermediate phase is the relative reduction of inflammation, which is evidenced by diminution of its five classic indicators: redness (rubor), heat (calor), pain (dolor), swelling (tumor), and loss of function (functio laesa). When the pain and inflammation are under control, emphasis shifts to restoring function because diminished pain does not imply that restoration of function has occurred.[50]

Subacute (Intermediate) Phase

As mentioned earlier, the subacute phase of soft tissue resolution begins as the effects of inflammation decrease.[49] In this phase the healing connective tissue is still immature and relatively fragile; therefore, therapeutic exercises used during this phase should be gentle and cause no pain. This phase is transitional to active movement. However, tissue may revert back to the acute stage if it is overstressed and inflammation recurs.[51] Nonetheless, an appropriate amount of stress is necessary in this phase to avoid understressing tissue. Inadequate stress applied to soft tissue diminishes its mobility, which not only delays restoration of range of motion but also potentially results in more severe consequences, such as the formation of adhesions.[30,52]

Joint range of motion should dramatically improve in the subacute stage and allow the rehabilitation specialist to advance the rehabilitation program to flexibility training and strengthening exercises.[44] Joint range of motion forms the basis for physical performance, and its improvement is paramount for successful rehabilitation.[44] To improve joint range of motion, specific joint motion must occur progressively and be in the form of accessory or physiologic movements (see the section on therapeutic exercise later in this chapter and in Chapter 6). Strengthening should also be increased progressively in a rehabilitation program during the subacute stage. A few methods that progressively increase strength training include the low-resistance, high-repetition method, the DeLorme and Watkins regimen, the Oxford technique, and daily adjustable progressive resistive exercise philosophies (see the section on progressive resistive exercise later in this chapter).[53-56] As range of motion and strength improve, coordination and agility activities begin to increase as rehabilitation progresses.

Coordination and agility are important for normal functioning, whether it be functional activities or performance-specific actions of a particular sport. Normal movement requires complex neuromuscular coordination between similar or opposing muscle groups (or both). Movement patterns are smoother and more fluidlike when the action of muscle groups is coordinated. The subacute (intermediate) stage plays a role in reestablishing neuromuscular control via progression of proprioceptive exercises (see Chapter 24).

The ultimate goal of the subacute stage is to prepare the athlete for the more complex activities that occur in the return-to-sport phase. Table 4-3 summarizes treatment considerations during the subacute stage of soft tissue healing.

The Chronic or Return-to-Sport Phase

Culmination of the earlier phases should provide the athlete with full range of motion and strength of the affected extremity. Connective tissue by this time has improved tensile strength, primarily because the orientation of its fibers is better suited to withstand tensile stress.[57] The intensity of the strengthening exercises increases in this phase. Agility, coordination, and plyometric activities are performed at a more intense level to prepare athletes for the demands of specific activities within their particular sport.[45] Table 4-4 summarizes treatment considerations during the chronic or return-to-sport stage of soft tissue healing.

Neurologic Considerations

The neurologic system transmits information, recognizes and interprets the information, and then formulates a response, if necessary.[58,59] Afferent neurons carry signals from the periphery to the central nervous system (brain and spinal cord) that deliver information about the body or environment, whereas efferent neurons carry impulses to effector organs or muscles to carry out a specific response.[58,59] Key concepts of neurologic physiology, particularly afferent activity, will now be reviewed because of its crucial role in rehabilitation. This discussion begins with a review of peripheral receptors and finishes with a review of the concepts of motor learning and voluntary neuromuscular activation.

Peripheral Receptors

Sherrington identified and categorized afferent receptors into three groups according to location: articular, deep (muscle-tendon related), and superficial (cutaneous).[60] Our attention now turns to the joint receptors, which have profound effects associated with neuromuscular function.

PERIPHERAL RECEPTORS: JOINTS

In 1863, Hilton described the innervation of joints by articular branches of nerves supplying the muscles of each articulation (Hilton's law).[61] Sherrington was the first to note the presence of receptors in pericapsular structures.[60] He coined the term "proprioception" to include all neural input originating from the joints, muscles, tendons, and associated deep tissues.[60]

Articular receptors are located within the joint capsule, ligaments, and any other joint structures within the body.[62-65] The human joint capsule has been studied extensively and contains four very distinct types of nerve endings: Ruffini corpuscles, Golgi receptors (also present within the Golgi tendon organ), pacinian corpuscles, and free nerve endings[66-68] (Table 4-5).

ARTHROGENIC INHIBITION

Afferent activity from arthrogenous receptors contributes to the manifestation of arthrogenic inhibition of an affected muscle group. Afferent activity may occur as a result of increased articular pressure or from the transmission of pain signals.[7-10,19] Joint trauma often causes fluid to collect inside the joint (effusion), which increases intraarticular pressure. Increased intraarticular pressure subsequently causes the joint capsule to stretch, which activates afferent joint receptors. Joint pain may occur with or without joint effusion and is typically associated with an increased firing rate of free nerve endings. Joint receptor afferents integrate with an inhibitory interneuron at the spinal cord. The interneuron releases an inhibitory neurotransmitter in

Table 4-3 Rehabilitation During the Subacute Phase of Soft Tissue Healing, From Days 4 to 21 of Recovery From Injury

Goals	Treatment
Continue to control inflammation	Protect the area with prophylactic devices, if necessary; gradually increase the amount of joint movement; and continuously monitor tissue response to progression of exercise and adjust the intensity/duration accordingly.
Progressively increase mobility	Progress from passive to more active ROM; gradually increase the intensity of tissue stretch for tight structures.
Progressively strengthen muscles	Progress from isometric to active ROM without resistance and gradually increase the amount of resistance; progress to isotonic exercise as joint integrity/kinematics allows.
Continue to maintain condition of noninjured areas	Progressively strengthen and/or recondition noninjured areas with increased intensity/duration of activity as healing of tissue allows.

Data from Kisner, C., and Colby, L.A. (2002): Therapeutic Exercise: Foundations and Techniques, 4th ed. Philadelphia, Davis.
ROM, Range of motion.

Table 4-4 Rehabilitation During the Chronic Phase of Soft Tissue Healing, From 21 Days up to 12 Months Following Injury

Goals	Treatment
Decrease pain from adhesions	Appropriate modalities when indicated, mechanical stretching of affected structures
Increase extensibility of other structures	Passive stretches, joint mobilizations, cross–soft tissue friction massage, flexibility exercises
Progress strengthening of affected and supporting musculature	Isotonic and isokinetic exercises of affected and supporting musculature when indicated
Progress proprioception, coordination, and agility	Balance activities, surface modification

Data from Kisner, C., and Colby, L.A. (2002): Therapeutic Exercise: Foundations and Techniques, 4th ed. Philadelphia, Davis.

Table 4-5 Nerve Endings Found in the Human Joint Capsule

Nerve Ending	Characteristics
Ruffini corpuscles	Sensitive to stretching of the joint capsule
Golgi receptors	Intraligamentous and become active when the ligaments are stressed at the extremes of joint movement
Pacinian corpuscles	Sensitive to high-frequency vibration
Free nerve endings	Sensitive to mechanical stress

Data from Gardner, E. (1948): The innervation of the knee joint. Anat. Rec., 101:109–130; Halata, F., Rettig, T., and Schulze, W. (1985): The ultrastructure of sensory nerve endings in the human knee joint capsule. Anat. Embryol., 172:265–275; and Schutte, M.J., Dabezies, E.J., and Zimny, M.L. (1987): Neural anatomy of the human anterior cruciate ligament. J. Bone Joint Surg. Am., 69:243–247.

response to increased activity from the joint afferents. Ultimately, this diminishes the activity of motor neurons supplying muscles that act on the affected joint (Fig. 4-3). Diminished motor unit activity results in atrophy and weakness, most commonly seen in the quadriceps and shoulder after surgery or gross articular trauma.[7-10,19] The body attempts to protect the associated joint by "shutting down" the associated musculature, but the resulting atrophy and weakness prolong recovery time unless the rehabilitation specialist takes proper steps to minimize and reverse the adverse effects of arthrogenic inhibition.

Neuromuscular Considerations

The motor cortex does not think in terms of activation of specific motor units; rather, our bodies attempt to achieve a specified movement by activating certain muscles or muscle groups.[69,70] Movements often require complicated neuromuscular coordination, which we learn over time through experience or practice.[71] However, injury often causes temporary loss of the ability to activate specific muscles or muscle groups.[7-10,19,69,70] Measures that directly improve volitional motor control and activation of

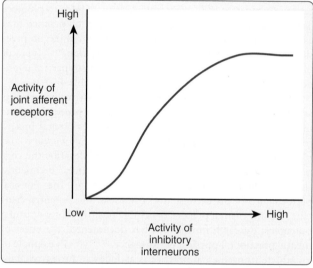

FIGURE 4-3 Increased activity of joint afferent nerve fibers as a result of pain or joint effusion concomitantly increases the activity of inhibitory interneurons. Increased activity of inhibitory interneurons contributes to muscle inhibition.

motor units while concomitantly decreasing arthrogenic inhibition by controlling joint effusion and pain are essential to rehabilitation. Physical training in conjunction with motor-learning principles assists the process of muscle reactivation and motor skill reacquisition.[71-74]

More complicated movement patterns associated with functional and sport-specific activities are not possible until muscle inhibition is reduced or removed.[7-10,19,69,70] Furthermore, performance of complex sport-specific activities in the advanced stages of rehabilitation ensures that athletes reacquire the motor skills inherent in their particular sport.

Many rehabilitation professionals often unknowingly use motor-learning concepts in one capacity or another during athletic rehabilitation. Whether the athlete is acutely recovering from surgical reconstruction or is in the final return-to-sport phase, it is imperative that the rehabilitation specialist use instructions, verbal or visual feedback, and practice conditions that match the learning needs of the athlete.[71] It is beyond the scope of this brief synopsis on motor learning to cover all theories and issues related to this important topic, and the reader is referred to other sources for more information.[71,75-82] Rather, key concepts pertinent to teaching athletes movement patterns related to therapeutic exercise, which should ultimately prepare them to return to their sport, are presented. Nonetheless, before discussing some of these concepts, two major theories concerning motor learning are briefly reviewed: the three-stage model and the two-stage model.

Three-Stage Model

In 1967, Paul Fitts and Michael Posner presented a classic motor-learning theory known as the three-stage model.[83] The three-stage model consists of the cognitive, associative, and autonomous stages[71,83] (Table 4-6).

The cognitive stage requires a great deal of attention from the athlete because of the need to focus on cognitively oriented problems.[81,83] In this stage, athletes must generally put forth conscious effort to either learn new movements or reacquire movements previously mastered. During rehabilitation, the athlete's neurologic system must "relearn" how to accomplish a given task as the appropriate movement patterns are selected and proper muscle groups are recruited to perform the task. Frequently, the athlete may be fearful of using the involved extremity, and the apprehension in doing so invokes cognitive activity on the task at hand. The athlete commits numerous errors while

Table 4-6 Comparison of the Three- and Two-Stage Motor-Learning Models

Three-Stage Model		Two-Stage Model	
Stage	**Characteristics**	**Stage**	**Characteristics**
Cognitive	Athlete puts forth conscious effort to either learn new movements or reacquire movements previously mastered.	"Getting the idea"	The correct movement pattern is selected on the basis of various regulatory conditions, such as distance, size, and shape of the object.
Associative	Athlete begins to associate certain environmental cues with the performance of movements.	Fixation and diversification	Fixation implies that the athlete performs the movement in a nonchanging environment.
Autonomous	Activity becomes automatic and requires very little cognitive processing for proper performance.		Diversification refers to a changing environment that requires the athlete to make modifications in the skill for proper performance.

performing the task but begins to get a "feel" for the activity with repetition and feedback.[82,83] Thus, the rehabilitation specialist plays an important role in this stage by providing appropriate extrinsic feedback.[44,71] As the athlete's practice level increases in this phase, the athlete begins to obtain a sense of correct and incorrect or safe and unsafe movements within the exercise or activity.[82]

Cognitive activity changes somewhat in the associative stage as the athlete begins to associate certain environmental cues with performance of the movements.[71,83] The athlete performs the task with fewer errors and refines the movement; in fact, Fitts and Posner refer to the associative stage as the refining stage.[83] The timing and distance of the movement are examples of how the athlete refines the activity or exercise and begins to decrease variability in performance. Coordination of muscle activity improves, which produces more efficient movements. Feedback is still important in the associative stage, but the athlete depends less on it for proper performance. The athlete begins to detect errors independently and make corrections in performance.[82,83] Additionally, as the practice level increases during this stage, the athlete may explore modifications of the movement, such as environmental variation.[81,83]

Finally, the athlete reaches the autonomous stage whereby the activity becomes automatic, with very little cognitive processing required for proper performance.[83] This allows the athlete to incorporate the activity into more complex exercises or to concentrate on other simultaneous tasks.[71,83] Variability in performance decreases tremendously, and the athlete consistently performs the task well in this stage. However, many healthy noninjured athletes may never reach this level of learning; therefore, it is rarely accomplished during rehabilitation because of the amount of practice time required to achieve it.[71] Nonetheless, the minimal goal of rehabilitation is to return the athlete to preinjury levels of motor functioning.

An important concept to consider is that one typically moves through the three stages in a continuum manner.[71] Consistent practice of the activity over time moves the athlete from the cognitive stage into the associative stage and finally into the autonomous stage. It may be difficult for the rehabilitation professional to determine exactly what stage an athlete is in at any given moment, especially because there is overlap to a degree across the continuum.[71]

Two-Stage Model

Another motor-learning theoretic model, the two-stage model, was described by Gentile in 1972 and 1987 (see Table 4-6).[72,73] In the two-stage model, the learner moves from "getting the idea" in the first stage to fixation and diversification in the second stage.[71-73] For the athlete to "get the idea" in the first stage, the correct movement pattern must be selected while taking into consideration the various regulatory conditions (environmental mandates). Regulatory conditions regulate performance based on certain variables: distance, speed, and the weight, size, and shape of the object.[72,73] Nonregulatory conditions pertain to environmental qualities that do not affect the movement strategy, such as whether the person uses a broomstick or a T-bar for active assisted shoulder range-of-motion exercises. As practice continues in the first stage, skills improve and the athlete gradually moves into the second stage.[72,73]

Fixation and diversification occur in the second stage. Briefly, fixation implies that the athlete refines the movement in a closed

(nonchanging) environment, whereas diversification occurs in an open or changing environment, which requires the athlete to make modifications in the skill for proper performance.[71-73]

Applying Principles of Motor Learning to Rehabilitation

Before injury, athletes attain the advanced motor-learning skills necessary to accomplish complex motor tasks. However, with injury, the athlete is unable (because of reflex inhibition) or unwilling (because of pain or guarding) to use an affected extremity, and motor skills become repressed. Motor-learning principles assist the rehabilitation professional in properly reintroducing the movement patterns to the athlete. The two primary motor-learning principles to consider during rehabilitation are the amount and type of practice and the feedback available to the athlete.[71,84]

PRACTICE

Practicing the activity or movement is perhaps the most important factor in the learning process.[71,80,81] The athlete should deliberately and purposefully practice to achieve optimal motor-learning results.[78] Additionally, the type of practice is also important to consider, as well as obtaining adequate sleep to promote "off-line learning."[85] Systematic manipulation of practice may assist the motor-learning process, especially variability in practice conditions in the later stages of rehabilitation.[86,87] Types of practice include mental and physical; whole versus part; and random, blocked, and random-blocked[44,81,87,88] (Table 4-7).

Physical practice implies that the athlete physically performs an exercise or activity during the rehabilitation process, whereas mental practice indicates that the athlete uses mental images to rehearse the movement.[71,75,77,81,89-91] *Mental imagery* and *visualization* are two common terms used to describe the cognitive processes that occur during mental practice.[92] Frequently, the rehabilitation specialist focuses more on the physical performance of an exercise and overlooks the potential benefits of using mental practice to achieve positive motor-learning outcomes. Research in this area has documented the effect of mental practice on physical performance.[75-77,89-92] An example of an athlete using mental practice is as follows: during rehabilitation an athlete recovering from a shoulder injury performs a

Table 4-7 **Types of Practice**

Type	Characteristics
Physical	Athlete physically performs an exercise or activity.
Mental	Athlete uses mental images to rehearse the movement.
Whole	Athlete performs the entire task from start to finish.
Part	Exercise is divided into different segments or phases.
Blocked	Practice or exercise conditions remain constant or unchanging.
Random	Practice or exercise conditions are randomly alternated, thereby introducing variability into the performance.
Random-blocked	Qualities of random and blocked practice both prevail within an exercise session.

unilateral active range-of-motion exercise with the unaffected extremity, and before performing the exercise with the affected shoulder, the athlete uses mental practice to rehearse the movement. The mental practice before actual performance with the affected upper extremity prepares the athlete by allowing him or her to gauge the requirements necessary for the movement. The specific preparation offered by mental practice relies on some type of movement experience; in this case it was from the unaffected shoulder.

Whole practice implies that the athlete performs the entire task from start to finish, whereas part practice occurs when the exercise is divided into different segments or phases.[88] Complicated movement tasks and activities occurring in the early phases of rehabilitation are usually divided into smaller, less complex activities for the athlete to practice.[88] When the athlete masters the smaller tasks, progression of activity occurs by adding the smaller tasks together to ultimately form the larger and more complex movement pattern.[88] For example, an athlete "relearns" how to voluntarily activate the quadriceps after knee surgery by first performing and mastering the basic quadriceps-setting exercise. As muscle control improves, the athlete builds on the basic quadriceps-setting exercise by lifting the lower extremity in a straight leg raise exercise. Straight leg raises require the isometric activity of quadriceps setting to maintain knee extension during the dynamic activity of hip flexion. In this simplified example, quadriceps-setting exercises could be considered "part practice," whereas the straight leg raises would be "whole practice."

As rehabilitation progresses, the athlete should be able to perform the newly acquired or reacquired task under more functional or sport-specific conditions because clinical situations often do not match those in real life.[86,93,94] The ability to perform the skill under different conditions, or practice variability, enforces retention of the motor skill and allows the athlete to "generalize" the skill to new conditions.[86,87,93,94] Examples of varying practice include alternating the surface, implementing distractions, and adding secondary tasks, such as an athlete progressing from stationary balance activities on one foot to throwing and catching a ball while balancing on one foot.[86]

Practice variability leads us to a brief definition of random, blocked, and random-blocked practice. Essentially, blocked practice implies that the practice or exercise conditions remain constant or unchanging.[87] Blocked practice is beneficial for enhancement of performance during the early phases of rehabilitation.[44] However, blocked practice is not necessarily best for retention of motor skills.[87] Random practice requires the rehabilitation specialist to randomly alternate practice conditions, thereby introducing variability into the performance.[87] Random practice, because of the inherent variability in practice, leads to better retention of motor skills.[44,81,87] Random-blocked practice implies that qualities of random and blocked practice both prevail within an exercise session.[44] Typically, in random-blocked practice, an exercise or activity is performed for more than one repetition before new conditions are implemented. This allows the athlete to correct errors before making adjustments to new practice conditions.[44] An example of random-blocked practice is having an athlete perform a task for two repetitions, followed by an adjustment in the conditions of the exercise, and then having the athlete perform the activity with the new practice conditions.

FEEDBACK

Feedback, or the information that an athlete receives during or after execution of a movement, is perhaps the second most important factor affecting motor learning.[44,71,81,95] Although many different types of feedback exist, only several specific types of feedback relevant to physical rehabilitation are presented here. The major types of feedback are intrinsic and extrinsic[44,71,95] (Table 4-8).

Intrinsic feedback is the information acquired by the athlete's own sensory system.[71,81] The senses most commonly used to acquire information during physical movement are the visual, proprioceptive, and auditory sensory systems.[71,81,96-98]

Vision provides a large amount of information to the human nervous system about movement and allows corrective actions to take place during performance of an exercise. We rely on our vision for many tasks, whether performing an activity of daily living or an activity specific to a given sport.[71,98] We use vision to aim and reach for objects, both in static and dynamic environments and during complex motor activities that involve walking, running, and jumping.[98] Because of vision's role in providing feedback during and after performance of an exercise, the rehabilitation specialist should incorporate visual stimuli into rehabilitation exercises. Visual targets on a wall that correspond to a targeted range of motion during active assisted shoulder exercise are an example of visual stimuli that allow the athlete to make adjustments during movement.

Proprioception offers the second greatest amount of information about movements during exercise.[97] This discussion of proprioceptive feedback is brief because Chapter 24 is devoted entirely to proprioception. We rely on proprioceptive feedback during motor learning to develop a "feel" for the exercise, which improves muscle activation during the movement.[96,97] An example would be having the athlete perform an exercise bilaterally and then instructing the athlete to concentrate on how each extremity feels during the movement. The athlete should understand that the goal is to attempt to have the involved side work or "feel" like the uninvolved extremity during the movement. This is accomplished by the athlete attempting to activate the function of the involved extremity similar to that of the uninvolved

Table 4-8 **Types of Feedback**

Intrinsic	Extrinsic
Information is acquired by the athlete's own sensory system.	Information about the performance of an exercise is derived from a source other than the athlete.
Usually, the visual, proprioceptive, and auditory sensory systems are involved.	This information can come from the clinician or a piece of equipment.
	Two types of extrinsic feedback: • Knowledge of performance (KP) provides information on movement characteristics that lead to a certain outcome. • Knowledge of results (KR) provides information relating the outcome of performance of the exercise to the goal for a particular exercise.

extremity by using proprioceptive discernment, or feedback, of the discrepancy in motor activation between the extremities.[96,97] Proprioceptive feedback also has an impact on spatial accuracy and the timing of motor commands.[71,99] However, proprioceptors may incur damage from soft tissue injury that diminishes their ability to transmit afferent information. Activities designed to restore and retrain proprioception in previously injured tissues are outlined in Chapter 24.

Auditory feedback is sound information associated with a movement or physical performance. The auditory feedback associated with rehabilitation is not usually intrinsic; that is, we do not rely on sound to gather information about our movements unless it comes from another source, which is technically extrinsic feedback. A biofeedback apparatus that interprets and then converts physiologic information into auditory information during an exercise is an example of auditory information assembled from an extrinsic source.[100]

Extrinsic feedback is information about the performance of an exercise that is derived from a source other than the athlete.[71,81] This extrinsic information is processed by the same intrinsic sensory systems of the athlete mentioned earlier for auditory feedback. When deciding whether feedback information is intrinsic or extrinsic to the athlete, it is important to remember who or what is providing the actual information about the performance and not necessarily what sensory registers of the athlete acquire the information. For example, an athlete uses vision to observe the rehabilitation professional providing an initial introductory demonstration. Similarly, the athlete observing his or her reflection in a mirror integrates visual information of the activity. In both cases, demonstration of the exercise and use of the mirror, information about the movement originated from an external source. We may not always have a demonstration or a mirror to use for feedback when we perform a given task.

The rehabilitation specialist or a sophisticated apparatus may provide extrinsic information about physical performance at different points in time in execution of the exercise.[100,101] Extrinsic feedback supplied during an activity is known as concurrent augmented feedback, whereas information occurring after the performance of an activity is terminal augmented feedback.[71]

The two primary types of extrinsic feedback are known as *knowledge of performance* (KP) and *knowledge of results* (KR).[71,79,95]

KP provides the athlete with information about the characteristics of movement that lead to a certain outcome, thus making it pertinent to physical rehabilitation.[71] KP is especially useful in identifying patterns of substitution or compensation during movements. The two types of KP are verbal and visual. Verbal KP includes the descriptive and prescriptive varieties.[71] Descriptive verbal KP merely identifies the error in performance of the exercise, whereas prescriptive KP identifies the error and then prescribes the remedy to correct the error.[71] Visual KP implies that the rehabilitation professional uses a visual display to provide information about the performance. The rehabilitation specialist typically acquires information about the performance and then passes along the information in some sort of visual display to the athlete. Another source of visual information during performance may arise from biofeedback equipment. Heart rate and electromyographic traces are two common types of biofeedback used in rehabilitation settings.[71,100,101]

When providing KP, the rehabilitation specialist must use some type of performance analysis to acquire information about the exercise. The analysis can be either quantitative or qualitative.[102] In quantitative analysis, certain characteristics of the performance are quantified; equipment such as high-speed cameras, motion analysis software packages, force platforms, and research-quality electromyographic equipment are required.[102] Qualitative analysis describes the qualities of the movement, and this is usually sufficient for rehabilitation.[102] Rehabilitation professionals must possess the ability to at least qualitatively analyze the movement patterns associated with performance of an exercise to provide this type of feedback. Videotaped rehabilitation sessions also allow qualitative analysis, which the rehabilitation professional may use as an educational tool to provide the athlete with KP feedback.[71] In later stages of rehabilitation, such as when an athlete begins sport-specific activities, quantitative analysis of an activity may be more appropriate.

KR feedback provides information relating the outcome of performance of an exercise to the goal for a particular exercise.[79,95] For example, the rehabilitation specialist provides an athlete with knowledge of the amount of knee flexion achieved during a rehabilitation session and relates it to the rehabilitation goal for knee flexion. However, Winstein defined KR feedback as the "augmented extrinsic information about task success provided to the performer."[95] She continued by stating that the information serves as a basis for correction of errors on the next trial and thus can be used to achieve more effective performance as practice continues. Several variables of KR feedback are important to consider when one uses it as a tool to enhance motor learning during rehabilitation: the form used (e.g., verbal or visual), the precision or amount of information contained in the KR, and the frequency or schedule of the KR.[79,95] The precision or amount of information contained in the KR feedback influences the number of performance errors: specifically, the greater the precision of the KR, the smaller the amount of performance errors. There is perhaps a ceiling effect with the amount of precision, and the optimal levels necessary to improve performance may depend on the type of performer (i.e., novice versus elite performers). Research has demonstrated that the frequency of KR feedback influences the acquisition and retention of a task.[79] Specifically, KR presented after every trial produces better acquisition of a skill, whereas KR presented after several trials actually produces better learning over time.[79] KR feedback presented after every trial leads the athlete to become sensory dependent on the externally presented information for improving performance and to ignore information available from intrinsic acquisition systems.[79] Decrements in performance occur when KR is removed as a source of feedback after the athlete becomes dependent on extrinsic feedback.[79,95]

Basic Strategies for Implementing Concepts of Motor Learning in Rehabilitation

Learning is not directly observable; rather, the effects of learning are manifested in certain types of behavior or performance characteristics. According to Kisner and Colby, several specific instructional strategies can be used by the rehabilitation specialist to maximize patient learning during exercise instruction.[44] First, select an environment that allows the athlete to pay attention to your instructions.[44] If it is not feasible or possible to interact one on one with the athlete without distractions, it may be necessary to schedule rehabilitation sessions at times when relatively fewer distractions or interruptions occur. Use clear and concise verbal instructions followed by proper demonstration of the exercise or activity.[44] The athlete should follow the demonstration with a performance of the exercise while the rehabilitation professional guides movements and provides feedback on the performance both during (KP) and after (KR) the exercise.[44] As exercises and activities become more complicated throughout the progression of rehabilitation, it may be useful to break down complex movements into simple ones. The athlete may then synthesize simple movements into more complex ones.[44]

Crossover Training Effect

A well-documented phenomenon, the crossover training effect or crossover education, associates improved muscle activation of an affected or unexercised extremity with physical exercise of the unaffected extremity.[103-108] Physical performance indices, such as strength, power, speed, endurance, and range of motion, may improve with crossover education.[103-109] An intriguing characteristic of the crossover effect is that it occurs not only in normal, unaffected extremities but also in extremities affected by immobilization, orthopedic surgery, and stroke.[103-105,107,108] Crossover training may occur in occupationally embedded tasks, as well with the untrained extremity, to improve the speed and accuracy of movement as a result of training the contralateral limb.[109]

CLINICAL IMPLICATIONS

Knowledge of the crossover effect offers several advantages for physical rehabilitation:

1. It prevents deconditioning of the unaffected extremity.
2. It augments early exercise efforts of the affected extremity.
3. It is useful for conditions in which movement of the affected extremity is contraindicated (e.g., it is beneficial for early postoperative rehabilitation of an extremity after surgical repair of muscles, tendons, or both).[105,107-109]

According to the work of Stromberg and others, the major benefit of using the crossover phenomenon resides in gains in strength.[103-105,107,108] Gains in muscle strength attributed to the crossover effect range from 30% to 50%,[107,108] although others report more modest improvements.[106] Nonetheless, any gain in muscle strength is advantageous for an affected extremity undergoing a rehabilitation program, especially when exercise of the affected side is contraindicated.

Using both extremities simultaneously at low levels (submaximal) of force intensity also promotes neuromuscular facilitation.[110,111] Simultaneous bilateral activation of the affected and unaffected extremities has implications for rehabilitation because the patient is able to "feel" the difference between the affected and unaffected muscle groups while also benefiting from the effects of crossover training. The patient's ability to detect differences during simultaneous bilateral muscle activation is a proprioceptive feedback mechanism that increases motor learning and control.[71]

As rehabilitation progresses and force intensity increases, specific training considerations may contraindicate performance of simultaneous bilateral activities to a degree. Deemphasis of bilateral actions later in rehabilitation may be necessary if the sport of interest requires maximal power of unilateral muscle activation and because higher intensities of resistance during bilateral homologous limb activity may actually inhibit relative force production.[110] Beutler and

associates[112] found that muscle activation increases when the affected extremity is exercised alone as opposed to when both extremities are exercised together during closed kinetic chain exercises, which is in agreement with data on the bilateral deficit phenomenon.[110,113,114]

TYPES OF THERAPEUTIC EXERCISE

Therapeutic exercise is physical activity prescribed to restore or favorably alter specific functions in an individual after injury. These specific physical functions include joint range of motion, soft tissue flexibility, muscle strength and power, and neuromuscular coordination and balance. Figure 4-4 classifies the various therapeutic exercises that a clinician can incorporate into a therapeutic rehabilitation program.

Joint Range-of-Motion Exercise

Passive Exercise

Passive exercise is carried out by the application of an external force with minimal participation of muscle action by the injured athlete (Fig. 4-5). Passive exercise can be forced or nonforced. Nonforced exercises are those used to help maintain normal joint motion and are usually kept within a painless range of motion, such as grade I joint mobilizations.[44] Conversely, forced passive exercises generally produce movement into tissue resistance and are associated with some discomfort by the individual. Forced passive exercises are aggressive and rarely indicated, and should be performed only by experienced clinicians.

The goal of passive exercise techniques is to restore accessory and physiologic joint motions. Accessory motions are necessary for physiologic motions to occur, yet accessory motions do not occur under volitional control of the athlete.[52] Restoration of accessory motions (spin, roll, and glide) is achieved by mobilization and manipulation techniques implemented by the clinician (see Chapter 6).[44] Passive restoration of physiologic motions is usually performed for the injured athlete by the clinician or a mechanical appliance, such as a continuous passive motion unit or isokinetic dynamometer set in the passive mode.

Active Exercise

Active and active-assisted exercises are beneficial for moving the associated joint, regaining neuromuscular control of an affected extremity, and allowing the patient to have control over the exercise.[44,115] Active exercise requires muscle activity, at least to some degree, during joint movement. In all cases, the athlete may not have complete neuromuscular control of the extremity, in which case some type of assistance may facilitate performance of the activity. Active and active-assisted exercises are generally safe unless a muscle or tendon has been repaired, and then active range of motion is initially contraindicated in the early phases of rehabilitation.[44,115]

Therapeutic Exercise for Neuromuscular Strength/Endurance

Essentially, natural progression to resistive exercise occurs as the athlete moves from early range-of-motion and flexibility exercises to active range of motion against gravity without assistance. When the athlete has noncompensatory active range of motion,

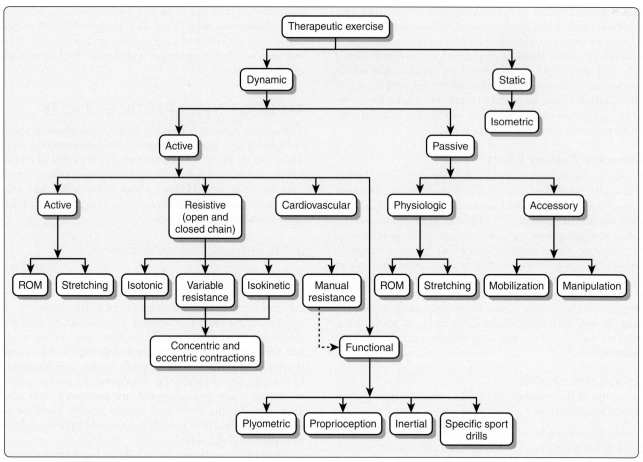

FIGURE 4-4 Classification of therapeutic exercise. *ROM*, Range of motion. *(Modified from Irrgang, J.J. [1995]: Rehabilitation. In: Fu, F.H., and Stone, D. [eds.]. Sports Injuries: Mechanisms, Prevention, Treatment. Baltimore, Williams & Wilkins.)*

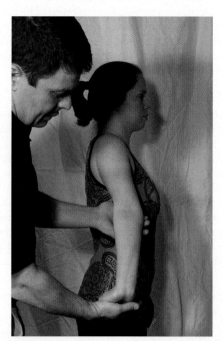

FIGURE 4-5 Passive range of motion. The athlete (standing) moves passively into wrist and elbow extension as a result of external forces at each joint (applied by the clinician).

resistance to the active range of motion is added to further strengthen the musculature involved.

Houglum described this natural rate of strength progression for individuals in a rehabilitation program.[116] The initial phase is characterized by relatively rapid improvement in strength, followed by a second phase in which the rate of improvement is slowing or tapering, and a third (final) phase consisting of progression toward a plateau state in which minimal or no improvement in strength occurs (Fig. 4-6).

Muscular strength and endurance increase with progressive resistive exercise (PRE), as long as it occurs in an orderly and progressive manner. PRE permits an ever-increasing overload to be applied to the musculature, which allows bones, ligaments, tendons, and muscles to adapt to the applied stress. This philosophy is based on the principle of specific adaptation to imposed demands (see the section on conditioning later in this chapter), which implies that the body responds to a given demand with a specific and predictable adaptation.[31] Stated another way, specific adaptation requires that a specific demand be imposed.[55] With rehabilitation, it is important that overload not be applied too quickly to avoid further damage to the healing tissue.

Rehabilitative strength training may involve static (isometric) or dynamic exercise. Types of dynamic resistive exercise include isotonic, isokinetic, and variable resistance. Box 4-6 summarizes factors related to the production of muscle force.

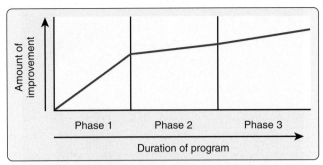

FIGURE 4-6 Typical progression during a rehabilitation program. *(Adapted from Houglum, P. [1977]: The modality of therapeutic exercise: Objectives and principles. Athl. Train. J. Natl. Athl. Train. Assoc., 12:43.)*

Box 4-6

Factors Affecting Production of Muscle Force

Muscle fiber type
Length-tension relationship
Number of motor units activated
Firing frequency
Muscle temperature
Elastic energy of muscle and type of muscle action
Force-velocity relationship
Size of muscle fibers (cross-sectional area)
Decreased activity of inhibitory reflexes
Angle of pull during muscle action

Data from Kreighbaum, E., and Barthels, K.M. (1996): Biomechanics: A Qualitative Approach for Studying Human Movement, 4th ed. Boston, Allyn & Bacon.

Static Exercise

Static exercises, or isometric actions, occur without joint movement. The activated muscle groups maintain a fixed length because the tension generated is equal to the resistance encountered.[117] Because gains in strength generally occur close to a specific angle in which the isometric exercise occurs, it is important for the athlete to perform the exercise at multiple joint angles.[118-121] For example, to strengthen elbow flexors throughout the full 150° of available motion, sets could be performed at 20°, 60°, 100°, and 140° of elbow flexion.[115] Generally, the muscle should remain under tension for 3 to 10 seconds.[44,115,118]

The clinician should ensure that the athlete does not strain during the holding period of the isometric action, particularly as the intensity of the action increases. Straining instinctively causes one to "hold one's breath," also known as the Valsalva maneuver, which is associated with momentary increases in arterial blood pressure.[122,123] For most athletes, this may not be a concern because the intensity of their normal weight-training bout far exceeds that of a rehabilitation program, but individuals suffering from hypertension may incur an adverse sequela when blood pressure rises to dangerous levels.[122] New research in this area shows that the body can adapt to the acute hypertensive response associated with careful isometric training and consequently lower resting blood pressure.[124]

A contemporary exercise modality is whole-body vibration, which could be used with isometric or dynamic exercise modes. Whole-body vibration exercise challenges the musculoskeletal

system by perturbations from a platform.[37,125-127] Emerging research is showing promising results in strength gains, possible improvement in bone mineral deposition, and enhancement of sports performance[37,125-127]; however, more research is warranted to better elucidate its effects on local tissue and its safety in general.[128]

Clinical Pearl #4

Have the athlete count out loud during isometric actions to relatively attenuate the increases in blood pressure associated with isometric actions. Blood pressure may still increase, but not to the extent that occurs during a Valsalva maneuver.

Dynamic Exercise

Dynamic exercise implies that movement occurs. Most types of dynamic exercise include isotonic, variable-resistance, manual, and isokinetic (accommodating variable-resistance) movements.[129] Additionally, dynamic exercise may be more functional in nature, some examples of which are plyometric, proprioceptive, and inertial exercises and sport-specific drills. Almost all dynamic exercises include concentric and eccentric movement phases.

CONCENTRIC AND ECCENTRIC ACTIONS

As mentioned earlier, the two types of muscle actions that occur during dynamic training are (1) concentric contractions, in which shortening of muscle fibers results in a decrease in the angle of the associated joint, and (2) eccentric actions, in which the muscle resists lengthening so that the joint angle increases during the action.[44,117] Concentric and eccentric actions are also referred to as positive and negative work, respectively.[130] Concentric contractions generally function to accelerate a limb; for example, the shoulder internal rotators accelerate the arm during the acceleration phase of throwing. Conversely, eccentric actions generally function to decelerate a limb and provide shock absorption; for example, the shoulder external rotators decelerate the shoulder during the follow-through phase of throwing.[131] Another interesting difference between concentric and eccentric muscle actions is their relative capabilities for production of force. A maximum eccentric action may generate forces 14% to 50% greater than a maximal concentric contraction of the same group.[130] How is this possible? There are at least two reasons: (1) the energy-consuming mechanical work of sliding actin and myosin together has already occurred and now allows the actin and myosin to "pull apart" under controlled tension, which takes less energy, and (2) some energy is conserved as a result of elongation of the elastic (parallel and series) components of muscle.[39] Training studies clearly demonstrate an association between eccentric actions and muscle hypertrophy and increases in strength versus concentric-only actions. In fact, it is advisable for individuals to use both concentric and eccentric actions to maximize the benefits derived from strength training.[29]

Besides advantages in production of force, another benefit of eccentric exercise is its positive effects on tendonitis and overuse syndromes.[132-136] Eccentric training may directly improve the integrity of musculotendinous structures by inducing hypertrophy and increased tensile strength or by lengthening the muscle-tendon unit, which induces relatively less strain during active motion.[133,136] It is conceivable that eccentric training may elicit its therapeutic effects by both proposed mechanisms. Nonetheless, rehabilitation involving eccentric actions is effective in restoring strength and function in athletes with tendinitis, as long as careful progression is ensured.

A major reason for eccentric exercise to progress slowly and carefully is its association with delayed-onset muscle soreness (DOMS).[137-139] DOMS is defined as muscular pain or discomfort occurring 1 to 5 days after unusual muscular exertion.[131] The syndrome of DOMS also includes joint swelling and weakness, and its timing of onset and severity are inversely proportional to the intensity of eccentric exercise; DOMS generally occurs in individuals unaccustomed to eccentric exercise.[131,137-139] Therefore, eccentric activities are important to include but should be progressed gradually during rehabilitation.

Clinical Pearl #5

Eccentric actions may be emphasized by having the athlete perform the activity with both extremities (bilateral) during the concentric phase but then use only the affected extremity (unilateral) during the eccentric phase.

Isotonic Exercise

Isotonic resistance activities are perhaps the most common type of dynamic exercise. With isotonic exercise, the actual muscle length changes as an external force causes a change in the joint angle.[129] In pure isotonic exercise, resistance remains constant, whereas the velocity of movement depends on the load, known as the force-velocity relationship.[129] Eccentric and concentric phases occur during isotonic exercise. Isotonic exercise has two inherent disadvantages: (1) the weight is fixed and does not adjust to the variation in expression of force present during speed work or at various ranges of motion, and (2) the momentum of weight propulsion diminishes the strength required at the extremes of joint motion. This type of exercise is readily available in the form of exercises performed with ankle weights, free weights, and weight machines (Fig. 4-7).

Variable-Resistance Exercise

Production of muscle force is less at extreme joint range of motion (e.g., the muscle is too short or excessively lengthened). Variable-resistance exercise machines address the relative decrements in force throughout the range of motion by a cam that varies the resistance to match the decrements in normal force during resisted exercise.[129] The cam varies the resistance by changing the length of the machine's lever arm of the weight being lifted (Fig. 4-8). Variable-resistance exercise machines are commonly used in rehabilitation and fitness settings. The machines usually have adjustments that allow proper joint alignment (the joint's axis of rotation should always be in alignment with the machine's axis of rotation), as well as range-of-motion limiters, which are beneficial for some types of rehabilitation.

Manual Resistance

Manual resistance is a variation of accommodating variable-resistance exercise.[115] The clinician provides the resistance with this mode of exercise and can modify the resistance and speed

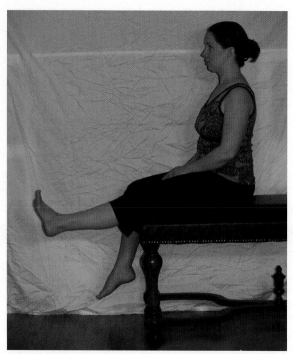

FIGURE 4-7 Long-arc knee extensions: isotonic exercise in which resistance remains constant and velocity is inversely proportional to the load.

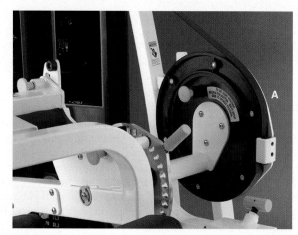

FIGURE 4-8 Variable-resistance exercise. A specialized cam (A) allows varied resistance during a specific motion. *(Photo courtesy Cybex International, Medway, MA.)*

during the exercise as the athlete's fatigue is recognized (Fig. 4-9). This exercise mode is applicable to an extent during all rehabilitation phases because it is capable of producing movement patterns that cannot be duplicated on machines (e.g., proprioceptive neuromuscular facilitation diagonals [see Chapter 6]).[115]

Isokinetic Exercise

Isokinetic exercise, or accommodating variable-resistance exercise, is performed at a fixed speed with the resistance matching the muscle force at that speed of movement.[140] As the muscle force input changes, the resistance changes because the speed remains constant. Application of the athlete's own muscular resistance is met with a proportional amount of resistance

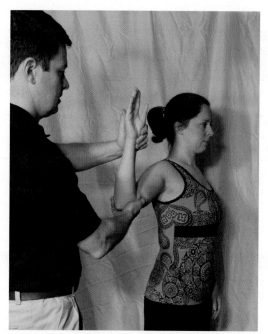

FIGURE 4-9 Manual resistance of the right external rotators. Note how the athlete's right arm is stabilized by the clinician (darker shirt) as resistance is applied by the clinician's left hand.

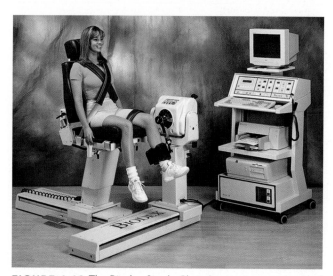

FIGURE 4-10 The Biodex Single Chair System is an example of isokinetic (accommodating variable resistance) equipment. The resistance changes to match the input, but the speed remains constant. *(Courtesy Biodex, Shirley, NY.)*

throughout a range of motion. Isokinetic machines may be set to offer concentric-concentric, concentric-eccentric, or eccentric-eccentric actions at various velocities (Fig. 4-10). Chapter 25 provides an in-depth discussion of isokinetics.

Inertial Exercise

Inertial loading is a relatively novel mode of exercise with respect to other forms of dynamic exercise.[141-144] This mode of exercise simulates the changes in momentum and velocity of functional activity through reciprocal acceleration and deceleration of a variable mass (Fig. 4-11).[144,145] Albert described the type of

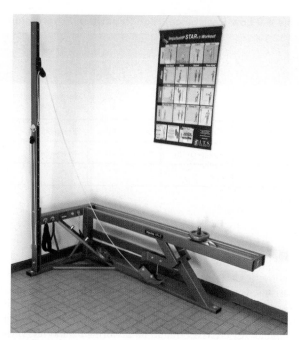

FIGURE 4-11 Impulse machine for inertial exercise. *(Courtesy Impulse Training Systems, Newnan, GA.)*

loading that the impulse machine produces as "horizontal, submaximal, gravity eliminated plyometrics."[141]

PROGRESSIVE RESISTIVE EXERCISE

Before an athlete begins a PRE program, functional range of motion must be present.[38] The theory behind resistance exercise is to apply an overload to increase muscular strength and, at the same time, to maintain integrity of the tissues of concern and not impede the healing process. Several progression philosophies are discussed in the literature, including the low-resistance, high-repetition method; the DeLorme and Watkins regimen; the Oxford technique; the daily adjustable progressive resistance exercise (DAPRE) method; and the Sanders program.

The Low-Resistance, High-Repetition Method

Before 1945, the traditional method of strength training during rehabilitation actually stressed muscle endurance more so than strength.[129] A low-resistance, high-repetition technique may be the best regimen for athletes with injuries of insidious onset and during the early postoperative period.[146] Exercise with high resistance or intensity could potentially cause the supporting structures to break down and exacerbate the inflammation associated with the condition. Use of smaller weights and submaximal intensities provides a therapeutic effect that stimulates blood flow, diminishes tissue breakdown, and promotes local muscle endurance.[146-148]

The PRE program outlined here can be carried out early in rehabilitation by using the low-resistance, high-repetition concept (Table 4-9). Early rehabilitation begins with an active range of motion of two or three sets of 10 repetitions (even up to 20 to 30 repetitions), with progression to five sets of 10 repetitions (up to 50 repetitions) as tolerated. When the athlete can perform 50 repetitions without stopping and without overcompensation of other muscle groups or joint actions, 1 lb of weight may be added

Table 4-9 Low-Resistance, High-Repetition Progression

Week	Day						
	Sun	Mon	Tues	Wed	Thurs	Fri	Sat
1			Surgery/injury	30 rep (no weight)	40 rep (no weight)	50 rep (no weight)	30 rep @1 lb
2	40 rep @1 lb	50 rep @1 lb	30 rep @2 lb	40 rep @2 lb	50 rep @2 lb	30 rep @3 lb	40 rep @3 lb
3	50 rep @3 lb	30 rep @4 lb	40 rep @4 lb	50 rep @4 lb	30 rep @5 lb	40 rep @5 lb	50 rep @5 lb
◆	etc.						

rep, Repetitions.

and the number of repetitions reduced to three sets of 10 to 30 repetitions. The cycle repeats when the athlete reaches 50 repetitions, and as another pound of weight is added, the repetitions are reduced to 10 to 30. The athlete progresses through the PRE program as tolerated, with emphasis placed on proper lifting technique. All exercises should be performed smoothly, with a pause at the terminal position. The athlete must also concentrate on lowering the weight in a controlled fashion.

Houglum outlined a program using a resistance that the athlete safely controls for two sets of 6 to 15 repetitions.[39] That resistance is continued until the athlete successfully performs three sets of 2 to 25 repetitions each. At this point, resistance increases and the number of repetitions decreases accordingly. As the athlete progresses into later stages of rehabilitation and the healing tissue is capable of tolerating increased stress, other more intense models of progression could be used, such as those of DeLorme and Watkins or DAPRE.

The DeLorme and Watkins Program

DeLorme first introduced the concept of PRE in 1945 as a challenge to the traditional concept of low-resistance, high-repetition exercise.[53,129] The rationale for using PRE is that it creates a condition in which an individual muscle or set of muscles must work against ever-increasing resistance in subsequent sets.[54,149]

DeLorme's concept of PRE was based on the amount of weight that could be carried through a full range of motion for 10 repetitions.[53] DeLorme referred to this as heavy-resistance exercise because the weights used were heavy in comparison to those used in previous strengthening methods, and all-out effort was necessary to lift them.[53] This mode of PRE, however, is not generally applicable to athletes in the early postoperative stages. Box 4-7 outlines the DeLorme and Watkins program.[54]

The Oxford Technique

The Oxford technique, developed by Zinovieff, also incorporates relatively heavy resistance after the determination of a 10 repetition maximum (RM).[56] However, unlike the DeLorme and Watkins regimen, the Oxford technique decreases exercise intensity with each new set to accommodate fatiguing muscle (Table 4-10).[56] Zinovieff suggested this modification after observing that most patients were excessively fatigued during the final set of repetitions with the DeLorme and Watkins technique.[56]

Box 4-7

The DeLorme and Watkins Progressive Resistance Exercise Program

1. First set of 10 repetitions: use one half of 10 RM
2. Second set of 10 repetitions: use three fourths of 10 RM
3. Third set of 10 repetitions: use full 10 RM

Modified from DeLorme, T.L., and Watkins, A. (1948): Techniques of progressive resistance exercise. Arch. Phys. Med., 29:263-268. *RM*, Repetition maximum.

Table 4-10 The Oxford Technique of Progressive Resistance Exercise

Set	Amount of Resistance (Intensity)	Repetitions (Duration)
1	100% of 10 RM	10
2	75% of 10 RM	10
3	50% of 10 RM	10

Data from Zinovieff, A.N. (1951): Heavy-resistance exercises: The "Oxford technique." Br. J. Phys. Med., 14(6):129–132.
RM, Repetition maximum.

The Daily Adjustable Progressive Resistance Exercise Technique

Knight's technique of DAPRE,[55] along with other modifications of DeLorme's PRE concept,[56,116,150] uses the same basic principles of PRE. According to Knight, the DAPRE technique allows individual differences in the rate at which a person regains strength in the muscle and provides an objective method for increasing resistance in accordance with increases in strength.[55] The key to the program is that athletes perform as many full repetitions as they can in the third and fourth sets.[55] These numbers of repetitions are then used to determine the amount of weight that is added to or removed from the working weight for the fourth set in the current bout and the first set of the next session. The working weight is estimated for the initial reconditioning session. A good

Table 4-11 Daily Adjustable Progressive Resistance Exercise

Set	Portion of Working Weight Used	Number of Repetitions
1	One half	10
2	Three fourths	6
3*	Full	Maximum
4†	Adjusted	Maximum

Data from Knight, K.L. (1985): Guidelines for rehabilitation of sports injuries. Clin. Sports Med., 4:413.

*The number of repetitions performed during the third set is used to determine the adjusted working weight for the fourth set according to the guidelines in Table 4-12.

†The number of repetitions performed during the fourth set is used to determine the adjusted working weight for the next day according to the guidelines in Table 4-12.

Table 4-12 General Guidelines for Adjustment of Working Weight

Number of Repetitions Performed During Set	Adjustment of Working Weight Fourth Set*	Next Day†
0-2	Decrease by 5-10 lb and perform the set over	
3-4	Decrease by 0-5 lb	Keep the same
5-7	Keep the same	Increase by 5-10 lb
8-12	Increase by 5-10 lb	Increase by 5-15 lb
13+	Increase by 10-15 lb	Increase by 10-20 lb

Data from Knight, K. (1985): Guidelines for rehabilitation of sports injuries. Clin. Sports Med., 4:414.

*The number of repetitions performed during the third set is used to determine the adjusted working weight for the fourth set according to the guidelines in Table 4-11.

†The number of repetitions performed during the fourth set is used to determine the adjusted working weight for the next day according to the guidelines in Table 4-11.

estimate would result in five to seven repetitions during the third set. More repetitions are performed if the estimate is low, and fewer are performed if it is too high.

During the first and second sets, the athlete performs 10 repetitions against one half of the estimated working weight and six repetitions against three quarters of the working weight (Tables 4-11 and 4-12). These sets warm up and educate the muscles and neuromuscular structures involved.

Emphasis during the third and fourth sets is on the athlete performing the greatest number of full repetitions possible. The full working weight is used in the third set, and the athlete performs as many repetitions as possible. The number of full repetitions performed in the third set is used to determine the adjusted working weight for the fourth set, and the number of full repetitions performed in the fourth set is used to determine the working weight for the next day.

Box 4-8

The Sanders Program of Progressing Resistance Exercise

Determining the initial resistance load (median starting points) for 10 repetitions:

- Universal leg extension: 15% of body weight
- Universal leg press: 50% of body weight
- Barbell squat: 45% of body weight
- Barbell bench press: 30% of body weight

Adapted from Sanders, M. (1990): Weight training and conditioning. In: Sanders, B. (ed.). Sports Physical Therapy. Norwalk, CT, Appleton & Lange, pp. 239–250.

The Sanders Program

Athletes tolerate higher intensities in advanced stages of rehabilitation, which is addressed in the Sanders program of resistance exercise progression.[151] The beginning intensity of resistance varies according to the athlete's body weight and the particular exercise (e.g., leg extension, squats, or bench press). The athlete exercises at high intensity (100% of a two to five RM) for three sessions per week. Box 4-8 summarizes the Sanders program.

NEUROMUSCULAR COORDINATION AND PROPRIOCEPTION

In a comprehensive rehabilitation program the clinician must not overlook the component of neuromuscular control, which is necessary for joint stability. Healing of static or dynamic restraints and strengthening of the appropriate muscles do not prepare a joint for the sudden changes in position that occur during sport-specific activities.[152-156] To adequately address this phenomenon, the rehabilitation specialist must be familiar with the structures contributing to proprioception, as well as the process by which articular sensations contribute to functional stability.

When joint sensation is described, the terms *proprioception* and *kinesthesia* are often interchanged erroneously. Proprioception describes the awareness of posture, movement, and changes in equilibrium and the knowledge of position, weight, and resistance of objects in relation to the body.[157] Kinesthesia, however, refers to the ability to perceive the extent, direction, or weight of movement.[157] These two definitions are combined into a comprehensive, operational definition: "Proprioception is considered a specialized variation of the sensory modality of touch and encompasses the sensations of joint movement (kinesthesia) and joint position (joint position sense)."[158] As Lephart and others assert, both conscious and unconscious proprioception is essential for proper joint function in sports and other daily tasks, as well as for stabilization of reflexes.[155,156,159-161] These articular sensations are the direct focus of proprioceptive rehabilitation and are crucial for efficient, noninjurious movement. Figures 4-12 and 4-13 provide examples of exercises used for proprioceptive training of the lower and upper extremities, respectively. Chapter 24 provides more detailed information on proprioception.

Improving neuromuscular coordination builds on the foundations of range of motion, strengthening, and proprioception. Athletic coordination, often an innate skill that is difficult to teach or coach, may be enhanced with training.[162] Most physical

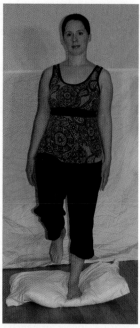

FIGURE 4-12 Proprioceptive exercise while standing: "stork stand." This athlete is standing on a pillow, which increases the difficulty of exercise versus standing on a firm surface.

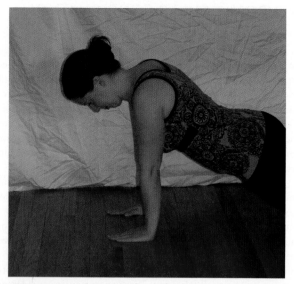

FIGURE 4-13 Closed kinetic chain exercise for the upper extremities. The push-up position incorporates joint compression and facilitates joint stability.

tasks require the actions of multiple joints and muscle groups; as the complexity of the task increases, so must coordination between the working muscle groups. Generally, complex tasks are composed of multiple smaller tasks. The athlete must be able to unconsciously carry out these tasks while concentrating mental attention on the outcome of the performance and using feedback to modify performance as necessary.[71] The physical act of practicing a given task increases the skill level at which it is performed and its automaticity (see the section on motor learning earlier in this chapter).[71]

Table 4-13 Three Phases of Plyometric Exercise

Phase	Characteristics
Eccentric	This is the preloading period in which the muscle spindle is prestretched before activation.
Amortization	This is the time between the eccentric contraction and initiation of a concentric force. The rate of the stretch is more critical than the duration of the stretch. Therefore, the more quickly an athlete can overcome the yielding eccentric force and produce a concentric force, the more powerful the response.
Concentric	This is a summation of the eccentric and amortization phases, with the product being an enhanced concentric contraction.

NEUROMUSCULAR POWER

Plyometrics

Plyometric training consists of drills or exercises that aim to link strength and speed of movement to produce an explosive-reactive type of muscle response.[24,163-165] The purpose of plyometric training is to heighten the excitability of neurologic receptors to achieve improved reactivity of the neuromuscular system.[24,166] By means of an eccentric muscle action, the muscle is fully stretched immediately preceding the concentric contraction. The greater the stretch placed on the muscle from its resting length immediately before the concentric contraction, the greater the load that the muscle can lift or overcome. Thus, plyometrics has been referred to as "stretch-shortening" drills or "reactive neuromuscular" training.[24,163] Wilk et al described the three phases of a plyometric exercise (Table 4-13).[24]

Plyometrics is implemented in the later stages of rehabilitation and should mimic a sport-specific skill. It must be used judiciously because of the relative stress placed on involved tissue. The clinician should remember that both postexercise soreness and DOMS are by-products of this type of exercise.

Absolute contraindications to plyometrics include the acute recovery period after surgery, gross instability, pain, and a state of unconditioning. Chapter 26 is devoted to plyometric exercise and the reader is referred to it for a more in-depth discussion of the topic.

Clinical Pearl #6

Plyometrics is a form of exercise that trains muscles to produce power. Power production also increases when the athlete performs repetitions at the same relative resistance (intensity) but at higher velocities. A metronome may be used to keep the athlete on a faster "pace" while performing repetitions within a set.

Kinetic Chain

The term *kinematic chain* was introduced by Reuleaux in 1875 to refer to a mechanical system of links in engineering.[167] In engineering, a kinematic chain is usually a closed system of links joined together so that if any free link is moved on a fixed link, all the other links move in a predictable pattern. Steindler first suggested the terms *open kinetic chain* (OKC) and *closed kinetic chain* (CKC).[168] He defined a kinetic chain in the human body as a combination of successively arranged joints that constitutes a complex motor unit.[168]

Steindler described an OKC as being characterized by the distal segment terminating freely in space, whereas in a CKC the distal segment of the joint is fixed and meets with considerable external resistance that prohibits or restrains its free motion.[169] CKC exercise (CKCE) is characterized by the distal segment being fixed and body weight being supported by the extremity, which is associated with considerable external resistance (see Fig. 4-13).[169] OKC exercise (OKCE), conversely, is associated with the distal segment not being fixed, body weight not being supported, and the affected muscles working against relatively less external resistance.[169] As researchers have examined CKCE and OKCE, the basic characteristics have expanded (Table 4-14).

Most of the research on CKCE has targeted the lower extremity, specifically the knee joint. With regard to the effect of CKCE on the knee, most investigations have examined anterior tibial displacement and the resultant stress placed on the anterior cruciate ligament. The advantages of CKCE over OKCE have been well reported in the literature and include a decrease in shear force, stimulation of proprioceptors, enhancement of joint stability, allowance of more functional patterns of movement, and greater specificity for athletic activities.[152,170-176]

Although the characterization of CKCE and OKCE has broadened, application of lower extremity CKCE principles to the upper extremity is still being debated. The upper extremity has unique anatomic, biomechanical, and functional features, especially the shoulder, which makes applying the traditional definitions of OKCE and CKCE difficult.[175] Wilk and Arrigo state the following[175]:

The conditions that apply to the lower extremity such as weight-bearing forces, which create a closed kinetic chain effect, do not routinely occur in the upper extremity. However, due to the unique anatomical configuration of the glenohumeral joint, whereas the stabilizing muscles contract producing a joint compression force that stabilizes the joint much to the same effect as closed kinetic chain exercise for the lower extremity. It is for this reason we believe that the principle of closed kinetic chain exercise as explained for the lower extremity may not apply for upper extremity exercises. Rather, we suggest specific terminology for the upper extremity exercise program under specific conditions, such as weight bearing or axial compression.

Because of incongruities between the lower and upper extremities, some authors have recommended different classification systems for describing OKCEs and CKCEs for the upper extremity.[177] Dillman et al proposed three classifications of OKCE and CKCE for the upper extremity based on mechanics.[178] Their system takes into account the boundary condition and the external load encountered at the distal segment. The boundary condition of the distal segment may be either fixed or

Table 4-14 Characteristics of Closed Kinetic Chain Exercise Versus Open Kinetic Chain Exercise

Closed Kinetic Chain Exercise	Open Kinetic Chain Exercise
Large-resistance and low-acceleration forces	Large-acceleration and low-resistance forces
Greater compressive forces	Distraction and rotatory forces
Joint congruity	Promotion of a stable base
Decreased shear	Joint mechanoreceptor deformation
Stimulation of proprioceptors	Concentric acceleration and eccentric deceleration
Enhanced dynamic stabilization	Assimilation of function

Data from Lephart, S.M., and Henry, T.J. (1995): Functional rehabilitation for the upper and lower extremity. Orthop. Clin. North Am., 26:579–592.

movable, and an external load may or may not exist at the distal link. Thus, the categories include a fixed boundary with an external load, a movable boundary with an external load, and a movable boundary with no external load.[178] The concepts fixed boundary with an external load and movable boundary with no external load correspond to the extremes of CKCEs and OKCEs, respectively, and movable boundary with an external load refers to the "gray" region between these two extremes. These authors suggest that the confusing terms *OKC* and *CKC* be eliminated and that the biomechanics, load, and muscular response to the exercises be used.

Lephart and Henry proposed a functional classification system for upper extremity rehabilitation with the objective of restoring functional stability of the shoulder by reestablishing neuromuscular control of overhead activities.[177] This system addresses three areas of the shoulder complex: scapulothoracic stabilization, glenohumeral stabilization, and humeral control. The functional classification system considers boundary, load, and the direction in which the load is applied. Table 4-15 summarizes the functional classification system.

There appears to be agreement that the traditional classification system of OKCEs and CKCEs, which considers fixation of the distal segment, body weight, and external resistance, is not adequate for describing exercises for the upper extremities. Nonetheless, both open and closed chain exercises have characteristics that are important in restoring strength and neuromuscular control to an injured upper extremity, and both should be incorporated into an upper extremity rehabilitation program.[175,177,179]

Physical Conditioning and Rehabilitation

General Considerations

Within the context of rehabilitation and conditioning, several considerations affect the quality of performance of exercises and the outcome of the program, including progression from general to specific exercises and the specific order of exercises.

Table 4-15 **Summary of the Upper Extremity Functional Classification System**

Classification	Characteristics	Examples
Fixed boundary: external, axial load	Considerable load, slow velocity	Axial loading in the tripod position
	NM reaction: active or reactive	Slide board
	MM action: coactivation, acceleration, deceleration	
	Coactivation of force couples	Unstable platform
	Joint compression	
	Minimal shear forces	
	Promotion of dynamic stability	
Movable boundary: external, axial load with variable velocity	Considerable load, variable velocity	Closed chain protraction/retraction on an isokinetic dynamometer
	MM action: coactivation, acceleration, deceleration	Traditional bench press
	Coactivation of force couples	Rhythmic stabilization activities
	Promotion of dynamic stability	
	Activation of prime movers	
	Minimal shear forces	
Movable boundary: external, axial load with functional velocity	Variable load, functional speeds	Isokinetic exercises in functional diagonal patterns
	NM reaction: active or reactive	Multiaxial machine
	MM action: coactivation, acceleration, deceleration	Resistance tubing exercise
	Stability of scapular and glenohumeral base	Proprioceptive neuromuscular facilitation exercise
	Activation of prime movers	
	Functional point kinematics	
	Functional motor patterns	
Movable boundary: no load	Negligible load, variable velocity	Joint sensibility training: active and passive
	NM reaction: active or passive	
	MM action: coactivation, acceleration, perceptual	
	Activation of muscles: proximal to distal	
	Low muscle activation without resistance	
	Functional significance	

From Lephart, S.M., and Henry, T.J. (1996): The physiological basis for open and closed kinetic chain rehabilitation for the upper extremity. J. Sports Rehabil., 5:77.
MM, Muscular; *NM,* neuromuscular.

Exercises should progress from general (simple) to specific (complex).[29] This consideration applies to initial conditioning programs, as well as to rehabilitation programs, because untrained or healing tissue may not tolerate the stress inherent in some types of specific exercises. Specific exercises are usually better tolerated as tissue integrity improves, which generally occurs in more advanced phases of rehabilitation. The concept of generalized adaptation relies on the premise that a bout of physical exercise affects more than one physiologic system simultaneously.[129] For instance, cardiovascular exercise specifically stresses the heart, lungs, and circulatory system and improves local muscle endurance in the extremities performing the mode of exercise. Even though the exercise bout specifically targets cardiovascular and muscular endurance, relative muscular force

production also improves when compared with previous force production capability.[129]

Another consideration that optimizes the outcomes of exercise is the specific order of exercises.[180] To minimize the deleterious effects of fatigue, higher-intensity exercises using larger muscle groups and multiple joints should be performed early in the exercise session.[29,180] Thus, exercises that use lower intensities and that stress single joints or smaller muscle groups (or both) are best performed at the end of the bout.

Physical conditioning and comprehensive athletic rehabilitation both stress multiple physiologic systems that influence athletic performance. These systems include the cardiovascular, neurologic, thermoregulatory, and musculoskeletal systems. The efficiency of operation of these systems is improved, which results in improved functioning and sports performance. The following discussion emphasizes the cardiovascular and neuromuscular systems.

Stress involving the aforementioned systems can be adjusted by changing one or more of the following conditioning parameters: intensity, duration, frequency, specificity, and progression of exercises. Incorporating knowledge of the various conditioning parameters allows systematic manipulation of physiologic stress.

Conditioning During Rehabilitation

A very challenging aspect of rehabilitation for the clinician is providing the athlete with a form of physical stress involving the noninjured extremities, especially the cardiovascular system, to minimize the deleterious effects of a relative decrease in activity.[181-183] Sport-specific activities are most desirable as long as they are not contraindicated during rehabilitation. The principles of generality and specificity are important to consider with physical conditioning during rehabilitation.

Cardiovascular fitness should be addressed, if possible, throughout the various rehabilitation phases. General adaptations occur within the cardiovascular system as a result of participation in nonspecific aerobic activity. For example, an athlete with a lower extremity injury may not be able to participate in running or cycle ergometry with the lower extremities but may be able to participate in aerobic activities with the upper extremities. General adaptations are useful in the early phases of rehabilitation because they allow injured tissue to recover from the mechanisms causing injury. General conditioning is beneficial up to a point, but it is rather unsatisfactory for returning an athlete to a given sport because the adaptations may not be sufficiently specific to the demands of the sport.

Specific conditioning, according to the demands of an athlete's sport, is relatively more stressful because it integrates the previously injured tissue into the activity or exercise. Therefore, sport-specific conditioning usually takes place later in the rehabilitation program because healing tissue needs to reach a maturation level that is able to withstand the specific stress incurred with a specific sport.

Prehabilitation

Prehabilitation describes one of two possible scenarios: preventive conditioning based on findings from a preparticipation examination (PPE)[184-186] or rehabilitation after an injury requiring surgical intervention that better prepares the patient for postsurgical rehabilitation. Although clinicians are quite familiar with the benefits of both types of prehabilitation, relatively few scientific data substantiate its practice.

Prophylactic Prehabilitation

Prehabilitation may mean that athletes continue with maintenance exercises/activities to prevent or avoid injury or reinjury. An example of this concept is a healthy baseball pitcher who incorporates specific rotator cuff exercises into his offseason workout regimen. It is beneficial to screen athletes during the preseason (e.g., with a PPE) to reveal a predisposition to injury.

PPE routinely evaluates flexibility, strength, power, and endurance of athletes during the preseason because vulnerability in these areas may predispose the athlete to injury.[186-192] Equally important, the rehabilitation specialist must understand the inherent demands of various sports to be able to provide a sound preventive conditioning program.[185] Together with the PPE, the prehabilitation program targets specific areas of vulnerability and addresses sport-specific requirements in an attempt to prevent injury.[192-194] Thus, in this context, prehabilitation is a type of conditioning program used to achieve physiologic adaptations for increasing neuromuscular activity and coordination, bone and joint integrity, metabolic capacity, recovery mechanisms, and joint stability-force coupling.[194] Generally, improvements in these areas will also correlate with improvements in physical performance, which is the typical goal of most regular conditioning programs.

Prehabilitation Preceding Surgery

Prehabilitation also refers to specific exercises and patient education before surgery.[192,195] It is thought to result in a decrease in morbidity and a reduction in the relative loss of muscular strength and endurance postoperatively.[195] Prehabilitation is also beneficial in that the individual has an understanding of what to expect in addition to beginning the postoperative period with a higher level of conditioning.

Patient education plays an integral role in prehabilitation and rehabilitation programs. Preoperative and postoperative education of the athlete is often taken for granted, and the surgical procedure, extent of damage, prognosis, and rehabilitation course are often not discussed with the athlete. Therefore, it is important to educate the athlete about the initial rehabilitation program and what is expected in the early phases of rehabilitation, to perform gait training, to take baseline measurements if indicated and tolerated by the athlete, and to fit any orthotic appliances that are to be used in the early postoperative phases. The athlete should also be informed about the surgical procedure to be performed, the prognosis after surgery, any potential complications, and precautions and limitations after surgery. The importance of rehabilitation, its function, and its approximate duration should also be discussed. Finally, it is beneficial for the clinician to involve athletes in goal setting, to allow them to have input into their rehabilitation program, and to be sure that they understand early rehabilitation restrictions and realize the consequences of noncompliance with rehabilitation.[44]

A long period of prehabilitation is not usually necessary for a conditioned athlete. In a deconditioned athlete or individual, initiation of a therapeutic exercise program 4 to 6 weeks before surgical intervention is preferable. Generally, the program focuses on regaining range of motion and on therapeutic exercises that do not exacerbate symptoms or further damage the injured area.

PARAMETERS OF CONDITIONING AND REHABILITATION

The functional capability developed by the athlete coincides with the progression of conditioning attained during the rehabilitation period. Progression of rehabilitation and conditioning depends on systematic manipulation of the following parameters: intensity, duration, frequency, specificity (such as the mode of exercise), speed of movement, and amount of rest and recovery within or between rehabilitation sessions. The clinician adjusts these parameters to ensure that the state of physical conditioning of the athlete continues to improve.

Intensity

The goal of the rehabilitation program is to overload, not overwhelm.[44,115] Generally, exercise intensity is less at the onset of rehabilitation and increases as the tissue becomes stronger. Higher intensities are demanding on the tissues and systems involved during physical activity. Thus, the rehabilitation professional modulates exercise intensity according to the injury time frame. In addition, intensity is inversely related to the duration of activity. As intensity increases, duration decreases and vice versa.

Strengthening Muscle and Connective Tissue

Muscle and connective tissue must be subjected to a load greater than that of the usual stresses of daily activity to induce hypertrophy and strengthening. Resistance training is the mode of exercise most often used to elicit these adaptive responses of muscle and connective tissue.[29,196] Increasing resistance linearly increases the intensity of the exercise bout. Generally speaking, the number of repetitions performed in each exercise set decreases as the intensity of the repetitions increases.[29,39,129]

Resistance training programs designed for gains in strength call for intensities ranging from 35% to 80% of a one RM, depending on the training status of the individual.[29,39,129] The intensity advocated to increase strength in healthy adults corresponds to resistance intensities that allow 8 to 12 repetitions.[29] However, rehabilitation intensity must also accommodate healing tissue to avoid reactive inflammation.[197] Rehabilitation programs incorporating resistance exercise must begin with relatively less weight to accommodate the fragility of healing tissue. The lower weight and higher repetitions improve local muscular endurance to a greater extent than muscular strength, but after the program is under way, an increase in exercise intensity (higher weight and lower number of repetitions) increases the rate of gain in strength.[29]

Cardiovascular Conditioning

Cardiovascular conditioning improves when the intensity of the exercise bout is equal to 60% to 90% of the maximum heart rate for trained individuals and 35% to 45% for relatively untrained individuals.[196] Barring contraindications as a result of impairment of the affected limb, athletes should exercise at intensities appropriate to maintain cardiovascular conditioning during rehabilitation.

Duration

The duration of an exercise bout or rehabilitation session pertains to the time that an athlete spends in an exercise or rehabilitation session. Similar yet technically different, the duration of exercise is the amount of time that the athlete spends performing a specific mode of exercise. This includes the number of repetitions and the time spent performing the repetition during a resistance-training bout. As discussed previously, duration inversely interacts with the intensity of the exercise bout. Generally, duration increases as intensity decreases and vice versa.

The duration of exercise necessary to improve cardiovascular conditioning during continuous exercise generally ranges from 20 to 60 minutes.[196] This is adjusted according to the intensity of the exercise bout, which is influenced by the integrity of healing tissue. It may be necessary for the athlete to perform several bouts of shorter duration (approximately 10 minutes) early in the rehabilitation program and gradually increase duration as tolerated.[196]

The duration of the entire rehabilitation program relates to how long it will take the athlete to return to full (100%) participation. Obviously, one of the major factors affecting the duration of rehabilitation programs is the individual healing rate of the injured tissue, which varies with the specific tissue type (see Table 4-1 and Chapter 2). Other factors affecting the duration of the rehabilitation program include the athlete's compliance, the number of incidents exacerbating inflammation, and the severity of tissue reinjury.

Frequency

Frequency refers to the number of exercise bouts within a given period (usually per day or week). Frequency is interdependent on the intensity and duration of exercise.[196] Recovery time, or the time between exercise bouts, increases concomitantly with increases in intensity and duration. Therefore, exercise performed more often must be of an appropriate intensity to allow adequate recovery.[198,199]

Muscle strengthening responds best to 2 to 4 days per week of resistance training in healthy individuals.[29,199] The training status of the individual largely determines the frequency of the bouts; less trained individuals need less frequent sessions to see improvement, whereas highly trained individuals have a better response with more frequent sessions.[29,199] However, this principle applies mostly to healthy individuals capable of sustaining intensities not yet tolerated by individuals undergoing rehabilitation.

Dickinson and Bennett reported that exercise performed twice daily in the early phases of rehabilitation yields greater improvement in strength than does exercise performed once per day.[197] When the athlete is in the early phases of rehabilitation, an exercise routine can be implemented twice daily (see Fig. 4-6).[44,115] When this concept is used, the athlete's performance should be monitored, and a reduction in exercise may be needed occasionally to thwart exacerbations of inflammation. As the athlete's condition improves and increased exercise intensity is tolerated, a once-daily exercise program is sufficient. This usually corresponds to a change in the PRE schedule toward increased resistance, lower repetitions, and advancement toward functional activities. The reduction in frequency should be instituted for two reasons: it helps minimize the athlete's chances of becoming bored and discontented with the program, and no reports have noted that exercising isotonically during advanced phases more than once per day produces any additional physical benefits.[116] When the athlete returns to participation, the maintenance program can be advanced to once or twice weekly. It is important that the athlete continue a rehabilitation maintenance program during the season, particularly if the regular weight room regimen does not specifically address the appropriate muscle groups or necessary movements.

The frequency advocated for improving cardiovascular function varies according to the training level, or functional capacity, of the individual. Frequencies range from one to two times per day for low-intensity and short-duration exercise up to three to five times per week for higher-intensity or long-duration exercise.[196]

Speed and Specificity

Speed or velocity refers to the rate at which the exercise is performed. The exercises should be performed in a slow and deliberate manner, with emphasis placed on concentric and eccentric contractions. The athlete should pause at the end of the exercise and should exercise through the full range of motion that is allowed while avoiding jerky movements.

In the late stages of rehabilitation, exercise speed should be varied. Traditional PREs are performed at a rate of about 60° per second, a speed that is not functional for attempts to return athletes to their sport.[200,201] For example, a pitcher's throwing arm travels at approximately 7000° to 10,000° per second.[202,203] Thus, continuation of a PRE program as the only tool in restoring this baseball pitcher to function does not prepare the pitcher for the great demands placed on the throwing arm on return to sport. As Costill et al noted, it is important to vary the type and speed of the exercise.[204] Surgical tubing can be used to implement a high-speed regimen to produce a concentric or eccentric synergistic pattern, and isokinetic units at the highest speeds on the spectrum can also be used.

The type of exercise performed elicits a specific response.[31] As discussed previously, the exercise program must be tailored to meet the specific needs of the individual. Activities or exercises that simulate part of the athlete's activity are ideal for this aspect of rehabilitation, and ultimately, the athlete should progressively perform sport-specific activities.[29] For example, a baseball pitcher should progressively return to throwing in a progressive throwing program.[46] Thus, the mode of exercise is important to consider, especially during the late phases of rehabilitation.

Rest and Recovery

The body needs time to recover from the stresses encountered during exercise. Relative recovery occurs in the rest periods between exercise sets. Recovery also occurs between exercise sessions within the same day or between sessions on multiple days of the week.

Longer periods of rest between exercises allow the anaerobic system to recharge.[29,199] The amount of rest should be greater than the amount of time spent during an activity, usually 3 to 20 times greater than that spent during exercise.[29] This allows the athlete to better tolerate performance of exercises at high intensity. Coincidentally, it improves anaerobic performance in both expression of cardiovascular performance and production of muscle force.[29]

Shorter rest periods between exercises, equal to 0.5 to 2 times that spent during the exercise bout, do not allow the anaerobic system to recharge and thereby cause the oxidative system to fuel the activity.[205] Thus, improvements in aerobic capability and endurance occur with the incorporation of shorter rest periods.

Interval training is an effective conditioning tool that manipulates work-to-rest ratios. Almost any type of repetitive exercise regimen may be manipulated to follow the principles of interval training. Such regimens include cardiovascular activities, PRE, and plyometrics.

FUNCTION-BASED REHABILITATION

If the rehabilitated athlete cannot perform activities specific to his or her sport on completion of the rehabilitation program, it does not matter whether the athlete regains normal range of motion and strength, agility, and power. The rehabilitation program would have failed if this were to happen; in fact, although we may have resolved many different problems inherent to the injury, technically we did not rehabilitate the athlete based on our earlier definition of rehabilitation.

Initial considerations for implementation of a functional progression program revolve around the physical parameters of the athlete's intended activity. This involves analysis of the demands of specific athletic endeavors, which are assessed for difficulty and complexity of response. The tasks are then placed on a continuum of difficulty with respect to the athlete's status. Overlaps occasionally occur as a particular task is accomplished but still remain in the athlete's program for solidification as the next task is begun. Because performing a specific motor skill involves a motor-learning component, rehabilitation should include activities specific to the athlete's sport.[71] Care should be taken to ensure that task progression is blended with specific restrictions concerning the nature of the pathologic condition.[44,45,115,206]

CONCLUSION

- Rehabilitation and physical conditioning are similar processes that evoke physiologic adaptation.
- The goals of rehabilitation are to (1) reverse and prevent adverse sequelae resulting from immobility or disuse and (2) facilitate tissue healing and avoid excessive stress on immature tissue.
- The general phases of rehabilitation include the acute, subacute (intermediate), and chronic (return-to-activity) phases.
- The neurologic system affects rehabilitation in a number of ways. Protective reflexes, such as arthrogenic inhibition, involuntarily diminish muscular activity. Therefore, the clinician should recognize arthrogenic inhibition as a threat to timely rehabilitation and treat the manifestations of pain, edema, and effusion as potential harbingers of impending muscle inhibition. Furthermore, the clinician should incorporate motor learning and facilitatory techniques, such as crossover education, to maximize recovery rates following injury.
- Types of therapeutic exercise used during rehabilitation include range of motion, strengthening, proprioceptive, and plyometric.
- Therapeutic exercises during rehabilitation may be open or closed chain activities.
- Methods of progressive resistive exercise include the low-resistance, high-repetition method, the DeLorme and Watkins regimen, the Oxford technique, the daily adjustable progressive resistive exercise method, and the Sanders program.
- Physical conditioning may occur as prehabilitation, which is preventive in nature, or may occur in unaffected extremities/physiologic systems as an adjunct during rehabilitation.
- Parameters of conditioning and rehabilitation include the intensity, duration, frequency, specificity and mode of exercise, and the speed of the movement.

REFERENCES

1. American Heritage College Dictionary (2006): Boston, Houghton Mifflin.
2. Cook, C., and Hegedus, E. (2008): Orthopedic Physical Examination Tests: An Evidence-Based Approach. Upper Saddle River, NJ, Pearson-Prentice Hall.
3. Evans, R. (2009): Illustrated Orthopedic Physical Assessment. St Louis, Mosby.
4. Giallonardo, L. (2001): Clinical decision making in rehabilitation. In: Prentice, W., and Voight, M. (eds.). Techniques in Musculoskeletal Rehabilitation. New York, McGraw-Hill.
5. Hughston, J.C. (1980): Knee surgery: A philosophy. Phys. Ther., 60:1611–1614.
6. Welch, B. (1986): The injury cycle. Sports Med. Update, 1:1.
7. Deandrade, J.R., Grant, C., and Dixon, A.S. (1965): Joint distension and reflex muscle inhibition in the knee. J. Bone Joint Surg. Am., 47:313–322.
8. Fahrer, H., Rentsch, H.U., Gerber, N.J., et al. (1988): Knee effusion and reflex inhibition of the quadriceps. A bar to effective retraining. J. Bone Joint Surg. Br., 70:635–638.

9. Iles, J.F., Stokes, M., and Young, A. (1990): Reflex actions of knee joint afferents during contraction of the human quadriceps. Clin. Physiol., 10:500–689.

10. Tsang, K., Hertel, J., Denegar, C., et al. (2002): The effects of induced effusion of the ankle on EMG activity of the lower leg muscles. J Athl. Train., 37:(S-25).

11. Palmieri, R.M., Tom, J.A., Edwards, J.E., et al. (2004): Arthrogenic muscle response induced by an experimental knee joint effusion is mediated by pre- and post-synaptic spinal mechanisms. J. Electromyogr. Kinesiol., 14:631–640.

12. Palmieri, R.M., Weltman, A., Edwards, J.E., et al. (2005): Pre-synaptic modulation of quadriceps arthrogenic muscle inhibition. Knee Surg. Sports Traumatol. Arthrosc., 13:370–376.

13. Palmieri-Smith, R.M., Kreinbrink, J., Ashton-Miller, J.A., and Wojtys, E.M. (2007): Quadriceps inhibition induced by an experimental knee joint effusion affects knee joint mechanics during a single-legged drop landing. Am. J. Sports Med., 35:1269–1275.

14. Dickerman, J. (1992): The use of pain profiles in clinical practice. Fam. Pract. Recertif., 14:35–44.

15. Bonica, J. (1990): The Management of Pain. Philadelphia, Lea & Febiger.

16. Mannheimer, J. (1984): Clinical Transcutaneous Electrical Nerve Stimulation. Philadelphia, Davis.

17. Bremander, A., Bergman, S., and Arvidsson, B. (2009): Perception of multimodal cognitive treatment for people with chronic widespread pain—changing one's life plan. Disabil. Rehabil. 31:1996–2004.

18. Young, A. (1993): Current issues in arthrogenous inhibition. Ann. Rheum. Dis., 52:829–834.

19. Hart, J.M., Pietrosimone, B., Hertel, J., and Ingersoll, C.D. (2010): Quadriceps activation following knee injuries: A systematic review. J Athl. Train., 45:87–97.

20. Knight, K. (1995): Cryotherapy in Sports Injury Management. Champaign, IL, Human Kinetics.

21. Wigerstad-Lossing, I., Grimby, G., Jonsson, T., et al. (1988): Effects of electrical muscle stimulation combined with voluntary contractions after knee ligament surgery. Med. Sci. Sports Exerc., 20:93–98.

22. Wilk, K.E., and Arrigo, C. (1993): Current concepts in the rehabilitation of the athletic shoulder. J. Orthop. Sports Phys. Ther., 18:365–378.

23. Wilk, K.E., Arrigo, C., and Andrews, J.R. (1993): Rehabilitation of the elbow in the throwing athlete. J. Orthop. Sports Phys. Ther., 17:305–317.

24. Wilk, K.E., Voight, M.L., Keirns, M.A., et al. (1993): Stretch-shortening drills for the upper extremities: Theory and clinical application. J. Orthop. Sports Phys. Ther., 17:225–239.

25. Wilmore, J.H. (1976): Athletic Training and Physical Fitness. Boston, Allyn & Bacon.

26. Fu, S.C., Hung, L.K., Shum, W.T., et al. (2010): In vivo low-intensity pulsed ultrasound (LIPUS) following tendon injury promotes repair during granulation, but suppresses decorin and biglycan expression during remodeling. J. Orthop. Sports Phys. Ther., 40:422–429.

27. Calle, M.C., and Fernandez, M.L. (2010): Effects of resistance training on the inflammatory response. Nutr. Res. Pract., 4:259–269.

28. Pezzullo, D.J., and Fadale, P. (2010): Current controversies in rehabilitation after anterior cruciate ligament reconstruction. Sports Med. Arthrosc., 18:43–47.

29. ACSM (2009): American College of Sports Medicine position stand. Progression models in resistance training for healthy adults. Med. Sci. Sports Exerc., 41:687–708.

30. Nash, C.E., Mickan, S.M., Del Mar, C.B., and Glasziou, P.P. (2004): Resting injured limbs delays recovery: A systematic review. J. Fam. Pract., 53:706–712.

31. Selye, H. (1978): The Stress of Life. New York, McGraw-Hill.

32. Bortz, W.M. 2nd. (1984): The disuse syndrome. West. J. Med., 141:691–694.

33. Adams, G.R., Hather, B.M., and Dudley, G.A. (1994): Effect of short-term unweighting on human skeletal muscle strength and size. Aviat. Space Environ. Med., 65:1116–1121.

34. Bamman, M.M., Clarke, M.S., Feeback, D.L., et al. (1998): Impact of resistance exercise during bed rest on skeletal muscle sarcopenia and myosin isoform distribution. J. Appl. Physiol., 84:157–163.

35. Bamman, M.M., Hunter, G.R., Stevens, B.R., et al. (1997): Resistance exercise prevents plantar flexor deconditioning during bed rest. Med. Sci. Sports Exerc., 29:1462–1468.

36. Cooper, D., and Fair, J. (1976): Reconditioning following athletic injuries. Phys. Sports Med., 4:125–128.

37. Mulder, E.R., Horstman, A.M., Stegeman, D.F., et al. (2009): Influence of vibration resistance training on knee extensor and plantar flexor size, strength, and contractile speed characteristics after 60 days of bed rest. J. Appl. Physiol., 107:1789–1798.

38. Houglum, P. (1992): Soft tissue healing and its impact on rehabilitation. J. Sports Rehabil., 1:19–39.

39. Houglum, P. (2005): Muscle strength and endurance. In: Houglum P. (ed.). Therapeutic Exercise for Athletic Trainers. 2nd ed. Champaign, IL, Human Kinetics.

40. Hoffmann, A., and Gross, G. (2009): Innovative strategies for treatment of soft tissue injuries in human and animal athletes. Med. Sport Sci., 54:150–165.

41. Sanchez, M., Anitua, E., Lopez-Vidriero, E., and Andia, I. (2010): The future: Optimizing the healing environment in anterior cruciate ligament reconstruction. Sports Med. Arthrosc., 18:48–53.

42. Pasternak, B., and Aspenberg, P. (2009): Metalloproteinases and their inhibitors—diagnostic and therapeutic opportunities in orthopedics. Acta Orthop., 80:693–703.

43. Woo, S. (1986): Biomechanics of tendons and ligaments. In: Fund, Y. (ed.). Frontiers in Biomechanics. New York, Schmid-Schonbein.

44. Kisner, C., and Colby, L. (2007): Therapeutic, Exercise: Foundations and Techniques 5th ed. Philadelphia, Davis.

45. Ellenbecker, T., De Carlo, M., and DeRosa, C. (2009): Effective Functional Progressions in Sport Rehabilitation. Champaign, IL, Human Kinetics.

46. Wilk, K.E., Meister, K., and Andrews, J.R. (2002): Current concepts in the rehabilitation of the overhead throwing athlete. Am. J. Sports Med., 30:136–151.

47. Kelln, B.M., Ingersoll, C.D., Saliba, S., et al. (2009): Effect of early active range of motion rehabilitation on outcome measures after partial meniscectomy. Knee Surg. Sports Traumatol. Arthrosc., 17:607–616.

48. Noyes, F., Mangine, R., and Barber, S. (1987): Early knee motion after open and arthroscopic anterior cruciate ligament reconstruction. Am. J. Sports Med., 15:149–160.

49. Gieck, J., and Saliba, E. (1988): The athletic trainer and rehabilitation. In: The Injured Athlete. Philadelphia, Lippincott, pp. 165–239.

50. Cole, A., and Herring, S. (1997): Lumbar spine pain: Rehabilitation and return to play. In: Sallis, R.E., and Massimino, F. (eds.). ACSM's Essentials of Sports Medicine. St. Louis, Mosby, pp. 396–402.

51. Zohn, D., and Mennell, J. (1976): Musculoskeletal Pain: Principles of Physical Diagnosis and Physical Treatment. Boston, Little-Brown.

52. Cyriax, J. (1982): Textbook of Orthopedic Medicine, Vol. 1, Diagnosis of Soft Tissue Lesions. London, Bailliere & Tindall.

53. DeLorme, T. (1945): Restoration of muscle power by heavy resistance exercise. J. Bone Joint Surg., 27:645–667.

54. DeLorme, T., and Watkins, A. (1948): Techniques of progressive resistance exercise. Arch. Phys. Med., 29:263–268.

55. Knight, K. (1985): Guidelines for rehabilitation of sports injuries. Clin. Sports Med., 4:405–416.

56. Zinovieff, A.N. (1951): Heavy-resistance exercises: The "Oxford technique." Br. J. Phys. Med., 14(6):129–132.

57. Kellett, J. (1986): Acute soft tissue injuries—a review of the literature. Med. Sci. Sports Exerc., 18:489–500.

58. Guyton, A. (1991): Basic Neuroscience: Anatomy and Physiology, 2nd ed. Philadelphia, Saunders.

59. Bear, M., Connors, B., and Paradiso, M. (2007): Neuroscience: Exploring the Brain. 3rd ed. Baltimore, Lippincott Williams & Wilkins.

60. Sherrington, C. (1906): On the proprioceptive system, especially in its reflex aspects. Brain, 29:467–479.

61. Hilton, J. (1863): On the Influence of Mechanical and Physiological Rest in the Treatment of Accidents and Surgical Diseases, and the Diagnostic Value of Pain. A Course of Lectures. London, Bell and Daldy.

62. Jimmy, M. (1988): Mechanoreceptors in articular tissues. Am. J. Anat., 182:16–32.

63. Kennedy, J.C., Alexander, I.J., and Hayes, K.C. (1982): Nerve supply of the human knee and its functional importance. Am. J. Sports Med., 10:329–335.

64. Norkin, C., and Levangie, P. (2001): Joint Structure and Function: A Comprehensive Analysis, 3rd ed. Philadelphia, Davis.

65. Schultz, R.A., Miller, D.C., Kerr, C.S., and Micheli, L. (1984): Mechanoreceptors in human cruciate ligaments. A histological study. J. Bone Joint Surg. Am., 66:1072–1076.

66. Gardner, E. (1948): The innervation of the knee joint. Anat. Rec., 101:109–130.

67. Halata, Z., Rettig, T., and Schulze, W. (1985): The ultrastructure of sensory nerve endings in the human knee joint capsule. Anat. Embryol. (Berl.), 172:265–275.

68. Schutte, M.J., Dabezies, E.J., Zimny, M.L., and Happel, L.T. (1987): Neural anatomy of the human anterior cruciate ligament. J. Bone Joint Surg. Am., 69:243–247.

69. Basmajian, J.V. (1970): Reeducation of vastus medialis: A misconception. Arch. Phys. Med. Rehabil., 51:245–247.

70. Basmajian, J.V. (1977): Motor learning and control: A working hypothesis. Arch. Phys. Med. Rehabil., 58:38–41.

71. Magill, R. (2010): Motor Learning: Concepts and Applications, 9th ed. Boston, McGraw-Hill.

72. Gentile, A. (1972): A working model of skill acquisition with application to teaching. Quest. Monogr., 17:3–23.

73. Gentile, A. (1987): Skill acquisition: Action, movement, and the neuromotor processes. In: Carr, J., Shepherd, R., Gordon, J., et al. (eds.). Movement Science: Foundations for Physical Therapy in Rehabilitation. Rockville, MD, Aspen.

74. Kraemer, W.J. (1994): General adaptations to resistance and endurance training programs. In: Baechle, T. (ed.). Essentials of Strengthening and Conditioning. Champaign, IL, Human Kinetics.

75. Gentili, R., Papaxanthis, C., and Pozzo, T. (2006): Improvement and generalization of arm motor performance through motor imagery practice. Neuroscience, 137:761–772.

76. Doheny, M.O. (1993): Mental practice: an alternative approach to teaching motor skills. J. Nurs. Educ., 32:260–264.

77. Kremer, P., Spittle, M., McNeil, D., and Shinners, C. (2009): Amount of mental practice and performance of a simple motor task. Percept. Mot. Skills, 109:347–356.

78. Ericcsson, K., Krampe, R., and Tesch-Romer, C. (1993): The role of deliberate practice in the acquisition of expert performance. Psychol. Rev., 100:363–406.

79. Hobbel, S.L., and Rose, D.J. (1993): The relative effectiveness of three forms of visual knowledge of results on peak torque output. J. Orthop. Sports Phys. Ther., 18:601–608.

80. Lee, T.D., Swanson, L.R., and Hall, A.L. (1991): What is repeated in a repetition? Effects of practice conditions on motor skill acquisition. Phys. Ther., 71:150–156.

81. Schmidt, R., and Lee, T.D. (2005): Motor Control and Learning: A Behavior Emphasis, 4th ed. Champaign, IL, Human Kinetics.

82. Sullivan, S., and Schmidt, T. (2006): Strategies to improve motor control. In: Sullivan, S., and Schmidt, T. (eds.). Physical Rehabilitation, 5th ed. Philadelphia, Davis.

83. Fitts, P., and Posner, M. (1967): Human Performance. Belmont, CA, Brooks/Cole.

84. Nicholson, D. (1997): Teaching psychomotor skills. In: Shepard, K., and Jensen, G. (eds.). Handbook of Teaching for Physical Therapists. Boston, Butterworth-Heinemann.

85. Siengsukon, C.F., and Boyd, L.A. (2009): Does sleep promote motor learning? Implications for physical rehabilitation. Phys. Ther., 89:370–383.

86. Mulder, T. (1991): A process-oriented model of human motor behavior: Toward a theory-based rehabilitation approach. Phys. Ther., 71:157–164.

87. Wrisberg, C.A., and Liu, Z. (1991): The effect of contextual variety on the practice, retention, and transfer of an applied motor skill. Res. Q. Exerc. Sport, 62:406–412.

88. Naylor, J.C., and Briggs, G.E. (1963): Effects of task complexity and task organization on the relative efficiency of part and whole training methods. J. Exp. Psychol., 65:217–224.

89. Maring, J.R. (1990): Effects of mental practice on rate of skill acquisition. Phys. Ther., 70:165–172.

90. McBride, E., and Rothstein, A. (1979): Mental and physical practice and the learning and retention of open and closed motor skills. Percept. Mot. Skills, 49:359–365.

91. Yoo, E., Park, E., and Chung, B. (2001): Mental practice effect on line-tracing accuracy in persons with hemiparetic stroke: A preliminary study. Arch. Phys. Med. Rehabil., 82:1213–1218.

92. Gabriele, T., Hall, C., and Lee, T. (1989): Cognition in motor learning: Imagery effects on contextual interference. Hum. Mov. Sci., 8:227–245.

93. Gouvier, W.D. (1987): Assessment and treatment of cognitive deficits in brain-damaged individuals. Behav. Modif., 11:212–328.

94. Wilson, B. (1989): Models of cognitive rehabilitation. In: Wood, R., and Eames, P. (eds.). Models of Brain Injury. London, Chapman and Hall.

95. Winstein, C.J. (1991): Knowledge of results and motor learning—implications for physical therapy. Phys. Ther., 71:140–149.

96. Newell, K., Sparrow, W., and Quinn, J. (1985): Kinetic information feedback for learning isometric tasks. J. Hum. Mov. Studies, 11:113–123.

97. Nyland, J., Brosky, T., Currier, D., et al. (1994): Review of the afferent neural system of the knee and its contribution to motor learning. J. Orthop. Sports Phys. Ther., 19:2–11.

98. Weir, P., and Leavitt, J. (1990): The effects of model's skill level and model's knowledge of results on the performance of a dart throwing task. Hum. Mov. Sci., 9:369–383.

99. Bard, C., Paillard, J., Lajoie, Y., et al. (1992): Role of afferent information in the timing of motor commands: A comparative study with a deafferented patient. Neuropsychologia, 30:201–206.

100. Sprenger, C.K., Carlson, K., and Wessman, H.C. (1979): Application of electromyographic biofeedback following medial meniscectomy: A clinical report. Phys. Ther., 59:167–169.

101. Levitt, R., Deisinger, J., Remondet, W., et al. (1995): EMG feedback–assisted postoperative rehabilitation of minor arthroscopic knee surgeries. J. Sports Med. Phys. Fitness, 35:218–223.

102. Neumann, D. (2009): Kinesiology of the Musculoskeletal System, 2nd ed. Philadelphia, Mosby.

103. Farthing, J.P. (2009): Cross-education of strength depends on limb dominance: Implications for theory and application. Exerc. Sport Sci. Rev., 37:179–187.

104. Farthing, J.P., Borowsky, R., Chilibeck, P.D., et al. (2007): Neuro-physiological adaptations associated with cross-education of strength. Brain Topogr., 20:77–88.

105. Farthing, J.P., Krentz, J.R., and Magnus, C.R. (2009): Strength training the free limb attenuates strength loss during unilateral immobilization. J. Appl. Physiol., 106:830–836.

106. Kannus, P., Alosa, D., Cook, L., (1992): Effect of one-legged exercise on the strength, power and endurance of the contralateral leg, et al. A randomized, controlled study using isometric and concentric isokinetic training. Eur. J. Appl. Physiol. Occup. Physiol., 64:117–126.

107. Stromberg, B.V. (1986): Contralateral therapy in upper extremity rehabilitation. Am. J. Phys. Med., 65:135–143.

108. Stromberg, B.V. (1988): Influence of cross-education training in postoperative hand therapy. South. Med. J., 81:989–991.

109. Nagel, M.J., and Rice, M.S. (2001): Cross-transfer effects in the upper extremity during an occupationally embedded exercise. Am. J. Occup. Ther., 55:317–323.

110. Archontides, C., and Fazey, J.A. (1993): Inter-limb interactions and constraints in the expression of maximum force: A review, some implications and suggested underlying mechanisms. J. Sports Sci., 11:145–158.

111. Asanuma, H., and Okuda, O. (1962): Effects of transcallosal volleys on pyramidal tract cell activity of cat. J. Neurophysiol., 25:198–208.

112. Beutler, A.I., Cooper, L.W., Kirkendall, D.T., Garrett, W.E., Jr. (2002): Electromyographical analysis of single-leg, closed chain exercises: Implications for rehabilitation after anterior cruciate ligament reconstruction. J. Athl. Train., 37:13–18.

113. Dale, R., Sirikul, B., and Bishop, P. (2001): Bilateral indices of knee extensors and flexors in males and females at 1 and 10 RM. J. Athl. Train, 36:(S-86).

114. Magnus, C.R., and Farthing, J.P. (2008): Greater bilateral deficit in leg press than in handgrip exercise might be linked to differences in postural stability requirements. Appl. Physiol. Nutr. Metab., 33:1132–1139.

115. Brody, L., and Hall, C. (2011): Therapeutic Exercise: Moving Toward Function, 3rd ed. Philadelphia, Lippincott Williams & Wilkins.

116. Houglum, P. (1977): The modality of therapeutic exercise. Athl. Train., 12:42–45.

117. Marino, M. (1986): Current concepts of rehabilitation in sports medicine: Research and clinical interrelationship. In: The Lower Extremity in Sports Medicine. St. Louis, Mosby.

118. Folland, J.P., Hawker, K., Leach, B., et al. (2005): Strength training: Isometric training at a range of joint angles versus dynamic training. J. Sports Sci., 23:817–824.

119. Graves, J.E., Pollock, M.L., Jones, A.E., et al. (1989): Specificity of limited range of motion variable resistance training. Med. Sci. Sports Exerc., 21:84–89.

120. Weir, J.P., Housh, T.J., and Weir, L.L. (1994): Electromyographic evaluation of joint angle specificity and cross-training after isometric training. J. Appl. Physiol., 77:197–201.

121. Weir, J.P., Housh, T.J., Weir, L.L., and Johnson, G.O. (1995): Effects of unilateral isometric strength training on joint angle specificity and cross-training. Eur. J. Appl. Physiol. Occup. Physiol., 70:337–343.

122. MacDougall, J.D., McKelvie, R.S., Moroz, D.E., et al. (1992): Factors affecting blood pressure during heavy weight lifting and static contractions. J. Appl. Physiol., 73:1590-1597.

123. Cobb, W.S., Burns, J.M., Kercher, K.W., et al. (2005): Normal intraabdominal pressure in healthy adults. J. Surg. Res., 129:231–235.

124. Owen, A., Wiles, J., and Swaine, I. (2010): Effect of isometric exercise on resting blood pressure: a meta analysis. J. Hum. Hypertens., 24:796–800.

125. Colson, S.S., Pensini, M., Espinosa, J., et al. Whole-body vibration training effects on the physical performance of basketball players. J. Strength Cond. Res., 24:999-1006.

126. Eckhardt, H., Wollny, R., Muller, H., et al. (2011): Enhanced myofiber recruitment during exhaustive squatting performed as whole-body vibration exercise. J. Strength Cond. Res., 25:1120–1125.

127. Petit, P.D., Pensini, M., Tessaro, J., et al. (2010): Optimal whole-body vibration settings for muscle strength and power enhancement in human knee extensors. J. Electromyogr. Kinesiol., 20:1186–1195.

128. Vela, J.I., Andreu, D., Diaz-Cascajosa, J., and Buil, J.A. (2010): Intraocular lens dislocation after whole-body vibration. J. Cataract Refract. Surg., 36:1790–1791.

129. McArdle, W., Katch, F., and Katch, V. (2009): Muscular strength: Training muscles to become stronger. In: McArdle, W., Katch, F., and Katch, V. (eds.). Exercise Physiology: Energy, Nutrition, and Human Performance, 7th ed. Baltimore, Lippincott Williams & Wilkins.

130. Dean, E. (1988): Physiology and therapeutic implications of negative work. A review. Phys. Ther., 68:233–237.

131. Keskula, D. (1996): Clinical implications of eccentric exercise in sports medicine. J. Sports Rehabil., 5:321–329.

132. Young, M.A., Cook, J.L., Purdam, C.R., et al. (2005): Eccentric decline squat protocol offers superior results at 12 months compared with traditional eccentric protocol for patellar tendinopathy in volleyball players. Br. J. Sports Med., 39:102–105.

133. Stanish, W.D., Rubinovich, R.M., and Curwin, S. (1986): Eccentric exercise in chronic tendinitis. Clin. Orthop. Relat. Res., 208:65–68.

134. Kjaer, M., Langberg, H., Heinemeier, K., et al. (2009): From mechanical loading to collagen synthesis, structural changes and function in human tendon. Scand. J. Med. Sci. Sports, 19:500–510.

135. Rees, J.D., Wolman, R.L., and Wilson, A. (2009): Eccentric exercises; why do they work, what are the problems and how can we improve them? Br. J. Sports Med., 43:242–246.

136. Alfredson, H., Pietila, T., Jonsson, P., and Lorentzon, R. (1998): Heavy-load eccentric calf muscle training for the treatment of chronic Achilles tendinosis. Am. J. Sports Med., 26:360–366.

137. Cleak, M.J., and Eston, R.G. (1992): Muscle soreness, swelling, stiffness and strength loss after intense eccentric exercise. Br. J. Sports Med., 26:267–272.

138. Dedrick, M.E., and Clarkson, P.M. (1990): The effects of eccentric exercise on motor performance in young and older women. Eur. J. Appl. Physiol. Occup. Physiol., 60:183–186.

139. Weber, M.D., Servedio, F.J., and Woodall, W.R. (1994): The effects of three modalities on delayed onset muscle soreness. J. Orthop. Sports Phys. Ther., 20:236–242.

140. Dvir, Z. (2004): Isokinetics: Muscle Testing, Interpretation, and Clinical Applications, 2nd ed. Edinburgh, Churchill Livingstone.

141. Albert, M. (1995): Inertial training concepts. In: Albert, M. (ed.). Eccentric Muscle Training in Sports and Orthopaedics. New York: Churchill Livingstone, pp. 89–113.

142. Albert, M.S., Hillegass, E., and Spiegel, P. (1994): Muscle torque changes caused by inertial exercise training. J. Orthop. Sports Phys. Ther., 20:254–261.

143. Caruso, J.F., Hernandez, D.A., Porter, A., et al. (2006): Integrated electromyography and performance outcomes to inertial resistance exercise. J. Strength Cond. Res., 20:151–156.

144. Norrbrand, L., Pozzo, M., and Tesch, P.A. (2010): Flywheel resistance training calls for greater eccentric muscle activation than weight training. Eur. J. Appl. Physiol., 110:997–1005.

145. Tracy, J., Obuchi, S., and Johnson, B. (1995): Kinematic and electromyographic analysis of elbow flexion during inertial exercise. J. Athl. Train., 30:254–258.

146. Blackburn, T.A., Jr. (1987): Rehabilitation of the shoulder and elbow after arthroscopy. Clin. Sports Med., 6:587–606.

147. Berger, R. (1982): Applied Exercise Physiology. Philadelphia, Lea & Febiger.

148. Moss, C., and Grimmer, S. (1993): Strength and contractile adaptations in the human triceps surae after isotonic exercise. J. Sports Rehabil., 2:104–114.

149. Hellebrandt, F.A. (1951): Physiological bases of progressive resistance exercise. In: DeLorme, T.L., and Watkins, A.L. (eds.). Progressive Resistive Exercise. New York, Appleton-Century-Crofts.

150. Knight, K. (1979): Rehabilitating chondromalacia patellae. Physician Sportsmed., 7:147–148.

151. Sanders, M. (1990): Weight training and conditioning. In: Sanders, B. (ed.). Sports Physical Therapy. Norwalk, CT, Appleton & Lange.

152. Harter, R. (1996): Clinical rationale for closed kinetic chain activities in functional testing and rehabilitation of ankle pathologies. J. Sports Rehabil., 5:13–24.

153. Harter, R., Osternig, L., and Singer, K. (1992): Knee joint proprioception following anterior cruciate ligament reconstruction. J. Sports Rehabil., 1:103–110.

154. Irrang, J. (1995): Rehabilitation. In: Fu, F., and Stone, D. (eds.). Sports Injuries: Mechanisms, Prevention, Treatment. Baltimore, Lippincott Williams & Wilkins.

155. Cooper, R.L., Taylor, N.F., and Feller, J.A. (2005): A systematic review of the effect of proprioceptive and balance exercises on people with an injured or reconstructed anterior cruciate ligament. Res. Sports Med., 13:163–178.

156. Batson, G. (2009): Update on proprioception: Considerations for dance education. J. Dance Med. Sci., 13:(2):35–41.

157. Taber's Cyclopedic Medical Dictionary, 21st ed. (2009): Philadelphia, Davis.

158. Lephart, S.M., Kocher, M., Fu, F., et al. (1992): Proprioception following anterior cruciate ligament reconstruction. J. Sports Rehabil., 1:188–196.

159. Niessen, M.H., Veeger, D.H., and Janssen, T.W. (2009): Effect of body orientation on proprioception during active and passive motions. Am. J. Phys. Med. Rehabil., 88:979–985.

160. Gross, M.T. (1987): Effects of recurrent lateral ankle sprains on active and passive judgements of joint position. Phys. Ther., 67:1505–1509.

161. Lephart, S.M., and Henry, T.J. (1995): Functional rehabilitation for the upper and lower extremity. Orthop. Clin. North Am., 26:579–592.

162. Filipa, A., Byrnes, R., Paterno, M.V., et al. (2010): Neuromuscular training improves performance on the star excursion balance test in young female athletes. J. Orthop. Sports Phys. Ther. 40:551–558.

163. Markovic, G., and Mikulic, P. (2010): Neuro-musculoskeletal and performance adaptations to lower-extremity plyometric training. Sports Med., 40:859–895.

164. Chu, D. (1984): Plyometric exercise. Natl. Strength Cond. Assoc. J., 6:56–62.

165. Chu, D. (1998): Jumping Into Plyometrics, 2nd ed. Champaign, IL, Human Kinetics.

166. Voight, M., Draovitch, P., and Tippett, S. (1998): Plyometrics. In: Albert, M., (ed.). Eccentric Muscle Training in Sports and Orthopedics. 2nd ed. New York, Churchill Livingstone.

167. Reuleaux, F. (1875): Theoretishce Kinematic: Grundigeine Theorie des Maschinenwessens [The Kinematic Theory of Machinery: Outline of a Theory of Machines]. London, MacMillan.

168. Steindler, A. (1955): Kinesiology of the Human Body. Springfield, IL, Charles C Thomas.

169. Steindler, A. (1970): Kinesiology of the Human Body Under Normal and Pathological Conditions. Springfield, IL, Charles C Thomas.

170. Bunton, E.E., Pitney, W.A., Cappaert, T.A., and Kane, A.W. (1993): The role of limb torque, muscle action and proprioception during closed kinetic chain rehabilitation of the lower extremity. J. Athl. Train., 28:10–20.

171. Bynum, E.B., Barrack, R.L., Alexander, A.H. (1995): Open versus closed chain kinetic exercises after anterior cruciate ligament reconstruction: A prospective randomized study. Am. J. Sports Med., 23:401–406.

172. Graham, V.L., Gehlsen, G.M., and Edwards, J.A. (1993): Electromyographic evaluation of closed and open kinetic chain knee rehabilitation exercises. J. Athl. Train., 28:23–30.

173. Snyder-Mackler, L. (1996): Scientific rationale and physiological basis for the use of closed kinetic chain exercise in the lower extremity. J. Sports Rehabil., 5:2–12.

174. Wawrzyniak, J.R., Tracy, J.E., Catizone, P.V., and Storrow, R.R. (1996): Effect of closed chain exercise on quadriceps femoris peak torque and functional performance. J. Athl. Train., 31:335–340.

175. Wilk, K.E., and Arrigo, C. (1996): Closed and open kinetic chain exercise for the upper extremity. J. Sports Rehabil., 5:88–102.

176. Yack, H.J., Collins, C.E., and Whieldon, T.J. (1993): Comparison of closed and open kinetic chain exercise in the anterior cruciate ligament–deficient knee. Am. J. Sports Med., 21:49–54.

177. Lephart, S.M., and Henry, T.J. (1996): The physiological basis for open and closed kinetic chain rehabilitation for the upper extremity. J. Sports Rehabil., 5:77.

178. Dillman, C., Murray, T., and Hintermeister, R. (1994): Biomechanical differences of open and closed chain exercises with respect to the shoulder. J. Sports Rehabil., 3:228–238.

179. Prentice, W. (2001): Open versus closed kinetic chain exercise in rehabilitation. In: Prentice, W., and Voight M. (eds.). Techniques in Musculoskeletal Rehabilitation. New York, McGraw-Hill.

180. Sforzo, G., and Touey, P. (1996): Manipulating exercise order affects muscular performance during a resistance exercise training session. J. Strength Cond. Res., 10:20–24.

181. Mackey, A.L., Donnelly, A.E., Swanton, A., et al. (2006): The effects of impact and non-impact exercise on circulating markers of collagen remodelling in humans. J. Sports Sci., 24:843–848.

182. Reilly, T., Dowzer, C.N., and Cable, N.T. (2003): The physiology of deep-water running. J. Sports Sci., 21:959–972.

183. Dale, R., Childress, R., and Riewald, S. (2002): Conditioning during rehabilitation of swimming injuries. In: Bourdreau, C., Riewald, S., Sokolovas, G., and Tuffey, S. (eds.). The Science in the Science and Art of Coaching. Colorado Springs, CO, Swimming Sport Science.

184. Friedman, M., and Nichaolas, J. (1984): Conditioning and rehabilitation. In: Scott, W., Nisonson, B., and Nichaolas, J. (eds.). Principles of Sports Medicine. Baltimore, Lippincott Williams & Wilkins.

185. Kibler, W., and Safran, M. (1994): Pediatric and adolescent sports injuries. Am. J. Sports Med., 22:424–432.

186. Rao, A.L., Standaert, C.J., Drezner, J.A., and Herring, S.A. (2010): Expert opinion and controversies in musculoskeletal and sports medicine: Preventing sudden cardiac death in young athletes. Arch. Phys. Med. Rehabil., 91:958–962.

187. Joy, E.A., Paisley, T.S., Price, R., Jr., et al. (2004): Optimizing the collegiate preparticipation physical evaluation. Clin. J. Sport Med., 14:183–187.

188. Garrick, J.G. (2004): Preparticipation orthopedic screening evaluation. Clin. J. Sport Med., 14:123–126.

189. Kibler, W.B., and Chandler, T.J. (1993): Preparticipation evaluations. In: Renstrom, P. (ed.). Sports Injuries: Basic Principles of Prevention and Care. Oxford, Blackwell.

190. Kibler, W.B., Chandler, T.J., Uhl, T., Maddux, R.E., A musculoskeletal approach to the preparticipation physical examination (1989): Preventing injury and improving performance. Am. J. Sports Med., 17:525–531.

191. Noble, R., Linder, M., Janssen, E., et al. (1997): Prehabilitation exercises for the lower extremities. Strength Cond., 19:25–33.

192. Ditmyer, M.M., Topp, R., and Pifer, M. (2002): Prehabilitation in preparation for orthopaedic surgery. Orthop. Nurs., 21:(5) 43–51; quiz 52-54.

193. Chandler, T.J., and Kibler, W.B. (1993): Muscle training in injury prevention. In: Renstrom, P. (ed.). Sports Injuries: Basic Principles and Care pp. 252–261. Oxford: Blackwell.

194. Kibler, W.B., and Chandler, T.J. (1994): Sport-specific conditioning. Am. J. Sports Med., 22:424–432.

195. Topp, R., Swank, A.M., Quesada, P.M., et al. (2009): The effect of prehabilitation exercise on strength and functioning after total knee arthroplasty. PMR, 1:729–735.

196. ACSM (2009): ACSM's Guidelines for Exercise Testing and Prescription, 8th ed, Baltimore, Lippincott Williams & Wilkins.

197. Dickinson, A., and Bennett, K.M. (1985): Therapeutic exercise. Clin. Sports Med., 4:417–429.

198. Jones, E.J., Bishop, P.A., Richardson, M.T., and Smith, J.F. (2006): Stability of a practical measure of recovery from resistance training. J. Strength Cond. Res., 20:756–759.

199. McLester, J.R., Bishop, P.A., Smith, J., et al. (2003): A series of studies—a practical protocol for testing muscular endurance recovery. J. Strength Cond. Res., 17:259–273.

200. Coyle, E.F., Feiring, D.C., Rotkis, T.C., et al. (1981): Specificity of power improvements through slow and fast isokinetic training. J. Appl. Physiol., 51:1437–1442.

201. Slawinski, J., Bonnefoy, A., Ontanon, G., et al. (2010): Segment-interaction in sprint start: Analysis of 3D angular velocity and kinetic energy in elite sprinters. J. Biomech., 43:1494–1502.

202. Werner, S.L., Suri, M., Guido, J.A., Jr., et al. (2008): Relationships between ball velocity and throwing mechanics in collegiate baseball pitchers. J. Shoulder Elbow Surg., 17:905–908.

203. Stodden, D.F., Fleisig, G.S., McLean, S.P., and Andrews, J.R. (2005): Relationship of biomechanical factors to baseball pitching velocity: within pitcher variation. J. Appl. Biomech., 21:44–56.

204. Costill, D., Fink, W., and Habansky, A. (1971): Muscle rehabilitation after knee surgery. Phys. Sports Med., 5:71–77.

205. Stone, M.H., and Conley, M.S. (1994): Bioenergetics. In: Baechle, T. (ed.). Essentials of Strengthening and Conditioning. Champaign, IL, Human Kinetics.

206. Christakou, A., and Lavallee, D. (2009): Rehabilitation from sports injuries: From theory to practice. Perspect. Public Health, 129:120–126.

Measurement in Rehabilitation

Elizabeth Swann, PhD, ATC, and Gary L. Harrelson, EdD, ATC

CHAPTER OBJECTIVES

- Explain and recommend various instruments and methods of measurement.
- Perform and interpret objective measurements of girth and joint motion.

- Discuss the reliability and validity of the various instruments used to measure girth and joint motion.
- Take appropriate actions to improve the reliability of girth and joint motion measurements.

Measurement has long been used to chart progress during the rehabilitation process. Therefore, it is important for all clinicians to be competent in performing and interpreting objective measurements of girth and joint motion. This chapter addresses the reliability and validity of these measurements, methods of ensuring reliable measurements, and various techniques for performing girth and joint motion assessments.

GIRTH MEASUREMENTS

In the clinical setting, objective measurements must be obtained when decision making is necessary for a therapeutic exercise program. A flexible tape measure can be used to measure the girth of a limb and is probably the most common clinical method for documenting muscle bulk and swelling. Girth assessment with the use of a tape measure is also referred to as girth measurement, circumferential measurement, and anthropometric measurement. Not only is this assessment technique used before a weight-training program is implemented to assess its impact on muscle hypertrophy, it is also used to assess muscle atrophy or joint swelling after injury or surgery and to determine the subsequent effect of a rehabilitation program on muscle hypertrophy and joint swelling. Girth measurements have been reported in the literature for documenting the effects of a rehabilitation program on muscle atrophy or hypertrophy and joint swelling[1] after injury,[2-4] surgery, or implementation of a rehabilitation program.[5-8]

The increase or decrease in girth measurement is thought to indicate a direct relationship between an increase or decrease in muscle strength. For example, as a muscle atrophies, the loss of strength is directly related to muscle size because the muscle fibers themselves are reduced in size; the outcome, therefore, is

a reduction in strength. However, some evidence does support the absence of a direct relationship between girth measurement and muscle size.[9]

Most of the variability in obtaining girth measurements arises from the use of different anatomic landmarks, tension placed on the tape measure by the clinician, and contraction of the muscle. The tension placed on the tape measure by a clinician when assessing girth does not appear to be as big an issue as was thought previously.[10,11] Box 5-1 lists recommendations to improve intraclinician and interclinician reliability during girth assessments.

Several investigators[10,11] have assessed the reliability of lower extremity girth measurements in young healthy patients. The data suggest that these measurements are reliable and can be reproduced with a high degree of accuracy, particularly when the same clinician takes the measurements. Measurements taken by different clinicians are not as reliable when a standard tape measure is used.[10] In addition, many times clinicians use a healthy extremity to determine the amount of atrophy that may have occurred as a result of trauma. Healthy right and left lower extremities appear to have similar circumferences, which should not vary more than 1.5 cm between the right and left sides.[11] Furthermore, comparisons between a standard flexible tape measure and a Lufkin tape measure with a Gulick spring-loaded end indicate that both intraclinician and interclinician reliability is better with the Gulick spring-loaded end than with a standard tape measure for lower extremity measurements in healthy subjects.[10]

Although girth measurements appear to be reproducible, the validity of measurement of thigh bulk has been questioned. Stokes and Young[12] were concerned that the tape measure was not sensitive and accurate enough for measuring selective wasting of the quadriceps. Doxey[13] reported that detection of changes in muscle bulk in nonsurgical subjects probably requires more sensitive methods than girth measurements, such as ultrasonography or computed tomography. Moreover, a small decrease (1%) in thigh measurement may be an indicator of a significant reduction (13%) in muscle bulk.[13] Research using ultrasonography[4,13] and computed tomography[9] has shown that muscle fiber atrophy is not adequately reflected by circumference measurements. Rather, extremity fat can mask such muscle atrophy. Thus, caution should be exercised when interpreting the results of girth measurements with regard to muscle strength and progression of individuals through a plan of care. In a rehabilitation setting, the clinician should keep accurate records of not only girth measurements but also the anatomic landmarks used so that consistency is maintained.

GONIOMETRY

Goniometry is the use of instruments to measure the range of motion of body joints. All clinicians should be able to competently perform and interpret objective measurements of joint motion. Initial range-of-motion measurements provide a basis for developing a treatment or therapeutic exercise plan, and repeated measurements throughout the course of rehabilitation help determine whether improvement has been made and the goals achieved.

Historical Considerations

The literature on goniometry is extensive and describes many aspects of goniometric measuring. Gifford, in 1914,[14] was probably the first to have reported on goniometric devices in the United States. Historically, various instruments and methods of measurement have been described and recommended.[15-22] The most common methods of measuring range of motion involve the use of a universal goniometer, an inclinometer, or a tape measure (Box 5-2). Special devices are also available for measuring specific joint motion, such as cervical and back motion, temporomandibular joint motion, and ankle motion.

Instruments for assessing joint motion are generally of two types: (1) devices with universal application (e.g., full-circle or half-circle universal goniometer), which remain the most versatile and popular (Fig. 5-1), and (2) goniometers designed to measure a single range of motion for a specific joint (Fig. 5-2). Although not as common as universal goniometers, gravity-dependent goniometers or inclinometers use the effect of gravity on pointers or fluid levels to measure joint position and motion

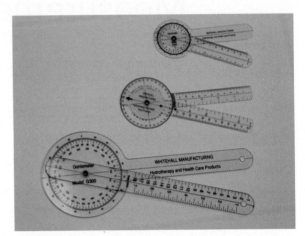

FIGURE 5-1 Full-circle manual universal goniometer.

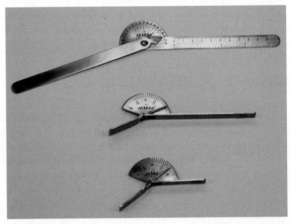

FIGURE 5-2 Goniometers for measuring a single joint motion.

and can either be mechanical or electronic.[23] Mechanical inclinometers are either (1) pendulum goniometers that consist of a 360° protractor with a weighted pointer hanging from the center of the protractor (Fig. 5-3, A) or (2) fluid goniometers that have a fluid-filled circular chamber containing an air bubble, similar to a carpenter's level (Fig. 5-3, B). Electrogoniometers, which convert angular motion of the joint into an electric signal, can also be used.[24] They are generally used for research purposes because of their expense and the time needed to calibrate and attach to a patient.

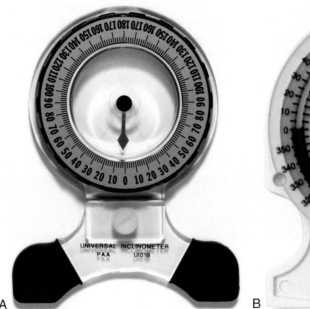
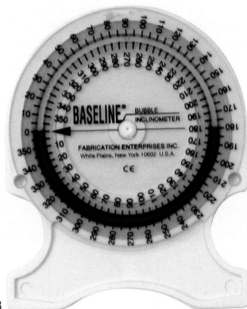

FIGURE 5-3 A, Universal inclinometer. **B,** Bubble inclinometer. (**A,** *Photo courtesy of Performance Attainment Associates, St. Paul, MN;* **B,** *photo courtesy of Fabrication Enterprises, White Plains, NY.)*

As goniometry evolved, efforts were focused on standardizing methods of measurement, including developing common nomenclature and definitions of terms, clearly defining movements to be measured, and establishing normal ranges of motion. In 1965, the American Academy of Orthopaedic Surgeons published a manual of standardized methods of measuring and recording joint motion; since then, the manual has been reprinted numerous times.[25] Norkin and White[23] and Reese and Bandy[24] have also provided thorough descriptions of goniometry.

Goniometric Assessment

Anatomic Zero Position

The anatomic zero position is the starting 0° orientation for most measurements.[17] The exceptions are shoulder rotation, hip rotation, and forearm pronation-supination, for which the starting position is between the two extremes of motion. If the individual to be measured cannot assume the starting position, the position of improvisation should be noted when joint motion is recorded. Normal range of motion varies among individuals and is influenced by factors such as age, gender, and whether the motion is performed actively or passively.

Three methods of recording range of motion are accepted: the 0°–180° system, which is the most common system used; the 180°–0° system; and the 360° system[23,24,26] (Box 5-3). In the 0°–180° system the neutral starting position is noted as 0°, and the degrees of joint motion are added in the direction of joint movement.[23] When a range of motion is documented, both the beginning (where the motion starts) and ending (where the motion ends) readings are reported. Motion that is beyond the anatomic zero position can be denoted with a plus (+) sign (hypermobility), and when motion is unable to reach the zero position, a minus (−) sign is used (hypomobility). Average ranges of motion for the upper and lower extremities are presented in Table 5-1.[27]

Box 5-3

Methods of Documenting Goniometry Readings

0°-180° SYSTEM

Determines the anatomic 0° starting point for all joints except the forearm, which is fully supinated. Extension of a joint is recorded as 0°, and as the joint flexes, motion progresses toward 180°.[24] It is the most common system used.

180°-0° SYSTEM

Neutral extension at each joint is recorded as 180°; movement toward flexion approaches 0°, and movement toward extension past neutral also approaches 0°.[24,26]

FULL 360° CIRCLE

The 0° position of each joint is full flexion, neutral extension is recorded as 180°, and motions toward extension past neutral approach 360°.[24]

Validity and Reliability of Goniometric Measurement

The purpose of goniometry is to measure the joint angle or range of motion.[23] It is assumed that the angle created by aligning the arms of a universal goniometer with bony landmarks truly represents the angle created by the proximal and distal bones composing the joint.[23] One infers that changes in goniometer alignment reflect changes in joint angle and represent a range of joint motion.[23] Additionally, goniometer measurements are generally compared with radiographs, which represent the "gold standard" for measurements. Several studies[28-30] have indicated a degree of relationship between measurements obtained with radiography and goniometry.

The reliability of goniometric joint motion measurements has been studied both within and between instruments/techniques, as well as clinicians. Several reports have noted that joint range of motion can be measured with good to excellent reliability.[31-34] Intratester reliability appears to be higher than intertester reliability regardless of the device used.[31,34-43] Additionally, it appears that upper extremity joint measurements are more reliable than those of the lower extremity joints,[35,40] and reliability can be less for different joints.[33,34,44-46] This may be due to the complexity of the joint or the difficulty in palpating anatomic landmarks.[23] Because reliability is different for each joint, the standard error of measurement can also differ for each joint. Norkin and White[23] and Reese and Bandy[24] documented the standard deviation and standard error of measurement for

Table 5-1 Average Ranges of Motion for the Upper and Lower Extremities

Joint	Motion	Range of Motion (°)	
		American Academy of Orthopaedic Surgeons	**Kendall and McCreary[27]**
Shoulder	Flexion	0-180	0-180
	Extension	0-60	0-45
	Abduction	0-180	0-180
	Internal rotation	0-70	0-70
	External rotation	0-90	0-90
Elbow	Flexion	0-150	0-145
Forearm	Pronation	0-80	0-90
	Supination	0-80	0-90
Wrist	Extension	0-70	0-70
	Flexion	0-80	0-80
	Radial deviation	0-20	0-20
	Ulnar deviation	0-30	0-35
Thumb			
CMC	Abduction	0-70	0-80
	Flexion	0-15	0-45
	Extension	0-20	0-45
MCP	Flexion	0-50	0-60
IP	Flexion	0-80	0-80
Digits 2 to 5			
MCP	Flexion	0-90	0-90
	Extension	0-45	
PIP	Flexion	–	–
DIP	Extension	–	–
Hip	Flexion	0-120	0-125
	Extension	0-30	0-10
	Abduction	0-45	0-45
	Adduction	0-30	0-10
	External rotation	0-45	0-45
	Internal rotation	0-45	0-45
Knee	Flexion	0-135	0-140
Ankle	Dorsiflexion	0-20	0-20
	Plantar flexion	0-50	0-45
	Inversion	0-35	0-35
	Eversion	0-15	0-20
Subtalar	Inversion	–	0-5
	Eversion	0-5	–

Adapted from Norkin, C.C., and White, D.J. (1985): Measurement of Joint Motion: A Guide to Goniometry. Philadelphia, Davis.
CMC, Carpometacarpal; *DIP,* distal interphalangeal; *IP,* interphalangeal; *MCP,* metacarpophalangeal; *PIP,* proximal interphalangeal.

each joint in their books on goniometry. Boone et al[35] indicated that the same individual should perform the goniometric measurements when the effects of treatment are evaluated. Visual estimation is used by some clinicians to assess joint positions. Investigations assessing the accuracy and reliability of visual estimation versus goniometer measurements report the latter to be more accurate and reliable.[34,38,39,44,46-48]

Synthesis of investigations evaluating the interchangeability of different types of goniometers shows that this is not an acceptable clinical practice.[49-52] Furthermore, the results of research assessing the interreliability and intrareliability and validity of inclinometers and electrogoniometers vary depending on the technique used and the joint measured.[49-52]

Technical Considerations

The positioning of the patient should be consistent. The prone or supine position provides greater stabilization through the patient's body weight. Measurements should be acquired with the use of passive range of motion when possible, and the body part should be uncovered for better accuracy. The goniometer is placed next to or on top of the joint whenever possible, and three landmarks are used for alignment.[24] The goniometer arms are placed along the longitudinal axis of the bones of the joint after the motion has occurred. The fulcrum of the goniometer is placed over a point that is near the joint's axis of rotation. Because this axis of rotation is not stationary during motion, this is the least important of the three landmarks, and emphasis is placed on proper alignment of the goniometer arms.[24]

In evaluating the joint and assessing range of motion, the clinician should view the affected joint from above and below to determine whether any additional limitations are present in the involved extremity. The opposite extremity must also be assessed to determine normal motion for that patient. Box 5-4 suggests guidelines to improve the reliability of goniometry. Box 5-5 describes the principles for measuring range of motion for joints.

Box 5-4

Suggested Guidelines to Improve the Reliability of Goniometry

Use consistent, well-defined testing positions and anatomic landmarks to align the arms of the goniometer.[23]

Do not interchange different types of goniometers for repeated measures from day to day on the same patient.[49-52]

The same clinician should measure the patient from day to day if possible.[49,52]

Use a standardized protocol for measuring joint motion.[23]

Take repeated measurements on a subject with the same type of measurement device.[23]

Use large universal goniometers when measuring joints with large body segments.[23]

Inexperienced examiners should take several measurements and record the average of those measurements to improve reliability, but one measurement is usually sufficient for more experienced examiners using good technique.[23]

Note: Successive measurements are more reliable if they are taken by the same clinician rather than by different clinicians.

Special Joint Considerations

Spine

The wide range of motion available in the spine can make measurement of cervical and lumbar motion challenging. Many instruments are advocated for measuring motion of these areas, including tape measures, universal goniometers, and inclinometers. Use of the double-inclinometer technique has also been suggested for measuring cervical and lumbar motion.[24] Specific devices are available to measure only the cervical and lumbar spine, such as cervical range-of-motion and back range-of-motion devices (Performance Attainment Associates, Roseville, MN) (Figs. 5-4 and 5-5). Lumbar and thoracolumbar motions are most commonly measured with a tape measure. Flexion and extension of the lumbar spine can be measured via the Schober technique, which has been revised over time to the modified Schober technique and the modified-modified Schober technique (Box 5-6).[53,54] Specific advantages and disadvantages of each technique, as well as a detailed description, can be found in other sources.[23,24]

The validity and reliability of the devices and techniques used for measuring spine range of motion have been investigated extensively, with comparisons of devices/techniques and intertester and intratester reliability. Research findings exhibit a fair amount of disparity, and the reader is urged to consult a more in-depth review of this literature to make an informed decision regarding the devices/techniques to incorporate into clinical practice.[23,24]

Box 5-5

Application Technique for Measuring Joint Range of Motion

1. The clinician places the patient in a posture that is closely related to an anatomic position.
2. It may be necessary to explain and demonstrate the procedure to the patient before the activity.
3. The clinician should make a visual estimate of the approximate range of motion that the joint will allow during active movement.
4. The clinician stabilizes the proximal segment of the joint to prevent error.
5. The landmarks are located and marked with a pen to ensure proper placement and alignment.
6. The axis of the joint is observed and the fulcrum of the goniometer is placed at this juncture. The goniometer is held 1 to 2 inches from the patient's body.
7. The stationary arm is aligned parallel to the longitudinal axis of the proximal limb segment and the appropriate anatomic landmarks.
8. After the goniometer is aligned properly, the patient is instructed to move the distal segment as far as it can go.
9. The movable arm is aligned parallel to the longitudinal axis of the distal limb segment and the appropriate anatomic landmarks.
10. The clinician reads the goniometer.
11. It is not necessary to move the stationary arm when the measurements are repeated.
12. The clinician records and reports the data.

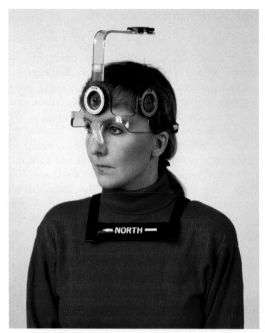

FIGURE 5-4 Cervical range-of-motion device for measuring cervical rotation. *(Photo courtesy of Performance Attainment Associates, St. Paul, MN.)*

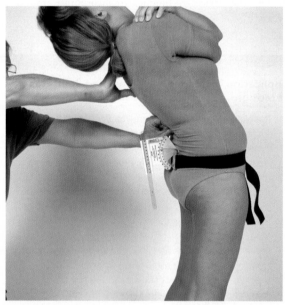

FIGURE 5-5 Back range-of-motion device for measuring lumbar flexion. *(Photo courtesy of Performance Attainment Associates, St. Paul, MN.)*

Scapular Position

Scapular position can have an effect on shoulder function. Thus, reliable methods of determining scapular position will allow clinicians to classify the degree of scapular abduction and the effect of therapeutic interventions.[55] Two primary methods of measuring scapular abduction are reported in the literature. DiVeta et al[56] described a technique that involves measurement from the inferior angle of the acromion to the spinous process of the third

---

Box 5-6

Schober Technique

SCHOBER TECHNIQUE
Two-mark method with the patient standing in a neutral posture:

1. Lumbosacral junction
2. 10 cm above the lumbosacral mark

The patient bends forward, and the increased distance between the first and second marks provides an estimate of spine flexion.

Because the technique relies on stretching or distraction of the skin overlying the spine, it is also referred to as the "skin distraction method."

MODIFIED SCHOBER TECHNIQUE[53]
Introduced a third mark placed 5 cm below the lumbosacral junction, along with the two marks described in the Schober technique.

The rationale for this third mark was the observation that during the Schober technique, the skin above and below the lumbosacral junction was distracted as the patient bent forward.

MODIFIED-MODIFIED SCHOBER TECHNIQUE[54]
Uses two landmarks:

1. A point bisecting a line that connects the two posterior superior iliac spines (PSISs)
2. A mark 15 cm superior to the PSIS landmark

The rationale was the difficulty palpating the lumbosacral junction. The PSISs are more readily palpated.

thoracic vertebra with patients standing in a relaxed position with their arms at their sides. This distance is referred to as the total scapular distance. Kibler[57] proposed what is known as the lateral scapular slide test (LSST) in which three measurements are made at 0°, 40°, and 90° of shoulder abduction. Scapular distance is measured from the inferior angle of the scapula to the T7 thoracic process.

Intertester and intratester reliability of the technique of DeVeta et al for measuring scapular distance (abduction) is high[55,56,58,59]; in addition, it appears to be a valid test for measuring scapular protraction.[59] Conversely, data on interreliability and intrareliablity for the LSST conflict, with the only strong indication being that intratester reliability seems to be better than intertester reliability.[58,60] It appears that both techniques may be promising, but more research is needed before definite conclusions can be drawn.

CONCLUSION

Girth

- A standard tape measure appears to be a reliable instrument for measuring girth, particularly when the same clinician makes all the measurements.
- There is no direct relationship between girth measurements and muscle size.

Goniometry

- The most common instruments used to measure joint motion are a universal goniometer, inclinometer, and tape measure.
- The most common system used to record joint motion is the 0°–180° system.
- In general, goniometric measurements of joint motion are considered valid and reliable, but validity and reliability vary depending on the instrument, technique, and joint measured.
- It appears that intraclinician reliability is better than interclinician reliability; therefore, when possible, the same clinician should make all the measurements.
- Different types of goniometers should not be interchanged for repeated measures from day to day on the same patient.

For examples of commonly used goniometry techniques, see Figures W5-1 through W5-30 (in Appendix W5) on Expert Consult @ www.ExpertConsult.com.

REFERENCES

1. Spencer, J.D., Hayes, K.C., and Alexander, I. J. (1984): Knee joint effusion and quadriceps reflex inhibition in man. Arch. Phys. Med. Rehabil., 65:171–177.
2. Fowler, P.J., and Regan, W.D. (1987): The patient with symptomatic chronic anterior cruciate ligament insufficiency. Am. J. Sports Med., 15:321–325.
3. Kirwan, J.R., Byron, M.A., Winfield, J., et al. (1979): Circumferential measurements in the assessment of synovitis of the knee. Rheumatol. Rehabil., 18:78–84.
4. Young, A., Stokes, M., and Iles, J. F. (1987): Effects of joint pathology on muscle. Clin. Orthop. Relat. Res., 219:21–27.
5. Morrissey, M.C., Brewster, C.E., Shields, C.L., and Brown, M. (1985): The effects of electrical stimulation on the quadriceps during postoperative knee immobilization. J. Sports Med., 12:40–45.
6. Noyes, F.R., Mangine, R.E., and Barber, S. (1987): Early knee motion after open and arthroscopic anterior cruciate ligament reconstruction. Am. J. Sports Med., 15:149–160.
7. Reynolds, N.L., Worrell, T.W., and Perrin, D.H. (1992): Effect of a lateral step-up exercise protocol on quadriceps isokinetic peak torque values and thigh girth. J. Orthop. Sports Phys. Ther., 15:151–155.
8. Romero, J.A., Sanford, T.L., Schroeder, R.V., and Fahey, T.D. (1982): The effects of electrical stimulation on normal quadriceps strength and girth. Med. Sci. Sports Exerc., 14:194–197.
9. Doxey, G. (1987): Assessing quadriceps femoris muscle bulk with girth measurements in subjects with patellofemoral pain. J. Orthop. Sports Phys. Ther., 9:177–183.
10. Harrelson, G.L., Leaver-Dunn, D., Fincher, A.L., and Leeper, J.D. (1998): Inter- and intratester reliability of lower extremity circumference measurements. J. Sport Rehabil., 7:300–306.
11. Whitney, S.L., Mattocks, L., Irrgang, J.J., et al. (1995): Reliability of lower extremity girth measurements and right- and left-side differences. J. Sport Rehabil., 4:108–115.
12. Stokes, M., and Young, A. (1984): The contribution of reflex inhibition to arthrogenous muscle weakness. Clin. Sci., 67:7–14.
13. Doxey, G. (1987): The association of anthropometric measurement of thigh size and B-mode ultrasound scanning of muscle thickness. J. Orthop. Sports Phys. Ther., 8:462–468.
14. Gifford, H.D. (1914): Instruments for measuring joint movements and deformities in fracture treatment. Am. J. Surg., 28:237–238.
15. Clark, W.A. (1921): A protractor for measuring rotation of joint. J. Orthop. Surg., 3:154–155.
16. Leighton, J.R. (1955): An instrument and technic for the measurement of range of joint motion. Arch. Phys. Med., 36:571–577.
17. Moore, M.L. (1949): The measurement of joint motion. Part I. Introductory review of the literature. Phys. Ther. Rev., 29:195–205.
18. Moore, M.L. (1949): The measurement of joint motion. Part II. The technic of goniometry. Phys. Ther. Rev., 29:256–264.
19. Parker, J.S. (1929): Recording arthroflexometer. J. Bone Joint Surg., 11:126–127.
20. West, C.C. (1945): Measurement of joint motion. Arch. Phys. Med., 26:414–425.
21. Wiechec, F.J., and Krusen, F.H. (1939): A new method of joint measurement and a review of the literature. Am. J. Surg., 43:659–668.
22. Wilson, J.D., and Stasch, W.H. (1945): Photographic record of joint motion. Arch. Phys., 27:361–362.
23. Norkin, C.C., and White, D.J. (1995): Measurement of Joint Motion: Guide to Goniometry, 2nd ed. Philadelphia, Davis.
24. Reese, N.B., and Bandy, W.D. (2002): Joint Range of Motion and Muscle Length Testing. Philadelphia, Saunders.
25. American Academy of Orthopaedic Surgeons. (1965): Joint Motion: Methods of Measuring and Recording. Chicago, American Academy of Orthopaedic Surgeons.
26. Clark, W. A. (1920): A system of joint measurements. J. Orthop. Surg., 2:687–700.
27. Kendall, F.P., and McCreary, E.K. (1983): Muscle Testing and Function, 3rd ed. Baltimore, Williams & Wilkins.
28. Ahlback, S.O., and Lindahl, O. (1964): Sagittal mobility of the hip joint. Acta Orthop. Scand., 34:310–314.
29. Enwemeka, C.S. (1986): Radiographic verification of knee goniometry. Scand. J. Rehabil. Med., 18:47–50.
30. Gogia, P.P., Braatz, J.H., Rose, S.J., and Norton, B. (1987): Reliability and validity of goniometric measurements of the knee. Phys. Ther., 67:192–195.
31. Ekstaund, J., Wiktorsson, M., and Oberg, B. (1982): Lower extremity goniometric measurements: a study to determine their reliability. Arch. Phys. Med., 63:171–175.
32. Gajdoski, R.L., and Bohannon, R.W. (1987): Clinical measurement of range of motion: Review of goniometry emphasizing reliability and validity. Phys. Ther., 67:1867–1872.
33. Lovell, F.W., Rothstein, J.M., and Personius, W.J. (1989): Reliability of clinical measurement of lumbar lordosis taken with a flexible rule. Phys. Ther., 69:96–101.
34. Low, J. L. (1976): The reliability of joint measurement. Physiotherapy, 62:227–229.
35. Boone, D.C., Azen, S.P., Linn, C.N., et al. (1978): Reliability of goniometric measurements. Phys. Ther., 58:1355–1360.
36. Grohmann, J.L. (1983): Comparison of two methods of goniometry. Phys. Ther., 67:192–195.
37. Hamilton, G.F., and Lachenbruch, P.A. (1969): Reliability of goniometers in assessing finger joint angle. Phys. Ther., 49:465–469.
38. Hellebradt, F.A., Duvall, E.N., and Moore, M.L. (1949): The measurement of joint motion. Part III. Reliability of goniometry. Phys. Ther. Rev., 29:302–307.
39. Mayerson, N.H., and Milano, R.A. (1984): Goniometric measurement reliability in physical medicine. Arch. Phys. Med. Rehabil., 65:92–97.
40. Pandya, S., Florence, J.M., King, W.M., et al. (1985): Reliability of goniometric measurement in patients with Duchenne muscular dystrophy. Phys. Ther., 65:1339–1345.
41. Riddle, D.L., Rothstein, J.M., and Lamb, R.L. (1987): Goniometric reliability in a clinical setting: Shoulder measurements. Phys. Ther., 67:668–673.
42. Rothstein, J.M., Miller, P.J., and Roettger, R.F. (1983): Goniometric reliability in a clinical setting: Elbow and knee measurement. Phys. Ther., 63:1611–1615.
43. Solgaard, S., Carlsen, A., Krauhoft, M., and Petersen, V. S. (1986): Reproducibility of goniometry of the wrist. Scand. J. Rehabil. Med., 18:5–7.
44. Fitzgerald, G.K., Wynveen, K.J., Rheault, W., and Rothschild, B. (1983): Objective assessment with establishment of normal values for lumbar spine range of motion. Phys. Ther., 62:1776–1781.
45. Tucci, S.M., Hicks, J.E., Gross, E.G., et al. (1986): Cervical motion assessment: A new, simple and accurate method. Arch. Phys. Med. Rehabil., 67:225–230.
46. Youdas, J.W., Bogard, C.L., and Suman, V.J. (1993): Reliability of goniometric measurements and visual estimates of ankle joint active range of motion obtained in a clinical setting. Arch. Phys. Med. Rehabil., 74:1112–1118.
47. Watkins, M.A., Riddle, D.L., Lamb, R.L., and Personius, W.J. (1991): Reliability of goniometric measurements and visual estimates of knee range of motion obtained in a clinical setting. Phys. Ther., 71:90–96.
48. Youdas, J.W., Carey, J.R., and Garrett, T.R. (1991): Reliability of measurement of cervical spine range of motion: Comparison of three methods. Phys. Ther., 71:2–7.
49. Goodwin, J., Clark, C., Deakes, J., et al. (1992): Clinical methods of goniometry: A comparative study. Disabil Rehabil., 14:10–15.
50. Petherick, M., Rheault, W., Kimble, S., et al. (1988): Concurrent validity and intertester reliability of universal and fluid-based goniometers for active elbow range of motion. Phys. Ther., 68:966–969.
51. Rheault, W., Miller, M., Nothnagel, P., et al. (1988): Intertester reliability and concurrent validity of fluid-based and universal goniometers for active knee flexion. Phys. Ther., 68:1676–1678.
52. Rome, K., and Cowieson, F. (1996): A reliability study of the universal goniometer, fluid goniometer and electrogoniometer for the measurement of ankle dorsiflexion. Foot Ankle Int., 17:28–32.
53. Macrae, I.F., and Wright, V. (1969): Measurement of back movement. Ann. Rheum. Dis., 28:584–589.
54. Williams, R., Binkley, J., Bloch, R., et al. (1993): Reliability of the modified-modified Schober and double inclinometer methods for measuring lumbar flexion and extension. Phys. Ther., 73:26–37.
55. Neiers, L., and Worrell, T.W. (1993): Assessment of scapular position. J. Sport Rehabil., 2:20–25.
56. DiVeta, J., Walker, M.L., and Skibinski, B. (1990): Relationship between performance of selected scapular muscles and scapular abduction in standing subjects. Phys. Ther., 70:470–476.
57. Kibler, W. B. (1991): Role of the scapula in the overhead throwing motion. Contemp. Orthop., 22:525–532.
58. Gibson, M.H., Goebel, G.V., Jordan, T.M., et al. (1995): A reliability study of measurement techniques to determine static scapular position. J. Orthop. Phys. Ther., 21:100–106.
59. Greenfield, B., Catlin, P.A., Coats, P. W., et al. (1995): Posture in patients with shoulder overuse injuries and healthy individuals. J. Orthop. Phys. Ther., 21:287–295.
60. Odom, C.J., Taylor, A.B., Hurd, C.E., and Denegar, C.R. (2001): Measurement of scapular asymmetry and assessment of shoulder dysfunction using the lateral scapular slide test: A reliability and validity study. Phys. Ther., 81:799–809.

6

Range of Motion and Flexibility

Jeff G. Konin, PT, PhD, ATC, FACSM, FNATA, and Brittany Jessee, PT, DPT

CHAPTER OBJECTIVES

- Recognize and describe methods of assessing and measuring range of motion and flexibility.
- Identify the principles associated with stretching of connective tissue structures.
- Explain the principles and techniques for active, active assisted, passive, and resistive stretching.

- Identify the basic principles of proprioceptive neuromuscular facilitation and recognize its benefits for the rehabilitation of athletes.
- Identify key principles of, indications for, and contraindications to joint mobilization.

Range of motion is the available amount of movement of a joint, whereas flexibility is the ability of soft tissue structures, such as muscle, tendon, and connective tissue, to elongate through the available range of joint motion. Whether it is undergoing therapeutic stretching during postinjury rehabilitation or during a routine flexibility program, connective tissue is the most important physical focus of range-of-motion exercises. For favorable physiologic potentials to exist, both range of motion and range of flexibility need to be optimized. The connective tissue involved in the body's reparative process after trauma or surgery often limits normal joint motion. Therefore, understanding the biophysical factors of connective tissue is important for determining optimal ways to increase range of motion because histologic evidence has shown that fibrosis can occur within 4 days of the onset of immobility.[1] To effectively maintain and improve range of motion and flexibility, knowledge of both the related tissue structures and the various techniques used to facilitate extensibility of these structures is imperative.

REASONS FOR LIMITATIONS IN RANGE OF MOTION

The physiologic conditions associated with limitations in range of motion may vary. Often, a single structural component may be the cause of restricted movement. However, it is not uncommon to have related concurrent limitations from more than one structure. Structures that play a role in limiting one's range of motion are summarized in Box 6-1. Limitations as a result of structural involvement may be

caused by a traumatic incident, such as surgery, or may develop over time from disuse, such as a lack of stretching. Furthermore, the pain associated with disruption of tissue or caused by joint swelling that becomes a space-occupying lesion and compresses against joint receptors and cutaneous nerves may inhibit one's ability to actively and passively generate joint movement.

STRETCHING

Biophysical Considerations

Properties of Connective Tissue

Connective tissue is composed of collagen and other fibers within a ground substance—a protein-polysaccharide complex. A thorough discussion of the composition of connective tissue is presented in Chapter 2. Connective tissue has viscoelastic properties, defined as two components of stretch that allow elongation of the tissue.[1-4] The viscous component permits a plastic stretch that results in permanent tissue elongation after the load is removed. Conversely, the elastic component allows an elastic stretch, or temporary elongation, with the tissue returning to its previous length when the stress is removed. Range-of-motion exercise techniques should be designed to primarily produce plastic deformation. Repetitive intervention that incorporates sustained tissue elongation with low loads of stress versus shorter-duration aggressive loads may be more beneficial in achieving the clinical outcome of plastic deformational changes.

Neurophysiology

All stretching techniques are based on the premise of the stretch reflex, which involves two muscle receptors—the Golgi tendon organ (GTO) and the muscle spindle—that are sensitive to changes in muscle length.[5] The GTO is also affected by changes in muscle tension. These receptors must be considered in the process of selecting any stretching procedure. The intrafusal muscle spindle responds to rapid stretch by initiating a reflexive contraction of the muscle being stretched.[5] If a stretch is held long enough (at least 6 seconds),[6] this protective mechanism can be negated by the action of the GTO, which can override the impulses from the muscle spindle.[5] The reflexive relaxation that results is referred to as *autogenic inhibition*, and it allows effective stretching of the muscle tissue. Additionally, isotonic contraction of an agonist muscle causes reflexive relaxation of the antagonist muscle, which allows it to stretch. This phenomenon is referred to as *reciprocal inhibition*. Conversely, a quick stretch of the antagonist muscle will cause a contraction of the agonist muscle. For example, when the quadriceps muscle contracts, reflexive relaxation of the hamstring muscles occurs. In other words, when a tight muscle or muscles have been identified, an isotonic contraction of its antagonist will result in relaxation of the tight muscles and an improved range of motion. Autogenic inhibition and reciprocal inhibition are two components on which proprioceptive neuromuscular facilitation (PNF) stretching is based.

Duration

The amount and duration of the force applied during performance of the stretch are some of the principal factors determining how much elastic or plastic stretch occurs when connective tissue is stretched. Elastic stretch is enhanced by high-force, short-duration stretching, whereas plastic stretch results from low-force, long-duration stretching. Numerous studies representing decades of research have noted the effectiveness of prolonged stretching at low to moderate levels of tension.[2-4,7-19] A precise time frame for holding a static stretch has not been determined. Research has suggested that static stretches be held between 6 and 60 seconds,[6] with 15- to 30-second holds most commonly being advocated. Some authors have proposed that a single static stretch of 15 to 30 seconds one time each day is sufficient for most people.[20]

Temperature of Connective Tissue

Research has shown that temperature has a significant influence on the mechanical behavior of connective tissue under tensile stretch.[4,21-24] Because connective tissue is composed of collagen, which is resistant to stretch at normal body temperature, the effect of increased tissue temperature on stretch has been studied. Synthesis of the body of research shows that higher therapeutic temperatures at low loads produce the greatest plastic tissue elongation with the least damage. Lentell et al[25] reported greater increases in the range of motion of healthy shoulders after the application of heat.

Increased connective tissue temperature decreases the resistance of connective tissue to stretch and promotes increased soft tissue extensibility.[12,23] It has been reported that collagen is very pliable when heated to a range between 102°F and 110°F.[4,21] The use of ultrasound before joint mobilization has proved effective in elevating deep tissue temperature and extensibility.[22] Draper and Ricard[26] demonstrated the presence of a "stretching window" after a 3-MHz ultrasound application. This window indicates that for optimal tissue elongation, stretching should be performed during ultrasound treatment or within 3.3 minutes after termination of the treatment.[26] In a follow-up study, Rose et al[27] reported that after a 1-MHz ultrasound application, the deeper tissues cooled at a slower rate than did the superficial tissues; thus, the stretching window was open longer for deeper structures than for superficial ones. Although superior stretching results have been reported with the application of heat before and during stretching, other studies have found greater increases in flexibility after the application of cold packs. Brodowicz et al[28] reported improved hamstring flexibility in healthy subjects after 20 minutes of hamstring stretching with an ice pack applied to the posterior aspect of the thigh when compared with subjects who received heat or who performed stretching without the application of any therapeutic agent. Kottke et al[3] have also shown that greater plastic stretch results if the tissue is allowed to cool before tension is released, whereas others[25] have reported that the use of cold during the end stages of stretching diminishes the cumulative gains in flexibility that occurred after the application of heat. Moreover, it appears that the use of either a superficial heat or a cold modality in conjunction with stretching results in greater improvements in flexibility than does stretching alone.[25,28] It remains to be seen whether increased extensibility is the sole result of a single structure or a combination of structural changes perhaps related to musculotendinous, capsuloligamentous, or fascial tissue.

Objectivity of Range-of-Motion and Flexibility Assessments

Range of motion and flexibility are measured in a number of different ways. Typically, the type of tissue being assessed will dictate the method of assessment, although some methods may be used for various tissues. The primary movements that are assessed are termed as being *physiologic* or *accessory*. Physiologic movement accounts for the major portion of the range and can be measured with a goniometer (see Chapter 5). Physiologic joint movements occur in the cardinal movement planes and include flexion-extension, abduction-adduction, and rotation.[29] Accessory motion, also referred to as *arthrokinematics*, is necessary for normal physiologic range of motion; it occurs simultaneously with physiologic motion and cannot be measured precisely.

The ability to accurately assess and measure physiologic range of motion appears to be dependent on the joint.[30-38] These findings are detailed in Chapter 5, and the reader is encouraged to be innovative in developing improved methods of measurement to enhance those that currently exist. Devices, such as a sit-and-reach tool, can be used to assess excursion of the hamstring muscles[39-41] (Fig. 6-1).

Accessory range of motion is much more difficult to assess and measure because it is often measured in units of millimeters. Experience in assessing both normal and abnormal joint accessory movement plays a critical role in one's ability to accurately process such movement. Studies have shown a clear difference between novice and expert clinicians in determining accessory range of motion.[42-45] Equipment can also be used to assess accessory joint motion, such as that seen when one is measuring the amount of anterior translation of the knee as a result of injury to the anterior cruciate ligament[46-50] (Fig. 6-2).

Types of Stretching Techniques

The limited joint range of motion caused by soft tissue restriction often inhibits initiation or completion of the rehabilitative process. Conservative treatment of contractures is only moderately successful, and overly aggressive stretching may result in undesired adverse effects. Optimal stretching is achieved only when voluntary and reflexive muscle resistance is overcome or eliminated and tissue elongation is facilitated. The main types of tissue that are stretched include musculotendinous, capsuloligamentous, and myofascial.

Three types of stretching techniques are generally recognized to facilitate musculotendinous flexibility: ballistic, static, and PNF.

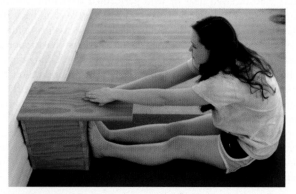

FIGURE 6-1 Assessing hamstring flexibility with a sit-and-reach box.

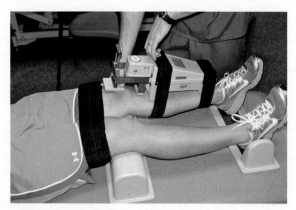

FIGURE 6-2 Assessment of anterior translation accessory motion of the knee with a knee arthrometer.

Ballistic stretching consists of repetitive bouncing movements that stretch a muscle group. Ballistic stretching has not been advocated because forces could be applied to a muscle that exceed its extensibility or that activate the muscle spindles described previously, with resultant microtrauma to the muscle fibers.[51-54] However, it has been reported that because many physical activities involve dynamic movement, ballistic stretching should follow a static stretching routine.[55] Static stretching involves stretching a muscle to a point of discomfort and holding the stretch for a length of time, followed by a return to normal resting muscle length. PNF involves alternating muscle contractions and stretching.[56] The efficacy of all three techniques has been evaluated, and it appears that each technique has the capacity to increase flexibility, with static stretching being the safest of the three.[9,57-72] In some cases static stretching has been advocated over PNF because it is easier to teach and perform.[72] Some clinicians prefer PNF stretching because it allows stretching to occur in functional planes of movement that more closely simulate activities. Each of the techniques should be performed with a prescribed set of repetitions while taking care to avoid overstretching. Contraindications to general stretching are indicated in Box 6-2.

Passive and Active Assisted Stretching Techniques

Various mechanical passive and active assisted techniques augment manual passive stretching. Methods of achieving the desired outcome are often limited only by creativity and improvisational skills. After the soft tissue restriction has been assessed, the clinician should analyze appropriate and effective ways of carrying out the treatment and rehabilitation plan. Several methods of stretching can be used, but a clinician should be careful to consider joint positioning when assessing extensibility and use standardized and consistent approaches to most accurately reflect reliable and valid measurements.

SPRAY AND STRETCH

This technique has been described in detail by Travell and Simons.[73,74] Spraying of Fluori-Methane* or ethyl chloride* cools taut muscle fibers and desensitizes palpable myofascial

---

*Available from Gebauer Chemical Co., Cleveland, OH.

trigger points, thereby facilitating stretching of the muscle to its full length. Passive stretch remains the central component in this technique. Concerns about the use of both vapocoolants have been documented. Travell and Simmons[73] advocated the use of Fluori-Methane spray. However, because Fluori-Methane is a chlorofluorocarbon, which destroys the atmospheric ozone layer, its use has been questioned.[75] Conversely, although ethyl chloride is not a chlorofluorocarbon, it is colder than Fluori-Methane, flammable, and explosive in a critical concentration with air. It is also a potent, readily acting general anesthesic[73,76] (see Chapter 8 for additional information on vapocoolants). Ice stroking has been advocated as an alternative to the use of vapocoolants.[73,76-78]

PROLONGED WEIGHTED STRETCH

The rationale for a prolonged-duration, low-load stretch has been discussed. Figure 6-3 illustrates a method of prolonged weighted stretching for the knee in which a small cuff weight is placed distally on the lower part of the leg to provide gentle passive stretching of the hamstring muscle group. Similar types of stretches can be performed for the upper extremity, as seen in Figure 6-4. The key to success with prolonged-duration, low-load types of stretches is to allow muscle relaxation and gentle overpressure. If not comfortable, an athlete will contract the muscles surrounding the joint and resist the overpressure, which results in no short- or long-term gains in flexibility.

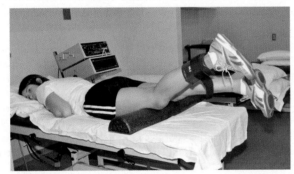

FIGURE 6-3 Prone low-load weighted stretch for the hamstring muscle group.

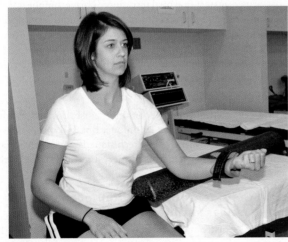

FIGURE 6-4 Weighted elbow stretch using a low-load, long-duration stretch.

ASSISTIVE DEVICES

These appliances aid in gaining and maintaining end range of motion. Assistive devices include pulleys, extremity traction,[4,23] T-bars or wands, and continuous passive range-of-motion units. Pulleys are commonly used for restriction of the shoulder (Fig. 6-5) and knee joints. Wands, T-bars, towels, sport sticks (Fig. 6-6), or other similar apparatus may be used for individual active assisted stretching of the upper extremities.

Continuous passive range-of-motion units are often valuable mechanical devices that can benefit various joints.[79-85] They can provide constant movement of a joint after surgical

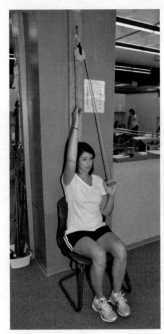

FIGURE 6-5 Active assisted range of motion of the shoulder with the use of pulleys.

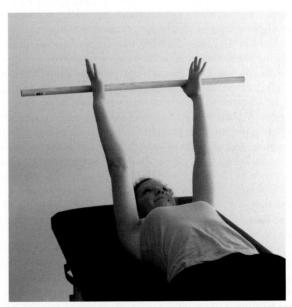

FIGURE 6-6 Active assisted range of motion of the shoulder with the use of a dowel.

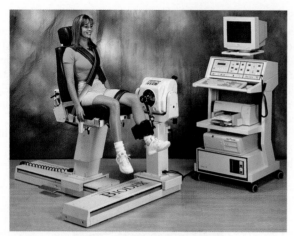

FIGURE 6-7 Isokinetic dynamometer unit set up in a passive mode.

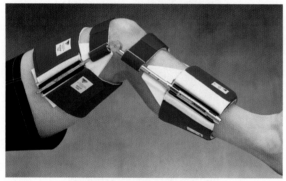

FIGURE 6-8 Knee Dynasplint. *(Photo courtesy Dynasplint Systems, Severna Park, MD.)*

intervention and are most helpful because longer durations of passive movement can be implemented. Postoperatively, most continuous passive range-of-motion units are not set within a range of motion that provides tissue stretching beyond even the slightest level of discomfort. Rather, movement is facilitated within the range of motion that currently exists, thereby allowing the device to serve as more of a passive component to maintain range of motion and promote joint nutrition. As joint range of motion gradually increases, the controls can be adjusted to allow movement within a larger range of motion. A passive mode can be used on other equipment, including isokinetic units, to permit controlled passive range of motion with a pause to provide a stretch at the end range of motion (Fig. 6-7). Some clinicians and patients alike do not promote the use of continuous passive range-of-motion and isokinetic units as a mechanism to maintain and gain joint range of motion for fear of the patient not being able to understand how to control the unit should any increase in pain be felt during use.

Adjustable dynamic splints can produce prolonged-duration, low-load force. The construction of these devices offers a lower progressive load that can be self-adjusted and graduated as orthotic tolerance time increases (Fig. 6-8). Dynamic splints have been used successfully for the treatment of restrictions in knee and elbow motion.[2,10,86]

Proprioceptive Neuromuscular Facilitation Techniques

PNF can be defined as a method of promoting or hastening the response of neuromuscular mechanisms through stimulation of mechanoreceptors.[56,87] PNF stretching techniques are based on a reduction in sensory activity through the spinal reflexes to cause relaxation of the muscle to be stretched. Sherrington's principle of reciprocal inhibition demonstrates relaxation of the muscle being stretched (agonist) through voluntary concentric contraction of its opposite (antagonist) muscle.[56,64,70] Many studies [58,59-61,64-68,70,71,88,89] support the efficacy of PNF and show greater increases in flexibility when PNF is used rather than static or dynamic stretching techniques. Other investigations [57,62,63,69,72] have found PNF to be at least as effective as other types of stretching. Originally, PNF was described as a rehabilitation technique for those recovering from neurologic disorders,[56] but the technique has the capability of being used for various orthopedic conditions as well.[66,68,90-97]

PNF patterns can be performed in a single plane, such as flexion-extension, or in rotational and diagonal patterns that incorporate multiple planes and synergistic patterns (Table 6-1). PNF techniques generally consist of five 5-second trials of passive stretching followed by a 5- to 10-second maximal voluntary contraction, as indicated by the technique used. The work of Cornelius et al[59] has shown that significant increases in systolic blood pressure occur after three trials consisting of a protocol of 5 seconds of passive stretching, followed by a 6-second maximal voluntary antagonist contraction. Thus, caution is warranted when one works with populations who have a predisposition to cardiovascular conditions.

CONTRACT-RELAX

The contract-relax technique[61,65,66,87,98] produces increased range of motion in the agonist pattern by using consecutive isotonic contractions of the antagonist. Box 6-3 outlines how this technique is performed.

The procedure is repeated several times, followed by the athlete moving actively through the obtained range (Fig. 6-9). When performing the contract-relax technique, the clinician must maintain proper stabilization to ensure that an isometric contraction occurs.

HOLD-RELAX

Hold-relax[56,58,59,98] is a PNF technique used to increase joint range of motion that is based on an isometric contraction of the antagonist performed against maximal resistance. This technique is done in the same sequence as the contract-relax technique, but because no motion is allowed on isometric contraction, this is the method of choice when joint restriction is accompanied by muscle spasm and pain. The intensity of each contraction is gradually increased with each successive repetition (Fig. 6-10).

SLOW REVERSAL HOLD-RELAX

The slow reversal hold-relax technique[56,87] uses reciprocal inhibition, as does the hold-relax technique. Box 6-4 outlines how this technique is performed. The technique is good for increasing range of motion when the primary limiting factor is the antagonist muscle group (Fig. 6-11).

Special Considerations for Proprioceptive Neuromuscular Facilitation

Proprioceptive neuromuscular feedback depends not only on the performance of an athlete but also on the ability of the clinician to provide appropriate and timely verbal and tactile commands.

Table 6-1 Upper and Lower Diagonal Proprioceptive Neuromuscular Facilitation Patterns

	Diagonal 1		Diagonal 2	
Extremity	Flexion	Extension	Flexion	Extension
Upper				
Scapula	Elevation	Depression	Elevation	Depression
Shoulder	Flexion	Extension	Flexion	Extension
	Adduction	Abduction	Abduction	Adduction
	External rotation	Internal rotation	External rotation	Internal rotation
Elbow	Flexion	Extension	Flexion	Extension
Forearm	Supination	Pronation	Supination	Pronation
Wrist	Radial deviation	Ulnar deviation	Radial deviation	Ulnar deviation
Fingers	Flexion	Extension	Extension	Flexion
Lower				
Pelvis	Elevation	Depression	Elevation	Depression
Hip	Flexion	Extension	Flexion	Extension
	Adduction	Abduction	Abduction	Adduction
	External rotation	Internal rotation	Internal rotation	External rotation
Knee	Flexion	Extension	Flexion	Extension
Ankle	Dorsiflexion	Plantar flexion	Dorsiflexion	Plantar flexion
Foot	Inversion	Eversion	Eversion	Inversion
Toes	Extension	Flexion	Extension	Flexion

Box 6-3

Contract-Relax Technique

1. The body part to be stretched is moved passively into the agonist pattern until limitation of range of motion is felt.
2. The athlete contracts isotonically into the antagonist pattern against strong manual resistance.
3. When the clinician realizes that relaxation has occurred, the body part is again moved passively into as much range of motion as possible until limitation is again felt.

Verbal commands, such as "contract" and "relax," must be made clear and at the precise moment to enhance gains in range of motion and minimize any associated discomfort. Hand placement by the clinician also provides tactile feedback and serves to inform the athlete into what direction a joint should be moving and with how much resistance. The limitations that exist will help dictate which PNF pattern is appropriate and how much resistance should be applied during performance of the technique.

Although specific patterns and techniques have been identified, it is also important for the athlete to progress through increasing levels of difficulty if one chooses to use a PNF technique to increase range of motion and muscle strength. Figure 6-12 demonstrates an upper extremity diagonal pattern that has been modified from the traditional supine position.

Although not in accordance with standard teachings of true PNF techniques, use of the PNF upper extremity diagonal "2" extension pattern in a seated position not only applies similar resistance as when it is performed supine but also requires the athlete to develop trunk control without the assistance of gravity or a table. This modification more closely resembles an individual who may be preparing to throw a baseball or football.

Clinical Pearl #1

Consider the activity and position when choosing PNF techniques for athletes in an attempt to closely simulate sport-specific function, proprioception, and gains in strength; clear and concise verbal commands will assist in optimal performance of an athlete during PNF exercises. To closely simulate sport performance, patterns and positioning may be modified.

JOINT MOBILIZATION

Techniques

Manual joint mobilization techniques are a form of passive range of motion used to improve joint arthrokinematics. Proper use of mobilization helps facilitate healing, reduce disability, relieve pain, and restore full range of motion.[99] The traditional approach to restoring loss of joint motion is to apply a passive sustained stretch without regard to a defined cause of limitation in motion. This can result in increased stimulation of pain receptors and reflexive contraction of muscles, which may interfere with attempts to increase motion.[100,101] The traditional approach is not necessarily effective if the joint restriction is related to capsuloligamentous adhesions. These adhesions need to be treated in a different manner that incorporates stretching of the joint capsule structures, referred to as accessory motion. Table 6-2 compares physiologic (stretching) and accessory (mobilization) movement techniques.[101]

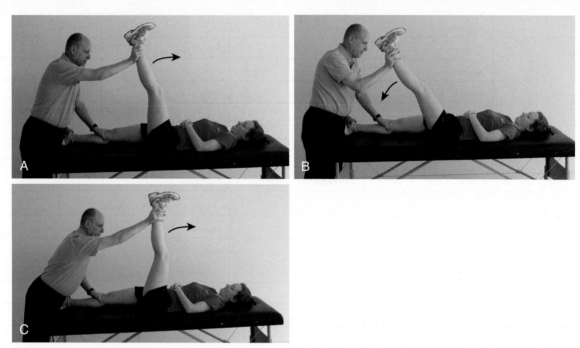

FIGURE 6-9 Contract-relax proprioceptive neuromuscular facilitation pattern for the hamstrings. **A,** The body part is moved passively by the clinician into the agonist pattern until limitation is felt. **B,** The athlete performs an isotonic contraction through the antagonist pattern. **C,** The clinician applies a passive stretch into the agonist pattern until limitation is felt. The procedure is repeated.

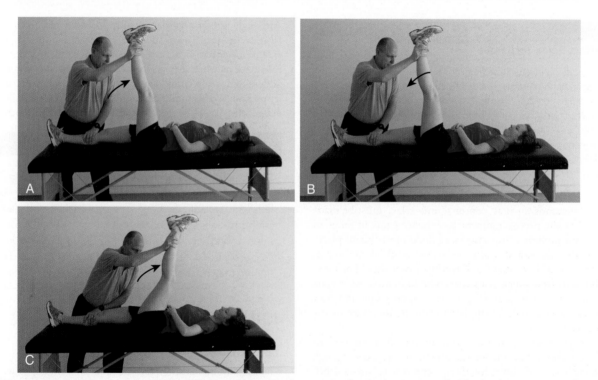

FIGURE 6-10 Hold-relax proprioceptive neuromuscular facilitation pattern for the hamstrings. **A,** The body part is moved passively by the clinician into the agonist pattern until limitation is felt. **B,** The athlete then performs an isometric contraction into the antagonist pattern. **C,** The clinician applies a passive stretch into the agonist pattern until limitation is felt. The procedure is repeated.

Joint mobilization techniques emphasize accessory motion. Accessory motion occurs between the two articulating surfaces and is described by the terms *roll*, *glide*, and *spin*. A roll involves multiple surfaces of a moving bone coming in contact with multiple surfaces of a stationary bone. A glide involves the same surface of a moving bone coming in contact with multiple surfaces of a stationary bone. A spin involves multiple surfaces of the moving bone coming in contact with the same surface of a stationary bone. Both rolling and gliding motions occur simultaneously at some point in the range of motion[29] (Fig. 6-13).

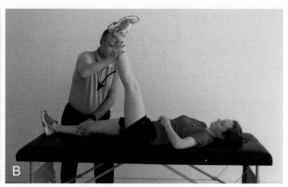

Box 6-4

Slow Reversal Hold-Relax Technique

1. The body part is moved actively into the agonist pattern to the point of pain-free limitation.
2. An isometric contraction is performed in the antagonist pattern for a 5- to 10-second hold.
3. The agonist muscle group actively brings the body part into a greater range of motion in the agonist pattern.
4. The process is repeated several times.

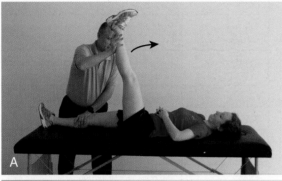

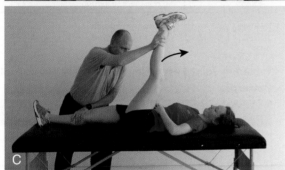

FIGURE 6-11 Slow reversal hold-relax proprioceptive neuromuscular facilitation pattern for the hamstrings. **A,** The athlete performs an active movement of the body part into the agonist pattern. **B,** The athlete then performs an isometric contraction into the antagonist pattern. **C,** The athlete next actively moves the body part further into the agonist pattern. The procedure is repeated.

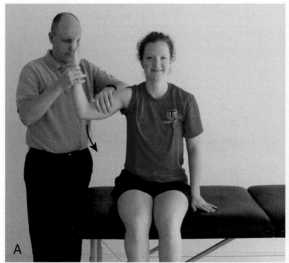

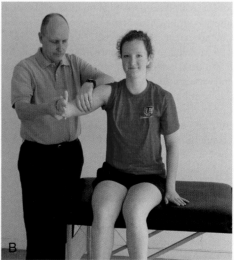

FIGURE 6-12 A and **B,** Demonstration of the proprioceptive neuromuscular facilitation upper extremity diagonal "2" pattern for extension with the athlete seated.

Table 6-2 Stretching Versus Mobilization

Stretching	Mobilization
Used when muscular resistance is encountered	Used when ligament or capsule resistance is encountered
Effective only at the end of the physiologic range of motion	Performed at any point in the range of motion
Limited to one direction	Can be done in any direction
Increased pain with increased range of motion	Decreased pain with increased range of motion
Used for tight muscular structures	Used for tight articular structures
Uses long–lever arm techniques	Safer—uses short–lever arm techniques

From Quillen, W.S., Halle, J.S., and Rouillier, L.H. (1992): Manual therapy: Mobilization of the motion-restricted shoulder. J. Sports Rehabil., 1:237–248.

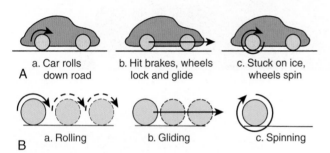

A
a. Car rolls down road   b. Hit brakes, wheels lock and glide   c. Stuck on ice, wheels spin

B
a. Rolling   b. Gliding   c. Spinning

FIGURE 6-13 A and **B,** Types of accessory motion: a, rolling; b, gliding; c, spinning. (From Konin, J.G. [1999]: Practical Kinesiology for the Physical Therapist Assistant. Thorofare, NJ, Slack, p. 37.)

Because accessory motion is necessary for physiologic motion to occur, an assessment to determine the cause of the restricted motion is necessary. When restriction of a joint is assessed on passive movement, it should be determined whether the restriction is in a capsular or noncapsular pattern. A capsular pattern is found only in synovial joints that are controlled by muscles.[102] Capsular patterns or restrictions indicate loss of mobility of the entire joint capsule as a result of fibrosis, effusion, or inflammation. Capsular and noncapsular patterns can be differentiated by noting the end-feel at the extremes of movement. The end-feels described in Table 6-3 may be normal or pathologic.[103] Joint restrictions from noncapsular patterns fall into three categories: ligament adhesions, internal derangement, and extraarticular limitations[103] (Table 6-4).

It is also important to recognize that an end-feel may be normal or abnormal depending on where it occurs within one's range of motion. For example, as the elbow moves into full extension, the resultant end range of motion should be a bony end-feel. However, if the athlete has a loose body floating in the joint, the elbow may be limited in achieving full range of motion. Although Cyriax[103] described this as being a form of internal derangement, it will nonetheless feel like a bony end-feel to the examining clinician. Likewise, elbow flexion normally has the end-feel of a soft tissue approximation when no restrictions exist. However, if the elbow joint has a significant amount of swelling within it after an acute injury, the total amount of elbow flexion may be limited, yet a soft tissue approximation end-feel may continue to exist.

Table 6-3 Normal and Pathologic End-Feel

End-Feel	Description and Example
Normal	
Capsular	Firm; forcing the shoulder into full external rotation
Bony	Abrupt; moving the elbow into full extension
Soft tissue	Soft; flexing the normal knee or elbow approximation
Muscular	Rubbery; tension of tight hamstrings
Pathologic	
Adhesions and scarring	Sudden; sharp arrest in one direction
Muscle spasm	Rebound; usually accompanies pain felt at the end of restriction
Loose	Ligamentous laxity; a hypermobile joint
Boggy	Soft, mushy; joint effusion
Internal derangement	Springy; mechanical block such as a torn meniscus
Empty	No resistance to motion

Data from Cyriax, J.H. (1975): Textbook of Orthopaedic Medicine, Vol. 1. Diagnosis of Soft Tissue Lesions, 6th ed. Baltimore, Williams & Wilkins.

Table 6-4 Joint Restrictions Caused by Noncapsular Patterns

Type	Description
Ligament adhesions	These occur when adhesions form about a ligament after an injury and may cause pain or a restriction in mobility. Some movements will be painful, some are slightly limited, and some are pain free.
Internal derangement	The restriction in joint mobility is the result of a loose fragment within the joint. The onset is sudden, pain is localized, and movements that engage against the block are limited, whereas all others are free.
Extraarticular limitation	The loss in joint mobility results from adhesions in structures outside the joint. Movements that stress the adhesion will be limited and painful.

Physiologic Effects

Joint mobilization techniques serve to restore the accessory motions. The effects of joint mobilization include mitigating capsular restrictions and breaking adhesions, distracting impacted tissue, and providing movement and lubrication for normal articular cartilage. Pain reduction and decreased muscle tension are achieved through the stimulation of fast-conducting fibers (type A-β and A-α fibers) to block small pain fibers (type C afferent fibers) and through the activation of dynamic mechanoreceptors to produce reflexive relaxation. Joint mobilization is indicated for the treatment of capsular restrictions. Contraindications and precautions are listed in Box 6-5.[71,102,104]

Box 6-5

Contraindications to and Precautions for Joint Mobilization

CONTRAINDICATIONS

Premature stressing of surgical structures
Vascular disease
Hypermobility
Advanced osteoarthritis
Acute inflammation
Neurologic signs
Infection
Congenital bone deformities
Fractures
Osteoporosis
Malignancy
Rheumatoid arthritis
Spondylolysis/spondylolisthesis
Paget disease
Tuberculosis
Vertebral artery insufficiency
Spinal cord instability

PRECAUTIONS

Unexplained pain
Onset of new symptoms
Joint ankylosis
Protective muscle spasm
Scoliosis
Pregnancy

Data from Barak, T., Rosen, E.R., and Sofer, R. (1990): Basic concepts of orthopaedic manual therapy. In: Gould, J.A. (ed.). Orthopaedic and Sports Physical Therapy. St. Louis, Mosby, pp. 195–211; Prentice, W.E. (1992): Techniques of manual therapy for the knee. J. Sport Rehabil., 1:249–257; Wadsworth, C.T. (1988): Manual Examination and Treatment of the Spine and Extremities. Baltimore, Williams & Wilkins, p. 27; and Edmond, S.L. (1993): Manipulation and Mobilization. St. Louis, Mosby, pp. 8–9.

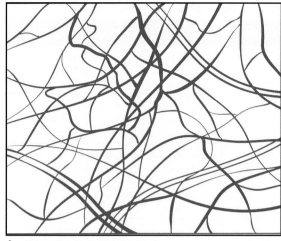

A   Wound collagen, unstressed

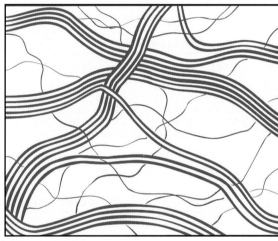

B   Wound collagen, stressed

FIGURE 6-14 Unstressed (**A**) and stressed (**B**) wound collagen. In the wound subject to stress, collagen reorganizes with larger, more parallel aligned fibers. *(From Hertling, D., and Kessler, R.M. [1996]: Management of Common Musculoskeletal Disorders: Physical Therapy Principles and Methods, 3rd ed. Philadelphia, Lippincott, p. 56.)*

One of the important factors that one should consider before the application of a joint mobilization technique is the underlying history. Many capsular and ligamentous adhesions form as a result of a traumatic injury and subsequently as a result of disuse of the joint. A common example is seen in the shoulder, where a person may have a rotator cuff tear. If not treated immediately, the individual may simply opt to not use the affected arm because raising it and performing daily activities are quite painful. As healing tissue forms, the fibers are "laid down" in close approximation to each other and not with optimal elasticity (nonbiased tissue formation) because the joint is not being moved under controlled circumstances.[55] With adequate and controlled movement and stress, the tissue would have a better chance of healing via joint nutrition and lubrication associated with movement and the application of gentle stress to the healing tissue to allow optimal growth and regeneration (biased tissue formation) (Fig. 6-14). In a case such as this, performance of joint mobilization to dissemble the resultant scar tissue would confer added risk because the underlying pathologic condition may be affected with use of a technique that is too aggressive. This becomes a more critical factor if the underlying pathologic condition is joint instability.

Clinical Pearl #2

Mobilization of any joint should be performed with extreme caution when the underlying pathologic condition is known to be instability.

Fundamentals

Systems of Grading Mobilization

Systems of grading joint mobilization have been described by Maitland,[105] Kaltenborn,[106] and Paris.[107] Maitland[105] described five grades of mobilization techniques (Table 6-5). Grade I and grade II mobilizations are used primarily for the treatment of pain, and grades III and IV are used for treating stiffness. It is necessary to treat pain first and stiffness second.[105]

Table 6-5 Grades of Mobilization Techniques

Grade	Description
I	Small-amplitude movement at the beginning of the range of motion that is used when pain and spasm limit movement early in the range of motion
II	Large-amplitude movement within the midrange of motion that is used when slowly increasing pain restricts movement halfway into the range
III	Large-amplitude movement up to the pathologic limit of the range of motion that is used when pain and resistance as a result of spasm, inert tissue tension, or tissue compression limit movement near the end of the range
IV	Small-amplitude movement at the very end of the range of motion that is used when resistance limits movement in the absence of pain and spasm
V	Small-amplitude, quick thrust delivered at the end of the range of motion that is usually accompanied by a popping sound called a cavitation

Data from Maitland, G.D. (1977): Extremity Manipulation, 2nd ed. London, Butterworth.

Table 6-6 Kaltenborn's Stages of Traction

Stage	Description
I (Piccolo)	This is traction that neutralizes pressure in the joint without actual separation of the joint surfaces. The purpose is to relieve pain by reducing grinding when performing mobilization techniques. This stage is analogous to a grade I mobilization.
II (Take up the slack)	This is traction that effectively separates the articulating surfaces and takes up the slack or eliminates play in the joint capsule. Stage II is used to relieve pain and is the same as a grade IV mobilization.
III (Stretch)	This is traction that involves actual stretching of the soft tissue surrounding the joint for the purpose of increasing mobility in a hypomobile joint.

Data from Kaltenborn, F.M. (1980): Mobilization of the Extremity Joints: Examination and Basic Treatment Techniques. Oslo, Olaf Noris Bokhandel; and Prentice, W.E. (1992): Techniques of manual therapy for the knee. J. Sport Rehabil., 1:249–257.

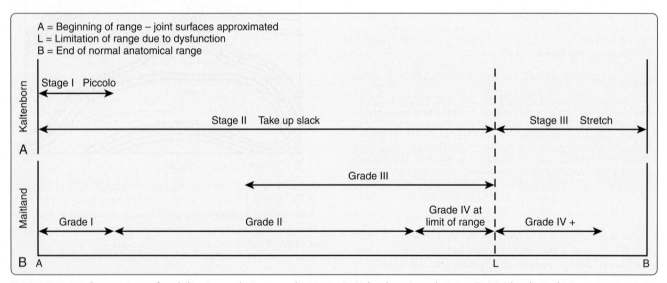

FIGURE 6-15 Comparison of mobilization technique applications. **A,** Kaltenborn's technique. **B,** Maitland's technique. *(From Barak, T., Rosen, E.R., and Sofer, R. [1990]: Basic concepts of orthopaedic manual therapy. In: Gould, J.A. [ed.], Orthopaedic and Sports Physical Therapy, 2nd ed. St. Louis, Mosby, pp. 195–211.)*

Traction is used to separate the joint surfaces to varying degrees into an open-packed position to increase the mobility of the joint.[29,108] Kaltenborn[106] proposed a system that uses traction combined with mobilization as a means of reducing pain or mobilizing hypomobile joints. All joints have some looseness that is described by Kaltenborn as slack, and some degree of slack is necessary for normal joint motion. Kaltenborn's stages of traction are described in Table 6-6.[106] It has been recommended that 10-second intermittent stage I and stage II traction be used, with distraction of the joint surfaces up to stage III and then releasing the distraction until the joint returns to its resting position.[108] Also, stage III traction should be used with mobilization glides to treat joint hypomobility.[106] Traction and translatory gliding can be applied separately or together in various mobilization techniques (Fig. 6-15).[102]

Joint Position and Application of Force

Successful joint mobilization depends on the position of the joint to be mobilized, the direction of the force, and the magnitude of the force applied. Correct positioning of a joint is

Clinical Pearl #3

When using joint mobilization to increase tissue extensibility, a clinician will often begin with a grade appropriate for pain relief, then move to a grade to increase tissue length, and conclude with a grade of mobilization to once again provide some pain relief.

critical when one mobilizes a joint. A joint may be in either a close-packed or an open-packed position. A joint is in a close-packed position when the joint surfaces are most congruent. In a close-packed position the major ligaments are maximally taut, the intracapsular space is minimal, and the surfaces cannot be pulled apart by traction forces.[102] This position is used as a testing position but is never used for mobilization because there is no freedom of movement.[102] The maximal open-packed position is known as the resting position and is characterized by the surrounding tissues being as lax as possible and the intracapsular space being its greatest.[102] The maximal open-packed position of a joint is the optimal position for joint mobilization.[55,99,102,105,106,109] The open-packed positions of joints have been described by many[71,104,106] and are summarized in Table 6-7.

The direction of the mobilizing force depends on the contour of the joint surface of the structure to be mobilized. In most articulations, one joint surface is considered to be concave and the other convex. The concave-convex rule[105,107] takes these joint surface configurations into account and states that when the concave surface is stationary and the convex surface is mobilized, gliding of the convex segment should be in the direction opposite the restriction in joint movement.[108,109] If the convex articular surface is stationary and the concave surface is mobilized, gliding of the concave segment should be in the same direction as the restriction in joint movement (Fig. 6-16). Typical treatment of a joint may involve a series of three to six mobilizations lasting up to 30 seconds, with one to three oscillations per second.[29] General principles for applying mobilizations are summarized in Box 6-6. The grades of mobilization and stages of traction were described earlier in this chapter. Traction should be used in conjunction with mobilization techniques to treat hypomobile joints. Prentice[108] reported that grade III traction stretches the joint capsule and increases the space between the articulating surfaces, which places the joint in an open-packed position. Applying grade III and grade IV oscillations within the athlete's pain limitations should maximally improve joint mobility.[108] For examples of commonly used joint mobilization techniques, see Figures W6-1 through W6-19 (in Appendix W6) on Expert Consult @ www.expertconsult.com.

Table 6-7 Open- and Closed-Pack Positions of Synovial Joints

Joint	Open Packed	Closed Packed
Facet	Midway between flexion and extension	Extension
TMJ	Mouth slightly open	Mouth closed with the teeth clenched
Glenohumeral	55° to 70° abduction, 30° horizontal adduction	Maximum abduction and external rotation
Acromioclavicular	Arm resting at the side	Arm abducted to 90°
Sternoclavicular	Arm resting at the side	Full coronal abduction, full external rotation
Humeroulnar	70° flexion, 10° supination	Full extension and supination
Humeroradial	70° flexion, 35° supination	90° elbow flexion, 5° supination
Proximal radioulnar	70° elbow flexion, 35° supination	5° supination and full extension
Distal radioulnar	10° supination	5° supination
Radiocarpal	Neutral, slight ulnar deviation	Full extension
Metacarpophalangeal	Slight flexion	Full flexion (2–5) Full extension (1)
Interphalangeal	PIP: 10° flexion DIP: 30°	Full extension
Hip	30° flexion, 30° abduction, and slight external rotation	Full extension, internal rotation, and abduction (ligamentous); 90° flexion, slight abduction, and internal rotation (bony)
Tibiofemoral	25° flexion	Full extension
Talocrural	10° plantar flexion, midway between inversion and eversion	Maximum dorsiflexion
Subtalar	10° plantar flexion and midway between inversion and eversion	Maximum inversion
Midtarsal	10° plantar flexion and midway between pronation and supination	Maximum supination
Tarsometatarsal	Midway between pronation and supination	Maximum supination
Metatarsophalangeal	Midway between flexion and extension, abduction and adduction	Full extension
Interphalangeal	Slight flexion	Full extension

Modified from Edmond, S.L. (1993): Manipulation and Mobilization. St. Louis, Mosby.
DIP, Distal interphalangeal; *PIP,* proximal interphalangeal; *TMJ,* temporomandibular.

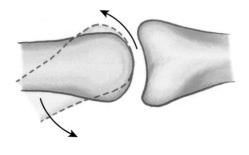

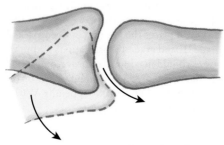

FIGURE 6-16 Convex-concave relationship of movement. *(From Konin, J.G. [1999]: Practical Kinesiology for the Physical Therapist Assistant. Thorofare, NJ, Slack, p. 37.)*

Box 6-6
Joint Mobilization Application Principles

Remove jewelry and rings.
Be relaxed (both the athlete and clinician).
Always examine the contralateral side.
Use an open-packed joint position.
Avoid pain.
Perform smooth, regular oscillations.
Apply each technique for 20-60 seconds.
Repeat each technique only 4-5 times per treatment session; it is easy to overmobilize.
Mobilize daily for pain and 2-3 times per week for restricted motion.
Follow mobilization with active range-of-motion exercises.

Myofascial Release Techniques

Myofascial release techniques have been anecdotally reported as being effective in relieving restrictions and increasing range of motion. These claims have not been well investigated in controlled settings. Hanten and Chandler[61] compared the effectiveness of the PNF contract-relax technique and the myofascial release leg pull technique in increasing hip flexion range of motion. Their results demonstrated significant gains in range of motion after the use of both techniques, but with significantly greater improvements achieved with the contract-relax stretch than with the leg pull.

The focus of myofascial release techniques is on the fascial system, which consists of embryologic tissue.[110] Fascial tissue is a tough connective tissue that assists the tissue that it surrounds in maintaining its shape.[111] Barnes and Smith[112] believed that gentle force applied to fascial tissue will elicit thermal changes

from a vasomotor response and lead to increased blood flow. As a result, they believed that lymphatic drainage improves and optimal structural alignment is allowed to occur.

Kostopoulos and Rizopoulos[113] described the use of myofascial tissue stretching after a trigger point acupressure intervention. Others have reported successful results on restricted soft tissue injuries treated with myofascial release techniques.[39,61,114-116] Myofascial release, like all other treatment interventions, requires that the clinician have a certain level of skill and experience. Effective treatments to achieve improved overall tissue enhancement also depend on the subject's ability to relax and "work" with the clinician.

Clinical Pearl #4

Myofascial release is a skill that requires knowledge of the body's inherent trigger points, awareness of normal versus abnormal tissue tension, and clinical practice to develop a level of expertise for successful treatment intervention.

CONCLUSION

- Changes in range of motion and flexibility can be improved with repetition, frequency, and consistency, which are key to making plastic deformation changes.
- Plastic deformation is achieved with low-force, long-duration stretching.
- Despite the absence of clear conclusive evidence regarding the duration of stretches, one should always keep in mind the practicality of performing too many stretches for too long a time frame, which could deter an athlete from proper technique and compliance.
- It appears that the application of a superficial heat or cold modality in conjunction with stretching results in greater improvements in flexibility than does stretching alone.
- To effectively measure progress, it is important to document on a regular basis changes in flexibility and range of motion.
- Although debate on various stretching techniques continues, ballistic stretching more closely simulates many athletic activities and, if done appropriately, may not pose any greater risk for injury to an athlete than static stretching does.
- Static stretching, ballistic stretching, and PNF can all improve flexibility, each with its own advantages and disadvantages.
- Scientific evidence suggests that PNF results in greater increases in flexibility than do static or dynamic stretching techniques.
- Joint mobilization techniques are used to restore the accessory motions of spin, glide, and roll and are performed with the joint in the open-packed position.
- PNF, joint mobilization, and myofascial release are techniques that can be initiated to complement methods of improving one's flexibility and range of motion. Each requires a sound base of anatomic knowledge combined with clinical experience before proper technique and optimal gains may be seen.

REFERENCES

1. Stap, L.J., and Woodfin, P.M. (1986): Continuous passive motion in the treatment of knee flexion contracture. Phys. Ther., 66:1720–1722.

2. Hepburn, G.R. (1987): Case studies: Contracture and stiff joint management with Dynasplint. J. Orthop. Sports Phys. Ther., 8:498–504.

3. Kottke, F.J., Pauley, D.L., and Ptak, K.A. (1966): The rationale for prolonged stretching for correction of shortening of connective tissue. Arch. Phys. Med. Rehabil., 47:345–352.

4. Sapega, A.A., Quendenfeld, T.C., Moyer, R.A., and Butler, R.A. (1981): Biophysical factors in range of motion exercise. Physician Sportsmed., 9:57–65.

5. Wallin, D., Ekblon, B., Grahn, R., and Nordenborg, T. (1985): Improvement of muscle flexibility. Am. J. Sports Med., 13:263–268.

6. Prentice, W.E. (1999): Restoring range of motion and improving flexibility. In: Prentice, W.E. (ed.), Rehabilitation Techniques in Sports Medicine. New York, McGraw-Hill, pp. 62–72.

7. Bandy, W.D., and Irion, J.M. (1994): The effect of time on static stretch on the flexibility of the hamstring muscles. Phys. Ther., 74:845–852.

8. Gillette, T.M., Holland, G.J., Vincent, W.J., and Loy, S.F. (1991): Relationship of body core temperature and warm-up to knee range of motion. J. Orthop. Sports Phys. Ther., 12:126–131.

9. Godges, J.J., MacRae, P.G., and Engelke, K.A. (1993): Effects of exercise on hip range of motion, trunk muscle performance, and gait economy. Phys. Ther., 73:468–477.

10. Hepburn, G.R., and Crivelli, K.J. (1984): Use of elbow Dynasplint for reduction of elbow flexion contractures: A case study. J. Orthop. Sports Phys. Ther., 5:269–274.

11. Kirkendall, D.T., and Garrett, W.E. (1997): Function and biomechanics of tendons. Scand. J. Med. Sci. Sports, 7:62–66.

12. Laban, N.M. (1962): Collagen tissue: Implications of its response to stress in vitro. Arch. Phys. Med. Rehabil., 43:461–466.

13. Light, K.E., Nuzik, S., Personius, W., and Barstrom, A. (1984): Low load prolonged stretch versus high load restretch in treating knee contractures. Phys. Ther., 64:330–333.

14. Noonan, T.J., Best, T.M., Seaber, A.V., and Garrett, W.E. (1994): Identification of a threshold for skeletal muscle injury. Am. J. Sports Med., 22:257–261.

15. Safran, M.R., Garrett, W.E., Seaber, A.V., et al. (1988): The role of warmup in muscular injury prevention. Am. J. Sports Med., 16:123–129.

16. Stromberg, D., and Wiederhielm, C.A. (1969): Viscoelastic description of a collagenous tissue in simple elongation. J. Appl. Physiol., 26:857–862.

17. Taylor, D.C., Dalton, J.D., Seaber, A.V., and Farrett, W.E. (1990): Viscoelastic properties of muscle-tendon units. The biomechanical effects of stretching. Am. J. Sports Med., 18:300–309.

18. Warren, C.G., Lehmann, J.F., and Koblanski, J.N. (1971): Elongation of rat tail tendon: Effect of load and temperature. Arch. Phys. Med. Rehabil., 52:465–474.

19. Warren, C.G., Lehmann, J.F., and Koblanski, J.N. (1976): Heat and stress procedures: An evaluation using rat tail tendon. Arch. Phys. Med. Rehabil., 57:122–126.

20. Shrier, M.D., and Gossal, K. (2000): Myths and truths of stretching. Phys. Sports Med., 28:1–11.

21. Lehmann, J.F., and DeLateur, B.J. (1982): Therapeutic heat. In: Lehmann J.F. (ed.). Therapeutic Heat and Cold. Baltimore, Lippincott Williams & Wilkins, pp. 404–405, 428.

22. Lehmann, J.F., DeLateur, B.J., and Silverman, D.R. (1966): Selective heating effects of ultrasound in human beings. Arch. Phys. Med. Rehabil., 47:331–339.

23. Lehmann, J.F., Masock, A.J., Warren, C.G., and Koblanski, J.N. (1970): Effect of therapeutic temperatures on tendon extensibility. Arch. Phys. Med. Rehabil., 51:481–487.

24. Wiktorsson, M.M., Oberg, B., Ekstrand, J., and Gillquist, J. (1988): Effects of warming up, massage, and stretching and range of motion for muscle strength in the lower extremity. Am. J. Sports Med., 11:249–252.

25. Lentell, G., Hetherington, T., Eagan, J., and Morgan, M. (1992): The use of thermal agents to influence the effectiveness of a low-load prolonged stretch. J. Orthop. Sports Phys. Ther., 16:200–207.

26. Draper, D.O., and Ricard, M.D. (1995): Rate of temperature decay in human muscle following 3 MHz ultrasound: The stretching window revealed. J. Athl. Train., 30:304–307.

27. Rose, S., Draper, D.O., Schulthies, S.S., and Durrant, E. (1996): The stretching window part two: Rate of thermal decay in deep muscle following 1-MHz ultrasound. J. Athl. Train., 31:139–143.

28. Brodowicz, G.R., Welsh, R., and Wallis, J. (1996): Comparison of stretching with ice, stretching with heat, or stretching alone on hamstring flexibility. J. Athl. Train., 31:324–327.

29. Prentice, W.E. (1992): Techniques of manual therapy for the knee. J. Sport Rehabil., 1:249–257.

30. Brosseau, L., Balmer, S., Tousignant, M., et al. (2001): Intra- and intertester reliability and criterion validity of the parallelogram and universal goniometers for measuring maximum active knee flexion and extension of patients with knee restrictions. Arch. Phys. Med. Rehabil., 82:396–402.

31. Ellis, B., Burton, A., and Goddard, J.R. (1997): Joint angle measurement: A comparative study of the reliability of goniometry and wire tracking for the hand. Clin. Rehabil., 11:314–320.

32. Gajdosik, R.L., and Bohannon, R.W. (1987): Clinical measurements of range of motion. Review of goniometry emphasizing reliability and validity. Phys. Ther., 67:1862–1872.

33. Goodwin, J., Clark, C., Deakes, J., et al. (1992): Clinical methods of goniometry: A comparative study. Disabil. Rehabil., 14:10–15.

34. Groth, G.N., VanDeven, K.M., Phillips, E.C., and Ehretsman, R.L. (2001): Goniometry of the proximal and distal interphalangeal joint. Part II: Placement preferences, interrater reliability and concurrent validity. J. Hand Ther., 14:23–29.

35. Hayes, K., Walton, J.R., Szomor, Z.R., and Murrell, G.A. (2001): Reliability of five methods of assessing shoulder range of motion. Aust. J. Physiother. 47:289–294.

36. MacDermid, J.C., Chesworth, B.M., Patterson, S., and Roth, J.H. (1999): Intratester and intertester reliability of goniometric measurement of passive lateral shoulder rotation. J. Hand Ther., 12:187–192.

37. Riddle, D.L., Rothstein, J.M., and Lamb, R.L. (1987): Goniometric reliability in a clinical setting: Shoulder measurement. Phys. Ther., 667:668–673.

38. Watkins, M.A., Riddle, D.L., Lamb, R.L., and Personius, W.J. (1991): Reliability of goniometric measurements and visual estimates of knee range of motion obtained in a clinical setting. Phys. Ther., 71:90–96.

39. Hui, S.S., and Yuen, P.Y. (2000): Validity of the modified back-saver sit-and-reach test: A comparison with other products. Med. Sci. Sports Exerc., 32:1655–1659.

40. Jones, C.J., Rikli, R.E., Max, J., and Noffal, G. (1988): The reliability and validity of a chair sit-and-reach test as a measure of hamstring flexibility in older adults. Res. Q. Exerc. Sport, 69:338–343.

41. Patterson, P., Wiksten, D.L., Ray, L., et al. (1996): The validity and reliability of the back saver sit-and-reach test in middle school girls and boys. Res. Q. Exerc. Sport, 67:448–451.

42. Cooperman, J.M., Riddle, D.L., and Rothstein, J.M. (1990): Reliability and validity of judgments of the integrity of the anterior cruciate ligament of the knee using the Lachman's test. Phys. Ther., 70:225–233.

43. Elveru, R.A., Rothstein, J.M., Lamb, R.L., and Riddle, D.L. (1988): Methods for taking subtalar joint measurements. A clinical report. Phys. Ther., 68:678–682.

44. Hayes, K.W., Peterson, C., and Falconer, J. (1994): An examination of Cyriax's passive motion tests with patients having osteoarthritis of the knee. Phys. Ther., 74:697–709.

45. McClure, P.W., Rothstein, J.M., and Riddle, D.L. (1989): Intertester reliability of clinical judgments of medial knee ligament integrity. Phys. Ther., 69:268–275.

46. Balasch, H., Schiller, M., Friebel, H., and Hoffman, F. (1999): Evaluation of anterior knee joint instability with the Rolimeter: A test in comparison with manual assessment knee joint instability with the KT-1000 arthrometer. Knee Surg. Traumatol. Arthrosc., 7:204–208.

47. Ganko, A., Engebretson, L., and Ozer, H. (2000): The Rolimeter: A new arthrometer compared with the KT-1000. Knee Surg. Sports Traumatol. Arthrosc., 8:36–39.

48. Kovaleski, J.E., Gurchiek, L.R., Heitman, R.J., et al. (1999): Instrumented measurement of anteroposterior and inversion-eversion laxity of the normal ankle joint complex. Foot Ankle Int., 20:808–814.

49. Muellner, T., Bugge, W., Johansen, S., et al. (2001): Inter- and intratester comparison of the Rolimeter knee tester: Effect of tester's experience and the examination technique. Knee Surg. Sports Traumatol. Arthrosc., 9:302–306.

50. Pizzari, T., Kolt, G.S., and Remedios, L. (1999): Measurement of anterior-to-posterior translation of the glenohumeral joint using the KT-1000. J. Orthop. Sports Phys. Ther., 29:602–608.

51. Beaulieu, L.A. (1981): Developing a stretching program. Phys. Sports Med., 9:59–65.

52. Shellock, F.G., and Prentice, W.E. (1989): Warming-up and stretching for improved physical performance and prevention of sports-related injuries. Sports Med., 2:267–278.

53. Stamford, B. (1984): Flexibility and stretching. Phys. Sports Med., 12:171.

54. Stark, S.D. (1997): Stretching techniques. In: Stark, S.D. (ed.). The Stark Reality of Stretching. Richmond, BC, Stark Reality Publishing, pp. 73–80.

55. Hertling, D., and Kessler, R.M. (1996): Management of Common Musculoskeletal Disorders: Physical Therapy Principles and Methods, 3rd ed. Philadelphia, Lippincott Williams & Wilkins, p. 19.

56. Knott, M., and Voss, D.E. (1968): Proprioceptive Neuromuscular Facilitation, 2nd ed. New York, Harper & Row.

57. Condom, S.M., and Hutton, R.S. (1987): Soleus muscle electromyographic activity and ankle dorsiflexion range of motion during four stretching procedures. Phys. Ther., 67:24–30.

58. Cornelius, W.L., Ebrahim, K., Watson, J., and Hill, D.W. (1992): The effects of cold application and modified PNF stretching techniques on hip joint flexibility in college males. Res. Q. Exerc. Sport, 63:311–314.

59. Cornelius, W.L., Jensen, R.L., and Odell, M.E. (1995): Effects of PNF stretching phases on acute arterial blood pressure. Can. J. Appl. Physiol., 20:222–229.

60. Etnyre, B.R., and Abraham, L.D. (1986): Gains in range of ankle dorsiflexion using three popular stretching techniques. Am. J. Phys. Med., 65:189–196.

61. Hanten, W.P., and Chandler, S.D. (1994): Effects of myofascial release leg pull and sagittal plane isometric contract-relax techniques on passive straight leg raise angle. J. Orthop. Sports Phys. Ther., 20:138–144.

62. Lucas, R.C., and Koslow, R. (1984): Comparative study of static, dynamic, and proprioceptive neuromuscular facilitation stretching techniques on flexibility. Percept. Motor Skills, 58:615–618.

63. Medeiros, J.M., Smidt, G.L., Burmeister, L.F., and Soderbert, G.L. (1977): The influence of isometric exercise and passive stretch on hip joint motion. Phys. Ther., 57:518–523.

64. Moore, M.A., and Hutton, R.S. (1980): Electromyographic investigation of muscle stretching technique. Med. Sci. Sports Exerc., 12:322–329.

65. Osternig, L.R., Robertson, R., Troxel, R., and Hansen, P. (1987): Muscle activation during proprioceptive neuromuscular facilitation (PNF) stretching techniques. Am. J. Phys. Med., 66:298–307.

66. Osternig, L.R., Robertson, R.N., Troxel, R.K., and Hansen, P. (1990): Differential responses to proprioceptive neuromuscular facilitation (PNF) stretch techniques. Med. Sci. Sports Exerc., 22:106–111.

67. Prentice, W.E. (1983): A comparison of static stretching and PNF stretching for improving hip joint flexibility. Athl. Train., 18:56–59.

68. Sady, S.P., Wortman, M., and Blanke, D. (1982): Flexibility training: Ballistic, static, or proprioceptive neuromuscular facilitation? Arch. Phys. Med. Rehabil., 63:261–263.

69. Sullivan, M., Dejulia, J.J., and Worrell, T.W. (1992): Effects of pelvic position and stretching method on hamstring muscle flexibility. Med. Sci. Sports Exerc., 24:1383–1389.

70. Tanijawa, M.D. (1972): Comparison of the hold relax procedure in passive immobilization on increasing muscle length. Phys. Ther., 52:725–735.

71. Wadsworth, C.T. (1988): Manual Examination and Treatment of the Spine and Extremities. Baltimore, Williams & Wilkins, p. 27.

72. Worrell, T.W., Smith, T.L., and Winegardner, J. (1994): Effect of hamstring stretching on hamstring muscle performance. J. Orthop. Sports Phys. Ther., 20:154–159.

73. Travell, J.G., and Simons, D.G. (1983): Myofascial Pain and Dysfunction: The Trigger Point Manual. Baltimore, Williams & Wilkins.

74. Travell, J.G., and Simons, D.G. (1992): Myofascial Pain and Dysfunction: The Trigger Point Manual. The Lower Extremity. Baltimore, Williams & Wilkins.

75. Vallentyne, S.W., and Vallentyne, J.R. (1988): The case of the missing ozone: Are physiatrists to blame? Arch. Phys. Med. Rehabil., 69:992–993.

76. Simons, D.G., Travell, J.G., and Simons, L.S. (1990): Protecting the ozone layer. Arch. Phys. Med. Rehabil., 71:64.

77. Houglum, P.A. (2001): Therapeutic Exercise for Athletic Injuries. Champaign, IL, Human Kinetics, p. 170.

78. Ingber, R. (1999): Myofascial Pain in Lumbar Dysfunction. Philadelphia, Hanley & Belfus.

79. Beaupre, L.A., Davies, D.M., Jones, C.A., and Cintas, J.G. (2001): Exercise combined with continuous passive motion or slider board therapy compared with exercise only: A randomized controlled trial of patients following total knee arthroplasty. Phys. Ther., 81:1029–1037.

80. Ferrari, J., Higgins, J.P., and Williams, R.L. (2000): Intervention for treating hallux valgus (abductovalgus) and bunions. Cochrane Database Syst. Rev., 2:CD000964.

81. Gasper, L., Farkas, C., Szepesi, K., and Csernatomy, Z. (1997): Therapeutic value of continuous passive motion after cruciate ligament replacement. Acta Chir. Hung., 36:104–105.

82. Lastayo, P.C., Wright, T., Jaffe, R., and Hartzel, J. (1998): Continuous passive motion after repair of the rotator cuff: A prospective outcome study. J. Bone Joint Surg. Am., 80:1002–1011.

83. Lau, S.K., and Chiu, K.Y. (2001): Use of continuous passive motion after total knee arthroplasty. J. Arthroplasty, 16:336–339.

84. McCarthy, M.R., Yates, C.K., Anderson, M.A., and Yates-McCarthy, J.L. (1993): The effects of immediate continuous passive motion on pain during the inflammatory phase of soft tissue following anterior cruciate ligament reconstruction. J. Orthop. Sports Phys. Ther., 17:96–101.

85. O'Driscoll, S.W., and Giori, N.J. (2000): Continuous passive motion (CPM): Theory and principles of clinical application. J. Rehabil. Res. Dev., 37:179–188.

86. Bonutti, P.M., Windau, J.E., Ables, B.A., and Miller, B.G. (1994): Static progressive stretch to reestablish elbow range of motion. Clin. Orthop. Relat. Res., 303:128–134.

87. Voss, D.E., Ionta, M.K., and Myers, B.J. (1985): Proprioceptive Neuromuscular Facilitation: Patterns and Techniques, 3rd ed. Philadelphia, Harper & Row.

88. Cornelius, W.L., and Craft-Hamm, K. (1988): Proprioceptive neuromuscular facilitation flexibility techniques: Acute effects on arterial blood pressure. Physician Sportsmed., 16:152–161.

89. Godges, J.J., MacRae, H., Longdon, C., et al. (1989): The effects of two stretching procedures on hip range of motion and gait economy. J. Orthop. Sports Phys. Ther., 11:350–357.

90. Galilee-Belfer, A. (1999): The Effect of Modified PNF Trunk Strengthening on Functional Performance in Female Rowers. Eugene, OR, University of Oregon, Microform Publications.

91. Havanloo, F., and Parkhotik, I. (2000): Rehabilitation process of patients with brachial plexus injury. Exerc. Soc. J. Sport Sci., 25:286.

92. McAttee, R.E. (1993): A variation of PNF stretching that's safer and more effective. Track Field Q. Rev., 93:53–54.

93. McCullen, J., and Uhl, T.L. (2000): A kinetic chain approach for shoulder rehabilitation. J. Athl. Train., 35:329–337.

94. Ninos, J. (2001): PNF-self stretching techniques. J. Strength Cond., 23:28–29.

95. Spernoga, S.G., Uhl, T.L., Arnold, B.L., and Gansneder, B.M. (2001): Duration of maintained hamstring flexibility after a one-time, modified hold-relax stretching protocol. J. Athl. Train., 36:44–48.

96. Stanley, S.N., Knappstein, A., and McNair, P.J. (1999): How long do the immediate increases in flexibility last after a PNF stretching session? Presented at the Fifth IOC World Congress on Sport Sciences, Canberra, Australia.

97. Surburg, P.R., and Schrader, J.W. (1997): Proprioceptive neuromuscular facilitation techniques in sports medicine: A reassessment. J. Athl. Train., 32:34–39.

98. Sullivan, P.E., and Markos, P.D. (1987): Clinical Procedures in Therapeutic Exercise. Norwalk, CT, Appleton & Lange.

99. Mennell, J. (1964): Joint Pain. Boston, Little, Brown.

100. Quillen, W.S., and Gieck, J.H. (1988): Manual therapy: Mobilization of the motion-restricted knee. Athl. Train., 23:123–130.

101. Quillen, W.S., Halle, J.S., and Rouillier, L.H. (1992): Manual therapy: Mobilization of the motion-restricted shoulder. J. Sport Rehabil., 1:237–248.

102. Barak, T., Rosen, E.R., and Sofer, R. (1990): Basic concepts of orthopaedic manual therapy. In: Gould J.A. (ed.). Orthopaedic and Sports Physical Therapy. St. Louis, Mosby, pp. 195–211.

103. Cyriax, J.H. (1975): Textbook of Orthopaedic Medicine, Vol. I, Diagnosis of Soft Tissue Lesions, 6th ed. Baltimore, Williams & Wilkins.

104. Edmond, S.L. (1993): Manipulation and Mobilization. St. Louis, Mosby, pp. 8–9.

105. Maitland, G.D. (1977): Extremity Manipulation, 2nd ed. London, Butterworth.

106. Kaltenborn, F.M. (1980): Mobilization of the Extremity Joints. Examination and Basic Treatment Techniques. Oslo, Olaf Noris Bokhandel.

107. Paris, S.V. (1979): Extremity Dysfunction and Mobilization. Atlanta, Institute Press.

108. Prentice, W.E. (1999): Mobilization and traction techniques in rehabilitation. In: Prentice, W.E. (ed.). Rehabilitation Techniques in Sports Medicine. New York, McGraw-Hill, pp. 188–197.

109. Kisner, C., and Colby, L. (2002): Therapeutic Exercise: Foundations and Techniques, 4th ed. Philadelphia, Davis.

110. Davis, C.M. (1997): Complementary Therapies in Rehabilitation. Thorofare, NJ, Slack, pp. 21–47.

111. Scott, J. (1986): Molecules that keep you in shape. New Scientist, 111:49–53.

112. Barnes, J.F., and Smith, G. (1987): The body is a self-correcting mechanism. Phys. Ther. Forum, July, p. 27.

113. Kostopoulos, D., and Rizopoulos, K. (2001): The Manual of Trigger Point and Myofascial Therapy. Thorofare, NJ, Slack, pp. 51–57.

114. Alvarez, D.J., and Rockwell, P.G. (2002): Trigger points: Diagnosis and management. Am. Fam. Physician, 15:653–660.

115. Han, S.C., and Harrison, P. (1997): Myofascial pain syndrome and trigger-point management. Reg. Anesth., 22:89–101.

116. Hanten, W.P., Olson, S.L., Butts, N.L., and Nowicki, A.L. (2000): Effectiveness of a home program of ischemic pressure followed by sustained stretch for treatment of myofascial trigger points. Phys. Ther., 80:997–1003.

7

Principles of Rehabilitation for Muscle and Tendon Injuries

Stacey Pagorek, PT, DPT, SCS, ATC, CSCS, Brian Noehren, PT, PhD, and Terry Malone, PT, EdD, ATC, FAPTA

CHAPTER OBJECTIVES

- Define the muscle-tendon unit.
- Describe the stages of tissue healing and the importance of application of this knowledge in rehabilitation.
- State the mechanism of injury for strains.
- Identify characteristics of the different grades of strains and application of this to rehabilitation.
- Describe the classifications of tendon pathology.

- State key aspects of the clinical evaluation.
- Identify rehabilitation principles for acute and chronic injuries and design appropriate rehabilitation interventions.
- Describe rehabilitation treatment techniques for common muscle-tendon pathologies.

Injury to muscle and tendon structures can substantially affect individual joint mobility and stability. Furthermore, muscle and tendon injuries can alter movement of the entire body and ultimately limit functional participation in life activities. The goal of this chapter is to aid the clinician in identifying and treating muscle and tendon injuries. Specifically, the objectives of this chapter are to (1) identify basic science components and healing parameters of the muscle-tendon unit, (2) differentially diagnose muscle and tendon pathologies, and (3) discuss evaluation considerations and rehabilitation principles for muscle and tendon injuries.

ANATOMIC COMPONENTS AND TISSUE RESPONSE TO INJURY

Muscles are composed of contractile tissue and are responsible for creating and dissipating force while enabling voluntary movement of the body. Movement of the skeletal system is made possible through the connection of muscle to bone via tendons. Together, muscles and tendons form a complex unit known as the muscle-tendon unit.

Muscle-Tendon Unit

The muscle-tendon unit is composed of a muscle with tendons at each end, and each tendon is attached to bone (Fig. 7-1). The point of connection between muscle and tendon is the myotendinous junction (MTJ), and the point of attachment of tendon to bone is the osseotendinous junction (OTJ). The entire muscle-tendon unit works to produce controlled movement, as well as to stabilize and protect joints. Therefore, when the musculotendinous unit sustains an injury, it often has an impact on joint stability and functional mobility. Injury to the muscle-tendon unit can occur within the body of the muscle or tendon or at their points of attachment. Frequently, the site of injury in the musculotendinous unit is at the MTJ.[1-3] When injury occurs near the OTJ, an avulsion fracture may result, with the bony insertion separated from the bone (Fig. 7-2).

A commonly seen clinical pathology, Osgood-Schlatter disease, occurs when activation of the quadriceps muscle-tendon unit causes the infrapatellar tendon to pull excessively at the OTJ on the tibia. The OTJ becomes inflamed, and contraction of the quadriceps muscle-tendon unit, especially against resistance, causes pain. The pull of the quadriceps muscle-tendon unit causes a small separation at the tibial tubercle, which then results in additional bone growth. Osgood-Schlatter disease is often seen in children who participate in running and jumping activities in which the quadriceps muscle is repeatedly activated. This pathology is also commonly seen during periods of rapid growth when appropriate flexibility of the quadriceps musculotendinous unit is not maintained. The enlargement of the tibial tubercle that occurs with Osgood-Schlatter disease remains even after the symptoms subside.

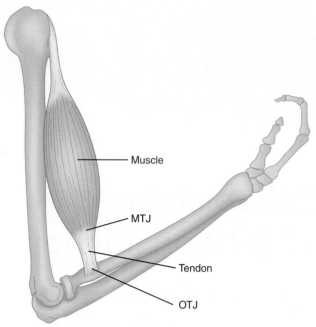

FIGURE 7-1 The biceps muscle-tendon unit. *MTJ,* Musculotendinous junction; *OTJ,* osseotendinous junction.

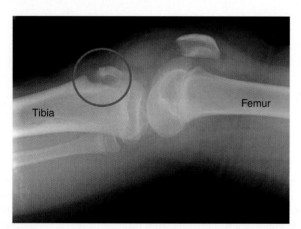

FIGURE 7-2 Radiographic image of an avulsion fracture near the osseotendinous junction of the infrapatellar tendon and tibia.

Clinical Pearl #1

When treating a patient with Osgood-Schlatter disease, care must be taken to prevent further tissue damage and protect the irritated structures until they heal. Initial treatment consists of rest and modification of activity to allow the inflammation to subside. Gentle, progressive stretching, particularly of the quadriceps musculature, will help improve musculotendinous flexibility. Use of a counter-force brace on the infrapatellar tendon may also be considered toward the end of the rehabilitation program to alter the application of force at the OTJ as the patient attempts to return to endurance activities and functional, sport-specific workout drills.

Stages of Healing

It is important to have a fundamental understanding of healing time frames before discussing pathology and ultimately deciding on appropriate treatment because knowledge of tissue-healing phases will help guide the decision-making process during patient progression. The stages of soft tissue healing consist of the inflammatory response phase, the fibroblastic-repair phase, and the maturation-remodeling phase.[4-9] Although the literature reports variations in the exact time frames for each phase, these phases of healing overlap and the time frames serve as general guidelines for the clinician because each soft tissue injury varies in severity and in the individual's response to injury.

The acute inflammatory phase begins immediately after tissue injury and is characterized by redness, swelling, increased temperature, and pain. The inflammatory phase involves capillary injury and vasodilation, which results in increased blood flow to the injured area. Neutrophils and macrophages are attracted to the site of injury to remove foreign debris and damaged tissue from the area and thereby improve the healing environment. The events in the inflammatory response phase last approximately 2 to 4 days.[4] During the fibroblastic-repair phase, which typically begins 3 days after injury and lasts approximately 2 weeks, new blood vessels form and fibroblasts migrate to the area to synthesize new ground substance and collagen.[7,9] The wound margins begin to contract in size and weaker type III collagen is deposited in an unorganized fashion to form scar tissue.[6] Finally, during the maturation-remodeling phase, ongoing synthesis and reorganization of collagen fibers take place. The continued collagen deposition transitions to mainly type I collagen, and the collagen fibers in the scar tissue become parallel in alignment as a result of tensile forces applied to the injured soft tissue. The parallel alignment of collagen fibers is usually achieved by 2 months after injury and allows the tissue to endure higher tensile loads.[8] However, this final healing phase is a long-term process that begins approximately 3 weeks after injury and may last up to 1 year.[5,10,11] While remodeling, the tensile strength of the wound continues to increase and at 3 months will have approximately 80% of normal tissue strength.[11] When the remodeling phase is complete, the damaged tissue has often not achieved the same tensile strength as uninjured tissue.[11-13] Luckily, the limitation in tensile strength does not typically affect function. The three phases of tissue healing overlap and represent a continuum of soft tissue healing (Fig. 7-3).

Injuries to muscles involve a similar process as just described, but unique to muscles are satellite cells, which are muscle-specific stem cells located on the border of muscle fibers.[14,15] With injury to muscle, the ruptured myofibers contract and the gap is filled with edema and eventually scar tissue. On the ends of the retracted muscle fibers, satellite cells are activated to proliferate and cause muscle regeneration. The newly regenerated myofibers on the end of the torn muscle project into the forming connective tissue scar.[14,15]

When compared with muscle, tendons have less vascularity and therefore less oxygen and nutrition after injury. As a result, tendons may be slower than muscles to recover after injury.[16] With tendons it is thought that healing may occur through intrinsic and extrinsic pathways.[8,9,16,17] The extrinsic mechanism involves inflammatory cells and fibroblasts from the surrounding area that enter to assist in tendon repair, whereas the intrinsic mechanism involves inflammatory cells and fibroblasts

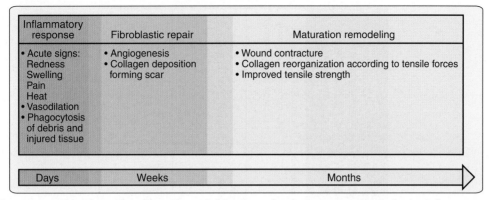

Inflammatory response	Fibroblastic repair	Maturation remodeling

• Acute signs:
  Redness
  Swelling
  Pain
  Heat
• Vasodilation
• Phagocytosis of debris and injured tissue
	• Angiogenesis
	• Collagen deposition forming scar
		• Wound contracture
		• Collagen reorganization according to tensile forces
		• Improved tensile strength

| Days | Weeks | Months |

FIGURE 7-3 Continuum of healing. The three phases of healing of soft tissue injury include the inflammatory response phase, fibroblastic-repair phase, and maturation-remodeling phase.

from within the tendon.[16,17] Within the tendon the reparative cell is the tenocyte, which may be activated to produce collagen.[8] Although collagen is needed to help repair the damaged tendon, fibrosis may develop and result in the formation of adhesions to surrounding tissue if excessive collagen synthesis occurs. Clinically, this is not ideal because limited mobility may occur as a consequence of the scar tissue adhesions.

MUSCLE-TENDON PATHOLOGIES

Muscle Strain

A muscle strain refers to pathology that involves some extent of disruption in the continuity and function of the muscle-tendon unit.[3,18] The mechanism of injury of muscle strains may be related to passive overstretching, excessive active loading, or repetitive loading of fatigued musculature.[3,18-21] In other words, the strain occurs when the amount of stretch exceeds the limits of flexibility, the amount of force exceeds the level of strength, or the duration of force exceeds the level of endurance of the involved muscle-tendon unit. In particular, eccentric repetitive loading is often a cause of muscle strain because muscle forces can be higher during the lengthening activation and lead to microscopic damage to the contractile element of the muscle.[21-23] A muscle strain can also be the result of an acute impact (direct blow) to the involved musculature, known as a contusion.

Clinically, strains are frequently seen in certain muscle groups. Strains commonly involve muscles that have a large percentage of type II fast-twitch muscle fibers and muscles that cross two joints, such as the hamstrings, gastrocnemius, and rectus femoris.[24,25] Muscles that span two joints are placed at risk through lengthening loads at both joints simultaneously and mixed demands during function. In sports medicine, muscle strains commonly occur in "speed athletes," such as sprinters and football, basketball, and soccer players.[26] Muscle strains also tend to occur during strenuous exercise, particularly during eccentric muscle activation or when the muscle is fatigued. At the end of practice or a training session, the musculature is more likely to be fatigued and the athlete is at an increased risk for an acute strain, especially if proper conditioning is not maintained.

Muscle strains should be differentiated from the exercise-induced muscle soreness that occurs after eccentric exercise or physical activity in naïve/unaccustomed individuals. Although both strains and exercise-induced muscle soreness occur with eccentric exercise and both produce pain with passive stretching or muscle activation (or both), a muscle strain is a painful event that is acute in nature and identified at the time of injury. In other words, the patient will report knowledge of the moment when the muscle strain was felt. In contrast, delayed-onset muscle soreness (or DOMS) typically peaks 24 to 72 hours after exercise. Importantly, DOMS occurs after bouts of eccentric exercise, especially in untrained muscle, but it typically resolves without intervention within a few days to a week.[3,20,27]

Grading of Strains

Strains range from damage to a limited number of muscle fibers or connective tissue to a complete muscle tear or tendon avulsion. Typically, strains are categorized as grade 1, grade 2, or grade 3 (Table 7-1). Determining the appropriate grade of strain will help guide the clinician through the rehabilitation process. A grade 1 strain may leave the athlete with slight discomfort and minimal swelling but full range of motion (ROM) and little functional deficit. A grade 2 strain is characterized by a small to moderate palpable area of involvement along with increased pain and swelling. An athlete with a grade 2 muscle strain will often demonstrate restricted ROM and impaired gait if the lower extremity musculature is involved. A grade 3 muscle strain is typified by a moderate to severe palpable area of involvement and sometimes a defect at the site of injury. The athlete will demonstrate significant deficits in ROM, and functional mobility will be severely impaired.

A grade 3 strain with a complete muscle or tendon rupture may require surgical repair, so correct assessment of an avulsion injury is critical. For example, a grade 3 muscle strain of the Achilles tendon is best evaluated with the Thompson test (Fig. 7-4). To perform this test, the patient should lie prone with the feet extended off the end of a treatment table while the clinician squeezes the belly of the gastrocnemius muscle. When the Achilles tendon is intact, the foot should move into plantar flexion. However, if the Achilles tendon is ruptured, the foot will not plantar-flex. A patient with an Achilles tendon rupture will often report the feeling of a "pop" or being kicked in the calf. Rupture of the Achilles tendon often occurs around 2 to 6 cm from its insertion site on the calcaneus, where the gastrocnemius and soleus tendons meet and which it is thought to be the area with the poorest blood supply.[9,24] Early diagnosis and treatment of this pathology are important. Treatment approaches can include either conservative or surgical management; however,

Table 7-1 Grading of Muscle Strains

| Grade | Structural Fiber Damage/Deformation | Impairments in Body Structure/Function | | | | Limitations in Ambulation (for Lower Extremity Strains) | Limitations in Participation in Sporting Activities (for Lower Extremity Strains) |
		Pain	Range of Motion	Strength	Swelling		
1	Some fibers stretched or actually torn, no gross disruption of the muscle-tendon unit	Pain or tenderness with AROM or stretching	No loss, full ROM possible	No loss, full strength	Minimal, localized edema	Minimal to no limitation in ambulation	Minimal limitations, may be able to participate by using equipment (wraps, bracing, taping)
2	Torn muscle/tendon fibers, palpable depression in the area of injury, some degree of disruption of the muscle-tendon unit	Pain with active contraction of the muscle-tendon unit	Loss of ROM because of swelling and bleeding, limitation in AROM	Some loss of strength	Moderate edema	Ambulation with a limp, may need crutches	Unable to participate but should be able to return to sport during the same season with appropriate rehabilitation
3	Complete rupture of the muscle belly, MTJ, or OTJ; noticeable defect in the muscle belly or evidence of a torn tendon	Intense pain that diminishes with damage and separation of nerve fibers	Severely limited ROM or total loss of ROM	Moderate to major loss of strength, unable to endure resisted motion	Moderate to major edema	Significant limitation in ambulation, likely to require crutches	Unable to participate; consider sitting out the season for conservative or operative treatment

AROM, Active range of motion; *MTJ,* myotendinous junction; *OTJ,* osseotendinous junction; *ROM,* range of motion.

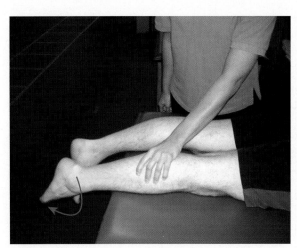

FIGURE 7-4 Thompson test. The Thompson test is a clinical test used to assess the integrity of the Achilles tendon. As the clinician squeezes the patient's calf musculature, an intact tendon will cause the foot to plantar-flex, whereas a ruptured tendon will not produce any movement of the foot.

surgical repair of an Achilles tendon rupture produces a lower rerupture rate and provides the patient with a quicker and more optimal return to function. One of the evolving rules in the treatment of these injuries is allowing ROM in the postoperative period or even with conservative care because ROM appears to be vital to long-term success.[24,28]

Contusions

A contusion injury may be caused by a direct hit or acute blow to the muscle belly. This impact results in muscle cell damage and bleeding into the muscle. Immediately following the injury, an acute inflammatory reaction takes place. Satellite cells on the membrane of muscle cells become new muscle cells, and connective tissue is formed in the damaged area.[14,15] The damaged tissue continues to progress through the stages of soft tissue healing as described earlier. The extent of muscle tissue damage with a contusion injury will determine the degree to which ROM, strength, and functional activity are impaired.

Contusion injuries are commonly seen in individuals engaging in athletic activities, such as football, where an athlete's helmet or shoulder pad may forcefully impact an opponent's quadriceps muscle, for example. Contusions can be classified as mild, moderate, or severe based on the amount of ROM allowed by the involved muscle in the adjacent joints (Table 7-2).[29,30] A mild contusion may cause a loss of one third of normal ROM, whereas a severe contusion may limit motion to less than one third of normal mobility.[29] Like strains, contusions may also lead to deficits in strength and functional limitations. A severe contusion is characterized by significant bleeding and a large palpable area of involvement, and the muscle may herniate through the fascia. Clinically, muscle strains and contusions are some of the most common injuries seen in sports participation.[24]

The clinician should also be aware of a condition known as myositis ossificans (also called heterotopic bone) that can develop after a severe muscle contusion (Fig. 7-5). It commonly occurs in the thigh musculature after a direct blow to the muscle causes tissue disruption and excessive bleeding that leads to ectopic bone formation in the area of the injured soft tissue. Initial

radiographs are negative, but after 4 to 6 weeks bone formation can be identified radiographically. Even though myositis ossificans can restrict mobility, it is not always treated surgically because the ectopic bone may not impair function and the body may eventually absorb the ossification. However, if surgical resection is indicated, it is performed only after the bone has fully matured because early surgery can exacerbate the condition.

Clinical Pearl #2

Proper treatment of a contusion can help decrease risk for the development of myositis ossificans. Immediately after a quadriceps contusion injury, the knee should be immobilized in flexion.[24,31,32] During this initial rest period, the knee is kept flexed to provide tension on the quadriceps muscle and inhibit blood pooling and muscle contracture.[24] While the leg is wrapped, ice is applied to the area of injury to limit excessive blood flow to the injured area, and nonsteroidal antiinflammatory medication may help in addressing the inflammation as well.[33] Typically, the leg is initially wrapped in flexion for the first 24 hours. Afterward, the patient can proceed through the rehabilitation process by beginning with isometric quadriceps-strengthening exercises and progressing to gentle, pain-free ROM and stretching. Reinjury, especially shortly after the initial injury, increases risk for the development of myositis ossificans. Therefore, it is important to avoid activities that may reinjure the muscle tissue, including aggressive overstretching, early aggressive massage, or trying to continue typical athletic activity with a grade 2 or 3 contusion. Heat or thermal modalities that increase blood flow to the area should also be avoided initially after injury.

Tendinopathy

The terminology involved in tendon injury is evolving and requires further clarification. In the past, *tendinitis* has been used as a catch-all term to describe all tendon pathologies. However, what is now known about the histologic differences in tendon pathologies requires further clarification of the language used when discussing tendon injuries. Several terms are used to describe various tendon pathologies. For example, *tenosynovitis* refers to inflammation of the synovial sheath that lines some tendons, and *enthesopathy* refers to a lesion at or near the enthesis or bony attachment. Therefore, new classification systems have been proposed to subgroup tendon pathologies.[8,9,34-36] For clarity, *tendinopathy* is used in this chapter as a broad term that refers to any pathology involving tendons and, as a result, is inclusive of several different tendon pathologies.

In this chapter, tendinopathies will be classified as *tendinitis*, *paratenonitis*, and *tendinosis* (Table 7-3). Tendinitis and paratenonitis are the earliest signs of tendon pathology and trigger an acute inflammatory response. However, if tendon damage continues, tendinosis, partial tears, or even tendon rupture may occur. Tendinitis, paratenonitis, and tendinosis may occur separately, or these pathologies may occur simultaneously, as is the case with paratenonitis and tendinosis.[9]

Table 7-2 Classification of Contusions with Emphasis on the Commonly Seen Quadriceps Contusion

| Grade | Impairments in Body Structure/Function | | | | | Limitations in Ambulation (for Quadriceps Contusions) | Limitations in Function and Participation in Sporting Activities (for Quadriceps Contusions) |
	Structural Fiber Damage/ Deformation	Pain	Range of Motion (for Quadriceps Contusions)	Strength	Swelling		
Mild	Muscle fiber damage, vascular hemorrhage, and hematoma formation	Localized tenderness	Knee ROM greater than 90°	Minimal to no loss of strength	Minimal, localized edema	Normal gait	Able to do deep knee bend, may be able to participate in sports but cautioned against risk for reinjury; protective pad used to cover the injured tissue
Moderate	Muscle fiber damage, vascular hemorrhage, and hematoma formation	Tender muscle mass	Knee ROM less than 90°	Moderate loss of strength	Moderate edema	Antalgic gait	Unable to climb stairs or rise from a chair without pain, unable to play sports
Severe	Muscle fiber damage, vascular hemorrhage, and hematoma formation; muscle may herniate through fascia	Marked tenderness	Knee ROM less than 45°	Moderate to major loss of strength	Marked edema, may be difficult to identify contours of defined musculature	Severe limp, likely to require crutches for ambulation	Unable to participate in sports, must take extreme caution to prevent aggravating the injury with functional activity

ROM, Range of motion.

Tendinopathies are often caused by repetitive tendon trauma, overuse, excessive loading, or preexisting tendon degeneration. Tendon overload is believed to be central to the pathologic process and may result in weakening and eventual failure of the tendon if it is unable to respond to the applied load. However, tendons are able to withstand some extent of tensile loading before injury (Fig. 7-6). At rest, the collagen fibers of the tendon are in a wavy, crimped formation. With slight elongation, the crimped fiber configuration straightens. As the tensile load increases, the collagen fibers continue to deform linearly.

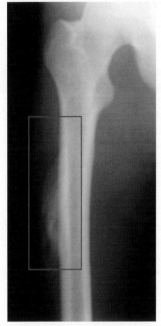

FIGURE 7-5 Myositis ossificans. A radiographic image shows ectopic bone formation in the thigh musculature.

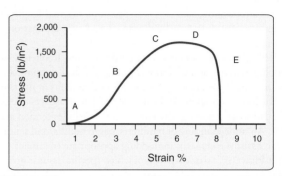

FIGURE 7-6 Stress-strain curve for tendon injury. The stress-strain curve represents the relationship for progressive loading of the tendon. The curve is divided into five different regions: toe region (*A*), linear region (*B*), progressive failure region (*C*), major failure region (*D*), and complete rupture region (*E*). The toe region represents a minimal amount of tissue elongation in which the crimped formation of collagen fibers straightens. In the linear region, the collagen fibers continue to deform linearly with increasing load but are able to return to their original configuration when the tension is removed. In the progressive failure and major failure regions (beyond 4% strain), increasing tendon damage occurs. At 8% elongation, the tendon ruptures.

Table 7-3 Classification of Tendon Injury

Pathology	Description	Nature of Onset	Inflammatory Process Present	Cause	Clinical Signs and Symptoms	Treatment
Tendinitis	Injury to the tendon itself involving partial or complete tearing, vascular disruption, acute inflammatory/ repair response; can involve symptomatic degeneration of the tendon when chronic	Acute	Yes (in tendon)	Macrotraumatic, strain or tear, repetitive loading/overuse	Swelling, pain, tenderness, warmth, (depending on the duration/severity of the pathology)	Ice, antiinflammatories, rest, modified activities, progressive ROM and strength exercises
Paratenonitis	Inflammation of only the paratenon, regardless of whether the paratenon is lined by synovium	Acute	Yes (in paratenon tissue)	Repetitive loading/overuse, irritation because of limited space	Swelling, pain, tenderness, warmth, crepitus (depending on the duration/ severity of the pathology)	Ice, antiinflammatories, rest, modified activities, progressive ROM and strength exercises
Tendinosis	Intratendinous degeneration, noninflammatory in nature	Chronic	No	Repetitive loading/overuse, "failed" healing response, vascular compromise, aging	No swelling of the tendon sheath, often palpable nodule that may or may not be tender, can occur asymptomatically	Eccentric exercises, stretching

ROM, Range of motion.

With tensile loading causing up to 4% elongation, the collagen fibers are able to return to their original configuration when the tension is released. However, tensile loading beyond 4% of its length will cause the collagen cross-links to fail, and the collagen fibers will slide past one another and cause injury to the tendon. The repetitive strain that occurs in tendon overuse injuries implies a repeated strain of 4% to 8% of its original length, and the tendon cannot endure further tension. At 8% elongation, the tendon ruptures.[5,9,17,37]

Tendinitis, paratenonitis, and tendinosis are frequently seen pathologies in the clinical setting. Specifically, these tendinopathies tend to commonly occur in the rotator cuff tendons at the shoulder, the forearm tendons at the medial and lateral aspects of elbow, the quadriceps tendon at the knee, and the Achilles tendon at the ankle. An understanding of tendinitis, paratenonitis, and tendinosis can assist the clinician in deciding appropriate treatment principles. However, a true diagnosis of which specific tissue is involved and the histopathologic factors present can be confirmed only with tissue biopsy, which is often performed only in the late stages of tendon injury when conservative treatment has failed.

Tendinitis

As mentioned previously, the term *tendinitis* has been used in the past to refer to any tendon pathology. However, clarification must be made that tendinitis refers to the presence of inflammation within the tendon tissue.[8,9,34,36,38] When initial overuse or a strain of the tendon occurs, microscopic tearing of the tendon results in inflammation, localized swelling, and complaints of pain.[9,38] As a result of the injury, the tendon will begin the healing process. In tendinitis, the initial inflammation occurs within the tendon itself, without inflammation of the surrounding paratenon.

Tendinitis is frequently caused by repetitive demands placed on the tendon during a period of overuse or during excessive acute strain, such as a recent increase in activity level. Applying a tensile load to the tendon will produce pain, and the inflamed tendon is often tender when palpated. Frequently, tendinitis occurs in individuals whose occupation requires repetitive motion or in sports-related repetitive loading of the muscle-tendon unit.

The initial response to acute microtrauma or strain takes place during the inflammatory phase, and the tendon continues to the fibroblastic-repair and maturation-remodeling phases of soft tissue healing. However, the typical healing process occasionally goes awry and chronic tendinitis persists. The exact mechanism that converts acute tendinitis to chronic tendinitis is unknown, but histologically, chronic tendinitis is characterized by increased collagen formation and fibrosis. Other characteristic signs similar to tendinosis and symptomatic degeneration of the tendon are also present.[9]

Paratenonitis

Tendons are covered by loose areolar connective tissue called the paratenon, which serves as an elastic sleeve to assist the tendon as it moves against surrounding tissue. Therefore, the term *paratenonitis* describes inflammation of the outer later of the tendon only, regardless of whether the paratenon is lined by synovium.[8,9,34,36,38] Collectively, paratenonitis includes the separate pathologies of peritendinitis, tenosynovitis, and tenovaginitis. Paratenonitis commonly occurs during repetitive motion when the tendon rubs over a bony prominence, is in a tight anatomic location, or is subjected to an external compressive force. For example, during a repetitive jumping motion, if the Achilles

tendon repeatedly slides against poor-fitting footwear as the gastrocnemius and soleus muscles contract, inflammation and irritation of the paratenon may occur. The limited space for the tendon to function during muscle contraction can result in friction as the tendon slides, and then it becomes inflamed. Paratenonitis is manifested as pain, swelling, warmth, and possibly crepitus over the inflamed paratenon. The crepitus is caused by the inflammatory products that accumulate on the irritated tendon and then cause adherence of the paratenon to surrounding structures as it slides back and forth during muscle activation.[36,37]

Clinical Pearl #3

In some tendons, the outermost lining is a synovial sheath that serves to decrease irritation in areas of high friction. Tenosynovitis, which is inflammation of this outer sheath, can be classified as paratenonitis and has symptoms similar to tendinitis: pain on movement, tenderness, and swelling. Crepitus may also occur with tenosynovitis because adhesions form to surrounding structures. Because the adhesions may restrict the gliding motion of the tendon and the space itself for the tendon to move may be diminished, the patient may also have greater limitation in ROM. Successful treatment of tenosynovitis is similar to treatment of tendinitis. Initial treatment focuses on addressing the inflammation and resting the injured tissue. Intrinsic and extrinsic factors that may be causing the inflammation should also be assessed. For example, intrinsic factors include structural malalignment, muscle weakness, and decreased flexibility, whereas extrinsic factors include poor equipment and training errors.

Tendinosis

Tendinosis describes degenerative changes within the tendon without histologic signs of an inflammatory response.[8,9,34,36,38] Whereas acute injuries are typified by inflammation, tendinosis has a slow, insidious onset because of chronic microtrauma and structural damage. With tendinosis, the tendon degeneration consists of loss of normal collagen structure and cell abnormality, but no inflammatory cellular response.[4,8,9,34,36,38] The histologic appearance of a normal tendon and one with tendinosis is shown in Figure 7-7. The degenerative tendon loses the parallel alignment of its collagen fibers and is therefore weaker and may be more vulnerable to injury.[8] Paratenonitis, as described earlier, can also occur with tendinosis. In this clinical scenario, inflammation of the outer paratenon with intratendinous degeneration is observed.

Tendinosis causes pain that often has a gradual onset and is commonly preceded by repetitive overloading of the tendon. The pain in the tendon results in a limitation in functional activity. However, tendinosis is not always symptomatic.[9] For example, the Achilles tendon can rupture without previous symptoms of injury or pain but still demonstrate histologic signs consistent with tendinosis degeneration. Because tendinosis may develop asymptomatically, it is unclear whether the acute inflammatory response always occurs before chronic degenerative changes. Regardless, the chronic degeneration seen with tendinosis has been associated with aging, vascular compromise, repetitive loading causing microtrauma to the tendon, and preexisting tendon injury.[9,39]

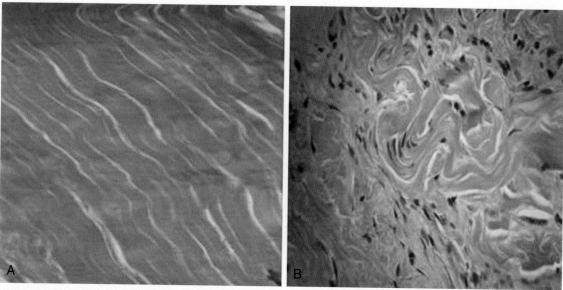

FIGURE 7-7 Histologic image of normal and pathologic tendon. **A,** Normal, healthy tendon with parallel alignment of collagen fibers. **B,** Pathologic tendinosis with disorganized structure.

Box 7-1

Questions That Should Be Included in a Patient's History

"What is the location, duration, and intensity of your pain?"

"What factors make the pain worse, and what factors make the pain better?"

"Has the pain progressively gotten better or worse over time?"

"Have you had any treatment for the current medical issue?"

"Have you had a similar injury in the past?"

"Are you currently taking any medications for the problem?"

"What are your functional limitations?"

CLINICAL EXAMINATION AND EVALUATION

Understanding of musculoskeletal anatomy and the mechanism of injury will provide the clinician with valuable knowledge during the clinical examination. In particular, a thorough and detailed history will help in discerning whether the injury is acute or chronic. Acute injuries occur as a result of a recent overstretch, recent overuse, or a single direct impact causing tissue damage. Conversely, chronic injuries are due to the accumulation of repeated small stresses over time, which ultimately results in tissue irritation and damage. For example, when assessing acute tendinitis, the patient may describe a recent activity involving repetitive motion or recent excessive stretching of the involved muscle-tendon unit. A "weekend warrior" often describes an acute injury with a history of suddenly increasing activity level and overexertion when proper training and conditioning have not been maintained.

After taking the patient's history, the clinician should supplement the history by asking questions that include those in Box 7-1. These questions will help provide further insight into the current injury for which the patent is seeking treatment.

In addition to eliciting a complete subjective history, palpation of the injured area will also provide the clinician with valuable information. For example, because most tendons are superficial and can be relatively easily palpated, the clinician can often accurately identify the specific location of the pain. When assessing acute muscle strains, the patient may report diffuse muscle pain or pain with muscle activation. Depending on the degree of strain, the clinician may be able to palpate the area of involvement or a defect in the muscle itself.

The next step in a comprehensive examination and evaluation includes performing static and dynamic assessments. The clinician should consider standard static measurements, including ROM, muscle girth for symmetry, strength testing, posture and alignment assessment, and balance and neuromuscular testing. If possible, it is also beneficial to assess dynamic tasks. This may be more realistic for an individual with a chronic versus acute injury, especially if evaluation of the acute injury takes place relatively soon after onset. Evaluation of dynamic mobility can include balance, gait, and a functional movement assessment. When assessing dynamic movement, it is important to identify faulty technique or other exacerbating factors for the particular movement pattern because they may play a causative role in the musculotendinous pathology.

Clinical Pearl #4

When assessing an individual's dynamic movement pattern, it is important to evaluate the entire kinetic chain. Weakness or dysfunction at any point throughout the kinetic chain may help determine one of the underlying causes of the individual's pathology. It is also beneficial to make the dynamic assessment as activity specific as possible. When evaluating athletes, it is important to consider any equipment they may use. Likewise, when evaluating an individual with an occupation-related problem, it is wise to observe movement pattern techniques for repetitive tasks, as well as long-duration static positioning.

Diagnostic testing can also aid the clinician in further identifying and understanding the extent of tissue pathology. Common diagnostic tests for individuals with muscle or tendon pathology include magnetic resonance imaging (MRI) and sonography.[40] Although MRI and sonography can assist in evaluating soft tissue injuries, radiographic imaging is also useful for assessing the attachment site of the tendon to bone. On MRI, first-degree strains are manifested as focal signal abnormalities without a tear, second-degree strains are seen as a partial tear, and third-degree strains are characterized by full-thickness tears with hemorrhage and muscle or tendon retraction.[25] However, because of the large cost associated with MRI, it is often not used for the diagnosis of acute grade 1 or 2 muscle strains or for acute tendinitis pathologies. Clinically, grade 1 or 2 strains can frequently be diagnosed by applying stretch to the injured muscle or by activating the muscle group against resistance. When a grade 3 strain is suspected or for chronic tendon pathologies that have failed conservative rehabilitation, MRI will probably be considered. In cases in which disruption of the tendon occurs at the bony attachment, radiographic images may be helpful in identifying an avulsion fracture but will provide limited information on the extent of soft tissue injury. Finally, ultrasound has been widely used for evaluation of tendon attachments and muscle tears.[25,41] In addition to being less costly than MRI, ultrasound is done in real time and allows dynamic assessment of the musculotendinous unit during muscle contraction.

REHABILITATION PRINCIPLES

As rehabilitation specialists, it is important to apply knowledge of anatomy and understanding of healing time frames to each unique muscle and tendon pathology. Additionally, each patient's personal characteristics, level of training, motivation, and other personal and external factors for the given scenario will influence individual rehabilitation programs. The following discussion covers rehabilitation principles for the acute, inflammatory-mediated and chronic, degenerative pathologies covered in this chapter.

Acute Inflammatory Injuries

One of the overlying principles for management of an acute injury involves applying the healing time frames for soft tissue injuries. Immediately after an acute injury, the inflammatory response process begins in the damaged tissue. As discussed earlier, the initial inflammatory response includes pain, heat, swelling, and redness. During this phase, the clinician should control pain and edema by using the principles of RICE (rest, ice, compression, elevation).[3,12,42,43] We like to use the principle PRICE because protection may play a larger role in an athletic population. Application of ice or cryotherapy is performed several times a day for a minimum of 48 hours to help limit the amount of bleeding from surrounding tissue. Compression wraps or bandages may also be used to help minimize the swelling.

Although the inflammatory phase of the healing response is important, rest and immobilization of the injured tissue should be limited and not last longer than 1 to 2 days. This is based on another principle of rehabilitation for acute injuries that involves early mobilization to restore tensile strength of the injured tissue. Soft tissue will respond to the physical demands placed on it; it will remodel or realign along the lines of tensile force, and

early motion that applies stress serves as a physical stimulus to aid in the formation and maintenance of collagen.[3,5,9] Prolonged immobilization and deprivation of stress lead to actual loss of collagen fibers. In other words, controlled mobilization is better than immobilization to restore the tensile properties of the tissue.[44] Additionally, immobilization may cause contractures, muscle atrophy, and disorganization of collagen fibers. The exception to this principle is complete muscle or tendon rupture, for which longer immobilization is necessary. In this case, conservative treatment involves immobilization with only controlled passive ROM for several weeks to allow the tissue to heal in proper alignment.

Early mobilization after injury is implemented through pain-free ROM exercises and should be initiated shortly after the initial inflammatory response phase. Both passive and active exercises that apply a longitudinal strain to the injured structure will help the tissue accommodate to the new stress.[44] When rehabilitating an acute injury, it is also important to prescribe exercises initially at a low load to stress the collagen fibers without overloading them and progressively increase the demands placed on the tissue. As the pain and swelling subside and the healing process continues, the patient can progress through ROM, flexibility, and strengthening exercises in a controlled fashion. The patient should begin with active ROM in the pain-free range. If mobility remains limited in the subacute stages of healing, heat modalities may be considered in combination with manual techniques to increase ROM and soft tissue mobility. Otherwise, isometric exercises can be prescribed for initial strengthening and should progress to isotonic strengthening. Balance activities can also be incorporated into the rehabilitation program because loss of proprioception often occurs with injury. Throughout the rehabilitation process, general conditioning exercises that do not aggravate the condition may be performed to maintain cardiovascular endurance, flexibility, and strength of the surrounding joints. While increasing tensile loading throughout the rehabilitation program, the clinician should continuously monitor for pain with progression of activity. Pain may indicate excessive loading and alert the clinician to alter the rehabilitation program.

The final phase of rehabilitation is return to functional participation in occupational, recreational, or athletic activities. This phase should include a gradual progression of functional or sport-specific training activities over a period of several weeks. As the level of functional activity progresses in difficulty, the clinician continues to monitor for pain or weakness as a sign to return to an easier level of physical activity. This is important because returning the patient to functional or athletic activity too soon may predispose the athlete to reinjury.[24,45]

The acute pathologies covered in this chapter include muscle strains, contusions, tendinitis, and paratenonitis. When addressing an acute muscle strain or contusion, one must first assess the severity of the injury. Although first- and second-degree strains are treated nonoperatively, a third-degree strain may require surgery. Likewise, contusions typically do not require surgery unless significant bleeding causes an acute compartment syndrome, which requires immediate surgical care involving a fasciotomy. After an acute strain and contusion, the initial treatment goals are to stop interstitial bleeding and prevent further injury to the muscle fibers. After the initial inflammatory response, the patient should begin early mobilization with gentle passive, pain-free stretching to improve ROM and flexibility. However,

Table 7-4 Management of First/Second-Degree Strains and Mild to Moderate Contusions

Phase	Goals	Treatment	Time Frame
I	Reduction of pain and edema	Immobilization, ice, rest, elevation	Days 1-2
II	ROM	Ice, modalities, pain-free ROM, isometric strength	Days 3-7
III	Strengthening, endurance	Progressive strengthening, isometrics to isotonics	Days 7-21
IV	Neuromuscular coordination, return to function/activity	Running, functional progression, sport-specific exercises	Days 21+

ROM, Range of motion.

care must be taken, especially after a contusion injury, to avoid reinjury of the muscle to limit risk for the development of further complications. Muscle strength and endurance are also important as the patient continues to progress through the rehabilitation program. Care must be taken to progress slowly and avoid reinjury to the tissue. Even though it is not recommended that a "cookbook approach" be taken when treating these pathologies, a general guideline for the management of grade 1 and 2 strains and mild to moderate contusions is provided in Table 7-4.

Initial treatment of acute tendonitis and paratenonitis involves rest, avoidance of repetitive motion, and removal of the external irritant that may be pressing or rubbing on tissue and causing inflammation. This means that patients need to avoid the irritant and modify their activity. Early treatment also includes ice or antiinflammatory medication to limit the amount of local inflammation in the tissue. ROM and strengthening exercises can then be introduced as the pain and swelling subside.

The process of rehabilitation for acute injuries involves several principles, including application of the soft tissue healing stages, early mobilization after injury with caution to avoid reinjury, and progressive strengthening for return to function. Specifically, the goals after an acute injury are to (1) control pain and edema; (2) restore normal ROM and flexibility; (3) reestablish normal strength, endurance, and neuromuscular control; and (4) achieve preinjury function and activity. Successful completion of the rehabilitation process is important because inappropriate management of injury may lead to exacerbating the pathology or may place the individual at risk for future injury.

Chronic Degenerative Injuries

The chronic pathology addressed in this chapter is tendinosis, which lacks the histologic inflammation seen with acute injuries. Therefore, different treatment principles apply when treating tendinosis. The overarching principle of management of tendinosis involves reducing tendon pain because it is the limiting factor for functional activity.

The most promising treatment of tendinosis is eccentric exercise, or active lengthening of the muscle-tendon unit. Eccentric

exercise has been shown to decrease pain and increase function in patients with tendinosis.[46-53] The basis of an eccentric exercise program is to place progressively increased stress on the tendon to ultimately improve its ability to withstand tensile loads. The eccentric loading may also lead to a more normalized tendon structure.[54] However, the specific mechanism that makes eccentric exercises effective has yet to be clearly described.

In addition to eccentric loading, stretching has also been shown to decrease pain and increase function in individuals with tendinosis.[49] Stretching works to lengthen the muscle-tendon unit, which improves flexibility and ROM. Moreover, if the resting length of the muscle-tendon unit increases, less joint strain may occur during loading. In other words, a regular stretching program will help decrease tension on the muscle-tendon unit.[49]

Finally, several other factors can be addressed to help decrease tendon pain. For example, rest periods or training modifications can be implemented. Additionally, external aids such as braces, orthotics, or taping can help alleviate the strain placed on the tendon. Antiinflammatory cortisone injections may also help relieve some of the pain with tendinosis; however, use of corticosteroids is controversial. Caution should be taken when working with a patient shortly after an injection because corticosteroids have also been associated with tissue damage and short-term decreased tensile strength of collagen.[55]

Prevention

Although the intent of this chapter is to focus on principles governing rehabilitation after muscle and tendon injuries, it is important to acknowledge the ability to educate patients on injury prevention principles as well. Important factors for preventing muscle strains include maintaining flexibility and proper conditioning, which is achieved through stretching and strengthening, respectively. First, the viscoelastic property of muscle is affected by warmth and can contribute greatly to changes in muscle length. Therefore, warm-up should facilitate stretching and thus prepare the muscle-tendon units for exercise.[3,20,42] Specifically, because strains are common in muscles that cross two joints, perhaps extra emphasis should be placed on stretching the hamstrings, rectus femoris, and gastrocnemius musculature in the lower extremities. In addition to stretching, proper conditioning and strengthening can aid in prevention of injuries.[3,56] Finally, fatigue may also play a role in injury, so proper training and conditioning are important for prevention of injuries. Unfortunately, in our experience prevention is more helpful in those who have not had a previous injury. It appears that once injured, individuals remain at a higher risk for reinjury than their not previously injured cohort.

CASE STUDIES

The following case studies are presented to provide the reader the opportunity to apply the information presented in this chapter. Specifically, the rehabilitation principles for acute and chronic injuries will be applied. For each case it will be assumed that a thorough examination has been completed, and in addition to the patient's history, a description of impairments and functional limitations will be provided. The aim of the case studies is to describe treatment examples for each unique patient scenario.

Hamstring Strain

History

A 16-year-old soccer player came to the clinic after sustaining a hamstring injury over the weekend. He reported that he was sprinting down the field and went to kick the ball when he felt an immediate "pull" in his hamstrings. He stopped playing and came out of the game to put ice on his injury.

Impairments/Functional Limitations

The patient complained of diffuse pain (4/10 rating) and was tender when palpated near his proximal hamstring. No palpable depression was noted in the area of injury and minimal localized edema. He had full knee flexion and extension, but limited hamstring flexibility. He was able to walk into the clinic without crutches but felt unable to take a full stride with gait and would not consider higher-demand activity. Unfortunately for this athlete, he appeared to have what we call a high hamstring strain, which typically requires longer to recover than more distal hamstring injuries.

Rehabilitation Program

Initial rehabilitation addressed the inflammatory factors of pain and edema. Treatment included cryotherapy to decrease the pain and reduce the swelling. The patient was also prescribed a thigh compression sleeve to help decrease the swelling and provide support. Gentle,

pain-free stretching exercises for the hamstring were initiated. One week later, the patient returned for follow-up care. He continued with the stretching exercises and started hamstring-strengthening exercises (isometric and isotonic). Typically, a progression of concentric to eccentric strengthening exercises is followed. Examples of exercises after a hamstring strain, including strengthening exercises (lunges, bridges on a stability ball, and hamstring curls on a stability ball) are shown in Figure 7-8. Two weeks after his injury, the patient reported no pain and demonstrated improved flexibility and good strength. He had also been performing endurance training on a bike with no restrictions. Therefore, he began functional exercises, such as agility drills and soccer-specific maneuvers. We also added kneeling assisted forward curls (also known as Russian hamstring curls) as shown in Figure 7-9. In the exercise the athlete leaned forward while keeping his trunk erect, which required the hamstrings to eccentrically control his forward motion. Typically a sport cord is attached around the trunk to enable control and assistance by the clinician. By 4 weeks after his grade 1 strain, he returned to running and was ready to play.

Achilles Tendinosis

History

A 55-year-old competitive runner complained of pain in the midportion of her Achilles tendon that was affecting her ability to run. She reported a gradual onset of dull pain that began

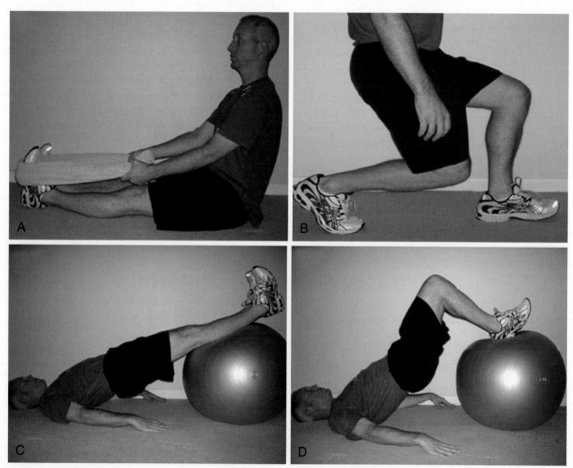

FIGURE 7-8 Exercises after a hamstring strain. Illustrated are just a few of the many exercises that can be performed during rehabilitation after a hamstring strain. **A,** Hamstring stretch. **B,** Forward lunge. **C,** Bridging on a stability ball. **D,** Hamstring curl on a stability ball.

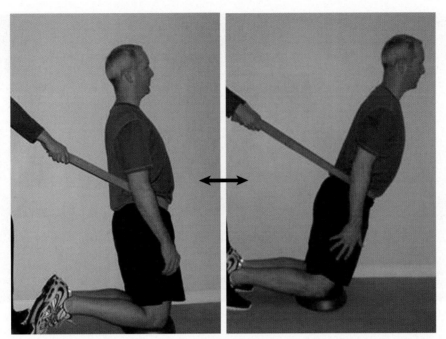

FIGURE 7-9 Russian hamstring curl. The patient starts in a kneeling position on a cushioned mat while the clinician braces the patient's feet and provides resistance by holding a support cord behind the patient. The patient then begins to lean forward to about 45° of knee flexion. The patient is instructed to maintain the trunk erect and to let the forward motion come from the knees. The patient then slowly returns to the upright starting position.

3 months ago after her long runs. Despite the pain, she continued with her competitive training. Now she reports pain during running and therefore decided to seek medical treatment at this time.

Impairments/Functional Limitations

Clinical evaluation revealed tenderness and local thickening of the Achilles tendon. Palpation revealed mild nodules and crepitus with active dorsiflexion and plantar flexion movement. Dorsiflexion ROM was limited, and the heel-raise motion was painful. The patient also had significant pes planus.

Rehabilitation Program

Treatment began with stretching of the Achilles tendon complex. Specifically, gastrocnemius (knee straight) and soleus (knee flexed) stretching was initiated. The patient was advised to hold the stretch for 20 to 30 seconds and repeat for three to five repetitions. The knee flexed stretching was accomplished by using a chair–foot flat–knee flexed–lean into the chair sequence. Eccentric strengthening exercises for the Achilles tendon were also started (Fig. 7-10). The eccentric exercises were repeated for three sets of 15 repetitions and were performed with the knee straight and again with the knee in a semiflexed position. Progressive loading of the eccentric exercises was continued for several weeks by slowly adding weight or use of a weighted vest. Finally, the patient was fitted with foot orthotics to correct the pes planus and improve alignment of the Achilles tendon. Because she had access to a leg press device, she was instructed in bilateral toe press with eccentric return via the involved single leg. She resumed a more competitive running sequence in 10 to 12 weeks.

CONCLUSION

Anatomic Components and Tissue Response to Injury

- The muscle-tendon unit is composed of the muscle, tendon, their attachment sites to each other (MTJ), and the tendon attachment site to bone (OTJ).
- Injury to the muscle-tendon unit can occur at any point in the musculotendinous unit, but it most commonly involves the MTJ.
- Injured muscle and tendon structures progress through the stages of soft tissue healing, which include the inflammatory response, fibroblastic-repair, and maturation-remodeling phases.
- The tensile strength of the damaged tissue increases with time as the collagen fibers remodel and become organized in a parallel alignment with the applied tensile force.
- Satellite cells are specific to muscles and aid in muscle fiber regeneration after injury, whereas tenocytes assist in tendon healing.

Muscle-Tendon Pathologies

- Muscle strains occur as a result of excessive passive stretching or during active eccentric loading. Muscles that cross two joints and muscles that are fatigued are at a higher risk for strain injury.
- Muscle strains can be categorized as grade 1, grade 2, or grade 3 based on the severity of the injury. Contusions can be categorized as mild, moderate, or severe based on the amount of ROM at the adjacent joint.

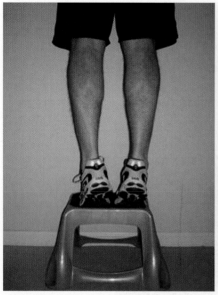
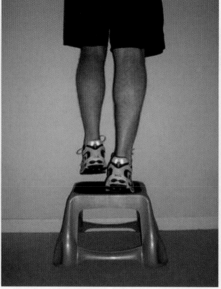
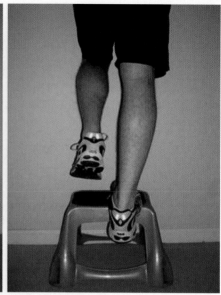

FIGURE 7-10 Eccentric strengthening of the Achilles tendon. The patient completes eccentric strengthening by rising up onto the toes of both feet, transferring the weight over to the involved leg, and then slowly eccentrically lowering the heel off the step until the ankle is in a maximal dorsiflexed position. This sequence is repeated for the prescribed repetitions.

- Tendinitis and paratenonitis refer to an inflammatory process taking place within either the tendon or paratenon, respectively. Tendinosis refers to a chronic degenerative noninflammatory process occurring within the tendon.
- Repetitive loading of the tendon is often the cause of tendon pathology. Tendons are able to withstand tensile loads causing up to 4% elongation, but tensile loads causing between 4% and 8% elongation result in tendon injuries.

Clinical Examination and Evaluation

- A thorough clinical examination consists of a detailed history, in-depth palpation, and static and dynamic clinical assessments.
- Diagnostic imaging of musculotendinous pathologies is often not indicated unless significant tissue damage is suspected or the patient has failed conservative treatment and is considering surgical measures. MRI and ultrasound can be used to identify soft tissue pathologies, whereas radiographic images can be used identify the extent of bony involvement if pathology at the OTJ is suspected.

Rehabilitation Principles

- The principles of rehabilitation for acute injuries include application of the soft tissue healing stages, early mobilization after injury, and progressive loading of the tissue for return to function.
- Goals after an acute injury are to (1) control pain and edema; (2) restore normal ROM and flexibility; (3) reestablish normal strength, endurance, and neuromuscular control; and (4) achieve preinjury function and activity.
- Management of tendinosis includes eccentric exercises and stretching. Other factors, such as modifications in training routines and the use of tape, braces, or orthotics, may also decrease pain and improve function.
- Strategies to prevent muscle-tendon injuries include flexibility and proper strength conditioning.

Case Studies

- Appropriate treatment of muscle and tendon pathologies involves application of the previously described principles of rehabilitation for acute and chronic pathologies.

REFERENCES

1. Garrett, W.E., Jr., Nikolaou, P.K., Ribbeck, B.M., et al. (1998): The effect of the muscle architecture on the biomechanical failure properties of skeletal muscle under passive extension. Am. J. Sports Med., 16:7–12.
2. Noonan, T.J., Best, T.M., Seaber, A.V., Garrett, W.E., Jr. (1994): Identification of a threshold for skeletal muscle injury. Am. J. Sports Med., 22:257–261.
3. Noonan, T.J., Garrett, W.E., Jr. (1999): Muscle strain injury: Diagnosis and treatment. J. Am. Acad. Orthop. Surg., 7:262–269.
4. Prentice, W.E., Jr. (2001): Understanding and managing the healing process through rehabilitation. In: Prentice, W.E., and Voight, M.I. (eds.). Techniques in Musculoskeletal Rehabilitation. New York, McGraw-Hill, pp. 17–41.
5. Tillman, L.J., and Chasan, N.P. (1996): Properties of dense connective tissue and wound healing. In: Hertling, D., and Kessler, R.M. (eds.). Management of Common Musculoskeletal Disorders. Philadelphia, Lippincott Williams & Wilkins, pp. 8–21.
6. Hardy, M.A. (1989): The biology of scar formation. Phys. Ther., 69:1014–1024.
7. Velnar, T., Bailey, T., and Smrkol, V. (2009): The wound healing process: An overview of the cellular and molecular mechanisms. J. Int. Med. Res., 37:1528–1542.
8. Leadbetter, W.B. (1992): Cell-matrix response in tendon injury. Clin. Sports Med., 11:533–578.
9. Jozsa, L., and Kannus, P. (1997): Human Tendons: Anatomy, Physiology, and Pathology. Champaign, IL, Human Kinetics.
10. Ramasastry, S.S. (1998): Acute wounds. Clin. Plast. Surg., 32:195–208.
11. Monaco, J.L., and Lawrence, W.T. (2003): Acute wound healing: An overview. Clin. Plast. Surg., 30:1–12.
12. Christensen-Holz, S., and Smuck, M. (2009): Tissue injury and healing. In: Buschbacher R.M., Prahlow N.D., and Dave S.J. (eds.). Sports Medicine & Rehabilitation: A Sport-Specific Approach. Philadelphia, Lippincott Williams & Wilkins, pp. 17–22.
13. Lawrence, W.T. (1998): Physiology of the acute wound. Clin. Plast. Surg., 25:321–340.
14. Ciciliot, S., and Schiaffino, S. (2010): Regeneration of mammalian skeletal muscle: Basic mechanisms and clinical implications. Curr. Pharm. Des., 16:906–914.

15. Lieber, R.L. (1992): Skeletal Muscle Structure and Function: Implications for Rehabilitation and Sports Medicine. Baltimore, Lippincott Williams & Wilkins.

16. Frank, C.B., Shrive, N.G., Lo, I.K.Y., and Hart, D.A. (2007): Form and function of tendon and ligament. In: Einhorn, T.A., O'Keefe, R.J., and Buckwalter, J.A. (eds.). Orthopaedic Basic Science: Foundations of Clinical Practice, 3rd ed. Rosemont, IL, American Academy of Orthopaedic Surgeons, pp. 191–222.

17. Fadale, P., Bluman, E., and Allen, S. (2006): Pathophysiology of muscle, tendon, and ligament injuries. In: Schepsis, A.A., and Busconi, B.D. (eds.). Sports Medicine. Philadelphia, Lippincott Williams & Wilkins, pp. 1–19.

18. Garrett, W.E., Jr. (1990): Muscle strain injuries: clinical and basic aspects. Med. Sci. Sports Exerc., 22:436–443.

19. Mair, S.D., Seaber, A.V., Glisson, R.R., Garrett, W.E., Jr. (1996): The role of fatigue in susceptibility to acute muscle strain injury. Am. J. Sports Med., 24:137–143.

20. Garrett, W.E., Jr. (1996): Muscle strain injuries. Am. J. Sports Med., 24(Suppl.):S2–S8.

21. Stauber, W.T. (1989): Eccentric action of muscles: Physiology, injury and adaptation. Exerc. Sport Sci. Rev., 17:157–185.

22. Friden, J., and Lieber, R.L. (1992): Structural and mechanical basis of exercise-induced muscle injury. Med. Sci. Sports Exerc., 24:521–530.

23. Lieber, R.L., and Friden, J. (1999): Mechanisms of muscle injury after eccentric contraction. J. Sci. Med. Sport., 2:253–265.

24. Miller, M.D., and Sekiya, J.K. (2006): Sports Medicine: Core Knowledge in Orthopaedics. Philadelphia, Mosby.

25. Eustace, S., Johnston, C., O'Neill, P., and O'Byrne, J. (2007): Sports Injuries: Examination, Imaging and Management. Philadelphia, Churchill Livingstone.

26. Kirkendall, D.T., Prentice, W.E., and Garrett, W.E. (2001): Rehabilitation of muscle injuries. In: Puddo, G., Giombini, A., and Selvanetti, A. (eds.). Rehabilitation of Sports Injuries. Berlin, Springer, pp. 185–193.

27. Stauber, W.T. (1996): Delayed-onset muscle soreness and muscle pain. In: Zachazewski, J.E., Magee, D.J., and Quillen, W.S. (eds.). Athletic Injuries and Rehabilitation. Philadelphia, Saunders, pp. 92–98.

28. Khan, R.J., Fick, D., Keogh, A., et al. (2005): Treatment of acute Achilles tendon ruptures. A meta-analysis of randomized, controlled trials. J. Bone Joint Surg. Am., 87:2202–2210.

29. Leadbetter, W.B. (2001): Soft tissue athletic injury. In: Fu, F.H., and Stone, D.A. (eds.). Sports Injuries: Mechanisms, Prevention, Treatment, 2nd ed. Philadelphia, Lippincott Williams & Wilkins, pp. 839–888.

30. Jackson, D.W., and Feagin, J.A. (1973): Quadriceps contusions in young athletes: Relation of severity of injury to treatment and prognosis. J. Bone Joint Surg. Am., 55:95–105.

31. Ryan, J.B., Wheeler, J.H., Hopkinson, W.J., et al. (1991): Quadriceps contusions: West Point update. Am. J. Sports Med., 19:299–304.

32. Aronen, J.G., Garrick, J.G., Chronister, R.D., and McDevitt, E.R. (2006): Quadriceps contusions: Clinical results of immediate immobilization in 120 degrees of knee flexion. Clin. J. Sport Med., 16:383–387.

33. Larson, C.M. (2002): Evaluating and managing muscle contusions and myositis ossificans. Physician Sportsmed., 30:41–50.

34. Clancy, W.G. (1990): Tendon trauma and overuse injuries. In: Leadbetter, W.B., Buckwalter, J.A., and Gordon, S.L. (eds.). Sports-Induced Inflammation: Clinical and Basic Science Concepts. Park Ridge, IL, American Academy of Orthopaedic Surgeons, pp. 609–618.

35. Nirschl, R.P., and Ashman, E.S. (2003): Elbow tendinopathy: Tennis elbow. Clin. Sports Med., 22:813–836.

36. Khan, K.M., Cook, J.L., Bonar, F., et al. (1999): Histopathology of common tendinopathies: Update and implications for clinical management. Sports Med., 6:393–408.

37. Curwin, S.L. (1996): Tendon injuries: Pathophysiology and treatment. In: Zachazewski, J.E., Magee, D.J., and Quillen, W.S. (eds.). Athletic Injuries and Rehabilitation. Philadelphia. Saunders, pp. 27–53.

38. Kaeding, C., and Best, T.M. (2009): Tendinosis: Pathophysiology and nonoperative treatment. Sports Health, 1:284–292.

39. Rees, J.D., Maffulli, N., and Cook, J. (2009): Management of tendinopathy. Am. J. Sports Med., 37:1855–1867.

40. Chang, A., and Miller, T.T. (2009): Imaging of tendons. Sports Health, 1:293–300.

41. Mitchell, A.W.M., Lee, J.C., and Healy, J.C. (2009): The use of ultrasound in the assessment and treatment of Achilles tendinosis. J. Bone Joint Surg. Br., 91:1405–1409.

42. Margherita, A. (2009): The sports medicine approach to musculoskeletal medicine. In: Buschbacher, R.M., Prahlow, N.D., and Dave, S.J. (eds.). Sports Medicine & Rehabilitation: A Sport-Specific Approach. Philadelphia, Lippincott Williams & Wilkins, pp. 23–30.

43. Jarvinen, T.A.H., Jarvinen, T.L.N., Kaariainen, M., et al. (2007): Muscle injuries: Optimizing recovery. Best Pract. Res. Clin. Rheumatol., 21:317–331.

44. Prentice, W.E., Jr. (2002): The healing process and guidelines for using modalities. In: Prentice, W.E., Jr. (ed.). Therapeutic Modalities for Physical Therapists. New York, McGraw-Hill, pp. 14–27.

45. Taylor, D.C., Dalton, J.D., Jr., Seaber, A.V., Garrett, W.E., Jr. (1993): Experimental muscle strain injury. Early functional and structural deficits and the increased risk for reinjury. Am. J. Sports Med., 21:190–194.

46. Stanish, W.D., Rubinovich, R.M., and Curwin, S. (1986): Eccentric exercise in chronic tendinitis. Clin. Orthop. Relat. Res., 208:65–68.

47. Alfredson, H., Pietila, T., Jonsson, P., and Lorentzon, R. (1998): Heavy-load eccentric calf muscle training for the treatment of chronic Achilles tendinosis. Am. J. Sports Med., 26:360–366.

48. Alfredson, H., and Lorentzon, R. (2000): Chronic Achilles tendinosis: Recommendations for treatment and prevention. Sports Med., 29:135–146.

49. Norregaard, J., Larsen, C.C., Bieler, T., and Langberg, H. (2007): Eccentric exercise in treatment of Achilles tendinopathy. Scand. J. Med. Sci. Sports, 17:133–138.

50. Wasielewski, N.J., and Kotsko, K.M. (2007): Does eccentric exercise reduce pain and improve strength in physically active adults with symptomatic lower extremity tendinosis? J. Athl. Train., 42:409–421.

51. Malliaras, P., Maffulli, N., and Garau, G. (2008): Eccentric training programmes in the management of lateral elbow tendinopathy. Disabil. Rehabil., 30:1590–1596.

52. Woodley, B.L., Newsham-West, R.J., and Baxter, G.D. (2007): Chronic tendinopathy: Effectiveness of eccentric exercise. Br. J. Sports Med., 41:188–198.

53. Andres, B.M., and Murrell, G.A.C. (2008): Treatment of tendinopathy: What works, what does not, and what is on the horizon. Clin. Orthop. Relat. Res., 466:1539–1554.

54. Ohberg, L., Lorentzon, R., and Alfredson, H. (2004): Eccentric training in patients with chronic Achilles tendinosis: Normalised tendon structure and decreased thickness at follow up. Br. J. Sports Med., 38:8–11.

55. Haraldsson, B.T., Langber, H., Aagaard, P., et al. (2006): Corticosteroids reduce the tensile strength of isolated collagen fascicles. Am. J. Sports Med., 34:1992–1997.

56. Hibbert, O., Cheong, K., Grant, A., et al. A systematic review of the effectiveness of eccentric strength training in the prevention of hamstring muscle strains in otherwise healthy individuals. N. Am. J. Sports Phys. Ther., 3:80-93.

8

Therapeutic Modalities As an Adjunct to Rehabilitation

Mark A. Merrick, PhD, ATC

CHAPTER OBJECTIVES

- Identify which modalities are effective and clinically useful for particular pathologies.
- Identify incorrect modality application techniques that can compromise clinical effectiveness.
- Choose the appropriate clinical use or uses for a specific modality.
- Explain the effect that cryotherapy has on certain biologic functions in the acute care of an injury.

- Explain the effect that compression and elevation have on certain biologic functions with an acute injury.
- Choose appropriate modalities based on their clinical efficacy for use during the rehabilitation process.
- Explain when to initiate, modify, and discontinue modality protocols based on patient needs and rehabilitative goals.

Optimal care of athletic injuries is different from the typical care that most musculoskeletal/orthopedic patients receive. Typical care of nonathletic patients with musculoskeletal injury produces good outcomes over time, but the time line is frustratingly slow for an athlete trying to return to full levels of play *this* season. Typical care takes too long to initiate, is reevaluated too infrequently, is too conservative in approach, and leads to considerable noncompliance by the patient. To meet the more aggressive time line and functional demands of an athletic patient, we must recognize the interrelated nature of evaluation, acute management, and rehabilitation and see them as a continuum. This continuum begins the moment the injury occurs, and immediate initiation of care for an athlete offers a critical time savings that is lost when care is delayed until the next day or next week. It is often the difference between returning to play in 2 weeks instead of 6.

Appropriate therapeutic techniques, when applied at appropriate times, can radically reduce complicating factors, such as edema and neuromuscular inhibition, which delay the patient's eventual return to normal function. Therapeutic modalities are one set of tools that can play a central role throughout the rehabilitative continuum but are most important early in the process. Like all tools, however, modalities have specific uses in specific situations. They are of little benefit when used for the wrong reason, with the wrong technique, or at the wrong time. At their

best, therapeutic modalities are an exceptionally useful complement to the rehabilitative process but are not a replacement for it. At their worst, therapeutic modalities can be blindly applied and ineffective tools that waste the time of both the patient and clinician. This chapter explores the general use, rehabilitative timing, and specific application of therapeutic modalities for the care of the injured athlete. More importantly, the literature on the clinical efficacy of common therapeutic modalities is examined to identify which appear to be effective and which do not.

GENERAL PRINCIPLES OF THEAPEUTIC MODALITIES

What Are Modalities and Why Use Them?

Simply stated, modalities are therapeutic techniques. They include such dissimilar things as surgery, medications, and psychologic counseling, none of which are appropriate for independent use by allied health practitioners, such as athletic trainers and physical therapists. The modalities with which we are more familiar and that are more appropriate for our use are generally referred to as *therapeutic modalities* and include primarily physical agents, such as heat, cold, sound, electromagnetic energy, and mechanical energy (such as massage and compression).

Modalities As Part of a Comprehensive Rehabilitative Program

The single most important point to remember about therapeutic modalities is that they are tools and should never be used as replacements for a comprehensive rehabilitative program. Modalities are an adjunct to rehabilitation. That is, they can *help* a clinician and patient to accomplish a goal, but therapeutic modalities are not usually capable of accomplishing goals in isolation. Instead, they should generally be combined with other rehabilitative techniques (especially therapeutic exercise) and should not be viewed as a substitute for these techniques. For example, using only ice massage before practice for someone with patellar tendinitis is not the same as using a comprehensive rehabilitative program that involves counteracting chronic inflammation; minimizing sclerosis; correcting biomechanics; improving strength, endurance, and power; and limiting overuse. Conversely, some practitioners will make statements such as, "I don't use modalities, I prefer exercise instead," as though their choices were *between* exercise and modalities. It is seldom correct to choose between these approaches because they are not used for the same purposes. Instead, it would be better to understand how each approach can be useful to achieve a goal and then choose a plan of care that combines the best available elements, often *both* exercise *and* modalities, to achieve the goal.

When to Use Modalities

Like any tool, a therapeutic modality should be used for a specific purpose and at a specific time. You would use a screwdriver to tighten a screw but not to drive in a nail. Likewise, you would use cryotherapy to counteract acute inflammation but not to counteract the loss of range of motion associated with prolonged immobilization. Although it seems obvious, the key to using modalities appropriately is to match the specific physiologic effects of the modality with the specific rehabilitative goal for the patient. The apparent corollary to this statement is that if the physiologic effects of the modality do not match the rehabilitative goals, the modality should not be used, or if the goals have been met, the modality should be discontinued. Even though these principles are almost self-evident, it is not uncommon for novice clinicians to make the mistake of using a modality without having a specific goal in mind or failing to discontinue a modality after the goal for which it was chosen has been achieved.

Most practitioners do a fine job of identifying patient problems, creating specific goals related to these problems, and choosing modalities to help achieve these goals. However, advanced practitioners are also skilled at determining *when* a modality should be initiated within the rehabilitative continuum. With modality use, the timing is often critical. If cryotherapy and compression are applied within the first few minutes following trauma, the secondary injury response can be substantially suppressed, thereby saving time and tissue. Waiting until the next day—or even perhaps just a few hours to begin such care—will almost certainly be pointless.

Likewise, it is critical to understand when use of a modality should be discontinued. In the current era in which health insurance providers are attempting to limit billed charges, it is important to be cost-effective in using rehabilitative programs, and efficient and effective use of therapeutic modalities is an important element of a cost-effective program. However, some

practitioners continue to use a modality even after the modality's goal has been achieved because they lack a goal-oriented focus in the use of modalities. To avoid this error, practitioners should ask themselves four questions before each modality treatment (Box 8-1).

How to Use Modalities

This chapter is not intended to be a substitute for a formal course in the application of therapeutic modalities. That topic is somewhat more comprehensive, and quite a few very good modalities texts[1-5] provide a greater level of instruction in the application of modalities. This chapter instead reviews the general elements common to all modality applications and discusses some specific aspects of the application and the efficacy of each modality presented.

Legal and Appropriate Use of Modalities

Physical agents are appropriate for application by clinicians in any of several different professions, such as physicians, athletic trainers, and physical therapists, although their actual use is generally governed by the practice acts of individual states. Consult your state's regulations before applying therapeutic modalities. A general provision in most practice acts is that practitioners are required to have specific training in both therapeutic modality theory and the application techniques for these modalities. A good principle to follow is that you should never use a therapeutic modality that you have not been specifically trained to use. Although this seems obvious, it is particularly relevant where students are concerned. Students should not apply therapeutic modalities until they have completed the relevant course work to support their modality use.

In addition to state regulation, many therapeutic modalities, including ultrasound, diathermy, lymphedema pumps, lasers, and others, are classified as medical devices and are therefore regulated in the United States by the Center for Devices and Radiological Health, part of the Food and Drug Administration (http://www.fda.gov/cdrh/consumer/mda/index.html). Different devices within the same category, such as lasers, may carry different classifications and be subject to different levels of regulation.

Another important aspect of the legal and appropriate use of modalities involves prescriptions for treatment. In most states, prescriptions for outpatient rehabilitation are required. Although specific prescriptions for each modality are sometimes required, frequently they are not, and use of therapeutic modalities is left to the professional judgment of the clinician. However, some modalities, particularly those involving pharmaceutical delivery (iontophoresis or phonophoresis), always require a specific prescription.

As is true with any rehabilitative procedure, practitioners assume some degree of liability with the use of therapeutic modalities. To maximize patient safety and minimize the liability associated with the use of therapeutic modalities, a number of policies and procedures should be adopted (Box 8-2).

General Application Procedures

Even though the specific application procedures for each therapeutic modality differ, all modality treatments have some commonalities. One of the most important, actively involving patients in their own care, is frequently overlooked. Before any modality is applied, it should be explained thoroughly to patients. Such explanations allow patients to make informed decisions about consent to treatment. Similarly, it also helps patients understand the specific goals and effects of the treatment. In addition, it helps patients understand any potentially harmful complications, such as excessive heating, and lets them know that the practitioner should be told if a treatment causes discomfort so that it can be modified before becoming a problem. Patients should also be asked whether they have any questions about the use of the modality in their treatment. An additional bonus of involving patients in their own care is that those who feel like a partner in their own care are frequently more compliant with their rehabilitative programs. Box 8-3 lists some common items that should be explained to patients before application of a modality.

In addition to making patients partners in their own care, another commonality with all modality treatments is in the actual setup for the treatment. The physical preparations for use of a modality involve two items. The first is preparation of the patient. Before any other aspect of patient preparation, you should determine whether a prescription for the modality treatment is required and present and whether the prescription has expired or the number of permissible treatments has been exceeded. When this step is completed, the remainder of patient preparation generally involves reviewing the specific goal of the treatment along with the indications for the modality to ensure

that no contraindications are present, review the patient's previous response to the treatment (ask the patient), and ensure that the patient consents to the treatment. The outcome of any previous treatments should also be reviewed. Physical preparation of the patient generally involves removing or adjusting clothing as necessary for the specific modality and positioning the patient as comfortably as possible. This last aspect is critically important when modality treatments are given for more than just a few minutes.

The second aspect of physical preparation is the physical setup of the modality equipment and treatment area. First and foremost, the patient's safety must be ensured through a quick but complete safety inspection of the equipment and area before use of any modality (Box 8-4). After the equipment safety inspection is completed, you should make sure that all the necessary accessories for the treatment are present before actually beginning the treatment.

Box 8-3
Patient Education Before Modality Treatments

State which modality is to be used: for example, "We're going to use some ice on your knee for about 20 minutes after your exercise today."

Inform the patient of the specific goal for the modality and what the modality does: for example, "The ice helps reduce any inflammation we may have caused today and it helps reduce your soreness."

Rule out contraindications: for example, "Do you have any circulatory or neurologic problems, such as Raynaud disease?"

Explain what the patient should expect: for example, "It will feel very cold and it'll probably be a little bit uncomfortable until you get used to it."

Explain the precautions and reasons to discontinue the treatment: for example, "You shouldn't feel any pain, numbness, or tingling down in your leg or foot, but if you do, let me know right away and I'll take the ice off."

Explain the criteria for discontinuing the use of this modality overall: for example, "We'll quit using the ice if it's not giving the result we want or when you quit having inflammation or soreness after your exercises."

Box 8-2
Suggested Policies and Procedures for the Application Modalities

Good professional judgment must be used. Exercise of good professional judgment and application of a modality that you have not been trained to use are mutually exclusive. Therefore, modalities should be used only by those formally trained (and legally permitted) to use them.

Every modality must be in good working order and have recently been calibrated to ensure safe use of it.

Every planned modality treatment for every patient should be evaluated to ensure that it is appropriate with regard to the indications and contraindications for use of the modality.

Every modality treatment should be monitored for both safety and efficacy throughout the treatment. Treatments causing adverse effects should be discontinued immediately, as should treatments that are not effective.

Unattended modality treatments are obviously to be avoided, as are patient self-applications of most modalities.

Box 8-4
Equipment Checklist Before Application of a Modality

Check the condition of any patient cables or electrodes and ensure that they meet the required standards.

Confirm that the equipment is operational.

Confirm that patient safety switches are operational.

For electrical modalities, ensure that the equipment is properly grounded and that the equipment is used only with outlets equipped with ground-fault circuit interrupters.

Evaluate the treatment area to make sure no hazards are present, such as standing water or unstable treatment tables.

Postapplication Procedures

Just as there are commonalities in the setup for all modality treatments, there are also commonalities in the posttreatment procedures. Most of these are obvious and include removing the patient from any equipment, returning the equipment to its appropriate storage area, and assisting the patient in wiping off any treatment-related water, gel, or other material as necessary. The most important aspects of the postapplication period are less obvious and often overlooked, particularly in competitive athletic settings. The first is record keeping. It is absolutely critical that practitioners record the treatment parameters used during application of the modality. Recording the parameters allows a different practitioner to continue the course of treatment if you are unavailable. Without such a record, other practitioners are either forced to guess your protocol or ask the patient what has been done. At no time should a practitioner ever have to ask the patient which treatment parameters have been used because even the most involved of patients cannot be expected to understand the parameters or explain them correctly. It is also important to make specific note of any complications that occurred during the treatment, as well as the patient's response to the treatment.

Another postapplication procedure often overlooked is reviewing the response to the modality treatment to determine whether the goal of the modality has been met, whether the treatment has been effective, or whether the treatment should be continued. A plan for discontinuing the modality treatment should be in place to help with this last issue.

SEPARATING FACTS FROM FICTION

Determining whether specific modalities are effective and clinically useful is often more difficult than it would outwardly appear. We will see that a number of clinically common modalities may not be as effective as once thought and that the clinical efficacy of modalities that are known to be useful can easily be compromised by incorrect application techniques. Unnecessary, incorrect, or inappropriate use of modalities has been a topic of discussion for clinicians and researchers, as well as for health insurance providers, who are carefully scrutinizing outcomes research to determine whether they should reimburse for certain modalities treatments. Unfortunately, poorly designed modality clinical trials or trials in which modalities are used incorrectly have led to poor outcomes that have negatively influenced the use of modalities in clinical practice. In addition, several very effective therapeutic modalities, such as short wave diathermy and low-power lasers, are not in common use because we are either not sufficiently aware of them, not trained to use them, or not able to afford to purchase them. To adequately examine the efficacy of therapeutic modalities, a few basics about modality research must first be reviewed.

Modality Research

In examining the history of modality use, one obvious trend is that clinical practice has almost always preceded scientific research. That is, clinicians pass along anecdotes about how they have used modalities and the results that they have observed. This has led to a great deal of modality folklore that in reality has very little basis in fact. We really did not see a meaningful body of scientific research on therapeutic modalities until the last few decades. This modality research has been conducted by scientists and clinicians from a number of different professional fields, including early work by physicians such as Lewis,[6] who examined cold, and Lehmann et al,[7-9] who examined heat. Most of the more recent research has been conducted by researchers from allied health fields, such as athletic training and physical therapy. In fact, the overwhelming majority of recent research on the clinical use of therapeutic modalities has been completed by athletic trainers, yet ironically, some states still prohibit athletic trainers from using these modalities.

The frequently observed trend of clinical practice preceding scientific inquiry with therapeutic modalities has greatly influenced research on modalities. Many, if not most modality researchers began their careers as clinicians. This clinician background has resulted in the use of many clinically relevant and relatively unsophisticated dependent variables in modalities research. Such clinical variables typically include range of motion, strength (usually isometric or isokinetic), swelling, pain/soreness, and various functional measures. There is also a body of research that has gone beyond clinical variables and examined slightly more basic variables, such as temperature, electromyographic activity, blood flow, and tissue stiffness. In recent years, a small number of laboratories have also examined very basic variables such as cell metabolism, protein expression, gene expression, enzyme activity, and cell proliferation.

The simpler and more clinical variables have obvious value to clinicians and are very useful in establishing outcomes, a type of research that is very helpful in supporting reimbursement activities. Unfortunately, these variables are generally less useful in helping establish modality theory. Most clinical variables are, at best, secondary manifestations of the effects of modalities. That is, modalities generally do not directly cause the effects seen in clinical variables, but instead they cause these clinical effects indirectly. For example, continuous ultrasound treatments do not improve range of motion directly or meaningfully. Instead, continuous ultrasound causes vibration between molecules in the tissue. The vibrations increase the temperature of the tissue,[7,9-11] and the increased tissue temperature may allow tissues to become more elastic.[8,12] In turn, increased elasticity may allow stretching techniques to be more effective. Finally, more effective stretching or joint mobilization may improve range of motion and do so more easily because of the improved elasticity. Without combining the stretching or mobilization with the ultrasound, the ultrasound is probably useless in this scenario.

The indirect relationship between most modalities and clinical variables presents problems in establishing theories because the clinical variables are easily confounded. That is, many factors might influence the clinical variables and can potentially mask or intensify the effects of the modality. The more steps between the modality's believed direct effect and the clinical variable, the greater the chance that something can become confounded along the way. If this happens, we may not be able to observe a strong effect that we can use to support or refute the underlying theory regarding the modality. Likewise, the more steps that the clinical variable is removed from the direct effect, the greater the number of opportunities for a methodologic mistake to prevent the desired outcome. When we are examining only a relatively limited number of modality protocols and do not see an effect, it is difficult and probably inappropriate to make broad generalizations about the modality. A classic example of this problem is an ultrasound review paper by Robertson and Baker[13] (Table 8-1). The conclusion drawn

Table 8-1 Robertson and Baker's "A Review of Therapeutic Ultrasound: Effectiveness Studies," *Physical Therapy,* **July 2001**

Robertson and Baker reviewed 35 ultrasound studies from peer-reviewed journals between 1975 and 1999. Because of small sample size or other problems, they were forced to discard 25 of the studies and therefore based their findings on 10 papers reporting clinical outcomes. Of these 10 papers, only 2 reported that ultrasound was better than placebo. Robertson and Baker concluded that the literature shows that ultrasound is no more effective than placebo.

At first glance, this study appears to be a redundant condemnation of the clinical use of ultrasound. On closer examination, however, this study actually becomes a good case in drawing poor conclusions because of poor data. In a letter to the editor in the February 2002 issue of *Physical Therapy,* Draper pointed out that 8 of the 10 studies used in this review had serious methodologic flaws that rendered them virtually useless for describing the clinical efficacy of ultrasound (see below). Just as an automobile appears to be useless as a means of transportation if you are stepping on the wrong pedal, ultrasound appears to be useless as a modality if you use the wrong parameters.

Problem Area	Problematic Protocol Used	Problem With the Protocol
Effective radiating area (ERA)	Thermal ultrasound applied to an area 5 times the size of the faceplate	The ERA is always smaller than the ultrasound faceplate, and the treatment area should be no larger than twice the ERA to induce an effective increase in temperature.
	Thermal ultrasound applied to an area 10-25 times the size of the faceplate	
	Thermal ultrasound applied to an area 10 times the size of the faceplate	
	Nonthermal ultrasound applied to an area 10 times the size of the faceplate	No published evidence has shown that nonthermal ultrasound applied to such a large area produces an increase in healing.
Ultrasound frequency	1-MHz ultrasound used to treat superficial tissues (epicondylalgia)	1-MHz ultrasound is effective at depths of 2.5 to 5 cm. The epicondyles are considerably more superficial and should have been treated with 3-MHz ultrasound.
Treatment time	1-MHz ultrasound applied for a 3-minute treatment to test joint mobility with a treatment size at least 12 times as large as the ERA	This would not have produced any meaningful change in temperature because of the huge treatment area. Even with an appropriate treatment area, it would be estimated to produce only a 1.2°C increase in temperature. An increase in temperature of at least 3°C to 4°C would be required to produce changes in elasticity.
	7 of the 10 studies used a 25% pulsed duty cycle, with treatment times varying from 2 to 15 minutes	The two studies that did show an effect of ultrasound both used 15-minute treatment times. The shorter treatment times very likely explain the lack of effect.

Data from Draper, D. (2002): Don't disregard ultrasound yet—the jury is still out. Phys. Ther., 82:190–191; Robertson, V., and Baker, K. (2001): A review of therapeutic ultrasound: Effectiveness studies. Phys. Ther., 81:1339–1350.

in this review was that therapeutic ultrasound is not an effective adjunct for improving range of motion or pain. The effect of this review was a reluctance by many to use therapeutic ultrasound because they feared that insurance providers, in the wake of this paper, might not reimburse for such treatments. Unfortunately, the research studies reviewed in this paper generally used clinical variables and rather ineffective ultrasound application protocols, and most did not observe a positive effect.[14] The use of substandard ultrasound protocols meant that the expected direct effect of ultrasound would have been smaller. A smaller than expected effect would have been further diluted because there were a number of physiologic steps between the presumed effect of ultrasound and the clinical variables studied. In fact, in examining the methods in the studies from this review, it is clear that most were wholly inappropriate and were very unlikely to cause a useful effect, and not surprisingly, no useful effects were seen.[14]

Although much of the research on the use of modalities has focused on clinical variables, a surprisingly large number of effects of modalities are commonly accepted by clinicians but have little, if any, scientific support. In some cases there is even scientific evidence to the contrary, yet these widely held clinical beliefs still persist. One common example of this is cold-induced vasodilation with cryotherapy. Similarly, incorrect beliefs still circulate regarding contrast baths for reduction of edema[15-18] and transcutaneously applied microcurrent for muscle injuries.[19-21]

Clinical Pearl #1

Cold-induced vasodilation, the notion that cryotherapy treatments can cause blood flow to increase above baseline levels, is still touted as an effect of cryotherapy by some clinicians.[6] In fact, you may still occasionally hear someone incorrectly suggest that cold should not be used for more than about 30 minutes to avoid this phenomenon. This is completely false. In reality, cryotherapy does not increase blood flow above baseline levels at all.[22] This has been repeatedly demonstrated[22-27] for more than 60 years!

Where to Go From Here

In the future, modality research needs to accomplish two important tasks. First, we need to establish a body of suitable outcomes research documenting the efficacy of our modality treatments.

Although we are continuing to learn about the physiologic effects of modalities, there is a wholly inadequate body of outcomes research related to the use of these modalities. Research is sorely needed to confirm whether our physiologically based treatments actually improve the outcomes of the patients whom we treat. This outcomes research must examine multiple protocols for each modality to refine our clinical techniques and maximize the benefits that our patients receive. Second, we need research that focuses more on the direct effects that we think are caused by the modalities. Generally, this means more research on the basic science variables that we think are the root of the clinical effects. When we establish and understand the very basic effects caused by our modalities, we will be better able to refine our treatments to maximize the clinical benefits of modality treatments. For example, we are very confident that cryotherapy is useful in minimizing the unwanted consequences of acute injury. However, we are not completely certain of the precise mechanisms by which this modality is effective. Even though a number of papers have proposed theories, these theories have yet to be confirmed. In fact, we do not yet know the answers to such basic cryotherapy questions as how cold the injured tissues need to be or how long the cold should be applied to be most effective. Answering the basic questions of how a modality works physiologically will allow us to better examine the clinically relevant questions of how to maximize the benefit of the modality.

MODALITIES FOR ACUTE CARE

Goals

The use of therapeutic modalities for acute injuries is governed by a specific set of clinical goals (Table 8-2). The most important of these goals is thought to be limiting the total quantity of tissue damage associated with the injury.[28,29] Because we know that the time required for tissue healing is partially dependent on the quantity of tissue damaged, a smaller amount of damaged tissue should translate into a quicker repair and faster return to sport.

When an injury occurs, the immediate tissue damage associated with that injury is referred to as the primary injury.[28-32] This damage includes disruption of a variety of structures, including ligamentous, tendinous, muscular, vascular, nervous, and bony tissues. Because primary injury occurs immediately with the trauma, it has already occurred before the injury is even evaluated. We can do nothing to limit the magnitude of this primary tissue damage apart from immobilizing the injured area to prevent further tearing of partially torn tissues. However, primary damage is not the end of the story. The pathophysiologic response to primary injury can lead to additional tissue damage, known as secondary injury, in tissues that were otherwise not initially injured.[28-32] For example, disruption of blood flow resulting from an injury to vascular tissue can lead to ischemic injury of the otherwise uninjured tissues that they supply. Although ischemia is probably one of the leading villains of secondary injury, there are actually a number of other suggested causes as well. Unlike primary injury, secondary injury may be inhibited by our acute interventions. For example, some evidence shows that immediate application of cryotherapy inhibits secondary injury following acute trauma.[33] By limiting secondary injury, the total quantity of injured tissue is limited, which should reduce the time necessary to repair the damage and return to sport.

Table 8-2 Goals and Modalities for Care of Acute Injuries

Acute Care Goal	Choice of Modality
Reduce pain	Cryotherapy, TENS
Minimize edema formation	Cryotherapy, compression, elevation, microcurrent(?)
Minimize bleeding	Cryotherapy, compression, elevation
Minimize secondary injury	Cryotherapy
Minimize acute inflammation	Cryotherapy, microcurrent(?)
Prevent further injury	Immobilization/protection

TENS, Transcutaneous electrical nerve stimulation.

A second but equally important goal of the acute use of modalities is to limit the sequelae of the acute inflammatory response. Because acute inflammation occurs with every injury to perfused tissues, all five signs of inflammation can be expected to occur to some extent.[34] These signs—redness, heat, pain, edema, and loss of function—can lead to an unnecessarily prolonged time needed for healing. By limiting these signs, particularly the pain and edema, function can be restored sooner and patients thereby returned to activity sooner. Likewise, the biochemical consequences of acute inflammation include the release of a number of damaging enzymes and radicals[34] that are capable of producing additional tissue damage (see Chapter 2). Obviously, limiting the quantity or activity of these damaging molecules could help reduce the total quantity of damaged tissue and therefore lead to quicker repair.

Cryotherapy

The traditional management of acute injuries is described by the acronym RICE, which stands for rest, ice, compression, and elevation.[1-5,35] Cryotherapy, or the therapeutic use of cold, is by far the most commonly used and probably the most effective modality for managing acute musculoskeletal injuries.[24,30-33,36-39] There is almost certainly no more familiar modality to practitioners than the ice bag; however, in clinical practice, cryotherapy takes many forms and can be used to help accomplish a variety of goals, both acute and postacute. From a scientific standpoint, there is perhaps no modality that we know more about; even so, our understanding of cryotherapy is somewhat more limited than probably imagined. This section discusses only the acute use of cryotherapy. Its postacute use in facilitating early exercise is discussed in conjunction with the other postacute modalities later in the chapter.

Description

Cryotherapy is one of the most broadly defined of the therapeutic modalities. Quite simply, it involves the therapeutic application of cold. Many different forms of cold therapy are commonly used in clinical practice, and new forms are being developed and marketed continually. Although one of the most common forms of cryotherapy is the ice bag, cold modalities also include ice massage, ice slush immersions, cold-water immersion, frozen gel

Table 8-3 Physiologic Effects and Clinical Uses of Cryotherapy

Physiologic Effect	Clinical Use
Reduced temperature	↓ secondary injury, ↓ edema formation, ↓ bleeding, ↓ pain
Reduced metabolic rate	↓ secondary injury
Reduced perfusion	↓ bleeding, ↓ edema formation
Reduced inflammation	↓ secondary injury, ↓ edema formation, ↓ pain

↓, Decrease.

packs, vapocoolant sprays, cold-compression devices, and even "instant" cold packs. Please note that virtually all of these involve the *local* use of cold rather than the *global* (whole body) application of cold. The physiology of local cooling is somewhat different from that of global cooling, and it is this local cooling that is of most interest in rehabilitation.

The wide array of cryotherapy options is reflective of both the obvious efficacy of this modality and our inadequate understanding of what constitutes an ideal treatment. All these various forms of cryotherapy are capable of cooling tissues to different extents; however, only limited data are available to suggest which of these forms of cryotherapy is the most effective.[40-45]

How We Think It Works

Like all modalities, cold treatments produce a variety of physiologic effects (Table 8-3). These physiologic effects can easily be translated into goals for cryotherapy treatments.[32] Although each of these effects is generally discussed separately, it should be remembered that they all occur simultaneously. Therefore, we need to consider all the effects of a modality when we use it, and we need to balance the desired effects with the unwanted effects to determine whether use of the modality is judicious or inadvisable.

REDUCTION IN TEMPERATURE

The most easily recognizable effect of cryotherapy is a reduction in tissue temperature. In fact, virtually all the effects observed with cryotherapy are a direct result of this change in tissue temperature. In the past 10 years alone, a great deal of cryotherapy research has used temperature reduction as the variable of interest.[15,16,18,39-57] Most of these studies have examined skin temperature (Fig. 8-1), but a growing body of literature is also reporting on deep temperatures during cryotherapy (Fig. 8-2). From this literature we know that during many forms of cryotherapy the skin can easily reach single-digit temperatures (°C) and that the change in intramuscular temperature is quite variable depending on the depth at which temperature is measured and the duration of the treatment. Typical intramuscular temperatures during most forms of cryotherapy are in the range of 25°C to 31°C.

The most important factor that determines the change in tissue temperature during cryotherapy is heat transfer.[32,41] An important concept to remember when we speak of tissue cooling is that cold cannot be transferred because cold is merely the absence of heat. Heat is transferred from one body to another, with the net transfer always being in the direction

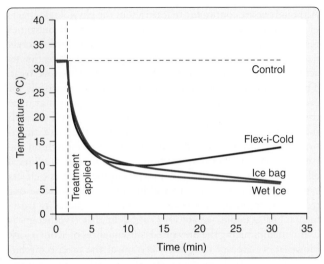

FIGURE 8-1 Skin temperatures during cryotherapy with various cold modalities. *(From Merrick, M., Jutte, L., and Smith, M. [2003]: Cold modalities with different thermodynamic properties produce different surface and intramuscular temperatures. J. Athl. Train., 38:28–33.)*

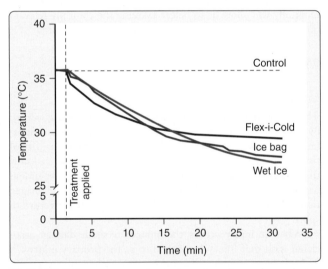

FIGURE 8-2 Temperatures 1-cm deep to adipose layer during cryotherapy with various cold modalities. *(From Merrick, M., Jutte, L., and Smith, M. [2003]: Cold modalities with different thermodynamic properties produce different surface and intramuscular temperatures. J. Athl. Train., 38:28–33.)*

of high heat moving toward lower heat. Therefore, body tissues (high heat) are cooled because they lose heat that is absorbed by the cold modality (low heat); the greater the ability of a cold modality to absorb heat, the greater the potential for reducing tissue temperatures.

The heat-absorbing capacity of cold modalities is determined by a number of factors (Box 8-5). Cold modalities with more mass can absorb more heat than those with a small mass. Similarly, the greater the contact area, the greater the heat transfer. Greater differences in temperature also lead to more rapid heat transfer. Conversely, the greater the tissue thickness, particularly adipose thickness, the slower the heat transfer.

One of the most important factors controlling heat transfer is the specific heat of the tissue and modality. *Specific heat* is

Factors That Determine the Heat-Absorbing Capacity of a Cold Modality

Patient's mass
Size of the contact area
Difference in temperature between the modality and the tissue
Distance across which heat must be transferred (tissue thickness)[32,41]

the amount of heat necessary to raise the temperature of 1 kg of the material by 1°K (or 1°C because the units are the same size).[32,41,58,59] The greater the specific heat, the more energy required to raise the temperature of the material. Therefore, material with a greater specific heat can absorb more heat energy per degree of change in temperature than can material with a lower specific heat. Perhaps even more important is whether the cold modality goes through a change of state (solid to liquid) when it absorbs heat. Changes in physical state occur at specific temperatures. For example, ice at 0°C becomes water at 0°C as it melts. The amount of heat required to cause this change in state during melting is known as the *heat of fusion* and is much higher than the material's specific heat.[32,41,58,59] For example, at 0°C the specific heat of ice is 2090 J/kg/°C, the specific heat of water at the same temperature is 4190 J/kg/°C, and the heat of fusion for ice melting to water is 333,000 J/kg. In other words, a cold modality changing from ice at 0°C to water at 0°C absorbs roughly 80 times as much heat as raising the temperature of cold water from 0°C to 1°C!

Clinical Pearl #2

From a thermodynamics standpoint, it is clear that modalities that undergo a phase change (e.g., ice) are capable of absorbing more heat than those that do not (e.g., frozen gel). This notion received some clinical support when it was demonstrated that lower skin and intramuscular temperatures are observed when using ice-based modalities than when using flexible gel cold packs.[41] Another important factor in reduction of tissue temperature is the use of compression. Cryotherapy used in combination with compression has been shown to produce greater reductions in temperature than cryotherapy used alone can.[40,42]

In addition to the thermodynamic properties of the modality itself, the tissue temperatures observed during cryotherapy are also largely dependent on factors related to the tissues being treated. Of these factors, the thickness of the adipose layer at the treatment site appears to be the most important.[49,53,55] In a noteworthy study, Otte et al[55] compared the duration of treatment required to produce a uniform change in temperature in patients with different adipose thickness (Fig. 8-3). Remarkably, to produce an identical 7°C drop in temperature of the quadriceps with the application of an ice bag, subjects with anterior thigh skinfolds of 11 to 20 mm required 23 minutes, whereas subjects with skinfolds of 31 to 40 mm required an almost unthinkable 59 minutes! Clearly, the days of "one duration fits all" for cryotherapy treatments are long gone.

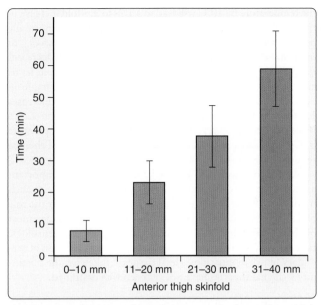

FIGURE 8-3 Duration of cryotherapy required to reduce thigh intramuscular temperature by 7°C in subjects with different adipose thickness. *(From Otte, J., Merrick, M., Ingersoll, C., and Cordova, M. [2002]: Subcutaneous adipose tissue thickness alters cooling time during cryotherapy. Arch. Phys. Med. Rehabil., 83:1501–1505.)*

REDUCTION IN METABOLIC RATE

Perhaps the most important goal of acute cryotherapy is a reduction in the metabolic rate of the cooled tissue. Such a reduction in metabolic rate would be quite beneficial in improving a tissue's ability to survive the proposed secondary injury events that follow primary trauma.[28-34] Although the exact mechanics of secondary injury is still being defined, it is clear that several of the mechanisms suggested would be altered by a change in temperature. For example, one of the two most common theories is that secondary injury results from the activity of damaging enzymes or free-radicals that are released during the inflammatory process.[28,29,32] We know that the rate of chemical reactions is reduced at lower temperatures,[60] so lowering a tissue's temperature with cryotherapy would reduce the rate of activity of the detrimental enzymes or radicals and thereby reduce the quantity of damage that they cause. Likewise, the other suggested principal mechanism of secondary injury is that it is the result of postinjury ischemia.[28,29,32] We know that without oxygen, tissues fail metabolically in a relatively short time.[34,60] A reduction in temperature and its related drop in metabolic rate have clearly been shown to reduce a tissue's demand for oxygen and thereby improve tissue survival under such conditions.[34,60,61]

The temperature-dependent alteration in metabolic rate is generally described by using a physical chemistry concept referred to as Q_{10}.[34,60] Q_{10} is simply the change in the rate of chemical reactions observed with a 10°C change in temperature as calculated with the Arrhenius equation. In physiology, Q_{10} is generally used to describe the metabolic rate and is most commonly determined by examining either O_2 consumption or NH_3 excretion. A common misconception among biologists is that $Q_{10} = 2$; that is, the rate of reaction doubles with each 10°C increase in temperature. In reality, Q_{10} is somewhat variable and depends on the organism, the specific temperature range, and the metabolic pathway of interest. It generally falls between 1.2 and 2.5. That is, increasing the temperature by 10°C will lead to a 1.2- to 2.5-fold increase in the reaction rate (i.e., a 20% to 150% increase). Though normally defined for an increase in temperature, we can also use Q_{10} to understand the physiologic effect of cryotherapy, which decreases temperature and therefore the metabolic rate. For example, let us arbitrarily say that the Q_{10} is 1.5 for temperature increasing from 27°C to 37°C. This would mean that the metabolic rate increases 1.5-fold for this increase in temperature (i.e., a 50% increase). If we were to apply cryotherapy to a tissue whose temperature is 37°C to decrease it to 27°C, the metabolic rate would then be reduced by 1.5-fold, or 50%.

Although a decline in metabolic rate is clearly an important aspect of the acute use of cryotherapy, we still do not know much in this area. For example, even though the arguments for the role of damaging enzymes and free radicals are getting stronger, most of this research has been performed on organs and neurologic tissues, and we still know very little about the progression of secondary injury in musculoskeletal tissues.[29] Likewise, the postinjury ischemia theories have not yet been well examined.

Clinical Pearl #3

The gaps in the area of research regarding ischemia lead to several significant shortcomings in our current understanding of cryotherapy. We do not yet have a definitive answer about the most effective tissue temperature, duration of cryotherapy, or on-off ratio for using cryotherapy for the treatment of acute injury. These questions are addressed later in the chapter.

PERFUSION/BLOOD FLOW

As is true with the metabolic rate, perfusion is also reduced with a decline in tissue temperature.[22,23,25-27,62] The decrease in blood flow is an effect of constriction of the vessel walls in response to cold. Some practitioners and even educators still suggest that cold can also cause dilation of blood vessels. This concept, known as cold-induced vasodilation,[6,22,32] does not occur and is discussed in Box 8-6.

As vessels become colder, their muscular walls begin to contract, which causes the vessel to constrict in diameter. The constriction is generally thought to be more pronounced in arteries and veins with smaller diameters and in arterioles and venules. It is important to note that constriction does not occur in capillaries because their walls are single-cell-thick endothelium and do not contain muscular tissue that can contract. Vasoconstriction causes a decrease in blood flow that has been well documented over the past few decades.[22-27,62] A decrease in blood flow is a mixed blessing and causes a bit of a dilemma for injury management theory. On the beneficial side, less blood flow would translate to less hemorrhaging from damaged vessels, less edema formation, and decreased accumulation of inflammatory cells that might cause secondary injury. These effects would all translate to improved outcomes of the injury. On the detrimental side, less blood flow would also mean less delivery of O_2 and nutrients and less removal of metabolic waste products. These effects could all worsen the secondary damage following injury. In reality, topical application of cold only reduces blood flow and does not completely prevent it. Therefore, we are probably not imposing too great of an ischemic stress, so the pros are thought to outweigh the cons.

Box 8-6

Facts Regarding Cold-Induced Vasodilation

As is the case with virtually every modality, a number of anecdotal beliefs about cryotherapy do not stand up to scrutiny in the laboratory. Unfortunately, modality myths have great tenacity and refuse to die quietly, and cold-induced vasodilation (CIVD) is no exception, even though the idea was discredited by Knight et al more than 20 years ago.[22] Some clinicians and even a few modality instructors still cite CIVD, sometimes called rebound vasodilation, as an important physiologic effect of cryotherapy. CIVD is generally described as an increase in blood flow, above baseline levels, that accompanies cryotherapy treatments. This phenomenon is often used as a rationale for limiting cryotherapy treatments to less than 20 to 30 minutes in duration. Originally, the notion of CIVD grew from a study by Lewis[6] in 1930 when he described cyclic fluctuations in finger temperature during immersion in ice water. He did not examine blood flow or vessel diameter, and his subjects were very likely hypothermic as a result of being underdressed in a very cold room. He observed that finger temperature fluctuated; it became warmer after a period immersed in cold water. This has been incorrectly translated to mean increased blood flow and was a popular rationale for the use of cryotherapy in rehabilitation for a number of years.

In reality, CIVD does not occur. Limb blood flow during cryotherapy is clearly depressed and never increases above baseline as long as the temperature is below normal.[22-27] However, as is often the case with misunderstood ideas, there is a hint of truth buried in the legend of CIVD. That hint is known as the hunting response.[179-181] During local hypothermic conditions, we see clear and profound vasoconstriction in vessels with muscular walls, such as arterioles. However, during prolonged local hypothermia, the degree of vasoconstriction in these vessels fluctuates and the resulting blood flow undergoes a cyclic increase and decrease. The important thing to note is that this cycling of blood flow occurs at flow levels that are considerably below their normal baseline.[22,32,63-65] Said another way, the cyclic increase in blood flow during prolonged hypothermia does not approach the precryotherapy baseline blood flow and certainly does not go above baseline levels. Therefore, practitioners can use cryotherapy for longer than 15 to 30 minutes without fear of hyperperfusing an acutely inflamed tissue.

INFLAMMATION

It is well accepted that cryotherapy inhibits inflammation,[24,30-33,36-38,54,66-68] but the specific effects of cold on inflammation are somewhat complex because inflammation itself is extremely complex. Most introductory texts[1-5,32,35,69] describe inflammation in terms of its vascular, chemical, and cellular events, and all three of these events are altered by acute cryotherapy. The vascular effects of inflammation, most notably vasodilation, are counteracted by the vasoconstriction that results from cold treatments, as already described. The chemical effects—release of more than 100 chemicals that mediate the inflammatory process—are also affected by cold.[34] Even though the effects of cold have not been explored for the majority of these inflammatory chemicals, we do know that the release or activity of several of the key inflammatory chemicals is inhibited during cryotherapy. The cellular events of inflammation are marked by the early activity of neutrophils, which gradually give way over a period of hours to the activity of macrophages.[34,60] Through a cold-induced reduction in metabolism, the activity of all these cells is reduced. This is thought to be quite beneficial in the early stages of inflammation in which neutrophils dominate but less useful later when macrophages are active in removing inflammatory debris in preparation for tissue repair. Neutrophils account for roughly 60% to 70% of all circulating white blood cells.[34,60] Their primary function is to fight an expanding bacterial infection by phagocytizing the bacteria and releasing a variety of damaging chemicals and free radicals—the immune system equivalent of hand grenades—to destroy additional bacteria. They are also very active in amplifying the overall immune response by releasing an assortment of chemical messengers. Because most musculoskeletal athletic injuries do not involve open wounds and infection, the activity of neutrophils with such injuries is generally greater than necessary and can lead to unwanted secondary damage to otherwise uninjured tissue[29,70] (see Chapter 2). The use of cryotherapy to retard neutrophil activity and thereby limit this damage is a promising area of future cryotherapy research.

EDEMA

One of the most important physiologic effects of acute cryotherapy is its ability to retard the formation of edema/effusion.[22,23,25-27,62] The primary mechanism by which cryotherapy retards edema formation is thought to be its effect on Starling forces.[31,32] These forces cause movement of fluid across the capillary wall, with two forces causing fluid to escape from the vessel and two forces attempting to retain fluid in the vessel. Under normal circumstances, the balance of these forces is such that a small amount of fluid is constantly escaping and being collected by the lymphatic system. When an injury occurs, tissue osmotic pressure, one of the escape forces, is thought to dramatically increase because of the release of free protein and other molecules from the damaged tissue. This would shift the balance of forces even further in the direction of fluid loss and edema formation. Cryotherapy is thought to minimize the total tissue damage and thereby hinder the release of free protein and thus the increase in tissue osmotic pressure. Coupled with the lowered blood flow resulting from vasoconstriction, cryotherapy results in a decrease in the other escape force, capillary hydrostatic pressure. With both escape forces reduced but not completely eliminated, the formation of edema or effusion is lessened, but not entirely prevented. Obviously, compression is a critical adjunct

to cold in limiting the formation of edema, but compression is discussed separately in this chapter.

The problem with the phrase "ice reduces swelling" is that it is misleading and frequently misunderstood. It is well accepted that cryotherapy retards the accumulation of fluid both intraarticularly and extraarticularly.[22,23,25-27,62] However, cryotherapy by itself is not effective in removing that fluid once it has accumulated. Cryotherapy and compression in combination are somewhat effective in removing accumulated fluid, but this is most likely a function of the compression and not the cold.[71-74]

PAIN

Aside from selected pharmaceuticals, no modality is more effective than cryotherapy in managing both the acute and chronic pain associated with athletic injuries.[32] Three primary theories attempt to explain cold's pain-relieving efficacy, and in reality, all three probably occur simultaneously (Box 8-7).[1-5,32]

Ironically, although cold is an outstanding pain control modality, its application can actually be quite painful. This is particularly true of cryotherapy treatments that involve immersion in ice water and patients who are not accustomed to the treatment. The pain with cold application can initially be intense but often subsides after several minutes. Repeated application over a period of days or weeks generally leads to better tolerance by patients as they grow accustomed to the treatment.[32,76,77]

NEUROMUSCULAR

The neuromuscular effects of cryotherapy are not generally used as a goal for cryotherapy treatment of acute injuries, but these effects can be quite useful in managing muscle spasms and in rehabilitation and are discussed with the rehabilitative use of cryotherapy.

Box 8-7

Three Theories That May Explain Cold's Pain-Relieving Efficacy

Gate Control Theory. The first and best known of these theories is gate control theory, in which the cold causes stimulation of Aβ afferent nerve fibers, which in turn inhibit transmission of pain to second-order neurons through gating at the substantia gelatinosa in the dorsal root ganglion of the spinal cord.

Reduction in Nerve Conduction Velocity. Nerve conduction velocity has been shown to be reduced by as much as 30% following typical cryotherapy treatments.[5,32,75] Slower conduction would translate into a diminished sensation of pain.

Reduction in Sensitivity to Pain Receptors. A lesser known theory is that local application of cold reduces the sensitivity of pain receptors much in the same way that it reduces the sensitivity of touch and pressure receptors.[32,60]

Table 8-4 Common Application Techniques for Acute Cryotherapy

Cold Modality	Application Technique	Comments
Ice bag	Apply directly to skin and use a compression wrap and elevation (ICE); the duration depends on adipose tissue and should be 20-40 minutes for most athletes.	Crushed ice conforms better than cubed. Ice from an unrefrigerated bin on an ice machine will not cause frostbite, but ice directly from a freezer may. Use appropriate caution.
Ice immersion	With submersion in water with ice, consider using a thin layer of elastic tape for compression (less insulating than elastic bandages).	Durations are not scientifically described, but most mimic ice bag durations.
Frozen gel pack	Do NOT apply directly to skin. Use a compression wrap and elevation. The duration should be 20-40 minutes for most athletes.	Because they are stored in a freezer at temperatures below 0°C, they can cause frostbite. They also rewarm much more quickly than ice bags.
Vapocoolant sprays	The spray and stretch technique is used for muscle spasms and trigger points.	Sprays are not used for most injuries (e.g., sprains, strains, fractures, contusions). They can quickly cause frostbite, so care must be exercised.

Techniques and Dosage

At the present time, we use cryotherapy under the assumption that colder tissue temperatures are better, provided that tissue freezing and frostbite does not occur. Therefore, cryotherapy treatment of acute injuries is aimed at reducing tissue temperature as greatly and quickly as possible.

TOPICAL APPLICATION AND INSULATING BARRIERS

The most common application technique for cryotherapy involves the direct application of a cold modality, generally an ice bag or frozen gel pack, to the injured area with some sort of a compressive wrap, usually an elastic bandage or plastic wrap (Table 8-4). As a general rule, cold packs made from ice are superior to frozen gel packs for the thermodynamic reasons discussed previously.[41] Ice-based cold packs are also generally safer than frozen gel packs. It is very possible to cause further injury with cryotherapy, and there are three primary ways that patients are injured (Box 8-8).

Typically, ice bags are filled with either cubed or crushed ice made by an ice machine and stored in an unrefrigerated hopper below the ice machine. Because this ice is not stored in a refrigerated container, it is continually melting. Because melting ice, by its very definition, has a temperature of 0°C and heat is being added to the ice from the tissues being treated, it is physically impossible for such ice to freeze the skin and cause frostbite.[32,44] For this reason, ice bags filled with ice stored in unrefrigerated

It is possible to cause injury by using too much compression over too small an area and create a tourniquet-like effect. For this reason, compression wraps should not be applied with more than moderate force, generally defined as 45 to 50 mm Hg.

Extended use of cryotherapy over superficial portions of peripheral nerves can cause further injury. In several cases, nerve palsy has resulted from cryotherapy treatments, typically over the common peroneal nerve on the lateral aspect of the knee or the ulnar nerve at the medial aspect of the elbow. When using cryotherapy over these areas, we must diligently monitor the treatment, control the compression, and limit the duration of treatment.

Cold-induced injury is frostbite. Frostbite occurs when tissue has been destroyed by freezing. For frostbite to occur, the tissues must be cooled to the point at which ice crystals begin to form. This occurs when the tissue temperature drops below 0°C and is accelerated by greater than required compression. Therefore, care must be used with cold modalities that are colder than 0°C, and compression should be applied carefully.

hoppers should be applied directly to the skin without the addition of an insulating layer. The same cannot be said for ice stored in a freezer or frozen gel packs, however. Because their temperatures will most likely be below 0°C, they pose a risk of causing frostbite and therefore require some type of barrier, such as a wet elastic wrap, between the pack and the skin.[32] Unfortunately, such barriers have been shown to severely limit the ability of the modality to cool the tissues and are therefore assumed to meaningfully impair the efficacy of the modality.[44]

Clinical Pearl #5

As a general rule, a barrier should be used only when applying a cold modality that has been stored at a temperature below 0°C; because cubed or crushed ice stored in an unrefrigerated hopper does not meet this criterion and is continually melting and heat is being added to the ice from the tissues being treated, no barrier should be used.

COLD COMBINED WITH COMPRESSION

One of the most overlooked aspects of applying ice packs for an acute injury is the use of compression. Practitioners are taught to treat injury with ice, compression, and elevation (ICE), with the compression and elevation being used to retard the formation of edema. However, we often overlook the fact that compression also plays a valuable role in cooling. When compression is used in combination with cryotherapy, we observe that deep tissues cool more rapidly and that lower temperatures can be achieved (Fig. 8-4).[40,42] Merrick et al[42] were the first to describe this combined effect on cooling, and they speculated that the improved cooling resulted from the combination of better contact between the tissue and the modality and compression-induced reduction in blood flow.

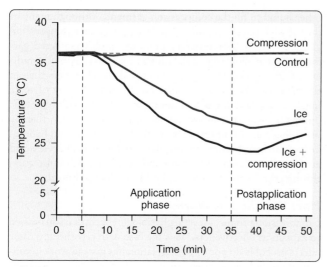

FIGURE 8-4 Compression improves the cooling ability of cryotherapy treatments. *(From Merrick, M., Knight, K., Ingersoll, C., and Potteiger, J. [1993]: The effects of ice and compression wraps on intramuscular temperatures at various depths. J. Athl. Train., 28:236–245.)*

Gaining in popularity are devices that automatically combine cryotherapy and compression. These devices, considered lymphedema pumps for regulatory purposes by the Food and Drug Administration, typically use a fluid-filled (hydraulic) sleeve that is filled with cold water to provide both cooling and compression. Many of these devices have partitioned sleeves that either fill sequentially in an effort to move edematous fluids proximally or use different pressure in each partition (gradient pressure) for the same purpose. Most devices allow the clinician to control the compression pressure, and some also allow control of the temperature of the water used for the compression. Although these devices make sense intuitively, like nearly all therapeutic modalities, few data describing their clinical outcomes are available.

COLD IMMERSION

Cold immersion treatments can be performed either with cold water, typically in the form of a cold whirlpool, or with an ice and water bath. Ice immersion has two important advantages over ice packs.[32] First, immersion treatments are able to treat larger areas and do so more uniformly. Second, immersion allows heat transfer through water, which has much greater thermal conductivity than ice packs do. This greater thermal conductivity may permit more rapid cooling. Cold immersion has disadvantages as well. The first is that it is nearly impossible to use elevation with immersion treatment. The second disadvantage of immersion treatment is that the water develops thermal gradients. Thermal gradients are regions where the water has been heated by the somewhat warmer tissues that are being immersed. The water around these tissues becomes warmer than the rest of the water in the immersion container. As these regions of water are warmed, they are less able to absorb heat and a reduction in cooling occurs. To avoid this gradient effect, the water should periodically be mixed throughout the treatment. Patients typically do not enjoy the mixing, however, because it brings colder water back into contact with their limb and is somewhat uncomfortable.

Ice and water baths, often referred to as ice slushes, are considerably more uncomfortable than cold water baths, but their

lower temperatures make them a more effective choice. Patient tolerance of ice slush treatments of the foot and ankle can be improved with the use of toe covers, which prevent the cold water from coming in direct contact with the toes.[72]

Clinical Pearl #6

When making an ice slush, a good analogy is to put the ice in first and then add water to the ice, just as you would add milk to breakfast cereal. The ice should just begin to float so that when the limb is added, the ice surrounds the area to be treated.

ICE MASSAGE

Ice massage, or rubbing a block of ice against the tissue, is an effective and common, but somewhat messy practice. Towels must be used beneath the treated tissue because the ice is constantly melting but the water is not collected in the ice bag. Ice massage treatments are generally of briefer duration than ice pack or cold immersion treatments and are capable of producing similar intramuscular temperatures. Care must be taken to avoid using excessive pressure over peripheral nerves.

SPRAY AND STRETCH

A somewhat different type of cryotherapy treatment known as spray and stretch is used to induce brief, intense cooling to relieve myofascial pain and spasm. The technique has also been used to treat muscle cramps, but this technique has not been examined in the literature. The spray and stretch technique involves the application of a vapocoolant spray, typically ethyl chloride or Pain Ease (Gebauer Company, Cleveland, OH), which rapidly cools the skin during evaporation. Ethyl chloride is very flammable and therefore nonflammable Pain Ease is becoming more popular and is just as effective.

The technique involves spraying the vapocoolant liquid in parallel strokes over the skin overlying a muscle with myofascial trigger points and then immediately stretching the muscle. The brief, intense cooling is thought to act as a distracting neurologic stimulus that may cause reflexive motor inhibition and thus allow more effective stretching. Amazingly, some recent work has demonstrated that skin temperatures can reach −10°C or colder with these products, yet they do not cause cold injury to the skin unless applied for a prolonged period (usually in excess of 8 seconds). A general guideline for their use is to stop applying the product when the skin surface "blanches" to a white color or when skin frosting begins to appear. Stopping at these points produces clinically meaningfully cooling without causing cold injury. In addition to spray and stretch, these products are commonly used to minimize the discomfort of needlesticks and venipuncture. They do cool deeply enough to be of much use in treating acute musculoskeletal injury.

Future Questions

For all that we have learned about cryotherapy, answers to the most important questions still elude us. The vast majority of cryotherapy research has used clinically convenient or easy-to-measure variables such as temperature. We now know a great deal about the response of skin and intramuscular tissue to cryotherapy. For example, we know that skin temperature drops almost immediately and that muscle temperature does not begin to fall until 3 to 5 minutes into the treatment. We also know that when the cold modality is removed, skin temperature begins to climb immediately but deep temperature actually continues to fall for nearly 5 minutes. We know that following cryotherapy treatments, temperature does not return to normal for more than an hour in resting subjects. However, we do not yet know the temperature that we need a tissue to reach to have a positive outcome with cryotherapy, and we certainly do not yet know the optimum intramuscular temperature for retarding secondary injury or inflammation. To answer these critically important questions, we will need to examine variables related to secondary injury or inflammation itself.

Because we do not yet know the optimum temperature that we need to reach during cryotherapy, we do not know how long our cryotherapy treatments should be applied to produce this temperature. We do know that there is a point of diminishing return with cryotherapy duration. In examining the time required for rewarming of the skin following cryotherapy, researchers have shown that longer, colder applications lead to longer rewarming periods only up to a point.[51,78] Applications that exceeded 30 minutes had nearly identical rewarming times as 30-minute applications. We also know that adipose thickness is an important factor that we need to consider when choosing the duration of applications. In fact, to produce a typical cryotherapy effect in many of our athletes, we need to double or even triple the treatment durations that are commonly in use now[55] (see Fig. 8-3). A third important question about cryotherapy is related to these first two. We do not yet know how often we need to reapply cold modalities. A typical recommendation is 20 minutes per hour for the first 5 or 6 hours following injury. Though typical, few data support any specific on-off cycling for cryotherapy.[56]

Compression

Compression, or the application of external pressure, is a commonly used adjunct to acute cryotherapy, but it also has usefulness in isolation. Compression, the "C" in RICE, is one of the cornerstones of traditional management of acute injury, although it has not been well studied. The effectiveness of compression is thought to largely be related to its effect on Starling forces, the forces governing transcapillary fluid movement,[62,72,79-81] although compression has other useful effects not related to these forces.[40,42,72,74,82] This section discusses only the acute use of compression. Its postacute use in resolving existing edema is discussed in conjunction with the other postacute modalities later in the chapter.

Description

Compression involves the application of external pressure to a tissue or tissues in either a circumferential or focal manner. Although the most common forms of compression involve circumferential application with either an elasticized bandage or elastic tape, quite a few other compression modalities are actually available.[83] Among the best of these are pneumatic or hydraulic lymphedema pumps, which provide circumferential compression in either a constant or intermittent manner. Pneumatic lymphedema pumps use air to fill a compression garment and provide nearly uniform circumferential compression. Hydraulic lymphedema pumps, in contrast, use water or some

other liquid to fill the compression garment. Although many of the early lymphedema pumps used single-chamber compression garments, most contemporary units use multichambered garments, which allow sequential filling (distal to proximal), gradient compression (more pressure in the distal chambers than in the proximal chambers), or both. For the management of acute injury, a large and important advantage is found with hydraulic pumps because they allow the use of precooled water, thereby providing concurrent cryotherapy. Both pneumatic and hydraulic lymphedema pumps are considered to be medical devices and are therefore regulated by the Food and Drug Administration through the Center for Devices and Radiological Health.

How We Think It Works

Compression produces several physiologic effects that can be used to explain its effectiveness. As is the case with cryotherapy, these effects probably do not work in isolation but instead work in concert to produce the desired outcome. Compression is thought to be effective in managing acute injuries by three primary means.[32] One is that compression increases the cooling efficacy of cryotherapy, as discussed previously in the cryotherapy section.[40,42] The other two mechanisms involve resisting the formation of edema. The first of these antiedema mechanisms entails a manipulation of Starling forces.[62,79,80] The second involves lessening bleeding from the vessels damaged during the injury.[84]

STARLING FORCES

The most common explanation for the obvious effects of compression on retarding the formation of edema is through its effect on Starling forces (Table 8-5).[32,34,60,85] These forces, sometimes called capillary filtration forces, govern movement of plasma from the vascular system into the extravascular space through the intact walls of capillaries.[34,60] Under normal homeostatic conditions, three forces, capillary hydrostatic, tissue hydrostatic, and tissue osmotic, cause fluid to migrate from the capillary into the extravascular space, and one force, capillary osmotic, resists the extravascular migration of fluid. Normally, a net loss of fluid from the vascular system occurs because of a slight imbalance in the Starling forces, with the "out" forces causing loss of fluid from the capillary being slightly larger than the "in" forces. As discussed in the cryotherapy section, acute injury causes a dramatic increase in the "out" forces through both a decrease in plasma osmotic pressure and an increase in interstitial osmotic pressure. These changes in pressure result from loss of plasma proteins into the surrounding tissues and from the release of free proteins from cells damaged by the injury.

External compression is thought to work primarily by increasing tissue hydrostatic pressure and thereby reducing the magnitude of the pressure gradient favoring the formation of edema. Reduction of this gradient would lessen fluid loss from the vascular system and consequently retard the formation of edema. Note, however, that it is unlikely that external pressure will completely compensate for the increase in tissue osmotic pressure, and therefore some edema can be expected to form even with the use of external compression.

PERFUSION/BLOOD FLOW

The edema or effusion associated with injury does not form solely from plasma fluid and protein that leak through intact capillary walls. A significant portion of the fluid accumulation associated with injury is from blood that spills out of blood

Table 8-5 Starling Equilibrium for Capillary Fluid Exchange*

Force	Description	Direction	Mean Value (mm Hg)	Effect of Injury (mm Hg)
Capillary hydrostatic	Fluid pressure from inside the capillary	Vascular fluid loss	−17.3	−17.3 (no change)
Interstitial osmotic	Osmotic pressure exerted by extravascular solutes	Vascular fluid loss	−8	−28
Interstitial hydrostatic	Extravascular fluid pressure in the tissue	Vascular fluid loss†	−3	+4
Capillary osmotic	Osmotic pressure exerted by interstitial fluid	Vascular fluid retention	+28	+14
Net force under normal conditions		Vascular fluid loss	−0.3	−27.3

Adapted from Guyton, A.C. (1991): Textbook of Medical Physiology, 8th ed. Philadelphia, Saunders, pp. 149–203; Knight, K.L. (1995): Cryotherapy in Sport Injury Management. Champaign, IL, Human Kinetics, pp. x, 301; and Majno, G., and Joris, I. (1996): Cells, Tissues, and Disease: Principles of General Pathology. Cambridge, MA, Blackwell Scientific.

* Negative values equal outward force; positive values equal inward force.

† Normally, a negative (outward) interstitial hydrostatic force (a partial vacuum) is present that helps hold tissue layers together, but as edema accumulates, this vacuum disappears, which allows tissues to separate and retain even more fluid. The fluid eventually develops positive pressure and can even occlude vessels if the pressure is great enough.

vessels damaged in the injury. It is this blood that causes most of the ecchymosis seen in the injured area over the days following the injury. Compression is effective in the management of this blood loss is several ways. First, it reduces the quantity of blood flow to the damaged vessels and therefore limits the volume of blood available to be spilled from these vessels. Second, compression slows the rate of flow and allows more rapid development of the fibrin scaffolding that eventually forms a clot and stops the blood loss.[34,60]

Technique and Dosage

Very little is found in the literature on the appropriate compression technique or dosage for managing acute injuries. Most often, compression is used in combination with cryotherapy, and the duration is based on the cryotherapy and not the compression. A small body of research examining typical compression pressures with elastic wraps and surface pressures of 40 to 50 mm Hg has been reported.[86] These pressures correspond to applying an elastic bandage at medium stretch in which roughly half the stretch capacity of the wrap is used during application. Some evidence has shown that compression in this pressure range improves the cooling observed with cryotherapy by producing both lower tissue temperatures and slightly faster cooling.[40,42] Other evidence, however, has shown that varying application pressures has little effect on tissue temperatures.[87]

The use of focal compression, such as that achieved with a felt or foam "horseshoe" pad around the malleolus in treating an acute ankle sprain, can provide increased compression. This type of focal compression can be very useful in limiting the accumulation of fluid at specific sites, such as around the malleoli with ankle injuries or in the peripatellar region with knee injuries.

In addition to compression wraps, the other common form of compression used with acute injuries involves the use of lymphedema pumps, typically combined with cryotherapy. The application parameters for these devices when used for acute injury management have also not been well described. Although ideal parameters have not yet been identified, typical guidelines include 20 to 40 minutes of intermittent compression consisting of a 30- to 40-second inflation time and a 20- to 30-second deflation or rest time. Appropriate application pressure for these devices is not yet clear, but manufacturers have recommended pressures between 50 and 90 mm Hg; however, these recommendations are generally intended for the postacute removal of

edema rather than retarding the formation of edema. On the other hand, there is a good argument for using pressures that are just below the patient's diastolic blood pressure in an effort to apply as much pressure as possible without occluding the vasculature.

Future Questions

Obviously, the acute use of compression is a very common clinical practice. As common as it is, very few studies have attempted to describe the physiologic effects of compression and even fewer that have examined its use for the management of acute injuries. This leaves many questions still unexamined. Among the most important would be the appropriate pressure, appropriate duration, use of intermittent versus continuous compression, intermittent cycling parameters, and whether compression or elevation is a more important factor in retarding the formation of edema.

Elevation

Description

Elevation, the "E" in RICE, is the least studied of the trio of ice, compression, and elevation, but its use is widespread in the management of acute injuries. Elevation of an injured body part can be accomplished in a variety of ways ranging from specially designed treatment tables to simple, on-the-field techniques, such as resting an injured ankle on a football helmet or equipment bag.

How We Think It Works

The underlying premise with elevation is that gravity will limit the amount of blood delivered to the acutely injured area. Limiting blood flow to the injured area immediately following the injury is perceived to have three benefits. First, it would help control bleeding from damaged vessels, and this would be a benefit in terms of limiting edema and hematoma formation, as described previously in this chapter. Second, it would alter the transcapillary Starling forces in the injured area by reducing capillary hydrostatic pressure, one of the major forces causing fluid to move from the vessel out into the extravascular space. This has obvious implications for retarding edema formation. The third and most often overlooked benefit is that the reduced blood flow and capillary hydrostatic pressure would also limit the transport of neutrophils to the injury site. The neutrophil is the most numerous leukocyte population and plays a vital role in early magnification of the inflammatory process. It is also thought to be among the most likely villains in secondary injury. Limiting the delivery of neutrophils and other proinflammatory agents to the injury site would be of potential benefit in limiting the total amount of tissue damage and inflammation that would have to be resolved before repair could take place.

Future Questions

Unfortunately, the magnitude of the actual benefits from elevation has not been described. Although the arguments for elevation are intuitive and make good physiologic sense, it is unclear whether elevation plays an important role, a minor role, or no role in improving outcomes after injury. Therefore, several important questions need to be examined, including the effects of elevation on edema formation, the magnitude and duration of elevation necessary, and a relative comparison of the importance of elevation and compression. For example, a number of clinicians treat acute ankle sprains by applying elastic tape compression wraps and then immersing the ankle in an ice bath. The more rapid cooling with an ice bath than with an ice bag may be of some benefit; however, the gravity-dependent position goes against the commonly accepted importance of elevation. The actual importance of elevation needs to be established to resolve this clinical dilemma.

Other Modalities?

Other modalities are claimed to be efficacious in the management of acute injuries, and some appear to hold some degree of promise. High-voltage electrical current has been proposed as an acute treatment and has been suggested to limit retraction of endothelial cells, thereby minimizing the increases in vascular permeability that accompany acute inflammation.[88-93] However, the efficacy of this approach in the actual management of acute musculoskeletal injuries in humans has not been well examined, and therefore claims about outcome must be made sparingly. Another valuable adjunct to acute injury management is transcutaneous electrical nerve stimulation.

MODALITIES FOR REHABILITATION

Goals

Whereas the goals for acute injury management were centered on minimizing the immediate sequelae of the injury, including limiting additional tissue damage, retarding the acute inflammatory process, slowing the formation of edema, and minimizing pain, goals for the rehabilitative use of modalities are somewhat different (Table 8-6). In postacute rehabilitation, the goals are focused mostly on removing the unwanted remnants of inflammation, repairing the tissue, and restoring more normal physiologic function of the repaired tissue. This is an important distinction that is sometimes lost on inexperienced practitioners. To make appropriate choices of modalities, you must first understand the patient's stage in the progression of injury and what the next logical stage would be. It is vital to understand that all injuries progress through a predefined set of stages and that these stages are sequential and progressive.

That is, you cannot truly begin to restore normal function to an acutely inflamed tissue until you first control the inflammation, second remove the inflammatory debris and fluid, and third repair the damage.

Generally, the goal should be to move to the next stage of the injury. When signs of acute inflammation are present, the choice of modalities should focus on minimizing the inflammation. When examination reveals that the acute phase of inflammation has been controlled, the choice of modalities should focus on removing the unwanted leftovers from inflammation and promoting tissue repair. When the debris has been removed successfully and tissue repair promoted, focus should be directed to remodeling the new tissue and restoring adequate function for mobility and activities of daily living. When these goals have been achieved, return to sport can be addressed. Fortunately, most athletic injuries are able to progress through the early phases quickly, and athletes are often able to begin addressing competitive function early in the postinjury time line. It should be kept in mind that the choice of modalities and goals of rehabilitation for each of these phases are not mutually exclusive. There is almost never a clear dividing point between these phases on examination of the patient, and likewise there is no clear dividing point between the rehabilitative goals and the modalities that can help in achieving these goals. There should often be a degree of overlap between goals and therefore an overlap in modalities. This is particularly true in the repair and remodeling phases. For example, we know that appropriate rehabilitation can influence both the quantity and orientation of scar tissue made by the body. It is of great benefit to use modalities and controlled exercise to minimize the quantity of scar tissue produced while at the same time improving the strength of that scar tissue.

It is also very important to note that the role of traditional therapeutic modalities is almost exclusively limited to the earlier phases of rehabilitation and that the later phases concerned with restoring athletic performance are almost exclusively dependent on exercise as the modality of choice (see Table 8-6). Modality use in the later phases of rehabilitation seldom consists of more than preactivity thermotherapy with the aim of increasing perfusion and decreasing stiffness or postactivity cryotherapy with the goal of minimizing any activity-related inflammation. This notion is very closely tied to concepts presented in the beginning of this chapter, where the importance of having criteria for discontinuation of a modality was discussed. When a modality is used to accomplish a specific goal, the modality can and should be discontinued when that goal has been accomplished or when the modality is proving to no longer be effective for the patient. For example, if electrotherapy is being used for muscle reeducation and to overcome postinjury inhibition, its use can be discontinued when neuromuscular function appears normal and the athlete is ready to begin resistance training.

Clinical Pearl #7

The hallmark of an experienced practitioner is using modalities for a specific purpose and replacing them with more appropriate measures when the goal has been met and they are no longer needed.

Table 8-6 Goals and Modalities for Rehabilitative Care

Rehabilitative Phase	Goals for Use of Modalities	Choices of Modalities
Postacute	Remove edema and inflammatory debris	Intermittent compression, thermotherapy, ultrasound, massage, electrotherapy, exercise
	Retard atrophy	Exercise, electrotherapy
Repair/regeneration	Increase perfusion/oxygen delivery	Thermotherapy, ultrasound, short wave diathermy, exercise, hyperbaric oxygen
	Increase healing stimulus	Exercise, ultrasound, low-power laser, microcurrent(?)
	Retard atrophy	Exercise, electrotherapy
Restore function (early)	Limit pain	Preactivity cryotherapy, cryokinetics, TENS, electrotherapy, microcurrent(?)
	Counteract neuromuscular inhibition	Preactivity cryotherapy, cryokinetics, electrotherapy
	Restore ROM	Thermotherapy, ultrasound, short wave diathermy, joint mobilization, ROM exercise
	Restore adequate muscular strength, power, and endurance for activities of daily living	Exercise, electrotherapy
	Minimize recurrence of inflammation following activity	Postactivity cryotherapy and compression
Restore function (middle)	Reduce preactivity stiffness as needed	Preactivity thermotherapy
	Increase muscular strength, power, and endurance to functional/competitive levels	Exercise only
	Restore muscular speed	Exercise only
	Restore cardiopulmonary endurance	Exercise only
	Minimize recurrence of inflammation following activity as needed	Postactivity cryotherapy and compression
Restore function (late)	Reduce preactivity stiffness as needed	Preactivity thermotherapy
	Restore agility	Exercise only
	Restore sport-specific skills	Exercise only
	Controlled sport activity	Exercise only
	Uncontrolled sport activity	Exercise only
	Minimize recurrence of inflammation following activity as needed	Postactivity cryotherapy and compression

ROM, Range of motion; *TENS,* transcutaneous electrical nerve stimulation.

Cryotherapy

Description

Cryotherapy for the management of acute injuries was addressed in great detail earlier in the chapter. The rehabilitative use of cryotherapy is somewhat different, however. Rehabilitatively, cryotherapy is used for two main purposes and at two different times in a rehabilitation session. First and most commonly, it is used to minimize any inflammation that develops as a result of the rehabilitation session and is applied following the session. For this purpose, use of cryotherapy is virtually identical to that already described for the management of acute injuries. The second use of cryotherapy rehabilitatively is to control pain and neuromuscular inhibition.[32,50,94,95] When used for this purpose, cryotherapy is typically used before activity or is alternated with activity, a highly effective technique known as cryokinetics.[32,96]

How We Think It Works

PAIN

Cryokinetics is perhaps the single most effective rehabilitative technique for the early restoration of function following joint injuries, particularly ankle sprains.[32] In this technique, several bouts of cryotherapy and exercise are alternated within a single rehabilitative session, usually very early following injury as discussed later. The preliminary rationale for the dramatic effectiveness of cryokinetics was that the cold reduced pain. Pain is thought to cause neuromuscular inhibition, and such inhibition is thought to be the primary limiting factor in the patient's ability to perform rehabilitative exercise in the early postinjury period. We know that early exercise is the most important modality in our arsenal, and the sooner that controlled rehabilitative exercise can be initiated, the faster the progression of the injury toward normal function and presumably the better the outcome. We know that cold is effective in reducing pain and most other sensations as well. Therefore, if cold reduces pain and pain causes inhibition, cold should help overcome inhibition and therefore allow the patient to begin controlled rehabilitative exercise at an earlier point in the rehabilitative process.

Cold actually plays a contradictory role with respect to pain. Anyone who has placed their bare feet into an ice slush can tell you in great detail that cold can absolutely cause pain. On the other hand, if you have ever burned your finger and then held it under running cold water, you can also testify to the fact that cold reduces pain. So how do we explain the contradiction? First, cold-induced pain seems to be much more common with ice slush immersions than with any other form of cryotherapy, although no explanation for this frequent observation has been offered. The magnitude of the pain also appears to be inversely related to the temperature of the ice bath. In addition, those with injury-related pain are often observed to tolerate cold applications better than do normal, uninjured subjects. It appears that when pain is already present, cold acts to inhibit that pain, whereas when cold is applied to patients without pain, the cold itself becomes uncomfortable.

The primary suggestions of how cryotherapy may inhibit pain lie in cold's effects on neurologic function. Cryotherapy has been shown to decrease nerve transmission in pain fibers and to decrease the excitability of free nerve endings, one of the most important pain receptors.[75] Cold also has been shown to cause asynchronous transmission in pain fibers, to induce the release of endorphins, and to inhibit spinal nerve conduction. All of these effects are capable of altering the perception of pain.[32]

NEUROMUSCULAR

Because cold reduces nerve conduction velocity on both afferent and efferent nerves, its effect is not limited to altering sensory function. Motor function is altered as well. The changes in motor function have often been overlooked but have some important implications for clinicians.

Among the more controversial neuromuscular effects of local cryotherapy is whether cold decreases maximal force production. The literature is mixed on the subject.[47,75,97-101] Decreased force production has been shown in a number of studies examining isometric force, as well as in some evaluating concentric and eccentric force. In a few studies examining isometric force, an increase in force production was noted roughly 60 to 80 minutes following treatment with cold, but this effect has not yet been examined adequately with regard to concentric or eccentric force. The authors speculated that the increase was the result of either increased temperature or increased blood flow to the limbs following removal of the cold. These explanations seem unlikely because intramuscular temperatures remain depressed for quite some time following cryotherapy.

The initial decrease in strength following cryotherapy has created concern in some clinicians regarding the appropriateness of preactivity cryotherapy. They have questioned whether athletes are being placed at risk for injury by having them practice or compete under circumstances in which nerve conduction velocity and maximal strength are diminished. In an effort to address this issue, a growing body of research is examining the effects of cryotherapy on proprioception.[75,97,100-104] As is often the case, the literature is divided, with studies some showing no alterations in proprioception or functional performance and others showing

a decline in functional performance. Unfortunately, the body of research in this area is still small, so a definitive answer has yet to be made. However, because maximal strength is seldom used and because a clear detriment in performance has not been shown, many believe that it is safe to use cryotherapy before activity.

Some of the most exciting new cryotherapy research relates to motor neuron pool availability.[50,94,95] Following injury, a period of neuromuscular inhibition occurs and results in motor weakness, impaired coordination of motor activities, and impaired proprioception. Clearly, these impairments present a significant hurdle in the early rehabilitation of injuries. One of the more common research strategies for examining inhibition is to look at the availability of the motor neuron pool. Under normal circumstances, we can voluntarily recruit only a portion of our total motor neuron pool. The body does not allow total recruitment of the pool because the forces that would be generated would cause us to pull muscles off their bony attachments and result in fractures and other injuries. During an injury and the subsequent postinjury rehabilitative period, the percentage of the motor neuron pool that can be recruited is less than normal and can be quantified by measurement of the Hoffmann reflex (H-reflex).[50,94,95]

In several studies, neuromuscular inhibition, as indicated by a diminished H-reflex, has been created artificially by inducing joint effusion via the injection of sterile saline into the synovial space.[94] This research strongly suggests that the neuromuscular inhibition following cryotherapy is not only related to pain (as suggested in cryokinetics theory) but also related to joint effusion. Interestingly, not only has the use of cryotherapy been shown to counteract this effusion-induced reduction in motor neuron pool availability, but cryotherapy has actually also led to motor neuron pool facilitation.[50,95] That is, the application of cold actually increased the amount of the motor neuron pool that was available for recruitment. This suggests that cryotherapy can be used not only to counter the pain that limits early rehabilitation following injury but also to overcome the neuromuscular inhibition following injury. Perhaps even more interesting, Krause et al[105] demonstrated that cryotherapy-induced facilitation also occurs when the cold modality is placed on a different body part, away from the injury (different dermatome). They showed that the knee effusion-induced reduction in motor neuron pool availability was counteracted by applying cryotherapy to the armpit! This suggests that facilitation is mediated by the central nervous system rather than by action on local nerves. On the other hand, members of this same research group[106] have also shown than artificial effusion-induced inhibition is not present in the contralateral limb, so there is still much to learn in this area.

Techniques and Dosage

Many cryotherapy techniques were discussed in the acute management section. Those presented here are more appropriate for rehabilitative use than for acute use.

COLD WHIRLPOOL

An old favorite among therapeutic modalities is the whirlpool, and virtually no athletic health care facility is without one. Cold whirlpools use water that is typically as cold as is available from the tap, usually around 50°F to 60°F.[1-5,32,107] Some clinicians add ice to the whirlpool to reduce its temperature, but to date no ideal temperature has been described in the literature. Whirlpools function by using a turbine to circulate the water around the body part, but they would probably be just as effective without the turbine. The key feature of the whirlpool is the water temperature itself and not the fact that the water is moving.[32] Cold whirlpools were not discussed in the acute management section of this chapter because most are probably too warm to work well for acute injuries and other cold modalities are more likely to be effective.[108-110] Cold whirlpools are very well suited to the rehabilitative use of cryotherapy, however, because emphasis is not placed on cooling a tissue as quickly as possible or to the greatest degree possible. Typical cold whirlpool treatments last from 15 to 30 minutes, thus mimicking the durations of other cold treatments, such as ice bags, but again, little evidence suggests that this duration is most appropriate.

An important safety consideration with whirlpools is that they should be appropriately grounded and connected to circuits only with a ground-fault circuit interrupter (GFCI). Whenever possible, it is recommended that an electrician be employed to disconnect the turbine on/off switch on the whirlpool and instead connect the whirlpool to a circuit with a GFCI and a timer switch that is out of reach of the patient in the whirlpool. This prevents the patient from operating the switch while standing in the water and provides an effective means of controlling the duration of the treatment. This second benefit is probably more important with warm whirlpool treatments, where athletes tend to not want to get out of the whirlpool.

CRYOKINETICS

Cryokinetics is a rehabilitative technique consisting of alternating bouts of cryotherapy and exercise (Table 8-7). The technique is used primarily in the early phases of a rehabilitative program in an attempt to allow exercise to be initiated sooner than might otherwise be possible because of pain and neuromuscular inhibition.[32,96] It is frequently started as soon as the day following the injury or even the day of the injury for relatively minor injuries. Cryokinetics is particularly useful for joint sprains, especially ankle sprains, but is not as effective for muscle injuries. The cold helps lessen the pain and reverse the inhibition so that exercise can take place. It has been suggested that early cryokinetics can cut days or even weeks from the rehabilitation of an ankle sprain. The real benefits from cryokinetics are found in the exercise because exercise is the single most important modality available to us in terms of its ability to cause positive changes following injury.

A typical cryokinetics regimen involves five bouts of exercise with cryotherapy treatments to produce numbing in between. The patient begins with a cryotherapy treatment, ideally an ice slush immersion, until the injured body part is numb. The initial bout of cryotherapy typically lasts 12 to 20 minutes. Following the initial cryotherapy, the patient completes an exercise bout until the numbness begins to wear off, usually 2 to 5 minutes. The patient then goes back in the ice slush until again numb, typically 5 minutes for these renumbing treatments. When numb again, the patient completes a second bout of exercise until the numbness begins to wear off, generally in 2 to 5 minutes. The patient continues this pattern of cold and exercise until five bouts of exercise have been completed, with each bout becoming progressively more difficult. When the exercise is completed, the session concludes with a final 5-minute ice immersion (see Table 8-7).

Knight suggests that the key to cryokinetics is not the time spent performing the activity or the number of repetitions, but instead the performance of progressively more difficult

Table 8-7 Typical Cryokinetics Protocol for an Ankle Sprain

Note that each exercise bout becomes progressively more difficult. When used correctly, by the 4th or 5th bout the patient should encounter exercises that he or she cannot complete. At that point, they should return to the most difficult task that they can complete and have them complete the bouts. Activities should mirror the actual requirements of the athlete's sport participation.[32]

Activity	Duration	Description
Ice slush immersion	15-20 minutes	Ice immersion until numb, 20 minutes maximum
Exercise bout 1	2-5 minutes	Non–weight-bearing exercise: PROM, AROM, and RROM as tolerated
Ice slush immersion	5 minutes	Ice immersion until numb, 5 minutes maximum
Exercise bout 2	2-5 minutes	Weight-bearing exercise: proprioceptive exercises, including weight shifting, wobble boards (two feet then one foot), in-line walking (without a limp)
Ice slush immersion	5 minutes	Ice immersion until numb, 5 minutes maximum
Exercise bout 3	2-5 minutes	More difficult weight-bearing exercise, including walking in curves or zigzags (without a limp), toe raises (two feet, then one foot), in-place hopping
Ice slush immersion	5 minutes	Ice immersion until numb, 5 minutes maximum
Exercise bout 4	2-5 minutes	More difficult weight-bearing activities, including in-line jogging and curve or zigzag jogging (without a limp), hopping over a line or in a square pattern
Ice slush immersion	5 minutes	Ice immersion until numb, 5 minutes maximum
Exercise bout 5	2-5 minutes	More difficult weight-bearing activities, including in-line running, curve running, running and cutting, sprint starts and stops, jump stops, backward running
Ice slush immersion	5 minutes	Ice immersion until numb

AROM, Active range of motion; *PROM*, passive range of motion; *RROM*, restricted range of motion.

exercises without pain.[32] Cryokinetics appears to work primarily by allowing the patient to overcome some of the neuromuscular inhibition produced by the injury. By completing progressively more difficult exercises, the neuromuscular system is forced to function at a higher and higher level, thereby reestablishing the motor control pathways that are so critical for return to normal function.

Superficial Thermotherapy

Description

Heating modalities are generally classified by their depth of effective heating and are considered to be superficial or deep.[1-5,66,107,111] Superficial thermotherapy, or the use of superficially applied heat, is an extremely common modality in the rehabilitative setting. In fact, it is so common that it may be our most overused rehabilitative modality. Like all modalities, superficial thermotherapy should be used to accomplish a specific goal and not be used as a "cure-all" modality. The goals most appropriately treated with superficial thermotherapy include improving range of motion, increasing circulation, and reducing pain or the sense of tightness that is frequently associated with injured tissues.

Clinical Pearl #8

Thermotherapy should be used only when examination of the patient suggests that the acute inflammation has passed and the patient is in the waste removal and repair phases or beyond.

How We Think It Works

RANGE OF MOTION

First coloquial, the range-of-motion effects for all thermal modalities are not a direct function of the modality itself. Instead, the thermal modality should be seen as an adjunct that allows other techniques, such as stretching or joint mobilization, to be more effective. In isolation, thermal modalities are not effective in altering limitations in range of motion. However, combining thermal modalities with specific techniques to improve range of motion can be effective when used correctly.

Correct use of thermal modalities for range of motion involves elevating the temperature of the tissue that is limiting the range of motion into a range where it becomes more elastic and its length can be effectively altered. This means that first, the choice of modality must be based on the depth of the limiting tissue and, second, the modality needs to be capable of producing adequate tissue temperatures. Superficial thermal modalities are generally capable of elevating tissue temperatures down to a depth of roughly 1 to 2 cm, thus making them appropriate for only the most superficial of tissues.[3,5,107] The tissue temperature required depends on the type of tissue. For collagenous tissues, such as tendon, ligament, and scar, tissue temperatures of between 39°C and 45°C (102°F and 113°F) are required.[8,12] Muscle tissue, in contrast, because it is able to change length easily, causes limitations in range of motion as a function of resting muscle tone rather than structural elements, such as with collagen fibers. To date, the appropriate temperature to best facilitate residual changes in muscle length have not

been described, but they are probably less than those required for collagenous tissues.

Achieving an elevated temperature is only a piece of the equation. The key to being effective is to apply the stretching or joint mobilization while the tissue is in the target temperature range, typically just 2 to 3 minutes.[112-114]

INCREASING THE CIRCULATION

Circulatory changes are observed with all thermal modalities, hot or cold. The degree of circulatory change is dependent on the tissue temperature achieved and the quantity of tissue being heated. Superficial thermotherapy increases tissue temperature and produces a vasodilation effect in small arteries and veins, arterioles, and venules. These vascular effects are seen only in superficial vessels.[60] There is some debate about the actual mechanism by which the vessels are induced to dilate, but the most commonly cited rationales involve local metabolites, nitric oxide signaling, and spinal reflexes.[60,115,116] A strong argument for spinal reflexes as an explanation is that some degree of dilation occurs in the contralateral limb during these treatments even though the metabolic demand of these contralateral tissues does not change.[60]

Dilation of vessels allows increased perfusion of the capillary beds fed by the arterioles. Note, however, that vasodilation does not occur in the capillary beds themselves. Capillaries have a vessel wall that is a single cell thick, and these cells are endothelium and not smooth muscle. Because capillaries have no muscular layer, they cannot actively dilate or constrict.

REDUCING PAIN

Pain reduction with superficial thermotherapy is perhaps the primary reason why this modality is so popular with patients. Hot packs simply feel good, and most patients enjoy them. This can lead to problems when athletes think that all they need is a hot pack before every practice. As is the case with any modality, superficial thermotherapy should be used only for a specific therapeutic goal rather than finding a goal to apply so the athlete can use thermotherapy.

Thermotherapy has many of the same effects on nerve function as cryotherapy treatments. They decrease peripheral nerve conduction velocity, inhibit most nerve receptors, and alter spinal nerve conduction.[2,3] Even with these changes, the most likely explanation for the pain-reducing effects of thermotherapy lies in their stimulation of cutaneous temperature receptors, which may help reduce pain through a gait control mechanism.[2,3]

Techniques and Dosage

HOT PACKS

The most common form of superficial thermotherapy is the application of moist heat packs, typically hot Hydrocollator packs. These canvas packs are partitioned into cells filled with silica gel or a similar substance that is capable of absorbing a large quantity of water. The packs are immersed in hot water (160°F to 170°F). By absorbing the hot water, the packs are able to retain heat for an extended period. Application of these packs necessitates some type of barrier between them and the skin because they will cause burns if applied directly. Generally, a terrycloth pack is used; however, towels also work nicely. Even with a Hydrocollator pack, towels are often used initially and are removed as the pack cools. The duration of application has not been well studied, but typical applications are in the range of 20 to 30 minutes and produce skin temperatures in excess of 40°C to 41°C and muscle temperatures in the range of 38°C.

Clinical Pearl #9

It is unlikely that Hydrocollator packs will produce adequate temperature to improve the elasticity of collagen in any tissues except the most superficial connective tissues with little overlying adipose tissue.

PARAFFIN BATH

Paraffin baths, or melted paraffin with a small amount of mineral oil (seven parts paraffin, one part mineral oil), are another common form of superficial thermotherapy. Paraffin, by nature of its low specific heat, allows considerably greater thermal conduction than does water of the same temperature. The mineral oil is used to lower the melting temperature of the paraffin to a point at which it can be used safely with patients. Paraffin baths are typically used to treat the hands or feet and are best for areas that can be dipped into the paraffin. Although some have suggested that paraffin can be applied with a brush to larger areas, these areas are better treated with hot packs. Paraffin bath temperatures are generally in the range of 118°F to 126°F, and the most common application technique involves dipping the hand or foot into the paraffin 7 to 12 times to form a wax "glove" and then covering the glove with a plastic bag and wrapping it with towels to help retain the heat. The duration with this method is generally 15 to 20 minutes. A less used but more effective alternative involves immersing the hand or foot directly in the bath for 5 to 15 minutes. This method is used less frequently because it presents an increased risk for burns.

WHIRLPOOLS

Warm whirlpools, like their cold counterparts, are extremely common in athletic health care settings. They are most beneficial in reducing the perception of soreness that occurs a few days after strenuous exertion or the stiffness in a recently immobilized body part, but they can be used for any superficial thermal modality purpose. The temperature of a warm whirlpool generally depends on the body part to be treated. Extremity whirlpool temperatures are usually hotter (102°F to 106°F) than whole-body immersion whirlpools (98°F to 102°F). They are sometimes used for cleaning skin wounds, and an anti-infective agent such as povidone-iodine solution is generally added for this purpose. When used for wound care, great diligence must be used in cleaning the whirlpool between patients.

FLUIDOTHERAPY

Although less common than moist heat techniques, such as hot packs or paraffin, fluidotherapy is another effective superficial thermal modality. Fluidotherapy involves the circulation of heated air and dry cellulose particles through a cabinet into which the body part is inserted through a nylon sleeve. The air and cellulose act as a fluid, with the body part floating as though it were in water and transferring heat to it through convection. The temperature used in fluidotherapy is typically in the range of 100°F to 118°F, and treatment durations are usually 20 minutes. Fluidotherapy devices come in a variety of sizes and configurations to accommodate different body parts, and many also have sleeves through which practitioners can insert their hands to perform manual therapy during the treatment.

Future Questions

Although the use of superficial thermal modalities is very common, very little good research about their specific physiologic effects has actually been conducted and even less about their efficacy in improving patient outcomes. The common 15- to 30-minute applications are more a matter of tradition than a data-driven guideline. The appropriate temperatures to use and the tissue target temperature sought are also an area for which few definitive data exist. These modalities are prime targets for future research to investigate their duration, frequency of use, and appropriate tissue temperatures.

Ultrasound

Description

Aside from cryotherapy, probably no other modality has had more research completed on it than therapeutic ultrasound. The unfortunate reality about this research, however, is that we still do not know a great deal about therapeutic ultrasound and there is a good amount of controversy about clinical outcomes.[13,14,117-120] Ultrasound, simply defined, is the use of acoustic energy at a frequency beyond the audible range (above 30,000 Hz). Ultrasonic energy is used for many different purposes, some of which, such as ultrasonic cleaning, have little to do with healing. Medical ultrasound is the application of ultrasonic energy for medical purposes, and it has two general categories. The first is imaging ultrasound, for which ultrasonic energy at frequencies between 1,000,000 Hz (1 MHz) and 10 MHz is used to image deep structures such as the heart or major blood vessels. A MEDLINE search using the term *ultrasound* will produce predominantly imaging ultrasound literature. Therapeutic ultrasound, in contrast, is the use of ultrasonic energy to cause specific changes in tissues in an effort to improve healing or alter their function.

Although therapeutic ultrasound can theoretically use any of thousands of frequencies between 800 and 3 MHz, two predominant frequencies, 1 and 3 MHz, are by far the most commonly used in the United States. A newer variant on ultrasound is long wave ultrasound, sometimes called *kilohertz* ultrasound to differentiate it from the more common *megahertz* ultrasound frequencies. Kilohertz ultrasound most commonly uses a frequency of 45 kHz instead of 1 or 3 MHz. The acoustic energy is created when an alternating electrical current is applied to a neutral crystal, usually lead zirconate-titanate, which causes the crystal to vibrate through a piezoelectric effect. The vibrating crystal is tightly adhered to a metal plate on the transducer of the ultrasound device, and sound waves are transmitted from the crystal through the metal plate and into the tissue. Generally, a coupling medium is used to facilitate the transmission of acoustic energy.

We tend to conceptualize therapeutic ultrasound as being either thermal or nonthermal based on the intensity and duty cycle parameters selected. In reality, the combination of intensity and duty cycle produces a continuum with thermal ultrasound at one end and nonthermal at the other. Most of the time, our treatments are somewhere in between. We collectively characterize thermal ultrasound as a deep heating modality, although this characterization may be misplaced for 3-MHz ultrasound because it is commonly thought to heat to depths between 0.8 and 1.6 cm.[11,107,121,122] For kilohertz ultrasound, the depth of heating is even less (almost no heating deeper than 1 cm),[123,124] which makes it essentially equivalent to a moist heat pack for thermal purposes.[125]

How We Think It Works

To answer the question about how we think therapeutic ultrasound works is somewhat complex because ultrasound is used for several different goals. We use thermal ultrasound for goals related to circulation, range of motion/tissue extensibility, reabsorption of calcium deposits, and driving medications through the skin. Nonthermal ultrasound is gaining popularity for goals related to resolution of edema, regeneration of tissue, and healing of fractures.

THERMAL ULTRASOUND

Because it is more commonly used, we will begin with thermal ultrasound, which is using ultrasound to cause an increase in temperature in tissues. For ultrasound to cause a rise in tissue temperature, the acoustic energy must be absorbed. Absorption of acoustic energy is greater in tissues with higher protein content and at the interface between different types of tissue, particularly between bone and muscle.[7-9] For the temperature to increase, the rise in temperature produced by ultrasound must be greater than removal of that heat by conduction to other tissues and by the influx of unheated blood and carrying away of heated blood. Typically, thermal ultrasound is produced by a combination of higher ultrasound intensity and greater duty cycle (the percentage of time that acoustic energy is being produced by the transducer).

The most common use of thermal ultrasound is to augment techniques to improve range of motion. As is the case with superficial thermal modalities, ultrasound by itself is not adequate to effect a change in range of motion. Instead, ultrasound is used in an attempt to alter the elasticity of restricting tissues so that efforts to stretch them will be more effective.[112-114,120]

Clinical Pearl #10

Ultrasound is not effective in producing changes in range of motion by itself; it is effective only as an adjunct to techniques, such as stretching or joint mobilization, and even then only if these techniques are performed while the tissue temperature is still elevated in the therapeutic range.

Many studies have investigated this therapeutic range and described the clinical parameters needed to produce therapeutic temperatures. Most of the early work was completed by Lehman et al in the 1960s through the early 1980s.[7-9,107] In several papers, they and others[8,12,107] attempted to identify the range of temperatures that produce changes in the elasticity of collagenous tissues and reported that the therapeutic range was somewhere between 39°C or 40°C and 45°C. Temperatures below 39°C or 40°C did not produce significant changes in elasticity, and temperatures higher than 45°C frequently caused tissue damage. Later, Lehmann paraphrased this range in relative terms; that is, he described it in terms of the change in temperature rather than absolute temperatures.[107] A very important and often overlooked aspect of this early temperature-defining work was that it was not studied in vivo or in humans and that the initial paper examining changes in elasticity and temperature did not use ultrasound![12] In reality, the therapeutic temperature range was determined by using excised sections of rat tail tendon in a heated bath at various temperatures. Although the data from this study are commonly applied to therapeutic ultrasound, we are actually making a relatively significant leap of faith that most clinicians do not realize they are making.

The relative description of change in temperature first suggested by Lehmann[107] has gained a great deal of popularity with the extensive work of Draper et al,[11,112-114,117,126-128] whose papers often cite that a "vigorous heating" temperature increase of 3°C to 4°C is required for changes in elasticity. As a general rule, thinking of relative change in temperature as a clinical goal may be problematic, however. Many tissues commonly treated with ultrasound have baseline temperatures in the neighborhood of 35.5°C, and some baseline temperatures have been recorded that are below 35°C.[120] For these tissues, a 4°C change in temperature barely reaches the lower bound of the therapeutic range or may not reach it at all. Merrick et al[121] observed that neurologically normal subjects reported that a distinct heating sensation was experienced with thermal ultrasound and that this sensation became uncomfortable to the point of discontinuing the treatments when temperatures exceeded 41°C. They speculated that this observation, though unconfirmed, may eventually form the basis of a clinical guideline for thermal ultrasound treatments, where the beginning of patient discomfort might serve as an indicator that the temperature has reached the therapeutic range.

The period when the temperature is in the therapeutic range has been described as the "stretching window."[113,114] The stretching window with ultrasound has been reported to last only 2 to 3 minutes, and researchers suggest that stretching should begin even before the conclusion of the ultrasound treatment. It has been clearly demonstrated that stretching at a lower magnitude for a longer period is more effective that shorter stretches of greater magnitude.[8,12,129] It has also been reported that the stretching window is briefer for superficial structures (3 MHz)[113] than it is for deeper structures (1 MHz).[114]

The literature directly examining ultrasound and stretching is very sparse, and in the small amount of research on the topic, very little promise is seen. Ultrasound applied to the calf of nonpathologic subjects produced little benefit during stretching when compared with stretching alone (only a 3° difference in dorsiflexion).[112] In addition, the benefits of ultrasound were not residual; that is, no difference was noted at the beginning of the session the next day. The lack of good findings here may be a function of how ultrasound was used in the study rather than failure of the modality.[118,120] The treatment area for ultrasound is normally limited to twice the effective radiating area of the crystal, and this generally represents a volume of tissue roughly the same as two rolls of 35-mm photographic film for 1-MHz ultrasound. This is a relatively small volume of tissue when compared with the total volume of the ankle plantar flexors. By heating only a portion of the total group and using subjects without an existing limitation in range of motion, it is quite possible that the lack of effect in this study was related to the methodology. Similarly, the heating took place mostly in muscle tissue rather than collagenous tissues such as the Achilles tendon, and there are presently no data to suggest how heating of muscle affects range of motion, particularly in normal subjects. For these reasons and because we know that temperature does indeed affect the elasticity of collagenous connective tissues, ultrasound should be further examined in range-of-motion studies in which the volume of tissue and the type of tissue are best suited to ultrasound treatments.

Thermal ultrasound, via its increase in temperature, can also lead to circulatory changes through vasodilation, and this increased blood flow may last as long as 45 to 60 minutes.[130] These circulatory changes, coupled with the case study–based notion that continuous ultrasound tends to cause reabsorption of calcium from bony deposits, has made ultrasound popular for the treatment of bone spurs and other bony deposits. This is particularly the case with bursitis and a variety of tendinopathies, as well as myositis ossificans. In reality, the actual efficacy of ultrasound for this purpose is still in question and has not been examined aside from the case study literature, where no specific cause for the resolution could be identified.[1]

NONTHERMAL ULTRASOUND

Nonthermal ultrasound is somewhat less familiar to most practitioners than its thermal counterpart, but it is gaining in popularity. By convention, most nonthermal ultrasound treatments are accomplished by using a pulsed duty cycle. That is, the acoustic energy emitted by the transducer is "pulsed" so that it has an "on" period in which acoustic energy is emitted and an "off" period in which no energy is emitted. A 20% duty cycle with relatively normal intensity is probably the most common protocol, but some machines allow a number of pulsed options. The idea is that the heat produced by ultrasound is allowed to dissipate before it induces a meaningful rise in tissue temperature. An alternative and increasingly more popular means of producing nonthermal ultrasound is to use a continuous (100% on time) duty cycle with a very low ultrasound intensity. To date, however, the data are inadequate to compare the two approaches.

Nonthermal ultrasound is used primarily when the goal is augmentation of a repair or regeneration of damaged tissue. Although the work is preliminary, a number of strong studies appear to support this use. Nonthermal ultrasound has been suggested to increase the regeneration of muscle and bony tissue and aid in the healing of slow-to-heal skin ulcers.[131-135] This work is still very preliminary, with much of it conducted in animal models or in patients who are very different from the athletic patients whom we typically see. Therefore, caution should be used in applying these findings to the sports medicine area. Likewise, we do not yet know whether nonthermal ultrasound is most effective when used in a pulsed protocol or a low-intensity continuous protocol, although investigations of this topic are under way.

KILOHERTZ ULTRASOUND

The newest trend in ultrasound devices is to use much lower frequencies. These devices produce sound waves in the kilohertz range rather than the more common megahertz range. Even so, the most common 45-kHz frequency is still more than twice the upper limit of human hearing. Because frequency and wavelength are inversely related, these kilohertz devices have much longer wavelengths than their megahertz-based cousins. In fact, typical wavelengths for 1- and 3-MHz ultrasound devices are 1.5 and 0.5 mm, respectively, whereas the wavelength for 45-kHz ultrasound is in the vicinity of 30 cm. Hence, they are often called *long wave* ultrasound.

Very little research[123-125,136,137] has been conducted on these devices, and therefore we know precious little about their physiology or clinical efficacy. The most commonly touted effect is that the long wavelength permits deeper penetration. However, it is important to recognize that these devices have an extremely short near field and much longer far field.[124,125,136] The far field is divergent, which means that it produces little to no thermal effects. Consequently, the thermal effects of kilohertz ultrasound appear to be limited to around 1 cm in depth and are much smaller in magnitude ($\approx 0.4°C$) than are the thermal effects of megahertz ultrasound ($\approx 10°C$ or higher). In fact, they are very similar to simply applying a hot water bottle.[125] It is likely that kilohertz ultrasound has little or no redeeming value as a thermal modality. However, some very interesting and compelling research suggests that it may be quite useful for stimulating bone healing.[137] Although most kilohertz devices are single frequency and not available from conventional ultrasound devices, multifrequency ultrasound devices, such as the Duo Son (S.R.A. Developments Ltd., South Devon, UK) are beginning to come to market.

PHONOPHORESIS

Another common use for therapeutic ultrasound is transcutaneous delivery of medications, a technique known as *phonophoresis*. Since its introduction in 1954, phonophoresis has become a very popular clinical technique for the management of musculoskeletal injuries in athletes.[116] Unlike its cousin iontophoresis, phonophoresis is thought to drive whole molecules through the skin and into the underlying tissue and bloodstream.[130] If effective, phonophoresis would have the benefit of providing local delivery of medication without the problems related to injection or the side effects often associated with oral medications. Transport of a drug across the skin barrier is limited by its ability to cross the outermost layer of the skin, the stratum corneum. Because this layer is composed of dead stratified squamous epithelial tissue, its permeability is greatly dependent on its level of hydration. Removal of a portion of the stratum corneum by abrasion greatly increases drug absorption until the layer is reestablished in 2 to 3 days. The easiest path for drug passage through the skin is through hair follicles, sebaceous glands, and sweat ducts, with the follicles serving as the primary route of transmission. Heating the skin before phonophoresis increases the rate of drug transmission, thereby enhancing local delivery.[119] Conversely, heating immediately following phonophoresis increases the rate of drug absorption by the vascular system, thereby decreasing local delivery but enhancing systemic delivery.

Phonophoresis is somewhat controversial, however.[119,138-142] In several studies, phonophoresis has been shown to increase the diffusion of hydrocortisone across the skin and into skeletal muscle and nervous tissue, and several studies have shown positive clinical effects. On the other hand, most hydrocortisone preparations for phonophoresis have been suggested to be poor transmitters of ultrasound (Table 8-8). In one abstract, however, ultrasound with hydrocortisone preparations was reported to produce intramuscular temperatures similar to those with standard ultrasound.[143] This leads to ongoing confusion about the efficacy of phonophoresis, and clearly, additional investigation is direly needed in this area.

Techniques and Dosage

To understand this section, a few ultrasound parameters should be discussed in relation to their effect on treatment. First, the frequency of the acoustic energy (usually 1 or 3 MHz) determines

Table 8-8 Ultrasound Transmission by Phonophoresis Media

Product	Transmission Relative to Water (%)
Media that Transmit Ultrasound (US) Well	
Lidex gel, fluocinonide 0.05%[a]	97
Thera-Gesic cream, methyl salicylate 15%[b]	97
Mineral oil[c]	97
US gel[d]	96
US lotion[e]	90
Betamethasone 0.05%[f] in US gel[d]	88
Media that Transmit US Poorly	
Diprolene ointment, betamethasone 0.05%[g]	36
Hydrocortisone (HC) powder 1%[h] in US gel[d]	29
HC powder 10%[b] in US gel[d]	7
Cortril ointment, HC 1%[i]	0
Eucerin cream[j]	0
HC cream 1%[k]	0
HC cream 10%[k]	0
HC cream 10%[k] mixed with equal weight US gel[d]	0
Myoflex cream, trolamine salicylate 10%[l]	0
Triamcinolone acetonide cream 0.1%[k]	0
Velva HC cream 10%[b]	0
Velva HC cream 10%[b] with equal weight US gel[d]	0
White petrolatum[m]	0
Other	
Chempad-L[n]	68
Polyethylene wrap[o]	98

Reprinted from Cameron, M.H., and Monroe, L.G. (1992): Relative transmission of ultrasound by media customarily used for phonophoresis. Phys. Ther., 72:147. With the permission of the American Physical Therapy Association.
[a] Syntex Laboratories Inc, 3401 Hillview Ave, PO Box 10850, Palo Alto, CA 94303.
[b] Mission Pharmacal Co, 1325 E Durango, San Antonio, TX 78210.
[c] Pennex Corp, Eastern Ave at Pennex Dr, Verona, PA 15147.
[d] Ultraphonic, Pharmaceutical Innovations Inc, 897 Frelinghuysen Dr, Newark, NJ 07114.
[e] Polysonic, Parker Laboratories Inc, 307 Washington St, Orange, NJ 07050.
[f] Pharmfair Inc, 100 Kennedy Dr, Hauppauge, NY 11788.
[g] Schering Corp, Galloping Hill Rd, Kenilworth, NJ 07033.
[h] Purepac Pharmaceutical Co, 200 Elmora Ave, Elizabeth, NJ 07207.
[i] Pfizer Labs Division, Pfizer Inc, 253 E 42nd St, New York, NY 10017.
[j] Beiersdorf Inc, PO Box 5529, Norwalk, CT 06856.
[k] E Fougera & Co, 60 Baylis Rd, Melville, NY 11747.
[l] Rorer Consumer Pharmaceuticals, Div of Rhône-Poulenc Rorer Pharmaceuticals Inc, 500 Virginia Dr, Fort Washington, PA 19034.
[m] Universal Cooperatives Inc, 7801 Metro Pkwy, Minneapolis, MN 55420.
[n] Henley International, 104 Industrial Blvd, Sugar Land, TX 77478.
[o] Saran Wrap, Dow Brands Inc, 9550 Zionsville Rd, Indianapolis, IN 46268.

the effective depth of the treatment. Lower-frequency ultrasound (i.e., 1 MHz) has a more collimated acoustic energy beam that results in a greater depth of heating than higher frequency (i.e., 3 MHz) does. We generally describe the effective depth of heating in terms of half-value depths. A half-value depth is the depth at which 50% of the ultrasound energy has been absorbed by the tissue. Ultrasound at 1 MHz has a greater half-value depth (2.3 cm) than 3 MHz (0.8 cm) does.[122] Ultrasound devices have been shown to produce effective heating at depths of at least up to twice the half-value depth (i.e., around 5 cm for 1 MHz and around 2 cm for 3 MHz).[11,122]

Other important parameters for ultrasound include the spatial averaged intensity, often referred to simply as intensity. The spatial averaged intensity is the total amount of acoustic energy emitted by the transducer averaged over the effective radiating area (ERA) of the transducer. The ERA is simply the area of the transducer that is actually emitting the acoustic energy. The ERA is related to the size of the crystal and not the area of the sound head that contacts the patient. In reality, the ERA is always smaller than the patient contact area of the sound head. The intensity of the ultrasound is one of two major factors that determine the rise in temperature. Higher intensities translate into higher temperatures. The other major determinant of rise in temperature is the duty cycle already discussed.

A final important parameter for ultrasound is the beam nonuniformity ratio (BNR). The BNR of an ultrasound transducer is simply the ratio of the peak intensity at any point on the sound head to the average intensity. Because ultrasound crystals do not have perfect structures, "hot spots" are produced on the crystal where more energy is emitted than in other spots. The lower the BNR, the more uniform the crystal and the more comfortable the treatment to the patient. BNRs greater than 5:1 are generally considered to be unacceptable in modern equipment, and BNRs lower than 4:1 should be sought. The BNR and ERA of the ultrasound device are generally found on a label on the transducer head or lead wire. Most ultrasound manufacturers report only the average BNR for a sample of their devices rather than reporting the BNR for each device.

Although not really considered a treatment parameter, another important consideration in ultrasound application is the coupling medium selected. Coupling media are used between the tissue being treated and the patient contact surface of the ultrasound transducer in an effort to facilitate the transfer of acoustic energy. Ultrasound is not well propagated through air, and without a coupling medium, a large amount of the energy is actually reflected at the transducer surface and may in fact cause damage to the ultrasound transducer. Although many types of coupling media are available, not all are equally effective. To allow comparison, the transmission capacity for media is usually expressed in terms relative to the transmission with distilled water (see Table 8-8). Some commonly used media, such as hydrocortisone powder in ultrasound gel, have actually been shown to exhibit poor transmission of ultrasound. Interestingly, although 10% hydrocortisone cream in ultrasound gel has been shown to transmit only 7% as much ultrasound as distilled water does, ultrasound treatments coupled with this medium appear to produce similar tissue temperature as ultrasound gel alone.[143] This apparent contradiction is puzzling and requires further study. Similarly, indirect ultrasound, in which the transducer and the body part are both immersed in water, has been shown to produce smaller temperature effects than directly coupled ultrasound. This may be a function of the temperature of the water and needs further exploration.

Perhaps more than any other research group, Draper et al have reported a great deal of information with regard to establishing guidelines for the use of thermal ultrasound.[11,113,114,117,127,144,145] Their findings and those of other laboratories are summarized in Box 8-9. In an often cited paper by Draper, Castel, and Castel,[11] changes in temperature with continuous ultrasound at both 1 MHz and 3 MHz, at different depths, and at different intensities were described. The observations from this study were that for 1-MHz ultrasound, an intensity of 2.0 W/cm^2 for 10 minutes was required to reach the therapeutic range and, for 3 MHz, an intensity of 2.0 W/cm^2 required only 3 minutes to reach the therapeutic range. An interesting set of observations was reported separately by Holcomb and Joyce[147] and by Merrick et al,[121] who used identical parameters to compare different brands of ultrasound devices. They each reported that not all devices produce the same results and that one brand in particular (Omnisound 3000) produced substantially greater increases in temperature than the others. Merrick et al[121] went

on to suggest that because the commonly accepted parameters described by Draper et al to produce therapeutic changes in temperature were determined with an Omnisound, these parameters may not be adequate for other brands and that either greater intensities or durations are probably required with other devices. Recommendations for effective ultrasound treatments are presented in Table 8-9.

Future Questions

Although several major questions still need to be answered regarding ultrasound, none are more important right now than the question of clinical outcome data. To date, virtually no quality outcome data are available for therapeutic ultrasound, as highlighted in a review by Robertson and Baker[13] earlier in the chapter (see Table 8-1). Even though they are to be commended for their attempts to describe the literature on outcomes with ultrasound, Robertson and Baker have created somewhat of a problem in that their review suggested that the data do not support the clinical efficacy of therapeutic ultrasound. Although they reviewed the available literature, the only studies available for their use had serious methodologic flaws that included dramatic problems in the size of the treatment area, the intensity used, and the duration used.[14] These flaws were of such magnitude that positive clinical outcomes could not have been expected to occur. Thus, when using data strictly from these problematic studies, the only logical conclusion would be that ultrasound is not effective. Since the publication of this review, a number of papers, editorials, and policy statements calling for the end of ultrasound as a clinical treatment have been made. However, these calls for the death of ultrasound are probably a bit premature. Evidence is mounting that when used appropriately, ultrasound does indeed cause some significant physiologic changes. However, quality clinical trials with good methodology are desperately needed to document whether these effects seen in the laboratory translate into positive outcomes for patients.

Box 8-9

Pertinent Research Findings Regarding the Clinical Use of Ultrasound for Thermal Purposes

Subcutaneous fat plays little or no role in determining the ultrasound dosage.[146]

Many (if not most) clinicians do not use an adequate intensity of ultrasound.[11,117]

Indirect (underwater) ultrasound does not produce the same temperature effect as direct ultrasound with coupling gel does.[145]

Precooling of tissues negates the thermal effects of ultrasound.[128]

Table 8-9 Recommendations for Effective Thermal Ultrasound Treatments

Parameter	Why It Is Important	Recommended Value
Sound frequency	It controls the depth of heating.	Use 1 MHz for tissues between 2.5 and 5 cm deep and 3 MHz for tissues up to 2.5 cm deep.
Duty cycle	It helps determine whether the heat can accumulate.	Continuous (100% duty cycle) should be used.
Treatment area	Diluting the treatment over too large an area negates the heating effect. It is like using a candle to heat a bathtub full of water.	The treatment area should be no larger than twice the effective radiating area (ERA) of the crystal. *Note:* the ERA is smaller than the patient contact area of the sound transducer.
Spatial averaged intensity	It determines the degree of heating. Higher intensities produce greater heating.	For 1-MHz ultrasound, the intensity should be at least 1.5 W/cm^2, with 2.0 W/cm^2 being recommended. For 3-MHz ultrasound, 1.5 W/cm^2 is recommended.
Treatment duration	It determines whether a thermal effect can be expected.	For 1-MHz treatments at 2.0 W/cm^2, the duration should be roughly 10 minutes. For 3-MHz treatments at 1.5 W/cm^2, the duration should be roughly 4-6 minutes. It may be possible to use patient sensation as a guide to duration. The patient should feel a heating sensation that approaches discomfort when the therapeutic range is reached.
Beam nonuniformity ratio (BNR)	It determines the patient's comfort and may contribute to the rate of heating.	Devices with lower BNRs are more comfortable and appear to heat tissue more quickly. Look for a BNR of 4:1 or less, and lower is better.

Short Wave Diathermy

Description

Short wave diathermy (SWD) is another deep-heating thermal modality, and it is probably the best thermal modality available to the practitioner.[148] It is also a modality about which many practitioners have significant reservations, some of which are well founded and others are not. SWD uses short wave (10 to 100 MHz) electromagnetic energy to cause an increase in tissue temperature. To avoid radiofrequency interference with communications frequencies, the Federal Communications Commission regulates the frequencies of SWD available and has allocated three frequencies for medical use (13.56, 27.12, and 40.68 MHz).

SWD devices are not commonly found in athletic health care facilities, and we rarely spend much time on these modalities in our education programs. In fact, many of those teaching modality courses have never used diathermy on a patient. In many cases, diathermy education consists of a brief discussion of indications and effects and a more pointed discussion of the risks, contraindications, and precautions. The net result is that many practitioners are unfamiliar with diathermy and are apprehensive about using it on their patients. Likewise, we have been taught (incorrectly) that ultrasound can produce similar effects with considerably more safety.

Clinical Pearl #11

SWD is probably safer than most practitioners suspect and appears to be considerably more effective than the other deep thermal modalities at our disposal.

How We Think It Works

All types of diathermy produce changes in temperature through resistance to the passage of electromagnetic energy through the tissue being treated.[127,148-152] In the case of SWD, the passage of energy can lead to therapeutic changes in temperature to depths up to 6 to 8 cm. As is the case with ultrasound, continuous SWD produces greater increases in temperature than does pulsed SWD.[152] However, unlike ultrasound, pulsed SWD can indeed cause therapeutic changes in temperature and is actually the most common form.

The effects of diathermy are essentially the same as those for any other deep thermal modality addressed in this chapter and include changes in temperature and their resulting changes in nerve function, circulation, tissue repair, and tissue elasticity. The real beauty of SWD is that it accomplishes all these effects to a much greater degree than do the other deep thermal modalities that we use.[151] For example, a typical 1-MHz therapeutic ultrasound treatment can cover a treatment area roughly the volume of two rolls of 35-mm photographic film. This is fine if something small is being treated, but it becomes a significant limitation if trying to treat an entire low back region or the hamstring of a running back. SWD, in contrast, is able to treat a volume of tissue roughly equivalent to a full bowl of breakfast cereal. The dramatic difference in the volume of tissue treated allows SWD to be effective in places where ultrasound cannot be.[112,144,151]

Techniques and Dosage

Although several application systems are available for pulsed SWD, the most common is the induction method. In this setup, an electromagnetic field is generated by passing an electrical current through a coiled cable electrode, and the patient is placed into this field. Unlike the conductance method of diathermy, the patient is not actually part of the electrical circuit. A tissue's resistance to the passage of this electromagnetic field causes the increase in temperature. The inductance method has two main configurations. One uses a cable electrode that is coiled on top of or around the body part. The other has the cable precoiled into a "drum" that is usually on a swing arm attached to the unit. The drum setup is very popular because it is the easiest and safest to use.

The most common frequency for pulsed SWD is 27.12 MHz, and quite a few devices are available on the market, although most are quite expensive and typically cost up to 10 times as much as a top-of-the-line ultrasound device. The parameters for most units are consistent and include a 20-minute treatment duration and pulsed delivery at 800 bursts per second with a 400-μsec burst width. Average outputs of less than 38 W are considered to be nonthermal, whereas higher outputs are thermal.

SWD is not without risks and drawbacks. Aside from the hefty price for the device, many practitioners have safety concerns related to both the patient and the clinician. Many safety concerns involve inadvertent burning of the patient. Patient burns typically result from clinician errors, including not checking the precautions and contraindications such as metal jewelry or implants, lack of sensation in the treatment area, or accumulation of perspiration (water heats preferentially). Burns are also more common with continuous SWD than with pulsed SWD, particularly when using capacitance-type electrodes, where the patient becomes part of an electrical circuit. Microwave diathermy, which is less common and not discussed in this chapter, can cause burns because the energy is reflected at tissue interfaces and forms standing waves that result in hot spots. Fortunately, most of the newer diathermy devices are pulsed SWD units operating at 27.12 MHz with induction electrodes that are no more likely to cause burns than are hot Hydrocollator packs.

A more pertinent safety-related concern with diathermy involves stray electromagnetic energy from the units.[148,153,154] Diathermy uses electromagnetic fields to produce thermal changes in the treated tissues. Unfortunately, these fields can extend beyond the area being treated. Martin et al[154] examined stray electromagnetic energy from both SWD and microwave diathermy units. They reported that continuous SWD units and microwave diathermy units have stray electromagnetic fields above the recommended levels for a distance of about 1 m surrounding cables and electrodes. Pulsed SWD units, which are more common, had stray fields above the recommended levels for a distance of about 0.5 m surrounding the electrodes. It has been suggested that repeated exposure to these stray fields may cause adverse health effects in clinicians, and thus appropriate care should be taken.

Electrical Stimulation

Description

People have been passing electrical currents through their bodies for healing purposes for thousands of years. In just the last century a systematic attempt has been made to describe the therapeutic effects of electricity and to organize them in such a way to make them useful. Much like the case with cryotherapy, we have collectively learned that there are a number of different forms and therapeutic uses of electricity, and their popularity in athletic health care facilities is growing. The recent growth in the use of electrotherapy is probably related to recent manufacturing improvements in electrotherapy devices that make them easier than ever to use and provide more treatment options than ever before. Although this has certainly bolstered the clinical use of electrotherapy, it has also created a strong tendency to use "cookbook" electrotherapy protocols rather than protocols based on specific goals for the patient. In fact, many clinicians now learn to use only preset protocols that are factory programmed into the machine, and they have great difficulty in creating a custom protocol to accomplish their goals. Worse yet, many of the factory preset protocols for electrotherapy devices have little or no basis in basic research or outcomes data and may not be effective at all. Similarly, because of a great deal of inconsistency in manufacturers' terminology, practitioners must first translate the instruction manuals into a common set of terms before they can understand them. For these reasons, it is important that practitioners have a good understanding of the basics of electrotherapy and the ability to apply these basics to produce the outcomes desired. This section provides a basic framework and description of electrotherapy, but it can not substitute for a comprehensive course in therapeutic modalities.

How We Think It Works

ELECTRICITY FUNDAMENTALS AND TERMINOLOGY

A basic familiarity with electricity is assumed for this discussion, but a brief review of a few essential concepts that influence the clinical use of electrotherapy is provided here.[58] First, *electricity* is the flow of electrons from an area of high concentration to an area of lower concentration. Because electrons carry a negative charge, the area of high electron concentration has a negative charge or negative polarity, and the area of low concentration has a positive charge or positive polarity. Therefore, electricity flows from a negatively charged area, called the *negative pole* or *cathode*, to a positively charged area, called the *positive pole* or *anode*. An electrically conductive pathway connecting the negative pole to the positive pole is called a *circuit*. Electrotherapy treatments work by making the targeted tissues a part of this circuit. The flow of electricity along a circuit is known as *current*. Electrical currents can be either continuous, like water constantly running through a garden hose, or interrupted, which is like turning the spigot for our garden hose on and off quickly and repeatedly so that separate spurts of water travel through the hose. The amount of electricity flowing along the circuit is measured in *amperes* and is analogous to the volume of water in the garden hose. The force that moves the electrons along the circuit is referred to as *voltage*, and it is analogous to water pressure in our garden hose. The relationship between force and flow (voltage and current) is describe by Ohm's law (Box 8-10).

For most of the things that clinical electrotherapy is used for, the direction of the current flow (i.e., which end of the circuit is positive or negative) is seldom as important as ensuring that current actually flows through the target tissue in a sufficient amount to cause the physiologic response being sought. The flow of current is always unidirectional, from the negative pole

---

Box 8-10

Ohm's Law

$$I = \frac{V}{R}$$

I = current flow (in amperes)
V = driving force (in volts)
R = resistance to current flow (in ohms).

Note: The greater the driving force, the greater the flow of current.

---

to the positive pole. If the two poles at the ends of the circuit never change polarity while the current is on, the direction of current flow is constant and is called *direct current* (DC). If the two poles at the ends of the circuit switch polarity, the direction of current flow also switches and is called *alternating current* (AC). AC is the type of current available from electrical wall outlets, and it switches direction at a constant rate of 60 cycles per second (60 Hz) in North America. DC is the type of current available from a battery.

By connecting the electrical circuit to an oscilloscope, we can visualize the shape, or waveform, of the current (Fig. 8-5). The waveform for DC would be entirely on one side of the horizontal baseline and would continue along indefinitely until the current is turned off (A). Because the current is always moving in one direction, the charge would always have the same polarity and would remain on one side of the baseline. DC can therefore be said to have a single phase and is often called *monophasic current*. With AC, the waveform would initially be on one side of the baseline and then switch to the other side when the direction of the current and therefore the polarity alternated (B). The graph would repeat this switching as long as the current is flowing. Thus, AC can be said to have two phases (one positive and one negative) and is therefore often called *biphasic current*. A third type of current, *polyphasic*, actually has three or more phases and is typically produced by simultaneously overlaying an interrupted current over a continuous biphasic current called a carrier frequency. Common examples of polyphasic waveform devices are interferential stimulators and Russian stimulators.[155]

If the current is turned on and off repeatedly, individual phases with periods of no current flow (no charge) between them (C) would occur, and this is often called *pulsed* or *interrupted current*. The majority of electrotherapy devices use interrupted current, although a few exceptions are discussed later in the chapter. Electrotherapy devices allow the practitioner to control the number of these individual pulses per second (pulse rate). With low pulse rates (below 30), pulsing muscle contractions can be induced. By increasing the pulse rate to somewhere between 30 and 50 pulses per second, the muscle contraction appears smooth and sustained. A muscle that is contracting in a smooth and sustained fashion is said to be in tetany. Even higher pulse rates are often used and also cause tetanic contractions. It should be noted (D to G) that by using different combinations of polarity, voltage, and phase duration, the shape of each phase can be controlled. Common phase shapes are rectangular or square (E), spiked or twin spiked (D), asymmetric (F and G) in which the positive phase and negative phase have different shapes, and sinusoidal (Fig. 8-6). If the positive phase and negative phase have the same voltage (height), the waveform is said to be balanced (G).

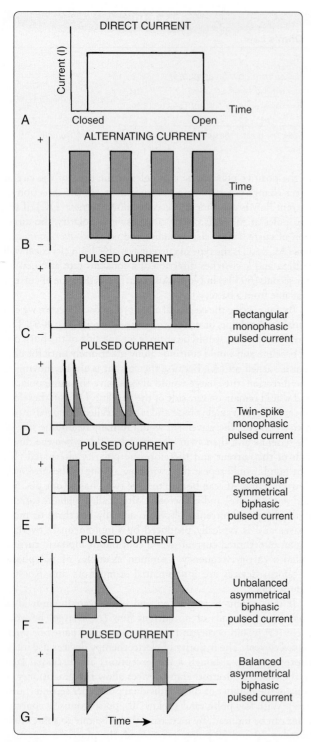

FIGURE 8-5 Graphic representation of the three types of electrical current. **A,** Direct current. **B,** Alternating current. **C** through **G,** Pulsed currents. *(Modified from Robinson, A.J. [1989]: Basic concepts and terminology in electricity. In: Snyder-Mackler, L., and Robinson, A.J. [eds.]. Clinical Electrophysiology. Baltimore, Williams & Wilkins, pp. 9, 11, 13.)*

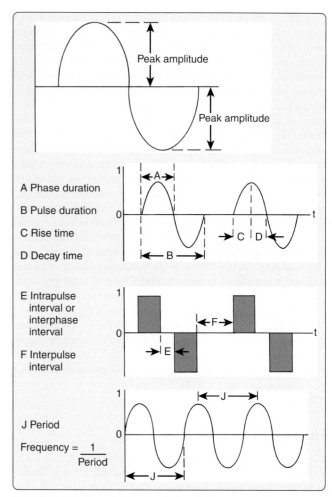

FIGURE 8-6 Characteristics of electricity. *(Modified from Robinson, A.J. [1989]: Basic concepts and terminology in electricity. In: Snyder-Mackler, L., and Robinson, A.J. [eds.]. Clinical Electrophysiology. Baltimore, Lippincott, Williams & Wilkins, p. 15.)*

In examining a waveform, a specific set of terms is used to describe the phases and pulses (see Fig. 8-6). A *phase* is a single positively or negatively charged bolus of current, whereas a *pulse* is several consecutive phases that are continuous. All currents have at least one phase, but pulses are seen only with interrupted current and are separated from each other by brief intervals when no phase is present. The height, or amplitude, of each phase represents the voltage (the driving force for the current). The width of each phase represents the phase duration or phase width, usually in milliseconds. A related concept is pulse width, or the combined duration of all of the phases within a single pulse of interrupted current. Related to phase and pulse widths are phase and pulse intervals, or the duration between phases when there is no current (phase interval) or between pulses where there is no current (pulse interval). *Phase interval* and *pulse interval* are terms that are sometimes used interchangeably.

The lack of consistency in terminology across manufactures and textbooks is an ongoing problem in electrotherapy, which leads us to a fourth and sometimes confusing waveform concept called *frequency*. The frequency of a waveform can mean two very different things. Technically, it represents the number of cycles per second for the current. A cycle, also called a period, is one complete waveform including all of its phases. In clinical usage, the term frequency more commonly means the number of pulses per second and is also called the pulse rate. Remember that a pulse consists of several consecutive cycles of a current in an interrupted current. For example, if you use the electricity

Table 8-10 **Common Therapeutic Goals for Electrotherapy**

Goal	Rationale
Muscle reeducation	Retrain firing patterns or overcome neuromuscular inhibition in intact muscles following injury or pathology. The mechanism is thought to be related to increasing the quantity of motor units recruited or decreasing the inhibition of the motor nerves that is preventing normal function
Retard atrophy	Cause the muscle to contract in an effort to reduce the effects of immobilization or paralysis on atrophy.
Retard edema formation	Limit the formation of edema during acute inflammation by inhibiting the increase in vascular permeability with sensory-level stimulation.
Remove edema	Remove edema that is already present through a muscle pump mechanism with motor-level stimulation.
Reduce pain	Interfere with the transmission or perception of pain through a variety of different electrotherapy approaches.
Reduce spasm	Reduce acute spasms by either decreasing the muscle's contraction frequency or by fatiguing the muscle until it fails (very uncomfortable). Electrotherapy can also be used to manage the spasticity associated with neuromuscular diseases or spinal cord trauma.
Increase strength	Increase muscle force output in nonpathologic tissue by causing hypertrophy of the muscle. Although muscular strength can be improved with motor-level stimulation, the protocols required are very uncomfortable and are not nearly as effective as resistance exercise. This is not generally an appropriate goal for electrotherapy.
Increase range of motion	A commonly cited but misleading goal. Electrotherapy can be effective in reducing muscle spasticity or edema and thereby countering loss of ROM associated with these conditions, but electrotherapy is not an effective means of improving ROM by itself.
Transport medications	Iontophoresis: deliver medications by driving electrically charged ions through the skin.
Tissue healing	Microcurrent: some evidence has shown that microcurrent may augment tissue repair in individuals with fractures or slow-healing skin ulcerations. The mechanism has yet to be described.

ROM, Range of motion.

coming from your wall outlet, it is a continuous sinusoidal biphasic current with a frequency of 60 Hz. Now, if you are using an outlet connected to a switch and you manually turn the current on and off 10 times per second, the resulting current would be an interrupted sinusoidal biphasic current with a frequency of 60 Hz and a pulse rate of 10 Hz. Obviously, this terminology can be somewhat confusing, and most clinicians and manufacturers generally use "frequency" to mean "pulse rate" and the actual frequency of the current being interrupted is ignored.

Although scientific study of electrotherapy is progressing, not as much is known about the physiology of this modality as is known about cryotherapy, superficial thermotherapy, or ultrasound, and the precise mechanisms by which electrotherapy is effective have not yet been described. As is the case for these better-studied modalities, electrotherapy is also characterized by a conspicuous lack of outcomes research. Even though the literature is still sparse, electrotherapy has been suggested to be effective in achieving a number of rehabilitative goals (Table 8-10), most of which are related to the ability of electricity to depolarize nerves. In addition, some the effects proposed are related to the electrical charge fields around the electrodes and do not rely on nerve depolarization.

MUSCLE REEDUCATION

Neuromuscular function is altered through inhibition following injury as discussed previously with regard to rehabilitative cryotherapy. In fact, the great majority of early muscular strength and power loss following an injury is thought to be the result of neurologic inhibition rather than more morphologic causes,

such as loss of muscle mass. Loss of muscular strength and power is seen immediately following injury before loss of muscle mass has even occurred. In fact, loss of muscle mass as an explanation for the loss of strength becomes valid only after several weeks have passed. The goal of muscle reeducation is to counteract postinjury inhibition in an attempt to allow more normal use of the surrounding musculature. By reducing the degree of inhibition seen in these muscles in the early period following injury, earlier and more functional exercise can begin, and it is this exercise that is the most important tool in returning the athlete to competition. This is sometimes thought of as helping a muscle "remember" how to contract. Similarly, reeducation can be used to help reestablish neuromuscular pathways after periods of immobilization or even to help correct pathologic neuromuscular patterns such as seen when a patient compensates for gait or postural abnormalities. An additional means by which electrotherapy can help in reeducation is by overcoming the inhibition associated with the injury.[90]

The primary means by which electrotherapy is thought to be an effective tool for muscle reeducation is through the recruitment of motor units that are not otherwise being recruited. The muscle tissue is not directly induced to contract, however. Instead, the electrical current stimulates motor neurons to depolarize and thereby causes contraction of their respective muscle fibers. By artificially recruiting these motor units through stimulation of the motor nerves it is thought that we may somehow overcome the inhibitory stimuli that are interfering with their voluntary recruitment at some location up the neurologic tree.[94] Despite common anecdotal agreement about the efficacy of muscle reeducation, very little research has directly examined its effects.

RETARD ATROPHY

As is the case with muscle reeducation, the use of electrotherapy to retard atrophy is based on the ability of electrical current to induce muscle contraction.[156,157] During disuse, immobilization, or paralysis, the relative inactivity of the muscles leads them to atrophy. Likewise, lack of muscle contraction–induced stress on the bones can also lead them to atrophy, eventually to the point where they can become fragile if the disuse is of sufficient duration. Electrotherapy is frequently used in cases in which prolonged immobilization is anticipated, such as with casting for fractures or with paralysis. The premise is that electrotherapy can be used to induce low-intensity isometric contractions of the muscle that can retard the progression of atrophy without compromising the immobilization. Note that the word *retard* was used rather than *prevent*. Prevention implies that we can completely counteract the atrophy that is occurring (Box 8-11). Instead, we are more likely to slow its progression.

Box 8-11

Three Reasons Why Electrotherapy Cannot Completely Prevent Atrophy

The scenario in which electrotherapy is typically used to retard atrophy involves prolonged and purposeful immobilization. In such situations, strong muscle contractions are generally to be avoided so that displacement of the immobilized structures does take place. Therefore, we tend to use mild isometric contractions that will retard atrophy, but not prevent it.

Second and probably more important, the pattern of motor unit recruitment with electrical stimulation appears to be quite different from that seen with voluntary contraction. In volitional contractions, smaller-diameter motor neurons supplying small muscle fibers of small motor units are recruited first, and larger neurons with larger and stronger motor units are recruited later as necessitated by the need for greater muscle force. With electrical stimulation, this order appears to be reversed, with larger-diameter motor neurons being recruited first and smaller-diameter fibers being recruited less and only when sufficient voltage is used.[1,2,4,5] This different pattern of muscle recruitment leads to a variable rate of atrophy in which the smaller motor neuron units, which are responsible for fine motor tasks, atrophy at a greater rate than do the larger motor neuron units, which are responsible for gross motor tasks.

A third reason why we appear to be unable to completely prevent atrophy is related to the athletic ability and training level seen in athletes. Even if we were not concerned about the consequences of displacing immobilized tissue with strong contractions, it is unlikely that strong enough contractions could be produced to prevent all muscle loss in injured athletes. By the nature of their extensive training and conditioning programs, athletes have considerably larger muscle mass and force-producing capacity than general patients do. The differential recruitment of motor units with electrical stimulation implies that we are unlikely to be able to generate sufficient muscle force with electrical stimulation to provide an adequate stimulus to retain the muscle mass that has been produced by extensive resistance training.

EDEMA MANAGEMENT

Management of edema with electrotherapy can take two different forms. The first is retarding the formation of edema. The second is removing edema that is already present. The technique is different for each strategy and should be used only in the correct situation. For example, electrotherapy should be used to retard the formation of edema only in the period while edema is forming immediately following the injury. Use of this approach after a large amount of edema is already present may actually inhibit removal of the edema.

Sensory-level, high-voltage pulsed electrical stimulation applied directly to the area of the injury has been shown to limit the volume of edema following uniform injuries in an animal model.[88,90-93] Two mechanisms have been proposed for this retarding of edema through the application of electrotherapy. The first is to combat the increasing permeability of the capillaries during the initial acute inflammatory response and thereby reduce the efflux of fluid from the circulatory system into the injured tissues. As explained in Chapter 2, one of the major events of the acute inflammatory response is a marked increase in capillary permeability that results from the release of numerous chemical mediators. The increase in permeability occurs when adjacent endothelial cells in capillaries do not adhere to each other as tightly as they normally do. This makes the capillaries "leaky" and allows the transcapillary Starling forces to exert an even greater influence. The second—and less accepted—of the proposed mechanisms is that pulsed monophasic current causes vascular spasm that limits delivery of fluid to the injured area. Regardless of the suggested physiologic explanations for the effectiveness of the technique, the protocol used is very specific, requires a specific waveform, and is outlined in the later section on technique and dosage. One of the key elements of the protocol is the timing in relation to injury. This approach is effective only when it is begun before meaningful edema has developed. Therefore, the time window for initiating this modality is quite literally the first few minutes following the injury.

In addition to retarding the formation of edema during acute inflammation, electrotherapy can also be a valuable adjunct in removal of the edema that is already present. The proposed mechanism by which existing edema is removed is somewhat different from that for retarding the formation of edema, however. Although retarding the formation of edema is based on limiting the permeability of the vasculature, such a strategy may actually hinder the ability to remove edema. When present, edema is removed by the lymphatic system rather than the circulatory system. Removal requires that the edematous fluid be absorbed into lymph capillaries, where it flows to larger collecting vessels and eventually to one of the lymphatic ducts, and the fluid is then returned to the circulatory system. If the permeability of the lymphatic capillaries is limited, a potential outcome of the edema retardation electrotherapy protocol, movement of fluid into the lymphatic system may actually be hindered and thus reduce the effectiveness of edema removal.

Instead of using protocols aimed at altering permeability, edema removal protocols focus on moving fluid into the lymphatic system and then moving it along the lymphatic vessels and away from the injury site.[158-163] This is accomplished by motor-level electrical stimulation in which the muscles are induced to contract in a pulsing fashion with interrupted current. Each muscle contraction exerts external pressure on the lymphatic vessels. Squeezing of the lymphatic vessels causes the fluid in them to move. This strategy for removal of edema is sometime called the "muscle pump" strategy. When fluid reaches the collecting vessels of the lymphatic system, its flow essentially becomes unidirectional because of the presence of one-way valves within the vessels. Much like the valves located in veins, pressure exerted on the lymphatic vessel from muscular contractions causes the upstream valve to close and the downstream valve to open, thereby allowing the fluid to flow back only toward the circulatory system. Because fluid moves with each muscular contraction, electrotherapy pulse rates that are below the level needed for tetany are used. Tetanic contractions would produce only a single pressure pulse and would not be expected to move as much fluid as would repetitive contractions.

Clinical Pearl #12

Even though electrotherapy can be a useful adjunct for removal of edema, the role of exercise in removing edema should not be overlooked. Exercise also induces muscle pumping, typically in more muscles than are used with electrotherapy alone.

PAIN MANAGEMENT

Management of pain with electrotherapy is among the most common, best documented, and most successful uses of this modality.[164-174] Much of the pain reduction literature deals with a subform of electrotherapy called transcutaneous electrical nerve stimulation (TENS). TENS typically involves the use of pulsed, sensory-level stimulation to interfere with the transmission of pain signals in the spinal cord through a mechanism known as gait control. Gait control uses sensory information on A-β afferent nerves to interfere with the transmission of pain on A-δ and C afferent fibers. To be effective, adequate stimulation of A-β fibers must occur. The literature suggests that this is most likely to occur at rates between 60 and 150 pulses per second, and rates of 100 to 150 pulses per second are most common.[1,2,5] The high pulse rates have led this protocol to be called *high-frequency TENS*. High-frequency TENS units generally use a short pulse duration (20 to 60 μsec) combined with a 50- to 100-Hz frequency of stimulation. Additionally, the combination of sensory-level TENS and cryotherapy has been shown to provide greater pain relief than with either of these modalities used individually.

Although the gait control strategy is certainly the most common, it is not the only strategy for controlling pain with electrotherapy. Motor-level stimulation with a high-voltage (>150 V) stimulator can be used to stimulate the release of endogenous opiate-like substances from nerve fibers. Sometimes this protocol is referred to as "low-frequency TENS" because of its low pulse rate (2 to 4 pulses per second). It is frequently uncomfortable during application but results in relief of pain following the treatment. This is somewhat different for conventional high-frequency TENS, in which pain relief is usually experienced during the treatment and for a short time thereafter. The release-of-opiates strategy is not as common as the gate control strategy; however, it may provide longer-lived pain relief.

Another pain relief technique with electrotherapy involves the use of a sensory-level polyphasic current known as *interferential*

current.[168,170,171] Interferential current is actually the combination of two different biphasic currents that are out of phase with each other. The two currents each have different frequencies and are carried on two different circuits (or channels) that are applied more or less perpendicular to each other. The differing frequencies of the currents and the fact that they are out of phase with each other produce a constantly changing waveform in the region where the currents cross. The key feature of interferential electrotherapy is this ever-changing waveform. Because the waveform is constantly changing, the body has a very difficult time accommodating to it. Accommodation is the process by which the sensory system learns to "ignore" sensory stimuli that are unchanging. For example, anyone married for more than a few months no longer senses the wedding ring against their finger. The body has a reasonably good ability to accommodate to electrotherapy, particularly sensory-level electrotherapy. This accommodation reduces the efficacy of the treatments. With interferential electrotherapy, the constantly changing waveform reduces the accommodation and allows the treatment be more effective than fixed-waveform treatments. The mechanism of pain relief is thought to be the same as for high-frequency TENS. In fact, many TENS units now use modulated waveforms that change throughout the treatment in an attempt to overcome accommodation.

SPASTICITY MANAGEMENT

Management of spasticity is among the more commonly cited uses of electrotherapy, although it is generally less applicable to athletic injuries than to other conditions, such as neurologic lesions. Management of the spasticity associated with neurologic lesions frequently involves stimulating the antagonist muscles and relying on reciprocal relaxation. In fact, the vast majority of the literature on the use of electrotherapy for spasticity focuses on the type of spasticity resulting from spinal cord trauma, cerebral vascular accidents, brain trauma, and disease.[175] Because these lesions are not common with athletic injuries, they will not be discussed further in this chapter. On the other hand, management of muscle spasm associated with athletic injuries is a common use of electrotherapy and needs to be addressed, although the literature describing such use is very sparse.

Two strategies are predominantly used for managing athletic injury–related acute muscle spasm with electrotherapy, although only one of them is very tolerable to the patient. The more tolerable of the two strategies involves using motor-level stimulation of the spastic muscles in an attempt to alter their frequency of contraction. Recall that the rate of firing of the motor units determines whether a muscle's contraction will be pulsing or smooth (tetanic). Smooth contractions occur with firing rates higher than 30 to 50 pulses per second. When a muscle is in spasm, it is generally contracting smoothly and continuously. By using a muscle stimulator with relatively high intensity and less than a tetanic pulse rate, it may be possible to slow the firing rate and cause the spasm to abate. The other and probably more effective strategy involves using the stimulator to fatigue the muscle to the point where the spasm ceases. This strategy has been shown to be effective, but it is not very comfortable and most patients may not tolerate it well. Generally, the technique involves using high–pulse rate, maximum tolerable intensity stimulation with a high-voltage stimulator to recruit as many motor units as possible. This will eventually lead to muscular fatigue, and the spasm will lessen or stop altogether. Although this technique is uncomfortable, it can be made more comfortable and more effective if it is combined with static stretching of the affected muscles. Cryotherapy is also a common adjunct with this technique.

INCREASING STRENGTH

Even though electrotherapy can indeed be used to improve strength, this is among the most often misused forms of this modality. To understand this use of electrotherapy, a distinction must first be made between using electrotherapy for muscle reeducation versus electrotherapy for increasing strength. As discussed earlier, muscle reeducation involves using electrotherapy to overcome the neuromuscular inhibition that is interfering with normal muscle function. Said another way, muscle reeducation uses an electrical stimulator in an attempt to improve pathologic muscle function by reestablishing the normal and appropriate neurologic pathways for muscle contraction. This is different from using a stimulator to improve muscle strength.

When a stimulator is used to improve strength, the goal is not to overcome inhibition or other neuromuscular pathology. Instead, electrotherapy is used to strengthen tissue that has normal neuromuscular function but is not as strong as desired. Said another way, muscle strengthening with electrotherapy involves causing the contractile elements within muscle to overload in an attempt to induce them to adapt by becoming stronger. This is precisely the same goal as used during resistance training to improve muscle strength, but the catch is that resistance training is considerably more effective in achieving this goal than electrotherapy is.

To strengthen muscle tissue, regardless of the method, the muscle must be made to exert more force than it is accustomed to exerting. This principle is known as *overload*. Overload of a muscle can be accomplished in two ways: increasing the rate of firing of motor units and recruiting a larger number of motor units.[60] During resistance training, the body's strategy is to do both, but to predominantly favor recruiting more motor units. In fact, during exercise the body varies its motor unit recruitment pattern. At the beginning of an exercise, the smaller-diameter motor neurons of the fine control motor units are recruited. If more force is required, the larger-diameter motor neurons controlling the stronger but less finely controlled motor units are recruited. As the muscle begins to fatigue, the fine control motor units fail first and additional large motor units are recruited until they eventually fail. This is why some shaking and less coordination are observed as someone fatigues during resistance training. When a muscle stimulator is used, however, a different pattern of recruitment takes place.[1,2,5]

Use of a muscle stimulator to improve strength also depends on overload, and both a high rate of motor unit firing and measures aimed at recruiting more motor units are used. In strengthening with electrotherapy, a pulse rate at or near the maximum available for the stimulator is used in an effort to produce as high a rate of motor unit firing as possible. In addition, as high an intensity (voltage) as tolerable is used because higher intensities lead to better penetration of the nerve by the electrical current and therefore recruitment of an increased number of motor units. The unfortunate catch in this strategy, however, is that recruitment of motor units with electrotherapy appears to be the reverse of normal voluntary recruitment. With electrotherapy, motor units that are of larger diameter and closer to the surface of the nerve are preferentially recruited. These same motor units appear to be stimulated over and over rather than recruiting different motor units as some of them fatigue, as is the case with normal exercise. This repeated firing of the same motor units is the reason that muscular fatigue is experienced so quickly with electrical stimulation and not as quickly with exercise. The repeated recruitment of a limited set of motor units also limits the effectiveness of electrotherapy-based strengthening programs. Strengthening adaptations are essentially limited to the motor units that are being recruited, and electrotherapy recruits fewer motor units than active exercise does. Although some degree of strengthening of normal tissue can occur with electrotherapy, the strengthening is not as effective as with active exercise in a resistance training program. Therefore, the use of electrotherapy for muscle reeducation is recommended in athletic therapy, but electrotherapy as a tool to strengthen muscles that have normal function is not.

INCREASING RANGE OF MOTION

Many modalities texts suggest that electrotherapy can be used to improve range of motion, and it most certainly can do so, but not in the way that we are usually seeking with athletic injuries. The use of electrotherapy to improve range of motion is appropriate and effective in only a few limited situations. The most common involves a patient with neurologic trauma or disease that results in spasticity. For example, it is not uncommon to see spasticity in the gastrocnemius and soleus of a spinal cord–injured patient. Such spasticity leads to lack of ankle dorsiflexion range of motion. Electrotherapy can be applied to the dorsiflexors to both stimulate them and inhibit the gastrocnemius and soleus. This would allow greater dorsiflexion range of motion because of the reduction in spasticity of the plantar flexors. Though useful in some cases for neurologic injuries and disease, this type of improvement in range of motion is of little value in the rehabilitation of common athletic injuries. Another limited situation that is of more use with athletic injuries would be improving range of motion that is limited by pain, edema, or both. As discussed earlier, electrotherapy can be used for the management of these conditions and may result in an indirect improvement in range of motion as well.

IONTOPHORESIS OF PHARMACEUTICALS

Iontophoresis, or the use of an electrical current to drive medications through the skin, is another common form of electrotherapy. This technique has some real advantages in that it can be used to deliver medications locally without having to inject them. This can be particularly useful for patients with fear of needles or for pediatric patients. In fact, iontophoresis with local anesthetics is gaining popularity as a preinjection technique to lessen the discomfort of pediatric immunizations. Though potentially advantageous, there is also some controversy over iontophoresis in the literature.[130,176-182] Reports conflict regarding whether iontophoresis delivers enough medication to a deep enough tissue depth to be effective for many conditions. Moreover, outcome data for iontophoresis are limited and have not yet adequately demonstrated that the technique is of much benefit to patients with musculoskeletal injuries.

Iontophoresis requires a very specific type of electrical current and is not possible with typical muscle stimulators. To use electrical current to move medications, the medications must dissociate into electrically charged ions in solution. When an electrical current is applied to the medication solution, the charge at each electrical pole repels the medication ions with like charges and attracts the ions with opposite charges. Therefore, it is critical to apply the medication to the electrode that has the same polarity as the ion of interest in the medication. Likewise, only direct (monophasic) current can be used because alternating (biphasic) current would both repel and retract the medication and produce no net transport through the skin. The current used also needs to be continuous. Interrupted currents do not repel the drug long enough for it to travel through the skin. For these reasons, iontophoresis stimulators are different from other electrotherapy devices and are designed expressly for use in iontophoresis. These devices are used with single-use electrodes and deliver low-intensity DC in a monopolar setup as described later. The dosage is typically the product of the duration of treatment and the amount of current used and is expressed in milliampere minutes (mA • min). The specific dosage depends on the medication being used, and treatments generally last between 10 and 20 minutes, although they can be longer if lower amounts of current must be used because the patient does not tolerate DC well. A new iontophoresis device, the IontoPatch, was introduced in April 2001 and is somewhat different. Instead of using the typical 10- to 20-minute treatment with low to moderate amounts of current, the IontoPatch uses a much longer duration (usually 24 hours) and an extremely low level of current delivered from a self-contained battery in the patch. The lower level of current means fewer complications in terms of skin burns, and anecdotal reports have been very favorable, although the device is new enough that research literature is lacking.

A relatively small number of medications, usually corticosteroids, are commonly used with iontophoresis in athletic medicine settings. However, from a technical standpoint, any medication that dissociates into ions in solution and produces the desired effects could be used. The most common medications are presented in Table 8-11.

Table 8-11 Nonsteroidal Ions and Radicals

Ion or Radical (Charge)	Features*
Magnesium (+)	From magnesium sulfate (Epsom salts), 2% aqueous solution; excellent muscle relaxant, good vasodilator, mild analgesic
Mecholyl (+)	Familiar derivative of acetylcholine, 0.25% ointment; powerful vasodilator, good muscle relaxant and analgesic; used for discogenic low back radiculopathies and sympathetic reflex dystrophy
Iodine (−)	From Iodex ointment, 4.7%; bactericidal, fair vasodilator, excellent sclerolytic agent; used successfully for adhesive capsulitis ("frozen shoulder"), scars
Salicylate (−)	From Iodex with methyl salicylate, 4.8% ointment (if desired without the iodine, can be obtained from Myoflex ointment—trolamine salicylate, 10%—or from a 2% aqueous solution of sodium salicylate powder); a general decongestant, sclerolytic, and antiinflammatory agent; used successfully for frozen shoulders, scar tissue, warts, and other adhesive or edematous conditions
Calcium (+)	From calcium chloride, 2% aqueous solution; believed to stabilize the irritability threshold in either direction, as dictated by the physiologic needs of the tissues; effective for spasmodic conditions, tics, "snapping joints"
Chlorine (−)	From sodium chloride, 2% aqueous solution; good sclerolytic agent; useful for scar tissue, keloids, burns
Zinc (+)	From zinc oxide ointment, 20%; trace element necessary for healing; especially effective for open lesions and ulcerations
Copper (+)	From 2% aqueous solution of copper sulfate crystals; fungicide, astringent, useful for intranasal conditions (e.g., allergic rhinitis—hay fever), sinusitis, and dermatophytosis (athlete's foot)
Lidocaine (+)	From Xylocaine, 5% ointment; anesthetic and analgesic, especially for acute inflammatory conditions (e.g., bursitis, tendinitis, tic douloureux, and temporomandibular joint pain)
Lithium (−)	From lithium chloride or carbonate, 2% aqueous solution; effective as an exchange ion for gouty tophi and hyperuricemia[†]
Acetate (−)	From acetic acid, 2% aqueous solution; dramatically effective as a sclerolytic exchange ion for calcific deposits[‡]
Hyaluronidase (+)	From Wydase crystals in aqueous solution, as directed; for localized edema
Tap water (+/−)	Usually administered with alternating polarity, sometimes with glycopyrronium bromide for hyperhidrosis
Ringer solution (+/−)	With alternating polarity; used for open decubitus lesions
Citrate (+)	From potassium citrate, 2% aqueous solution; reported effective for rheumatoid arthritis
Priscoline (+)	From benzazoline hydrochloride, 2% aqueous solution; reported effective for indolent ulcers
Antibiotics: gentamicin sulfate (+)	8 mg/mL; for suppurative ear chondritis

From Kahn, J. (1987): Non-steroid iontophoresis. Clin. Manage., 7:15. Reprinted from *Clinical Management* with the permission of the American Physical Therapy Association.

* All solutions are 2%; ointments are also low-percentage compounds. The literature and clinical reports agree that the lower the percentage, the more effective the ionic exchange and transfer. Whether this is purely a physical chemistry phenomenon or an example of the Arndt-Schultz law, which states that "the smaller the stimulant, the greater the physiologic response," remains to be proved.

† The lithium ion replaces the weaker sodium ion in the insoluble sodium urate tophus and converts it to soluble lithium urate.

‡ The acetate radical replaces the carbonate radical in the insoluble calcium carbonate calcific deposit and converts it to soluble calcium acetate.

Clinical Considerations

The specific waveform chosen for electrotherapy can be absolutely critical in some cases and can make very little difference in others. One of the hallmarks of a skilled practitioner is to understand the difference. To understand this difference, some familiarity with the electricity fundamentals and terminology discussed earlier is required, as is understanding of the following concepts. First, it has already been discussed that waveforms can be monophasic (also known as DC current), biphasic (also known as AC current), or polyphasic (a mixed waveform, such as interferential current). It has also been discussed that waveforms can be either continuous or interrupted. These features can be combined to produce some general classes of waveforms that have an impact on clinical treatments.

CONTINUOUS VERSUS INTERRUPTED CURRENT

Continuous currents are found in only very few devices and are used in very specific situations. The first of these situations is for iontophoresis, where a continuous monophasic current is used. Continuous currents must be used in this case because interrupted currents do not have a sufficient duration of current flow to move ions across the skin. A second situation in which continuous current is used involves the stimulation of denervated muscle to prevent disuse atrophy. In this case, continuous current is used because the longer current duration makes it easier to induce depolarization of what little remains of the motor nerves or perhaps even the muscle itself. Aside from these two situations, continuous currents are normally found only as biphasic carrier frequencies in polyphasic currents. In these situations, they are normally used to help create a perpetually changing waveform to help overcome accommodation, as is the case with both interferential current and a waveform used for strengthening known as MFBurstAC, or Russian current.[155]

POLARITY

Electrotherapy devices that offer monophasic waveforms can readily be distinguished from biphasic or polyphasic waveforms by nature of the ability to select a polarity for the treatment electrodes. Because biphasic and polyphasic waveforms have both positively and negatively charged phases that alternate, no specific polarity can be assigned to the electrodes. In reality, only in very few situations does the specific polarity of the electrodes make a clinical difference; however, it makes a very big difference in a few. For example, iontophoresis can be accomplished only with a continuous monophasic current and, even then, only when the drug is applied to the correct electrode. The other situation in which polarity clearly matters involves the stimulation of denervated muscle for preventing disuse atrophy; however, this application is less important in the rehabilitation of athletic injuries. Another situation in which polarity has been suggested to make a difference involves the use of electrotherapy to retard the formation of edema. In this case, cathodal (negative polarity) stimulation has been shown to be effective, as discussed later. There is little evidence to suggest that polarity is an important consideration in the management of pain or in the ability to produce contractions in innervated muscle tissue.

UNIPOLAR VERSUS BIPOLAR

One of the easiest to understand yet most misunderstood application technique related to electrotherapy is unipolar versus bipolar electrode configuration. A unipolar electrode configuration means that the active effects of the stimulator are seen only in the electrodes attached to one of the two electrical poles. Bipolar configuration means that the active effects of the stimulator are seen in the electrodes attached to both poles. Recall that to have an electrical circuit, the electricity must have a pathway to flow from one pole (negative) to another pole (positive). In DC these poles maintain constant polarity, and in AC they switch polarity. For purposes of electrode configuration, the actual polarity of the electrode does not matter except in the cases discussed earlier. Whether an electrode displays "active effects" of the current depends on the current density under the electrode, and this is determined by the combination of current intensity and size of the electrode. For a given amount of current, a bigger electrode will have the current spread over a larger area, and a smaller electrode will have the current spread over a smaller area. The amount of current per unit of area is the current density. To have an active effect, such as inducing sensory or motor stimulation, the current density must be adequate. The smaller the electrode, the greater the current density, and therefore greater stimulation effects will be seen. Conversely, the larger the electrode, the smaller the current density, and therefore little or no stimulation effect will occur.

In a unipolar configuration, current density is manipulated by using electrode size. One pole has a relatively small electrode (or several small electrodes), and the other pole has a relatively large electrode, usually called a dispersive electrode. Because a dispersive electrode has a large area, it has a small current density that does not produce active effects. Unipolar configurations are standard on monophasic high-voltage stimulators and are very useful in situations in which you want to move the active electrode, such as with trigger point stimulation. Bipolar configurations use similarly sized electrodes at both poles, so similar effects are seen at both electrodes. Bipolar configurations are more common on newer devices and biphasic stimulators. Bipolar configurations are useful for situations in which you do not plan to move the electrodes or when exposure of enough skin to use a dispersive electrode can compromise a patient's modesty.

The names *unipolar* and *bipolar* can sometimes be confusing because they sound similar to polarity. In reality, unipolar and bipolar configurations have absolutely nothing to do with the polarity of the electrical current under the electrode. Although unipolar arrangements are typically the standard electrode setup on monophasic high-voltage stimulators, this is actually a matter of convention rather than necessity. In reality, any stimulator can be used in either a unipolar or bipolar configuration. The choice is really a matter of clinical convenience rather than association with a specific stimulator. To convert a unipolar configuration to a bipolar configuration, the large dispersive electrode would simply be replaced with an electrode similar in size to the other active electrode. Similarly, a greater effect can be produced with the stimulator by merely using smaller electrodes. To convert a bipolar configuration to a unipolar configuration, one of the active electrodes would simply be replaced with a larger dispersive electrode. One unique case of a unipolar setup involves using electrotherapy while immersed in water, such as a whirlpool or ice slush. In this case, a relatively small electrode is attached to a motor point of a body part that is immersed in water (e.g., the gastrocnemius). This small (active) electrode must be attached to a motor point that is out of the water. The other electrode lead wire is immersed in the water along with the body part.

The water acts as a very large dispersive electrode, and the small electrode acts as an active electrode. This technique is generally used for edema retardation or removal protocols.

CURRENT MODULATION

In addition to the manipulations of electrical currents already discussed, a number of other current modulations are also common. Current modulation is simply an alteration in the current's waveform. It includes applications already discussed, such as using interrupted current, as well as a few other alterations that will be discussed here. It is used for a variety of reasons, such as counteracting accommodation, increasing patient comfort, minimizing fatigue, or making contraction easier.

Among the most common modulations is varying the pulse rate of an interrupted current to minimize accommodation. Most contemporary stimulators have built-in presets to modulate the pulse rate. Typically, these presets vary the pulse rate up and down within a specific band of frequencies that corresponds to a desired effect. For example, among the more common presets is one that varies the pulse rate up and down between 1 and 10 pulses per second, obviously in the subtetanic range if used with muscle contraction. With sufficient intensity, this setting would cause the muscle to visibly twitch at a varying rate that would not become a tetanic contraction. Similar presets can be found in the pulse rate range just above the threshold for tetany and also at much higher frequencies such as those commonly used for pain management or muscle strengthening.

Another common modulation is ramping the intensity with an interrupted current. When using a ramp setting, the current is not at its maximum intensity when it first comes on. Instead, each successive pulse of current increases slightly in intensity until the desired maximum is reached. The ramp setting allows the user to specify the time that it takes for the maximum to be reached. Some devices also allow a ramp setting for when the current is ending. Ramp settings are used to increase patient comfort, with it generally being more comfortable to ramp up to the maximum rather than being hit with it all at once.

Another modulation related to patient comfort is controlling the pulse width. There is an indirect relationship between the pulse duration (width) and the pulse amplitude (the intensity) when inducing a muscle contraction. For patients who have a hard time tolerating high amplitudes, the amplitude can be reduced to tolerable levels and the pulse width increased to still induce muscle contraction. Increasing pulse width can also improve the ability to induce a contraction in other situations as well.

The use of "on-time" and "off-time" is another common modulation with electrotherapy. Recall that muscle stimulators induce recruitment of the same set of motor units over and over. Because this does not match the normal physiologic recruitment pattern for motor units, it often leads to rapid fatigue in the muscle. Although in some protocols fatigue is desirable, such as when trying to overcome spasticity, muscle fatigue is to be avoided with most electrotherapy protocols. For this reason, many stimulators provide the practitioner with the ability to have either "continuous" current flow or current flowing for a certain period followed by a rest period with no flow of current. This type of modulation is often called *interrupted*, but it should not be confused with interrupted current as discussed previously. Normally, when we speak of current interruption, we mean that

discreet pulses of current alternate with brief (microseconds to milliseconds) intervals of no current. When on and off modulation is used, current flows during the on-time, and this current is almost pulsed at whatever pulse rate setting is chosen. Likewise, the continuous setting on most stimulators means that the flow of interrupted (pulsed) current is constant rather than meaning a noninterrupted current. Obviously, the terminology gets to be confusing and becomes worse when different manufacturers use their own terminology. There is little consensus on the correct durations for on-time or off-time or even the correct on-off ratio. Even though research is required to better explore this parameter, many clinicians anecdotally report using a 1:1 ratio or less of on-time to off-time.

INTENSITY

The intensity setting controls the amplitude (voltage) of the waveform and therefore controls the quantity of current flowing through the circuit. Recall that the relationship between force and flow (voltage and current) is describe by Ohm's law (see Box 8-10). The greater the intensity, or driving force, the greater the flow of current. Although most contemporary stimulators provide the user with a readout of intensity or current levels, use of a numerical value can be misleading. Because of variability in electrode placement, electrode size, skin conductivity, moisture, and other factors, the voltage used for one treatment to induce muscle contraction would not necessarily induce the same degree of contraction with a different treatment for the same patient. For this reason, it is more useful to think of intensity levels in terms of their effects rather than their numerical value. Perhaps the easiest scheme involves classifying intensity progressively as subsensory, sensory, motor, and noxious (Table 8-12). Subsensory levels are obviously not perceived by the patient and are rarely used outside microcurrent electrotherapy. Sensory levels of intensity imply that the patient can feel the current but the current does not cause muscle contraction. Motor levels of intensity cause muscle contractions. As the name implies, noxious levels of intensity are rather uncomfortable and are rarely if ever used, but they provide the maximum tolerable level of muscle contraction.

Techniques and Dosage

This chapter presents only a general framework for electrotherapy techniques. For more complete and detailed information, a full text on modalities should be consulted. To simplify this section, general strategies and parameters are summarized

Table 8-12 Classification of Intensity Level by Its Effects

Subsensory level	The level is not perceived by the patient and is rarely used outside microcurrent electrotherapy.
Sensory level	The patient can feel the current but the current does not cause muscle contraction.
Motor level	Motor levels of intensity cause muscle contractions. As the name implies, noxious levels of intensity are rather uncomfortable and are rarely if ever used, but they provide the maximum tolerable level of muscle contraction.

Table 8-13 General Electrotherapy Parameters Common in Rehabilitation of Athletic Injuries

Goal	Waveform	Pulse Rate*	Intensity†	On-Time/Off-Time
Muscle reeducation	Interrupted, shape matters little	Subtetanic	Motor	Yes
Retard atrophy in innervated tissue	Interrupted, shape matters little	Tetanic	Motor	Yes
Retard edema formation	Interrupted monophasic	Supertetanic (120 pps reported)	Sensory (10% below motor threshold)	Use recurrent 30-minute bouts with 60 minutes in between
Remove edema	Interrupted, shape matters little	Subtetanic (usually <10 pps)	Motor	Yes
Reduce pain	High TENS	Tetanic to supertetanic (50-100 pps)	Sensory	No
	Low TENS (45 min +)	Subtetanic (2-4 pps)	Motor/noxious	No
	Interferential	Variable, see device instructions	Sensory	No
Reduce spasm	Interrupted, shape matters little	Subtetanic	Motor	No
	Interrupted, shape matters little	Supertetanic	Motor/noxious	No
Improve strength	Interrupted or MFBurstAC (Russian)	Supertetanic	Noxious	Yes
Iontophoresis	Continuous monophasic	N/A	As tolerated	N/A

* Pulse rates are as follows: subtetanic, less than 30 pps; tetanic, 30 to 50 pps and produces smooth contraction; supertetanic, 100 pps and higher.

† Intensity levels are as follows: sensory, perceived by the patient; motor, causes strong but tolerable contraction; noxious, maximum tolerable intensity.

N/A, Not applicable; *pps*, pulses per second; *TENS*, transcutaneous electrical nerve stimulation.

in Table 8-13. Very few data are available regarding appropriate treatment durations for most protocols. By convention, most are 15 to 30 minutes in duration unless otherwise noted.

Future Questions

Many questions are still unanswered about electrotherapy because very little research has actually has examined specific combinations of parameters to determine their efficacy. Similarly, very few quality outcomes studies are available. Currently, some very promising work is being conducted in the areas of retarding edema formation and in the management of pain. Similarly, iontophoresis also receives sporadic and conflicting examinations. As a general statement, electrotherapy as a whole remains a vast and little explored area with many areas for further study.

CONCLUSION
Introduction

- Modalities have specific uses in specific situations and are of little benefit when used for the wrong reason, with the wrong technique, or at the wrong time. At their best, therapeutic modalities are an exceptionally useful complement to the rehabilitative process but are not a replacement for it.
- The key to using modalities appropriately is to match the specific physiologic effects of the modality with the specific rehabilitative goal for the patient.

- Practitioners should familiarize themselves with the specific details of their state practice acts before using any therapeutic modalities.

Research Regarding Modalities

- A number of clinically common modalities may not be as effective as once thought, and the clinical efficacy of modalities that are known to be useful can easily be compromised by incorrect application techniques.
- The general trend is that clinical practice almost always precedes scientific research in regard to the use of modalities.
- Most research concerning the therapeutic value of modalities has concentrated on clinically relevant types of data, which are indirect measures of a modality's effectiveness and important in establishing outcomes data, versus the direct effect, which is important in establishing modality theory.
- A number of modality effects are commonly accepted by clinicians but have little scientific support. In some cases there is even scientific evidence to the contrary, yet these widely held clinical beliefs still persist.

Modalities for Acute Care

- The two primary goals of using modalities for acute injures are restricting the total quantity of tissue damage associated with an injury and limiting sequelae of the acute inflammatory response.

Cryotherapy

- Data support the application of cold in reducing local skin and intramuscular temperature, the metabolic rate of the cooled tissue, and blood flow; inhibiting inflammation; retarding the formation of edema/effusion; and helping manage pain.
- We do not yet have a definitive answer about the most effective tissue temperature, duration of cryotherapy, or on-off ratio for using cryotherapy for the treatment of acute injury.
- Cold-induced vasodilation is a misnomer; in reality, cryotherapy does not increase blood flow above baseline levels at all.
- Cryotherapy used in combination with compression has been shown to produce greater reductions in temperature than cryotherapy used alone.
- Ice bags made from ice stored in unrefrigerated hoppers should be applied directly to the skin without the addition of an insulating layer. Frozen gel packs or ice stored in a freezer, however, should have some type of appropriate barrier between them and skin.

Compression

- It is believed that compression is effective in managing acute injuries by increasing the cooling efficacy of cryotherapy, manipulating Starling forces, and reducing bleeding from vessels damaged during the injury.
- Little scientific evidence supports a specific pressure and duration, intermittent versus continuous compression, intermittent cycling parameters, and whether compression or elevation is a more important factor in retarding edema formation.

Elevation

- The premise for elevation is based on gravity limiting the amount of blood delivered to an acutely injured area, which would result in several positive physiologic events. Unfortunately, the magnitude of the actual benefits from elevation has not been described in the literature.

Modalities for Rehabilitation

- In postacute rehabilitation, the goals are focused mostly on removing the unwanted remnants of inflammation, repairing tissue, and restoring more normal physiologic function of the repaired tissue.
- When a modality is used to accomplish a specific goal, the modality can and should be discontinued when that goal has been accomplished or when the modality is no longer proving to be effective for the patient.

Cryotherapy

- Cold reduces pain and pain is one cause of inhibition; therefore, cold should help overcome inhibition and allow the patient to begin controlled rehabilitative exercise at an earlier point in the rehabilitative process. This is also the primary basis for the efficacy of cryokinetics.
- Some early evidence indicates that cryotherapy facilitates the motor neuron pool, which helps overcome neuromuscular inhibition following injury.

Superficial Thermotherapy

- Superficial thermotherapy should be used as an adjunct, along with stretching or joint mobilization techniques, to improve range of motion.

- These types of modalities do increase the superficial circulation and reduce pain.
- Further research still needs to address the duration of thermal modalities, frequency of use, and appropriate tissue temperatures.

Ultrasound

- Thermal ultrasound is used primarily to augment techniques for improving range of motion, although the literature directly examining the efficacy of ultrasound and stretching is very sparse.
- Nonthermal ultrasound is used primarily when the goal is to augment the repair or regeneration of damaged tissue, and scientific evidence supports such use.
- Not all coupling media for ultrasound are equally effective.

Phonophoresis

- Research regarding the efficacy of phonophoresis is mixed at this point.

Short Wave Diathermy

- This is probably the best thermal modality available to the practitioner today and is capable of therapeutically treating a much larger area than possible with ultrasound.

Electrical Stimulation

- The most promising uses of electrical stimulation appear to be managing pain, reeducating muscle, and aiding in retarding the formation and removal of edema.
- Some degree of strengthening of normal tissue can occur with electrotherapy, but the strengthening is not as effective as with active exercise in a resistance program.

Iontophoresis

- Reports conflict regarding whether iontophoresis delivers enough medication to a deep enough tissue depth to be effective for many conditions. In addition, outcomes data for iontophoresis are limited, and it has not yet been adequately demonstrated that the technique is of much benefit to patients with musculoskeletal injuries.

REFERENCES

1. Cameron, M. (1999): Physical Agents in Rehabilitation: From Research to Practice. Philadelphia: Saunders.
2. Denegar, C. (2000): Therapeutic Modalities for Athletic Injuries. Champaign IL, Human Kinetics.
3. Michlovitz, S.L. (1996): Thermal Agents in Rehabilitation, 3rd ed. Philadelphia, Davis, pp. xxvi, 405.
4. Prentice, W. (1999): Therapeutic Modalities in Sports Medicine, 4th ed. Boston, McGraw-Hill.
5. Starkey, C. (1999): Therapeutic Modalities, 2nd ed. Philadelphia, Davis, p. 397.
6. Lewis, T. (1930): Observations upon the reactions of the vessels of the human skin to cold. Heart, 15:177–208.
7. Lehmann, J., deLateur, B., Stonebridge, J., and Warren, C. (1967): Therapeutic temperature distribution produced by ultrasound as modified by dosage and volume of tissue exposed. Arch. Phys. Med. Rehabil., 47:662–666.
8. Lehmann, J., Masock, A., Warren, C., and Koblanski, J. (1970): Effect of therapeutic ultrasound on tendon extensibility. Arch. Phys. Med. Rehabil., 51:481–487.
9. Lehmann, J.F., deLateur, B., and Warren, C. (1967): Heating produced by ultrasound in bone and soft tissue. Arch. Phys. Med. Rehabil., 48:397–401.
10. Chan, A., Myrer, J., Measom, G., and Draper, D. (1998): Temperature changes in human patellar tendon in response to therapeutic ultrasound. J. Athl. Train., 33:130–135.
11. Draper, D., Castel, J., and Castel, D. (1995): Rate of temperature increase in human muscle during 1 MHz and 3 MHz continuous ultrasound. J. Orthop. Sports Phys. Ther., 22:142–150.
12. Gersten, J. (1959): Effect of ultrasound on tendon extensibility. Am. J. Phys. Med., 34:662.

13. Robertson, V., and Baker, K. (2001): A review of therapeutic ultrasound: Effectiveness studies. Phys. Ther., 81:1339–1350.

14. Draper, D. (2002): Don't disregard ultrasound yet—the jury is still out. Phys. Ther., 82:190–191.

15. Higgins, D., and Kaminski, T. (1998): Contrast therapy does not cause fluctuations in human gastrocnemius intramuscular temperature. J. Athl. Train., 33:336–340.

16. Myrer, J., Draper, D., and Durrant, E. (1994): Contrast therapy and intramuscular temperature in the human leg. J. Athl. Train., 29:318–322, 376–377.

17. Myrer, J., Higgins, D., and Kaminski., T. (1999): Some concerns—"Contrast therapy does not cause fluctuations in human gastrocnemius intramuscular temperature" (J. Athl. Train. 1998;33:336-340). J. Athl. Train, 34:231.

18. Myrer, J., Measom, G., Durrant, E., and Fellingham, G. (1997): Cold- and hot-pack contrast therapy: Subcutaneous and intramuscular temperature change. J. Athl. Train., 32:238–241.

19. Byl, N.N., McKenzie, A.L., West, J.M., et al. (1994): Pulsed microamperage stimulation: A controlled study of healing of surgically induced wounds in Yucatan pigs. Phys. Ther., 74:201–213; discussion 213-208.

20. Merrick, M. (1999): Research digest. Unconventional modalities: Microcurrent. Athl. Ther. Today, 4:53–54.

21. Weber, M., Servedio, F., and Woodall, W. (1994): The effects of three modalities on delayed onset muscle soreness. J. Orthop. Sports Phys. Ther., 20:236–242.

22. Knight, K.L., Aquino, J., Johannes, S.M., and Urban, C.D. (1980): A re-examination of Lewis' cold-induced vasodilatation in the finger and the ankle. Athl. Train. J. Natl. Athl. Train. Assoc., 15:238–250.

23. Barcroft, H., and Edholm, O.G. (1943): The effect of temperature on blood flow and deep temperature in the human forearm. J. Physiol., 102:5–20.

24. Curl, W.W., Smith, B.P., Marr, A., et al. (1997): The effect of contusion and cryotherapy on skeletal muscle microcirculation. J. Sports Med. Phys. Fitness, 37:279–286.

25. Ho, S., Coel, M., Kagawa, R., and Richardson, A. (1994): The effects of ice on blood flow and bone metabolism in knees—including commentary by Johnson RJ with author response. Am. J. Sports Med., 22:537–540.

26. Ho, S., Illgen, R., Meyer, R., et al. (1995): Comparison of various icing times in decreasing bone metabolism and blood flow in the knee—presented at the 19th Annual Meeting of the AOSSM, Sun Valley, Idaho, July 12, 1993 and at the AOSSM/JOSSM Transpacific Meeting, Maui, Hawaii, March 21 through 25, 1993. Am. J. Sports Med., 23:74–76.

27. Karunakara, R., Lephart, S., and Pincivero, D. (1999): Changes in forearm blood flow during single and intermittent cold application. J. Orthop. Sports Phys. Ther., 29:177–180.

28. Knight, K.L. (1976): Effects of hypothermia on inflammation and swelling. Athl. Train. J. Natl. Athl. Train. Assoc., 11:7–10.

29. Merrick, M. (2002): Secondary injury after musculoskeletal trauma: A review and update. J. Athl. Train., 37:209–217.

30. Knight, K., Brucker, J., Stoneman, P., and Rubley, M. (2000): Muscle injury management with cryotherapy. Athl. Ther. Today, 5:26–30, 32-23, 64.

31. Knight, K.L. (1985): Cryotherapy: Theory, Technique, and Physiology, 1st ed. Chattanooga, TN, Chattanooga Corp. Education Division, pp. ix, 188.

32. Knight, K.L. (1995): Cryotherapy in Sport Injury Management. Champaign, IL, Human Kinetics, pp. x, 301.

33. Merrick, M., Rankin, J., Andres, F., and Hinman, C. (1999): A preliminary examination of cryotherapy and secondary injury in skeletal muscle. Med. Sci. Sports Exerc., 31:1516–1521.

34. Majno, G., and Joris, I. (1996): Cells, Tissues, and Disease: Principles of General Pathology. Cambridge, MA, Blackwell Scientific.

35. Hecox, B., Andemicael Mehreteab, T., and Weisberg, J. (1994): Physical Agents: A Comprehensive Text for Physical Therapists. Norwalk, CT, Appleton & Lange, pp. xv, 473.

36. Knight, K.L., Thoma, D.B., Fink, D., et al. (1996): Cryotherapy for First Aid. Champaign, IL, Human Kinetics.

37. Knight, K.L., Thoma, D.B., Fink, D., et al. Cryotherapy for Rehabilitation. Champaign, IL, Human Kinetics.

38. Lessard, L., Scudds, R., Amendola, A., and Vaz, M. (1997): The efficacy of cryotherapy following arthroscopic knee surgery. J. Orthop. Sports Phys. Ther., 26:14–22.

39. Martin, S., Spindler, K., Tarter, J., et al. (2001): Cryotherapy: An effective modality for decreasing intraarticular temperature after knee arthroscopy. Am. J. Sports Med., 29:288–291.

40. Barlas, D., Homan, C., and Thode, H.J. (1996): In vivo tissue temperature comparison of cryotherapy with and without external compression. Ann. Emerg. Med., 28:436–439.

41. Merrick, M., Jutte, L., and Smith, M. (2003): Cold modalities with different thermodynamic properties produce different surface and intramuscular temperatures. J. Athl. Train., 38:28–33.

42. Merrick, M., Knight, K., Ingersoll, C., and Potteiger, J. (1993): The effects of ice and compression wraps on intramuscular temperatures at various depths. J. Athl. Train., 28:236–245.

43. Myrer, J., Measom, G., and Fellingham, G. (1998): Temperature changes in the human leg during and after two methods of cryotherapy. J. Athl. Train., 33:25–29.

44. Tsang, K., Buxton, B., Guion, W., et al. (1997): The effects of cryotherapy applied through various barriers. J. Sport Rehabil., 6:343–354.

45. Zemke, J., Andersen, J., Guion, W., et al. (1998): Intramuscular temperature responses in the human leg to two forms of cryotherapy: Ice massage and ice bag. J. Orthop. Sports Phys. Ther., 27:301–307.

46. Chesterton, L., Foster, N., and Ross, L. (2002): Skin temperature response to cryotherapy. Arch. Phys. Med. Rehabil., 83:543–549.

47. Cornwall, M. (1994): Effect of temperature on muscle force and rate of muscle force production in men and women. J. Orthop. Sports Phys. Ther., 20:74–80.

48. Holcomb, W., Mangus, B., and Tandy, R. (1996): The effect of icing with the Pro-Stim Edema Management System on cutaneous cooling. J. Athl. Train., 31:126–129.

49. Jutte, L., Merrick, M., Ingersoll, C., and Edwards, J. (2001): The relationship between intramuscular temperature, skin temperature, and adipose thickness during cryotherapy and rewarming. Arch. Phys. Med. Rehabil., 82:845–850.

50. Krause, B., Hopkins, J., Ingersoll, C., et al. (1998): The relationship of ankle temperature during cooling and rewarming to the human soleus H reflex. J. Sport Rehabil., 9:253–262.

51. Mancuso, D.L., and Knight, K.L. (1992): Effects of prior physical activity on skin surface temperature response of the ankle during and after a 30-minute ice pack application. J. Athl. Train., 27:242–249.

52. Myrer, J., Measom, G., and Fellingham, G. (2000): Exercise after cryotherapy greatly enhances intramuscular rewarming. J. Athl. Train., 35:412–416.

53. Myrer, J., Myrer, K., Measom, G., et al. (2001): Muscle temperature is affected by overlying adipose when cryotherapy is administered. J. Athl. Train., 36:32–36.

54. Ohkoshi, Y., Ohkoshi, M., Nagasaki, S., et al. (1999): The effect of cryotherapy on intraarticular temperature and postoperative care after anterior cruciate ligament reconstruction. Am. J. Sports Med., 27:357–362.

55. Otte, J., Merrick, M., Ingersoll, C., and Cordova, M. (2002): Subcutaneous adipose tissue thickness alters cooling time during cryotherapy. Arch. Phys. Med. Rehabil., 83:1501–1505.

56. Palmer, J., and Knight, K. (1996): Ankle and thigh skin surface temperature changes with repeated ice pack application. J. Athl. Train., 31:319–323.

57. Rimington, S., Draper, D., Durrant, E., and Fellingham, G. (1994): Temperature changes during therapeutic ultrasound in the precooled human gastrocnemius muscle. J. Athl. Train., 29:325–327, 376–377.

58. Halliday, D., and Resnick, R. (1988): Fundamentals of Physics, 3rd ed. New York, John Wiley & Sons, pp. 464–475.

59. Lide, D. (ed.). (1994): CRC Handbook of Chemistry and Physics, 74th ed. Boca Raton, FL, CRC Press.

60. Guyton, A.C. (1991): Textbook of Medical Physiology, 8th ed. Philadelphia, Saunders, pp. 149–203.

61. Merrick, M. (1999): Research digest. Unconventional modalities: Therapeutic magnets. Athl. Ther. Today, 4:56–57.

62. Meeusen, R., Van der Veen, P., Joos, E., et al. (1998): The influence of cold and compression on lymph flow at the ankle. Clin. J. Sports Med., 8:266–271.

63. Brown, R.T., and Baust, J.G. (1980): Time course of peripheral heterothermy in a homeotherm. Am. J. Physiol., 239:R126–R129.

64. Daanen, H.A., Van de Linde, F.J., Romet, T.M., and Ducharme, M.B. (1997): The effect of body temperature on the hunting response of the middle finger skin temperature. Eur. J. Appl. Physiol. Occup. Physiol., 76:538–543.

65. Gardner, C.A., and Webb, R.C. (1986): Cold-induced vasodilatation in isolated, perfused rat tail artery. Am. J. Physiol., 251:H176–H181.

66. Chapman-Jones, D., and Hill, D. (2002): Novel microcurrent treatment is more effective than conventional therapy for chronic Achilles tendinopathy: Randomised comparative trial. Physiotherapy, 88:471–480.

67. Edwards, D., Rimmer, M., and Keene, G. (1996): The use of cold therapy in the postoperative management of patients undergoing arthroscopic anterior cruciate ligament reconstruction. Am. J. Sports Med., 24:193–195.

68. Konrath, G., Lock, T., Goitz, H., and Scheidler, J. (1996): The use of cold therapy after anterior cruciate ligament reconstruction: A prospective, randomized study and literature review—presented at the 22nd Annual Meeting of the AOSSM, Lake Buena Vista, Florida, June 1996. Am. J. Sports Med., 24:629–633.

69. Bracciano, A.G. (2000): Physical Agent Modalities: Theory and Application for the Occupational Therapist. Thorofare, NJ, Slack, pp. viii, 160.

70. Matthews, J., Fisher, B., Magee, D., and Knight, K. (2001): Lipid peroxidation and protein turnover after trauma and cold treatment in skeletal muscle of exercise-trained rats. J. Phys. Ther. Sci., 13:21–2601.

71. Kraemer, W., Bush, J., Wickham, R., et al. (2001): Continuous compression as an effective therapeutic intervention in treating eccentric-exercise–induced muscle soreness. J. Sport Rehabil., 10:11–23.

72. Kraemer, W., Bush, J., Wickham, R., et al. Influence of compression therapy on symptoms following soft tissue injury from maximal eccentric exercise. J. Orthop. Sports Phys. Ther., 31:282-290.

73. Smith, J., Stevens, J., Taylor, M., and Tibbey, J. (2002): A randomized, controlled trial comparing compression bandaging and cold therapy in postoperative total knee replacement surgery. Orthop. Nurs., 21:61–66.

74. Webb, J., Williams, D., Ivory, J., et al. (1998): The use of cold compression dressings after total knee replacement: A randomized controlled trial. Orthopedics, 21:59–61.

75. Knight, K., Okuda, I., Ingersoll, C., and Edwards, J. (1997): The effects of cold applications on nerve conduction velocity and muscle force [abstract]. J. Athl. Train., 32:S-5.

76. Misasi, S., Morin, G., Kemler, D., et al. (1995): The effect of a toe cap and bias on perceived pain during cold water immersion. J. Athl. Train., 30:49–52.

77. Streator, S., Ingersoll, C., and Knight, K. (1995): Sensory information can decrease cold-induced pain perception. J. Athl. Train., 30:293–296.

78. Mlynarczyk, J. (1984): Temperature Changes During and After Ice Pack Application of 10, 20, 30, 45, and 60 Minutes. Terre Haute, IN: Indiana State University, Dept. of Physical Education.

79. Angus, J.C. (1993): Intermittent Compression and Cold and Their Effects on Edema in Postacute Ankle Sprains [thesis]. University of North Carolina at Chapel Hill.

80. Brewer, K.D. (1992): The Effects of Intermittent Compression and Cold on Edema in Postacute Ankle Sprains [thesis]. University of North Carolina at Chapel Hill.

81. Gilbart, M., Oglivie-Harris, D.J., Broadhurst, C., and Clarfield, M. (1995): Anterior tibial compartment pressures during intermittent sequential pneumatic compression therapy. Am. J. Sports Med., 23:769–772.

82. Dervin, G., Taylor, D., and Keene, G. (1998): Effects of cold and compression dressings on early postoperative outcomes for the arthroscopic anterior cruciate ligament reconstruction patient. J. Orthop. Sports Phys. Ther., 27:403–406.

83. Whitelaw, G., DeMuth, K., Demos, H., et al. (1996): The cryo/cuff versus ice and elastic wrap: postoperative care of knee arthroscopy patients. Reprinted with permission from The American Journal of Knee Surgery. 1995;8:28–31. Today's OR Nurse, 18:31–34.

84. Mayrovitz, H., Delgado, M., and Smith, J. (1997): Compression bandaging effects on lower extremity peripheral and sub-bandage skin blood perfusion. Wounds, 9:146–152.

85. Dawson, D. (1997): Pathophysiology of focal ischemic injury: An overview. Top. Emerg. Med., 19:63–78.

86. Varpalotai, M., and Knight, K. (1991): Pressures exerted by elastic wraps applied by beginning and advanced student athletic trainers to the ankle and the thigh with and without an ice pack. Athl. Train. J. Natl. Athl. Train. Assoc., 26:246–250.

87. Serwa, J., Rancourt, L., Merrick, M., et al. (2001): Effect of varying application pressures on skin surface and intramuscular temperatures during cryotherapy [abstract]. J. Athl. Train., 36:S-90.

88. Bettany, J.A., Fish, D.R., and Mendel, F.C. (1990): High-voltage pulsed direct current: Effect on edema formation after hyperflexion injury. Arch. Phys. Med. Rehabil., 71:677–681.

89. Dolan, M., Thornton, R., Fish, D., and Mendel, F. (1997): Effects of cold water immersion on edema formation after blunt injury to the hind limbs of rats. J. Athl. Train., 32:233–237.

90. Karnes, J., Mendel, F., Fish, D., and Burton, H. (1995): High-voltage pulsed current: Its influence on diameters of histamine-dilated arterioles in hamster cheek pouches. Arch. Phys. Med. Rehabil., 76:381–386.

91. Mendel, F., and Fish, D. (1993): New perspectives in edema control via electrical stimulation. J. Athl. Train., 28:63–64, 66-70, 72 passim.

92. Taylor, K., Mendel, F., Fish, D., et al. (1993): Effect of high-voltage pulsed current and alternating current on macromolecular leakage in hamster cheek pouch microcirculation. Phys. Ther., 77:1729–1740.

93. Thornton, R., Mendel, F., and Fish, D. (1998): Effects of electrical stimulation on edema formation in different strains of rats. Phys. Ther., 8:386–394.

94. Hopkins, J., Ingersoll, C., Edwards, J., and Klootwyk, T. (2002): Cryotherapy and transcutaneous electric neuromuscular stimulation decrease arthrogenic muscle inhibition of the vastus medialis after knee joint effusion. J. Athl. Train., 37:25–31.

95. Hopkins, J., and Stencil, R. (2002): Ankle cryotherapy facilitates soleus function. J. Orthop. Sports Phys. Ther., 32:622–627.

96. Pincivero, D., Gieck, J., and Saliba, E. (1993): Rehabilitation of a lateral ankle sprain with cryokinetics and functional progressive exercise. J. Sport Rehabil., 2:200–207.

97. Benoit, T., Martin, D., and Perrin, D. (1996): Hot and cold whirlpool treatments and knee joint laxity. J. Athl. Train., 31:242–244, 286–287.

98. Burke, D., MacNeil, S., Holt, L., et al. (2000): The effect of hot or cold water immersion on isometric strength training. J. Strength Cond. Res., 14:21–25.

99. Jameson, A., Kinzey, S., and Hallam, J. (2001): Lower-extremity-joint cryotherapy does not affect vertical ground-reaction forces during landing. J. Sport Rehabil., 10:132–142.

100. Kimura, I., Gulick, D., and Thompson, G. (1997): The effect of cryotherapy on eccentric plantar flexion peak torque and endurance. J. Athl. Train., 32:124–126.

101. Kinzey, S., Cordova, M., Gallen, K., et al. (2000): The effects of cryotherapy on ground-reaction forces produced during a functional task. J. Sport Rehabil., 9:3–14.

102. Rivers, D.A., Kimura, I., Sitler, M., and Kendrick, Z. (1995): The influence of cryotherapy and Aircast bracing on total body balance and proprioception [abstract]. J. Athl. Train., 30:S-15.

103. Thieme, H., Ingersoll, C., Knight, K., and Ozmun, J. (1996): Cooling does not affect knee proprioception. J. Athl. Train., 31:8–11.

104. Uchio, Y., Ochi, M., Fujihara, A., et al. (2003): Cryotherapy influences joint laxity and position sense of the healthy knee joint. Arch. Phys. Med. Rehabil., 84:131–135.

105. Krause, B., Hopkins, J., Ingersoll, C., et al. (2000): The effects of ankle and axillary cooling on the human soleus Hoffman reflex [abstract]. J. Athl. Train, 35:S-58.

106. Palmieri, R., Ingersoll, C., Edwards, J., et al. (2003): Arthrogenic muscle inhibition is not present in the limb contralateral to a simulated knee joint effusion [abstract]. J. Athl. Train, 38:S-35.

107. Lehmann, J.F. (1982): Therapeutic Heat and Cold, 3rd ed. Baltimore, Williams & Wilkins, pp. xiv, 641.

108. McCulloch, J., and Boyd, V. (1992): The effects of whirlpool and the dependent position on lower extremity volume. J. Orthop. Sports Phys. Ther., 16:169–173.

109. Meeker, B.J. (1994): Description of the Effects of Whirlpool Therapy on Postoperative Pain and Surgical Wound Healing [thesis]. Louisiana State University Medical Center, New Orleans School of Nursing, p. 109.

110. Meeker, B. (1998): Whirlpool therapy on postoperative pain and surgical wound healing: An exploration. Patient Educ. Couns., 33:39–48.

111. Robinson, V., Brosseau, L., Casimiro, L., et al. (2002): Thermotherapy for treating rheumatoid arthritis. Cochrane Database Syst. Rev., 2:CD002826.

112. Draper, D., Anderson, C., Schulthies, S., and Ricard, M. (1998): Immediate and residual changes in dorsiflexion range of motion using an ultrasound heat and stretch routine. J. Athl. Train., 33:141–144.

113. Draper, D., and Ricard, M. (1995): Rate of temperature decay in human muscle following 3 MHz ultrasound: The stretching window revealed. J. Athl. Train., 30: 304–307.

114. Rose, S., Draper, D., Schulthies, S., and Durrant, E. (1996): The stretching window part two: Rate of thermal decay in deep muscle following 1-MHz ultrasound. J. Athl. Train., 31:139–143.

115. Bickford, R., and Duff, R. (1953): Influence of ultrasonic irradiation on temperature and blood flow in human skeletal muscle. Circ. Res., 1:534–538.

116. Crockford, G., Hellon, R., and Parkhouse, J. (1962): Thermal vasomotor response in human skin mediated by local mechanisms. J. Physiol., 161:10–15.

117. Draper, D. (1998): Guidelines to enhance therapeutic ultrasound treatment outcomes. Athl. Ther. Today, 3:7–11, 28-29, 55.

118. Merrick, M. (2001): Research digest. Does 1-MHz ultrasound really work? Athl. Ther. Today, 6:48–49.

119. Merrick, M. (2000): Research digest. Does phonophoresis work? Athl. Ther. Today, 5:46–47.

120. Merrick, M. (2000): Research digest. Ultrasound and range of motion examined. Athl. Ther. Today, 5:48–49.

121. Merrick, M., Bernard, K., Devor, S., and Williams, J. (2003): Identical 3-MHz ultrasound treatments with different devices produce different intramuscular temperatures. J. Orthop. Sports Phys. Ther., 33:379–385.

122. Stewart, H. (1982): Ultrasound therapy. In: Respacholi, M., and Benwell, D. (eds.). Essentials of Medical Ultrasound. Clifton, NJ, Humana Press, p. 196.

123. Robertson, V., and Ward, A. (1997): 45kHz (longwave) ultrasound. Physiotherapy, 83:271–272.

124. Robertson, V., and Ward, A. (1997): Longwave ultrasound reviewed and reconsidered. Physiotherapy, 83:123–130.

125. Meakins, A., and Watson, T. (2006): Longwave ultrasound and conductive heating increase functional ankle mobility in asymptomatic subjects. Phys. Ther. Sport, 7:74–80.

126. Draper, D., Harris, S., Schulthies, S., et al. (1998): Hot-pack and 1-MHz ultrasound treatments have an additive effect on muscle temperature increase. J. Athl. Train., 33:21–24.

127. Draper, D., Knight, K., Fujiwara, T., and Castel, J. (1999): Temperature change in human muscle during and after pulsed short-wave diathermy—including commentary by Byl N with author response. J. Orthop. Sports Phys. Ther., 29:13–22.

128. Draper, D., Schulties, S., Sorvisto, P., and Hautala, A. (1995): Temperature changes in deep muscles of humans during ice and ultrasound therapies: An in vivo study. J. Orthop. Sports Phys. Ther., 21:153–157.

129. Peres, S., Draper, D., Knight, K., and Ricard, M. (2002): Pulsed shortwave diathermy and prolonged long-duration stretching increase dorsiflexion range of motion more than identical stretching without diathermy. J. Athl. Train., 37:43–50.

130. Byl, N. (1995): The use of ultrasound as an enhancer for transcutaneous drug delivery: Phonophoresis. Phys. Ther., 75:539–553.

131. Byl, N.N., McKenzie, A., Wong, T., et al. (1993): Incisional wound healing: A controlled study of low and high dose ultrasound. J. Orthop. Sports Phys. Ther., 18:619–628.

132. Byl, N.N., McKenzie, A.L., West, J.M., et al. (1992): Low-dose ultrasound effects on wound healing: A controlled study with Yucatan pigs. Arch. Phys. Med. Rehabil., 73:656–664.

133. Gum, S.L., Reddy, G.K., Stehno-Bittel, L., and Enwemeka, C. (1997): Combined ultrasound, electrical stimulation, and laser promote collagen synthesis with moderate changes in tendon biomechanics. Am. J. Phys. Med. Rehabil., 76:288–296.

134. Houghton, P. (1999): Effects of therapeutic modalities on wound healing: A conservative approach to the management of chronic wounds. Phys. Ther. Rev., 4:167–182.

135. Kloth, L., and McCulloch, J. (1996): Promotion of wound healing and electrical stimulation. Adv. Wound Care, 9:42–45.

136. Bradnock, B., Law, H.T., and Roscoe, K. (1996): A quantitative comparative assessment of the immediate response to high frequency ultrasound and low frequency ultrasound ("longwave therapy") in the treatment of acute ankle sprains [corrected] [published erratum appears in Physiotherapy 1996 Mar;82(3):216]. Physiotherapy, 82:78–84.

137. Maddi, A., Hai, H., Ong, S.T., et al. (2006): Long wave ultrasound may enhance bone regeneration by altering OPG/RANKL ratio in human osteoblast-like cells. Bone, 39:283–288.

138. Bare, A., McAnaw, M., Pritchard, A., et al. (1996): Phonophoretic delivery of 10% hydrocortisone through the epidermis of humans as determined by serum cortisol concentrations—including commentary by Robinson AJ, and Echternach JL with author response. Phys. Ther., 76:738–749.

139. Byl, N.N., McKenzie, A., Halliday, B., et al. (1993): The effects of phonophoresis with corticosteroids: A controlled pilot study. J. Orthop. Sports Phys. Ther., 18:590–600.

140. Conner-Kerr, T., Franklin, M., Kerr, J., et al. (1998): Phonophoretic delivery of dexamethasone to human transdermal tissues: A controlled pilot study. Eur. J. Phys. Med. Rehabil., 8:19–23.

141. Darrow, H., Schulthies, S., Draper, D., et al. (1999): Serum dexamethasone levels after Decadron phonophoresis. J. Athl. Train., 34:338–341.

142. Klaiman, M., Shrader, J., Danoff, J., et al. (1998): Phonophoresis versus ultrasound in the treatment of common musculoskeletal conditions. Med. Sci. Sports Exerc., 30:1349–1355.

143. Fahey, S., Smith, M., Merrick, M., et al. (2000): A comparison of hydrocortisone cream to powder in increasing intramuscular tissue temperature during phonophoresis treatments [abstract]. J. Athl. Train, 35:S-47.

144. Draper, D., Miner, L., Knight, K., and Ricard, M. (2002): The carry-over effects of diathermy and stretching in developing hamstring flexibility. J. Athl. Train., 37:37–42.

145. Draper, D., Sunderland, S., Kirkendall, D., and Ricard, M. (1993): A comparison of temperature rise in human calf muscles following applications of underwater and topical gel ultrasound. J. Orthop. Sports Phys. Ther., 17:247–251.

146. Draper, D., and Sunderland, S. (1993): Examination of the law of Grotthus-Draper: Does ultrasound penetrate subcutaneous fat in humans? J. Athl. Train, 28:246, 248-250, 278-279.

147. Holcomb, W., and Joyce, C. (2003): A comparison of temperature increases produced by 2 commonly used ultrasound units. J. Athl. Train., 38:24–27.

148. Merrick, M. (2001): Research digest. Do you diathermy? Athl. Ther. Today, 6:55–56.

149. Birkett, J. (1996): Soft tissue healing and the physiotherapy management of lower limb soft tissue injuries. Phys. Ther. Rev., 4:251–263.

150. Bricknell, R., and Watson, T. (1995): The thermal effects of pulsed shortwave therapy—BJTR pull-out physiotherapy supplement on electrotherapy. Br. J. Ther. Rehabil., 2:430–434.

151. Garrett, C., Draper, D., and Knight, K. (2000): Heat distribution in the lower leg from pulsed short-wave diathermy and ultrasound treatments. J. Athl. Train., 35:50–55.

152. Kitchen, S., and Partridge, C. (1992): Review of shortwave diathermy continuous and pulsed patterns. Physiotherapy, 78:243–252.

153. Lerman, Y., Jacubovich, R., Caner, A., and Ribak, J. (1996): Electromagnetic fields from shortwave diathermy equipment in physiotherapy departments. Physiotherapy, 82:456–458.

154. Martin, C., McCallum, H., Strelley, S., and Heaton, B. (1991): Electromagnetic fields from therapeutic diathermy equipment: A review of hazards and precautions. Physiotherapy, 77:3–7.

155. Ward, A., and Shkuratova, N. (2002): Russian electrical stimulation: The early experiments. Phys. Ther., 82:1019–1030.

156. Baldi, J., Jackson, R., Moraille, R., and Mysiw, W. (1998): Muscle atrophy is prevented in patients with acute spinal cord injury using functional electrical stimulation. Spinal Cord, 36:463–469.

157. Oldham, J., Howe, T., Petterson, T., et al. (1995): Electrotherapeutic rehabilitation of the quadriceps in elderly osteoarthritic patients: A double blind assessment of patterned neuromuscular stimulation. Clin. Rehabil., 9:10–20.

158. Cook, H., Morales, M., La, R.E., et al. (1994): Effects of electrical stimulation on lymphatic flow and limb volume in the rat. Phys. Ther., 74:1040–1046.

159. Faghri, P., Hovorka, C., and Trumbower, R. (2002): From the field. Reducing edema in the lower extremity of hemiplegic stroke patients: A comparison of non-pharmacological approaches. Clin. Kinesiol., 56:51–60.

160. Giudice, M. (1990): Effects of continuous passive motion and elevation on hand edema. Am. J. Occup. Ther., 44:914–921.

161. Holcomb, W. (1997): A practical guide to electrical therapy. J. Sport Rehabil., 6:272–282.

162. Norwig, J. (1997): Injury management update. Edema control and the acutely inverted ankle sprain. Athl. Ther. Today, 2:40–41.

163. Ogiwara, S. (2001): Calf muscle pumping and rest positions during and/or after whirlpool therapy. J. Phys. Ther. Sci., 13:99–105.

164. Ardic, F., Sarhus, M., and Topuz, O. (2002): Comparison of two different techniques of electrotherapy on myofascial pain. J. Back Musculoskel. Rehabil., 16:11–16.

165. Brosseau, L., Milne, S., Robinson, V., et al. (2002): Efficacy of the transcutaneous electrical nerve stimulation for the treatment of chronic low back pain: A meta-analysis. Spine, 27:596–603.

166. Carroll, D., Moore, R., McQuay, H., et al. (2001): Transcutaneous electrical nerve stimulation (TENS) for chronic pain. Cochrane Database Syst. Rev, 3:CD003222.

167. Ellis, B. (1996): A retrospective study of long-term users of transcutaneous electrical nerve stimulators. Br. J. Ther. Rehabil., 3:88–93.

168. Hou, C., Tsai, L., Cheng, K., et al. (2002): Immediate effects of various physical therapeutic modalities on cervical myofascial pain and trigger-point sensitivity. Arch. Phys. Med. Rehabil., 83:1406–1414.

169. Hsueh, T., Cheng, P., Kuan, T., and Hong, C. (1997): The immediate effectiveness of electrical nerve stimulation and electrical muscle stimulation on myofascial trigger points. Am. J. Phys. Med. Rehabil., 76:471–476.

170. Johnson, M., and Tabasam, G. (1999): A double-blind placebo controlled investigation into the analgesic effects of inferential currents (IFC) and transcutaneous electrical nerve stimulation (TENS) on cold-induced pain in healthy subjects. Physiother. Theory Pract., 15:217–233.

171. Johnson, M., and Tabasam, G. (2003): An investigation into the analgesic effects of interferential currents and transcutaneous electrical nerve stimulation on experimentally induced ischemic pain in otherwise pain-free volunteers. Phys. Ther., 83:208–223.

172. Milne, S., Welch, V., Brosseau, L., et al. (2001): Transcutaneous electrical nerve stimulation (TENS) for chronic low back pain. Cochrane Database Syst. Rev., 2:CD003008.

173. Osiri, M., Welch, V., Brosseau, L., et al. (2000): Transcutaneous electrical nerve stimulation for knee osteoarthritis. Cochrane Database Syst. Rev., 4:CD002823.

174. Proctor, M., Smith, C., Farquhar, C., and Stones, R. (2002): Transcutaneous electrical nerve stimulation and acupuncture for primary dysmenorrhoea. Cochrane Database Syst. Rev.,1:CD002123.

175. Seib, T., Price, R., Reyes, M., and Lehmann, J. (1994): The quantitative measurement of spasticity: Effect of cutaneous electrical stimulation. Arch. Phys. Med. Rehabil., 75:746–750.

176. Anderson, C., Morris, R., Boeh, S., et al. (2003): Effects of iontophoresis current magnitude and duration on dexamethasone deposition and localized drug retention. Phys. Ther., 83:161–170.

177. Costello, C., and Jeske, A. (1995): Iontophoresis: Applications in transdermal medication delivery. Phys. Ther., 75:554–563.

178. Li, L., Scudds, R., Heck, C., and Harth, M. (1996): The efficacy of dexamethasone iontophoresis for the treatment of rheumatoid arthritic knees: A pilot study. Arthritis Care Res., 9:126–132.

179. Perron, M., and Malouin, F. (1997): Acetic acid iontophoresis and ultrasound for the treatment of calcifying tendinitis of the shoulder: A randomized control trial. Arch. Phys. Med. Rehabil., 78:379–384.

180. Smutok, M., Mayo, M., Gabaree, C., et al. (2002): Failure to detect dexamethasone phosphate in the local venous blood postcathodic iontophoresis in humans. J. Orthop. Sports Phys. Ther., 32:461–468.

181. Van, H.G. (1997): Iontophoresis: A review of the literature. N. Z. J. Physiother., 25:16–17.

182. Wallace, M., Ridgeway, B., Jun, E., et al. (2001): Topical delivery of lidocaine in healthy volunteers by electroporation, electroincorporation, or iontophoresis: an evaluation of skin anesthesia. Reg. Anesth. Pain Med., 26:229–238.

Rehabilitation Considerations for the Female Athlete

Timothy E. Hewett, PhD, FACSM, and Bohdanna T. Zazulak, DPT, MS, OCS

CHAPTER OBJECTIVES

- Explain the biomechanical and neuromuscular factors that predispose females to lower extremity injury.

- Relate biomechanical and neuromuscular factors to the lower extremity injuries more commonly experienced by females.

- Describe specific rehabilitation interventions targeting the neuromuscular and biomechanical risk factors associated with lower extremity injury in female athletes.

Women have become more involved in both recreational and competitive sports since enactment of Title IX and are therefore receiving more attention in the sports medicine literature. Recent studies suggest that some lower extremity injuries are encountered more often by female athletes. Most impressive is the two to eight times higher risk for noncontact anterior cruciate ligament (ACL) tears in females than in male basketball and soccer players.[1-3] Women runners are also reported to sustain twice as many overall lower extremity injuries as their male counterparts.[4] In addition, studies indicate that stress fractures[5,6] and patellofemoral dysfunction are twice as likely to develop in female runners as male runners.[7,8] The injury patterns in women may be a consequence of structural, mechanical, neuromuscular, hormonal, or some combination of these factors.

Rehabilitation programs for the injured female athlete, in addition to resolving impairments, should include therapeutic exercises to alter the factors that may have led to the injury. Although it may not be possible to alter structure, normalization of mechanical and neuromuscular problems is necessary to decrease the possibility of reinjury. In this chapter, an overview of the structural, biomechanical, and neuromuscular factors that may predispose females to injury and a summary of gender differences in movement are presented, followed by descriptions of specific rehabilitation programs and techniques that may be useful in minimizing the influence of these factors.

GENDER DIFFERENCES

Structural Differences

Several differences in lower extremity structure have been noted between males and females (Fig. 9-1). When compared with men, women exhibit greater amounts of static external knee rotation alignment[9] and active hip internal rotation,[10] which may result in greater rotational motion and work at both the hip and knee. In addition, women have been shown to exhibit a greater interacetabular distance[11] and increased hip width when normalized to femoral length than seen in men.[12] Greater pelvic width and increased knee external rotation have been suggested to contribute to greater amounts of standing genu valgum alignment in women than in men[9,13] (see Fig. 9-1). In addition, the structural combination of increased hip adduction, femoral anteversion, and genu valgum may explain, in part, the well-documented larger Q angle in women than in men[12,14-16] (Fig. 9-2).

A more valgus knee position has been suggested to increase frontal plane motion at the knee and increase the risk for lower extremity overuse injuries.[17-19] Cowan et al[17] found that subjects with a Q angle greater than 15° had a significantly increased risk for overuse injury and that the risk for lower extremity stress fractures was significantly higher in participants with the most valgus knee positions.[17] An increased knee valgus angle also increases the Q angle, which is thought to lead to patellofemoral disorders (see Fig. 9-2). Mizuno et al[20] investigated the relationship between

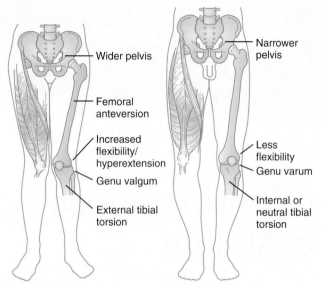

FIGURE 9-1 Structural differences between men and women. Women *(left)* typically exhibit a wider pelvis, femoral anteversion, greater tibial external rotation, and genu valgum. *(Adapted from Ireland, M.L., and Hutchinson, M.R. [1995]: Women. In: Griffin, L.Y. [ed.]. Rehabilitation of the Injured Knee. St. Louis, Mosby, p. 298.)*

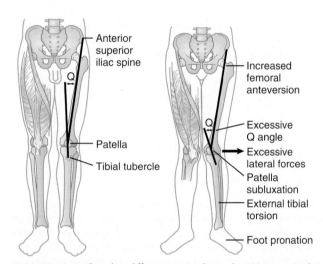

FIGURE 9-2 Gender differences in Q angle. Women *(right)* exhibit a greater Q angle, increased external tibial torsion, and increased femoral anteversion. The combination of these structural differences can lead to increased lateral patellar compressive forces and patellar subluxation. *(Adapted from Ireland, M.L., and Hutchinson, M.R. [1995]: Women. In: Griffin, L.Y. [ed.]. Rehabilitation of the Injured Knee. St. Louis, Mosby, p. 299.)*

Q angle and patellofemoral kinematics. Through manipulation of the Q angle in vitro, these authors reported that a larger Q angle may lead to greater lateral patellar contact forces and increase the potential for patellofemoral pain syndrome and lateral patellar dislocations. In support of this hypothesis, runners with patellofemoral pain were found to exhibit a significantly greater Q angle than did a group of healthy control subjects.[19]

Intercondylar notch size and shape (Fig. 9-3) have been proposed as a potential contributor to the greater incidence of ACL injury in women.[21,22] It has been suggested that women have

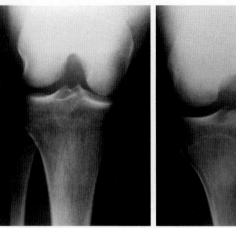

FIGURE 9-3 Radiographs of the intercondylar notch from a male *(right)* and female *(left)*. Note that the shape and size of the female's notch is markedly smaller and narrower than that of the male. *(From Ireland, M.L., and Hutchinson, M.R. [1995]: Women. In: Griffin, L.Y. [ed.]. Rehabilitation of the Injured Knee. St. Louis, Mosby, p. 301.)*

a narrower notch width than men do, and some investigators have reported that this contributes to a smaller and potentially weaker ACL.[21,22] Lund-Hanssen et al[23] found that women with a narrow notch width were six times more likely to rupture their ACL than were women with larger notch widths. However, more recent work has suggested that there are no differences in intercondylar notch width between males and females.[24,25] Ireland et al[24] performed a retrospective investigation and measured the notch width of males and females with and without ACL injuries and reported that smaller notch widths were associated with previous ACL injury regardless of gender or notch shape. Thus, further investigation is warranted to better determine the influence of femoral intercondylar notch width and shape on the incidence of ACL injury.

Clinical Pearl #1

Gender differences in lower extremity structure include increased pelvic and hip width, static knee external rotation, genu valgum, increased Q angle, and decreased intercondylar notch size in females.

Differences in Mechanics

It is believed that structural differences may lead to different movement patterns, which in turn place women at risk for injury in comparison to their male counterparts. Although relatively few studies have been performed in the area of gender differences in lower extremity mechanics during functional tasks, the studies that have been conducted show that females may perform some tasks differently from males. The following sections address each of these activities with respect to possible gender-related differences.

Running

Gender differences during running have received little attention in the scientific literature, but the studies that have been conducted show that women have different running mechanics than men. Similar to the results of landing studies (see later), women tend to run with less knee flexion.[26] Women also exhibit a significantly greater knee valgus angle throughout stance than men do and demonstrate significantly greater peak hip adduction and hip internal rotation angles, which may be the result of a greater Q angle.[26] Hip frontal and transverse plane negative work is greater in women than in men, which suggests that the muscles controlling hip adduction and internal rotation are under greater eccentric loading while running. These gender differences in running mechanics may lend insight into the greater incidence of specific lower extremity injuries seen in women, such as patellofemoral pain.

The greater femoral internal rotation and tibial external rotation exhibited by female runners may also place them in a biomechanical dilemma with respect to the patellofemoral joint. Tiberio[27] suggested that excessive femoral internal rotation might result in malalignment of the patellofemoral joint and lead to anterior knee pain. It has also been suggested that abnormal tibial rotation results in subsequent interruption of the normal tibiofemoral rotational relationship and an alteration in normal patellofemoral mechanics.[18] The increased femoral internal rotation observed in female athletes, coupled with the increased tibial external rotation position, may result in a greater Q angle, thereby increasing the risk for patellofemoral disorders in females.

Clinical Pearl #2

The hip adduction and hip internal rotation angles and the frontal and transverse planes work are greater in females than in males during running.

Cutting

Another common noncontact mechanism of injury is performance of a cutting maneuver while running. It has been suggested that when the knee approaches a valgus position, the load experienced by the ACL may be five times greater than that when the knee is aligned in the frontal plane.[28] Women tend to exhibit less knee flexion and greater knee valgus during side-cutting and cross-cutting tasks,[26] which in turn may place the knee in a position in which significant ACL strain can occur. No differences were found between males and females in knee rotation during cutting; however, females have greater intertrial variability in femoral rotation patterns.[29] This amount of variability was most strongly influenced by the level of experience, with less experienced female athletes exhibiting greater knee rotation variability. Thus, it may be possible to train female athletes to use specific lower extremity movement patterns that do not predispose them to lower extremity injury or reinjury.

Clinical Pearl #3

During cutting maneuvers, females exhibit greater dynamic valgus and a dependence of knee rotation variability on the level of experience in performing cutting.

Landing

Landing from a jump results in forces between 3 and 14 times body weight that must be attenuated by the lower extremity.[30] One of the most common noncontact mechanisms of lower extremity injury is landing from a jump, and it has been reported that women are more likely than men to injure themselves during sports that involve jumping and landing.[31] Huston et al[32] studied the landing patterns of males and females and reported that females land with less knee flexion than men do and thus experience greater ground reaction force vertical loading rates. Specifically, women experienced a 9% increase in loading rate per unit of body weight when compared with men.[32] Lephart et al[33] found that females land with less knee flexion and with greater femoral internal and tibial external rotation than males do. The decreased amount of knee flexion exhibited by females may reduce their ability to attenuate the impact forces experienced during landing. Furthermore, because ACL strain has been found to be greatest when the knee is near or at full extension, the extended knee position during landing may predispose female athletes to greater ACL strain.[34] Recent video analysis of the mechanics of ACL injury reveals four common components, especially apparent in women.[35,36] As a female athlete lands, her knee buckles inward into a valgus position, the injured knee is relatively straight, and her trunk tends to be tilted laterally with the center of mass displaced from the plantar aspect of the foot. Female athletes display different neuromuscular strategies than do male athletes during landing. These gender differences in muscle recruitment and timing of muscle activation may affect dynamic lower extremity stability and contribute to injury.[37]

Clinical Pearl #4

Females experience higher ground reaction force and have increased femoral rotation motion during landing.

Neuromuscular Differences

Ligament Dominance

A potential contributor to the greater incidence of lower extremity injury in females than in males is the gender difference in joint stability as a result of active muscle stiffness. Stiffness has been defined as the resistance exerted by the soft tissue structures in response to a force that may result in joint stress, and active joint stiffness can be modulated through voluntary muscle contraction.[38] In addition, it has been suggested that individuals who are less able to voluntarily contract their muscles in response to an external force or perturbation may be more likely to sustain an injury. Wojtys et al[38] used a dynamic stress test to measure anterior tibial translation and simultaneous muscular response to an externally applied stress. It was reported that muscle cocontraction significantly decreases anterior tibial translation in both men and women. However, men exhibited significantly greater stiffness than women, thus suggesting that women have a reduced ability to actively protect the knee in response to an anteriorly applied force. Other studies measuring active muscle stiffness in males and females during isometric knee flexion and extension contractions and during functional hopping tasks have been conducted.[39] During either task, females demonstrated reduced active muscle stiffness in comparison to males.[39] Thus, it is possible that reduced active muscle stiffness may lead to reduced joint stability and predispose females to lower extremity joint injury. Because the muscles in female athletes do not adequately absorb ground reaction forces, the joints and ligaments are forced to absorb high amounts of force over short periods. This ligament dominance creates higher impulse forces and probably results in ligament injury. Ligament dominance is characterized by the use of anatomic bone structures, articular cartilage, and ligament to absorb ground reaction forces during athletic maneuvers rather than the active musculature of the lower extremity. Especially important for lower extremity dynamic control is the musculature of the posterior kinetic chain (gluteals, hamstrings, gastrocnemius, and soleus).[40]

Quadriceps Dominance

Considerable attention has been focused on how the muscles surrounding the knee joint react during joint loading and to unexpected perturbations. This area of research is particularly important because failure of the ACL occurs when large mechanical loads exceed the capacity of the stabilizing ligaments.[41,42] In addition, whereas the ACL provides significant static restraint to anterior tibial translation, active muscle recruitment can assist the ACL in maintaining joint stability and preventing injury.[41] Thus, gender-related differences in muscle activation in response to joint loading and unexpected perturbations may shed light on the gender bias of lower extremity injury. Previous work by Huston and Wojtys[43] indicated that female athletes initially use their quadriceps muscles for knee stabilization in response to anterior tibial translation whereas female nonathletes and males initially rely on their hamstring muscles. In addition, female athletes took significantly longer to generate maximum hamstring muscle torque during isokinetic testing than did males.[43] Females, unlike males, do not increase hamstring-to-quadriceps torque ratios at velocities approaching those of functional activities.[44] Female athletes exhibit reduced hamstring and greater quadriceps electromyographic activity during landing, running, side-cutting, and cross-cutting tasks.[26,45] These muscle recruitment patterns, in combination with less knee flexion and greater loading rates exhibited by female athletes, certainly increase the potential for ACL strain. The combination of these muscle activation patterns may produce excessive strain on the ACL. In addition, it has been reported that females exhibit hamstring muscle onset that is less coincident with anterior tibial shear forces during landings, thereby increasing the potential for ACL injury.[46]

Leg Dominance

Female athletes tend to be more one leg dominant than their male counterparts. Leg dominance refers to a measurable imbalance between right and left lower extremity muscle strength or relative recruitment. This imbalance is particularly important in tasks that normally require side-to-side symmetry of the lower extremities.[40] In single-leg jump tasks, it is known that most athletes have a favored plant or kick leg. However, the difference between limbs in muscle recruitment patterns, muscle strength, and muscle flexibility tends to be greater in women than in men.[40,47-51] Hewett et al[52] have shown that those who have greater asymmetry in these force and torque profiles have greater risk for future injury and should be targeted for interventional neuromuscular training to equalize bilateral lower extremity muscular recruitment, strength, and flexibility.

Trunk Dominance

Impaired trunk neuromuscular control, or trunk dominance, appears to increase the risk for lower extremity injury in female athletes.[53] Prospective evidence suggests a correlation between trunk neuromuscular control and lower extremity injury. In studies performed by Zazulak et al in which the association between trunk neuromuscular control and injury was examined in 277 collegiate varsity athletes, trunk proprioception and trunk displacement after quick release predicted risk for future ligament injury in female athletes but not in male athletes.[54,55] Trunk dominance may be exaggerated by growth and maturation factors. After puberty, females have increased trunk mass with a higher center of gravity but do not experience a "neuromuscular spurt" of muscular development and increase power as males do.[56] Video analysis of the mechanism of knee injuries reveals a common position of trunk leaning, with the center of mass being displaced from the plantar aspect of the foot, thus indicating an inability to precisely control the trunk in three-dimensional space.[35,57]

This excessive uncontrolled lateral motion creates medial-lateral torque on the knee, which increases the risk for injury.[40]

Clinical Pearl #5

Neuromuscular responses that may predispose females to injury include ligament dominance, quadriceps dominance, leg dominance, and trunk dominance.

Hormonal Influences

Although not a structural difference, the most obvious differences between males and females are reproductive hormones and the menstrual cycle exhibited by women. The menstrual cycle ranges from 24 to 35 days, with an average of 28 days, and can be broken down into three phases with varying levels of reproductive hormones within each stage. The first phase is the menstrual phase (days 1 to 5) and is marked by low estrogen and progesterone levels. The follicular phase (days 6 to 13) is marked by rising levels of estrogen and leads to ovulation, which occurs immediately after a surge in estrogen. Finally, the luteal phase lasts approximately 14 days, during which progesterone is the dominant hormone, but estrogen is also increased to approximately half the value of the late follicular phase surge.[58]

The physiologic link between surges in estrogen levels and ACL laxity has been the topic of recent research because some studies have identified estrogen receptors on the human ACL.[59] Thus, it has been suggested that based on in vitro data, the higher rates of ACL injury in women may be due to decreased fibroblastic proliferation and decreased procollagen synthesis in the human ACL caused by increases in estrogen concentration.[60] Whether increasing levels of estrogen cause females to have a greater risk for ACL injury remains debatable. A systematic review of the literature analyzed the effect of the menstrual cycle on anterior knee laxity. Six of nine studies reported no significant effect of the menstrual cycle on anterior knee laxity in women. However, three studies observed significant associations between the menstrual cycle and anterior knee laxity. These studies all reported that laxity increased during the ovulatory or postovulatory phases of the cycle. A metaanalysis that included data from all nine reviewed studies corroborated this significant effect of cycle phase on knee laxity (F value = 56.59, $P = .0001$). In the analyses, the knee laxity data measured at 10 to 14 days were greater than that at 15 to 28 days, which in turn were greater than that at 1 to 9 days. Although hormone confirmation was provided in many of the studies that selected specific days to depict a particular cycle for all women, it is unknown from these data whether they truly captured times of peak hormone values in all women. This combined systematic review and metaanalysis of the literature indicate that the menstrual cycle may have an effect on anterior-posterior laxity of the knee; however, further investigation is needed to confirm or reject this hypothesis.[61]

Several studies have investigated the effect of the menstrual cycle on ACL injury. In a prospective study, Myklebust et al[62] reported that 14 women suffered injury in the late follicular or menstrual phases in a group of 17 female handball players with ACL injuries. The most notable limitation of this study was the lack of stratification of the athletes taking oral contraceptives. However, a more recent study by this same group analyzed the distribution of ACL injuries in 46 subjects and found that most ACL injuries occurred during the menstrual phase.[63] Arendt et al corroborated the trend of increased ACL injury during the first half of the menstrual cycle in two studies that retrospectively studied collegiate female athletes.[64,65] Wojtys et al[66] also attempted to determine the menstrual phase in which ACL injury occurred by using a retrospective approach up to 3 months after injury. These authors reported a significantly higher frequency of ACL injury than expected during the late follicular phase and a significantly lower frequency of ACL injury than expected in the early follicular phase. However, the phase of the menstrual cycle was self-reported in these investigations and not confirmed by direct hormone measurements. More recently, Slauterback et al[67] studied the relationship between ACL injury and serum estrogen levels in women within 48 hours after ACL injury. These authors stated that a significant number of ACL injuries occurred on days 1 and 2 of the menses, when estrogen levels were lowest. A systematic review of these seven studies revealed a consistent trend of increased ACL injury during the preovulatory phase of the menstrual cycle.[68]

Clinical Pearl #6

The presence of estrogen receptors on the ACL and the prevalence of ACL injuries in certain phases of the menstrual cycle may indicate a link between hormones and injury in female athletes.

Summary

Many differences exist between males and females, and the differences appear to influence injury patterns in females. Females have a different structural alignment of the lower extremities, and this alignment may predispose them to specific injuries. The structural alignment also has the potential to influence mechanics, thus further predisposing females to specific injuries. Although relatively little information is available on gender differences during functional, sport-specific activities, it appears that females may perform tasks differently, regardless of their alignment, and

the manner in which they perform these tasks may make them susceptible to injury. Two areas receiving greater attention in recent years are the influence of neuromuscular responses and hormones on injuries in female athletes. Further research is warranted to determine the magnitude of their influence.

SCREENING FOR THE HIGH-RISK ATHLETE

Measures related to lower extremity valgus angles at the knee were found to be highly predictive of risk for noncontact ACL injury in female athletes.[52] More recently, biomechanical measures during landing studied in subjects after ACL reconstruction were found to be predictors of a second ACL injury in athletes after being released to return to sport.[53] Furthermore, Zazulak et al discovered that measures of trunk proprioception and displacement are predictive of knee injury with high sensitivity and moderate specificity.[54,55] The predictive screening tools used in these studies included motion analysis to measure lower extremity kinematics, stabilimetry to measure postural sway, a trunk proprioception apparatus that measures the athlete's ability to detect trunk rotation, and a trunk quick-release apparatus that measures trunk displacement. These are sophisticated laboratory tools that many clinicians may not be privy to. Hence, Hewett et al developed a clinic-based neuromuscular screening tool.[40] The assessment algorithm identifies female athletes with neuromuscular deficits in the clinic or in the field (Fig. 9-4). This algorithm delineates five biomechanical factors, including tibia length, knee valgus motion, knee flexion range of motion, mass, and quadriceps-hamstring ratio, and has been validated by the highly accurate laboratory assessment instruments. Although a valuable tool, it does not readily allow immediate feedback for correction of neuromuscular deficits.[40]

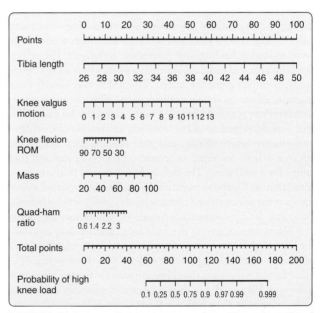

FIGURE 9-4 Injury prediction nanogram. *ham*, Hamstring; *Quad*, quadriceps; *ROM*, range of motion. *(Reproduced from Myer, G.D., Ford, K.R., Khoury, J. et al. [2010]: Clinical correlates to laboratory measures for use in non-contact anterior cruciate ligament injury risk prediction algorithm. Clin. Biomech. [Bristol Avon]. 25:693–699. Used with permission, Clinical Biomechanics.)*

Tuck Jump Assessment	Pre	Mid	Post	Comments
Knee and Thigh Motion				
① Lower extremity valgus at landing	☐	☐	☐	
② Thighs do not reach parallel (peak of jump)	☐	☐	☐	
③ Thighs not equal side to side (during flight)	☐	☐	☐	
Foot Position During Landing				
④ Foot placement not shoulder width apart	☐	☐	☐	
⑤ Foot placement not parallel (front to back)	☐	☐	☐	
⑥ Foot contact timing not equal	☐	☐	☐	
7 Excessive landing contact noise	☐	☐	☐	
Plyometric Technique				
8 Pause between jumps	☐	☐	☐	
9 Technique declines prior to 10 seconds	☐	☐	☐	
10 Does not land in same footprint (excessive in-flight motion)	☐	☐	☐	
	Total _____	Total _____	Total _____	

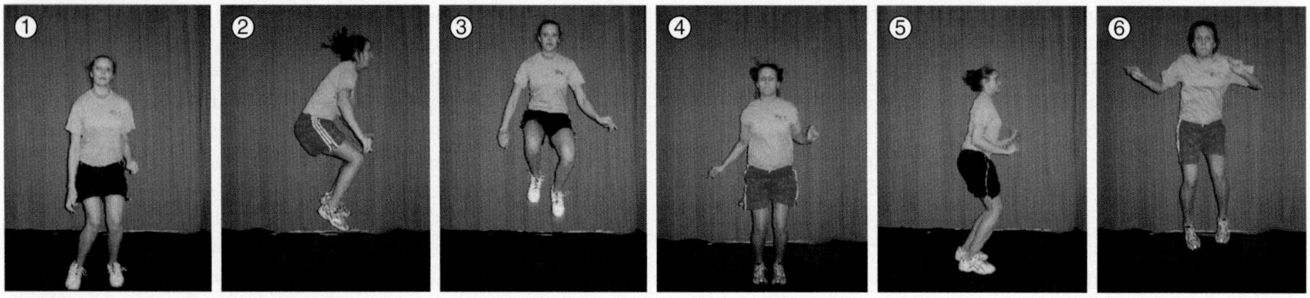

FIGURE 9-5 Tuck jump assessment: six common mistakes that clinicians should aim to correct in athletes while they perform the tuck jump exercise. *1.* Athlete displays unwanted medial knee collapse. *2.* Athlete does not achieve the desired knees-parallel position at the top of flight. *3.* Athlete does not display synchronized lower limb positions during flight. *4.* Athlete lands with the feet too close together. *5.* Athlete lands in an undesirable staggered position. *6.* Athlete does not land with both feet at the same time. *(Reproduced from Myer, G.D., Ford, K.R., and Hewett, T.E. [2008]: Tuck jump assessment for reducing anterior cruciate ligament injury risk. Athl. Ther. Today, 13[5]:39–44 with permission from the editor.)*

The functional performance and technique assessment is a useful clinician-friendly, real-time, field-based tool for identifying the four neuromuscular flaws that can occur during a functional task.[40,69] The criteria evaluated are knee and thigh motion, foot position during landing, and plyometric technique. The athlete performs repeated tuck jumps for 10 seconds, which allows the clinician to visually grade the criteria. The athlete may initially focus cognitive efforts on simply completing the difficult task, so faulty technique can readily be revealed to the examiner. An assessment tool was developed to allow clinicians to monitor the athlete's performance before, during, and after training (Fig. 9-5).[70] The athlete's deficits are rated as present (checked) or not and then tallied for a total score. The deficits found should be the focus of correction, and improvement can be tracked by repeated assessments at the midpoint and conclusion of training or rehabilitation programs. If improvements are made in neuromuscular control and biomechanics during the tuck jump and landing sequence, the learned skill may be transferred to competitive play.[40] Empiric laboratory evidence suggests that athletes who demonstrate six or more flawed techniques should be targeted for further training in technique. Pilot work has shown intrarater reliability of the tuck jump assessment to be high, r = 0.84 (range, 0.72 to 0.97).[40]

REHABILITATION INTERVENTIONS

The majority of rehabilitation programs developed specifically for female athletes have been designed to decrease risk for ACL injury. Although these programs have been designed with injury prevention in mind, the principles behind these programs can be implemented during postinjury rehabilitation for females as a means of preventing future injury. This section presents specific exercises, along with published programs, that can be implemented during rehabilitation for the injured female athlete to address the four predominant deficits in neuromuscular control: ligament dominance, quadriceps dominance, leg dominance, and trunk dominance.

Core Stability Training

Core stability training is gaining popularity in rehabilitation as clinicians become more aware of the influence of weakness in the "core" of the body on lower extremity mechanics and performance. The lumbar, pelvic, and hip region together are considered to be the core of the body and are collectively called the lumbopelvic-hip complex (LPHC). Optimal core function involves both trunk mobility and stability. When the core is functioning efficiently, advantageous length-tension relationships are maintained that allow the athlete to produce strong movements in the extremities.[71] Core stability may also be important in allowing an athlete to maintain the center of gravity over the base of support.[72]

Core stability training may be particularly important for the female athlete because weakness in the core could alter posture, thereby exacerbating factors that are believed to contribute to injury. For example, weakness of the hip abductors and external rotators could result in greater hip adduction and femoral internal rotation, which could contribute to increased knee valgus and thus possibly result in patellofemoral injury. In addition, weakness of the gluteal musculature has been hypothesized to cause tightness in the tensor fasciae latae and a more erect hip and trunk, which could result in greater loads across the knee.[71,73] To create a comprehensive core stability training program, the practitioner must first understand the functional anatomy of the core.

Clinical Pearl #7

A weak and underrecruited core may result in inefficient movements and altered postures that can lead to injury.

Many muscles in the core region are important for postural alignment and dynamic postural equilibrium during activities.[71,74] A summary of these muscles and their functions is presented in Table 9-1. In the lumbar region, the main muscles include the transversospinalis group, erector spinae, quadratus lumborum, and latissimus dorsi. The transversospinalis group is mainly responsible for dynamic stabilization of the LPHC during movement and plays a very small role in producing movement. In addition, the transversospinalis muscles have been found to contain two to six times the number of muscle

Table 9-1 Muscles of the Core and Their Function in Providing Core Stability

Muscle Group	Muscle	Function
Lumbar spine	Transversospinalis group	Intersegmental stabilization Proprioceptive feedback
	Erector spinae	Intersegmental stabilization Back extension
	Quadratus lumborum	Frontal plane stabilization
	Latissimus dorsi	Dynamic stabilization
Abdominal muscles	Rectus abdominus	Trunk flexion
	External oblique	Lateral trunk flexion Contralateral rotation
	Internal oblique	Lateral trunk flexion Ipsilateral rotation
	Transversus abdominis	Increased abdominal pressure Dynamic stabilization
Hip muscles	Gluteus maximus	Hip extension Femoral external rotation Stabilize sacroiliac joint
	Gluteus medius	Frontal plane stabilization Femoral external rotation Femoral abduction
	Psoas major	Hip flexion Trunk extension

Data from Clark, M.A., Fater, D., and Reuteman, P. (2000): Core (trunk) stabilization and its importance for closed kinetic chain rehabilitation. Orthop. Phys. Ther. Clin. North Am., 9:119–135.

spindles as other muscles, thus providing a significant amount of proprioceptive feedback to the central nervous system.[74] The erector spinae muscles contract to produce trunk extension and also serve to provide dynamic intersegmental stabilization, whereas the quadratus lumborum muscles provide frontal plane stabilization along with the gluteus medius and tensor fasciae latae muscles.

Clinical Pearl #8

The initial difficulty of exercises in core stability training should be adapted to the level of proficiency of the patients.

The abdominal muscles include the rectus abdominis, external oblique, internal oblique, and transversus abdominis.[74] Although the rectus abdominis is mainly responsible for trunk flexion, the internal and external oblique muscles produce lateral trunk flexion. In addition, the internal and external oblique muscles produce ipsilateral and contralateral trunk rotation, respectively. The transversus abdominis is perhaps the most important of the abdominal muscles because contraction of this muscle dramatically increases intraabdominal pressure and provides the greatest degree of LPHC stability during dynamic movement. In addition, it has been reported that contraction of the transversus abdominis, similar to the multifidus muscle of the transversospinalis group, precedes initiation of limb movement.[75]

The core hip muscles are primarily the gluteus maximus, gluteus medius, and psoas major.[74] The gluteus maximus contracts to produce hip extension and external rotation and provides dynamic stability to the sacroiliac joint during movment.[74] The gluteus medius muscle provides frontal plane stabilization and causes femoral abduction and external rotation, and the psoas major muscle produces hip flexion and assists in trunk extension.[74]

Various rehabilitation interventions are specifically designed for improving core stability. Most notable are Pilates, Swiss ball, and medicine ball exercises. Regardless of the specific exercise initiated for core stabilization training, several principles should be followed in developing a core stability training program to produce the best outcome. First, the training program should be systematic, and in each phase of training, specific goals should be met.[71] Second, the program should be progressive.[71] This includes progression from straight plane to multiplane movements, from isometric to concentric and eccentric contractions, from slow to fast movements, from nonresisted to resisted movements, from no limb movement to the addition of limb movement, and from lying-down positions to standing. Finally, the program should be functional.[71] Isolated movements may be proficient for targeting specific muscles, but the gains may not carry over into functional movement.

Clinical Pearl #9

Exercises should be progressed only when the patient is able to maintain spinal stability and a normal breathing pattern.

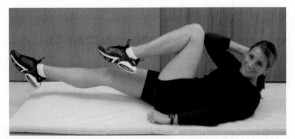

FIGURE 9-6 Bicycle exercise for core stability training. When properly performed, the pelvis should not move as leg movements are alternated.

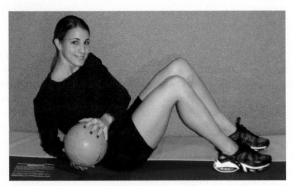

FIGURE 9-7 Side-to-side rotation with a medicine ball. The pelvis and low-back position should remain stable as the upper part of the body is rotated from side to side.

In the initial phases of core stability training, the focus should be to increase the base level of strength and endurance in muscles of the core region. Slow, controlled, isometric movements may be necessary initially, depending on the starting level of strength and control in the patient. Pelvic tilting and isometric transversus abdominis exercises are very basic exercises that may be prescribed. The isometric transversus abdominis exercise requires the athlete to draw the navel in by contracting the muscles and hold the contraction with a normal breathing pattern and without global muscle activation.[76] When the athlete is able to perform these exercises correctly and can maintain a normal breathing pattern during the exercises, the difficulty may be progressed as noted earlier. Exercises that may be prescribed include leg slides, prone arm or leg raises, abdominal crunches on a Swiss ball, or a bicycle exercise (Fig. 9-6). It is imperative that the athlete maintain spinal stabilization during each exercise, and if the athlete cannot do so, the difficulty of the exercise should be decreased. Next, resistance should be added to further increase muscular strength, and the duration of the exercises should be increased to enhance muscular endurance. Potential exercises in this phase include crunches with a ball toss into a rebounder or trunk rotation with a medicine ball (Fig. 9-7). Finally, exercises that closely mimic movements during the athlete's sport should be incorporated into training (Fig. 9-8), or sports activities should be performed with an emphasis on maintaining core stability.

Jump or Plyometric Training

Studies that document gender differences in landing provide support for including jump or plyometric training in rehabilitation programs for female athletes. A 6-week training program

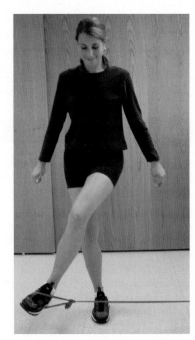

FIGURE 9-8 Soccer kicking is performed with resistance from a Thera-Band attached to the leg. The athlete is instructed to maintain stability through the trunk as the kicking motion is performed.

developed by Hewett et al[77] includes jump training in addition to stretching and strengthening exercises (Table 9-2). After participating in the training program, female athletes had decreased knee abduction and adduction moments, predictors of peak landing force, and lower peak vertical ground reaction force than did males.[77] A prospective investigation using a similar program demonstrated that fewer knee injuries were experienced by female athletes who had participated in the training program than by untrained female athletes.[77] The Prevent Injury and Enhance Performance program was modeled after the program of Hewett et al[77] but was designed specifically for female soccer players.[78] The program includes a series of stretching, strengthening, agility training, and jumping exercises. Preliminary results, reported in an abstract presented at the 2002 Annual Meeting of the American Academy of Orthopaedic Surgeons, showed 88% fewer ACL injuries in female soccer players who participated in this program than in untrained female soccer players. Another program, the Frappier Acceleration Sports Training Program (available from Frappier Accelerations, Fargo, ND) combines graded incline treadmill running with plyometric jump training. Female high school soccer players who participated in the 7-week program had a significantly reduced incidence of injuries in their lower extremities than untrained athletes did.[79] Although each of the aforementioned programs includes components other than jump training, jump training is a critical component. The combined results of these reports support plyometric training as a means of normalizing mechanical differences and preventing future knee injury.

Clinical Pearl #10

Plyometric training can be used to decrease force on the knee and normalize lower limb alignment when landing.

Table 9-2 Jump Training Program

Exercise	Repetitions/Time	
Phase I		
Wall jumps	20 seconds	25 seconds
Tuck jumps	20 seconds	25 seconds
Broad jumps, stick land	5 repetitions	10 repetitions
Squat jumps	10 seconds	15 seconds
Double-leg cone jumps (side to side, back to front)	30 seconds each	30 seconds each
180° jumps	20 seconds	25 seconds
Bounding in place	20 seconds	25 seconds
Phase II		
Wall jumps	30 seconds	30 seconds
Tuck jumps	30 seconds	30 seconds
Jump, jump, jump, vertical jump	5 repetitions	8 repetitions
Squat jumps	20 seconds	20 seconds
Bounding for distance	1 run	2 runs
Double-leg cone jumps	30 seconds each	30 seconds each
Scissor jump	30 seconds	30 seconds
Hop, hop, stick	5 repetitions/leg	5 repetitions/leg
Phase III		
Wall jumps	30 seconds	30 seconds
Step, jump up, down, vertical	5 repetitions	10 repetitions
Mattress jumps (side to side, back to front)	30 seconds	30 seconds
Single-leg jumps distance	5 repetitions/leg	5 repetitions/leg
Squat jumps	25 seconds	25 seconds
Jump into bounding	3 runs	3 runs
Single-leg hop, hop, stick	5 repetitions/leg	5 repetitions/leg

Adapted from Hewett, T.E., Stroupe, A.L., Nance, T.A., and Noyes, F.R. (1996): Plyometric training in female athletes. Decreased impact forces and increased hamstring torques. Am. J. Sports Med., 24:765–773.

Instruction by clinicians can be used to increase the effectiveness of jump training. Patients should be instructed to land on the balls of the feet, as opposed to flat-footed, and with a flexed knee and hip close to a 90/90 position to encourage recruitment of the posterior chain and core musculature. Verbally instructing subjects to land on the balls of their feet with flexed knees has been found to be effective in decreasing impact landing force.[77,80] Instructing subjects to use the sound made at impact as a guide to decreasing impact force has likewise been found to be effective.[81,82] Clinicians should also cue patients on alignment, such as avoiding increased knee valgus when landing (Fig. 9-9). Inability to maintain alignment may also indicate a need for core stability training.

Clinical Pearl #11

Verbal feedback by clinicians can enhance jump training technique.

Balance Training

Balance training is implemented into many postinjury rehabilitation programs as a mechanism for improving proprioception, or joint awareness, after injury. Decreased proprioception has been found after such injuries as ACL rupture and ankle sprain[83-85] and is attributed to altered mechanoreceptor afferent input after injury.[86] Because reflex pathways, including those responsible for postural sway, depend on afferent input, loss of afferent input or altered afferent input after injury can also influence postural sway.[87] Increased sway during single-leg standing has been found in subjects with ACL deficiency, reconstructed ACLs, and lateral ankle sprains.[88-91] The sensory input achieved during balance training may restore neuromuscular pathways.

A variety of therapeutic exercise techniques can be categorized under balance training. Some exercises involve primarily maintenance of balance without applied disturbance, for example, single-leg standing exercises on an unstable board (Fig. 9-10). Maximum crossover effect is achieved when single-limb activities are alternately performed by both lower extremities. Other exercises involve maintenance of balance in response to an applied postural disturbance (Fig. 9-11). These exercises may not be equivalent; however, research is needed to determine whether they produce similar outcomes.

Research on the ability of training on unstable boards to prevent lower extremity injury is conflicting; however, some positive adaptations can be made for muscular reflexes. Male soccer players who performed single-leg standing and step-up exercises on wobble boards for 20 minutes per day during preseason training had fewer ACL injuries than untrained players did,[92] and female handball players who used an ankle disk for 10 to 15 minutes during practice sessions over a 10-month season had significantly fewer ankle injuries and fewer traumatic lower extremity injuries overall than control subjects did.[93] In contrast, no difference was found in the occurrence of traumatic lower extremity injuries between female soccer players who participated in a program of 10 to 15 minutes of training on a balance board during the season and those who did not.[94] Differences in instruction to subjects and progression of the exercises may explain the conflicting results of these studies. Osborne et al[95] found that control subjects and subjects with ankle sprains who participated in 8 weeks of ankle disk training had decreased tibialis anterior onset in response to an inversion perturbation, thus suggesting that balance training on an unstable disk may be able to induce changes in neuromuscular response. More research is necessary, though, to identify the effect of this type of training on neuromuscular responses in other muscles and the relationship of the change to function.

Another type of balance training involves the application of a perturbation to the surface on which the patient stands. Subjects with ACL deficiency who participated in rehabilitation with perturbation training have been found to be more successful in returning to sports without knee instability[96] and have a faster hamstring reaction time to forward movement of an isokinetic dynamometer arm after training.[97,98] Coordination of muscle

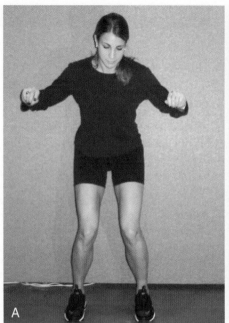 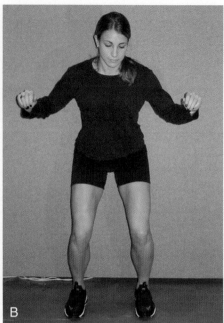

FIGURE 9-9 A, Improper knee alignment during jump training. **B,** The athlete should be instructed to maintain a knee position that is over the feet when landing.

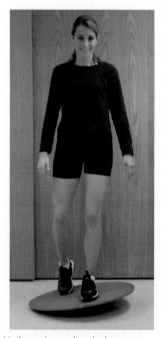

FIGURE 9-10 Unilateral standing balance on an unstable board.

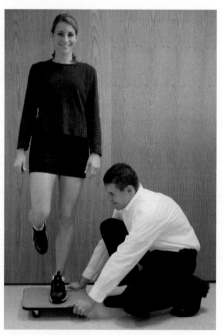

FIGURE 9-11 A perturbation training technique. The athlete stands in a unilateral stance on a rolling board and attempts to maintain balance as the therapist applies a disturbance to the rolling board.

activity during walking is also altered after this type of training in ways that are consistent with improved dynamic knee stability.[99] These results demonstrate that training with perturbations in the support surface changes neuromuscular control in the ACL-deficient knee. However, to date, no study has been published on the effect of this type of training on injury prevention or postoperative rehabilitation or the differential effect of this training in males versus females.

Clinical Pearl #12

Balance training may normalize afferent input after injury, which in turn can normalize postinjury sway and alter neuromuscular responses.

Perturbation training, similar to the other rehabilitation interventions presented in this chapter, should follow a logical progression. Fitzgerald et al[96] described the initial application of support surface perturbations with upper limb support provided and verbal cues given for the onset of the perturbation. When the patient demonstrated the ability to maintain balance without difficulty, the support and verbal cues were removed and the perturbations were progressed by randomizing the timing, direction, and force of application.[96] During perturbation training, if a patient demonstrates an inability to maintain balance, it is likely that the progression was too difficult, and this often occurs when many variables (magnitude of force, direction, and timing) are progressed simultaneously. At least one variable should be reduced in difficulty so that the patient is sufficiently challenged but is able to perform the task. Perturbation training should also be progressed to include sport-specific tasks to encourage carryover to functional activity.[96] An example of such progression would be adding chest passes with a basketball while perturbations are being applied.

CONCLUSION

- Anatomically, females exhibit a wider pelvis, greater Q angle, greater femoral anteversion, a more externally rotated position of the tibia, and greater genu valgum than males do.
- During athletic movements, females exhibit less knee flexion, greater genu valgum, greater femoral anteversion and hip abduction, and greater tibial external rotation than do males performing the same tasks.
- When compared with males, females exhibit reduced lower extremity active muscle stiffness; females also demonstrate earlier recruitment of the quadriceps muscle and slower onset of hamstring activity after an unexpected force applied to the knee.
- Female reproductive hormones may potentially influence ligament laxity.
- Core stability training improves dynamic lower extremity alignment, produces more efficient movements, and maintains the center of gravity over the base of support.
- Plyometric training improves dynamic lower extremity alignment, improves neuromuscular response time, and decreases landing forces.
- Balance training improves neuromuscular response time, improves muscular coordination, and improves functional ability.
- Teach athletes the following concepts for correction of neuromuscular deficits during athletic maneuvers: minimize lateral trunk sway, avoid valgus collapse of the knee, recruit the posterior chain musculature by maintaining controlled hip and knee flexion, and encourage equal bilateral use of the lower extremities.

ACKNOWLEDGMENTS

The authors would like to thank Terese Chmielewski, Ph.D., P.T., S.C.S., Reed Ferber, Ph.D., C.A.T., and Jeanette Vitello, D.P.T., O.C.S., for their contributions to this chapter.

REFERENCES

1. Arendt, E., and Dick, R. (1995). Knee injury patterns among men and women in collegiate basketball and soccer. NCAA data and review of literature. Am. J. Sports Med., 23:694–701.
2. Gray, J., Taunton, J.E., McKenzie, D.C., et al. (1985): A survey of injuries to the anterior cruciate ligament of the knee in female basketball players. Int. J. Sports Med., 6:314–316.
3. Hutchinson, M.R., and Ireland, M.L. (1995): Knee injuries in female athletes. Sports Med., 19:288–302.
4. Knapik, J.J., Sharp, M.A., Canham-Chervak, M., et al. (2001): Risk factors for training-related injuries among men and women in basic combat training. Med. Sci. Sports Exerc., 33:946–954.
5. Pester, S., and Smith, P.C. (1992): Stress fractures in the lower extremities of soldiers in basic training. Orthop. Rev., 21:297–303.
6. Reinker, K.A., and Ozburne, S. (1979): A comparison of male and female orthopaedic pathology in basic training. Mil. Med., 144:532–536.
7. Almeida, S.A., Trone, D.W., Leone, D.M., et al. (1995): Gender differences in musculoskeletal injury rates: A function of symptom reporting? Med. Sci. Sports Exerc., 31:1807–1812.
8. DeHaven, K.E., and Lintner, D.M. (1986): Athletic injuries: Comparison by age, sport, and gender. Am. J. Sports Med., 14:218–224.
9. Yoshioka, Y., Siu, D.W., Scudamore, R.A., and Cooke, T.D. (1989): Tibial anatomy and functional axes. J. Orthop. Res., 7:132–137.
10. Simoneau, G.G., Hoenig, K.J., Lepley, J.E., and Papanek, P.E. (1998): Influence of hip position and gender on active hip internal and external rotation. J. Orthop. Sports Phys. Ther., 28:158–164.
11. Kersnic, B., Iglic, A., Kralj-Iglic, V., et al. (1996): Determination of the femoral and pelvic geometrical parameters that are important for the hip joint contact stress: Differences between female and male. Pflugers Arch., 431:207–208.
12. Horton, M.G., and Hall, T.L. (1989): Quadriceps femoris muscle angle: Normal values and relationships with gender and selected skeletal measures. Phys. Ther., 69:897–901.
13. Hsu, R.W., Himeno, S., Coventry, M.B., and Chao, E.Y. (1990): Normal axial alignment of the lower extremity and load-bearing distribution at the knee. Clin. Orthop. Relat. Res., 255:215–227.
14. Aglietti, P., Insall, J.N., and Cerulli, G. (1983): Patellar pain and incongruence. I: Measurements of incongruence. Clin. Orthop. Relat. Res., 176:217–224.
15. Livingston, L.A. (1998): The quadriceps angle: A review of the literature. J. Orthop. Sports Phys. Ther., 28:105–109.
16. Woodland, L.H., and Francis, R.S. (1992): Parameters and comparisons of the quadriceps angle of college-aged men and women in the supine and standing positions. Am. J. Sports Med., 20:208–221.
17. Cowan, D.N., Jones, B.H., Frykman, P.N., et al. (1996): Lower limb morphology and risk of overuse injury among male infantry trainees. Med. Sci. Sports Exerc., 28:945–952.
18. James, S.L., Bates, B.T., and Osternig, L.R. (1978): Injuries to runners. Am. J. Sports Med., 6:40–50.
19. Messier, S.P., Davis, S.E., Curl, W.W., et al. (1991): Etiologic factors associated with patellofemoral pain in runners. Med. Sci. Sports Exerc., 23:1008–1015.
20. Mizuno, Y., Kumagai, M., Mattessich, S.M., et al. (2001): Q-angle influences tibiofemoral and patellofemoral kinematics. J. Orthop. Res., 19:834–840.
21. Good, L., Odensten, M., and Gillquist, J. (1991): Intercondylar notch measurements with special reference to anterior cruciate ligament surgery. Clin. Orthop. Relat. Res., 263:185–189.
22. Shelbourne, K.D., Facibene, W.A., and Hunt, J.J. (1997): Radiographic and intraoperative intercondylar notch width measurements in men and women with unilateral and bilateral anterior cruciate ligament tears. Knee Surg. Sports Traumatol. Arthrosc., 5:229–233.
23. Lund-Hanssen, H., Gannon, J., Engebretsen, L., et al. (1994): Intercondylar notch width and the risk for anterior cruciate ligament rupture. A case-control study in 46 female handball players. Acta Orthop. Scand., 65:529–532.
24. Ireland, M.L., Ballantyne, B.T., Little, K., and McClay, I.S. (2001): A radiographic analysis of the relationship between the size and shape of the intercondylar notch and anterior cruciate ligament injury. Knee Surg. Sports Traumatol. Arthrosc., 9:200–205.
25. Teitz, C.C., Hu, S.S., and Arendt, E.A. (1997): The female athlete: Evaluation and treatment of sports-related problems. J. Am. Acad. Orthop. Surg., 5:87–96.
26. Malinzak, R.A., Colby, S.M., Kirkendall, D.T., et al. (2001): A comparison of knee joint motion patterns between men and women in selected athletic tasks. Clin. Biomech., 16:438–445.
27. Tiberio, D. (1987): The effect of excessive subtalar joint pronation on patellofemoral mechanics: A theoretical model. J. Orthop. Sports Phys. Ther., 9:160–165.
28. Bendjaballah, M.Z., Shirazi-Adl, A., and Zukor, D.J. (1997): Finite element analysis of human knee joint in varus-valgus. Clin. Biomech., 12:139–148.
29. McLean, S.G., Neal, R.J., Myers, P.T., and Walters, M.R. (1999): Knee joint kinematics during the sidestep cutting maneuver: Potential for injury in women. Med. Sci. Sports Exerc., 31:959–968.
30. Dufek, J.S., and Bates, B.T. (1991): Biomechanical factors associated with injury during landing in jump sports. Sports Med., 12:326–337.
31. Ferretti, A., Papandrea, P., Conteduca, F., et al. (1992): Knee ligament injuries in volleyball players. Am. J. Sports Med., 20:203–207.
32. Huston, L.J., Vibert, B., Ashton-Miller, J.A., and Wojtys, E.M. (2001): Gender differences in knee angle when landing from a drop-jump. Am. J. Knee Surg., 14:215–220.
33. Lephart, S.M., Ferris, C.M., Riemann, B.L., et al. (2002): Gender differences in strength and lower extremity kinematics during landing. Clin. Orthop. Relat. Res., 401:162–169.
34. Beynnon, B.D., and Johnson, R.J. (1996): Anterior cruciate ligament injury rehabilitation in athletes. Biomechanical considerations. Sports Med., 22:54–64.
35. Hewett, T.E., Torg, J.S., and Boden, B.P. (2009): Video analysis of trunk and knee motion during non-contact anterior cruciate ligament injury in female athletes: lateral trunk and knee abduction motion are combined components of the injury mechanism. Br. J. Sports Med., 43:417–422.

36. Myer, G.D., Ford, K.R., Khoury, J., et al. (2011): Biomechanics laboratory–based prediction algorithm to identify female athletes with high knee loads that increase risk of ACL injury. Br. J. Sports Med., 45:245–252.

37. Hewett, T.E., Zazulak, B.T., Myer, G.D., and Ford, K.R. (2005): A review of electromyographic activation levels, timing differences, and increased anterior cruciate ligament injury incidence in female athletes. Br. J. Sports Med., 39:347–350.

38. Wojtys, E.M., Ashton-Miller, J.A., and Huston, L.J. (2002): A gender-related difference in the contribution of the knee musculature to sagittal-plane shear stiffness in subjects with similar knee laxity. J. Bone Joint Surg. Am., 84:10–16.

39. Granata, K.P., Wilson, S.E., and Padua, D.A. (2002): Gender differences in active musculoskeletal stiffness. Part I. Quantification in controlled measurements of knee joint dynamics. J. Electromyogr. Kinesiol., 12:119–126.

40. Hewett, T.E., Ford, K.R., Hoogenboom, B.J., and Myer, G.D. (2010): Understanding and preventing ACL injuries: Current biomechanical and epidemiological considerations—Update 2010. North Am. J. Sports Phys. Ther., 5:234–250.

41. Renstrom, P., Arms, S.W., Stanwyck, T.S., et al. (1986): Strain within the anterior cruciate ligament during hamstring and quadriceps activity. Am. J. Sports Med., 14:83–87.

42. Solomonow, M., Baratta, R., Zhou, B.H., et al. (1987): The synergistic action of the anterior cruciate ligament and thigh muscles in maintaining joint stability. Am. J. Sports Med., 15:207–213.

43. Huston, L.J., and Wojtys, E.M. (1996): Neuromuscular performance characteristics in elite female athletes. Am. J. Sports Med., 24:427–436.

44. Hewett, T.E., Myer, G.D., and Zazulak, B.T. (2008): Hamstrings to quadriceps peak torque ratios diverge between sexes with increasing isokinetic angular velocity. Sci. Med. Sport, 11:452–459.

45. Zazulak, B.T., Ponce, P.L., Straub, S.J., et al. (2005): Gender comparison of hip muscle activity during single-leg landing. J. Orthop. Sports Phys. Ther., 35:292–299.

46. Cowling, E.J., and Steele, J.R. (2001): Is lower limb muscle synchrony during landing affected by gender? Implications for variations in ACL injury rates. J. Electromyogr. Kinesiol., 11:263–268.

47. Ford, K.R., Myer, G.D., and Hewett, T.E. (2003): Valgus knee motion during landing in high school female and male basketball players. Med. Sci. Sports Exerc., 35:1745–1750.

48. Hewett, T.E., Myer, G.D., and Ford, K.R. (2006): Anterior cruciate ligament injuries in female athletes: Part 1, mechanisms and risk factors. Am. J. Sports Med., 34:299–311.

49. Myer, G.D., Ford, K.R., and Hewett, T.E. (2011): New method to identify high ACL injury risk athletes using clinic based measurements and freeware computer analysis. Br. J. Sports Med., 45:238–244.

50. Myer, G.D., Ford, K.R., Khoury, J., et al. (2010): Development and validation of a clinic-based prediction tool to identify female athletes at high risk for anterior cruciate ligament injury. Am. J. Sports Med., 38:2025–2033.

51. Paterno, M.V., Schmitt, L.C., Ford, K.R., et al. (2010): Biomechanical measures during landing and postural stability predict second anterior cruciate ligament injury after anterior cruciate ligament reconstruction and return to sport. Am. J. Sports Med., 38:1968–1978.

52. Hewett, T.E., Myer, G.D., Ford, K.R., et al. (2005): Biomechanical measures of neuromuscular control and valgus loading of the knee predict anterior cruciate ligament injury risk in female athletes: A prospective study. Am. J. Sports Med., 33:492–501.

53. Zazulak, B., Cholewicki, J., and Reeves, N.P. (2008): Neuromuscular control of trunk stability: Clinical implications for sports injury prevention. J. Am. Acad. Orthop. Surg., 16:497–505.

54. Zazulak, B.T., Hewett, T.E., Reeves, N.P., et al. (2007): The effects of core proprioception on knee injury: a prospective biomechanical-epidemiological study. Am. J. Sports Med., 35:368–373.

55. Zazulak, B.T., Hewett, T.E., Reeves, N.P., et al. (2007): Deficits in neuromuscular control of the trunk predict knee injury risk: A prospective biomechanical-epidemiologic study. Am. J. Sports Med., 35:1123–1130.

56. Hewett, T.E., Myer, G.D., and Ford, K.R. (2004): Decrease in neuromuscular control about the knee with maturation in female athletes. J. Bone Joint Surg. Am., 86:1601–1608.

57. Krosshaug, T., Nakamae, A., Boden, B.P., et al. (2007): Mechanisms of anterior cruciate ligament injury in basketball: Video analysis of 39 cases. Am. J. Sports Med., 35:359–367.

58. Heitz, N.A. (1999): Hormonal changes throughout the menstrual cycle and increased anterior cruciate ligament laxity in females. J. Athl. Train., 34:144–149.

59. Liu, S.H. (1997): Estrogen affects the cellular metabolism of the anterior cruciate ligament: A potential explanation for female athletic injury. Am. Orthop. Soc. Sports Med., 25:704–709.

60. Yu, W.D. (2001): Combined effects of estrogen and progesterone on the anterior cruciate ligament. Clin. Orthop. Relat. Res., 383:268–281.

61. Zazulak, B.T., Paterno, M., Myer, G.D., et al. (2006): The effects of the menstrual cycle on anterior knee laxity: A systematic review. Sports Med., 36:847–862.

62. Myklebust, G., Maehlum, S., Holm, I., and Bahr, R. (1998): A prospective cohort study of anterior cruciate ligament injuries in elite Norwegian team handball. Scand. J. Med. Sci. Sports, 8:149–153.

63. Myklebust, G., Engebretsen, L., Braekken, I.H., et al. (2003): Prevention of anterior cruciate ligament injuries in female team handball players: A prospective intervention study over three seasons. Clin. J. Sport Med., 13:71–78.

64. Arendt, E.A., Agel, J., and Dick, R. (1999): Anterior cruciate ligament injury patterns among collegiate men and women. J. Athl. Train., 34:86–92.

65. Arendt, E.A., Bershadsky, B., and Agel, J. (2002): Periodicity of noncontact anterior cruciate ligament injuries during the menstrual cycle. J. Gend. Specif. Med., 5:19–26.

66. Wojtys, E.M., Huston, L.J., Lindenfeld, T.N., et al. (1998): Association between the menstrual cycle and anterior cruciate ligament injuries in female athletes. Am. J. Sports Med., 26:614–619.

67. Slauterback, J.R., Fuzie, S.F., Smith, M.P., et al. (2002): The menstrual cycle, sex hormones, and anterior cruciate ligament injury. J. Athl. Train., 37:275–280.

68. Hewett, T.E., Zazulak, B.T., and Myer, G.D., Effects of the menstrual cycle on anterior cruciate ligament injury risk: A systematic review. Am. J. Sports Med., 35:659–668.

69. Myer, G.D., Ford, K.R., and Hewett, T.E. (2004): Rationale and clinical techniques for anterior cruciate ligament injury prevention among female athletes. J. Athl. Train., 39:352–401.

70. Myer, G.D., Ford, K.R., and Hewett, T.E. (2003): Tuck jump assessment for reducing anterior cruciate ligament injury risk. Athl. Ther. Today, 13(5):39–44.

71. Clark, M.A., Fater, D., and Reuteman, P. (2000): Core (trunk) stabilization and its importance for closed kinetic chain rehabilitation. Orthop. Phys. Ther. Clin. North Am., 9:119–135.

72. Roetert, P. (2001): 3-D balance and core stability. In: Foran, B. (ed.). High Performance Sports Conditioning. Champaign, IL., Human Kinetics, p. 126.

73. Toth, A.P., and Cordasco, F.A. (2001): Anterior cruciate ligament injuries in the female athlete. J. Gend. Specif. Med., 4:25–34.

74. Porterfield, J.A., and DeRosa, C. (1991): Mechanical Low Back Pain: Perspectives in Functional Anatomy. Philadelphia, Saunders.

75. Cresswell, A.G., Grundstrom, H., and Thorstensson, A. (1992): Observations on intra-abdominal pressure and patterns of abdominal intra-muscular activity in man. Acta Physiol. Scand., 144:409–418.

76. Johnson, P.J. (2002): Training the trunk in the athlete. Strength Cond. J., 24:52–59.

77. Hewett, T.E., Stroupe, A.L., Nance, T.A., and Noyes, F.R. (1996): Plyometric training in female athletes. Decreased impact forces and increased hamstring torques. Am. J. Sports Med., 24:765–773.

78. Roniger, L.R. (2002): Training improves ACL outcomes in female athletes. Biomechanics, January, pp. 51–57.

79. Heidt, R.S., Jr., Sweeterman, L.M., Carlonas, R.L., et al. (2000): Avoidance of soccer injuries with preseason conditioning. Am. J. Sports Med., 28:659–662.

80. Mizrahi, J., and Susak, Z. (1982): Analysis of parameters affecting impact force attenuation during landing in human vertical free fall. Eng. Med., 11:141–147.

81. McNair, P.J., Prapavessis, H., and Callender, K. (2000): Decreasing landing forces: Effect of instruction. Br. J. Sports Med., 34:293–296.

82. Prapavessis, H., and McNair, P.J. (1999): Effects of instruction in jumping technique and experience jumping on ground reaction forces. J. Orthop. Sports Phys. Ther., 29:352–356.

83. Beynnon, B.D., Ryder, S.H., Konradsen, L., et al. (1999): The effect of anterior cruciate ligament trauma and bracing on knee proprioception. Am. J. Sports Med., 27:150–155.

84. Friden, T., Roberts, D., Zatterstrom, R., et al. (1996): Proprioception in the nearly extended knee. Measurements of position and movement in healthy individuals and in symptomatic anterior cruciate ligament injured patients. Knee Surg. Sports Traumatol. Arthrosc., 4:217–224.

85. Lentell, G., Baas, B., Lopez, D., et al. (1995): The contributions of proprioceptive deficits, muscle function, and anatomic laxity to functional instability of the ankle. J. Orthop. Sports Phys. Ther., 21:206–215.

86. Lephart, S.M., Pincivero, D.M., Giraldo, J.L., and Fu, F.H. (1997): The role of proprioception in the management and rehabilitation of athletic injuries. Am. J. Sports Med., 25:130–137.

87. Wooley, S.M., Rubin, A.M., Kantner, R.M., et al. (1993): Differentiation of balance deficits through examination of selected components of static stabilometry. J. Otolaryngol., 22:368–375.

88. Chmielewski, T.L., Wilk, K.E., and Snyder-Mackler, L. (2002): Changes in weight-bearing following injury or surgical reconstruction of the ACL: Relationship to quadriceps strength and function. Gait Posture, 16:87–95.

89. Leanderson, J., Wykman, A., and Eriksson, E. (1993): Ankle sprain and postural sway in basketball players. Knee Surg. Sports Traumatol. Arthrosc., 1:203–305.

90. Lysholm, M., Ledin, T., Odkvist, L.M., and Good, L. (1998): Postural control—A comparison between patients with chronic anterior cruciate ligament insufficiency and healthy individuals. Scand. J. Med. Sci. Sports, 8:432–438.

91. Shiraishi, M., Mizuta, H., Kubota, K., et al. (1996): Stabilometric assessment in the anterior cruciate ligament–reconstructed knee. Clin. J. Sport Med., 6:32–39.

92. Caraffa, A., Cerulli, G., Projetti, M., et al. (1996): Prevention of anterior cruciate ligament injuries in soccer. A prospective controlled study of proprioceptive training. Knee Surg. Sports Traumatol. Arthrosc., 4:19–21.

93. Wedderkopp, N., Kaltoft, M., Lundgaard, B., et al. (1999): Prevention of injuries in young female players in European team handball. A prospective intervention study. Scand. J. Med. Sci. Sports, 9:41–47.

94. Soderman, K., Werner, S., Pietila, T., et al. (2000): Balance board training: Prevention of traumatic injuries of the lower extremities in female soccer players? A prospective randomized intervention study. Knee Surg. Sports Traumatol. Arthrosc., 8:356–363.

95. Osborne, M.D., Chou, L.S., Laskowski, E.R., et al. (2001): The effect of ankle disk training on muscle reaction time in subjects with a history of ankle sprain. Am. J. Sports Med., 29:627–635.

96. Fitzgerald, G.K., Axe, M.J., and Snyder-Mackler, L. (2000): The efficacy of perturbation training in nonoperative anterior cruciate ligament rehabilitation programs for physical active individuals. Phys. Ther., 80:128–140.

97. Beard, D.J., Kyberd, P.J., Fergusson, C.M., et al. (1993): Proprioception after rupture of the anterior cruciate ligament. An objective indication of the need for surgery? J. Bone Joint Surg. Br., 75:311–315.

98. Ihara, H., and Nakayama, A. (1986): Dynamic joint control training for knee ligament injuries. Am. J. Sports Med., 14:309–315.

99. Chmielewski, T.L., Rudolph, K.S., and Snyder-Mackler, L. (2002): Development of dynamic knee stability after acute ACL injury. J. Electromyogr. Kinesiol., 12:267–274.

Biomechanical Implications in Shoulder and Knee Rehabilitation

Michael M. Reinold, PT, DPT, SCS, ATC, CSCS, and Charles D. Simpson II, DPT, CSCS

CHAPTER OBJECTIVES

- Summarize the importance of thorough knowledge of the biomechanical factors associated with rehabilitation.
- Describe the best rehabilitation exercises to elicit recruitment of the glenohumeral and scapulothoracic musculature.
- Explain the normal function of the supraspinatus and deltoid musculature during various ranges of motion.
- Identify which shoulder exercises produce the most amount of supraspinatus activity with the least amount of deltoid activity.
- Explain the effect of pathologic changes on shoulder biomechanics.
- Identify which exercises produce cocontraction of the quadriceps and hamstrings musculature.

- Explain the tibiofemoral shear forces observed during open kinetic chain and closed kinetic chain exercises.
- Describe the in vivo forces on the anterior cruciate ligament during open kinetic chain, closed kinetic chain, bicycle, and stair-climbing exercises.
- Explain the normal arthrokinematics of the patellofemoral joint.
- Summarize the stress on the patellofemoral joint during open kinetic chain and closed kinetic chain exercises.
- Select safe and appropriate exercises for the glenohumeral musculature, scapulothoracic musculature, anterior cruciate ligament, posterior cruciate ligament, and patellofemoral joint.

Biomechanical analysis of rehabilitation exercises has gained recent attention in sports medicine and orthopedic practice. Several investigators have sought to quantify the kinematics, kinetics, and electromyographic (EMG) activity during common rehabilitation exercises in an attempt to fully understand the implications of each exercise on the arthrokinematics and soft tissues of the shoulder and knee. Advances in understanding the biomechanical factors associated with rehabilitation have led to enhancement of rehabilitation programs that place minimal strain on specific healing structures while returning the injured athlete to competition as quickly and safely as possible. The purpose of this chapter is to provide an overview of the biomechanical implications associated with rehabilitation of the athlete's shoulder and knee.

BIOMECHANICAL IMPLICATIONS OF SHOULDER REHABILITATION

The glenohumeral joint exhibits the greatest amount of motion of any articulation in the human body, although little inherent stability is provided by its osseous configuration. Functional stability is accomplished through the integrated functions of the joint capsule, ligaments, and glenoid labrum, as well as through neuromuscular control and dynamic stabilization of the surrounding musculature, particularly the rotator cuff muscles.[1-4] The rotator cuff musculature maintains stability of the glenohumeral joint by compressing the humeral head into the concave glenoid fossa during upper extremity motion.[5] Thus, the glenohumeral muscles play a vital role in normal arthrokinematics and asymptomatic shoulder function.

Rehabilitation programs for the shoulder joint often focus on restoring maximum strength and muscular balance, particularly of the rotator cuff and scapulothoracic joint. The majority of research on shoulder biomechanics has focused on quantifying the EMG activity of particular muscles during common rehabilitation exercises, the goal of which is to determine the most optimal exercise to recruit specific muscle activity and maximize shoulder strength and efficiency.

ELECTROMYOGRAPHIC ANALYSIS OF SHOULDER EXERCISES

Townsend et al[6] conducted one of the first comprehensive studies analyzing EMG activity in the shoulder musculature during rehabilitation exercises. Dynamic fine-wire EMG activity in the four rotator cuff muscles, pectoralis major, latissimus dorsi, and the three portions of the deltoid was studied in 15 healthy male subjects during 17 common shoulder exercises. The authors quantified the exercises that produced the most activity in each specific muscle (Table 10-1).

For the anterior deltoid, exercises involving elevation of the shoulder, such as scaption with internal rotation (empty can), scaption with external rotation (full can), and forward flexion, produced the greatest amount of activity at approximately 70% manual muscle test activity (70% MMT). This was also consistent with results for the middle deltoid, although exercises in the prone position involving horizontal abduction produced approximately 80% MMT. The posterior deltoid showed the greatest amount of activity in the prone position during such exercises as horizontal abduction and rowing at approximately 90% MMT.

Similar to the anterior deltoid, the supraspinatus muscle was most active during shoulder elevation movements, although the military press (from 0° to 30°) produced the greatest amount of supraspinatus activity at 80% MMT.

Table 10-1 Electromyographic Analysis of Glenohumeral Musculature*

Muscle	Exercise	Peak (% MMT ± SD)	Duration (% Exercise)	Peak Arc Range (°)
Anterior deltoid	Scaption IR	72 ± 23	50	90-150
	Scaption ER	71 ± 39	30	90-120
	Flexion	69 ± 24	31	90-120
	Military press	62 ± 26	50	60-90
	Abduction	62 ± 28	31	90-120
Middle deltoid	Scaption IR	83 ± 13	70	90-120
	Horiz. abd. IR	80 ± 23	38	90-120
	Horiz. abd. ER	79 ± 20	57	90-120
	Flexion	73 ± 16	31	90-120
	Scaption ER	72 ± 13	58	90-120
	Rowing	72 ± 20	43	90-120
	Military press	72 ± 24	38	90-120
	Abduction	64 ± 13	31	90-120
	Deceleration	58 ± 20	27	90-60
Posterior deltoid	Horiz. abd. IR	93 ± 45	63	90-120
	Horiz. abd. ER	92 ± 49	57	90-120
	Rowing	88 ± 40	57	90-120
	Extension	71 ± 30	44	90-120
	External Rot.	64 ± 62	43	60-90
	Deceleration	63 ± 28	27	60-90
Supraspinatus	Military press	80 ± 48	50	0-30
	Scaption IR	74 ± 33	40	90-120
	Flexion	67 ± 14	31	90-120
	Scaption ER	64 ± 28	25	90-120

Table 10-1 Electromyographic Analysis of Glenohumeral Musculature*—cont'd

Muscle	Exercise	Peak (% MMT ± SD)	Duration (% Exercise)	Peak Arc Range (°)
Subscapularis	Scaption IR	62 ± 33	22	120-150
	Military press	56 ± 48	50	60-90
	Flexion	52 ± 42	23	120-150
	Abduction	50 ± 44	23	120-150
Infraspinatus	Horiz. abd. ER	88 ± 25	71	90-120
	External rot.	85 ± 26	43	60-90
	Horiz. abd. IR	74 ± 32	38	90-120
	Abduction	74 ± 23	31	90-120
	Flexion	66 ± 15	23	90-120
	Scaption ER	60 ± 21	38	90-120
	Deceleration	57 ± 17	27	90-60
	Push-up (hands together)	54 ± 31	38	90-60
Teres minor	External rot.	80 ± 14	57	60-90
	Horiz. abd. ER	74 ± 28	57	60-90
	Horiz. abd. IR	68 ± 36	43	90-120
Pectoralis major	Press-up	84 ± 42	75	½ pk-pk
	Push-up (hands apart)	64 ± 63	50	60-30
Latissimus dorsi	Press-up	55 ± 27	50	pk-1 sec

Data from Townsend, H., Jobe, F.W., Pink, M., and Perry, J. (1991): Electromyographic analysis of the glenohumeral muscles during a baseball rehabilitation program. Am. J. Sports Med., 19:264–272.
* Ranked by intensity of peak arc.
ER, External rotation; *Horiz. abd.,* horizontal abduction; *IR,* internal rotation; *MMT,* manual muscle test; *pk,* peak; *SD,* standard deviation.

Comparing the empty can and full can exercises, the authors found 74% MMT during the empty can and 64% MMT during the full can.

The exercises with the most activity in the subscapularis muscle also included those involving shoulder elevation, though at a moderate intensity of approximately 55% MMT. Interestingly, the side-lying internal rotation exercise was not found to produce significant activity in the subscapularis, although the similar exercise of internal rotation at 0° abduction with exercise tubing was shown to have 52% maximal voluntary contraction by Hintermeister et al.[7] Others have recommended motions involving lifting the hand off the lower part of the back and motions that replicate a tennis forehand with internal rotation and horizontal adduction.

The infraspinatus and teres minor muscles showed similar results with high activity during the side-lying external rotation exercise (85% for the infraspinatus and 80% for the teres minor). Exercises in the prone position involving horizontal abduction also produced high activity in the external rotators, with up to 88% MMT (range, 68% to 88% MMT) in the infraspinatus during prone horizontal abduction with external rotation.

The press-up exercise was found to elicit the most activity in the latissimus dorsi (55% MMT) and the pectoralis major (84%). This is consistent with the prime function of shoulder depression for each of these muscles. In comparison, the push-up produced 64% MMT in the pectoralis major.

Townsend et al[6] studied 17 exercises and recommended inclusion of the empty can exercise, shoulder flexion, prone horizontal abduction with external rotation, and the press-up in shoulder rehabilitation programs based on the high activity in each muscle examined during these exercises.

Several research studies have since expanded on the work of Townsend et al.[6] In particular, researchers have sought to compare the effectiveness of several exercises for the external rotators, supraspinatus, deltoid, and scapulothoracic musculature. The following sections discuss each one in detail.

External Rotators

An overhead throwing athlete requires the rotator cuff to maintain an adequate amount of glenohumeral joint congruency for asymptomatic function.[8] Strength of the infraspinatus and teres minor is integral during the overhead throwing motion to develop a compressive force equal to body weight (BW) at the shoulder joint to prevent distraction.[9] Andrews and Angelo[10] found that overhead throwers most often have rotator cuff tears located from the mid–supraspinatus posterior to the midinfraspinatus area, which they believed to be a result of the compressive force produced to resist distraction, horizontal adduction, and internal rotation at the shoulder during arm deceleration. Thus, the external rotators are muscles that often appear weak and are affected by different pathologic shoulder conditions, such as internal impingement,[11,12] joint laxity, labral lesions, and rotator cuff lesions,[13,14] particularly in overhead throwing athletes.[15,16] Consequently, many authors have advocated emphasis on strengthening of external rotation during rehabilitation or athletic conditioning programs to enhance muscular strength, endurance, and dynamic stability in overhead throwing athletes.

Several studies have documented the EMG activity in the glenohumeral musculature during specific shoulder exercises.[6,17-25] Variations in experimental methodology have resulted in conflicting outcomes and controversy in the selection of exercises. As discussed previously, Townsend et al[6] evaluated infraspinatus and teres minor activity during 17 shoulder exercises. The authors determined that the exercise eliciting the most EMG activity in the infraspinatus muscle was prone horizontal abduction with external rotation (88% MMT) and that the most effective exercise for the teres minor muscle was side-lying external rotation (80% MMT).

Similarly, Blackburn et al[18] performed EMG analysis of the rotator cuff muscles in 28 healthy subjects during a series of 23 common posterior rotator cuff–strengthening exercises. The authors reported high levels of EMG activity in the infraspinatus (80% EMG activity) and teres minor (70% EMG activity) when the prone horizontal abduction movement at 90° and 100° of abduction with full external rotation was performed by 28 healthy subjects.

Conversely, Greenfield et al[20] compared shoulder rotational strength in the scapular and frontal planes during isokinetic testing in 20 healthy subjects. The authors reported that no significant differences were found in internal rotation strength between positions; however, external rotation strength was significantly higher in the scapular plane, thus suggesting that the plane of the scapula may be a more effective position to exercise the external rotators.

Ballantyne et al[17] compared EMG activity in the external rotators during side-lying external rotation and during external rotation in the prone position at 90° of abduction in 40 subjects. The authors reported similar EMG findings for the infraspinatus and teres minor during both exercises, with approximately 50% normalized activity for each muscle. Conversely, in the previously cited study by Blackburn et al,[18] the authors compared side-lying external rotation and prone external rotation exercises and noted greater EMG activity during prone external rotation in the infraspinatus (prone, 80%; side lying, 30%) and teres minor (prone, 88%; side lying, 45%).

Reinold et al analyzed several different exercises commonly used to strengthen the external rotators to determine the most effect exercise and position to recruit muscle activity in the posterior rotator cuff.[26] Integrated EMG activity in the infraspinatus, teres minor, supraspinatus, posterior deltoid, and middle deltoid in 10 asymptomatic subjects (5 male and 5 female subjects; mean age, 28.1 years; range, 22 to 38 years) was analyzed during seven exercises: prone horizontal abduction at 100° of abduction, full external rotation and prone external rotation at 90° of abduction, standing external rotation at 90° of abduction, standing external rotation at 45° in the scapular plane, standing external rotation at 0° of abduction, standing external rotation at 0° of abduction with a towel roll, and side-lying external rotation at 0° of abduction.

Based on the results of this study, the exercise that elicited the most combined EMG activity in the infraspinatus and teres minor was side-lying external rotation (infraspinatus, 62% maximum voluntary isometric contraction [MVIC]; teres minor, 67%), followed closely by external rotation in the scapular plane (infraspinatus, 53%; teres minor, 55%), and finally prone external rotation in the 90° abducted position (infraspinatus, 50%; teres minor, 48%) (Table 10-2).

Exercises in the 90° abducted position are often incorporated to simulate the position and strain on the shoulder during similar overhead activities such as throwing. This position produced moderate activity in the external rotators but also increased activity in the deltoid and supraspinatus to stabilize the shoulder. It appears that the amount of infraspinatus and teres minor activity progressively decreases as the shoulder moves into an abducted position whereas activity in the supraspinatus and deltoid increases. This may imply that as the arm moves into a position of less shoulder stability, the supraspinatus and deltoid are active to assist in the external rotation movement while providing some degree of glenohumeral stability through muscular contraction.

Table 10-2 Peak Muscle Activity During External Rotation Exercises (% MVIC, Mean ± SD)

Muscle	Prone Horizontal Abduction (100°, Full ER)	Prone ER (90° Abduction)	Standing ER 90° (90° Abduction)	Standing ER Scapular Plane	Standing ER 0°	Standing ER 0° with Towel	Side-Lying ER	Significance*
Supraspinatus	82 ± 37	68 ± 33	57 ± 32	32 ± 24	41 ± 39	41 ± 37	51 ± 47	a, c, d, e
Middle deltoid	82 ± 32	49 ± 15	55 ± 23	38 ± 19	11 ± 7	11 ± 6	36 ± 23	a, b, c, f
Posterior deltoid	88 ± 33	79 ± 31	59 ± 33	43 ± 30	27 ± 27	31 ± 27	52 ± 42	a, c, d, f, g
Infraspinatus	39 ± 17	56 ± 30	59 ± 38	53 ± 24	40 ± 15	51 ± 14	62 ± 13	h
Teres minor	41 ± 24	41 ± 22	33 ± 18	64 ± 51	34 ± 14	46 ± 22	62 ± 31	

* Significant finding for the exercises (P < .050).

a, Prone horizontal abduction > ER 90°, ER scapular plane, ER 0°, ER 0° with towel, side-lying ER; *b*, prone horizontal abduction > prone ER; *c*, prone ER > ER 0° and ER 0° with towel; *d*, prone ER > ER scapular plane; *e*, prone ER > side-lying ER; *f*, 90° ER > ER 0° and ER 0° with towel; *g*, side-lying ER > ER 0° and ER 0° with towel; *h*, side-lying ER > prone horizontal abduction.

ER, External rotation; *MVIC*, maximum voluntary isometric contraction.

In the standing position, external rotation at 90° of abduction may have a functional advantage over 0° of abduction, and in the scapular plane, because of the close replication of this position in sporting activities the combination of abduction and external rotation places strain on the shoulder's capsule, particularly the anterior band of the inferior glenohumeral ligament.[27,28] When the arm is not in an abducted position, external rotation places less strain on this portion of the joint capsule. Therefore, although muscle activity was low to moderate during external rotation at 0° of abduction, this rehabilitation exercise may be worthwhile when strain of the inferior glenohumeral ligament is a concern. Side-lying external rotation may be the most optimal exercise to strengthen the external rotators based on the highest amount of EMG activity observed during this study.

Theoretically, external rotation at 0° of abduction with a towel roll provides both low capsular strain and also good balance between the muscles that externally rotate the arm and the muscles that adduct the arm to hold the towel. Our clinical experience has shown that adding a towel roll to the external rotation exercise provides assistance to the patient by ensuring that proper technique is observed without muscle substitution (Fig. 10-1). With the addition of a towel roll to the exercise, a tendency toward higher activity in the posterior rotator cuff was consistently seen as well. An approximately 20% to 25% increase in infraspinatus and teres minor EMG activity was noted with the use of a towel roll.

Furthermore, external rotation in the scapular plane may be an effective exercise during rehabilitation because of the moderate amount of muscular activity in each of the muscles tested, with a moderate amount of capsular strain occurring in the 45° abducted position (Fig. 10-2). This exercise may offer a compromise between strengthening and stabilization.

Clinical Pearl #1

The exercises that produced the greatest amount of activity in the external rotators were side-lying external rotation, external rotation in the scapular plane, and external rotation at 90° of abduction (both standing and in the prone position).

Clinical Pearl #2

As the angle of arm elevation increases during shoulder external rotation exercises, the amount of supraspinatus and deltoid activity increases, whereas the amount of infraspinatus and teres minor activity decreases.

Clinical Pearl #3

Adding a towel roll to external rotation at 0° of abduction results in higher EMG activity in the infraspinatus and teres minor.

Supraspinatus and Deltoid

Numerous investigators have studied EMG activity in the supraspinatus during rehabilitation exercises. Controversy exists regarding the optimal exercise to elicit muscle activity. Jobe and Moynes[29] were the first to recommend elevation in the scapular plane with internal rotation, or the empty can exercise. The authors recommended this exercise for strengthening the

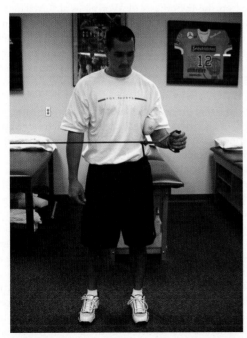

FIGURE 10-1 External rotation at 0° of abduction with a towel roll placed between the arm and body.

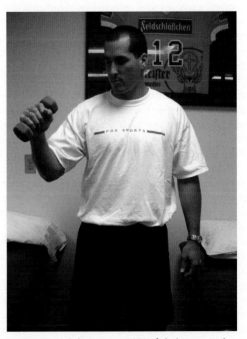

FIGURE 10-2 External rotation at 45° of abduction in the scapular plane.

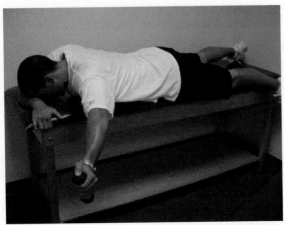

FIGURE 10-3 Prone horizontal abduction at 100° of abduction and full external rotation.

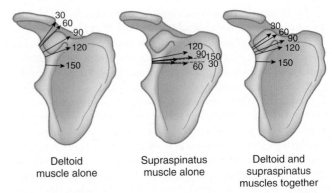

Deltoid muscle alone   Supraspinatus muscle alone   Deltoid and supraspinatus muscles together

FIGURE 10-4 Direction of the magnitude of the resultant force vector for different glenohumeral joint positions as a function of different muscle activity. *(From Morrey, B.F., Itoi, E., and An, K.N. [1998]: Biomechanics of the shoulder. In: Rockwood, C.A., and Matsen, F.A. [eds]. The Shoulder, 2nd ed. Philadelphia, Saunders, pp. 233–276.)*

supraspinatus because of the high EMG activity observed during this movement. The recommendation for the empty can exercise was further strengthened by the work of Townsend et al,[6] who reported greater amounts of EMG activity in the supraspinatus and deltoid muscles during the empty can exercise than during exercises consisting of elevation in the scapular plane with external rotation, or the full can exercise, although statistical analysis was not performed to compare the exercises (see Table 10-1).

In clinical studies, numerous authors have suggested that the empty can exercise may provoke pain in many patients by encroaching on soft tissue within the subacromial space during this impingement-type maneuver. Numerous authors have since compared the empty can exercise with several other common supraspinatus exercises to determine whether exercises that place the shoulder in less of a disadvantageous position elicit similar amounts of supraspinatus activity.

Blackburn et al[18] compared EMG activity in the rotator cuff during several exercises and reported no significant differences in supraspinatus activity during the empty can and full can exercises. However, the authors did report a statistically significant increase in supraspinatus activity during prone horizontal abduction at 100° with full external rotation (Fig. 10-3).

Worrell et al[25] compared the amount of supraspinatus activity during the empty can exercise recommended by Jobe and Moynes[29] and the prone horizontal abduction exercise recommended by Blackburn and associates.[18] The authors performed fine-wire EMG and handheld dynamometer measurements in 22 healthy subjects and reported greater supraspinatus activity during the prone exercise but less total force production than during the empty can exercise. The authors hypothesized that although supraspinatus activity was greater in the prone position, a greater amount of surrounding muscular activity was noted during the empty can exercise.

The effect of increased deltoid activity during arm elevation is a concern for the rehabilitation specialist, especially when a patient with subacromial impingement or pathologic rotator cuff conditions is being rehabilitated. Morrey et al[30] examined the resultant force vectors of the deltoid and supraspinatus during arm elevation at various degrees of motion. Deltoid activity alone exhibited a superiorly orientated force vector from 0° to 90° and a compressive force on the glenohumeral joint at 120° to 150°. Conversely, the supraspinatus muscle produced a

consistent compressive force throughout the range of elevation (Fig. 10-4). In patients with subacromial impingement, weak posterior rotator cuff muscles, inefficient dynamic stabilization, or pathologic changes in the rotator cuff, exercises that produce high levels of deltoid activity may be detrimental because of the amount of superior humeral head migration observed when the rotator cuff does not efficiently compress the humeral head within the glenoid fossa. Superior humeral head migration may be disadvantageous to patients with rotator cuff pathology or decreased stability of the glenohumeral joint. Superior humeral head migration may result in subacromial impingement, subdeltoid bursa trauma, and bursal thickening. The previously mentioned pathologies can result in tendon degeneration and eventually failure of the rotator cuff. Therefore, exercises are often chosen that minimize the opportunity for the deltoid to overpower the rotator cuff musculature during arm elevation.[31]

Based on the hypothesis of Worrell et al,[25] Malanga et al[22] examined EMG activity in the supraspinatus and deltoid muscles during the empty can and prone exercises in 17 healthy subjects. The authors reported no significant differences in supraspinatus EMG activity during the two exercises (empty can, 107%; prone, 94%). However, a statistically significant increase in posterior deltoid EMG activity was observed during the prone exercise (empty can, 76%; prone, 96%) and significantly greater anterior deltoid EMG activity during the empty can exercise (empty can, 96%; prone, 65%). Middle deltoid EMG activity was high during both exercises (empty can, 104%; prone, 111%).

In a similar study, Kelly et al[32] compared isometric EMG activity in the supraspinatus and deltoid muscles during the full can and empty can exercises in 11 healthy subjects. The authors again reported no significant difference in supraspinatus activity; however, they did note that the least amount of surrounding muscle activity was observed during the full can position and therefore recommended this position for manual muscle testing of the supraspinatus.

Takeda et al[33] examined the most effective exercise for strengthening the supraspinatus by comparing magnetic resonance imaging (MRI) T2 relaxation times in the shoulders of six healthy subjects. The authors reported an increase in relaxation time that correlated well with concentric and eccentric muscle contractions. Subjects performed the empty can, full can, and prone

Table 10-3 **Peak Muscle Activity During Supraspinatus Exercises (Mean % MVIC ± SD)**

Muscle	Full Can	Empty Can	Prone
Supraspinatus	62.2 ± 39.9	62.7 ± 45.2	66.8 ± 50.1
Middle deltoid	52.2 ± 26.6	76.9 ± 43.9*	63.1 ± 30.8*
Posterior deltoid	37.8 ± 32.0	54.1 ± 28.3*	86.7 ± 52.7*

* Significantly greater muscle activity in comparison to the full can exercise (P = .017).

Empty can, Scaption with internal rotation; *full can,* scaption with external rotation; *prone,* prone horizontal abduction at 100° with external rotation.

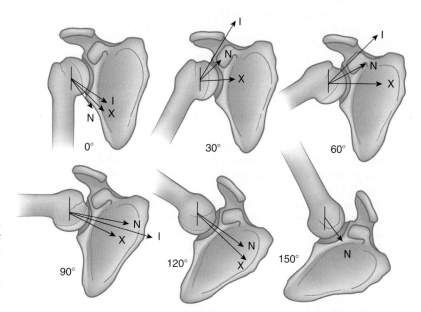

FIGURE 10-5 Position of the resultant force vector of the shoulder for different positions of arm elevation in (*N*) neutral rotation, (*I*) internal rotation, and (*X*) external rotation. *(From Poppen, N.K., and Walker, P.S. [1978]: Forces at the glenohumeral joint in abduction. Clin. Orthop. Relat. Res., 135:165–170.)*

exercises, and MRI scans were obtained immediately before and after each exercise. The change in relaxation in the supraspinatus was significantly higher during the empty can (10.5 msec) and full can (10.5 msec) exercises than during the prone exercise (3.6 msec). The least amount of deltoid activity was observed during the full can exercise.

Reinold et al[34] were the first to examine both supraspinatus and deltoid muscle activity dynamically during all three exercises—empty can, full can, and prone. The authors measured fine-wire EMG activity in the dominant shoulder of 22 healthy subjects (15 male and 7 female subjects; mean age, 27 ± 5 years) (Table 10-3). EMG activity was normalized to MVIC and analyzed with a one-way repeated measures analysis of variance. The authors reported no significant difference in supraspinatus activity, which ranged from 62% to 67% MVIC during each exercise. However, post hoc analysis revealed significant differences in deltoid activity during the three exercises. The posterior deltoid showed the greatest activity during the prone full can exercise, whereas the middle deltoid displayed the greatest activity during the empty can and prone full can exercises. This information is important to consider when creating a strength program to maximize strength gains in the supraspinatus.

Biomechanically, Poppen and Walker[35] examined the resultant force vectors of the glenohumeral joint during elevation with the arm positioned in neutral, internal rotation, and external rotation, similar to the empty can and full can exercises, respectively. The authors reported that at angles below 90° of abduction, the empty can position resulted in a superiorly orientated force vector whereas the full can position produced a compressive force from 0° to 120° (Fig. 10-5). These results of Poppen and Walker[35] may correlate well with the previously mentioned studies reporting increased deltoid activity and thus superior humeral head migration during the empty can exercise.

The empty can and full can exercises have also been examined to determine the accuracy of each when lesions of the supraspinatus tendon are detected. Itoi et al[36] performed the two tests in 143 shoulders before MRI scans to detect a full-thickness tear of the rotator cuff. The authors considered a test positive if the subject exhibited pain, weakness, or both. The authors reported 75% accuracy with the full can test versus 70% with the empty can test. However, the empty can test also provoked greater pain.

Anatomically, internal rotation of the humerus during the empty can exercise does not allow the greater tuberosity to clear from under the acromion during arm elevation, which may increase risk for subacromial impingement because of decreased acromial space width. Biomechanically, shoulder abduction performed in extreme internal rotation progressively decreases the abduction moment arm of the supraspinatus from 0° to 90° of abduction. A diminished mechanical advantage may result in the supraspinatus needing to generate more force, thereby increasing tensile stress on an injured or healing tendon. This may also make the exercise more challenging for patients with weakness and facilitate compensatory movements such as the shoulder shrug.[31]

Scapular kinematics is also different between these exercises. Scapular internal rotation, or "winging" (which occurs in the transverse plane with the scapular medial border moving posteriorly away from the trunk) and anterior tilt (which occurs in the sagittal plane with the scapular inferior angle moving posteriorly away from the trunk), is greater with the empty can exercise than with the full can exercise. This occurs in part because internal rotation of the humerus in the empty can position places tension on both the posteroinferior capsule of the glenohumeral joint and the rotator cuff (primarily the infraspinatus). Tension in these structures contributes to anterior tilt and internal rotation of the scapula, both of which contribute to scapular protraction. This is clinically important because scapular protraction has been shown to decrease the width of the subacromial space and thereby increase risk for subacromial impingement. In contrast, scapular retraction has been shown to increase the width of the subacromial space and supraspinatus strength potential (enhanced mechanical advantage) when compared with a more protracted position. These data also emphasize the importance of strengthening the scapular retractors and maintaining a scapular retracted position during shoulder exercises. We routinely instructed patients to emphasize an upright posture during shoulder exercises.[31]

Therefore, based on the numerous EMG investigations, the full can exercise may be the best exercise for the supraspinatus because it produces moderate amounts of muscle activity with the least amount of pain provocation and surrounding muscle activation.

Clinical Pearl #4

The full can position is recommended for strengthening the supraspinatus muscle because the amount of muscle activity is similar to that for the empty can and prone exercises, with less activity in the deltoid and surrounding muscles, which possibly minimizes the amount of superior humeral head migration.

Scapulothoracic Joint

The scapulothoracic joint is often overlooked; however, it plays a critical role in movement of the upper extremity. During humeral elevation, the scapula rotates upwardly in the frontal plane at a ratio of 1° for every 2° of humeral elevation. After 120° of elevation, the scapula and humerus elevate at a 1:1 ratio. Total scapula upward rotation is minimal at 45° to 55°. A properly functioning scapula also tilts posteriorly (20° to 40°) and rotates externally (15° to 35°).[31]

EMG activity in muscles of the scapulothoracic joint have also been studied by several authors. Moseley et al[37] examined eight muscles—the upper, middle, and lower trapezius, levator scapula, rhomboids, pectoralis minor, and middle and lower serratus anterior—during 16 commonly performed exercises in nine healthy subjects (Table 10-4). The authors reported the peak EMG activity in each muscle and noted that the majority of the muscles had assisted in more than one scapular function.

Table 10-4 **Electromyographic Analysis of Scapulothoracic Musculature**

Muscle	Exercise	Duration Qualified (% of Exercise)	Peak Arc (% MMT ± SD)	Peak Arc Range	Function
Upper trapezius	Rowing	75	112 ± 84	Isometric*	Retraction
	Military press	27	64 ± 26	150-peak	Upward rotation
	Horiz. abd. with ER	33	75 ± 27	Isometric*	Retraction
	Horiz. abd. (neutral)	33	62 ± 53	90-peak	Retraction
	Scaption	23	54 ± 16	120-150	Upward rotation
	Abduction	31	52 ± 30	90-120	Upward rotation
Middle trapezius	Horiz. abd. (neutral)	78	108 ± 63	90-peak	Retraction
	Horiz. abd. with ER	67	96 ± 73	Peak-90	Retraction
	Extension (prone)	27	77 ± 49	Neutral-30	Retraction
	Rowing	33	59 ± 51	90-120	Retraction
Lower trapezius	Abduction	50	68 ± 53	90-150	Upward rotation
	Rowing	50	67 ± 50	120-150	Retraction
	Horiz. abd. with ER	33	63 ± 41	90-peak	Retraction
	Flexion	23	60 ± 18	120-150	Upward rotation
	Horiz. abd. (neutral)	33	56 ± 24	90-peak	Retraction
	Scaption	23	60 ± 22	120-150	Upward rotation

Based on the results of the study, the authors recommended that a core program of exercises, including shoulder scaption, prone rowing, push-ups with a plus, and press-ups, should be included in shoulder and scapular rehabilitation programs.

More specifically, Decker et al[38] documented the EMG activity in the serratus anterior during several different scapulohumeral rehabilitation exercises. The authors analyzed serratus anterior activity during eight common rehabilitation exercises in 20 healthy subjects. The authors developed a rank order of exercises that elicited the greatest amount of serratus activity. The three exercises that were suggested were the push-up with a plus (Fig. 10-6), the dynamic hug (Fig. 10-7), and a standing serratus anterior punch exercise (Fig. 10-8).

Ekstrom et al[39] also looked at serratus activity during common exercises. The results of his study suggested that the serratus anterior has increased activity when performing movement that causes simultaneous upward rotation and protraction. A good example of this is the serratus anterior punch performed at 120° of abduction (Fig. 10-9) and during diagonal exercises that involve protraction with shoulder flexion, horizontal adduction, and external rotation.[31]

Table 10-4 Electromyographic Analysis of Scapulothoracic Musculature—cont'd

Muscle	Exercise	Duration Qualified (% of Exercise)	Peak Arc (% MMT ± SD)	Peak Arc Range	Function
Levator scapulae	Rowing	78	114 ± 69	Isometric*	Retraction
	Horiz. abd. (neutral)	67	96 ± 57	Isometric*	Retraction
	Shrug	63	88 ± 32	Isometric*	Elevation
	Horiz. abd. with ER	33	87 ± 66	Isometric*	Retraction
	Extension (prone)	36	81 ± 76	Isometric*	Elevation
	Scaption	46	69 ± 46	120-150	Retraction
Rhomboids	Horiz. abd. (neutral)	33	66 ± 38	90-peak	Retraction
	Scaption	25	65 ± 79	120-150	Retraction
	Abduction	31	64 ± 53	90-150	Retraction
	Rowing	30	56 ± 46	Isometric*	Retraction
Middle serratus anterior	Flexion	69	96 ± 45	120-150	Up. rot./protract.
	Abduction	54	96 ± 53	120-150	Up. rot./protract.
	Scaption	58	91 ± 52	120-150	Up. rot./protract.
	Military press	64	82 ± 36	150-peak	Up. rot./protract.
	Push-up with a plus	28	80 ± 38	Plus man.	Up. rot./protract.
	Push-up hands apart	21	57 ± 36	Last arc of push up	Up. rot./protract.
Lower serratus anterior	Scaption	50	84 ± 20	120-150	Up. rot./protract.
	Abduction	54	74 ± 65	120-150	Up. rot./protract.
	Flexion	31	72 ± 46	120-150	Up. rot./protract.
	Push-up with a plus	67	72 ± 3	Chest moving away from floor	Up. rot./protract.
	Push-up hands apart	21	69 ± 31	Isometric as the chest was near the floor	Up. rot./protract.
	Military press	36	60 ± 42	120-150	Up. rot./protract.
Pectoralis minor	Press-up	75	89 ± 62	Isometric*	Depression
	Push-up with a plus	34	58 ± 45	Plus man.	Protraction
	Push-up with hands apart	50	55 ± 34	2nd to last arc	Protraction

Data from Moseley, J.B., Jr, Jobe, F.W., Pink, M., et al. (1992): EMG analysis of the scapular muscles during a shoulder rehabilitation program. Am. J. Sports Med., 20:128–134.

* Isometric contractions were at the extreme of the range of motion.

ER, External rotation; *Horiz. abd.,* horizontal abduction; *IR,* internal rotation; *MMT,* manual muscle test; *SD,* standard deviation; *Up. rot./protract.,* upward rotation and protraction.

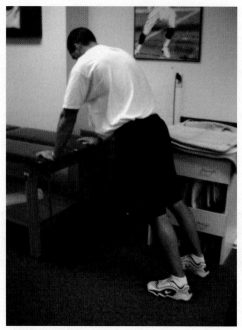

FIGURE 10-6 Push-up on a tabletop with a plus. The patient is instructed to fully protract the shoulder blade at the top of the push-up.

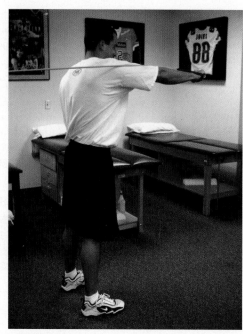

FIGURE 10-8 Standing serratus anterior punch exercise. The patient protracts the shoulder blade against resistance.

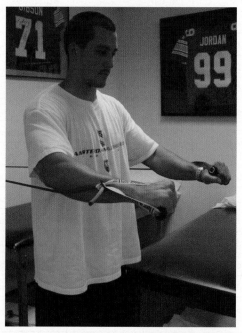

FIGURE 10-7 Dynamic hug exercise. Using resistance, the patient horizontally adducts the shoulder at 60° of elevation while protracting the scapula.

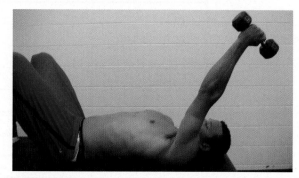

FIGURE 10-9 Supine punch performed at 120° of shoulder flexion to increase activation of the serratus anterior.

the wall might also compress the humeral head into the glenoid and thus improve glenohumeral stability during the early phases of rehabilitation.[31]

BIOMECHANICAL EFFECTS OF PATHOLOGIC SHOULDER CONDITIONS

Although the majority of biomechanical research on shoulder rehabilitation has involved healthy subjects, certain pathologic conditions may affect biomechanical function of the shoulder and require modification of the rehabilitation program.

Reddy et al[41] evaluated EMG activity in the four rotator cuff and middle deltoid muscles in 15 healthy subjects and 15 subjects with subacromial impingement during elevation in the scapular plane. The diagnosis of impingement was based on radiographic evidence and confirmed after testing at the time of arthroscopic subacromial decompression. The authors reported an overall decrease in EMG activity in each muscle throughout the exercise in patients with impingement. A statistically significant decrease in EMG activity was observed in

Hardwick et al[40] looked at serratus anterior activity during the wall slide, wall push-up with a plus, and the full can exercise. The wall slide (Fig. 10-10, *A* to *C*) produced similar serratus anterior activity as did scapular abduction above 120° with no resistance. The wall slide might be advantageous in that patients report that it is less painful to perform. This may be due to the support that the upper extremities have when placed against the wall during the exercises. Placing the upper extremities against

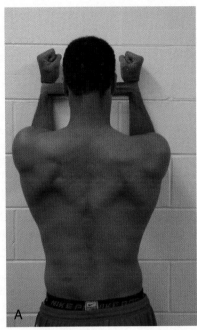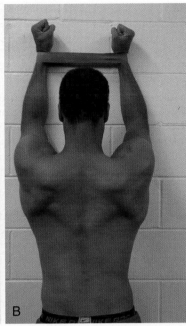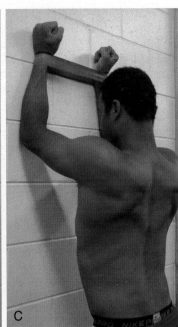

FIGURE 10-10 Wall slides performed with use of a Thera-Band to promote contraction of the external rotators of the glenohumeral joint. **A,** The patient begins the exercises with the elbows bent and shoulders below 90°. **B,** and **C,** Keeping the shoulders externally rotated, the patient slides his arms vertically up the wall as high as possible while maintaining both forearm contact with the wall and external rotation of the glenohumeral joint.

the infraspinatus, subscapularis, and middle deltoid from 30° to 60° of elevation. In addition, the infraspinatus muscle demonstrated a statistically significant decrease in EMG activity from 60° to 90° of elevation in patients with impingement.

The authors suggested that the decreased EMG activity in the shoulder musculature observed during arm elevation may lead to subacromial impingement. Furthermore, the decreased activity of the infraspinatus and subscapularis force couple along with normal activity of the supraspinatus may allow superior migration of the humeral head rather than glenohumeral joint compression and cause impingement within the subacromial space.

McMahon et al[42] compared EMG activity in the rotator cuff and scapulothoracic muscles in 15 normal shoulders and 23 shoulders with anterior instability. EMG testing of abduction, scaption, and forward flexion was performed before surgical intervention for unidirectional anterior stabilization. The authors reported a statistically significant decrease in supraspinatus activity during abduction and scaption from 30° to 60° in subjects with instability. During all three movements, a statistically significant decrease in serratus anterior activity was also observed in subjects with instability. This occurred in the range of 30° to 120° of abduction and at 0° to 120° of scaption.

The authors suggested that the decreased amount of supraspinatus activity may result in disadvantageous superior humeral head migration and affect the amount of abnormal glenohumeral translation. Blasier et al[43] reported that the supraspinatus muscle is highly active in stabilization of the shoulder joint, with an 18% reduction in force needed for subluxation of the glenohumeral joint when the supraspinatus muscle was not active.

Furthermore, the finding of decreased serratus anterior activity is also important in patients with shoulder instability. Decreased serratus anterior activity has likewise been observed

in baseball pitchers with anterior instability[44] and in swimmers with shoulder pain.[28] The authors suggested that the decreased amount of serratus anterior activity may result in an inability to place the scapula in an upward position during shoulder elevation and thus alter the position and length-tension relationship of the static and dynamic stabilizers of the shoulder.

Clinical Pearl #5

EMG activity in the rotator cuff is decreased in shoulders with subacromial impingement and anterior shoulder instability.

Clinical Pearl #6

Based on the EMG results of these studies, the Thrower's Ten Exercise Program (see Appendix A [online]) is recommended for athletes to strengthen the glenohumeral and scapulothoracic muscles so that they can perform competitively.

BIOMECHANICAL IMPLICATIONS OF KNEE REHABILITATION

Several methods of biomechanical analysis have been used to study rehabilitation of the knee, including cadaveric, EMG, kinematic, kinetic, mathematic modeling, and in vivo strain gauge measurements. To best evaluate these studies, it is helpful to delineate the findings based on the tissue or structure being examined, such as the anterior cruciate ligament (ACL), posterior cruciate ligament (PCL), and patellofemoral joint.

Anterior Cruciate Ligament

The majority of biomechanical research during rehabilitation of the knee has focused on the ACL. The efficacy of open kinetic chain (OKC) and closed kinetic chain (CKC) exercises has been heavily scrutinized after years of theoretic and anecdotal assumptions. Markolf et al[45] examined the effect of compressive loads on cadaveric knees to simulate BW. The authors reported that when compared with OKC exercises, compressive forces reduce strain on the ACL, thus providing a protective mechanism. Fleming et al[46] investigated this theory with in vivo strain gauge measurements within the ACL. The use of in vivo strain gauge measurements within the ACL has allowed a method to directly measure ACL strain during activity. The authors noted that strain on the ACL increased from −2.0% during non–weight bearing to 2.1% in a weight-bearing position. Although an increase in ACL strain was observed in a weight-bearing position, it is still unclear whether a 2% strain is detrimental to the healing ACL graft, although clinical experience has shown that early weight bearing has not resulted in poor functional outcomes of ACL reconstructions postoperatively.

CKC exercises have also been theorized to reduce ACL strain by providing cocontraction of the hamstrings and quadriceps. Wilk et al[47] examined EMG activity in the quadriceps and hamstrings during CKC squat, leg press, and OKC knee extension. The authors noted that cocontraction occurred from 30° to 0° during the ascent phase of the squat, when the body is positioned directly over the knees and feet, but did not occur at other ranges of motion or during the CKC leg press or OKC knee extension. Thus, not all CKC exercises produce cocontraction of the quadriceps and hamstrings. Rather, it appears that several factors affect muscle activation during CKC exercises, including knee flexion angle, body position relative to the knee, and direction of movement (ascending or descending). Clinically, exercises performed in an upright and weight-bearing position with the knee flexed to approximately 30°, such as squats and lateral lunges, may be used during knee rehabilitation to promote cocontraction of the quadriceps and hamstrings.

Wilk et al[47] also used mathematic modeling to estimate the shear forces at the tibiofemoral joint during the squat, leg press, and knee extension exercise (Fig. 10-11). The authors reported that a posterior tibiofemoral shear force was observed throughout the entire range of motion during both CKC squatting and leg press (peak, 1500 N) and during deep angles of OKC knee extension from 100° to 40° (peak, 900 N). Anterior tibiofemoral shear force (peak, 250 N) and theoretically ACL strain were observed during the OKC knee extension exercise from 40° to 10°.

Similar to the results of Wilk et al,[47] Beynnon et al[48] reported that the greatest amount of ACL strain (2.8%) occurred from 40° to 0° during OKC knee extension using in vivo strain gauge measurements. This strain was found to significantly increase in a linear fashion with the application of an external 45-N boot (3.8%). However, the authors also reported ACL strain of 3.6% during the CKC squat exercise. In contrast, application of external loading did not significantly increase the amount of strain on the ACL (4.0%). Based on the results of these studies,[46-48] both OKC and CKC exercises are performed, although the patient is often limited to 90° to 40° during the OKC knee extension when heavy resistance is applied.

Recent research has looked at the different stresses placed on the ACL during some common exercises used during the rehabilitation process to strengthen the lower extremity. Escamilla et al[49] investigated the strain placed on the ACL during lunges with different step lengths. They found that minimal strain was placed on the ACL during both long- and short-stride lunges. ACL loading occurred only during lunges with a short stride (0 to 50 N between 0° and 10° of flexion). In a different study, Escamilla et al[50] examined ACL forces during the side lunge and compared them with the forward lunge. They found that side lunges placed no additional strain on the ACL. Thus, both forward and side lunges appear to be safe and effective methods of strengthening the lower extremity during all phases of ACL rehabilitation.

Additionally, Escamilla studied the impact of different squat variations on the ACL. He showed that low anterior shear forces occur during the dynamic squat, especially in the early ranges of motion (0° to 60°) of knee flexion.[51] Furthermore, Escamilla et al[49] also assessed anterior shear forces in the knee during one-legged squats and wall squats. They found that wall squats with both legs close to the wall and with the legs farther away from the wall yielded

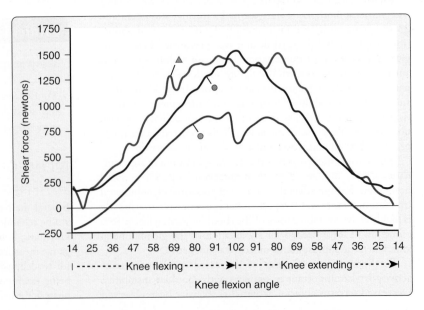

FIGURE 10-11 Shear forces at the tibiofemoral joint during the squat (*triangle*), leg press (*blue circle*), and knee extension exercises (*red circle*). *(Data from Wilk, K.E., Escamilla, R.F., Fleisig, G.S., et al. [1996]: A comparison of the tibiofemoral joint forces and electromyographic activity during open and closed kinetic chain exercises. Am. J. Sports Med., 24:518–527.)*

no increased strain on the ACL. Anterior shear forces did increase during the one-legged squat from 0° to 40° of knee flexion (59 ± 52 N).

Also commonly used during ACL rehabilitation are the bicycle and stair-climbing machines. Fleming et al[52] analyzed six different bicycle-riding conditions induced by manipulating speed and power. The authors found no significant differences between conditions, with a minimal mean ACL strain of 1.7%. The greatest amount of strain was observed when the knee reached the greatest amount of extension. Similarly, Fleming et al[53] analyzed two cadences of stair climbing (80 and 112 steps per minute) and noted a similar 2.7% strain on the ACL. Again, the most amount of strain was observed during terminal knee extension. Thus, when compared with other rehabilitation exercises, both bicycling and stair climbing are safe exercises that place low strain on the ACL (Table 10-5). Furthermore, the greatest amount of strain was observed as the knee moved into terminal knee extension, similar to the results of Wilk et al[47] and Beynnon et al[48] during OKC and CKC exercises.

Clinical Pearl #7

OKC knee extension may be performed from 90° to 40° with progressive resistance to minimize strain on the ACL.

Table 10-5 In Vivo Strain on the Anterior Cruciate Ligament

Exercise	Strain (%)
Isometric quadriceps contraction at 15°	4.4
Squatting with resistance	4.0
Active knee flexion with resistance	3.8
Lachman test (150 N of anterior shear at 30°)	3.7
Squatting without resistance	3.6
Active knee flexion without resistance	2.8
Quadriceps and hamstring cocontraction at 15°	2.7
Isometric quadriceps contraction at 30°	2.7
Stair climbing	2.7
Anterior drawer test (150 N of anterior shear at 90°)	1.8
Stationary bicycle	1.7
Quadriceps and hamstrings cocontraction at 30°	0.4
Passive knee range of motion	0.1
Isometric quadriceps contraction at 60° and 90°	0.0
Quadriceps and hamstrings cocontraction at 60° and 90°	0.0
Isometric hamstring contraction at 30°, 60°, and 90°	0.0

Modified from Fleming, B.C., Beynnon, B.D., Renstrom, P.A., et al. (1999): The strain behavior of the anterior cruciate ligament during stair climbing: An in vivo study. Arthroscopy, 15:185–191.

Clinical Pearl #8

Weight bearing and CKC exercises may be performed immediately without placing excessive strain on the ACL.

Clinical Pearl #9

CKC exercise in the upright position with the knee flexed to 30° (such as squatting and lateral lunges) may be used to promote cocontraction of the quadriceps and hamstrings.

Clinical Pearl #10

Bicycling and stair climbing may be performed with minimal strain on the ACL.

Posterior Cruciate Ligament

Historically, the results of rehabilitation after PCL injury have been mixed. Poor functional outcomes have often been attributed to the residual laxity present after surgical reconstruction. The biomechanics of the tibiofemoral joint during exercise must be understood so that the rehabilitative process will not create deleterious effects on the PCL. The posterior tibiofemoral shear forces that occur during specific activities, such as level walking,[54] ascending and descending stairs,[55] and resisted knee flexion exercises[56,57] have previously been documented.[58,59] Level walking and descending stairs produce a relatively low posterior tibiofemoral shear force of 0.4 × BW and 0.6 × BW, respectively (Table 10-6). However, high posterior shear force has been noted during several commonly performed activities of daily living, such as climbing stairs (1.7 × BW at 45° of knee flexion)[55,60] and squatting (3.6 × BW at 140° of knee flexion), and may have an effect on residual laxity postoperatively. Further studies show that isometric knee flexion at 45° places a posterior shear force of 1.1 × BW on the tibiofemoral joint.[57]

Tremendous shear forces on both the PCL and the tibiofemoral joint occur during OKC resisted knee flexion. Posterior tibial displacement is attributed to the high EMG activity in the hamstring muscle while resistive knee flexion is performed. Lutz et al reported a maximum shear force of 1780 N at 90° of flexion, 1526 N at 60°, and 939 N at 30° during isometric knee flexion (Fig. 10-12). Kaufman et al[56] also noted a PCL load of 1.7 × BW at 75° of flexion during the isokinetic knee flexion exercise. Because PCL stress increases with knee flexion angle, isolated OKC knee flexion exercises should be avoided for at least 8 weeks postoperatively and until symptoms subside in nonoperative cases.

Excessive stress on the PCL has also been observed during deeper angles of OKC knee extension. Several studies have proved that resisted knee extension at 90° of flexion causes a posterior tibiofemoral shear force and potential stress on the PCL.[47,56,61-63] Wilk et al[47] documented a posterior shear force from 100° to 40° with resisted OKC knee extension (see Fig. 10-11). The highest

Table 10-6 Posterior Tibiofemoral Shear Forces

Source	Activity	Knee Angle (°)	Force (× Body Weight)
Kaufman et al[54]	60°/sec flexion isokinetic	75	1.7
	180°/sec flexion isokinetic	75	1.4
Morrison[52]	Level walking	5	0.4
Morrison[53]	Descending stairs	5	0.6
	Ascending stairs	45	1.7
Smidt[55]	Isometric flexion	45	1.1

amount of stress on the PCL was found at angles of 85° to 95° during knee flexion. Conversely, the lowest amount of posterior shear force occurred from 60° to 0° of resisted knee extension.[47] Kaufman et al[56] also reported that posterior shear forces take place until 50° to 55° of knee flexion. Furthermore, Jurist and Otis[62] also documented stress on the PCL at 60° of flexion during an isometric knee extension exercise when resistance was applied at the proximal end of the tibia. To reduce the excessive posterior shear force placed on the PCL, OKC resisted knee extension should be performed from 60° to 0°.[58,59]

The stress applied to the PCL while CKC exercises are performed is relative to the knee flexion angle produced during the exercise. Wilk et al[47,64] reported an increase in posterior shear force as the knee flexion angle increases during CKC exercise (see Fig. 10-11). Meglan et al[65] also documented a linear increase in posterior shear force from 40° to 100° of knee flexion during the front squat maneuver. Escamilla et al[49] assessed the load applied to the PCL during the wall and single-leg squat. They found that the wall squat with the legs farther away from the wall and thus a greater flexion angle was associated with significantly greater posterior shear force than was the wall squat with the feet closer to the wall and less knee flexion. The wall squat with a greater flexion angle of the knee also produced higher posterior shear forces than did the one-legged squat. Therefore, to reduce PCL stress during CKC exercises, leg presses and squats are performed from 0° to 60° of knee flexion.[58,59]

Escamilla et al investigated the tension placed on the PCL during forward lunge with a short step, forward lunge with a long step, and side lunge.[47,48] They found that PCL tension increased as the stride became longer in the forward lunge, which resulted in deeper knee flexion angles. They also determined that as knee flexion increased in the side lunge, so did posterior shear forces at the knee. It is recommended that clinicians use caution when prescribing both forward and side lunges during PCL rehabilitation, especially during the early phases of rehabilitation. It is crucial to monitor and limit the amount of knee flexion that occurs during the lunge exercise when rehabilitating the PCL.

Clinical Pearl #11

OKC knee flexion produces high posterior tibiofemoral shear forces and should initially be limited to minimize strain on the PCL.

Clinical Pearl #12

OKC knee extension may be performed from 60° to 0° to minimize strain on the PCL.

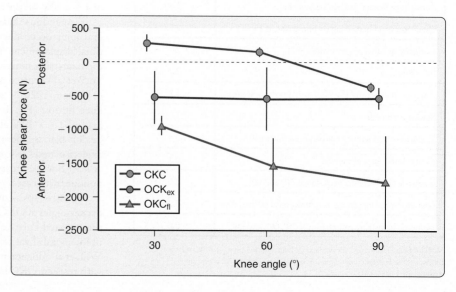

FIGURE 10-12 Shear force at the tibiofemoral joint during squatting, knee extension, and knee flexion. *CKC,* Closed kinetic chain; *OKC_ex,* open kinetic chain extension; *OKC_fl,* open kinetic chain flexion. *(Data from Lutz, G.E., Palmitier, R.A., An, K.N., and Chao, E.Y. [1993]: Comparison of tibiofemoral joint forces during open and closed kinetic chain exercises. J. Bone Joint Surg. Am., 75:732–735.)*

Clinical Pearl #13

CKC exercise may be performed from 0° to 30° and progress to 0° to 45° and to 0° to 60° as the patient's condition improves to minimize strain on the PCL.

Patellofemoral Joint

When one is rehabilitating a patient with a known lesion of the patellofemoral joint, it is important to first understand normal patellofemoral joint arthrokinematics. Articulation between the inferior margin of the patella and the femur begins at approximately 10° to 20° of knee flexion.[66] As the knee proceeds into greater degrees of knee flexion, the contact area of the patellofemoral joint moves proximally along the patella. At 30°, the area of patellofemoral contact is approximately 2.0 cm.[1,66] The area of contact gradually increases as the knee is flexed. At 90° of knee flexion the contact area increases up to 6.0 cm.[1,66]

Alterations in the Q angle are often associated with patellofemoral disorders and may change the contact areas and thus the amount of joint reaction forces on the patellofemoral joint. Huberti and Hayes[67] examined in vitro patellofemoral contact pressures at various degrees of knee flexion from 20° to 120°. The maximum contact area occurred at 90° of knee flexion with a force estimated to be 6.5 × BW. An increase or decrease in the Q angle of 10° resulted in increased maximum contact pressure and a smaller total area of contact throughout the range of motion. This information may be applied when one prescribes rehabilitation interventions so that the exercises are performed in ranges of motion that place minimal strain on damaged structures.

The effectiveness and safety of OKC and CKC exercises during patellofemoral rehabilitation have been heavily scrutinized in recent years. Whereas CKC exercises replicate functional activities such as ascending and descending stairs, OKC exercises are often desired for isolated muscle strengthening when specific muscle weakness is present.[68]

Steinkamp et al[69] analyzed patellofemoral joint biomechanics during leg press and extension exercises in 20 normal subjects. Patellofemoral joint reaction force, stress, and moments were calculated during both exercises (Fig. 10-13). From 0° to 46° of knee flexion, patellofemoral joint reaction force was less during the CKC leg press. Conversely, from 50° to 90° of knee flexion, joint reaction forces were lower during the OKC knee extension exercise. Joint reaction forces were minimal at 90° of knee flexion during the knee extension exercise.

Escamilla et al[70] observed the patellofemoral compressive forces during OKC knee extension and CKC leg press and vertical squat. The results were similar to the findings of Steinkamp et al[69]; OKC knee extension produced significantly greater force at angles less than 57° of knee flexion, whereas both CKC activities produced significantly greater force at knee angles greater than 85°.

Escamilla et al[71,72] studied compressive force on the knee during the lunge exercise both with and without a stride. The results of their study showed a direct relationship between knee force and the amount of knee flexion performed during the lunge exercise. As knee flexion increases, the amount of patellofemoral compressive force increases linearly, and compressive

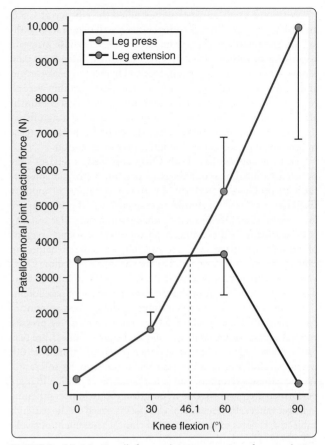

FIGURE 10-13 Patellofemoral joint reaction forces during leg press and leg extension exercises. *(Data from Steinkamp, L.A., Dillingham, M.F., Markel, M.D., et al. [1993]: Biomechanical considerations in patellofemoral joint rehabilitation. Am. J. Sports Med., 21:438–444.*

force decreases as knee flexion decreases. Furthermore, they found that knee compressive force is greater in lunges performed with a stride than in lunges performed without a stride. The side lunge caused more compressive force on the patellofemoral joint than the forward lunge did.[71]

When analyzing the biomechanics of OKC knee extension, Grood et al[73] reported that quadriceps force was greatest near full knee extension and increased with the addition of external loading. The small patellofemoral contact area observed near full extension, as discussed previously, and the increased amount of quadriceps force generated at these angles may make the patellofemoral joint more susceptible to injury. As the knee approaches terminal extension, the large magnitude of quadriceps force is focused onto a more condensed location on the patella. When one applies the results of Steinkamp et al,[69] Escamilla et al,[70] and Grood et al,[73] it appears that during OKC knee extension, as the contact area of the patellofemoral joint decreases, the force of quadriceps pull subsequently increases, thereby resulting in a large magnitude of patellofemoral contact stress being applied to a focal point on the patella. In contrast, during CKC exercises, quadriceps force increases as the knee continues into flexion. However, the area of patellofemoral contact also increases as the knee flexes, which leads to wider dissipation of contact stress over a larger surface area.

Witvrouw et al[74] prospectively studied the efficacy of OKC and CKC exercises during nonoperative patellofemoral rehabilitation. Sixty patients participated in a 5-week exercise program consisting of either OKC or CKC exercises. Subjective pain scores, functional ability, quadriceps and hamstring peak torque, and hamstring, quadriceps, and gastrocnemius flexibility were all recorded before and after rehabilitation, as well as at 3 months after intervention. Both treatment groups reported a significant decrease in pain, an increase in muscle strength, and an increase in functional performance 3 months after intervention.

Thus, it appears that both OKC and CKC exercises may be used to maximize outcomes in patients with patellofemoral joint problems if performed within a safe range of motion. Exercises are based on clinical assessment. If CKC exercises are less painful than OKC exercises, that form of muscular training is encouraged. Additionally, in postoperative patients, regions of articular cartilage wear are carefully considered before an exercise program is designed. For the most part, we allow OKC exercises such as knee extension from 90° to 40° of knee flexion. This range of motion provides the lowest amount of patellofemoral joint reaction force while exhibiting the greatest amount of patellofemoral contact area. CKC exercises, such as leg presses, vertical squats, lateral step-ups, and wall squats (slides), are performed initially from 0° to 30° and then progressed from 0° to 60° when patellofemoral joint reaction forces can be tolerated. As the patient's symptoms subside, the ranges of motion that are performed are progressed to allow greater muscle strengthening in larger ranges. Progression of exercises is based on the patient's subjective reports of symptoms and clinical assessment of swelling, range of motion, and painful crepitus.

Clinical Pearl #14

OKC knee extension may be performed from 90° to 40° to produce the lowest amount of patellofemoral joint reaction force with the greatest amount of patella surface contact.

Clinical Pearl #15

CKC exercise may be performed initially at 0° to 45° and be progressed to 0° to 60° as the patient's condition improves to produce the lowest amount of patellofemoral joint reaction force.

Clinical Pearl #16

Exercise prescription should be based on the location of the symptoms and symptom reproduction during exercises.

A thorough understanding of the biomechanical factors associated with rehabilitation is necessary to return the injured athlete to competition as quickly and safely as possible. Various factors are associated with specific pathologic conditions that will alter the rehabilitation program to minimize stress on healing structures. Knowledge of the biomechanical implications discussed in this chapter may be used when rehabilitation programs are designed for patients with pathologic rotator cuff, ACL, PCL, and patellofemoral joint conditions.

CONCLUSION

Overview

- Knowledge of the biomechanical implications for rehabilitation is a vital component in successful treatment prescription.
- Exercises vary according to the specific pathologic conditions.

Shoulder Rehabilitation

- Several exercises may be effective in strengthening the rotator cuff, glenohumeral, and scapulothoracic musculature.
- Shoulder rehabilitation exercises may be adjusted or performed in different positions to minimize the activity of and strain on specific healing structures.
- The diagnosis of specific pathologic shoulder conditions may have an effect on the biomechanics of the shoulder.

Knee Rehabilitation

- Not all CKC exercises produce cocontraction of the quadriceps and hamstring muscles.
- The amount of cocontraction depends on several factors, including body position and direction of movement (ascent and descent phases).
- Use of both OKC and CKC exercises may be advantageous in the rehabilitation of pathologic ACL, PCL, and patellofemoral joint conditions if performed in safe ranges of motion that apply minimal stress to the injured structures.

REFERENCES

1. Apreleva, M., Hasselman, C.T., Debski, R.E., et al. (1998): A dynamic analysis of glenohumeral motion after simulated capsulolabral injury. J. Bone Joint Surg. Am., 80:474–480.
2. Cain, P.R., Mutsehler, T.A., and Fu, F. H. (1987): Anterior stability of the glenohumeral joint. A dynamic model. Am. J. Sports Med., 15:144–148.
3. Harryman, D.T., II, Sidles, J.A., Clark, J.A., et al. (1990): Translation of the humeral head on the glenoid with passive glenohumeral motion. J. Bone Joint Surg. Am., 72:1334–1343.
4. Saha, A.K. (1971): Dynamic stability of the glenohumeral joint. Acta Orthop. Scand., 42:491–505.
5. Wilk, K.E., Arrigo, C.A., and Andrews, J.R. (1997): Current concepts: The stabilizing structures of the glenohumeral joint. J. Orthop. Sports Phys. Ther., 25:364–379.
6. Townsend, H., Jobe, F. W., Pink, M., and Perry, J. (1991): Electromyographic analysis of the glenohumeral muscles during a baseball rehabilitation program. Am. J. Sports Med., 19:264–272.
7. Hintermeister, R.A., Lange, G.W., Schultheis, J.M., et al. (1998): Electromyographic activity and applied load during shoulder rehabilitation exercises using elastic resistance. Am. J. Sports Med., 26:210–220.
8. Wilk, K. E., and Arrigo, C. (1993): Current concepts in the rehabilitation of the athletic shoulder. J. Orthop. Sports Phys. Ther., 18:365–378.
9. Fleisig, G.S., Barrentine, S.W., Escamilla, R.F., and Andrews, J.R. (1996): Biomechanics of overhand throwing with implications for injuries. Sports Med., 21:421–437.
10. Andrews, J.R., and Angelo, R.L. (1988): Shoulder arthroscopy for the throwing athlete. Tech. Orthop., 3:75.
11. Jobe, F.W., Kvitne, R.S., and Giangarra, C.E. (1989): Shoulder pain in the overhand or throwing athlete. The relationship of anterior instability and rotator cuff impingement. Orthop. Rev., 18:963–975.
12. Walch, G., Boileau, P., Noel, E., and Donell, T. (1992): Impingement of the deep surface of the infraspinatus tendon on the posterior glenoid rim. J. Shoulder Elbow Surg., 1:239–245.
13. Neer, C.S., II, Craig, E.V., and Fukuda, H. (1983): Cuff tear arthropathy. J. Bone Joint Surg. Am., 65:1232.

14. Rockwood, C.A., and Matsen, F.A., eds. (1990): The Shoulder. Philadelphia, Saunders, pp. 755–795.

15. Wilk, K.E., Andrews, J.R., Arrigo, C.A., et al. (1993): The internal and external rotator strength characteristics of professional baseball pitchers. Am. J. Sports Med., 21:61–66.

16. Wilk, K.E., Meister, K., and Andrews, J.R. (2002): Current concepts in the rehabilitation of the overhead throwing athlete. Am. J. Sports Med., 30:136–151.

17. Ballantyne, B.T., O'Hare, S.J., Paschall, J.L., et al. (1993): Electromyographic activity of selected shoulder muscles in commonly used therapeutic exercises. Phys. Ther., 73:668–677.

18. Blackburn, T.A., McLeod, W.D., and White, B. (1990): EMG analysis of posterior rotator cuff exercises. Athl. Train., 25:40–45.

19. Bradley, J.P., and Tibone, J.E. (1991): Electromyographic analysis of muscle action about the shoulder. Clin. Sports Med., 10:805.

20. Greenfield, B.H., Donatelli, R., Wooden, M.J., and Wilkes, J. (1990): Isokinetic evaluation of shoulder rotational strength between the plane of the scapula and the frontal plane. Am. J. Sports Med., 18:124–128.

21. Kronberg, M., Nemeth, G., and Brostrom, L.A. (1990): Muscle activity and coordination in the normal shoulder—An electromyographic study. Clin. Orthop. Relat. Res., 257:76–85.

22. Malanga, G.A., Jenp, Y.N., Growney, E.S., and An, K.A. (1996): EMG analysis of shoulder positioning in testing and strengthening the supraspinatus. Med. Sci. Sports Exerc., 28:661–664.

23. McCann, P.D., Wootten, M.E., Kadaba, M.P., and Bigliani, L.U. (1993): A kinematic and electromyographic study of shoulder rehabilitation exercises. Clin. Orthop. Relat. Res., 288:179–188.

24. Moynes, D.R., Perry, J., Antonelli, D.J., et al. (1986): Electromyographic motion analysis of the upper extremity in sports. Phys. Ther., 66:1905–1911.

25. Worrell, T.W., Corey, B.J., York, S.L., and Santiestaban, J. (1992): An analysis of supraspinatus EMG activity and shoulder isometric force development. Med. Sci. Sports Exerc., 24:744–748.

26. Reinold, M.M., Wilk, K.E., Fleisig, G.S., et al. (2004): Electromyographic analysis of the rotator cuff and deltoid musculature during common shoulder external rotation exercises. J. Orthop. Sports Phys. Ther., 34:385–394.

27. O'Brien, S.J., Neves, M.C., Arnoczky, S.P., et al. (1990): The anatomy and histology of the inferior glenohumeral ligament complex of the shoulder. Am. J. Sports Med., 18:449–456.

28. Scovazzo, M.L., Browne, A., Pink, M., et al. (1991): The painful shoulder during freestyle swimming. An electromyographic cinematographic analysis of twelve muscles. Am. J. Sports Med., 19:577–582.

29. Jobe, F.W., and Moynes, D.R. (1982): Delineation of diagnostic criteria and a rehabilitation program for rotator cuff injuries. Am. J. Sports Med., 10:336–339.

30. Morrey, B.F., Itoi, E., and An, K.N. (1998): Biomechanics of the shoulder. In: Rockwood, C.A., and Matsen, F.A. (eds.). The Shoulder, 2nd ed. Philadelphia, Saunders, pp. 233–276.

31. Reinold, M.M., Escamilla, R.F., and Wilk, K.E. (2009): Current concepts in the scientific and clinical rationale behind exercises for glenohumeral and scapulothoracic musculature. J. Orthop. Sports Phys. Ther., 39:105–117.

32. Kelly, B.T., Kadrmas, W.R., and Speer, K.P. (1996): The manual muscle examination for rotator cuff strength: An electromyographic investigation. Am. J. Sports Med., 24:581–588.

33. Takeda, Y., Kashiwaguchi, S., and Endo, K. (2002): The most effective exercise for strengthening the supraspinatus muscle: Evaluation by magnetic resonance imaging. Am. J. Sports Med., 30:374–381.

34. Reinold, M.M., Ellerbusch, M.T., Barrentine, S.W., et al. (2002): Electromyographic analysis of the supraspinatus and deltoid muscles during rehabilitation exercises. J. Orthop. Sports Phys. Ther., 32: A-43.

35. Poppen, N.K., and Walker, P.S. (1978): Forces at the glenohumeral joint in abduction. Clin. Orthop. Relat. Res., 135:165–170.

36. Itoi, E., Kido, T., Sano, A., et al. (1999): Which is more useful, the "full can test" or the "empty can test," in detecting the torn supraspinatus tendon. Am. J. Sports Med., 27:65–68.

37. Moseley, J.B., Jr., Jobe, F.W., Pink, M., et al. (1992): EMG analysis of the scapular muscles during a shoulder rehabilitation program. Am. J. Sports Med., 20:128–134.

38. Decker, M.J., Hintermeister, R.A., Faber, K.J., and Hawkins, R.J. (1999): Serratus anterior muscle activity during selected rehabilitation exercises. Am. J. Sports Med., 27:784–791.

39. Ekstrom, R.A., Donatelli, R.A., and Soderberg, G.L. (2003): Surface electromyographic analysis of exercises for the trapezius and serratus anterior muscles. J. Orthop. Sports Phys. Ther., 33:247–258.

40. Hardwick, D.H., Beebe, J.A., McDonnell, M.K., and Lang, C.E. (2006): A comparison of serratus anterior muscle activation during a wall slide exercise and other traditional exercises. J. Orthop. Sports Phys. Ther., 36:903–910.

41. Reddy, A.S., Mohr, K.J., Pink, M.M., et al. (2002): Electromyographic analysis of the deltoid and rotator cuff muscles in person with subacromial impingement. J. Shoulder Elbow Surg., 9:519–523.

42. McMahon, P.J., Jobe, F.W., Pink, M.M., et al. (1996): Comparative electromyographic analysis of shoulder muscles during planar motions: Anterior glenohumeral instability versus normal. J. Shoulder Elbow Surg., 5:118–123.

43. Blasier, R.B., Guldberg, R.E., and Rothman, E.D. (1992): Anterior shoulder stability: Contributions of rotator cuff forces and the capsular ligaments in a cadaveric model. J. Shoulder Elbow Surg., 1:140.

44. Glousman, R., Jobe, F., Tibone, J., et al. (1988): Dynamic electromyographic analysis of the throwing shoulder with glenohumeral instability. J. Bone Joint Surg. Am., 70:220–226.

45. Markolf, K.L., Gorek, J.F., Kabo, J.M., and Shapiro, M.S. (1990): Direct measurement of resultant forces in the anterior cruciate ligament. An in vitro study performed with a new experimental technique. J. Bone Joint Surg. Am., 72:557–567.

46. Fleming, B.C., Renstrom, P.A., Beynnon, B.D., et al. (2001): The effect of weightbearing and external loading on anterior cruciate ligament strain. J. Biomech., 34:163–170.

47. Wilk, K.E., Escamilla, R.F., Fleisig, G.S., et al. (1996): A comparison of the tibiofemoral joint forces and electromyographic activity during open and closed kinetic chain exercises. Am. J. Sports Med., 24:518–527.

48. Beynnon, B.D., Johnson, R.J., Flemming, B.C., et al. (1997): The strain behavior of the anterior cruciate ligament during squatting and active flexion-extension: A comparison of an open and closed kinetic chain exercise. Am. J. Sports Med., 25:823–829.

49. Escamilla, R.F., Zheng, N., Imamura, R., et al. (2009): Cruciate ligament force during the wall squat and the one-leg squat. Med Sci Sports Exerc., 41:408–417.

50. Escamilla, R.F., Zheng, N., MacLeod, T.D., et al. (2002). Cruciate ligament tensile forces during the forward and side lunge. Clin. Biomech. (Bristol, Avon), 25:213–221.

51. Escamilla, R.F. (2001): Knee biomechanics of the dynamic squat exercise. Med. Sci. Sports Exerc., 33:127–141.

52. Fleming, B.C., Beynnon, B.D., Renstrom, P.A., et al. (1998): The strain behavior of the anterior cruciate ligament during bicycling: An in vivo study. Am. J. Sports Med., 26:109–118.

53. Fleming, B.C., Beynnon, B.D., Renstrom, P.A., et al. (1999): The strain behavior of the anterior cruciate ligament during stair climbing: An in vivo study. Arthroscopy, 15:185–191.

54. Morrison, J.B. (1970): The biomechanics of the knee joint in relation to normal walking. J. Biomech., 3:51.

55. Morrison, J.B. (1969): The biomechanics of the knee joint in various knee activities. Biomech. Eng., 4:573–578.

56. Kaufman, K.R., An, K.N., Litchy, W.J., et al. (1991): Dynamic joint forces during knee isokinetic exercise. Am. J. Sports Med., 19:305–316.

57. Smidt, G.L. (1973): Biomechanical analysis of knee extension and flexion. J. Biomech., 6:79–83.

58. Wilk, K.E. (1994): Rehabilitation of isolated and combined posterior cruciate ligament injuries. Clin. Sports Med., 13:649–677.

59. Wilk, K.E., Andrews, J.R., Clancy, W.G., et al. (1999): Rehabilitation programs for the PCL-injured and reconstructed knee. J. Sport Rehabil., 8:333–361.

60. Clancy, W.G. (1988): Repair and reconstruction of the posterior cruciate ligament. In: Chapman, M.W. (ed.). Operative Orthopaedics. Philadelphia, Lippincott Williams & Wilkins, pp. 2093–2107.

61. Daniel, D.M., Stone, M.L., Barnett, P., et al. (1988): Use of quadriceps active test to diagnose posterior cruciate ligament disruptions and measure posterior laxity of the knee. J. Bone Joint Surg. Am., 70:386–390.

62. Jurist, K.A., and Otis, J.C. (1985): Anteroposterior tibiofemoral displacements during isometric extension efforts. Am. J. Sports Med., 13:254–258.

63. Lutz, G.E., Palmitier, R.A., An, K.N., and Chao, E.Y. (1993): Comparison of tibiofemoral joint forces during open and closed kinetic chain exercises. J. Bone Joint Surg. Am., 75:732–735.

64. Wilk, K.E., Zheng, N., Fleisig, G.S., et al. (1997): Kinetic chain exercise: Implication for the ACL patient. J. Sport Rehabil., 6:125–143.

65. Meglan, D., Lutz, G., and Stuart, M. (1993): Effects of closed kinetic chain exercises for ACL rehabilitation upon the load in the capsular and ligamentous structures of the knee. Presented at the Orthopedic Research Society Meeting, San Francisco, February 15–18.

66. Hungerford, D.S., and Barry, M. (1979): Biomechanics of the patellofemoral joint. Clin. Orthop. Relat Res., 144:9–15.

67. Huberti, H.H., and Hayes, W.C. (1984): Patellofemoral contact pressures. J. Bone Joint Surg. Am., 66:715–724.

68. Wilk, K.E., and Reinold, M.M. (2001): Closed kinetic chain exercises and plyometric activities. In: Bandy, W. D., and Sanders, B. (eds.). Therapeutic Exercise: Techniques for Intervention. Baltimore, Lippincott Williams & Wilkins, pp. 179–211.

69. Steinkamp, L.A., Dillingham, M.F., Markel, M.D., et al. (1993): Biomechanical considerations in patellofemoral joint rehabilitation. Am. J. Sports Med., 21:438–444.

70. Escamilla, R.F., Fleisig, G.S., Zheng, N., et al. (1998): Biomechanics of the knee during closed kinetic chain and open kinetic chain exercises. Med. Sci. Sports Exerc., 30:556–569.

71. Escamilla, R.F., Zheng, N., MacLeod, T.D., et al. (2008): Patellofemoral compressive force and stress during the forward and side lunges with and without a stride. Clin. Biomech. (Bristol, Avon), 23:1026–1037.

72. Escamilla, R.F., Zheng, N., MacLeod, T.D., et al. (2008): Patellofemoral joint force and stress between a short- and long-step forward lunge. J. Orthop. Sports Phys Ther., 38:681–690.

73. Grood, E.S., Suntay, W.J., Noyes, F.R., and Butler, D.L. (1984): Biomechanics of the knee-extension exercise. Effect of cutting the anterior cruciate ligament. J. Bone Joint Surg. Am., 66:725–734.

74. Witvrouw, E., Lysens, R., Bellemans, J., et al. (2000): Open versus closed kinetic chain exercises for patellofemoral pain. A prospective, randomized study. Am. J. Sports Med., 28:687–694.

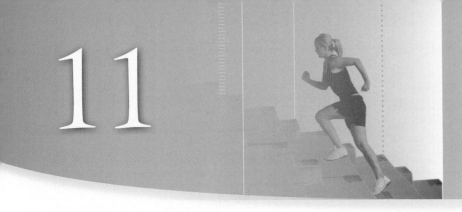

11

Aquatic Rehabilitation

Jill M. Thein-Nissenbaum, PT, DSc, SCS, ATC

CHAPTER OBJECTIVES

- Explain the physical properties of water, including buoyancy, hydrostatic pressure, viscosity, and fluid dynamics.
- Identify the effect of immersion on weight bearing and appropriately apply weight-bearing guidelines in a clinical situation.
- Explain the physiologic responses of water immersion.

- Compare and contrast the physiologic response of exercise on land and in water.
- Identify and apply recommended guidelines for cardiovascular conditioning in water.
- Design a comprehensive aquatic-based rehabilitation program for an athlete that uses the principles of stretching, strengthening, balance, and aerobic conditioning.

INTRODUCTION

Since the earliest recording of history, water has offered a healing environment. Accordingly, it has been used throughout history to treat diseases and illnesses and for recreation. Although commonly used in Europe, aquatic-based rehabilitation in the United States did not begin until the early 1900s.[1] Today, patients participating in aquatic rehabilitation benefit from a marriage of many different approaches, including the Bad Ragaz Ring method (Switzerland) and the Halliwick method (London).[1] Although once viewed as a tool to be used solely in the acute stages of rehabilitation, where land-based rehabilitation was of limited use, aquatic-based rehabilitation has evolved considerably. It is now used throughout the rehabilitation process and serves as a component of prevention and wellness programs.

The purpose of this chapter is to discuss aquatic-based rehabilitation and training for the athlete. The physical properties of water are reviewed, and current research regarding aquatic-based cardiovascular conditioning programs is discussed. Extremity-, spine-, and core body–strengthening exercises are reviewed, as are balance and coordination exercises. Finally, recommendations regarding the transition from aquatic-based programs to resumption of competitive sports are made, and sample training programs are suggested.

PHYSICAL PROPERTIES OF WATER

Almost all of the biologic effects of immersion are related to the principles of water; a thorough understanding of these principles and their effect on the body is essential to support and provide a rationale for the use of aquatic-based rehabilitation. The key characteristics of water that affect the physiology of the human body include buoyancy and specific gravity, hydrostatic pressure, viscosity, and fluid dynamics.

Buoyancy and Specific Gravity

Archimedes' principle states that when a body is immersed in a fluid, it will experience an upward thrust equal to the weight of the fluid that was displaced.[2] Buoyancy is the upward thrust acting in the opposite direction of gravity; it is related to the specific gravity of the immersed object. By definition, the specific gravity of water is 1.0; the specific gravity of a human averages 0.974, which implies that on average, humans float when immersed.[2] However, lean body mass (bone, muscle, and organs) has a specific gravity of 1.1, whereas fat has a specific gravity of 0.9.[2] Therefore, lean athletes may have difficulty floating because of their body composition, which causes them to rest slightly below the water's surface, or their lean extremities may sink while their trunk remains at the surface. Consequently, buoyant equipment may be necessary on the trunk or at various points along the limb to maintain buoyancy of a lean athlete in the pool.

Buoyancy has numerous clinical implications. Buoyancy-assisted exercises, which are movements toward the surface of the water, increase mobility and range of motion (ROM).[3] Buoyancy-supported exercises are movements that are perpendicular to the upward thrust of buoyancy and parallel to the bottom of the pool. When performing buoyancy-supported exercises, buoyancy neither assists nor impedes the movement; it is similar to active ROM on land. Finally,

Table 11-1 Buoyancy-Related Movements and Exercises

Movement	Examples
Buoyancy assisted (PROM, AAROM)	Standing shoulder abduction from 0° to 90° In the prone position, shoulder flexion from 90° to 180° Standing knee extension from 90° to 0° (with the hip in 90° of flexion) Standing knee flexion from 0° to 90° (with the hip in neutral)
Buoyancy supported (AROM)	Trunk lateral flexion or hip abduction in the supine position (with flotations supporting the body) Standing shoulder horizontal adduction
Buoyancy resisted (RROM)	Standing elbow extension (with the shoulder in neutral) Standing knee extension (from 90° of knee flexion with the hip in neutral) Shoulder flexion from 0° to 90° in the prone position

AAROM, Active assisted range of motion; *AROM,* active range of motion; *PROM,* passive range of motion; *RROM,* resisted range of motion.

buoyancy-resisted exercises directly oppose the upward thrust of buoyancy and are directed toward the bottom of the pool. They are similar to resisted exercises on land. Buoyancy-related movements and sample exercises are summarized in Table 11-1.

Clinical Pearl #1

Because athletes are often very lean, they may have difficulty maintaining buoyancy. To properly position the athlete in the water, the clinician may need to strategically place buoyant equipment along the athlete's limbs, trunk, or both.

Hydrostatic Pressure

Pascal's law of hydrostatic pressure states that at any given depth, the pressure from the liquid is exerted equally on all surfaces of the immersed object.[2] As the depth of the liquid increases, so does hydrostatic pressure. Water exerts a pressure of 22.4 mm Hg/ft of water depth. At a water depth of 4 feet, the force from hydrostatic pressure is 89.6 mm Hg, which is slightly greater than diastolic pressure.[2] Therefore, hydrostatic pressure may be used in rehabilitation to control effusion in an injured extremity while allowing the athlete to exercise. The effects of hydrostatic pressure occur immediately on immersion; blood is pushed proximally from the lower extremities, the chest wall is compressed, and the diaphragm is displaced upwardly.[2] These changes have a significant impact on exercise training parameters.

Viscosity

Viscosity is defined as the friction occurring between individual molecules in a liquid, and it is responsible for resistance to flow.[4] Resistance occurs as the molecules adhere to the surface of the

Clinical Pearl #2

In general, in water greater than 4 feet in depth, hydrostatic pressure will exceed the athlete's diastolic pressure. Therefore, hydrostatic pressure may allow an athlete with an ankle injury to exercise acutely without increasing effusion.

moving object. Consequently, viscosity is noticeable only with motion through the liquid. Because of viscosity, all fast movements are subject to resistance in water, even in a buoyancy-assisted direction. In addition, when a patient who experiences pain with movement decreases the speed of movement, resistance also decreases, thereby allowing the patient to control the intensity of exercise.

Fluid Dynamics

Two different types of water flow exist: laminar flow and turbulent flow. Laminar flow is the smooth, streamlined flow of water molecules. It has the least amount of resistance because the water molecules are all traveling the same speed and direction. In contrast, turbulent flow is interrupted flow, as when laminar flow encounters an object, which causes the water molecules to rebound in all directions. As an object moves through water, resistance is created from pressure. Positive pressure exists in front of a moving object and impedes movement. The area immediately behind a moving object, the wake, is an area of low pressure and can hold the object back. This drag force created behind the object produces the majority of resistance to movement.[2]

The shape of the object moving the water affects drag. A tapered, streamlined object will produce minimal disruption of flow, whereas an unstreamlined object will create rapid disruption of flow and cause turbulence.[2] For example, forward walking is more resistive than walking sideways (Fig. 11-1, *A* and *B*).

Resistance is an important variable that clinicians can use when designing a rehabilitation program for an athlete. Resistance can be modified in three ways. First, resistance is affected by speed of movement. Drag force is proportional to the velocity of movement: the faster the movement, the greater the drag force and resistance to movement.[2] For example, standing knee flexion and extension at 45°/sec will not be as challenging as performing the same movement at 120°/sec. Second, the frontal surface area of the object is directly proportional to the drag force produced and may be used to alter resistance. For instance, shoulder internal and external rotation with the forearms pronated creates less drag than performing the same exercise with the forearm neutral (Fig. 11-2, *A* and *B*). Finally, the flow of the water is another factor that affects resistance.[2] Turbulent water flow increases the friction between molecules and therefore increases resistance to movement. This is the theory behind competitive swimmers' preference to race through "still" water; resistance is less in nonturbulent water, which makes it easier for athletes to "pull" themselves through the water. All these factors and their effects on movement must be taken into consideration when designing a rehabilitation program for athletes. Table 11-2 summarizes methods to alter resistance in the pool.

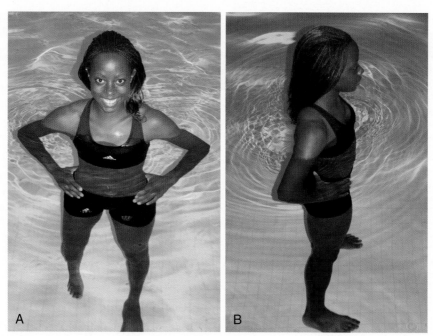

FIGURE 11-1 A, Resistance is increased by walking in the sagittal plane because of increased surface area (thereby creating turbulent flow). **B,** Resistance is decreased when walking in the frontal plane because of decreased surface area.

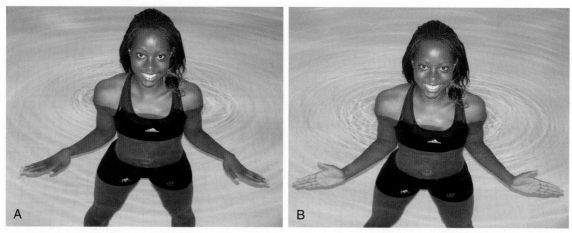

FIGURE 11-2 A, Performing rotator cuff strengthening with the forearms pronated. **B,** Performing the same exercises with the forearms in neutral, which is more challenging due to increased surface area.

The type of muscle contraction is also an important consideration when designing a resistance program. Exercises performed against the water's resistance almost always elicit concentric muscle contractions. Consider performance of shoulder internal and external rotation with the shoulder in neutral; the movements elicit concentric contractions of the rotator cuff muscles in a reciprocal fashion. However, it is possible to elicit eccentric muscle contractions in two ways: by using large pieces of buoyant equipment or with the use of a current. For example, an eccentric contraction of the hamstrings can be achieved when performing knee extension from 90° to 0° (with the hip in 90° of flexion) if a large flotation device is placed on the ankle. The athlete must eccentrically contract the hamstrings in a controlled fashion (Fig. 11-3). In addition, eccentric contractions can be generated with the use of a current, as with the Swim Ex or

Hydro Track AquaCiser III. For example, eccentric contractions of the left infraspinatus/teres minor can be accomplished by having athletes stand with the left side of their body against the current. They can achieve an eccentric contraction by holding a piece of equipment that increases surface area while allowing their shoulder to go from external rotation (in 0° shoulder abduction) to internal rotation in a controlled fashion. The faster the current, the greater the eccentric contraction generated.

Effect of Depth of Immersion on Weight Bearing

The depth of water affects weight bearing because of the buoyancy of water. This is an important issue when designing a rehabilitation program, specifically for the lower extremities, for

Table 11-2 Strategies to Alter Resistance in the Pool

Methods to Alter Resistance	Effect	
	To Make an Exercise More Challenging	To Make an Exercise Less Challenging
Speed of movement	↑ Speed	↓ Speed
Object surface area	↑ Surface area	↓ Surface area
Water flow	Turbulent flow	Streamlined flow

Table 11-3 Static Weight-Bearing Percentages for Males and Females

Anatomic Landmark	Weight-Bearing Percentages	
	Males	Females
Seventh cervical vertebrae	8	8
Xiphoid process	35	28
Anterior superior iliac spine	54	47

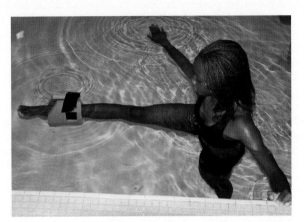

FIGURE 11-3 Eccentric contraction of the hamstrings can be achieved by using buoyant equipment as the knee extends from a flexed position.

Table 11-4 Summary of Cardiovascular Responses That Occur at Rest

Measure	Response
Right atrial venous pressure	Increases (8-12 mm Hg)
Heart blood volume	Increases (180-250 mL)
Cardiac output	Increases (25% +)
Stroke volume	Increases (25% +)
Central venous pressure	Increases
Heart rate	Remains the same or decreases slightly
Systemic blood pressure	Remains the same or increases slightly

From Thein, J.M., and Brody, L.T. (1998): Aquatic-based rehabilitation and training for the elite athlete. J. Orthop. Sports Phys. Ther., 27:32–41. Reprinted with permission.

which weight bearing may be a concern. General weight-bearing percentages for males and females are listed in Table 11-3.[5] These numbers reflect static weight bearing; increasing the activity level to a fast walk can increase weight bearing by as much as 76%.[5] Consequently, two options for progression of lower extremity weight bearing are available: decreasing the depth of the water and increasing the amount of impact at any given depth.

Clinical Pearl #3

Resistance can be increased in three ways: by increasing the speed of movement, by increasing the frontal surface area of the object, and by performing exercises in turbulent (versus "still") water. The clinician must choose the most appropriate progression based on the athlete's functional needs.

PHYSIOLOGIC RESPONSES TO AQUATIC EXERCISE

Responses to Water Immersion

Physiologic changes occur when immersed in water, both at rest and during exercise. It is imperative that the clinician be aware of these changes to modify rehabilitation programs appropriately. Changes that occur at rest during water immersion are the result of hydrostatic pressure. Most importantly, a cephalad redistribution of blood flow of approximately 0.7 L occurs.[6] Of the 0.7 L redistributed proximally, one third of the blood is redistributed to the heart and two thirds to the pulmonary arterial circulation.[6] Because of the increase in blood volume, the heart distends and myocardial wall tension increases, which results in a Frank-Starling reflex and a subsequent increase in stroke volume (SV) by approximately 35%.[6-11] Diuresis and hormonal changes have also been observed with sustained periods of water immersion (Table 11-4).[12-15]

Immersion and Response to Exercise

Several studies have been conducted to determine whether cardiovascular training can be performed effectively in the water.[16-19] Davidson[17] performed a study to determine the effects of deep water running (DWR) and road running (RR) on the maximal oxygen consumption ($\dot{V}o_2$max) of untrained females in a crossover design. They determined that $\dot{V}o_2$max values did not differ between groups and concluded that both DWR and RR can improve cardiovascular fitness in young, sedentary women.[17]

Byrne et al[16] compared heart rate (HR), SV, and cardiac output ($\dot{Q}$) when 20 subjects ambulated at 2 and 3 mph on a dry land treadmill and an underwater treadmill. Underwater treadmill walking resulted in greater $\dot{Q}$ and SV at both speeds. When oxygen consumption ($\dot{V}o_2$) levels for land and water were matched, the underwater treadmill session demonstrated a significantly lower HR and higher SV. The authors concluded that underwater treadmill walking may be beneficial and that HR may be a poor indicator of aquatic exercise intensity.[16]

Robertson and Factora[18] compared heart rates during DWR and shallow water running (SWR) at the same rate of perceived exertion. The authors found a significant difference of 10 beats/min between mean DWR (145 beats/min) and mean SWR (155 beats/min). The authors concluded that clinicians should not prescribe SWR at HR values obtained from DWR exercise.[18]

To determine whether a water running program could maintain aerobic performance, Wilber et al[19] studied 16 trained male runners. The runners were assigned to either a treadmill running or a water running group and trained five times per week for 6 weeks. The results showed no group differences. The authors concluded that DWR may serve as an effective alternative to land running to maintain aerobic performance.[19]

Based on these studies and others, it has been determined that in general, $\dot{V}o_2$ is approximately three times greater at a given speed in water than on land. Therefore, a training effect can be achieved at a lower intensity in water than on land.[20,21] In addition, HR during cardiovascular training will be approximately 10 beats/min lower than values attained during comparable exercise on land.[6]

Effects of Water Temperature

Water temperature can have a profound effect on the cardiovascular response to exercise. Water is an effective conductor, with heat transferred 25 times faster than in air.[2] Avellini et al[22] studied three groups of males: one group exercising on land and one group each exercising in 32°C (90°F) or 20°C (68°F) water, respectively. Based on their findings, the authors concluded that training in cold water enhances SV and decreases HR, thereby increasing exercise efficiency.[22]

In contrast, exercising in warm water can increase cardiovascular demands above those of exercise alone. Choukroun and Varene[23] studied the effects of water temperature on the cardiovascular system of resting subjects immersed to the neck in 25°C (77°F), 34°C (93°F), and 40°C (104°F) water while measuring cardiovascular demands. $\dot{Q}$ increased significantly at 40°C (104°F).[23] Because of the potential for heat-associated illness, temperature recommendations for intense training of athletes should be between 26°C and 28°C (79°F and 82°F) to prevent any heat-related complications.

REHABILITATION

As a result of the unique properties of water, aquatic rehabilitation offers advantages over land-based rehabilitation. It is imperative that the clinician apply aquatic principles appropriately when designing a rehabilitation program for an injured athlete. Buoyancy decreases weight bearing and joint compressive forces, which may be an important consideration with lower extremity rehabilitation. Buoyancy also allows exercises to be progressed from assisted, to supported, to resisted by simply changing the position of the athlete in the water. Because of viscosity, resistance is encountered in all directions of movement, and it can be modified by adjusting the lever arm, the speed of movement, or the turbulence of the water. Because resistance increases as the speed of movement increases, water provides an accommodating resistance to exercise and makes rehabilitation programs safe for an injured athlete.

Water also makes an ideal environment for cardiovascular conditioning. Training can be performed in a non–weight-bearing or partial–weight-bearing environment to allow the athlete to begin conditioning sooner. For example, an athlete with a lower extremity injury (e.g., an inversion ankle sprain) may perform DWR without the deleterious effects of increased edema because of the hydrostatic pressure of water. As healing continues, the athlete may be progressed to SWR, which minimizes the impact in comparison to land-based running.[24]

Similar to land-based programs, the principles of tissue healing and exercise progression must be respected when designing an aquatic-based rehabilitation program for an athlete to prevent delayed healing and further injury. Cardiovascular conditioning should be addressed as soon as possible to prevent deconditioning. Stretching and ROM may be started when indicated, and strengthening, gait training, and increased weight bearing are initiated and progressed as tolerated with respect to tissue-healing constraints. The later phases of aquatic rehabilitation involve specific cardiovascular-conditioning drills combined with functional movement patterns, balance, impact loading, plyometrics, and sport-specific drills.[25,26] An aquatic-based program can also be used to add variety to a maintenance program.

Cardiovascular Conditioning

Cardiovascular conditioning is a key component of a comprehensive rehabilitation program. With proper use of a pool, athletes can maintain or improve their cardiovascular function while resting an injury. This is particularly useful for athletes with a lower extremity injury, who may have weight-bearing or impact restrictions.

Appropriate warm-up and cool-down periods are fundamental components of the rehabilitation program. These activities should be performed in the water and may include walking, jogging, bicycling, or calisthenics; stretching should complement the warm-up and cool-down sessions. Many different cardiovascular activities may be performed. Depending on the stage of rehabilitation, the clinician may have the athlete rest the affected area or may choose to challenge muscles specific to the sport or activity. For example, a basketball player with a subacute knee injury may perform deep water cross-country skiing (possibly with a knee immobilizer to minimize knee motion). In the later phases of rehabilitation, SWR with impact may be appropriate. Both running and cross-country skiing may be performed in shallow or deep water, and the athlete may be tethered to the side of the pool in either depth. When teaching these techniques, the clinician should encourage proper form. The athlete is encouraged to maintain an upright posture and avoid excessive leaning, which mimics a swimming stroke. Running involves a small amount of ROM of the upper extremity but requires hip and knee flexion in the lower extremity. In contrast, cross-country skiing requires a large amount of hip and shoulder flexion and extension. Techniques may be modified to protect an injured area. When performing drills or cardiovascular conditioning in shallow water, the athlete may want to use aqua shoes or wear an old pair of running shoes in the pool. This will minimize foot irritation while offering support to the foot.

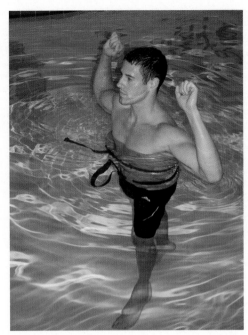

FIGURE 11-4 Vertical kicking using a flotation vest with the arms out of the water.

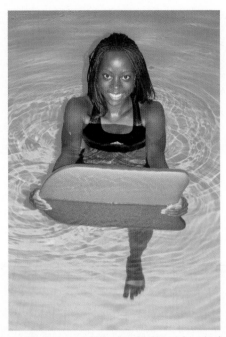

FIGURE 11-5 Lineman drills with kickboards, which increase surface area, will make the exercise functional and challenging.

When basic cardiovascular-conditioning techniques have been mastered, advanced techniques such as vertical kicking may be incorporated, if indicated. Vertical kicking in deep water may be performed with or without fins and should be initiated with a small flutter kick. The athlete may initially require a flotation vest as well (Fig. 11-4). The athlete may be progressed to a dolphin kick, which is used with the butterfly stroke but performed in an upright position, especially if dynamic lumbar stabilization is indicated. Ideally, kicking should be performed without upper extremity assistance, with the arms held behind the back or out of the water.

Flotation vests may be used when initially instructing an athlete in a technique, if safety is a concern, or if the athlete is very lean. If possible, the flotation device should be discontinued to increase the difficulty of the workout. When selecting a belt or vest, the device needs to be assessed regarding its primary location of flotation or buoyancy. To maintain the athlete in a vertical position, a vest or belt that provides flotation uniformly around the entire circumference of the belt is recommended.

The fundamental guidelines for cardiovascular training should be at the core of program design. Twenty-five minutes five times per week or more is recommended as a minimum, but many athletes will need a longer training period, depending on the season and sport. The intensity and duration should mimic the athlete's particular sport. Ankle floats, arm paddles or gloves, and fins will increase the lever arm and resistance, and discontinuing use of the flotation vest will also make the activity more challenging. The athlete may increase speed to further increase resistance.

Like land-based exercise, the program should be as sport specific as possible. For example, a marathon runner might perform low-intensity, long-duration running and cross-country skiing, with the workload maintained at 70% to 80% $\dot{V}o_2$max. In contrast, a volleyball player can perform interval jumping drills and work near peak $\dot{V}o_2$, with intermittent jogging and shuffling drills used for recovery. Likewise, a football lineman may perform shallow water sprints with a resistive board for 6- to 10-second intervals, with light jogging during recovery, to replicate the demands of his sport (Fig. 11-5). A number of stations or a variety of exercises performed during a single session can alleviate boredom and ensure a well-rounded workout.

Stretching

Mobility may be impaired following an injury or surgery or can result from the pain of overuse injuries, such as tendinitis or tendinosis. The impaired mobility may be manifested as altered biomechanics, and a goal of rehabilitation may be restoration of normal osteokinematics and joint arthrokinematics. The pool is an ideal medium to improve mobility of the upper extremity. Because upward movement of the glenohumeral joint is assisted by buoyancy, the athlete may discover that normal shoulder movement patterns occur earlier in the pool than on land. This movement is similar to active assisted ROM on land, but instead of having the limb supported by a pulley or cane, the buoyancy of the water now supports the extremity. Accordingly, the athlete can position himself or herself in a sport-specific position to restore familiar muscle length-tension relationships in the upper extremity and trunk. Buoyant equipment may assist the movement initially and may be discontinued as active and resistive ROM exercises are initiated (Fig. 11-6).

Lower extremity stretching can also be performed successfully in the pool. Large muscle groups, such as the hamstrings, gluteals, adductors, and quadriceps, may be stretched in a buoyancy-assisted fashion. Functional positions and length-tension relationships can be restored sooner in the pool than on land (Figs. 11-7 and 11-8).

A warm water pool (32°C to 35°C [90°F to 95°F]) provides a relaxing environment, which may allow increased soft tissue extensibility. Thus, athletes may find themselves performing

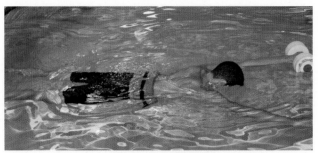

FIGURE 11-6 Stretching of the latissimus dorsi is achieved via buoyancy-assisted shoulder flexion to 180°. The athlete is prone in the water and may need cuing to bias the spine into a posterior pelvic tilt; this can be achieved by placing buoyant equipment under the abdomen. The athlete may wear a snorkel to breathe if a prolonged stretch is desired.

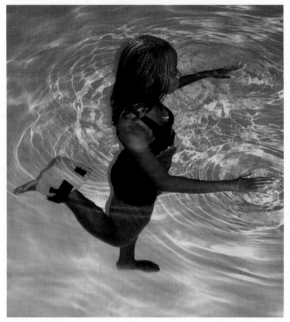

FIGURE 11-7 Buoyancy-assisted stretching of the quadriceps muscle. The athlete may require verbal cuing to maintain the pelvis in a slightly posterior pelvic tilt to provide optimal lengthening of the rectus femoris.

their warm-up and cool-down routines in a warm water pool and performing the cardiovascular and strength-training portion of their program in cooler water. When stretching, the duration of the stretch can vary, but to promote tissue elongation and permanent structural changes, a low-intensity, long-duration (20 to 30 seconds) stretch has proved to be beneficial. However, ballistic stretching may be indicated after the muscle is adequately warmed up.[27] Stretching should be performed as indicated throughout the rehabilitation process.

Resistance Training and Functional Progression

Upper Extremity

Restoration of loss of strength is crucial for any athlete, and strength training is a large component of any rehabilitation program. The clinician may prescribe a comprehensive aquatic

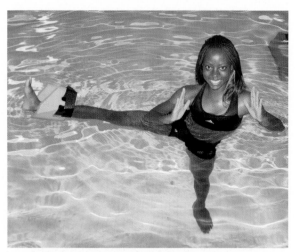

FIGURE 11-8 An athlete participating in martial arts may find prolonged stretch of the hip adductors in a functional position beneficial. Buoyant equipment may be placed anywhere along the affected extremity.

strengthening program for the athlete by using equipment and implementing the basic principles of aquatics. The program should be sport specific as much as possible and consider the intensity, duration, and type of muscular contraction that the athlete will incur in the particular sport.

The viscosity of water provides resistance, and exercises consist of isometric or dynamic contractions. Isometric contractions require the athlete to stabilize against movement of the water, whereas dynamic exercises produce either a concentric or eccentric muscle contraction. The type of contraction required by the exercise should reflect the type of contraction needed during the sport. For example, resisted walking with the arms in various positions will generate isometric contractions of the scapular stabilizers (Fig. 11-9, *A* and *B*). Dynamic contractions in the pool typically consist of reciprocal concentric contractions, which is different from what occurs on land. In the pool, the athlete typically performs a concentric contraction of the agonist followed by a concentric contraction of the antagonist. Eccentric contractions can be performed via various methods as described previously; the clinician should design a program specific to the individual.

Shoulder-strengthening exercises that are performed on land can be performed in the pool. Examples include glenohumeral flexion/extension and abduction/adduction from 0° to 90° in shoulder-deep water, horizontal abduction/adduction, elbow flexion and extension, and shoulder internal and external rotation. In addition, diagonal patterns, such as those implemented in proprioceptive neuromuscular facilitation, may be used. As with stretching activities, resistive exercise can be performed through only partial ROM (if indicated). Another consideration with upper extremity strengthening is that the mechanics is different for some exercises when compared with their land-based counterparts. For example, shoulder horizontal abduction and adduction performed at 90° of abduction is resisted in the transverse plane but supported in the sagittal plane. That is, the athlete no longer has to hold the arm abducted against gravity while performing the horizontal component of the exercise. The clinician must be cognizant of these changes to appropriately use the principles of aquatics (Fig. 11-10).

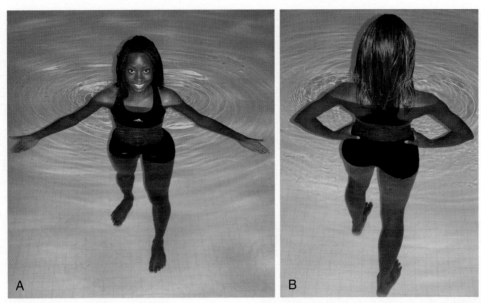

FIGURE 11-9 Walking with the upper extremities in various positions will challenge the scapular stabilizers. **A,** Forward walking with the arms in the scapular plane. **B,** Backward walking with the arms in 60° of abduction. The scapular stabilizers must contract isometrically to maintain the scapula in proper position.

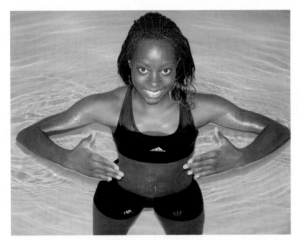

FIGURE 11-10 Buoyancy-supported elbow flexion and extension.

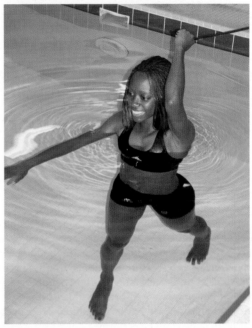

FIGURE 11-11 Performing sport-specific drills, such as a tennis serve, can be done in the pool with resistive bands. The water will offer additional resistance to the trunk and core body. The clinician must be certain that the line of pull of the resistive band is similar to the resistance experienced during the sport.

Overhead activity can be performed in the pool. Resistive tubing may be used in the pool just as it is on land. An added advantage of performing the exercise in the pool is that the water will provide additional resistance to the trunk and core, thereby requiring the athlete to recruit core stabilizers. For example, an athlete may practice the motion of a tennis serve while standing in chest-deep water and using resistive bands. The water is providing core body resistance, whereas the band resists arm movement (Fig. 11-11). Second, exercise may be performed while supine, while prone with a snorkel, or while standing forward flexed in shallow water with the face turned and out of the water. A wide range of resistive and stabilization activities can be performed in these positions. For example, while supine with the arms abducted 90°, rapid alternating movements of shoulder internal and external rotation can be performed (Fig. 11-12). This may be a very functional beginning exercise for a middle or outside blocker in volleyball. The athlete may perform rapid alternating small movements of shoulder flexion and extension with the arms flexed to 150° to 180° and the elbow extended to increase the length of the lever arm (Fig. 11-13). Both exercises require muscular cocontraction for stabilization. Athletes should perform sport-specific repetitions and sets, such as sets of 30 to 50 repetitions until fatigue ensues, to ensure quality of movement and proper form.

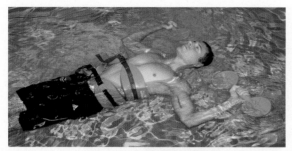

FIGURE 11-12 Rapid alternating movements elicit cocontraction of the glenohumeral musculature, which enhances stability. This is a functional position for an overhead athlete.

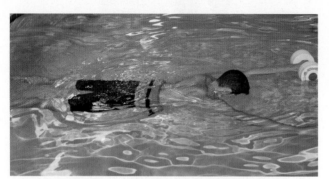

FIGURE 11-13 Eccentric contractions are achieved with the use of buoyant equipment. In the prone position with the arm overhead, the buoyant equipment forces the glenohumeral joint into overhead flexion; the athlete is required to eccentrically control the movement. This can be followed by a concentric contraction of the same muscle group. When performed rapidly, this exercise requires stabilization of the glenohumeral joint and proves to be beneficial for volleyball players, particularly middle and outside blockers. Notice that this is the same position as in Figure 11-6, but the intent is entirely different.

Upper extremity closed kinetic chain exercises are beneficial for athletes whose sports require such activities, such as gymnasts and wrestlers, and may be performed in the pool. Dips at the side of the pool, which use triceps, deltoid, and scapular stabilizers, may be performed more easily because of the buoyancy-assisted upward movement of the body. Buoyancy-assisted pull-ups can be performed with an overhead railing or ladder. Overhead push-pull in the buoyancy-supported supine or prone position may be specific to the athlete's sport.

Upper extremity impact may be introduced in the pool. Wall push-ups with impact can be performed safely because viscosity will slow the body's movement through water. The athlete may start in chest-deep water and progress by moving to more shallow water and by standing farther away from the wall.

When performing open chain upper extremity training, surface area will be increased substantially with equipment such as gloves, paddles, and resistive bells. Resistive boards may also be used and held under water in front of the athlete while performing a "push-pull" motion for scapular protraction/retraction to strengthen the rhomboids, trapezius, and serratus anterior. The clinician must remember that a small increase in surface area will translate into a significant increase in resistance in the upper extremity. Other equipment specific to the athlete's sport should be used throughout the rehabilitation process.

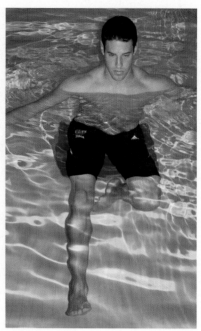

FIGURE 11-14 Seated open chain knee flexion and extension exercises challenge lower extremity endurance and core body strength and may be performed with or without fins.

For example, a baseball player may use an old bat to mimic the swinging motion, whereas a tennis player may practice forehand and backhand with an old racket.

Lower Extremity

The lower extremity functions in both the open and closed chain during activities of daily living and sporting activities. Consequently, it is imperative that the athlete's rehabilitation program consist of both types of exercises. Lower extremity–strengthening exercises can be performed completely non–weight bearing in the open chain. Examples include hip flexion/extension and abduction/adduction and knee flexion/extension. More advanced activities, such as vertical kicking, are especially effective for increasing lower extremity muscle endurance (see Fig. 11-4). Another excellent lower extremity endurance exercise is kicking while prone or supine with fins. These exercises require concentric contractions at the hip and isometric contractions at the knee. Sitting on a flotation device while performing repetitive knee flexion and extension with or without fins is a very fatiguing open chain quadriceps and hamstring exercise and proves beneficial for those involved in kicking sports, such as football and soccer. This activity also requires trunk stabilization because the athlete is sitting on a dynamic surface (Fig. 11-14). Fins, which increase surface area, or ankle cuffs, which increase buoyancy, are effective means of increasing resistance in an open chain. Resistive boots can increase resistance as much as fourfold, and exercises using boots are useful in sports requiring explosive power such as figure skating and gymnastics.[28,29]

To strengthen the quadriceps and gluteals in a closed kinetic chain, such exercises as lunges, step-downs, and squats may be incorporated. Because of buoyancy, the eccentric work with most aquatic exercise is decreased relative to comparable land-based exercise. Floating squats, in which the athlete stands on

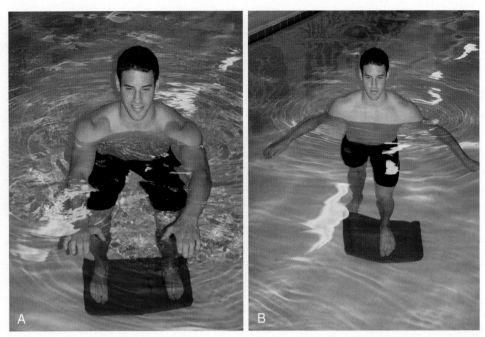

FIGURE 11-15 Floating squats can be performed with the athlete using a flotation board. **A,** Double-leg squats. **B,** Single-leg squats.

a flotation board and pushes down, require coordination and eccentric control. This drill can also be performed while standing with only one leg on the board (Fig. 11-15, *A* and *B*).

Lower extremity balance and proprioception are important to any athlete, and a well-designed rehabilitation program should address all impairments in balance. Balance is controlled by sensory input, central processing, and neuromuscular responses.[30] Any self-perturbation activity, such as hip flexion/extension and circumduction in waist-deep water while standing on the injured leg, will challenge balance. Other examples include single-leg balance on the injured leg while altering the center of gravity by moving the upper extremity, as in a push-pull motion with a kickboard, or rotation of the upper extremity while using water paddles as resistance. Increasing knee flexion on the weight-bearing leg will increase the challenge for these muscles. Additionally, athletes may close their eyes and rely more heavily on neuromuscular than on visual input (Fig. 11-16).

If impact is required for return to sport, jumping and hopping drills may be introduced in the pool. The viscosity of water allows jumping drills to be introduced while minimizing impact. Athletes who require explosive push-offs for sports such as track and baseball, as well as athletes in jumping sports, will benefit from jumping drills and plyometric drills.[25,26] In a study of female high school volleyball players, one group performed aquatic-based plyometric drills in approximately 4 feet of water, whereas another group performed the same exercises on land. The aquatic-based plyometric group had a larger increase in their vertical jump than did the land-based group.[25] In a similar study, college athletes were divided into an aquatic-based plyometric group, a land-based plyometric group, and a control group. Posttesting demonstrated that the two plyometric groups improved more than the control group did, with no difference seen between the two plyometric groups. However, the aquatic-based plyometric group performed their exercises in knee-deep water, which was most likely not deep enough to obtain the benefits of buoyancy.[26] When instructing an athlete in jumping

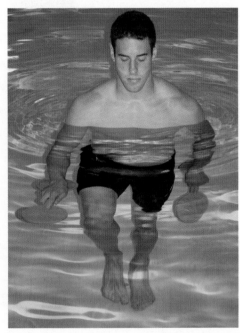

FIGURE 11-16 Single-leg balance with the eyes closed and the use of upper extremity self-perturbation. The arms are moving rapidly in a reciprocal fashion.

and plyometric drills, appropriate landing techniques in which the athlete works on bent-knee landings and "sticking" their landings should be emphasized. Examples of jumping progression include two-footed jumping in the sagittal plane progressed to single-leg hopping and eventually to hopping with 90° turns (Fig. 11-17, *A* and *B*). These drills are beneficial for figure skaters, gymnasts, and volleyball, soccer, and basketball players, for whom jumping and turning are essential skills. The athlete may jump from different heights as well (Fig. 11-18, *A* and *B*).

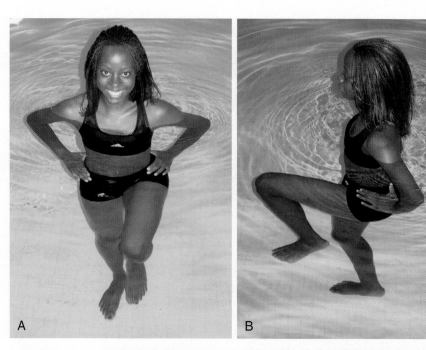

FIGURE 11-17 Shallow water single-leg hopping drills with 90° turns. **A,** Start position. **B,** End position.

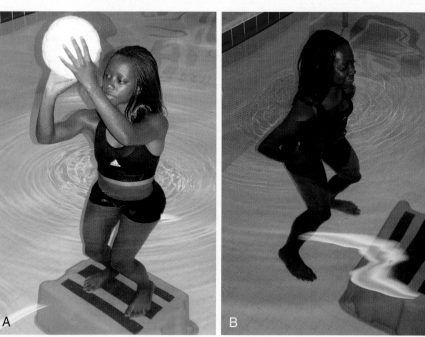

FIGURE 11-18 Box jumping with 180° turns. The athlete shoots the ball while turning 180°. **A,** Start position. **B,** End position.

Bounding and leaping drills may also be introduced in the pool. All impact drills may be made more challenging by performing the drills with the eyes closed, by decreasing the depth of the water, by progressing to single-leg jumps, and by incorporating upper extremity activities such as shooting a basketball or playing catch while performing the activity. Shock absorptive shoes may be necessary for these activities.

Spine

Strengthening of the spinal musculature can be accomplished successfully with use of the pool. Numerous pathologies, such as mechanical low back pain, disk herniation, spondylolysis, and spondylolisthesis, can be managed in the pool.[31-33] Disk herniation is typically treated with an exercise program biased toward

extension.[32] Exercises, such as backward walking, backward lunges, and hip extension, while standing may prove beneficial. In addition, the front crawl biases the spine into extension and may prove to be a successful means of providing some cardiovascular conditioning in an athlete with a herniated disk. Lying supine in the pool with a flotation device, such as a noodle or buoyant belt under the low back region, may minimize radicular symptoms (Fig. 11-19).

For athletes with spondylolysis or spondylolisthesis, a program biased toward flexion will be most beneficial. Such exercises as a single knee to chest while standing with the use of buoyant equipment may be beneficial (Fig. 11-20). In addition, hip flexion, such as when marching, may decrease symptoms. Performing lower extremity–strengthening exercises in a seated position, as described previously, will provide an athlete with

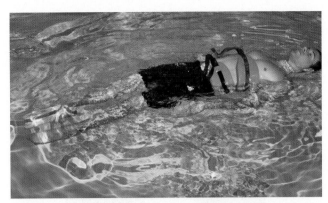

FIGURE 11-19 Supine lying with buoyant equipment under the lumbar spine to bias the athlete into extension may be beneficial for disk herniation.

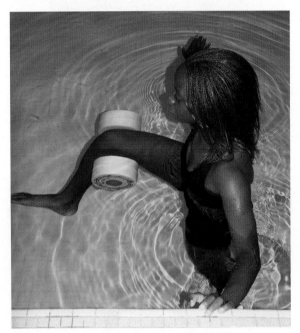

FIGURE 11-20 Standing single knee to the chest with the use of buoyant equipment will bias the spine into flexion.

spondylolysis or spondylolisthesis an opportunity to maintain or improve lower extremity strength without increasing symptoms in the low back region.

As an athlete with lumbar spine pathology improves, introducing impact in the pool will provide the athlete with a safe, controlled environment. The athlete may perform cross-country skiing, jogging, and brisk walking as described previously. In the case of an athlete with spinal pathology, the activity can be biased into flexion or extension, depending on the athlete's condition.

Clinical Pearl #4

The pool is an excellent environment to introduce impact loading and landing techniques into the rehabilitation program. Because of buoyancy, eccentric contractions are minimized with landings and closed kinetic chain activities.

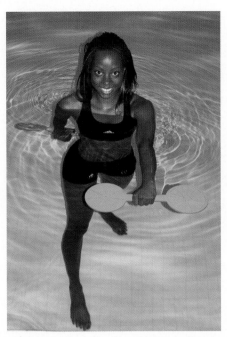

FIGURE 11-21 Reciprocal shoulder flexion and extension with paddles require isometric stabilization via the internal and external obliques.

Core Body Strengthening

Core body strength and postural control are critical for any athlete. Baseball players must be able to transfer kinetic energy from their lower extremity to the arm via their trunk musculature. A soccer player must be able to twist and rotate at the trunk while kicking or passing the soccer ball. A pole vaulter must be able to stabilize the trunk and lower extremity while rotating the body around the shoulder to clear the bar. Core body strength can easily be addressed in the pool and makes a nice addition to a rehabilitation program in the area of maintenance and prevention. Because any extremity movement must be counterbalanced by a stabilizing force in the trunk, most extremity exercises also train the core body. For example, standing leg kicks in a sagittal plane require both single-leg balance and core strength to avoid being displaced by the movement of the leg against the water. Similarly, bilateral shoulder flexion and extension cause posterior and anterior displacement of the body, respectively, which must be counteracted by the rectus abdominis and trunk extensor muscles. Alternating shoulder flexion and extension challenges the internal and external obliques as they stabilize the rotational forces created by the arm motion (Fig. 11-21).

The previous examples require the core body to perform as a static stabilizer; however, in most sporting activities, the trunk musculature, including the transversus abdominis, must be engaged during dynamic activity. Accordingly, incorporating dynamic exercises, as previously mentioned, is a crucial part of any athlete's rehabilitation program. Therefore, it is imperative that the clinician properly instruct the athlete in core recruitment of the abdominal musculature in conjunction with instruction for any extremity-strengthening exercise or cardiovascular exercise. For example, before performing alternating biceps curls with paddles, the athlete should be instructed in proper recruitment of the core musculature. Cues such as "pull your belly button back to your spine" and "lift the floor of your pelvis up by contracting the muscles you would use to stop the flow of urine" may

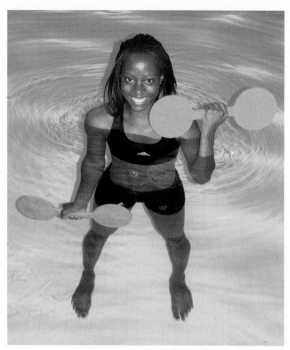

FIGURE 11-22 Alternating biceps/triceps with paddles while performing core recruitment. This concept superimposes movement on a stable base of support.

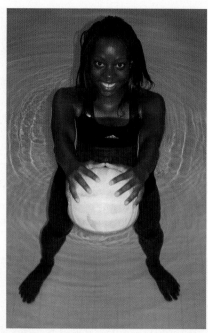

FIGURE 11-23 Eccentric abdominal strengthening with a buoyant ball. This exercise may be performed in the sagittal plane to focus on the rectus abdominis or with trunk rotation to incorporate the obliques.

be helpful (Fig. 11-22). Athletes should be reminded frequently to maintain low-grade muscle contraction of their core musculature throughout their rehabilitation program while performing all exercises. If specific strengthening of the rectus abdominis is indicated, eccentric work can be achieved with use of a buoyant ball by performing trunk flexion/extension while slowly allowing the ball to return to the surface of the water (Fig. 11-23). Sport-specific exercises, such as trunk rotations with the arms abducted, may benefit soccer players, golfers, or quarterbacks, who require a lot of rotation for their sport (Fig. 11-24). Resisted water walking/jogging with kickboards may be helpful for football linemen. Figure skaters, as well as long and triple jumpers, may increase core body strength via pike jumping.

Return to Sport

Although aquatic-based programs may be made very sport specific for an injured athlete, many athletes have difficulty mentally if they cannot train specifically for their particular sport. The biggest mistake made by most athletes is failing to allow adequate recovery time and returning too quickly after injury. An extensive, intense rehabilitation program that incorporates aquatics and challenges the athlete will permit the athlete to train and condition while allowing adequate recovery time. Some injuries, such as stress fractures and postoperative rehabilitation protocols, may have specific guidelines for return to sport and impact activities. Others, including overuse injuries, are often limited by symptoms. Consequently, the clinician must rely on subjective input and the athlete's response to functional testing to determine readiness to return to sport. Regardless of the injury, gradual return to sport and impact activities is crucial to prevent reinjury.

Before resuming land activities, the athlete should be put through a battery of sport-specific tests to assess readiness. An athlete with a lower extremity or spine injury may be assessed by observing response to activities in shallow water. Athletes

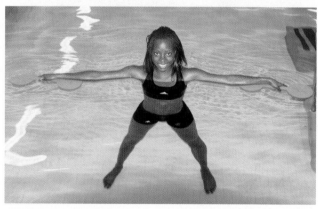

FIGURE 11-24 Trunk rotation with the arms abducted and paddles to increase surface area is a beneficial exercise for an athlete who requires rotation for a particular sport.

should be able to complete any testing with proper form and without a significant increase in pain, muscle soreness, or swelling. When the athlete tolerates the battery of tests, a land-based program may be initiated; such a program may or may not include impact, depending on the response to shallow water impact. The athlete may perform the water-based program on alternate days. Ideally, the athlete should increase time on land slowly, with no increase in pain, altered biomechanics, or significant muscle soreness. Land-based programs may continue to be complemented by pool programs indefinitely. Frequently, even on returning to preinjury status, an athlete may enjoy continuing to train in the pool one to two times per week for variety and to give their extremities a much needed break, especially from impact. Sample training programs for various athletes are presented in Tables 11-5 to 11-7.

Table 11-5 Sample Training Program for a Gymnast

Area of Focus	Activity
Upper extremity training	Standing shoulder horizontal abduction/adduction Standing shoulder PNF D1 and D2 to 90° of flexion Standing rows Standing wall push-ups with impact (double and single arm) Supine rapid shoulder IR/ER at 90° of abduction Supine overhead push-pull Prone rapid shoulder flexion/extension at 135° of abduction Elbow flexion and extension
Lower extremity training	Standing shallow water lunge jumps Vertical kicking with fins Seated knee flexion/extension sprints with fins Standing buoyancy-resisted knee extension Seated buoyancy-resisted knee flexion Standing hip adduction/abduction
Core training	Pike jumps Tuck jumps Side-to-side hops Leg lifts Ball push-downs Trunk rotations with paddles
Balance training	Eyes closed hip flexion/extension Eyes closed hip abduction/adduction, circumduction Leaping and bounding in all directions with single-leg landings (cannot use arms) Single-leg hopping with 90° and 180° turns
Cardiovascular training	½-Mile swim Deep water running and cross-country skiing Tethered shallow water sprints (10 seconds with jogging for recovery)

ER, External rotation; *IR*, internal rotation; *PNF*, proprioceptive neuromuscular facilitation.

CONCLUSION

Principles of Aquatics

Buoyancy
- Buoyancy can be used with assisted (passive), active assisted, supported (active), or resisted range of motion.

Specific Gravity
- Athletes who are very lean may require flotation devices to remain at the water's surface.

Hydrostatic Pressure
- Lower extremity effusion can be controlled with the hydrostatic pressure of water.

Viscosity
- Viscosity causes resistance to movement by adhering to the surface of the moving object.

Fluid Dynamics
- The pressure immediately behind a moving object, the wake, produces the majority of resistance to movement.

Table 11-6 Sample Training Program for a Football Lineman With a History of Low Back Pain

Area of Focus	Activity
Cardiovascular training	Shallow water interval sprints 1:2 work-rest intervals (15-second interval)
Flexibility	Stretching of the hamstrings, quadriceps, hip flexors, and gastrocnemius
Stabilization	Single-leg balance and shoulder horizontal abduction/adduction with paddles Single-leg balance and shoulder flexion/extension with paddles Kicking with fins sitting on a flotation device with the arms flexed forward as though blocking Standing trunk twists with paddles Floating squats without arm support
Core training	Straddle jumps Lunge jumps Explosive push-offs from a stance position
Sport specific	Standing explosive 10-second plow pushes forward and back Direction change sprinting drill Frontal and sagittal plane jump drills on aqua step Coordination drills over pool lines (such as carioca)

Weight Bearing
- Static weight-bearing percentages change significantly (by as much as 76%) with impact.

Physiologic Responses to Aquatic Exercise

Physiologic Responses to Water Immersion
- Numerous changes occur in the body when submersed in water, including a cephalad shift in blood flow, increase in heart blood volume, and increased cardiac output and stroke volume.

Immersion and Response to Exercise
- The pool can be used successfully to maintain or improve aerobic conditioning.
- Heart rate in the pool differs from heart rate on land.

Water Temperature
- The temperature of the water can have a significant effect on heart rate response; intense training of the athlete should be in water that is between 26°C and 28°C (79°F and 82°F)

Rehabilitation

Cardiovascular Conditioning
- Aerobic conditioning is a critical component of any rehabilitation program and can be performed successfully in the pool.
- Monitor technique if the athlete is a novice.

Table 11-7 Sample Training Program for a Basketball Player

Area of Focus	Activity
Upper extremity training	Prone overhead flexion/extension with paddles, small movements Standing abduction/adduction with gloves Standing kickboard plows (scapular protraction/retraction) Prone overhead wall push-ups Standing wall push-ups Elbow flexion/extension with gloves
Lower extremity training	Resisted hip flexion/extension, abduction/adduction, and circumduction Floating squats Resisted double/single-leg jumping (all planes, tethered to the side of the pool) Scissors jumping Shallow water lunges Buoyancy-resisted hip extension
Core training	Tuck jumps Leg lifts in deep water with the trunk supported by a flotation device Interval shallow water plow running (forward/backward) Ball push-downs
Balance training	Eyes closed single-leg box jumping with holding landing pose Eyes closed double-leg jumping with 90°, 180° turns Single-leg stance and trunk rotations with paddles
Combination drills	Tuck jumps with rotation Straddle/split jumps Vertical kicking without a flotation vest Sprint kickboard laps (supine and prone)
Cardiovascular training	Shallow water running, backpedaling, and shuffling with tuck jumping intervals $^{3}/_{4}$-Mile swim with fins Deep water cross-country skiing

Stretching

- The athlete may be able to achieve optimal length-tension relationships in the pool to allow prolonged stretching because of buoyancy.
- Use buoyant equipment and lever arms as necessary to maintain appropriate positioning.

Resistance Training and Functional Progression

- Resistance training can be performed successfully in the pool with buoyancy-resisted movements.
- Training can be progressed by increasing the speed of movement and surface area.
- Impact loading can be introduced in the pool before the athlete is ready for impact on land.
- Activities should be as sport specific as possible with the use of sports equipment.

Core Body Strengthening

- All movements of the extremities require static stabilization of the trunk via the core body musculature.
- Dynamic strength is required in all sports and can easily be addressed in the pool.

Return to Sport

- As on land, the late phases of an aquatic-based rehabilitation program should be as sport specific as possible.
- The pool provides a medium for maintenance programs.

REFERENCES

1. Martin, J. (2009): The Halliwick method. Physiotherapy, 67:288–291.
2. Becker, B.E. (2009): Aquatic therapy: Scientific foundations and clinical rehabilitation applications. PMR, 1:859–872.
3. Golland, A. (1981): Basic hydrotherapy. Physiotherapy, 67:258–262.
4. Poyhonen, T., Keskinen, K.L., Hautala, A., et al. (2000): Determination of hydrodynamic drag forces and drag coefficients on human leg/foot model during knee exercise. Clin. Biomech. (Bristol, Avon), 15:256–260.
5. Thein, J.M., and Brody, L.T. (1998): Aquatic-based rehabilitation and training for the elite athlete. J. Orthop. Sports Phys. Ther., 27:32–41.
6. Arborelius, M., Jr., Ballidin, U.I., Lilja, B., et al. (1972): Hemodynamic changes in man during immersion with the head above water. Aerosp. Med., 43:592–598.
7. Begin, R., Epstein, M., Sackner, M.A., et al. (1976): Effects of water immersion to the neck on pulmonary circulation and tissue volume in man. J. Appl. Physiol., 40:293–299.
8. Echt, M., Lange, L., and Gauer, O.H. (1974): Changes of peripheral venous tone and central transmural venous pressure during immersion in a thermo-neutral bath. Pflugers Arch., 352:211–217.
9. Farhi, L.E., and Linnarsson, D. (1977): Cardiopulmonary readjustments during graded immersion in water at 35 degrees C. Respir. Physiol., 30:35–50.
10. Lange, L., Lange, S., Echt, M., et al. (1974): Heart volume in relation to body posture and immersion in a thermo-neutral bath. A roentgenometric study. Pflugers Arch., 352:219–226.
11. Risch, W.D., Koubenec, H.J., Beckmann, U., et al. (1978): The effect of graded immersion on heart volume, central venous pressure, pulmonary blood distribution, and heart rate in man. Pflugers Arch., 374:115–118.
12. Epstein, M. (1978): Renal effects of head-out water immersion in man: Implications for an understanding of volume homeostasis. Physiol. Rev., 58:529–581.
13. Epstein, M., Preston, S., and Weitzman, R.E. (1981): Isoosmotic central blood volume expansion suppresses plasma arginine vasopressin in normal man. J. Clin. Endocrinol. Metab., 52:256–262.
14. Greenleaf, J.E., Shevartz, E., and Keil, L.C. (1981): Hemodilution, vasopressin suppression, and diuresis during water immersion in man. Aviat. Space Environ. Med., 52:329–336.
15. Lin, Y.C. (1984): Circulatory functions during immersion and breath-hold dives in humans. Undersea Biomed. Res., 11:123–138.
16. Byrne, H.K., Craig, J.N., and Willmore, J.H. (1996): A comparison of the effects of underwater treadmill walking to dry land treadmill walking on oxygen consumption, heart rate, and cardiac output. J. Aquatic Phys. Ther., 4:4.
17. Davidson, K. (2000): Deep water running and road running training improve Vo$_2$max in untrained women. J. Strength Cond. Res., 14:191.
18. Robertson, J.M., and Factora, K.I. (2001): Comparison of heart rates during water running in deep water and shallow water at the same rating of perceived exertion. J. Aquatic Phys. Ther., 9:21.
19. Wilber, R.L., Moffatt, R.J., Scott, B.E., et al. (1996): Influence of water run training on the maintenance of aerobic performance. Med. Sci. Sports Exerc., 28:1056–1062.
20. Evans, B.W., Cureton, K.J., and Purvis, J.W. (1978): Metabolic and circulatory responses to walking and jogging in water. Res. Q., 49:442–449.
21. Gleim, G.W., and Nicholas, J.A. (1989): Metabolic costs and heart rate responses to treadmill walking in water at different depths and temperatures. Am. J. Sports Med., 17:248–252.
22. Avellini, B.A., Shapiro, Y., and Pandolf, K.B. (1983): Cardio-respiratory physical training in water and on land. Eur. J. Appl. Physiol. Occup. Physiol., 50:255–263.
23. Choukroun, M.L., and Varene, P. (1990): Adjustments in oxygen transport during head-out immersion in water at different temperatures. J. Appl. Physiol., 68:1475–1480.
24. Harrison, R.A., and Bulstrode, S. (1992): Loading of the lower limb when walking partially immersed. Physiotherapy, 78:164.
25. Martel, G.F., Harmer, M.L., Logan, J.M., et al. (2005): Aquatic plyometric training increases vertical jump in female volleyball players. Med. Sci. Sports Exerc., 37:1814–1819.
26. Stemm, J.D., and Jacobson, B.H. (2007): Comparison of land- and aquatic-based plyometric training on vertical jump performance. J. Strength Cond. Res., 21:568–571.
27. Bandy, W.D., Irion, J.M., and Briggler, M. (1998): The effect of static stretch and dynamic range of motion training on the flexibility of the hamstring muscles. J. Orthop. Sports Phys. Ther., 27:295–300.
28. Law, L.A., and Smidt, G.L. (1996): Underwater forces produced by the hydro-tone bell. J. Orthop. Sports Phys. Ther., 23:267–271.

29. Svedenhag, J., and Seger, J. (1992): Running on land and in water: Comparative exercise physiology. Med. Sci. Sports Exerc., 24:1155–1160.
30. Wegener, L., Kisner, C., and Nichols, D. (1997): Static and dynamic balance responses in persons with bilateral knee osteoarthritis. J. Orthop. Sports Phys. Ther., 25:13–18.
31. Dundar, U., Solak, O., Yigit, I., et al. (2009): Clinical effectiveness of aquatic exercise to treat chronic low back pain: A randomized controlled trial. Spine, 34:1436–1440.
32. Kim, Y.S., Park, J., and Shim, J.K. (2010): Effects of aquatic backward locomotion exercise and progressive resistance exercise on lumbar extension strength in patients who have undergone lumbar diskectomy. Arch. Phys. Med. Rehabil., 91:208–214.
33. Waller, B., Lambeck, J., and Daly, D. (2009): Therapeutic aquatic exercise in the treatment of low back pain: A systematic review. Clin. Rehabil. 23:3–14.

Upper Extremity

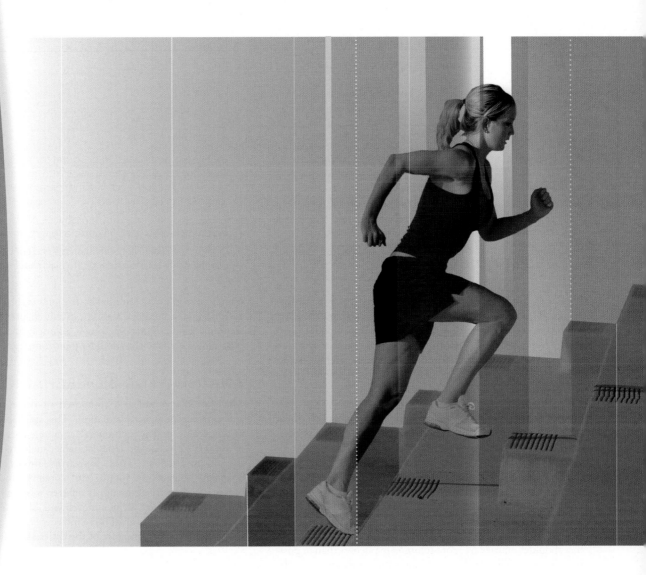

12

Shoulder Rehabilitation

Kevin E. Wilk, PT, DPT, Leonard C. Macrina, MSPT, SCS, CSCS,
and Christopher Arrigo, PT, MS, ATC

CHAPTER OBJECTIVES

- Incorporate biomechanical principles of the shoulder as they relate to prevention and postinjury or postsurgical rehabilitation for specific injuries.

- Associate anatomic structures of the shoulder to particular injuries based on function of the structures during the pitching act.

- Explain the role of the rotator cuff in shoulder arthrokinematics and prevention of injury.

- Develop a rehabilitation program for specific pathologic shoulder conditions that takes into account the biomechanical function and healing parameters for the anatomic structures involved.

- Advance an athlete through phases of shoulder rehabilitation based on specific criteria for progression.

- Incorporate rehabilitation limitations and concerns for specific postinjury and postsurgical pathologic shoulder conditions.

Most athletic shoulder injuries are due to one of two mechanisms: (1) repetitive overhead activity (microtrauma) or (2) a significant force (macrotrauma) applied to the shoulder complex. The violent act of throwing and other similar overhead movements results in the repeated application of high stress to both the shoulder and the elbow. Most of these injuries can be classified as microtraumatic and result from repetitive overuse mechanisms. Tullos and King[1] reported that at least 50% of all baseball players experience sufficient shoulder or elbow joint symptoms to keep them from throwing for varying periods during their careers. Conte et al[2] reported that 28% of all injuries sustained by professional baseball pitchers occurred in the shoulder joint. McFarland and Wasik[3] found that upper extremity injuries in collegiate baseball players accounted for 75% of the time lost from the sport because of injury, with the pitcher being the most frequently injured player (69%). The most common injury cited was rotator cuff tendinitis. It has been reported that shoulder injuries are more common in pitchers than in position players.[2,3] The synchronous kinematics of throwing can be influenced by a number of factors, including glenohumeral and scapulothoracic motion, connective tissue flexibility, osseous structure, and dynamic muscle balance and symmetry. The glenohumeral joint complex is also susceptible to traumatic injuries such as dislocations, subluxations, acromioclavicular joint sprains, soft tissue injuries, and other types of injuries that commonly occur during collision and contact sports. The shoulder region is further predisposed to athletic injury because the

tremendous mobility afforded by the joint is the result of inherently poor glenohumeral stability. In this chapter we discuss the anatomy, biomechanics, common injuries, and rehabilitation programs specific to the shoulder joint complex.

ANATOMY AND BIOMECHANICS

The shoulder complex is composed of three synovial joints and one physiologic articulation. The sternoclavicular, acromioclavicular, and glenohumeral components are true joints, whereas the physiologic articulation is usually referred to as the scapulothoracic joint. These four articulations, along with the ligaments (Fig. 12-1), rotator cuff complex, and the primary mover musculature of the upper quarter, work in unison to produce and control the various movements of the shoulder complex. Dysfunction in any of these interdependent structures can result in limited performance of the entire shoulder complex.

Sternoclavicular Joint

Functionally, the sternoclavicular joint is the only bony articulation connecting the shoulder complex to the thorax. It is a modified saddle joint with a joint capsule, three major ligaments, and an intraarticular disk. The costoclavicular ligament is the primary stabilizer of the joint. It stabilizes the clavicle against the pull of the sternocleidomastoid muscle and controls motion about the joint that produces elevation-depression and

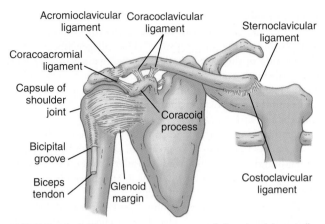

FIGURE 12-1 Ligamentous structures of the shoulder girdle. *(From O'Donoghue, D.H. [1984]: Treatment of Injuries to Athletes, 4th ed. Philadelphia, Saunders, p. 119.)*

Box 12-1
Passive and Active Mechanisms for Glenohumeral Joint Stability

PASSIVE MECHANISMS
Bony
Glenoid labrum
Intraarticular pressure
Joint cohesion
Glenohumeral capsule
Glenohumeral ligaments

ACTIVE MECHANISMS
Joint compression
Dynamic ligament
Tension
Neuromuscular control
Scapulothoracic joint

---

protraction-retraction.[4] The costoclavicular ligament also functions to check elevation of the clavicle.[5] The sternoclavicular ligament stabilizes the joint anteriorly and posteriorly by controlling anterior and posterior movements of the clavicular head on the sternum. The proximal end of the clavicle is separated from the sternal manubrium by an intraarticular disk or meniscus. This joint disk helps absorb centrally directed forces transmitted along the clavicle and improves the incongruence of the articular surfaces, thus decreasing the tendency of the clavicle to dislocate medially on the manubrium.[6]

Acromioclavicular Joint

The acromioclavicular joint is a plane joint that consists of two major ligament complexes and an intraarticular meniscus. The two primary functions of the acromioclavicular joint are (1) to maintain the appropriate clavicle-scapula relationship during the early stages of upper limb elevation and (2) to allow the scapula additional range of rotation on the thorax in the later stages of limb elevation.[4]

The integrity of the articulation between the acromion and the distal end of the clavicle is maintained by the surrounding ligaments rather than by the bony configuration of the joint. The coracoclavicular ligaments are the stabilizers of the primary acromioclavicular joint. The ligaments consist of a lateral portion, the trapezoid ligament, and a medial portion, the conoid ligament. It is these ligaments that are responsible for controlling the longitudinal rotation of the clavicle that is necessary for full unrestricted upper extremity elevation. The joint capsule is reinforced by the anterior, inferior, posterior, and superior acromioclavicular ligaments. The fibers of the deltoid and upper trapezius muscles, which attach to the superior aspect of the clavicle and acromion process, function to reinforce the acromioclavicular ligaments and further stabilize the joint.

A fall onto an outstretched arm tends to translate the scapula medially, and the small acromioclavicular joint alone cannot adequately control scapular motion, which frequently results in joint dislocation. As the scapula and its coracoid process attempt to move medially, the trapezoid ligament tightens, thereby shifting the force to the clavicle and, ultimately, to the strong sternoclavicular joint.[4] Therefore, anterior-posterior stability of

the acromioclavicular joint is maintained by the joint capsule, whereas vertical stability is provided by the coracoclavicular ligaments.

Glenohumeral Joint

The glenohumeral joint is the most mobile and the least stable of all the joints in the human body.[7] It is also the most commonly dislocated major joint in the human body.[8-11] Even though the glenohumeral joint exhibits significant physiologic motion, only a few millimeters of humeral head displacement occur during any of these movements in normal individuals.[12-18] Conversely, on clinical examination, Matsen[19] demonstrated excessive passive displacement consisting of 10 mm inferiorly and 8 mm anteriorly in normal asymptomatic shoulders. Therefore, stabilization of the humeral head within the glenoid is accomplished via the combined effort of the static and dynamic glenohumeral stabilizers. These two categories of joint stabilizers can be classified into passive and active stabilizing mechanisms (Box 12-1).

The Static Stabilizers: Bony Geometry

The bony geometry of the glenohumeral joint sacrifices osseous stability to facilitate excessive joint mobility. The articular surface of the glenoid is pear-shaped, with the inferior half being 20% larger than the superior half.[20] Additionally, the articular surface of the glenoid is much smaller than the articular surface of the humeral head, which is approximately three to four times that of the glenoid.[21] At any given time during normal motion, only 25% to 30% of the humeral head is actually in contact with the glenoid.[22-24] This lack of articular contact contributes to the inherent instability of the glenohumeral joint.[25]

The glenoid faces superiorly, anteriorly, and laterally. The superior tilt of the inferior glenoid limits inferior translation of the humeral head on the glenoid.[26] The glenoid articular surface is within 10° of being perpendicular to the blade of the scapula; thus, the glenoid fossa is retroverted approximately 6°.[27] Excessive retroversion of the glenoid is considered a primary cause predisposing an individual to posterior glenohumeral instability, and increased glenoid anteversion is found in individuals suffering from recurrent anterior dislocations.[27,28]

The areas of contact between the articular surfaces of the humeral head and the glenoid vary depending on arm position, with the greatest amount of articular contact occurring in the midpoint of elevation between 60° and 120°.[21] With increasing arm elevation, contact points on the humeral head move from inferior to posterosuperior while the glenoid contact shifts from a central location posteriorly.

At the extremes of normal motion the glenohumeral joint does not function in a strict ball-and-socket fashion. In these extremes, rotation is coupled with humeral head translation on the glenoid.[16,29,30] Normally, external rotation (ER) produces posterior translation and vice versa, whereas subjects with known anterior instability demonstrate anterior humeral head translation in extreme ER.[15,29,31]

Bony defects on either the humeral head or the glenoid are commonly associated with glenohumeral instability.[32] With recurrent anterior instability, an osseous defect is commonly noted on the posterolateral portion of the humeral head (Hill-Sachs lesion).[33] In contrast, an anteromedial lesion is often noted with recurrent posterior instability (reverse Hill-Sachs lesion). Bony defects of the anterior or posterior glenoid rim may also occur with recurrent glenohumeral instability.[34-36] Both these lesions represent impaction fractures and occur as the humeral head subluxates and then reduces repetitively over the glenoid rim.

The Glenoid Labrum

The glenoid labrum is a fibrous rim that serves to slightly deepen the glenoid fossa and allows attachment of the glenohumeral ligaments on the glenoid. The superior attachment of the labrum is loose and approximates the mobility of the meniscus within the knee joint, whereas the inferior attachment is firm and unyielding.[37] The labrum functions to deepen the glenoid anywhere from 2.5 to 5 mm.[29] The labrum may function in tandem with joint compression forces to stabilize the joint in the midrange of glenohumeral motion, where the ligamentous structures are lax.[38,39] The labrum also serves as a buttress that assists in controlling glenohumeral translation, similar to a chock, which would prevent a wheel from rolling downhill. Finally, Bowen et al[31] noted that the labrum also contributes to glenohumeral joint stability by increasing the surface area and acting as a load-bearing structure for the humeral head. In addition, the long head of the biceps brachii muscle inserts into the superior portion of the labrum. The vascular supply to the labrum arises mostly from its peripheral attachment to the capsule and is derived from a combination of the suprascapular circumflex scapular branch of the subscapular and the posterior circumflex humeral arteries.[40,41] The anterosuperior labrum appears to generally have a poor blood supply, whereas the inferior labrum exhibits significant blood flow.[40] The vascularity of the labrum decreases with increasing age.[11] No mechanoreceptors have been identified within the glenoid labrum.[42,43] However, free nerve endings have been isolated in the fibrocartilaginous tissue of the labrum, the biceps-labrum complex, and the connective tissue surrounding the labrum.[42,44]

Shoulder Capsule and Ligaments

The shoulder joint capsule is large, loose, and redundant, which also allows the large range of glenohumeral motion naturally available at the glenohumeral joint. The capsule is composed of multilayer collagen fiber bundles of differing strength and orientation. The anteroinferior capsule is the thickest and strongest portion of the joint capsule.[45] The collagen fibers within this portion of the joint capsule have two distinct orientations, radial fibers that are linked to each other by circular fibers. In this manner, rotational forces create tension within the fibers that produces compression on the joint surfaces while centering the articular surfaces.[45]

The glenohumeral joint capsule is reinforced with capsular ligaments that contribute greatly to joint stability. The size, strength, and orientation of these capsular ligaments vary widely, and they typically function when the joint is placed in extremes of motion to protect against instability.[46-48]

The anterior glenohumeral joint capsule consists of three distinct ligaments: the superior glenohumeral ligament, the middle glenohumeral ligament, and the inferior glenohumeral ligament complex.[46,48,49] The superior glenohumeral ligament arises from the anterosuperior labrum anterior to the biceps tendon and inserts superiorly into the lesser tuberosity of the humerus. The middle glenohumeral ligament originates adjacent to the superior glenohumeral ligament and extends laterally to attach onto the lesser tuberosity with the subscapularis tendon. The inferior glenohumeral ligament complex is composed of three functional portions: an anterior band, a posterior band, and an axillary pouch. These structures exhibit tremendous variation, with the middle glenohumeral ligament having the greatest degree of variation.[46,50] Posteriorly, the capsule is the thinnest and has no distinct capsular ligaments except for the posterior band of the inferior glenohumeral ligament complex.

The anterior glenohumeral ligaments function as primary restrains to anterior translation of the humerus on the glenoid.[51,52] The superior and middle glenohumeral ligaments are the primary restraints to anterior translation with the arm completely abducted.[53] The middle glenohumeral ligament plays a significant role in limiting translation of the humeral head in the midrange of shoulder abduction.[50,54,55] The inferior glenohumeral ligament complex, particularly the anterior band, is responsible for preventing translation of the humeral head with the arm abducted to 90° and beyond.[51,56,57]

The constraints to posterior translation are also based on arm position. The posteroinferior portion of the inferior glenohumeral ligament complex is the primary passive stabilizer against posterior instability with the arm in 90° of abduction. At less than 90° of abduction, the posterior capsule is the primary restraint against posterior forces.

During the combined motion of abduction and ER, the anterior band of the inferior glenohumeral ligament complex fans out and surrounds the anteroinferior aspect of the humeral head like a hammock restraining anterior displacement while the posterior band provides inferior support.[37] During abduction and internal rotation (IR), the anterior band of the inferior glenohumeral ligament complex moves inferiorly to resist inferior displacement, and the posterior band shifts posterosuperiorly to prevent posterior translation.[37] Additionally, when the arm is positioned in 90° of abduction and 30° of extension, the anterior band of the inferior glenohumeral ligament complex becomes the primary stabilizer to both anterior and posterior forces. Finally, as a general rule, the superior capsular structures play significant roles in glenohumeral joint stability when the arm is adducted, whereas the inferior structures are the primary providers of joint stability between 90° of abduction and full elevation.

Table 12-1 Three Types of Bankart Lesions

Grade	Definition	Instability Present Under Anesthesia
I	Capsular tears without labral lesions	Stable
II	Capsular tears with partial labral detachments	Mildly unstable
III	Complete capsular-labral detachments	Grossly unstable

From Baker, C.L., Uribe, J.W., and Whitman, C. (1990): Arthroscopic evaluation of acute initial anterior shoulder dislocations. Am. J. Sports Med., 18:25–28.

The forces required to dislocate the shoulder change with age. Less force is required in individuals younger than 20 and older than 40 years of age.[58-60] Bankart described the "essential lesion" responsible for shoulder instability as detachment of the labrum and capsule from the glenoid (referred to subsequently as a Bankart lesion). It is interesting to note that a Bankart lesion is not one specific anatomic defect, but rather a wide spectrum of pathologic conditions related to detachment of the capsulolabral complex of the glenohumeral joint. Baker et al[61] identified three types of Bankart lesions initially caused by acute anterior glenohumeral dislocation (Table 12-1). It is also interesting to note that the degree of instability present during examination under anesthesia varies depending on the grade of the lesion (see Table 12-1).[61] Approximately 85% of patients with traumatic anterior glenohumeral dislocations exhibit detachment of the glenoid labrum from the anterior glenoid rim, whereas the remaining individuals show interstitial stretch or rupture of the capsule without loosening or detachment of the labrum.[62]

Intraarticular Pressure and Joint Cohesion

Normally, the capsule of the glenohumeral joint is sealed airtight and contains very little (less than 1 mL) fluid.[62] This limited fluid volume contributes to joint stability in a manner similar to syringe-type suction and serves to hold the articular surfaces together with viscous and intermolecular forces.[62] The normal intraarticular pressure of the glenohumeral joint is negative, which creates a relative vacuum that also helps resist translation.[63-65] This force is relatively small, with only approximately 20 to 30 lb of stabilizing pressure being exerted, but when these properties are disrupted via capsular puncture or tear, subluxation tends to occur.[62,63] In an unstable shoulder this vacuum effect of viscous and intermolecular forces is lost because the labrum is no longer able to function as a seal or gasket.[66]

The Dynamic Stabilizers: Neuromuscular Control

The primary active stabilizers of the glenohumeral joint and the secondary stabilizers are listed in Box 12-2. The most important function that the primary glenohumeral stabilizers provide is the production of a combined muscular contraction that enhances humeral head stability during active arm movements. These muscles act together in an agonist/antagonist relationship to both effect movement of the arm and at the same time stabilize the glenohumeral joint. The combined effect of the rotator cuff

Box 12-2

Dynamic Stabilizers of the Shoulder

PRIMARY STABILIZERS
Rotator cuff muscles (supraspinatus, infraspinatus, teres minor, subscapularis)
Deltoid
Long head of the biceps brachii

SECONDARY STABILIZERS
Teres major
Latissimi dorsi
Pectoralis major

musculature is a synergistic action that creates humeral head compression within the glenoid and counterbalances the shearing forces generated by the deltoid.[67,68]

The second method of active glenohumeral joint stability is provided through blending of the rotator cuff tendons in the shoulder capsule, which produces tension with the capsular ligaments. This tension serves to actively tighten the glenohumeral ligamentous capsule and thereby accentuates centering of the humeral head within the glenoid fossa.

The third component that contributes to dynamic shoulder stability is neuromuscular control.[69,70] This refers to the continuous interplay of afferent input and efferent output in an individual's awareness of joint position (proprioception) and the ability to produce a voluntary muscular contraction to stabilize the joint or alter joint position so that excessive humeral head translation can be prevented. The ability to control the shoulder joint during active motion is referred to as *reactive neuromuscular control*. This factor is more important to normal shoulder function than joint position or repositioning ability.[70] Reactive neuromuscular control is an individual's ability to integrate proprioceptive information and motor control to react to the information.

Scapulothoracic Joint

The scapulothoracic joint is not a true anatomic joint because it has none of the usual joint characteristics, such as a joint capsule. However, it is a free-floating physiologic joint without any ligamentous restraints, except where it pivots about the acromioclavicular joint.[71] According to Steindler,[72] the primary force holding the scapula to the thorax is atmospheric pressure. The ultimate function of scapular motion is to orient the glenoid fossa for optimal contact with the maneuvering arm and to provide a stable base of support for controlled rolling and gliding of the articular surface of the humeral head.[4] This relationship allows optimal function of the upper extremity in space by continually adjusting the length-tension relationships of all vital musculature as the scapula constantly repositions itself on the thoracic wall. The muscles of the scapulothoracic joint play a significant role in maintaining optimal scapular position and posture. Five muscles directly control the scapula: the trapezius (upper, middle, and lower), the rhomboids, the levator scapulae, the serratus anterior, and to a lesser extent, the pectoralis minor. These muscles act in a synchronous fashion to provide both mobility and stability to the scapulothoracic joint.

Coracoacromial Arch

The coracoacromial arch, or subacromial space, has also been considered a physiologic joint by some authors.[73] It provides protection against direct trauma to the subacromial structures and prevents the humeral head from dislocating superiorly. It is bordered by the acromion process and acromioclavicular joint superiorly; the coracoid process anteromedially; and the rotator cuff and greater tuberosity of the humeral head inferiorly. The coracoacromial ligament, which serves as a "roof" over the greater tubercle of the humerus, rotator cuff tendons, portions of the biceps tendon, and the subdeltoid bursa, further decreases the available space within the arch. The space between the humeral head and the inferior aspect of the acromion depends on arm position and varies from approximately 30 ± 4.9 mm (when the arm is at $0°$ of abduction) and 6 ± 2.4 mm (when the arm is at $90°$ of abduction).[31] Additionally, this space can be decreased in shoulders with inflamed or swollen soft tissues. Soft tissue structures such as the supraspinatus and infraspinatus tendons, which lie between the two unyielding joint borders, are at risk for impingement or compressive injuries in individuals with abnormal glenohumeral joint mechanics or trauma.

Rotator Cuff

The supraspinatus, infraspinatus, teres minor, and subscapularis muscles make up the rotator cuff (Fig. 12-2). Collectively, each tendon blends with and reinforces the glenohumeral capsule, and all contribute significantly to dynamic stability of the glenohumeral joint.[74] The rotator cuff muscles could be considered the fine tuners of the glenohumeral joint and shoulder girdle, whereas the latissimus dorsi, teres major, deltoid, and pectoralis muscles are the prime movers.[75] All the rotator cuff muscles contribute in some degree to glenohumeral abduction, with the

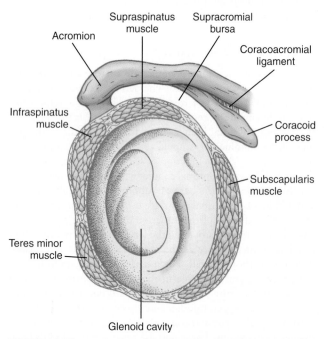

Acromion

Supraspinatus muscle

Supracromial bursa

Coracoacromial ligament

Infraspinatus muscle

Coracoid process

Subscapularis muscle

Teres minor muscle

Glenoid cavity

FIGURE 12-2 Anatomic view of the glenoid cavity with its surrounding structures. *(From Hill, J.A. [1988]: Rotator cuff injuries. Sports Med. Update, 3:5.)*

supraspinatus and deltoid muscles functioning as the primary abductors. The rotator cuff muscles also function to compress the glenohumeral joint and act to reduce or control vertical shear imparted onto the humeral head.[76,77] The infraspinatus is considered the next most active rotator cuff muscle, after the supraspinatus.[78-80] Selective nerve blocks have shown that the supraspinatus and infraspinatus muscles are responsible for 90% of the ER strength of the shoulder.[44] The teres minor also contributes to ER of the glenohumeral joint. The subscapularis is the primary internal rotator, with abduction activity peaking at around $90°$.[44]

SHOULDER ELEVATION

Most glenohumeral motion occurs around the plane of the scapula. This plane of motion is approximately $30°$ to $45°$ anterior to the frontal plane.[16] Codman[81] first reported that abduction of the humerus to $180°$ overhead requires that the clavicle, scapula, and humerus move through essentially their full range of motion (ROM) in a specific pattern of interaction. When internally rotated, the humerus can abduct on the scapula to approximately $90°$ before the greater tubercle strikes up against the acromion. If the humerus is fully externally rotated, however, the greater tubercle and accompanying rotator cuff tendons clear the acromion, coracoacromial ligament, and superior edge of the glenoid fossa,[82-84] thereby allowing another $30°$ of abduction. Thus, the glenohumeral joint contributes $90°$ to $120°$ of shoulder abduction, depending on the rotational position of the humeral head.[5,83,85] The remaining $60°$ is supplied by scapular elevation. This combined motion between the scapula and the humerus is known as scapulohumeral rhythm. During the first $30°$ of glenohumeral abduction, the contribution of scapular elevation is negligible and is not coordinated with movement of the humerus.[83,85] This is referred to as the setting phase, during which the scapula is seeking a position of stability on the thoracic wall in relation to the humerus.[85] The purpose of scapular rotation is twofold[4]: (1) to achieve a ratio of motion for maintaining the glenoid fossa in an optimal position to receive the head of the humerus, thus increasing ROM, and (2) to ensure that the accompanying motion of the scapula permits muscles acting on the humerus to maintain a satisfactory length-tension relationship. After the initial $30°$ of humeral elevation, scapular motion becomes better coordinated. Toward the end range of glenohumeral elevation, however, the scapula contributes more motion and the humerus less.[82,86] In gross terms, it is generally agreed that every $1°$ of scapular motion is accompanied by $2°$ of humeral elevation. Scapulohumeral rhythm is therefore considered to be a ratio of 1:2.[85] If scapular movement is prevented, only $120°$ of passive abduction and $90°$ of active motion are possible.[83]

Clavicular motion at both the acromioclavicular and sternoclavicular joints is essential for full shoulder elevation. Inman and Saunders[86] demonstrated that for full abduction of the arm to occur, the clavicle must rotate $50°$ posteriorly. Surgical pinning of the clavicle to the coracoid process, which has been performed in some cases in which a complete tear of the coracoclavicular ligament is present, dramatically limits shoulder abduction.

Glenohumeral elevation in abduction is the primary function of the deltoid and supraspinatus muscles. The contribution of the deltoid and supraspinatus to shoulder abduction has been investigated extensively. It was commonly assumed that abduction of the arm is initiated by the supraspinatus and is continued by the deltoid.[75] Studies in which selective nerve blocks were used to deactivate the deltoid and supraspinatus muscles have shown that complete abduction still occurs, though with a 50% loss in power, when one or the other muscle is deactivated.[42,87] Simultaneous nerve blocks of both these muscles result in an inability to raise the arm.[87] Thus, each muscle can elevate the arm independently, but there is a resultant loss of approximately 50% of the normal power generated in abduction.[88]

Additionally, the other three rotator cuff muscles—the teres minor, infraspinatus, and subscapularis—are active to some degree throughout the full abduction ROM.[83] These three rotator cuff muscles work as a functional unit to compress the humeral head and counteract the superior shear of the deltoid during arm elevation.[82,85]

THROWING MECHANISM

Throwing is an integral part of many sports, but different techniques are required, depending on the endeavor. High-speed motion analysis has allowed investigators to slow down the pitching act and examine the kinetics and kinematics involved (Fig. 12-3). The throwing act, as performed by a baseball pitcher, is a series of complex and synchronized movements involving both the upper and lower extremities. As described by several authors,[6,89] the throwing mechanism can be divided into five phases (Fig. 12-4): (1) windup, (2) cocking, (3) acceleration, (4) release and deceleration, and (5) follow-through. Injuries to the shoulder joint can occur during the cocking, acceleration, or deceleration phases. The overhead throw is the fastest human movement and takes approximately 0.5 second to complete.

Windup

The purpose of the windup is to put the athlete in an advantageous starting position from which to throw. In addition, it can serve as a distraction to the hitter. The windup is a relatively slow maneuver that prepares the pitcher for correct body posture and balance while leading the body into the cocking phase (see Fig. 12-4). It can last from 0.5 to 1.0 second[90] and is characterized by shifting of the shoulder away from the direction of the pitch, with the opposite leg being cocked quite high and the baseball being removed from the glove.[6] It is also during this phase that the head of the humerus can wear and roughen from leverage on the posterior glenoid labrum.

Cocking

The cocking phase is most often divided into early and late cocking phases. During the cocking phase (see Fig. 12-4), the shoulder is abducted to approximately 90°, externally rotated 90° or more, and horizontally abducted to approximately 30°.[6,89] This is primarily accomplished by the deltoid and stabilized by the rotator cuff muscles, which pull the humeral head into the glenohumeral joint.[91] The anterior, middle, and posterior deltoids reach peak electromyographic (EMG) activity in the early cocking phase when the arm is abducted to 90°.[92] During late cocking, the activity of the deltoids decreases as the rotator cuff musculature becomes more dominant. Additionally, the pectoralis major, subscapularis, and latissimus dorsi act eccentrically to stabilize the humeral head during the late cocking phase. This position places the anterior joint capsule and internal rotators, which are used to accelerate the ball, in maximum tension. In addition, the opposite leg is kicked forward and placed directly in front of the body. Kinetic energy begins to be transferred from the lower extremities and trunk to the arm and hand in which the ball is held.[90] Because of the significant stress placed

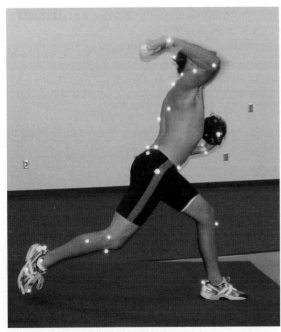

FIGURE 12-3 High-speed photography allows investigators to slow down the pitching act and examine the arthrokinematics involved. *(Courtesy American Sports Medicine Institute, Birmingham, AL.)*

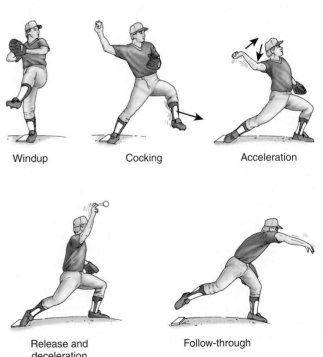

Windup Cocking Acceleration

Release and deceleration Follow-through

FIGURE 12-4 Dynamic phases of pitching. *(From Walsh, D.A. [1989]: Shoulder evaluation of the throwing athlete. Sports Med. Update, 4:24.)*

on the anterior shoulder capsule, the capsule may "stretch out" with continuous throwing. If the anterior capsule is significantly stretched out, increased humeral head displacement during the late cocking phase can occur. This may be manifested clinically as "internal impingement" and is discussed in detail later. Furthermore, this extreme ER position (late cocking) may also lead to glenoid labrum lesions. This type of glenoid labrum lesion has been referred to as a *peel-back lesion* and is also discussed later.

Acceleration

The acceleration phase (see Fig. 12-4) begins at the point of maximal ER and ends at ball release.[93] This phase lasts an average of 50 msec, approximately 2% of the duration of the pitching act.[89,94] Muscles that once were placed on stretch in the cocking phase become the accelerators in a powerful concentric muscular contraction. The body is brought forward, with the arm following behind. The energy developed by the body's forward motion is transferred to the throwing arm to accelerate the humerus.[1] This energy is enhanced via contraction of the internal rotators (primarily the subscapularis) as the humerus is rotated internally from its previously externally rotated position, and the ball is accelerated to delivery speed.[6] During this phase the maximum IR angular velocity is approximately $7365 \pm 1503°/\text{sec}$.[89] An anterior displacement force of approximately 50% of body weight also occurs during this phase. Rotatory torque at the shoulder can start at approximately 14,000 inch-pounds and builds up to approximately 27,000 inch-pounds of kinetic energy at ball release.[91]

During the acceleration phase, the pectoralis major and latissimus dorsi are the main muscles that actively generate velocity and arm speed.[95] The subscapularis muscle is active in steering the humeral head. At ball release, the throwing shoulder should be abducted about 90° to 100°, regardless of the type of pitch being thrown or the style of the thrower. The difference between an "overhead" and a "sidearm" baseball pitcher is not the degree of glenohumeral abduction, but rather the degree of lateral tilt at the trunk.[89] Because of the tremendous force acting at the glenohumeral joint, numerous injuries can result during this phase of overhead throwing, such as instability, labral tears, overuse tendinitis, and tendon ruptures.[87]

Release and Deceleration

In the release and deceleration phases of throwing, the ball is released, and the shoulder and arm are decelerated (see Fig. 12-4). Generally, deceleration forces are approximately twice as great as acceleration forces but act for a shorter period (approximately 40 msec).[6] Initially in the deceleration phase, the humerus has a relatively high rate of IR, and the elbow extends rapidly.[6] Great eccentric force is applied to the posterior rotator cuff muscles to slow the IR and horizontal adduction of the humerus and to stabilize the humeral head within the glenoid cavity. Jobe et al[10,96] analyzed the throwing mechanism with electromyography and found that the muscles of the rotator cuff are extremely active during the deceleration phase. It has been reported that the posterior rotator cuff must resist as much as 200 lb of distraction force that is attempting to pull the arm out of the glenohumeral joint in the direction that the ball has been thrown.[97] Labral tears at the attachment of the long head of the biceps, subluxation of the long head of the biceps as a result of tearing of the transverse

ligament, and various lesions of the rotator cuff, such as tearing of the undersurface or tensile overload, can be incurred during this phase of throwing.[90]

Follow-Through

During the follow-through phase (see Fig. 12-4), the body moves forward with the arm, thereby effectively reducing the distraction force applied to the shoulder.[98] This results in relief of tension on the rotator cuff muscles.

Because of the repetitive action of throwing, a baseball pitcher's shoulder undergoes adaptive changes that should be recognized and distinguished from pathologic lesions. The throwing shoulder has significantly increased ER and decreased IR in comparison to that on the nonthrowing side. This is considered a functional adaptation to throwing but may lead to specific pathologic conditions as discussed later. The various shoulder injuries that can occur in each phase of throwing are summarized in Table 12-2.

Glousman et al[99] compared the EMG activity of the shoulder girdle muscles in pitchers with isolated anterior glenohumeral instability and in normal subjects. In pitchers, the supraspinatus and serratus anterior exhibited increased activity throughout late cocking and acceleration, the infraspinatus exhibited enhanced activity during early cocking and acceleration, and the biceps brachii was noted to have an increase in activity during the acceleration phase. Additionally, the subscapularis, latissimus dorsi, and pectoralis major demonstrated less EMG activity in subjects with anterior instability during all phases of the throwing motion.

Wick et al[100] noted numerous significant differences between throwing a baseball overhead and throwing a football. During the acceleration phase, the angular velocity for throwing a baseball was $7365° \pm 1503°/\text{sec}$ versus $4586° \pm 843°/\text{sec}$ for throwing a football. At ball release, the shoulder was externally

Table 12-2 Potential Shoulder Injuries Associated With Each Throwing Phase

Phase	Potential Injuries
Windup	None that are common
Cocking	Anterior subluxation Internal impingement Glenoid labrum lesions
Acceleration	Shoulder instability Labral tears Overuse tendinitis Tendon ruptures
Release and deceleration	Labral tears at the attachment of the long head of the biceps Subluxation of the long head of the biceps by tearing of the transverse ligament Lesions of the rotator cuff, such as undersurface tears or tensile overload
Follow-through	Tear of the superior aspect of the glenoid labrum at the origin of the biceps tendon Abnormal glenohumeral kinematics caused by tight posterior shoulder structures forcing the humeral head anteriorly and superiorly into the acromial arch during this phase

rotated approximately 21° more for throwing a football. Also at ball release, shoulder abduction was calculated to be 99° during baseball throwing and 114° during football throwing. The duration of the football throw was also significantly longer (0.20 second) than a baseball throw (0.15 second).

OVERVIEW OF THE REHABILITATION PROGRAM

The shoulder rehabilitation program presented in this chapter is designed to restore shoulder ROM and strength in a functional and progressive manner. The exercises may be implemented with specific limitations of certain motions, depending on the injury sustained or surgical procedure performed. Frequently, emphasis is placed on the rotator cuff musculature and the scapular stabilizers. Rehabilitation exercises that concentrate on the rotator cuff musculature are paramount after any shoulder injury. With shoulder rehabilitation the clinician should concentrate on increasing dynamic stability, particularly that of the rotator cuff, because of the relatively weak nature of the static restraints of the glenohumeral joint.

The entire upper kinematic chain should be evaluated when a shoulder rehabilitation program is designed because of the importance of proximal stability for distal mobility. Synchronous interplay among each of the joints of the shoulder complex is vital for active, balanced joint stability and normal glenohumeral function. The scapular stabilizers (e.g., trapezius, latissimus dorsi, rhomboids, and serratus anterior) are often overlooked when shoulder injuries are addressed. The scapular stabilizers maintain the appropriate scapula–glenohumeral joint relationship, thereby allowing normal kinematics during functional activities. This is particularly true in the pitching motion, in which these muscles play a large role during the deceleration phase of throwing.

Strengthening exercises for the shoulder musculature, especially the rotator cuff, have been critically analyzed by numerous investigators.[101] Jobe and Moynes[102] first examined the effect of specific exercises on the rotator cuff musculature. They reported that the supraspinatus can best be exercised apart from the other cuff muscles with the arm abducted to 90°, horizontally adducted to 30°, and fully internally rotated, which is referred to as the *empty can* position. The infraspinatus and teres minor can be exercised in the side-lying position with the arm held close to the side and the elbow flexed to 90°. The subscapularis can be strengthened with the individual in the supine position, the affected arm held close to the side, and the elbow flexed to 90°.

Since the study of Jobe and Moynes,[102] Blackburn et al[71] investigated rotator cuff activation with intramuscular electromyography while subjects performed specific rotator cuff exercises. Although Jobe and Moynes[102] reported that the supraspinatus is best isolated and exercised with the arm abducted to 90°, horizontally flexed 30°, and fully internally rotated, Blackburn et al[71] noted that the supraspinatus is involved whenever the arm is elevated, whether the subject is standing or prone. Isolation of supraspinatus function appears to occur during pure abduction with neutral rotation of the arm while standing. In addition, Blackburn et al[71] noted that a significant increase in supraspinatus function can be achieved in the prone position with the arm in maximal ER and 100° of horizontal abduction (Fig. 12-5). Malanga et al[103] analyzed the EMG activity of the rotator cuff and deltoid muscles in the empty can and prone positions advocated by Blackburn et al.[71] The empty can position produced high levels of EMG activity in the supraspinatus (107% maximum voluntary isometric contraction), but the middle deltoid (104%) and anterior deltoid (96%) were also extremely active. Conversely, during prone horizontal abduction (at approximately 100°) with ER, the most active muscles were the middle deltoid (111%), the posterior deltoid (96%), and the supraspinatus (94%). The investigators concluded that neither position isolated the supraspinatus but that both positions could be used for exercising. In addition, Kelly et al[104] reported that the best test position to isolate the supraspinatus with the least activation of the infraspinatus is with the arm positioned at 90° of elevation in the scapular plane and 45° of humeral ER. This position is referred to as the *full can* position. We recommend this position for manual muscle testing of the supraspinatus (Fig. 12-6). Townsend et al[105] studied seven glenohumeral muscles during 17 traditional shoulder exercises and reported that certain exercises were better for recruiting selected muscles. For instance, the best exercise noted in the study to recruit the teres minor muscle was side-lying ER followed by prone horizontal abduction with ER. Table 12-3 provides detailed information about specific exercises and muscular activity.

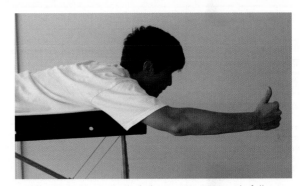

FIGURE 12-5 Horizontal abduction at 100° with full external rotation.

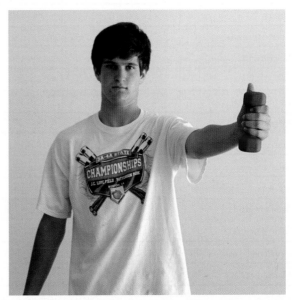

FIGURE 12-6 The "full can" position. This position has been suggested to be the best way to isolate the supraspinatus muscle while producing minimal activation of the surrounding muscles.

In a recent study performed at our center, Fleisig[101] reported that the exercise movement that produced the highest EMG activity in the posterior rotator cuff was side-lying ER, followed by prone ER, and then standing ER at 90° of abduction. Furthermore, the investigators noted that use of a towel roll between the humerus and body enhanced EMG activity of the infraspinatus and teres minor by 18% to 20%. Moreover, they showed via an indwelling

Table 12-3 Electromyographic Activity of Specific Muscles During Selected Exercises

Muscle and Exercise	Electromyographic Activity (% MVIC ± SD)	Peak Arc Range (°)
Anterior Deltoid		
Scaption, IR	72 ± 23	90–150
Scaption, ER	71 ± 39	90–120
Flexion	69 ± 24	90–120
Middle Deltoid		
Scaption, IR	83 ± 13	90–120
Horizontal abduction, IR	80 ± 23	90–120
Horizontal abduction, ER	79 ± 20	90–120
Posterior Deltoid		
Horizontal abduction, IR	93 ± 45	90–120
Horizontal abduction, ER	92 ± 49	90–120
Rowing	88 ± 40	90–120
Supraspinatus		
Military press	80 ± 48	0–30
Scaption, IR	74 ± 33	90–120
Flexion	67 ± 14	90–120
Subscapularis		
Scaption, IR	62 ± 33	90–150
Military press	56 ± 48	60–90
Flexion	52 ± 42	120–150
Infraspinatus		
Horizontal abduction, ER	88 ± 25	90–120
ER	85 ± 26	60–90
Horizontal abduction, IR	74 ± 32	90–120
Teres Minor		
ER	80 ± 14	60–90
Horizontal abduction, ER	74 ± 28	60–90
Horizontal abduction, IR	68 ± 36	90–120

Modified from Townsend, H., Jobe, F.W., Pink, M., et al. (1992): EMG analysis of the glenohumeral muscles during a baseball rehabilitation program. Am. J. Sports Med., 19:264–269.

ER, External rotation; *IR*, internal rotation; *MVIC*, maximum voluntary isometric contraction.

EMG study that the full can exercise produced significantly less activity of the middle and posterior deltoid muscles and may be the optimal position to recruit the supraspinatus muscle for rehabilitation and manual muscle testing.

After injury or surgery, modalities may be used as needed. Cryotherapy both before and after exercise is recommended in the acute stages of healing to reduce the inflammatory process. Cryotherapy may also be used prophylactically after the acute phase has subsided. Iontophoresis, moist heat, or ultrasound may be indicated for chronic overuse injuries of the shoulder to promote blood flow and a healing response in the tissue.

Therapeutic exercises for the shoulder should address strength, endurance, and dynamic stability. A variety of machines, dumbbells, and manual techniques can be used to accomplish specific goals. An upper body ergometer can be used in the early phases of rehabilitation for restoration of ROM and in the later phases for muscular endurance. Exercises that result in an eccentric contraction are particularly important for athletes performing overhead movements, especially for the muscles involved in deceleration movements of the shoulder. Manual resistance exercises, such as rhythmic stabilization exercises, can be used to promote cocontractions and facilitate muscle synergy (Fig. 12-7). Finally, surgical tubing is a versatile tool that can be used for strengthening in diagonal patterns or simulating the throwing act (Figs. 12-8 and 12-9). Use of each of these exercise types during the rehabilitation process depends on the goals of the particular phase. Specific uses for each exercise are explained throughout the treatment sections.

Glenohumeral mobilization techniques (see Figs. A6-1 through A6-5 [in Chapter 6 Appendix] on Expert Consult @ www.ExpertConsult.com) are important for attaining accessory motion in the early stages of healing without subjecting the joint to the high forces involved in passive stretching. Grade I or II anterior-posterior, inferior-superior, and long arm distraction mobilizations can be used early in the rehabilitation program

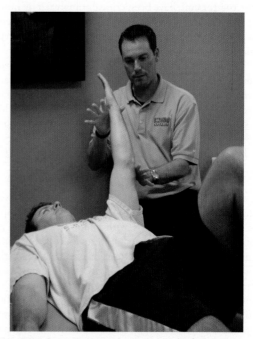

FIGURE 12-7 Proprioceptive neuromuscular facilitation patterns being performed against manual resistance.

to neuromodulate the athlete's pain. Grade III or IV mobilizations can be added in later phases of rehabilitation to increase flexibility within the capsule. In older patients (aged 45 to 60), it is imperative to restore inferior capsular mobility early in the rehabilitation process (especially after rotator cuff repair).

Glenohumeral flexibility, particularly flexibility of the posterior shoulder structures, is paramount for athletes using overhead movements. This is particularly evident with inflexibility of the posterior capsule and musculature, which is manifested as decreased motion in horizontal adduction and IR. Tightness in the posterior aspect of the shoulder leads to increased stress on the posterior shoulder structures during the follow-through phase of pitching. Tight posterior shoulder structures can also cause abnormal glenohumeral kinematics by forcing the humeral head anteriorly and superiorly into the acromial arch.[106] The flexibility exercises illustrated in Chapter 12 Appendix (see Figs. A12-1 through A12-40 on Expert Consult @ www. ExpertConsult.com) should be undertaken not only after injury or surgery but also during the off-season to help prevent posterior glenohumeral restriction and injury (Fig. 12-10, *A* and *B*).

Muscular strength and endurance of the scapular stabilizing musculature are important for maintaining correct joint arthrokinematics. The role of the scapulothoracic joint and surrounding musculature in maintaining a normally functioning shoulder is critical. Muscular spasm, weakness, and poor neuromuscular coordination of these stabilizing muscles directly affect glenohumeral motion. If the scapula cannot rotate on the thoracic cage, maintain the correct length-tension muscular relationship, or properly orient the glenoid fossa with the humeral head, asynchronous motion at the shoulder complex will lead to injury. Scapula stabilizers can be strengthened by having the athlete perform push-ups, prone horizontal abduction, scapular retraction exercises, and neuromuscular control drills.

Because the rotator cuff muscles are mainly endurance-type muscles, the progressive resistance exercise (PRE) program is based on low weight and high repetition.[107] This not only increases muscular endurance but also decreases the potential for perpetuating the inflammatory process by performing the exercises with too much weight. A common view held by numerous clinicians is that the PRE program should be progressed by

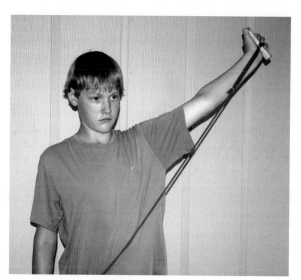

FIGURE 12-8 Proprioceptive neuromuscular facilitation pattern performed with surgical or exercise tubing.

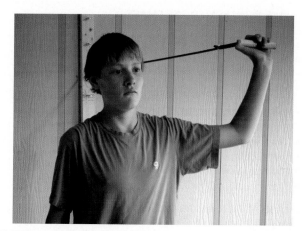

FIGURE 12-9 Exercise tubing being used to simulate the throwing motion.

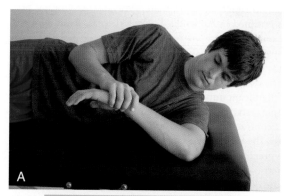

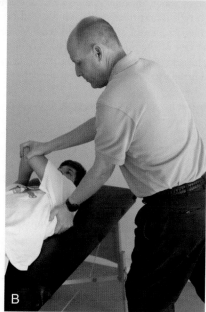

FIGURE 12-10 A, Sleeper stretch. **B,** Supine horizontal adduction stretch.

having the athlete work from 30 to 50 total repetitions and not add weight until 50 repetitions can be performed comfortably (see Chapter 4). The PRE program is begun with a gradual progression toward more dynamic exercises as healing progresses. This decreases the chance of rotator cuff inflammation and trauma while still producing muscle strength and endurance of the rotator cuff.

On the basis of numerous studies and EMG recordings during specific movements, Wilk et al[108] developed a core exercise program for athletes who use overhead movements called the Throwers' Ten Exercise Program (see Figs. A-1 through A-10 [in Appendix A] on Expert Consult @ www.ExpertConsult.com). The program emphasizes the key muscles and muscle groups responsible for the throwing motion. The goal of this exercise program is to reestablish dynamic stability of the glenohumeral joint by strengthening the rotator cuff musculature and achieving neuromuscular control. Athletes should begin with a traditional PRE program and stretching exercises and gradually progress to eccentric and isokinetic exercises and then into a more dynamic program consisting of high-speed movements performed to muscular fatigue, proprioception exercises, use of inertia machines (see Fig. 4-11), and upper extremity plyometrics. The athlete should return to throwing gradually by progressing through an appropriate interval rehabilitation program, as outlined in Appendix B (on Expert Consult @ www.ExpertConsult.com).

A plyometric exercise program can be extremely useful in the advanced phases of rehabilitation of an injured athlete. Plyometric exercise combines strength with speed of movement and has significant implications for overhead throwers.[109,110] The drills apply a stretch-shortening cycle to the muscle, that is, an eccentric contraction followed by a concentric contraction. This stimulates the neurophysiologic components of the muscle to produce greater force. Table 12-4 presents the three phases of a plyometric drill. Successful plyometric training relies heavily on the rate of stretch rather than on the length of stretch. With plyometric exercise the neuromuscular system is trained by using the stretch reflex, proprioceptive stimulus, and muscular activation. Plyometrics should be performed only two or three times weekly because of the microtrauma that may occur with this type of aggressive exercise. Performing plyometrics daily can result in additional trauma to a healing shoulder in some athletes.

The upper extremity plyometric program is organized into four different exercise groupings: (1) warm-up drills, (2) throwing movements, (3) trunk drills, and (4) wall drills. Some of the plyometric drills are illustrated in Appendix C (on Expert Consult @ www.ExpertConsult.com), and others can be found in Chapter 26. For a complete description, the reader is encouraged to review several articles.[109-112]

Table 12-4 Three Phases of a Plyometric Drill

Phase	Description
I	Stretch phase or the eccentric muscle loading that activates the muscle spindle
II	Amortization phase, which represents the time between the eccentric and concentric phases
III	Shortening phase or the response or concentric phase

The nonoperative rehabilitation program for an overhead thrower can be divided into four distinct phases. Each phase should represent specific goals and contain various exercises to accomplish these goals. Box 12-3 provides an overview of the program.

NONOPERATIVE REHABILITATION GUIDELINES

Range of Motion

Most throwers exhibit an obvious disparity in motion in which ER is excessive and IR is limited in 90° of abduction.[113-116] Several investigators have documented the fact that pitchers have greater ER than position players do.[114,116] Brown et al[114] reported that professional pitchers exhibited 141° ± 15° of ER measured at 90° of abduction. This was approximately 9° more than the ER of the nonthrowing shoulder and approximately 9° more than that of the throwing shoulder of positional players measured in 90° of abduction. Bigliani et al[113] examined the ROM of 148 professional players. They reported that a pitcher's ER at 90° of abduction averaged 118° (range, 95° to 145°) on the dominant shoulder whereas the ER of a position player's dominant shoulder averaged 108° (range, 80° to 105°). In an ongoing study of professional baseball players, Wilk et al[116] assessed the ROM of 369 professional baseball pitchers. They noted that pitchers exhibit an average of 132.9° of ER and 52° of IR when passively assessed at 90° of abduction. In pitchers, ER is approximately 7° greater in the throwing shoulder than in the nonthrowing shoulder, whereas IR is 7° greater in the nonthrowing shoulder. They also noted that pitchers exhibit the greatest total arc of motion

---

Box 12-3

Nonoperative Rehabilitation of Overhead Throwers

PHASE I: ACUTE PHASE

Goals:
- Diminish pain and inflammation
- Normalize or improve motion and flexibility
- Retard muscular atrophy
- Enhance dynamic stabilization

PHASE II: INTERMEDIATE PHASE

Goals:
- Improve muscular strength and endurance
- Maintain or improve flexibility
- Promote concentric-eccentric muscular training
- Maintain dynamic stabilization

PHASE III: ADVANCED PHASE

Goals:
- Initiate sport-specific training
- Enhance power and speed (plyometrics)
- Maintain a rotator cuff strengthening program
- Improve muscular endurance

PHASE IV: RETURN-TO-SPORT PHASE

Goals:
- Gradually return to sports activities
- Maintain gains in strength, power, endurance, and flexibility

(i.e., ER and IR at 90° abduction), followed closely by catchers, then outfielders, and finally infielders. Furthermore, when left-handed pitchers are compared with right-handed pitchers, left-handed throwers exhibit approximately 7° more ER and 12° more total motion than right-handed throwers. These findings were statistically significant ($P < .01$).

Recently, the disparity between IR of the dominant and nondominant shoulder has received increased attention from numerous clinicians.[117-121] This difference, evidenced as less IR in the throwing shoulder, has been referred to as *glenohumeral joint IR deficit* (GIRD). GIRD, as defined by Burkhart et al,[117,118,122] is a loss of IR of the throwing shoulder of 20° or greater in comparison to the nonthrowing shoulder and may be a cause of specific shoulder injuries. In addition to the GIRD principle, Wilk et al[116] proposed the *total rotational motion* (TRM) concept, in which the amount of ER and IR at 90° of abduction is added together and a TRM arc is determined. The authors reported that the TRM in the throwing shoulders of professional baseball pitchers is within 5° of the nonthrowing shoulder.[116] Furthermore, the authors suggested that a TRM arc outside the 5° range may be a contributing factor to shoulder injuries in the presence or absence of GIRD.

As a result of the repetition of such high forces generated during the throwing motion, an overhead-throwing athlete can exhibit numerous and substantial adaptations. Some of the most common adaptations seen occur at the glenohumeral joint. Most throwers have an obvious motion disparity whereby ER is excessive and IR is limited at 90° of abduction.[113-116,123-125] The loss of IR has been reported in the literature by numerous authors.[43,113,115,123,124,126-129] Numerous reasons have been proposed for the motion adaptations, including osseous adaptations (increased retroversion),[124,128-130] posterior musculature,[116,123,131] and soft tissue adaptations of the capsule.[115,127] Crockett et al[124] tested dominant and nondominant shoulder retroversion in 25 professional pitchers and compared them with a control group of nonthrowers' shoulders. They reported that the humeral head of the throwing shoulder had an 17° increase in retroversion in comparison to the nonthrowing shoulders. Reinold et al[131] reported that after a pitching performance, there is 9.5° loss of glenohumeral joint IR that lasts for 24 hours. Burkhart et al[122] suggested that GIRD is the result of posterior capsular tightness. They concluded that stretching is the most appropriate treatment to address the IR deficit. They went on to recommended a posterior capsular release should an aggressive stretching program not improve IR passive range of motion (PROM).

Borsa et al[123,126] documented that pitchers have greater posterior translation than anterior translation. Furthermore, they reported that some individuals with very small amounts of IR PROM exhibit considerable posterior glenohumeral laxity on objective testing. They have also proposed that the loss of IR is the result of muscular tightness and humeral head retroversion and not posterior capsular tightness. Crockett et al[124] and others[128-130] documented greater retroversion in throwers' dominant shoulder than in their nondominant shoulder. Thus, the primary and most frequent cause of the change in IR is the result of osseous adaptation, muscular tightness of the external rotators, and scapular positioning. Consequently, if the loss of IR is the result of osseous adaptation and muscular tightness, a stretching program directed toward the tightened posterior rotator cuff muscles appears to be most appropriate for treating GIRD. In this review we reported that pitchers exhibited greater glenohumeral

ER and less IR on the throwing side than on the nonthrowing side. This is consistent with previous research.[113,114,116,124,125] Furthermore, the average TRM was within 6°, nearly the same as reported by Wilk et al[116] in a previously published article.

There appears to be increasing concern regarding the correlation between sustaining a shoulder injury and the loss of IR and GIRD.[117,118,122] In a study looking at the relationship between ROM and injury rates in professional baseball pitchers, we found that pitchers with GIRD had almost twice the risk of sustaining a shoulder injury than did pitchers without GIRD.[132] Pitchers whose TRM comparison was outside the acceptable 5° difference range had a 2.5 times higher risk of sustaining a shoulder injury. Clinically, we believe that pitchers with GIRD and TRM differences outside the 5° window are at greater risk for injury.

Laxity

Most throwers have significant laxity of the glenohumeral joint, which permits excessive ROM. The hypermobility of the thrower's shoulder has been referred to as *thrower's laxity*.[133] The laxity of the anterior and inferior glenohumeral joint capsule can be recognized by the clinician during assessment of the stability of the overhead thrower's shoulder joint. Posteriorly, however, Borsa et al[126] documented that pitchers exhibit greater posterior translation than anterior translation. Furthermore, they reported that some individuals with very small amounts of IR PROM are found to have considerable posterior glenohumeral laxity on objective testing. They have also proposed that the loss of IR is the result of muscular tightness and humeral head retroversion and not posterior capsular tightness. Some clinicians have reported that the excessive laxity exhibited by throwers is the result of repetitive throwing and have referred to this as *acquired laxity*,[134] whereas others have documented that overhead throwers have *congenital laxity*.[113] Bigliani et al[113] examined glenohumeral laxity in 72 professional baseball pitchers and 76 position players. They noted a high degree of inferior glenohumeral joint laxity, with 61% of pitchers and 47% of position players exhibiting a positive sulcus sign in the throwing shoulder. Additionally, in the players who exhibited a positive sulcus sign in the dominant shoulder, 89% of the pitchers and 100% of the position players had a positive sulcus sign in the nondominant shoulder. Thus, it would appear that some baseball players have inherent congenital laxity, with superimposed acquired laxity occurring as a result of adaptive changes from throwing.

Muscular Strength

Several investigators have examined muscular strength parameters in overhead-throwing athletes[135-140] with varying results and conclusions. Wilk et al[139,140] performed isokinetic testing on professional baseball players as part of their physical examination during spring training (Table 12-5). They demonstrated that the ER strength of a pitcher's throwing shoulder is significantly weaker ($P > 0.05$) than that of the nonthrowing shoulder by 6%. Conversely, the IR strength of the throwing shoulder was significantly stronger ($P < 0.05$) by 3% than that of the nonthrowing shoulder. In addition, adduction strength of the throwing shoulder was also significantly stronger than that of the nonthrowing shoulder by approximately 9% to 10%. The authors believe that important isokinetic values are the unilateral muscle ratios, which describe the antagonist/agonist muscle strength relationship. A proper balance between agonist and antagonist muscle groups is thought to provide dynamic stabilization to the shoulder joint. To provide proper muscular balance, the ERs should be at least 65% of the strength of the IRs.[139] Optimally, the external-to-internal rotator muscle strength ratio should be 66% to 75%.[116,139,140] This provides proper muscular balance. Magnusson et al[141] measured the isometric muscular strength values of professional pitchers with a handheld dynamometer and compared them with the values in a control group of non–throwing, nonathletic individuals. In pitchers, the supraspinatus muscle was significantly weaker on the throwing side than on the nonthrowing side when measured by an isometric manual muscle test (the empty can maneuver).[141] Additionally, shoulder abduction, ER, IR, and the supraspinatus muscle were weaker in pitchers than in the control group of non–baseball players.

The scapular muscles play a vital role during the overhead-throwing motion.[95] Proper scapular movement and stability are imperative for asymptomatic shoulder function.[142,143] These muscles work in a synchronized fashion and act as force couples about the scapula to provide both movement and stabilization. Wilk et al[140] documented the isometric scapular muscular strength values of professional baseball players. Their results

Table 12-5 Muscular Strength Values in Professional Baseball Players

A. Bilateral Comparisons—Glenohumeral Joint

	180°/sec (%)	300°/sec (%)	450°/sec (%)
ER	95–105	85–95	75–85
IR	105–120	100–115	100–110
Abd	100–110	100–110	—

B. Unilateral Muscle Ratios—Glenohumeral Joint

	180°/sec (%)	300°/sec (%)	450°/sec (%)
ER/IR	63–70	65–72	62–70
Abd/Add	82–87	92–97	—
ER/Abd	64–69	66–71	—

C. Isokinetic Torque/Body Weight Ratios—Glenohumeral Joint

	180°/sec (%)	300°/sec (%)	
ER	18–23	15–20	—
IR	27–33	25–30	—
Abd	26–32	20–26	—
Add	32–36	28–33	—

D. Scapular Muscle

	Protract		Retract		Elevation		Depression	
	D	ND	D	ND	D	ND	D	ND
Catchers	71 ± 10	74 ± 13	62 ± 8	60 ± 7	83 ± 14	84 ± 5	22 ± 6	18 ± 5
Position players	68 ± 10	73 ± 10	63 ± 5	59 ± 7	88 ± 15	85 ± 8	21 ± 4	16 ± 5

E. Unilateral Muscle Ratios—Scapular

	Protraction/Retraction		Elevation/Depression	
	D (%)	ND (%)	D (%)	ND (%)
Pitchers	87	81	27	21
Catchers	93	81	24	19
Position players	98	94	29	27

Data condensed from Wilk, K.E., Andrews, J.R., Arrigo, C.A., et al. (1993): The strength characteristics of internal and external rotator muscles in professional baseball pitchers. Am. J. Sports Med., 21:61–69; and Wilk, K.E., Andrews, J.R., Arrigo, C.A. (1995): The abductor and adductor strength characteristics of professional baseball pitchers. Am. J. Sports Med., 23:307–311.

Abd, Abduction; *Add*, adduction; *D*, dominant; *ER*, external rotation; *IR*, internal rotation; *ND*, nondominant.

indicated that pitchers and catchers exhibit a significantly different increase in strength of the scapular protractors and elevators than position players do (see Table 12-5). All players (except infielders) had significantly stronger scapular depressors on the throwing side than on the nonthrowing side. In addition, they believed that optimal agonist/antagonist muscular ratios are important for the scapular muscles in providing stability, mobility, and symptom-free shoulder function. It is often clinically beneficial to enhance the ratio of lower trapezius to upper trapezius strength.[144] In the opinion of the authors, the poor posture and muscle imbalance commonly seen in patients with a variety of shoulder pain pathology are often a result of poor muscle balance between the upper and lower trapezius, with the upper trapezius being more dominant. A study by McCabe et al[145] reported that bilateral ER at 0° of abduction resulted in the greatest lower trapezius–to–upper trapezius ratio when compared with several other similar trapezius exercises (Fig. 12-11). Cools et al[144] also identified side-lying ER and prone horizontal abduction at 90° and ER as two beneficial exercises to enhance the ratio of lower to upper trapezius activity.

Relatively high lower trapezius activity occurs in prone rowing; prone horizontal abduction at 90° and 135° with ER and IR; prone and standing ER at 90° of abduction; D$_2$ diagonal pattern flexion and extension; proprioceptive neuromuscular facilitation (PNF) scapular clock; standing high scapular rows; and scaption, flexion, and abduction below 80° and above 120° with ER.[146-149] Lower trapezius activity tends to be relatively low at less than 90° of scaption, abduction, and flexion and then increases exponentially from 90° to 180°.[146,148-152] Significantly greater lower trapezius activity has been reported with prone ER at 90° of abduction than with the empty can exercise.[153] As mentioned previously, the lower trapezius is an extremely important muscle in shoulder function because of its role in scapular upward rotation, ER, and posterior tilt.

The serratus anterior works with the pectoralis minor to protract the scapula and with the upper and lower trapezius muscles to upwardly rotate the scapula. The serratus anterior is an important muscle because it contributes to all components of normal three-dimensional scapular movements during arm elevation, including upward rotation, posterior tilt, and ER.[154,155] The serratus anterior is likewise important in athletics, such as

during overhead throwing, to accelerate the scapula during the acceleration phase of throwing. The serratus anterior also helps stabilize the medial border and inferior angle of the scapula and thereby prevent scapular IR ("winging") and anterior tilt.

Several exercises elicit high serratus anterior activity, such as D$_1$ and D$_2$ diagonal pattern flexion; D$_2$ diagonal pattern extension; supine scapular protraction; supine upward scapular punch; military press; push-up plus; IR and ER at 90° of abduction; and flexion, abduction, and scaption above 120° with ER.[146-148,156,157] Serratus anterior activity tends to increase in a somewhat linear fashion with arm elevation.[146,148,150,151,154] However, increasing arm elevation increases risk for subacromial impingement,[158,159] and arm elevation at lower abduction angles also generates relatively high serratus anterior activity.[146]

Not surprising is high serratus anterior activity generated during the push-up. When performing the standard push-up, push-up on knees, and wall push-up, serratus activity is greater when full scapular protraction occurs after the elbows fully extend (push-up plus) (Fig. 12-12).[160] Moreover, serratus anterior activity was lowest in the wall push-up plus, exhibited moderate activity during the push-up plus on knees, and had relatively high activity during the standard push-up plus.[156,160] When compared with the standard push-up, performing a push-up plus with the feet elevated produced significantly greater serratus anterior activity.[161] These findings demonstrate that serratus anterior activity increases in a linear manner as the positional challenge increases.

Proprioception

Proprioception is defined as the conscious or unconscious awareness of joint position, whereas neuromuscular control is the efferent motor response to afferent (sensory) information.[162] The thrower relies on enhanced proprioception to influence the neuromuscular system to dynamically stabilize the glenohumeral joint because of significant capsular laxity and excessive ROM.

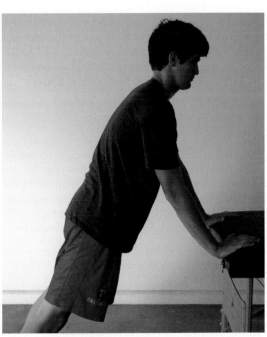

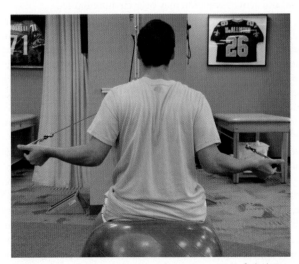

FIGURE 12-11 Bilateral external rotation at 0° of abduction.

FIGURE 12-12 Push-up plus.

Allegrucci et al[163] tested shoulder proprioception in 20 healthy athletes participating in various overhead sports. Testing of joint proprioception was performed on a motorized system with the subject attempting to reproduce a specific joint angle. These investigators noted that the dominant shoulder exhibited diminished proprioception in comparison to the nondominant shoulder. They also noted improved proprioception near end ROM in comparison to that at the starting point. Blasier et al[164] reported that individuals who have clinically appreciable generalized joint laxity are significantly less sensitive during proprioceptive testing. Wilk et al (unpublished data, 2000) studied the proprioception capability of 120 professional baseball players. They passively positioned the players at a documented point within the players' ER ROM. The athletes were then instructed to actively reposition the shoulder in the same position. The researchers noted no significant difference between the throwing shoulder and nonthrowing shoulder. In addition, Wilk et al (unpublished data, 2000) compared the proprioception ability in 60 professional baseball players with that of 60 non–overhead-throwing athletes. They noted no significant differences between baseball players and non–overhead-throwing athletes. However, baseball players exhibited slightly improved proprioception abilities at ER ROM than did non–overhead-throwing athletes, but these results were not significantly different. See Chapter 24 for an in-depth discussion of proprioception and neuromuscular control.

Painful Arc

A painful arc or "catching point," particularly with shoulder abduction (but also possibly present in other planes), is characterized by specific points throughout ROM at which pain intensifies but dissipates once past that point. As many as three or four catching points may be present through an arc of motion. The most common ROM in which patients demonstrate a painful arc is from 70° to 120° of arm elevation.[165] The athlete may attempt to exercise through these points of pain, which often dissipate within 5 to 7 days after initiation of treatment. Painful arcs in a young athlete can develop as a result of structural factors such as a hooked acromion, fracture malunion, or bursal swelling, or they may develop from loss of dynamic humeral head stability, which can cause the humeral head to displace superiorly during arm elevation. If the clinician determines the latter to be the cause, exercises that enhance dynamic stability should be emphasized immediately.

Crepitus

Crepitus within the shoulder joint is a common occurrence and is usually asymptomatic. Generally, crepitus can be detected after shoulder surgery or rotator cuff tendinitis. If the crepitus remains asymptomatic, the athlete should attempt to exercise through it. Crepitus should also dissipate within 7 to 10 days after initiation of an appropriate rotator cuff exercise program.

Middle Deltoid and Elbow Pain

Middle deltoid and elbow pain can be referred from the shoulder, often from a tight shoulder capsule. It is usually exacerbated with ER in the supine position with 90° of abduction and 90° of elbow flexion (90/90 position). This pain is generally seen in individuals with chronic shoulder problems or in those who have undergone prolonged immobilization. Frequently, the elbow pain at the end range of shoulder ER may be greater than that of the actual shoulder pain. This condition usually responds well to moist heat, application of ultrasound to the shoulder capsule, and glenohumeral joint mobilization. A shoulder with a limitation in ER should not be stretched aggressively in the 90/90 position because this will tend to exacerbate the elbow pain. Most patients can tolerate long arm distraction with imposed ER better than aggressive ER stretching in the 90/90 position. As treatment proceeds and normal synchronous glenohumeral motion is restored, the athlete should report a decrease in elbow and middle deltoid pain.

Pain Beyond 90° of Elevation

If impingement or rotator cuff tendinitis is present, pain beyond 90° of elevation is a common occurrence. Athletes with this complaint should begin active assisted range-of-motion (AAROM) exercises through full ROM, and joint mobilization techniques should be used as indicated. The pain is often propagated by a decrease in muscular strength and generally improves with a rotator cuff therapeutic exercise program. If symptoms are severe and the athlete has radiographic changes indicative of a grade III (or hooked acromion) type of injury, the prognosis is poor with nonoperative therapy.[166]

SHOULDER INJURIES

Scapulothoracic Joint Lesions

The scapulothoracic joint should also be assessed after any shoulder injury or surgery. Pathologic scapulothoracic conditions occur in chronic pain states in which glenohumeral motion has gradually decreased or the glenohumeral joint has been immobilized for a long period. In most instances the scapulothoracic joint becomes involved as a secondary problem. Increased shoulder pain can result in muscle spasm within the supraspinatus, trapezius, rhomboids, latissimus dorsi, and subscapularis. As mentioned earlier, for every 2° of glenohumeral abduction, approximately 1° of associated scapular motion must take place to achieve 180° of arm elevation. If the scapulothoracic joint is not functioning properly, the athlete may be able to attain only 100° to 120° of passive abduction, and active abduction may be even more limited.

The scapulothoracic joint should be evaluated for spasm in the rhomboids, latissimus dorsi, upper and lower trapezius, subscapularis, teres minor, infraspinatus, and supraspinatus muscles. These areas should also be assessed for active trigger points, as discussed by Travell and Simons.[167] Activation of trigger points in these muscles may refer pain to the middle deltoid and elbow and, with severe spasm, down the arm. In addition, the clinician may find that the vertebral scapular border cannot be distracted off the thoracic cage, which results not only in increased pain for the athlete but also in an increase in localized muscle spasm.

Before decreased glenohumeral motion can be treated, scapulothoracic motion must be restored. This is usually accomplished by reducing the muscle spasm with moist heat, ultrasound, soft tissue mobilization, trigger point release, and scapular mobilization (Fig. 12-13). With severe spasm, the spray-and-stretch technique of Travell and Simons,[167] which uses Fluori-Methane spray* to desensitize the trigger points,

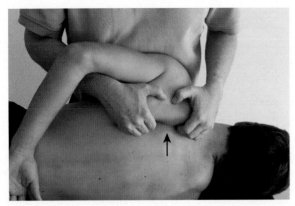

FIGURE 12-13 Scapula mobilization by distraction of the vertebral border of the scapula and lateral glide.

may be indicated. Trigger point injection may also be considered.[167] As trigger points are diminished, the athlete should report a decrease in shoulder pain, neck stiffness, and referred pain, along with an associated increase in glenohumeral abduction. A careful cervical (see Chapter 16) and thoracic spine evaluation is necessary any time that a patient has scapular pain and muscle spasm.

Rotator Cuff Lesions

The rotator cuff can become injured through a variety of mechanisms. Most commonly, the cuff can become frayed, which can progress to a full-thickness tear after repetitive wear, and it gradually degenerates. However, in young athletes the cuff most commonly exhibits partial tearing or fraying with symptoms of tendinitis. Andrews and Meister[168] classified rotator cuff lesions into categories based on the specific pathomechanics (Table 12-6). A few of these categories will be briefly discussed as they pertain to an athlete with a shoulder injury. First, an athlete involved in overhead sports (i.e., thrower or swimmer) is prone to capsular laxity, which contributes to the clinical syndrome referred to as *posterior impingement*. In addition, such athletes are susceptible to undersurface rotator cuff tearing (tensile overload) and occasionally to compressive cuff disease. In contrast, athletes involved in collision sports such as football, lacrosse, or hockey are more likely to sustain a traumatic rotator cuff tear because of the athlete's arm being forcefully abducted or violently pulled away from the body. Full-thickness tears of the rotator cuff are unusual in young athletes.

Impingement Syndrome

The term *impingement syndrome* was popularized by Neer in 1972.[169] He emphasized that both the supraspinatus insertion to the greater tubercle and the bicipital groove lie anterior to the coracoacromial arch with the shoulder in the neutral position and that with forward flexion of the shoulder, these structures must pass beneath the coracoacromial arch, thereby providing the opportunity for impingement.[170] He introduced the concept of a continuum in the impingement syndrome from chronic bursitis to partial or complete tears of the supraspinatus tendon, which may extend to involve ruptures of other parts of the rotator cuff.[167]

*Available from Gebauer Chemical Co., Cleveland, Ohio.

Table 12-6 Classification of Rotator Cuff Disease

Type	Classification
1	Primary compressive disease
2	Instability with secondary compressive disease
3	Primary tensile overload
4	Tensile overload because of capsular instability
5	Rotator cuff tear
6	Primary internal impingement
7	Calcific tendinitis
8	Partial articular-sided tendon avulsion (PASTA) lesion
9	Partial articular tear with intratendinous extension (PAINT) lesion
10	Secondary internal impingement with primary hypermobility
11	Secondary tensile overload with primary hypermobility

Impingement of the rotator cuff may occur in some athletes such as baseball players, quarterbacks, swimmers, and others whose activities involve repetitive use of the arm at or above 90° of shoulder abduction. Matsen and Arntz[170] defined impingement as encroachment of the acromion, coracoacromial ligament, coracoid process, or acromioclavicular joint on the rotator cuff mechanism, which passes beneath them as the glenohumeral joint is moved, particularly in flexion and IR. Impingement usually involves the supraspinatus tendon. When the supraspinatus muscle assists in stabilizing the head of the humerus within the glenoid, the greater tubercle cannot butt against the coracoacromial arch.[77] Whether impingement is the primary event causing rotator cuff tendinitis or whether rotator cuff impingement results from rotator cuff disease is undetermined.[77] In all likelihood both mechanisms of injury can occur.

Approximately 5 to 10 mm of space lies between the humeral head and the undersurface of the acromial arch at 90° of shoulder abduction (depending on the anatomy).[171] Thus, whenever the arm is elevated, some degree of rotator cuff impingement may occur.[75,168] The shoulder is most vulnerable to impingement when the arm is at 90° of abduction and the scapula has not rotated sufficiently upward to free the rotator cuff of the overhanging acromion and coracoacromial ligament.[172] Impingement of the glenohumeral joint can occur with horizontal adduction of the arm, which causes impingement against the coracoid process.[169] Forward flexion with IR of the humerus also jams the greater tubercle under the acromion, the coracoacromial ligament, and at times, the coracoid process.[33] If the arm is raised in ER, however, the greater tubercle is turned away from the acromial arch, and the arm can be elevated without impingement.

Impingement syndrome is perpetuated by the cumulative effect of many passages of the rotator cuff beneath the coracoacromial arch. This results in irritation of the supraspinatus and, possibly, the infraspinatus tendons, as well as in enlargement of the subacromial bursa, which can become fibrotic and thus further decrease the already compromised subacromial space. Furthermore, with time and progression of wearing and attrition, microtears and partial-thickness rotator cuff tears may result. If these continue, secondary bony changes (osteophytes) can develop under the acromial arch and propagate full-thickness rotator cuff tears.

Secondary factors may also contribute to the development of subacromial impingement. Issues of capsular hypomobility or hypermobility may result in altered glenohumeral arthrokinematics. The altered mechanics may overly stress the surrounding soft tissue structures, particularly the rotator cuff, and cause tendinopathy. Scapula position on the rib cage has also been implicated as a source of glenohumeral dysfunction.[142,143,122,173,174] The term *scapular dyskinesis* describes an alteration in the normal position or motion of the scapula during coupled scapulohumeral movements.[173] The altered scapula position may contribute to pathology of the rotator cuff, bursa, and surrounding structures. Rehabilitation is directed toward improving the scapula's position and affording a normal scapulohumeral coupling motion, particularly with overhead movements.

The cause of impingement syndrome is usually multifocal, and the supraspinatus tendon is the structure most likely to be involved. Several factors have been proposed as contributing to the development of impingement syndrome. Tendon avascularity has long been thought to contribute to impingement. In 1939, Lindblom[175] first reported avascularity of the rotator cuff at the supraspinatus attachment to the greater tubercle and described this as the "critical zone"[23] in which many lesions occur. However, from their work, Moseley and Goldie[176] concluded that the critical zone is no more avascular than the rest of the rotator cuff. Finally, Iannotti et al,[177] using laser Doppler technology, reported substantial blood flow in the critical zone of the rotator cuff.

Although it now appears that the rotator cuff is not a completely avascular structure, Rathbun and Macnab[178] and Sigholm et al[179] proposed two mechanisms that may compromise supraspinatus blood flow. Rathbun and Macnab[178] noted that shoulder adduction places the supraspinatus under tension and "wrings out" its vessels, thereby resulting in tissue necrosis. Sigholm et al[179] demonstrated that active forward flexion increases subacromial pressure to a level sufficient to reduce tendon microcirculation substantially. However, in interpreting these findings, Matsen and Arntz[170] point out that "since the shoulder is frequently moved, it is unclear whether either of these mechanisms could produce ischemia of sufficient duration to cause tendon damage." Brewer[180] reported that the blood supply to the critical zone diminishes with age. The relationship among cuff vascularity, impingement, and rotator cuff lesions is still speculative, and more research is needed. However, it appears that the critical zone is an area of hypovascularity and is prone to impingement and thus to tendon damage, especially in aging patients with a shoulder injury.

The shape of the acromion has been studied in individuals with impingement syndrome.[166,169] Figure 12-14 illustrates the three types of acromial shape. It appears that rotator cuff lesions are more likely to occur if a hooked acromion is present,[166,169] but it cannot be determined whether the acromial shape is caused by or results from a cuff tear.[170,181]

Finally, a weakened rotator cuff mechanism can predispose an athlete to rotator cuff impingement. The rotator cuff functions to stabilize the shoulder against the actions of the deltoid and pectoralis major muscles. In the presence of a weakened cuff mechanism, contraction of the deltoid causes upward displacement of the humeral head, which squeezes the remaining cuff

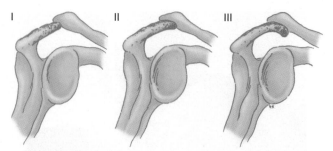

FIGURE 12-14 Biglianni et al[166] identified three different shapes of the acromion: type I, smooth; type II, curved; and type III, hooked. *(From Jobe, C.M. [1990]: Gross Anatomy of the Shoulder. In Rockwood, C.A., Jr., and Matsen, F.A., III [eds.]: The Shoulder. Philadelphia, Saunders, p. 45.)*

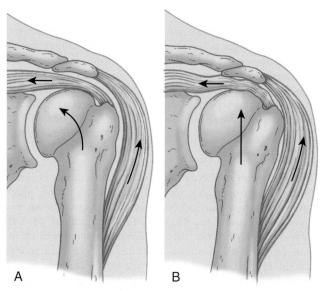

FIGURE 12-15 The supraspinatus helps stabilize the head of the humerus against upward pull of the deltoid. **A,** Subacromial impingement is prevented by normal cuff function. **B,** Deep surface tearing of the supraspinatus weakens the ability of the cuff to hold the humeral head down, thereby resulting in impingement of the tendon against the acromion. *(Redrawn from Matsen, F.A., III, and Arntz, C.T. [1990]: Subacromial impingement. In Rockwood, C.A., Jr., and Matsen, F.A., III [eds.]: The Shoulder. Philadelphia, Saunders, p. 624.)*

against the coracoacromial arch (Fig. 12-15).[182] Other factors that can result in rotator cuff impingement include degenerative spurs, chronic bursal thickening, rotator cuff thickening related to chronic calcium deposits, tightness of the posterior shoulder capsule, and capsular laxity.[170]

Neer[74] has described three progressive stages of impingement syndrome (Fig. 12-16). Stage I is a reversible lesion usually seen in individuals younger than 25 years of age. These patients have an aching type of discomfort in the shoulder. This stage usually involves only inflammation of the supraspinatus tendon and long head of the biceps brachii. Stage II is generally seen in individuals 24 to 40 years of age and involves fibrotic changes in the supraspinatus tendon and subacromial bursa. Again, an aching type of pain is present, which may increase at night, and individuals may be unable to perform the movement that produces the impingement syndrome. Injuries in this stage sometimes

Stage I: Edema and hemorrhage

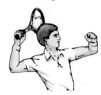

Typical age: <25 years
Differential diagnosis: Subluxation;
                        A/C arthritis
Clinical course: Reversible
Treatment: Conservative

Stage II: Fibrosis and tendinitis

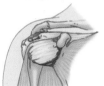

Typical age: 25–40 years
Differential
diagnosis: Frozen shoulder;
                        calcium deposits
Clinical course: Recurrent pain
                        with activity
Treatment: Consider bursectomy;
                        C/A ligament division

Stage III: Bone spurs and tendon rupture

Typical age: >40 years
Differential
diagnosis: Cervical radiculitis;
                        neoplasm
Clinical course: Progressive disability

Treatment: Anterior acromioplasty;
                        rotator cuff repair

FIGURE 12-16 Neer's three-stage classification of impingement syndrome. *A/C,* Acromioclavicular; *C/A,* coracoacromial. *(Reprinted with permission from Neer, C.S. [1983]: Impingement lesions. Clin. Orthop. Relat. Res., 173:70.)*

respond to conservative treatment, but surgical intervention may be required. Stage III seldom occurs in those younger than 40 years of age. In this stage the individual has had a long history of shoulder pain, and osteophyte formation, a partial-thickness or eventually a full-thickness rotator cuff tear,[183] and obvious wasting of the supraspinatus and infraspinatus muscles are often present. Injuries in this stage do not generally respond well to conservative treatment.

Rotator cuff impingement is a self-perpetuating process. Matsen and Arntz[170] noted the following: (1) muscle or cuff tendon weakness causes impingement from loss of the humeral head stabilizing function, which leads leading to tendon damage, disuse atrophy, and additional cuff weakness; (2) bursal thickening causes impingement as a result of subacromial crowding, which produces greater thickening of the bursa; and (3) posterior capsular tightness can lead to impingement, disuse, and stiffness because the tight capsule forces the humeral head to rise up against the acromion. Numerous factors, both structural and functional, contribute to impingement,[88] especially in young athletes. Additionally, if the capsule is especially lax and if the dynamic stabilizers are not sufficient, the humeral head may displace anterosuperiorly and lead to complaints of impingement.

The goal in treating athletes with impingement syndrome, either nonoperatively or surgically, is to reduce compression and friction between the rotator cuff and subacromial space. Box 12-4 lists several factors[170,184] that are necessary to minimize the compression. The primary complication of impingement syndrome is a rotator cuff tear. If impingement syndrome is diagnosed in its early stages, the prognosis is encouraging.

Box 12-4

Factors Necessary to Minimize Compression in the Subacromial Space

Shape of the coracoacromial arch, which allows passage of the adjacent rotator cuff mechanism
Normal undersurface of the acromioclavicular joint
Normal bursa
Normal function of the humeral head stabilizers (rotator cuff)
Normal capsular laxity
Smooth upper surface of the rotator cuff mechanism
Normal function of the scapular stabilizers

Data from Matsen, F.A., III, and Arntz, C.T.: Rotator cuff tendon failure. In Rockwood, C.A., Jr., and Matsen, F.A., III (eds.): The Shoulder, Vol. II. Philadelphia, Saunders, pp. 647–677; and Matsen, F.A., III, and Arntz, C.T. (1990): Subacromial impingement. In Rockwood, C.A., Jr., and Matsen, F.A., III (eds.): The Shoulder, Vol. II. Philadelphia, Saunders, pp. 623–646.

With acute impingement syndrome, time, rest from noxious stimuli, nonsteroidal antiinflammatory drugs, local modalities (e.g., cold, heat, and electrical stimulation), and a general shoulder rehabilitation program of flexibility and a PRE program (see Figs. A12-1 through A12-40 in Chapter 12 Appendix [on Expert Consult @ www.expertconsult.com]) are indicated.

On evaluation, active ROM may be limited with an empty or muscular guarding end-feel as a result of pain. This may be caused by posterior capsule stiffness. In such instances, moist heat, ultrasound, joint mobilization, and a general shoulder flexibility program with emphasis on supine IR and ER and horizontal adduction are appropriate. Most young throwers will exhibit functional loss of IR and therefore have decreased flexibility of the posterior musculature or, less likely, a tight posterior capsule. It is important to stretch the posterior capsule (if tight) and inferior capsule and normalize the degree of IR. Box 12-5 provides an outline of the rehabilitation protocol after nonoperative treatment of shoulder impingement syndrome.

Injection of the subacromial space with lidocaine in an athlete with impingement syndrome decreases pain. Steroid injections into the tendons of the rotator cuff and biceps tendon may result in tendon atrophy or reduce the ability of a damaged tendon to repair itself.[170] Kennedy and Willis[185] found a degenerative effect in the rabbit Achilles tendon after steroid injection. They concluded that physiologic doses of local steroids injected directly into a normal tendon weaken it significantly for up to 14 days after injection. This weakness was attributed to cellular necrosis. When developing a rehabilitation program, the clinician must be aware of the potential effects of steroid injection.

Surgical intervention for patients with grade III impingement syndrome or for those who do not respond to nonoperative care consists of subacromial decompression, referred to as *acromioplasty.* The goal in performing subacromial decompression is to relieve the mechanical impingement and prevent wear at the critical areas of the rotator cuff. Subacromial decompression consists of resection of the anteroinferior acromial undersurface to increase the space between the undersurface of the acromion and the rotator cuff/humeral head. Frequently, partial or complete resection of the coracoacromial ligament is also performed to further increase the available space. Acromioplasty may be performed in conjunction with débridement or repair of the rotator cuff.

Box 12-5

Rehabilitation Protocol After Nonoperative Treatment of Subacromial Impingement

Subacromial impingement is a chronic inflammatory process produced by one of the rotator cuff muscles and the subdeltoid bursa "pinching" against the coracoacromial ligament and/or anterior acromion when the arm is raised above the head. The supraspinatus portion of the rotator cuff is the most common area of impingement. This syndrome is commonly seen in individuals who use their arms repetitively in a position above shoulder height. It also occurs in golfers, tennis players, and swimmers.

This four-phase program can be used for conservative management of impingement. The protocol is designed to attain maximal function in minimal time. This systematic approach allows specific goals and criteria to be met and ensures safe progression of the rehabilitation process. Client compliance is critical.

MAXIMAL PROTECTION—ACUTE PHASE

Goals:
1. Relieve pain and inflammation
2. Normalize range of motion
3. Reestablish muscular balance
4. Educate the patient and improve posture

Avoidance:
- Elimination of any activity that causes an increase in symptoms

Range of Motion:
- L-bar
  - Flexion
  - Elevation in the scapular plane
  - External and internal rotation in the scapular plane at 45° of abduction
    - Progress to 90° of abduction
  - Horizontal abduction/adduction
  - Pendulum exercises
  - Active assisted range of motion—limited symptom-free available range of motion
    - Rope and pulley
      - Flexion

Joint Mobilization:
- Emphasize inferior and posterior glides in the scapular plane
- Goal is to establish balance in the glenohumeral joint capsule

Modalities:
- Cryotherapy
- Iontophoresis

Strengthening Exercises:
- Rhythmic stabilization exercises for external/internal rotation
- Rhythmic stabilization drills: flexion/extension
- External rotation strengthening
- Submaximal isometrics (external rotation, internal rotation, abduction)
- Scapular strengthening
- Retractors
- Depressors
- Protractors

Patient Education:
- Activity level, activities
- Pathologic condition of avoidance of overhead reaching and lifting activities
- Correct seating posture (consider a lumbar roll)
- Seated posture with shoulder retraction

Guideline for Progression:
1. Decreased pain and/or symptoms
2. Normal range of motion
3. Elimination of painful arc
4. Muscular balance

INTERMEDIATE PHASE

Goals:
1. Reestablish nonpainful range of motion
2. Normalize athrokinematics of shoulder complex
3. Normalize muscular strength
4. Maintain reduced inflammation and pain

Range of Motion:
- L-bar
- Flexion
  - External rotation at 90° of abduction
  - Internal rotation at 90° of abduction
  - Horizontal abduction/adduction at 90°
- Rope and pulley
  - Flexion
  - Abduction (symptom-free motion)

Joint Mobilization:
- Continue joint mobilization techniques for the tight aspect of the shoulder (especially the inferior)
- Initiate self–capsular stretching
- Grade II/III/IV
- Inferior, anterior, and posterior glides
- Combined glides as required

Modalities (As Needed):
- Cryotherapy
- Ultrasound/phonophoresis
- Iontophoresis

Strengthening Exercises:
- Progress to complete shoulder exercise program
- Emphasize rotator cuff and scapular muscular training
- External rotation tubing
- Side-lying external rotation
- Full can
- Shoulder abduction
- Prone horizontal abduction
- Prone rowing
- Prone horizontal abduction with external rotation
- Biceps/triceps
- Standing lower trapezius muscular strengthening

Functional Activities:
- Gradually allow increase in functional activities
- No prolonged overhead activities
- No lifting activities overhead

Box 12-5

Rehabilitation Protocol After Nonoperative Treatment of Subacromial Impingement—cont'd

ADVANCED STRENGTHENING PHASE

Goals:

1. Improve muscular strength and endurance
2. Maintain flexibility and range of motion
3. Gradual increase in functional activity level

Flexibility and Stretching:

- Continue all stretching and range-of-motion exercises
- L-bar external/internal rotation at 90° of abduction
- Continue capsular stretch
- Maintain/increase posterior/inferior flexibility

Strengthening Exercises:

- Start fundamental shoulder exercises:
  - Tubing external/internal rotation
  - Lateral raises to 90° with dumbbell
  - Full can with dumbbell
  - Side-lying external rotation
  - Prone horizontal abduction
  - Prone extension
  - Push-ups
  - Biceps/triceps

Guideline for Progression:

1. Full nonpainful range of motion
2. No pain or tenderness

3. Strength test fulfills criteria
4. Satisfactory clinical examination

RETURN-TO-SPORT PHASE

Goal:

1. Unrestricted symptom-free activity

Initiate Interval Sport Program:

- Throwing
- Tennis
- Golf

Maintenance Exercise Program:

- Flexibility exercises
  - L-bar
    - Flexion
    - External rotation and internal rotation at 90° of abduction
    - Self–capsular stretches
- Isotonic exercises
  - Fundamental shoulder exercises
    - Perform 3 times per week

Impingement syndrome can be corrected surgically by arthroscopy or arthrotomy. With open subacromial decompression, use of a technique that does not compromise the deltoid attachments is recommended rather than separating the deltoid from its insertion during the surgical procedure. This approach results in less morbidity and allows early postoperative motion, with almost no need for postoperative immobilization.[170] If the deltoid is detached from the acromion and distal end of the clavicle, the rehabilitation program should proceed more slowly to allow healing of the deltoid.[186]

Modalities can be used initially after surgery to help control pain and inflammation, along with the concurrent initiation of early ROM exercises. In the early stages the athlete may complain of joint crepitus and a painful arc or catching points; these problems should be worked through as tolerated. The crepitus and painful arc should subside in 7 to 10 days after the initiation of exercises. We expect full PROM or AAROM to be restored in 2 to 3 weeks after arthroscopic decompression. As active ROM is restored, a PRE program can be initiated. Resection of the coracoacromial ligament has no effect on the course of the rehabilitation. If a rotator cuff repair is performed in conjunction with acromioplasty, a rotator cuff repair rehabilitation protocol should be followed.

Internal impingement has been described in the literature by Walch et al.[187] Andrews and colleagues[40] originally identified the lesion in overhead throwers. This cuff lesion develops when the arm is abducted and externally rotated, such as in the cocking phase of throwing. During this movement the humeral head tends to glide anteriorly (especially when the

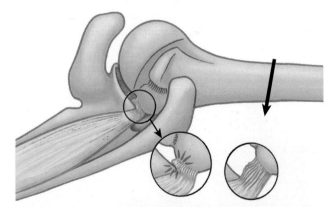

FIGURE 12-17 Posterior shoulder impingement. This occurs when the arm is abducted and externally rotated; the supraspinatus and infraspinatus muscles impinge (rub) on the posterosuperior rim of the glenoid cavity, which leads to fraying of the cuff or labrum. *(From Walch, G., Boileau, P., Noel, E., and Donell, T. [1992]: Impingement of the deep surface of the supraspinatus tendon on the glenoid rim. J. Shoulder Elbow Surg., 1:239–245.)*

anterior capsule is hypermobile). As this motion takes place, the supraspinatus and infraspinatus impinge (or produce friction) on the posterosuperior edge of the glenoid rim, which results in tearing of undersurface of the rotator cuff and fraying of the posterosuperior glenoid labrum (Fig. 12-17). This lesion is extremely common in athletes using overhead movements.

Posterosuperior glenoid impingement, often referred to as internal impingement, is one of the most commonly observed injuries in overhead-throwing athletes.[40,133,187-191] We believe that one of the underlying causes of symptomatic internal impingement is excessive anterior shoulder laxity. One of the primary goals of the rehabilitation program is to enhance the athlete's dynamic stabilization capacity and thus control anterior humeral head translation. In addition, another essential goal is to restore flexibility to the posterior rotator cuff muscles of the glenohumeral joint. We strongly caution against aggressive stretching of the anterior and inferior glenohumeral structures, which may result in increased anterior translation. Additionally, the program should emphasize muscular strengthening of the posterior rotator cuff to reestablish muscular balance and improve joint compression ability. The scapular muscles must be an area of increased focus as well. Restoration of dynamic stabilization is an essential goal to minimize anterior translation of the humeral head during the late cocking and early acceleration phases of throwing. Exercise drills such as PNF patterns with rhythmic stabilization are incorporated.[70,116] In addition, stabilization drills performed at the end range of ER are beneficial in enhancing dynamic stabilization (Fig. 12-18). Perturbation training of the shoulder joint is performed to enhance proprioception, dynamic stabilization, and neuromuscular control during this phase (see Chapter 24). It is the authors' opinion that this form of training has been extremely effective in treating a thrower with posterior/superior impingement.

After the clinician has restored posterior flexibility, normalized glenohumeral strength ratios, enhanced scapular muscular strength, and diminished the patient's symptoms, an interval throwing program may be initiated (see Appendix B [online]). Jobe[190] suggested abstinence from throwing for 2 to 12 weeks, depending on the thrower's symptoms. When the thrower begins an interval throwing program, the clinician or pitching coach should observe the athlete's throwing mechanics often. Occasionally, a thrower who exhibits internal impingement will allow the arm to lag behind the scapula, thus throwing with excessive horizontal abduction and not throwing with the humerus in the plane of the scapula. Jobe[133,190,191] referred to this as hyperangulation of the arm. This type of fault leads to excessive strain on the anterior capsule and internal impingement of the posterior rotator cuff.[133,190] Correction of throwing pathomechanics is critical to return the athlete to asymptomatic and effective throwing.

Rotator Cuff Tears

The primary function of the rotator cuff is to provide dynamic stabilization and steer the humeral head. It appears that the cuff is well designed to bear tension and resist upward displacement of the humerus.[25,192] The cuff balances the major forces applied by the prime mover muscles during motions such as flexion and abduction.

The role of the rotator cuff in shoulder movements has long been and still remains somewhat controversial. Poppen and Walker[16,17] reported that the pull of the supraspinatus is fairly constant throughout ROM and actually exceeds that of the deltoid until 60° of shoulder abduction has been reached. Norkin and Levangie[4] found that the EMG activity of the deltoid in abduction shows a gradual increase, with a peak at 90° of humeral abduction and no plateau until 180° has been reached. Colachis et al[42,87] used selective nerve blocks and noted that the supraspinatus and infraspinatus provide 45% of abduction and 90% of ER strength. Additionally, Howell et al[193] measured the torque produced by the supraspinatus and deltoid in the forward flexion and elevation planes. They found that the supraspinatus and deltoid muscles are equally responsible for producing torque about the shoulder joint in functional planes of motion. Currently, it appears that both the deltoid and the supraspinatus contribute to abduction throughout the full ROM. Active abduction is possible with loss of the deltoid or supraspinatus, with a corresponding loss of power.[42,87]

The cause of rotator cuff tears can be one or a combination of the following: repetitive microtrauma, disuse, overuse tendinitis, anatomic factors, and attrition. Neer[74] reported that acute cuff tears occurring as a result of trauma account for approximately 3% to 8% of all tears. It has been postulated that rotator cuff tears result after the commonly diagnosed "cuff tendinitis" and that rotator cuff tears may actually represent failure of the rotator cuff fibers. This may explain why individuals with this injury usually recover with time and conservative treatment.[184] Matsen and Arntz[184] suggested the following explanation for perpetuation of rotator cuff failure:

The traumatic and degenerative theories of cuff tendon failure can be synthesized into a unified view of pathogenesis. Let us assume that the normal cuff starts out well vascularized and with a full complement of fibers. Through its life it is subjected to various adverse factors such as traction, contusion, impingement, inflammation, injections, and age-related degeneration. Each of these factors places fibers of the cuff tendons at risk. Even though laboratory studies show that normal tendon does not fail before failure of the musculotendinous junction or the tendon bone junction, in the clinical situation the rotator cuff tendon ruptures both at its insertion to bone and in its mid-substance. With the application of loads (whether repetitive or abrupt, compressive, or tensile), each fiber fails when the applied load exceeds its strength.

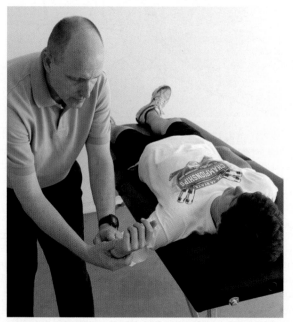

FIGURE 12-18 Manual rhythmic stabilization in the end range of glenohumeral external rotation.

Fibers may fail a few at a time or in mass. Because these fibers are under load even with the arm at rest, they retract after their rupture. Each instance of fiber failure has at least three adverse effects: (1) it increases the load on the neighboring fibers (fewer fibers to share the load); (2) it detaches muscle fibers from bone (diminishing the force that the cuff muscles can deliver); and (3) it risks the vascular elements in close proximity by distorting their anatomy (a particularly important factor owing to the fact that the rotator cuff tendons contain the anastomoses between the osseous and muscular vessels). Thus, the initially well-vascularized rotator cuff tendon becomes progressively less vascular with succeeding injuries. Although some tendons, such as the Achilles tendon, have a remarkable propensity to heal after rupture, cuff ruptures communicate with joint and bursal fluid, which removes any hematoma that could contribute to cuff healing. Even if the tendon could heal with scar, scar tissue lacks the normal resilience of tendon and is, therefore, under increased risk for failure with subsequent loading (minor or major). These events weaken the substance of the cuff, impair its function, and render the cuff weaker, more prone to additional failure with less load, and less able to heal.

Arthroscopy has allowed investigators to examine rotator cuff lesions and make observations regarding these lesions (Box 12-6).

Athletes with rotator cuff tendinitis generally respond favorably to a well-designed rehabilitation program. The involved shoulder is usually stiff, especially in the posterior capsule, with appreciable glenohumeral crepitus being present. The stiffness limits one or a combination of the following motions: forward flexion, IR and ER, and horizontal adduction. The emphasis of the program is to correct any asymmetric capsular tightness. The athlete may also have difficulty reaching behind the back because this movement elongates the musculotendinous unit and compresses it as it is pulled under the coracoacromial arch with IR.[197] Modalities (such as moist heat, iontophoresis, and ultrasound), mobilization, and stretching exercises for the posterior capsule and muscles may be indicated. Rest from noxious stimuli and the use of nonsteroidal antiinflammatory drugs are also appropriate. Initiation of a general shoulder flexibility program and a rotator

cuff PRE program (see Figs. A12-1 through A12-40 in Chapter 12 Appendix [online]) is necessary to prevent progressive cuff degradation. The PRE program should concentrate on the posterior rotator cuff muscles because these muscles are responsible for depression of the humeral head and contract eccentrically to slow the arm down during the deceleration phase of throwing. Strengthening exercises are initially performed with submaximal, subpainful isometric contractions to initiate muscle recruitment and retard muscle atrophy. Electrical stimulation of the posterior cuff musculature may also be incorporated to enhance this muscle fiber recruitment process early in the rehabilitation process and also in the next phase when the patient initiates isotonic strengthening activities (Fig. 12-19). Reinold et al[198] believe that the use of electrical stimulation may improve force production of the rotator cuff, particularly the external rotators immediately after an acute injury. Electrical stimulation of the posterior rotator cuff may be used throughout the rehabilitation process as the athlete performs isotonic and manual resistance strengthening.

Return to throwing should not begin until the entire rehabilitation program has been completed. The patient must exhibit specific criteria before a throwing program is initiated. The criteria used by the authors include full nonpainful ROM, satisfactory muscular strength, satisfactory findings on clinical examination, and appropriate progression through the rehabilitation program. When these criteria have been satisfied, an interval throwing program (see Appendix B [online]) may be initiated. The athlete should continue with a program that includes strengthening and flexibility exercises after the throwing program has been initiated.

Anterior Instability

Shoulder instability is a common clinical problem, with anterior instability occurring most commonly. The anatomy of the glenohumeral joint predisposes the shoulder to instability. The glenoid cavity is relatively small and shallow, and the capsule tends to be loose in young, athletic individuals. These factors

---

Box 12-6

Arthroscopy Observations Regarding Rotator Cuff Lesions

Failure of the musculotendinous cuff is almost always peripheral, near the attachment of the cuff to the greater tuberosity, and it nearly always begins in the supraspinatus part of the cuff near the biceps tendon.[170]

Partial-thickness tears appear to be 2 to 3 times as common as full-thickness lesions.[74,194]

Partial tears often occur on the joint side and not on the bursal side.[98,194]

Rotator cuff tears frequently begin deep and extend outward, thus challenging the concept of subacromial impingement as the primary cause of defects.[183,195,196]

Full-thickness cuff tears appear to occur in tendons that are weakened by some combination of age, repeated small episodes of trauma, steroid injections, subacromial impingement, hypovascularity of the tendon, major injury, and previous partial tearing.[183]

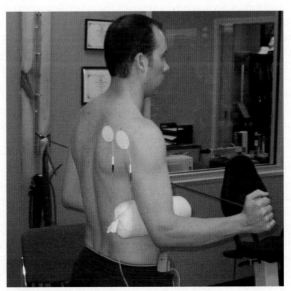

FIGURE 12-19 Electrical stimulation of the posterior cuff musculature.

combine to make the shoulder susceptible to dislocations anteriorly.[5,77,85,199] Anterior glenohumeral instability can be divided into acute traumatic dislocation and recurrent dislocation or subluxation. Most acute anterior dislocations occur with the arm abducted to 90°, extended, and externally rotated, such as when an athlete is attempting an arm tackle in football or when an abnormal force is applied to an arm that is executing a throw. The dislocated shoulder is characterized by a flattened deltoid contour, an inability to move the arm, and severe pain. With this injury the head of the humerus is forced out of its articulation, past the glenoid labrum and then upward, to rest under the coracoid process.[200]

The dislocated shoulder is usually readily detectable, but symptoms of a subluxating shoulder can be more subtle and may be overlooked. Anterior subluxation of the glenohumeral joint may develop without a history of trauma and is common in throwers. The subluxating shoulder is often referred to as the *dead arm syndrome* because it is characterized by loss of shoulder strength and power. Rowe[35,77] reported that in 60 instances of dead arm syndrome, 26 patients were aware of shoulder subluxation and 32 patients were not aware of its occurrence. Clinically, the athlete has soreness over the anterior aspect of the shoulder and reports reproduction of the signs and symptoms in the cocking or acceleration phase of the throwing act. Athletes may also report loss of shoulder strength and power and a feeling of clicking or sliding within the shoulder.

Several mechanisms of injury can explain the insidious onset of anterior instability. One of the most prevalent views is that in the cocking phase of throwing, extreme ER places repeated stress on the anterior capsule that results in capsule attenuation and, ultimately, anterior instability.

Weakness of the scapula stabilizers is also believed to contribute to anterior instability.[201] The function of the scapula rotators (e.g., trapezius, rhomboids, and serratus anterior) is to place the glenoid in the optimal position for the activities being performed. The rotator cuff seeks to stabilize the humeral head, and the glenohumeral ligament, particularly the inferior aspect, provides a static restraint at the margins of the joint.[202] Damage to the static restraints (gradual attenuation) results in instability and causes asynchronous firing of the scapular rotators and rotator cuff muscles. Greater stress is placed on the rotator cuff muscles in an attempt to stabilize the humeral head, which produces rotator cuff damage and leads to rotator cuff impingement (described earlier). Thus, Jobe et al[202] reported that impingement problems are due to the primary lesion, glenohumeral instability.

Shoulder instability can be associated with an anterior glenoid labrum tear as the humeral head slips past the anterior aspect of the labrum and then reduces itself. A small portion of the anterior labrum may be torn, especially with recurrent episodes of instability. Additionally, Hill-Sachs and Bankart lesions (Fig. 12-20) are common with anterior instability, and their presence can be used to confirm this diagnosis. Bankart lesions are caused by avulsion of the capsule and labrum from the glenoid rim and occur as a result of traumatic glenohumeral joint dislocation. Individuals who have had a subluxation generally do not have a Bankart lesion. A Hill-Sachs lesion is a bony injury involving the posterolateral aspect of the humeral head as it strikes the rim of the glenoid at the time of dislocation.[203] Therefore, greater force is required to dislocate a shoulder than to subluxate it, and greater tissue damage results.

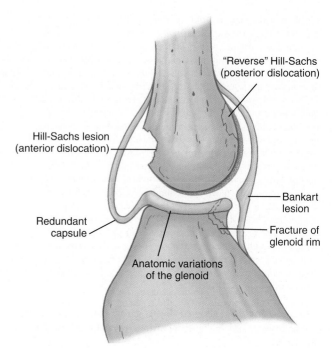

FIGURE 12-20 Anatomic lesions produced as a result of shoulder instability. *(From Rowe, C.R. [1988]: The Shoulder. New York, Churchill Livingstone, p. 177.)*

Whether the injury is a subluxation or a dislocation, nonoperative treatment is often attempted first. The success of nonoperative care varies,[183,204-206] and it most often consists of conservative treatment with immobilization in a sling and early controlled PROM exercises, especially with first-time dislocations. The incidence of recurrent dislocation ranges from 17% to 96% with a mean of 67% in patient populations between the ages of 21 and 30 years.[10,11,206] Therefore, the rehabilitation program should progress cautiously in young athletic individuals. It should be noted that Hovelius et al[10,110,206] demonstrated that the rate of recurrent dislocations is based on the patient's age and is not affected by the length of postinjury immobilization. Individuals between 19 and 29 years of age are the most likely to experience multiple episodes of instability. Hovelius et al[10,11,206] noted that patients in their 20s exhibited a recurrence rate of 60% whereas patients in their 30s to 40s had less than a 20% recurrence rate. In adolescents, the recurrence rate is as high as 92% and 100% with open physes.[71]

Athletes who have dislocated their shoulder and thus have Bankart lesions are less likely to return to unrestricted sports participation than are individuals who do not have Bankart lesions. Rehabilitation should initially concentrate on decreasing the acute inflammation and pain and then gradually restoring full shoulder motion. A short period of immobilization in a sling to control pain and allow scar tissue to form for enhanced stability may be necessary for 7 to 14 days, although no long-term benefits regarding recurrence rates and immobilization have been reported in younger patients between 17 and 29 years of age.[61,107] Individuals older than 29 are usually immobilized for 2 to 4 weeks to allow scarring of the injured capsule. The ideal position to immobilize the glenohumeral joint has traditionally been in IR with the arm close to the body. A study by Itoi et al[207] examined different positions of immobilization and compared the rates of recurrent dislocations. The authors concluded that immobilization in ER significantly reduced the recurrence rate of instability in chronic and first-time dislocators. Itoi et al[207] recommended immobilization with the arm in 30° of abduction and ER, as opposed to immobilization in IR. The results indicated a 0% recurrence rate in ER and a 30% incidence of instability in the group immobilized in IR. The authors stated that the resultant Bankart lesion had improved coaptation to the glenoid rim with immobilization in ER versus conventional immobilization in a sling. Potential complications with immobilization may include a decrease in joint proprioception, muscle disuse and atrophy, and loss of ROM in specific age groups. Therefore, prolonged use of immobilization following a traumatic dislocation may not be recommended for all patients. After normal motion is restored, an aggressive shoulder flexibility program is contraindicated because of attenuation of the tissues. A strengthening program for the rotator cuff with a focus on the rotator cuff muscles and scapular stabilizers should be implemented.[208] Historically, nonanatomic extraarticular surgical procedures such as the Bristow, Magnuson-Stack, and Putti-Platt have been performed with limited success in addressing glenohumeral listability.[54,209-215] These procedures have largely been replaced by the anatomic stabilization techniques detailed later in this chapter, which restore normal anatomy and facilitate early aggressive rehabilitation.

In some athletes who exhibit recurrent anterior instability and are not required to abduct and externally rotate their arms above shoulder height, a shoulder brace may be used. The SAWA shoulder orthosis* is an off-the-shelf brace made of cotton and rubber that has Velcro straps to limit motion. The Sully Brace† is another off-the-shelf brace made of neoprene. Use of these types of braces has proved to be beneficial in athletes such as interior linemen, hockey players, and soccer players, but their use has been completely unsuccessful in athletes who have to throw or catch a ball.

Posterior Instability

Posterior dislocation or subluxation is not as common as anterior instability, but it does occur. Usually, posterior subluxation results from traumatic forces that injure the posterior capsule. This can occur in football linemen who use their hands during blocking or rushing; with the elbow locked in extension and the shoulder flexed, the arm can be forcefully pushed posteriorly. For example, in professional or collegiate football, the incidence of posterior shoulder instability appears to be higher than in the general population, especially in linemen.

Again, nonoperative treatment using a balanced strengthening program for the anterior and posterior rotator cuff musculature should be attempted first. Strengthening of the posterior rotator cuff should be accomplished without placing the shoulder in a subluxated or apprehensive position.[216] An aggressive shoulder flexibility regimen is contraindicated because of the attenuated tissues. Engle and Canner[217] reported success with a rehabilitation program that emphasizes PNF exercise techniques centered around development of the posterior cuff muscles. Success of the nonoperative program depends greatly on the type of athlete and the sport. Athletes who use their arms in an extended position in front of their body are more susceptible to recurrent symptoms.

Surgical management of athletes whose injuries do not respond to nonoperative care is controversial. The results after surgical reconstruction for posterior instability are not as good as the results after anterior stabilization procedures.[218-225] Surgical techniques include shifting of the posterior capsule (capsulorrhaphy), posterior Bankart repair, or posterior osteotomy to help prevent dislocation. The posterior capsule tends to be much thinner than the anterior capsule and is thus prone to stretch out, which may contribute to the diminished surgical success.

Rehabilitation after posterior capsulorrhaphy advances more slowly than rehabilitation after anterior capsulorrhaphy. The most significant differences from the anterior capsulorrhaphy rehabilitation program include (1) immobilization using an abduction pillow in 15° to 30° of ER, (2) no forward flexion above 90° and no horizontal adduction for 6 weeks to avoid stress on the repaired capsule, (3) delay restoring IR in the 90/90 position until 6 weeks after surgery, and (4) slower return to functional or sports activities.

Multidirectional Instability

Athletes who exhibit atraumatic (congenital), multidirectional instability pose a difficult problem, not only to the clinician but also to the surgeon. These individuals typically have generalized ligamentous and capsular laxity.[226] Most frequently, these athletes are swimmers, gymnasts, and occasionally overhead-throwing athletes. The most common treatment plan for these individuals is a thorough nonoperative strengthening program. Although the program is usually successful, it is not uncommon for the athlete to intermittently experience symptoms.

Nonoperative treatment focuses on dynamic stabilization, proprioception, and neuromuscular control exercises. Rehabilitation techniques such as rhythmic stabilization, cocontractions, proprioceptive training, and motor control drills are the hallmark of a well-structured program. In the rehabilitation program the posterior and anterior musculature should be balanced in an attempt to control and stabilize the glenohumeral joint. In patients with atraumatic instability, it is critical that scapular muscle strength be improved through an aggressive rehabilitation program.

If nonsurgical treatment fails and the athlete is unable to participate in sports, surgical intervention may be indicated. Bigliani[227] suggested that a capsular shift procedure may correct redundancy on all three sides: anterior, posterior, and inferior.

Glenoid Labrum Lesions

In recent years, increasing attention has been paid to the glenoid labrum. Lesions involving the glenoid labrum are extremely common in athletes and can be classified as either atraumatic or traumatic. Traumatic injuries to the glenoid capsulolabral complex are known to occur with glenohumeral dislocations or subluxations. With this mechanism of injury, a wide spectrum of glenoid labral injuries may occur, including detachment of the labrum from the glenoid, a frank tear, or a combination of these lesions. Additionally, the labrum can be injured as a result of repetitive stress during the throwing motion. Andrews et al[40,188] described a tear of the superior aspect of the glenoid labrum at the origin of the biceps tendon. The authors theorized that this lesion may be due to repetitive forceful contraction of the biceps brachii during the follow-through phase of throwing.

Snyder et al[228] described an anterosuperior labral complex lesion. This superior labrum, anterior to posterior (SLAP) lesion

---

*Available from Brace International, Scottsdale, Arizona.
†Available from The Saunders Group, Chaska, Minnesota.

begins posteriorly, extends anteriorly, and involves the "anchor" of the long head of the biceps brachii to the labrum. Numerous mechanisms may produce this lesion. A labral tear may result from a fall onto an outstretched arm, from forceful muscular contraction of the biceps, or from repetitive strenuous overhead sport movements. Snyder et al[228] classified SLAP lesions into four types (Fig. 12-21 and Table 12-7). Specific treatment recommendations are based on the type of labral lesion present. The rehabilitation program for these pathologic conditions is discussed later in this chapter.

Acromioclavicular Separation

Injuries involving the acromioclavicular joint can occur insidiously from activities requiring repetitive overhead activity. Acute injuries occur either as a result of direct trauma, in which the athlete falls on the tip of the shoulder and depresses the acromion process inferiorly, or as a result of a fall on the outstretched arm, in which the forces are transmitted superiorly through the acromion process. The extent of acromioclavicular sprain or separation depends on whether the coracoclavicular ligaments are traumatized or the main stabilizing acromioclavicular ligaments are damaged. Rockwood and Young[229] identified six types of acromioclavicular joint sprains (Fig. 12-22 and Table 12-8).

Treatment of grade I and grade II injuries is nonoperative, but treatment of grade III injuries is still controversial. Many physicians elect to treat grade III injuries nonoperatively in the belief that outcomes are better with nonoperative management,[202,230] whereas others believe that the joint needs to be stabilized surgically. Depending on the extent of damage, a number of surgical measures are available, including (1) stabilization of the

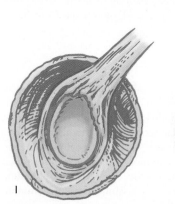
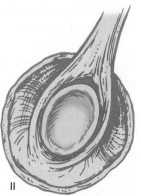
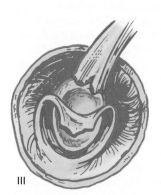
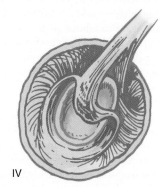

I   II   III   IV

FIGURE 12-21 Classification of superior labrum, anterior and posterior lesions according to Snyder et al.[228] *(From Zuckerman, J.D. [1993]: Glenoid labrum lesions. In Andrews, J.R., and Wilk, K.E. [eds.]: The Athlete's Shoulder. New York, Churchill Livingstone, p. 232.)*

Table 12-7 Classification of Superior Labrum, Anterior to Posterior (SLAP) Lesions

Type	Description	Treatment Recommendations
I	Superior labrum markedly frayed but attachment of the labrum and biceps remains intact	Débride the labrum to intact labrum.
II	Similar in appearance to type I except that the attachment of the superior labrum is compromised, which results in instability of the biceps-labral complex	Débride and reattach the superior labrum back to the glenoid rim with a bioabsorbable suture anchor. *Note:* Within the type II SLAP lesion group is a subgroup referred to as a peel-back lesion.[51] A peel-back lesion most commonly occurs in an overhead athlete as a result of the extreme of external rotation.[51]
III	Bucket handle tear of the labrum, which can displace into the joint	The bucket handle tear is excised.
IV	Similar to type III, except that the labral tear extends into the biceps tendon, which allows it to sublux into the joint	The tear is excised and a biceps repair or tenodesis is performed.
V	Anterior inferior Bankart lesion that propagates into the biceps tendon	Repair the labrum and biceps and possibly perform tenodesis.
VI	Unstable flap tear of the labrum with separation of the biceps anchor	Débride the flap tear and repair the attachment.
VII	Superior biceps-labral detachment that extends anteriorly beneath the middle glenohumeral ligament (MGHL)	Perform a SLAP and MGHL repair.
VIII	SLAP tear with extension into the posterior labrum as far as the 6-o'clock position	Perform a SLAP and posterior labral repair.
IX	Pan-labral SLAP lesion encompassing the entire circumference	Perform a 360° labral repair.
X	Superior labral tear with a posterior-inferior labral tear (reverse Bankart lesion)	Perform a SLAP and posterior labral repair.

Data from Snyder, S.J., Karzel, R.P., DelPizzo, W., et al. (1990): SLAP lesions of the shoulder. Arthroscopy, 6:274–276.

clavicle to the coracoid process with a screw, (2) transarticular fixation of the acromioclavicular joint with pins after reduction, (3) resection of the outer end of the clavicle, and (4) transposition of the coracoacromial ligament to the top of the acromioclavicular joint. Biomechanical studies[231] have indicated that the superior acromioclavicular ligament is the most important for stabilizing the acromioclavicular joint for normal daily activities. The conoid ligament is the most important for supporting the joint against significant injury.

Rehabilitation after first- and second-degree acromioclavicular separations consists of advancing motion as tolerated and beginning a PRE program when active ROM is equal bilaterally. Modalities may be used in the early stages of healing to help decrease inflammation and pain. Third-degree separations treated nonoperatively usually require 2 to 4 weeks of immobilization, with gradual progression of motion and strengthening exercises after immobilization. Pendulum exercises, elbow ROM exercises, isometrics in all planes, and rope-and-pulley exercises for shoulder flexion and abduction can be initiated as tolerated after immobilization. Precautions during rehabilitation after surgical repair of the acromioclavicular joint are similar to those after conservative care of grade III injuries and include

limitation of abduction and flexion to 90° for approximately 3 to 4 weeks. Pendulum and isometric exercises in all planes are encouraged in the initial stages of postsurgical rehabilitation. ROM is progressed to 90° in all planes as tolerated after 4 weeks. Rehabilitation should concentrate on strengthening the rotator cuff and scapula stabilizers and on restoring neuromuscular control and arthrokinematics, not unlike rehabilitation after other shoulder injuries.

GENERAL REHABILITATION GUIDELINES AFTER SURGERY

Injuries that do not respond to nonoperative care may require surgical intervention. Acromioplasty is commonly performed in conjunction with a rotator cuff repair. Rotator cuff tears treated arthroscopically are most often incomplete tears located on the undersurface of the muscle. Larger lesions may require repair with an open procedure. Numerous surgical techniques can be used to repair a full-thickness rotator cuff tear. The deltoid-splitting procedure is recommended to decrease morbidity and promote early ROM. It typically involves arthroscopic débridement and open rotator cuff repair via a deltoid-splitting or arthroscopy-assisted surgical procedure. The rehabilitation approach that we take following arthroscopic rotator cuff repair is depicted in Box 12-7. An abduction pillow (Fig. 12-23) can be used after rotator cuff repair to alleviate stress on the cuff repair because the adducted position may cause undue early stress on the repair, especially with large to massive tears. Lesion size and the extent of repair determine whether an abduction pillow will be used and the duration of use. In most patients, an abduction pillow or splint is not used after rotator cuff repair (except for large tears). The duration of use of the pillow can range from 2 to 5 weeks. Immediately after the repair, PROM exercises should be performed to minimize the development of adhesive capsulitis or a stiff shoulder. AAROM may be initiated when the physician believes that the repair has healed adequately. As active ROM is restored, a PRE program should be initiated with a focus on strengthening of the posterior cuff and scapular stabilizer muscles. Postoperative rehabilitation depends on the

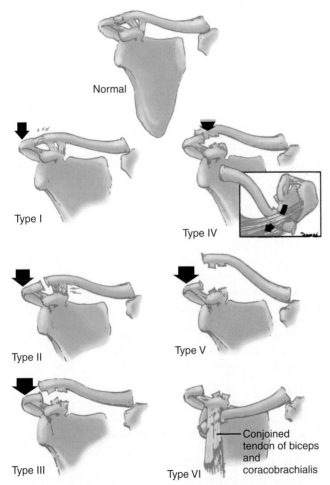

FIGURE 12-22 Rockwood classification of acromioclavicular joint sprains. *(From Rockwood, C.A., and Young, D.C. [1990]: Disorders of the acromioclavicular joint. In Rockwood, C.A., and Matsen, F.A. [eds.]: The Shoulder. Philadelphia, Saunders, pp. 413–468.)*

Table 12-8 Six Types of Acromioclavicular Joint Sprains

Type	Description
I	Injury to the acromioclavicular ligament
II	Injury to the acromioclavicular ligament and sprain of the coracoclavicular ligament
III	Disruption of the acromioclavicular and coracoclavicular ligaments and some detachment of the deltoid and upper trapezius muscles from the distal end of the clavicle
IV	Similar to type III injuries, except that in type IV acromioclavicular joint sprains, the clavicle displaces posteriorly through the trapezius muscle and the deltoid and trapezius are detached
V	Significant displacement of the clavicle by 100%–300%
VI	Involves the distal end of the clavicle displacing inferiorly under the acromion

---

Box 12-7

Rehabilitation Following Arthroscopic Repair of Medium to Large Rotator Cuff Tears

PHASE I: IMMEDIATE POSTSURGICAL PHASE (DAYS 1–10)

Goals:
- Maintain integrity of the repair
- Gradually increase PROM
- Diminish pain and inflammation
- Prevent muscular inhibition

Days 1–6
- Abduction pillow brace
- Pendulum exercises
- AAROM exercise (L - bar)
  - ER/IR in scapular plane at 45° of abduction (pain-free ROM)
- PROM
  - Flexion to tolerance (painful ROM)
  - ER/IR in scapular plane at 45° of abduction (pain-free ROM)
- Elbow/hand gripping and ROM exercises
- Submaximal pain-free isometrics (initiate on days 4–5)
  - Flexion with elbow bent to 90°
  - ER
  - IR
  - Elbow flexors
- Cryotherapy for pain and inflammation
  - Ice 15–20 minutes every hour
- Sleeping
  - Sleep in a pillow brace

Days 7–14
- Continue use of the pillow brace
- Pendulum exercises
- Advance PROM to tolerance
  - Flexion to at least 115°
  - ER in scapular plane at 45° of abduction to 20°–25°
  - IR in scapular plane at 45° of abduction to 30°–35°
- AAROM exercises (L - bar)
  - ER/IR in scapular plane at 45° of abduction
  - Flexion to tolerance (therapist provides assistance with supporting arm, especially with arm lowering)
- Continue elbow/hand ROM and gripping exercises
- Continue isometrics (submaximal and subpainful)
  - Flexion with bent elbow
  - Extension with bent elbow
  - Abduction with bent elbow
  - ER/IR with arm in scapular plane
  - Elbow flexion
- Initiate rhythmic stabilization ER/IR at 45° of abduction
- Continue use of ice for pain control
  - Use ice at least 6–7 times daily
- Sleeping
  - Continue sleeping in brace until physician instructs

Precautions:
1. No lifting of objects
2. No excessive shoulder extension
3. No excessive stretching or sudden movements
4. No supporting of body weight by hands
5. Keep incision clean and dry

PHASE II: PROTECTION PHASE (DAY 15–WEEK 6)

Goals:
- Allow healing of soft tissue
- Do not overstress healing tissue
- Gradually restore full PROM (weeks 4–5)
- Reestablish dynamic shoulder stability
- Decrease pain and inflammation

Days 15–21
- Continue use of sling or brace (physician or therapist will determine when to discontinue)
- PROM to tolerance
  - Flexion to 140°–155°
  - ER at 90° of abduction to at least 45°
  - IR at 90° of abduction to at least 45°
- AAROM to tolerance
  - Flexion (continue use of arm support)
  - ER/IR in scapular plane at 45° of abduction
  - ER/IR at 90° of abduction
- Dynamic stabilization drills
  - Rhythmic stabilization drills
    - ER/IR in scapular plane
    - Flexion/extension at 100° of flexion and 25° of horizontal abduction
- Continue all isometric contractions
- Initiate scapular isometrics
- Continue use of cryotherapy as needed
- Continue all precautions
  - No lifting
  - No excessive motion

WEEKS 4–5
- Patient should exhibit full PROM by week 4
- Continue all exercises listed above
- Initiate ER/IR strengthening with exercise tubing at 0° of abduction (use a towel roll)
- Initiate manual resistance ER supine in scapular plane (light resistance)
- Initiate prone rowing to neutral arm position
- Initiate prone shoulder extension
- Initiate ER strengthening exercises
- Initiate isotonic elbow flexion
- Continue use of ice as needed
- May use heat before ROM exercises
- May use pool for light AAROM exercises
- Rhythmic stabilization exercises (flexion of 45°, 90°, 125°) (ER/IR)

Weeks 5–6
- May use heat before exercises
- Continue AAROM and stretching exercises
  - Especially for movements that are not full
    - Shoulder flexion
    - ER at 90° of abduction
- Initiate AROM exercises
  - Shoulder flexion in scapular plane
  - Shoulder abduction

Box 12-7

Rehabilitation Following Arthroscopic Repair of Medium to Large Rotator Cuff Tears—cont'd

- Advance isotonic strengthening exercise program
  - ER tubing
  - Side-lying IR
  - Prone rowing
  - Prone horizontal abduction (bent elbow)
  - Biceps curls (isotonics)

Precautions:
1. No heavy lifting of objects
2. No excessive behind-the-back movements
3. No supporting of body weight with hands and arms
4. No sudden jerking motions

PHASE III: INTERMEDIATE PHASE (WEEKS 7–14)

Goals:
- Full AROM (weeks 8–10)
- Maintain full PROM
- Dynamic shoulder stability
- Gradual restoration of shoulder strength
- Gradual return to functional activities

Week 7
- Continue stretching and PROM (as needed to maintain full ROM)
- Continue dynamic stabilization drills
- Advance strengthening program
  - ER/IR tubing
  - Side-lying ER
  - Lateral raises*
  - Full can in scapular plane*
  - Prone rowing
  - Prone horizontal abduction
  - Prone extension
  - Elbow extension

Week 8
- Continue all exercise listed above
- If physician permits, may initiate *light* functional activities

Week 10
- Continue all exercise listed above
- Progress to fundamental shoulder exercises

- Clinician may initiate isotonic resistance (1-lb weight) during flexion and abduction (if nonpainful normal motion is exhibited!)

Weeks 11–14
- Advance all exercises
  - Continue ROM and flexibility exercises
  - Advance strengthening program (increase 1 lb/10 days if nonpainful)

PHASE IV: ADVANCED STRENGTHENING PHASE (WEEKS 15–22)

Goals:
- Maintain full nonpainful ROM
- Enhance functional use of the upper extremity
- Improve muscular strength and power
- Gradual return to functional activities

Week 15
- Continue ROM and stretching to maintain full ROM
- Self–capsular stretches
- Advance shoulder-strengthening exercises
  - Fundamental shoulder exercises
- Initiate interval golf program (if appropriate)

Weeks 20–22
- Continue all exercises listed above
- Advance golf program to playing golf (if appropriate)
- Initiate interval tennis program (if appropriate)
- May initiate swimming

PHASE V: RETURN-TO-SPORT PHASE (WEEKS 23–36)

Goals:
- Gradual return to strenuous work activities
- Gradual return to recreational sport activities

Week 23
- Continue fundamental shoulder exercise program (at least 4 times weekly)
- Continue stretching, if motion is tight
- Continue progression to sport participation

---

*Patient must be able to elevate the arm without shoulder or scapular hiking before initiating isotonics; if unable, continue glenohumeral joint exercises.
AAROM, Active assisted range of motion; *AROM,* active range of motion; *ER,* external rotation; *IR,* internal rotation; *PROM,* passive range of motion; *ROM,* range of motion.

---

extent of the cuff lesion, the tissue quality, and the procedure used for the repair. In the early 2000s, arthroscopic rotator cuff repair became more popular because of less scarring and loss of motion. However, we believe that the fixation currently available is not as secure as that for an open procedure; consequently, rehabilitation is slower.

In all of our rehabilitation programs after shoulder stabilization surgery, we take a multiple-phase approach, with each phase consisting of specific goals and exercises (Box 12-8). We also use a criteria-based rehabilitation approach to help guide the rate of progression of rehabilitation.

In the first phase, the immediate postoperative period, rehabilitation goals are to (1) protect the healing soft tissues, (2) prevent the negative effects of immobilization, (3) reestablish dynamic joint stability, and (4) diminish postoperative pain and inflammation. Thus, during this maximal-protection phase we use early motion in a restricted and protected arc of motion. This early motion is intended to nourish the articular cartilage, assist

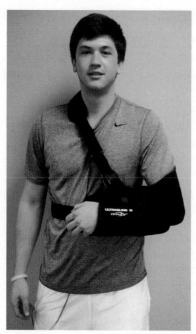

FIGURE 12-23 Use of an abduction pillow after rotator cuff repair can help alleviate stress on the repair.

in the synthesis and organization of collagen tissue, and promote healing. Early motion will assist in decreasing the patient's pain through neuromuscular modulation.[232-235] Depending on the type of surgical procedure, method of fixation, and the patient's tissue status, a prescribed ROM is outlined. The primary goal of this phase is to prevent excessive scarring but not allow too aggressive motion to compromise the surgical repair. Often after anterior stabilization, motions such as extension and ER are limited or restricted because of the anterior capsule, whereas shoulder elevation in the scapular plane is encouraged instead of shoulder abduction. Dynamic stabilization exercises are performed to reestablish dynamic joint stability. These stability drills are performed with the patient maintaining a static position as the clinician facilitates a muscular cocontraction (Figs. 12-24 and 12-25). The static joint position should be chosen carefully by the clinician to prevent excessive stress on the stabilization procedure. Submaximal isometrics for the rotator cuff are performed to initiate voluntary muscular contractions of these muscles, which aids in preventing muscular atrophy and loss of motor control. Wickiewicz et al[236] reported that most human shoulder musculature is roughly a 50:50 mixture of slow- and fast-twitch muscle fibers. Because immobilization has been shown to have a greater effect on slow-twitch fibers, it is important for the patient to perform submaximal isometrics

---

Box 12-8

Rehabilitation Phases and Goals

PHASE I: ACUTE PHASE

Goals:

- Diminish pain and inflammation
- Normalize motion
- Retard muscular atrophy
- Reestablish dynamic stability
- Control functional stress/strain

Exercises and Modalities:

- Cryotherapy, ultrasound, electrical stimulation
- Flexibility and stretching of the posterior shoulder muscles
- Rotator cuff strengthening (especially the external rotators)
- Scapular muscle strengthening (especially the retractors, protractors, depressors)
- Dynamic stabilization exercises (rhythmic stabilization)
- Closed kinetic chain exercises
- Proprioception training
- Abstain from throwing

PHASE II: INTERMEDIATE PHASE

Goals:

- Advance the strengthening exercise
- Restore muscular balance (external/internal rotation)
- Enhance dynamic stability
- Control flexibility and stretches

Exercises:

- Continue stretching and flexibility
- Advance isotonic strengthening
  - Complete shoulder program
  - Throwers' Ten Exercise Program

- Rhythmic stabilization drills
- Initiate core strengthening program
- Initiate leg program

PHASE III: ADVANCED STRENGTHENING PHASE

Goals:

- Aggressive strengthening
- Progressive neuromuscular control
- Improve strength, power, and endurance
- Initiate light throwing activities

Exercises:

- Flexibility and stretching
- Rhythmic stabilization drills
- Throwers' Ten Exercise Program
- Initiate plyometric program
- Initiate endurance drills
- Initiate short-distance throwing program

PHASE IV: RETURN-TO-SPORT PHASE

Goals:

- Progress to throwing program
- Return to competitive throwing
- Continue strengthening and flexibility drills

Exercises:

- Stretching and flexibility drills
- Throwers' Ten Exercise Program
- Plyometric program
- Advance the interval throwing program to competitive throwing

to prevent muscular atrophy. During this first week we attempt to control the patient's pain and inflammation through guarded motion and isometric exercises and the judicious use of various therapeutic modalities (e.g., ice, electrical stimulation).

Phase II, the intermediate phase, emphasizes advancement of shoulder mobility. Before the patient enters phase II, the following criteria must be met: (1) satisfactory static stability, (2) diminishing pain and inflammation, and (3) adequate muscular control and dynamic stability. During this phase the patient's ROM is gradually increased by using AAROM and PROM exercises, stretching, and joint mobilization techniques. Guidelines for progression of motion are based on the surgical procedure, method of fixation, and the patient's tissue status; they are discussed throughout this chapter. Additionally, the rate of progression is based on the clinician's assessment of the quantity and end-feel of motion. For example, in a patient with less motion than desirable at that time and a firm or hard end-feel, stretch is more aggressive than in a patient who has a capsular or soft end-feel. Joint mobilization techniques are used to restore normal motion and to correct asymmetric capsular tightness; thus, the anterior capsule and posterior capsule should exhibit comparable flexibility. If one side of the capsule is excessively tight in comparison to the opposite side, the humeral head will displace excessively in the opposite direction, away from the tightness.[29,116] Hence, if the anterior capsule is excessively tight with respect to the posterior capsule (after anterior stabilization surgery), the humeral head will tend to displace posteriorly during arm movements.[237] Correcting asymmetric capsular tightness should be a critical goal for the clinician. Other goals during this phase include improving muscular strength and enhancing neuromuscular control. To achieve these objectives, we use PNF techniques with rhythmic stabilization,[70] neuromuscular control drills (Fig. 12-26),[70,116] and isolated muscular strengthening exercises for the rotator cuff and scapular muscles. In an overhead-throwing athlete, toward the end of this phase the clinician can begin aggressive stretching techniques to gradually increase motion past 90° of ER. ER of approximately 115° ± 5° is necessary for these athletes to be able to begin throwing. Strengthening exercises are focused on reestablishing muscular balance, particularly the ER/IR unilateral muscle ratio. During this phase we usually initiate the Throwers' Ten Exercise Program (see Appendix A [online]).

The third phase, the dynamic strengthening phase, is focused on improving the patient's strength, power, and endurance while maintaining functional ROM of the shoulder joint.

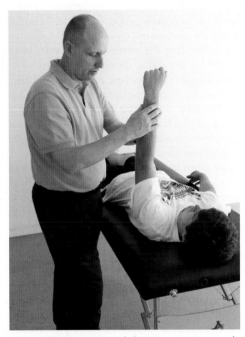

FIGURE 12-24 Dynamic stabilization training with manual resistance in the balanced shoulder position.

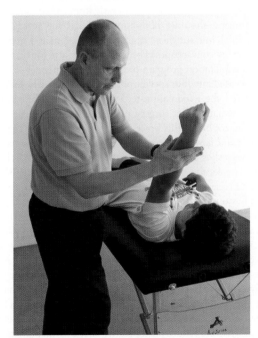

FIGURE 12-25 Dynamic stabilization training with manual resistance in 120° of glenohumeral elevation.

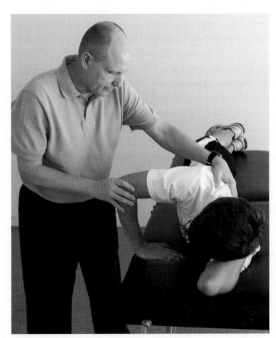

FIGURE 12-26 Side-lying manual neuromuscular control drills for scapulothoracic control.

The criteria that should be met before entering phase III are (1) full nonpainful functional motion, (2) muscular strength of at least 4 out of 5 or of the "good" grade (manual muscle test), (3) satisfactory static stability on clinical examination, and (4) dynamic joint stability. Resistance exercises are progressed during this phase. The goal of this phase is to reestablish significant strength for the desired functional activities but also to reestablish muscular balance. Thus, a suitable ratio should exist between the posterior and anterior muscles, rotator cuff and deltoid muscles, and retractor and protractor scapular muscles. The muscular ratios that we strive for are ER/IR ratios of 62% to 70%, posterior rotator cuff (external rotation)-to-deltoid (abduction) ratio of 66% to 72%, and scapular retractor-to-protractor ratio of approximately 100%.[238] Muscular balance and dynamic joint stability should be achieved before aggressive strengthening exercises such as plyometrics or functional activities such as throwing and swimming are initiated to ensure that dynamic joint stability has been accomplished. During this phase, eccentric muscle training and proprioceptive training are emphasized. Muscular endurance training is also emphasized in this phase. This is a critical element in the rehabilitation program. Wickiewicz et al[239] showed that once the rotator cuff muscles have reached a significant level of fatigue, the humeral head displaces superiorly with simple arm movements such as shoulder abduction. The rehabilitation program should emphasize muscular endurance training to enhance dynamic functional joint stability and to prevent fatigue-induced subluxation.[240] Plyometric training drills are used in this phase to generally increase the athlete's shoulder motion and to gradually increase functional stress on the shoulder joint.

Phase IV is referred to as the return-to-sport phase. The goal of this phase is to gradually and progressively increase the functional demands on the shoulder to return the patient to full, unrestricted sport or daily activities. The criteria established before a patient's return to sport activities are (1) full functional ROM, (2) adequate static stability, (3) satisfactory muscular strength and endurance, (4) adequate dynamic stability, and (5) satisfactory findings on clinical examination. When these criteria have been met successfully, the patient may initiate gradual return to sports activity in a controlled manner. Healing constraints based on surgical technique and fixation, as well as the patient's tissue status, should be considered before a functional program is initiated. Other goals of this phase are to maintain the patient's muscular strength, dynamic stability, and shoulder functional motion established in the previous phase. A stretching and strengthening program should be performed on an ongoing basis to maintain and continue to improve on these goals.

Rehabilitation After Arthroscopic Stabilization Procedures

Another surgical procedure performed on overhead throwers is an arthroscopic stabilization technique to either repair a Bankart-type lesion or tighten the capsule. At our center we use either a suture anchor device or a cannulated absorbable fixation device* in the arthroscopic stabilization technique for repair of a Bankart lesion as described by Warner and Warren.[241] An overhead-throwing athlete must exhibit specific criteria to be considered a candidate for arthroscopic stabilization.

The rehabilitation program after arthroscopic stabilization is significantly different from that after open stabilization. The rate of progression immediately after surgery is much slower in an arthroscopically stabilized shoulder because of the method of fixation used. Shall and Crowley[242] reported the pull-out strength of various soft tissue fixation devices. The Suretac was found to fail ultimately at approximately 122 N (27 lb), with the majority of failures (94%) occurring because of the tack pulling out of the bone. The investigators reported that the suture anchor (Mitek super-anchor)* was almost twice as strong (failing at 217 N). The Suretac is made of polyglyconate polymer, which loses its strength over a 4- to 6-week period and gradually becomes reabsorbed during the next several months.[241] It is important for the clinician to realize that the strength of the arthroscopic tissue fixation method is somewhat tenuous for the first 4 to 6 weeks and that care should be taken to not disturb the soft tissue repair. For that reason the initial postoperative rehabilitation is much slower for a shoulder undergoing arthroscopic stabilization than for a shoulder on which an open procedure was performed.

Several authors have briefly outlined their postoperative rehabilitation programs after arthroscopic stabilization.[243-246] Some of them have advocated postoperative immobilization for 4 to 6 weeks and a guarded motion program with a gradual restoration of motion. Wickiewicz et al[236] suggested 4 weeks of immobilization followed by AAROM and PROM exercises from week 4 and full motion by approximately 8 to 10 weeks. Various authors have suggested several time frames for immobilization. Some authors suggested 3 weeks of immobilization,[243-245] others 4 weeks,[244] and others 6 weeks[247] after arthroscopic stabilization. Grana et al[244] noted that some patients may not comply with long periods of strict immobilization because of minimal pain and less operative morbidity. These patients may return to some activities prematurely. Grana et al[244] reported on 27 patients who underwent arthroscopic suture stabilization. The authors noted that 10 patients admitted removal of the immobilizer after the first week; in 8 of 10 of these patients the results were rated poor because of recurrent instability. Most investigators agree on restricting or limiting shoulder abduction and ER for several weeks (4 to 6 weeks), initiating a strengthening program at 4 to 8 weeks, and restricting contact sports or strenuous sports for 6 months.

The rehabilitation program of two of the authors (K.E.W. and C.A.) is divided into four specific phases (Box 12-9). The first phase is considered the maximal-protection phase or restricted-motion phase. Immediately after surgery, the patient's shoulder is placed in an immobilizer brace; this brace is used consistently for the first 2 to 3 weeks and is worn during sleep for 4 weeks after surgery. The patient uses a sling during daily activities from weeks 2 to 4. During the first 2 weeks the patient is allowed to perform AAROM and PROM exercises. The active assisted motion is restricted to 60° of forward flexion, 45° of IR, and 5° to 10° of ER with the arm placed in 20° of abduction. Additionally, PROM is performed for shoulder flexion and abduction to a maximum of 90° while ER is limited to 20° of PROM while in the plane of the scapula. These ranges are strictly enforced to prevent potentially deleterious force from being exerted on the anteroinferior aspect of the glenohumeral capsule where the surgical procedure has been performed. During this phase the patient also performs submaximal and subpainful isometrics for the shoulder musculature. Additionally, cryotherapy and other modalities may be used to reduce postoperative pain and inflammation.

---

*Available from Suretac, Acufex Microsurgical, Inc., Mansfield, Massachusetts.

*Available from Mitek Surgical Products, Westwood, Massachusetts.

Box 12-9

Rehabilitation Protocol After Arthroscopic Anterior Bankart Repair

PHASE I: IMMEDIATE POSTOPERATIVE PHASE—RESTRICTED-MOTION PHASE (WEEKS 1–6)

Goals:
1. Protect the anatomic repair
2. Prevent the negative effects of immobilization
3. Promote dynamic stability and proprioception
4. Diminish pain and inflammation

Weeks 1–2
- Sling for 2–3 weeks
- Sleep in an immobilizer for 4 weeks
- Elbow/hand range of motion
- Hand-gripping exercises
- Passive and gentle active assisted range of motion exercises
- Flexion to 70° week 1
- Flexion to 90° week 2
- External/internal rotation with the arm in 30° of abduction
  - External rotation to 5°–10°
  - Internal rotation to 45°

No active external rotation or extension or abduction
- Submaximal isometrics for the shoulder musculature
- Rhythmic stabilization drills: external/internal rotation
- Proprioception drills
- Cryotherapy, other modalities as indicated

Weeks 3–4
- Discontinue use of the sling
- Use an immobilizer for sleep (physician decision)
- Continue gentle range-of-motion exercises (passive range of motion and active assisted range of motion)
  - Flexion to 90°
  - Abduction to 90°
  - External/internal rotation at 45° of abduction in the scapular plane
  - External rotation in the scapular plane to 15°–20°
  - Internal rotation in the scapular plane to 55°–60°

Note: Rate of progression based on evaluation of the patient
- No excessive external rotation, extension, or elevation
- Continue isometrics and rhythmic stabilization (submaximal)
- Core stabilization program
- Initiate scapular strengthening program
- Continue use of cryotherapy

Weeks 5–6
- Gradually improve range of motion
  - Flexion to 145°
  - External rotation at 45° of abduction: 55°–50°
  - Internal rotation at 45° abduction: 55°–60°
- May initiate stretching exercises
- Initiate exercise tubing external/internal rotation (arm at side)
- Scapular strengthening
- Proprioceptive neuromuscular facilitation against manual resistance

PHASE II: INTERMEDIATE PHASE—MODERATE-PROTECTION PHASE (WEEKS 6–13)

Goals:
1. Gradually restore full range of motion (week 10)
2. Preserve integrity of the surgical repair
3. Restore muscular strength and balance
4. Enhance neuromuscular control

Weeks 7–9
- Gradually advance range of motion
- Flexion to 160°
- Initiate external/internal rotation at 90° of abduction
  - External rotation at 90° of abduction: 70°–80° at week 7
  - External rotation to 90° at weeks 8–9
  - Internal rotation at 90° of abduction: 70°–75°
- Continue to advance isotonic strengthening program
- Continue proprioceptive neuromuscular facilitation strengthening

Weeks 10–13
- May initiate slightly more aggressive strengthening
- Advance isotonic strengthening exercises
- Continue all stretching exercises

Advance Range of Motion to Functional Demands (i.e., Overhead Activity)
- Progress to isotonic strengthening (light and restricted range of motion)

PHASE III: MINIMAL-PROTECTION PHASE (WEEKS 14–20)

Goals:
1. Maintain full range of motion
2. Improve muscular strength, power, and endurance
3. Gradually initiate functional activities

Criteria to Enter Phase III:
1. Full nonpainful range of motion
2. Satisfactory stability
3. Muscular strength (good grade or better)
4. No pain or tenderness

Weeks 15–18
- Continue all stretching exercises (capsular stretches)
- Continue strengthening exercises:
  - Throwers' Ten Exercise Program or fundamental exercises
  - Proprioceptive neuromuscular facilitation against manual resistance
  - Endurance training
  - Restricted sport activities (light swimming, half golf swings)
- Initiate interval sport program (weeks 16–18)

Weeks 18–21
- Continue all exercises listed above
- Advance interval sport program (throwing, etc.)

(Continued)

Box 12-9

Rehabilitation Protocol After Arthroscopic Anterior Bankart Repair—cont'd

PHASE IV: ADVANCED STRENGTHENING PHASE (WEEKS 22–26)

Goals:
1. Enhance muscular strength, power, and endurance
2. Advance functional activities
3. Maintain shoulder mobility

Criteria to Enter Phase IV:
1. Full nonpainful range of motion
2. Satisfactory static stability
3. Muscular strength 75%–80% of contralateral side
4. No pain or tenderness

Weeks 22–26
- Continue flexibility exercises
- Continue isotonic strengthening program
- Neuromuscular control drills
- Plyometric strengthening
- Advance interval sport programs

PHASE V: RETURN-TO-SPORT PHASE (MONTHS 7–9)

Goals:
1. Gradual return-to-activities
2. Maintain strength, mobility, and stability

Criteria to Enter Phase V:
1. Full functional range of motion
2. Satisfactory isokinetic test that fulfills criteria
3. Satisfactory shoulder stability
4. No pain or tenderness

Exercises:
- Gradually advance sport activities to unrestricted participation
- Continue stretching and strengthening program

At weeks 3 to 4, use of the sling is generally discontinued; this is based on clinical assessment of the stability of the joint and the patient's response to surgery and pain level. Occasionally, the patient is encouraged to continue use of the shoulder immobilizer while sleeping to restrict excessive uncontrolled shoulder motions and positioning. At this time, AAROM and PROM exercises are continued gradually to improve abduction and external rotation, as well as flexion and IR. At 4 weeks we increase but restrict active assisted and passive abduction and flexion motion to 90° of shoulder abduction, which are limited to 15° to 20° and 60°, respectively. In addition, the patient will perform light strengthening exercises such as rhythmic stabilization exercises for the ER/IR muscles and submaximal isometrics for all the shoulder musculature, both to restore dynamic joint stability.

At weeks 5 to 6, the goal is to gradually restore motion. The ER/IR stretching and motion exercises are performed at 45° of abduction, which produces a mild stretch on the inferior capsule (during ER motion). The patient is encouraged to gradually improve shoulder flexion by progressing to 135° to 140° at 6 weeks. Also at this time we allow the patient to begin light-resistance isotonic strengthening exercises. The ER/IR muscles are exercised by using exercise tubing. Additionally, a light weight (1 to 2 lb) can be used to perform abduction to 90°, flexion to 90°, and scapular musculature strengthening.

During the first 6 weeks we restrict motion to prevent overloading or overstressing the repaired capsule. Furthermore, we attempt to allow gradual restoration of motion, which helps prevent the negative effects of immobilization and assists in collagen formation and organization. During these first 6 weeks care must be taken by the clinician to not overstress the healing tissue and the soft tissue fixation.

Phase II, the moderate-protection phase, begins at week 6 and progresses to week 14. The goals of this phase are to (1) gradually restore full, nonpainful ROM, (2) preserve the integrity of the surgical repair, (3) restore muscular strength and endurance, and (4) allow some functional activities.

During this phase, all motions gradually progress. Shoulder flexion and abduction progress to 180°. Shoulder IR and ER motion exercises are performed at 90° of abduction, and at 7 to 8 weeks the patient should have 75° to 80° of ER and full IR (70° to 75°). At weeks 9 to 10 we expect full ROM; ER should be approximately 85° to 90°. At week 12 we begin to aggressively stretch the thrower's shoulder past 90° of ER with the goal of 115° to 125° of ER. During this phase, all strengthening exercises gradually progress with the goal of improving rotator cuff and scapular strength, restoring muscular balance, and enhancing dynamic stabilization of the glenohumeral joint complex. The patient is not allowed to perform isotonic exercises on weight-lifting equipment such as the bench press, pullovers, and so on.

Phase III, the minimal-protection phase, extends from weeks 14 through 20. The goals of this phase are to (1) establish or maintain full ROM, (2) improve strength and endurance, and (3) initiate functional activities gradually. At approximately 14 to 16 weeks, activities such as light swimming exercises at 90° of abduction, plyometrics, and golf swings are permitted. An interval throwing program or other interval sport programs may be initiated at week 18 if the criteria (see Appendix B [online]) have been met by the patient.

The advanced strengthening phase extends from weeks 22 through 26. This phase is characterized by aggressive strengthening exercises such as plyometrics, PNF drills, isotonic strengthening, and functional sports activities. In an overhead-throwing athlete, throwing from a pitching mound may be initiated. Contact sports may also be permitted during this period. Competitive throwing is not usually permitted until 7 to 9 months after surgery.

In summary, progression of the rehabilitation program after arthroscopic stabilization is much slower than that after open stabilization (Box 12-10), especially during the early phase, in

Box 12-10

Rehabilitation Protocol After Open Anterior Bankart Repair

PHASE I: IMMEDIATE POSTOPERATIVE PHASE

Goals:
1. Protect the surgical site
2. Minimize the effects of immobilization
3. Diminish pain and inflammation
4. Establish baseline proprioception and dynamic stabilization

Weeks 1–2
- Use a sling for comfort (1 week)
- May wear an immobilizer during sleep (2 weeks) (physician decision)
- Elbow/hand range of motion
- Gripping exercises
- Passive range of motion and active assistive range of motion (L-bar)
  - Flexion to tolerance: 0°–90° week 1, 0°–100° week 2
  - External/internal rotation at 45° of abduction in the scapular plane
- Submaximal isometrics
- No internal rotation strengthening for 2–3 weeks
- Rhythmic stabilization
- External/internal rotation proprioception drills
- Cryotherapy modalities as needed

Weeks 3–4
- Gradually advance range of motion
  - Flexion to 120°–140°
  - External rotation at 45° of abduction in the scapular plane to 35°–45°
  - Internal rotation at 45° of abduction in the scapular plane to 45°–60°
- Initiate light isotonics for shoulder musculature
  - Tubing for external/internal rotation
  - Abduction, full can, side-lying external rotation, prone rowing, biceps
  - Dynamic stabilization exercises, proprioceptive neuromuscular facilitation
- Initiate self–capsular stretching
- Core stabilization program

Weeks 5–6
- Advance range of motion as tolerated
  - Flexion to 160° (tolerance)
  - External/internal rotation at 90° of abduction:
    - Internal rotation to 75°
    - External rotation to 70°–75°
- Joint mobilization as necessary
- Continue self–capsular stretching
- Advance all strengthening exercises
- Continue proprioceptive neuromuscular facilitation diagonal patterns
- Throwers' Ten Exercise Program
- Continue isotonic strengthening
- Dynamic stabilization exercises
- Initiate internal rotation strengthening

- Closed kinetic chain exercises
- Push-up on ball
- Wall stabilization
- Advance range of motion:
  - External rotation at 90° of abduction: 80°–85°
  - Internal rotation at 90° of abduction: 70°–75°
  - Flexion: 165°–175°

PHASE II: INTERMEDIATE PHASE

Goals:
1. Reestablish full range of motion
2. Normalize arthrokinematics
3. Improve muscular strength
4. Enhance neuromuscular control

Weeks 8–10
- Progress to full range of motion (weeks 7–8)—flexion to 180°, external rotation at 90°–100°, internal rotation to 75°
- Continue all stretching exercises
  - Joint mobilization, capsular stretching, passive and active stretching
  - In overhead-throwing athletes, maintain 90°–100° external rotation
  - Continue strengthening exercises
- Throwers' Ten Exercise Program (for overhead-throwing athletes)
- Isotonic strengthening for the entire shoulder complex
- Proprioceptive neuromuscular facilitation against manual resistance
- Neuromuscular control drills
- Isokinetic strengthening

Weeks 10–14
- Continue all flexibility exercises
- Continue all strengthening exercises
- Two-hand plyometrics (week 10)
- Chest pass
- Overhead
- Side to side
- One-hand plyometrics (week 12)
- 90/90 position
- Dribble
- May initiate light isotonic machine weight training (weeks 12–14)

PHASE III: ADVANCED STRENGTHENING PHASE (MONTHS 4–6)

Goals:
1. Enhance muscular strength, power, and endurance
2. Improve muscular endurance
3. Maintain mobility

Criteria to Enter Phase III:
1. Full range of motion
2. No pain or tenderness
3. Satisfactory stability
4. Strength 70%–80% of contralateral side

(Continued)

Weeks 16–20

- Continue all flexibility exercises
- Perform self–capsular stretches (anterior, posterior, and inferior)
- Maintain external rotation flexibility
- Continue isotonic strengthening program
- Emphasize muscular balance (external/internal rotation)
- Continue proprioceptive neuromuscular facilitation against manual resistance
- May continue plyometrics
- Initiate interval sport program (physician approval necessary) (week 16)

Weeks 20–24

- Continue all exercise listed above
- Continue and advance all interval sport program (throwing off mound)

IV. PHASE IV: RETURN-TO-SPORT PHASE (AFTER MONTH 6)

Goals:
1. Gradual return-to-sport activities
2. Maintain strength and mobility of shoulder

Criteria to Enter Phase IV:
1. Full nonpainful range of motion
2. Satisfactory stability
3. Satisfactory strength (isokinetics)
4. No pain or tenderness

Exercises:

- Continue capsular stretching to maintain mobility
- Continue strengthening program
- Either Throwers' Ten Exercise Program or a fundamental shoulder exercise program
- Return to sport participation (unrestricted)
- For contact sports, consider shoulder brace

---

which soft tissue healing to bone occurs. A period of immobilization is often advocated and has been shown to be a critical factor in preventing recurrent instability.[244] We have noted significantly less postoperative scarring after arthroscopic stabilization than after open stabilization procedures. Additionally, slower rehabilitation and progression are encouraged because of the somewhat weaker fixation methods currently used in arthroscopic stabilization procedures and the significantly weaker than normal appearance of the capsulolabral complex tissue. A period of strict immobilization for at least 3 to 4 weeks appears to be sufficient to allow adequate tissue healing after arthroscopic stabilization.[163,245,248,249] We advocate relative immobilization with early restricted and protected motion to expedite functional return of the arm. We expect full motion at approximately 10 weeks after arthroscopic stabilization. The ultimate goals are similar to those of the open stabilization technique, with a return of the full ER necessary to simulate the throwing motion at weeks 12 to 14. Return to strenuous and contact sports is usually permitted 7 to 9 months after surgery, with return to competitive throwing occurring slightly later (9 to 12 months).

Rehabilitation After an Anterior Capsular Shift Procedure

An open capsular shift procedure may be another type of surgical procedure performed in an overhead-throwing athlete. This procedure requires a delicate balance between the surgical procedure and the postoperative rehabilitation program. In our experience with this type of surgical procedure, postoperative management can be more aggressive. We use what we refer to as an accelerated rehabilitation approach, which is based on immediate restricted motion and a gradual return to the motion necessary for throwing activities (Box 12-11). Immediately after surgery the patient's shoulder is moved passively, and the patient performs active assisted motion. In the first phase, the protected-motion phase lasting from weeks 1 through 6, the primary goals

are to (1) restore motion gradually, (2) protect the repaired capsule, and (3) reestablish dynamic stability. During weeks 1 through 3, AAROM for ER/IR is performed with the arm in 30° of abduction to patient tolerance. Shoulder flexion is also performed to tolerance, usually 100° to 125° by week 2. During the first 2 weeks, isometrics and rhythmic stabilization exercises are also performed.

During weeks 2 to 4, ROM and stretching gradually progress. Active assisted ER and IR ROM exercises are performed at 45° of abduction, with the goal of 45° of motion (ER and IR) by week 4. During this time, tubing exercises may be initiated for the shoulder internal and external rotators; rhythmic stabilization drills and cocontraction are also performed.

At weeks 4 to 5, ER/IR stretching is performed at 90° of abduction. This progression is based on clinical assessment (degrees of motion and end-feel). At approximately 4.5 to 5 weeks, ER motion progresses more aggressively. By the end of week 6, our goal is 75° of ER in an overhead-throwing athlete. The rate of progression (aggressiveness) of the stretching is determined by clinical assessment and is based on evaluation of motion, stability, and end-feel. If the patient appears to be progressing slowly toward these goals, the program must be adjusted at week 6. In our opinion, all of these stretches are safe if performed with a gradual force—the force should not be applied rapidly. Stretches are usually initiated during week 7, and the clinician should consult the physician before their use. During this phase, isotonic strengthening exercises are performed for the entire shoulder complex. During weeks 3 to 4, rhythmic stabilization drills are emphasized with the goal of restoring dynamic stability.

The intermediate phase, weeks 7 through 12, is characterized by establishing full motion at week 8 and improving muscular strength and endurance. At week 8, the patient should exhibit full motion (90° of ER and 45° to 55° of horizontal abduction). From weeks 8 to 12, an overhead-throwing athlete's stretching exercises progress to the amount of ER necessary

Box 12-11

Anterior Open Capsular Shift Rehabilitation Protocol (Accelerated)

The goal of this rehabilitation program is to return the patient/athlete to activity/sport as quickly and safely as possible while maintaining a stable shoulder. The program is based on muscle physiology, biomechanics, anatomy, and the healing process after capsular shift surgery.

In the capsular shift procedure, the orthopedic surgeon makes an incision in the ligamentous capsule of the shoulder, pulls the capsule tighter, and then sutures the capsule together.

The ultimate goal is a functional stable shoulder and return to a preoperative functional level.

PHASE I: PROTECTION PHASE (WEEKS 1–6)
Goals:
- Allow healing of the sutured capsule
- Begin early protected range of motion
- Retard muscular atrophy
- Decrease pain/inflammation

Weeks 1–2
Precautions:
1. Sleep in an immobilizer for 2 weeks
2. No overhead activities for 4 weeks
3. Wean from the immobilizer and into a sling as soon as possible (orthopedist or clinician will tell the athlete when), usually 2 weeks

Exercises:
- Wrist/hand range of motion and gripping
- Elbow flexion/extension and pronation/supination
- Pendulum exercises (nonweighted)
- Rope-and-pulley active assisted exercises
  - Shoulder flexion to 90°
  - Shoulder abduction to 60°
- T-bar exercises
  - External rotation to 15°–20° with the arm in the scapular plane
  - Internal rotation to 25° with arm abduction at 40°
  - Shoulder flexion to 90°
- Active range of motion of the cervical spine
- Isometrics
  - Flexion, extension, external rotation, internal rotation, abduction
  - Rhythmic stabilization drills

Weeks 2–4
Goals:
- Gradual increase in range of motion
- Normalize arthrokinematics
- Improve strength
- Decrease pain/inflammation

Range-of-Motion Exercises:
- L-bar active assisted exercises
- External rotation at 45° of abduction to 45°
- Internal rotation at 45° abduction to 45°
- Shoulder flexion to tolerance
- Shoulder abduction to tolerance

- Rope-and-pulley flexion
- Pendulum exercises

All Exercises Performed to Tolerance:
- Take to point of pain and/or resistance and hold
- Gentle self–capsular stretches

Gentle Joint Mobilization to Reestablish Normal Arthrokinematics in:
- Scapulothoracic joint
- Glenohumeral joint
- Sternoclavicular joint

Strengthening Exercises:
- Active range of motion week 3
- May initiate tubing for external/internal rotation at 0° on week 3
- Dynamic stabilization drills

Conditioning Program for:
- Trunk
- Lower extremities
- Cardiovascular system

Decrease Pain/Inflammation:
- Ice, nonsteroidal antiinflammatory drugs, modalities

Weeks 4–5
- Active assisted range of flexion motion to tolerance (145°)
- External/internal rotation at 90° of abduction to tolerance
- External rotation at 90°, abduction 60°
- Internal rotation at 90°, abduction 45°–50°
- Initiate isotonic (light weight) strengthening
- Gentle joint mobilization (grade III)

Week 6
- Active assisted range of motion; continue all stretching exercises
- Advance external/internal rotation at 90° of abduction
- External rotation at 90°, abduction 75°
- Internal rotation at 90°, abduction 65°
- Advance shoulder flexion to 165°–170°
- Progress to Thrower's Ten Exercise Program

PHASE II: INTERMEDIATE PHASE (WEEKS 7–12)
Goals:
- Full nonpainful range of motion at week 8
- Normalize arthrokinematics
- Increase strength
- Improve neuromuscular control

Weeks 7–10
Range-of-Motion Exercises:
- Shoulder flexion to 180°
- External rotation at 90°, abduction 90°
- Internal rotation at 90°, abduction 65°
- Horizontal adduction/abduction motion
- L-bar active assisted exercises
- Continue all exercises listed above
- Gradually increase range of motion to full range of motion week 8

(Continued)

Box 12-11

Anterior Open Capsular Shift Rehabilitation Protocol (Accelerated)—cont'd

- External rotation at 90°, abduction 85°–90°
- Internal rotation at 90°, abduction 70°–75°
- Continue self–capsular stretches
- Continue joint mobilization

Strengthening Exercises:
- Throwers' Ten Exercise Program
- Continue dynamic stabilization
- Closed kinetic chain exercises
- Core stabilization drills

Initiate Neuromuscular Control Exercises for Scapulothoracic Joint:
- Scapular muscular training

Weeks 10–12
- Continue all exercises listed above
- Continue all stretching exercises
  - Advance range of motion to thrower's motion
  - External rotation to 110°–115°
  - Flexion to 180°
- Continue strengthening exercises
  - Initiate progressive resistance exercise weight training

PHASE III: DYNAMIC (ADVANCED) STRENGTHENING PHASE (WEEKS 12–20)

Weeks 12–16
Goals:
- Improve strength, power, and endurance
- Improve neuromuscular control
- Maintain shoulder mobility
- Prepare the athlete to begin to throw

Criteria to Enter Phase III:
1. Full nonpainful range of motion
2. No pain or tenderness
3. Strength 70% or better than that on the contralateral side

Exercises:
- Continue all stretching and range-of-motion exercises
- Continue all strengthening
  - Throwers' Ten Exercise Program
- Initiate plyometrics:
  - Two-hand drills (week 12)
  - One-hand drills (weeks 13–14)
- Continue core stabilization drills

Weeks 16–20
- Continue all exercises above
- Continue stretching and range-of-motion exercises
- Initiate interval sport program (week 16)

PHASE IV: FUNCTIONAL ACTIVITY PHASE (WEEKS 21–26)
Goal:
- Progressively increase activities to prepare patient for full functional return

Criteria to Progress to Phase IV:
1. Full range of motion
2. No pain or tenderness
3. Isokinetic test that fulfills criteria to throw
4. Satisfactory clinical examination

Exercises:
- Continue interval sport program
- Continue Throwers' Ten Exercise Program
- Continue plyometric five exercises

Interval Throwing Program:
1. Long-toss program (phase I) (week 16)
2. Off-the-mound program (phase I) (week 22)

---

to throw, usually a minimum of 115° to 120° of ER. This is generally accomplished with physiologic stretching, capsular stretching, low-load long-duration stretches, and controlled plyometric activities. During this phase all strengthening exercises, muscular balance, scapular strengthening, and endurance are emphasized.

The advanced strengthening phase begins at week 12 and progresses through week 20. The primary goals are to enhance muscular strength, power, and endurance while maintaining capsular mobility and glenohumeral joint stability. The patient is instructed to continue stretching to prevent capsular or muscular tightening, or both, caused by the aggressive strengthening exercises. The strengthening exercises consist of PNF, the Throwers' Ten Exercise Program (see Appendix A [online]), plyometrics, and neuromuscular control drills.[137,140,240] At this time the patient is carefully evaluated and it is determined when a throwing program can be initiated. A gradual throwing or sport program can usually be initiated between 14 and 16 weeks, depending on patient variables and progression in rehabilitation.

The return-to-sport phase is initiated at 21 weeks after surgery and represents a gradual return to activities. During this time it is imperative that the athlete continue all strengthening and stretching exercises outlined in the previous phase. Return to unrestricted sports usually occurs between 6 and 9 months, depending on the patient's sport, position, skill level, and rate of progression.

Altchek et al[248] reported on 40 patients (42 shoulders) in whom surgical stabilization consisting of a T-plasty modification was performed for multidirectional instability. Thirty-eight of 40 patients returned to sports at an average of 6.5 months (range, 5 to 10 months). Only three patients in the series were throwers; all three reported that they were unable to throw as fast as before the operation. Bigliani et al[250] reported the results of an anteroinferior capsular shift performed on 63 athletic patients (68 shoulders). Of the 63 patients, 31 were overhead activity athletes, with 16 baseball players. The results indicated that 50% returned to the same competition level. Kvitne et al[251] reported on 105 patients who had undergone anterior capsulolabral reconstruction. In this series 52 were baseball players, 35 of whom were pitchers, and 60% of the professional baseball pitchers were able to return to the same competition level.

The rehabilitation process after capsular tensioning in an overhead activity athlete is challenging to the clinician. Success rates vary greatly, depending on the sport and position. The reasons for failure are multifactorial. One commonly seen reason is loss of ER. The rehabilitation program must be aggressive in restoring ER motion in a throwing athlete. Fleisig[252] determined the total arc of motion (late cocking [ER] to follow-through) to be one of the critical factors in a pitcher's effectiveness. Thus, one of the primary and critical postoperative goals is restoration of glenohumeral motion, particularly ER.

Rehabilitation After Glenoid Labrum Procedures

Labral lesions occur often in overhead-throwing athletes because of the extremes in motion and tremendous muscular forces. The specific rehabilitation program after surgical intervention involving the glenoid labrum depends on the severity of the pathologic condition. For type I and type III SLAP lesions, simple arthroscopic débridement of the frayed labrum is performed, and the rehabilitation program is similar. Because the biceps labral anchor is intact and no anatomic repair is necessary, the rehabilitation program is somewhat aggressive in restoring motion and function. Full ROM is expected by 10 to 14 days postoperatively. IR and ER tubing exercises are initiated at day 10, with gradual isotonic strengthening occurring between weeks 2 and 8. The athlete is allowed to begin an interval throwing program, usually at weeks 8 to 12. This start date for throwing is often variable based on the time of season. An athlete who is undergoing rehabilitation during the sport season will begin throwing at an earlier date than an athlete who is undergoing rehabilitating during the off-season. Ultimate success depends on dynamic stabilization of the athlete's glenohumeral joint.

Overhead-throwing athletes are commonly seen with a type II SLAP lesion with the biceps tendon detached from the glenoid rim. Usually, a peel-back lesion is present. Postoperative rehabilitation is delayed to allow healing of the anatomic repair to reattach the tendon. No isolated biceps strengthening is permitted for 6 to 8 weeks postoperatively to permit adequate healing. The athlete sleeps in a sling and swathe immobilizer and wears a sling in the daytime for the first 4 weeks. Protected ROM activity at less than 90° of elevation is allowed for the first 4 weeks. During the first 2 weeks, IR and ER are performed passively in the scapular plane to approximately 10° to 15° of ER and 45° of IR. No excessive ER, extension, or abduction is permitted until weeks 5 to 6, when a light isotonic strengthening program is initiated. IR and ER ROM is progressed to 90° of abduction at weeks 5 to 6. Motion is gradually increased to restore full range by 8 to 10 weeks and progressed to a thrower's motion through weeks 10 to 12. Restriction of motion is usually accomplished with little to minimal difficulty. Plyometric exercises are initiated at week 12 and an interval throwing program at week 16. Return to sport after surgical repair of a type II SLAP lesion occurs at approximately 9 to 11 months.

CONCLUSION

Shoulder Injuries

- Mobility of the shoulder joint is acquired at the expense of stability.
- Shoulder injuries can be induced acutely through traumatic injuries, or they may arise with an insidious onset as a result of repetitive stress over time.
- Overuse injuries of the shoulder are common in athletes whose endeavors require repetitive overhead activities, particularly throwers and swimmers.
- Most shoulder injuries occur during the late cocking, acceleration, and deceleration phases of throwing.
- The most common shoulder injuries include rotator cuff tendinitis or partial tears, compressive cuff disease, internal impingement syndrome, and shoulder instability (usually anterior).

Goals of Shoulder Rehabilitation

- The goals of shoulder rehabilitation are to prevent injuries through off-season and in-season conditioning programs that address flexibility, rotator cuff strength, scapular stability, and neuromuscular control of the shoulder girdle.
- The rehabilitation program should be progressive and systematic and use the principles of periodization.

General Shoulder Rehabilitation Principles

- Rehabilitation of shoulder injuries should concentrate on developing dynamic joint stability.
- Athletes who are susceptible to pathologic shoulder conditions should participate in an off-season shoulder flexibility and rotator cuff strengthening program to help prevent shoulder problems, and they should continue this stretching and strengthening program two or three times weekly during the season.
- Preventive and postinjury exercises that strengthen the rotator cuff muscles should be performed to dynamically stabilize the glenohumeral joint and the scapular stabilizers that help orient the glenoid fossa with the humeral head to maintain stability.
- Weakness of the scapula stabilizers can predispose the athlete to a variety of pathologic shoulder conditions.
- After shoulder surgery or injury, emphasis should be placed on addressing the inflammation process and restoring motion.
- After initiation of a rotator cuff strengthening program, PNF techniques may be implemented to help restore neuromuscular control.
- In the late phases of rehabilitation, eccentric, isokinetic, and plyometric exercises may be initiated.
- In the advanced strengthening phase, the goals of the program are to initiate sport-specific types of training for the shoulder joint complex.

REFERENCES

1. Tullos, H.S., and King, J.W. (1973): Throwing mechanism in sports. Orthop. Clin. North Am., 4:709–721.
2. Conte, S., Requa, R.K., and Garrick, J.G. (2001): Disability days in major league baseball. Am. J. Sports Med., 29:431–436.
3. McFarland, E.G., and Wasik, M. (1998): Epidemiology of collegiate baseball injuries. Clin. J. Sport Med., 8:10–13.
4. Norkin, C., and Levangie, P. (1983): Joint Structure and Function: A Comprehensive Analysis. Philadelphia, Davis.
5. Caillet, R. (1966): Shoulder Pain. Philadelphia, Davis.
6. McLeod, W.D. (1985): The pitching mechanism. In Zarins, B., Andrews J.R., and Carson, W.G. (eds.): Injuries to the Throwing Arm. Philadelphia, Saunders, pp. 22–29.
7. Williams, P.L., and Warwick, R. (1986): Gray's Anatomy, 36th ed. (British). Philadelphia, Saunders.
8. Cave, E.F., Burke, J.F., and Boyd, R.J. (1974): Trauma Management. Chicago, Year Book Medical, p. 437.
9. Kazar, B., and Relouszky, E. (1969): Prognosis of primary dislocation of the shoulder. Acta Orthop. Scand., 40:216–219.
10. Hovelius, L., Augustini, B.G., Fredin, H., et al. (1996): Primary anterior dislocation of the shoulder in young patients. A ten-year prospective study. J. Bone Joint Surg. Am., 78:1677–1684.
11. Hovelius, L., Nilsson, J.A., and Nordqvist, A. (2007): Increased mortality after anterior shoulder dislocation: 255 patients aged 12-40 years followed for 25 years. Acta Orthop., 78:822–826.
12. Altchek, D.W., Schwartz, E., and Warren, R.F. (1990): Radiologic measurement of superior migration of the humeral head in impingement syndrome. Presented at the annual meeting of the American Shoulder and Elbow Surgeons, New Orleans, LA, February 8–12.
13. Harryman, D.T., II, Sidles, J.A., Harris, S.L., and Matsen, F.A. (1992): Laxity of the normal glenohumeral joint: A qualitative in vivo assessment. J. Shoulder Elbow Surg., 1:66–76.
14. Harryman, D.T., II, Sidles, J.A., Harris, S.L., and Matsen, F.A. (1992): Role of the rotator interval capsule in passive motion and stability of the shoulder. J. Bone Joint Surg. Am., 74:53–66.
15. Howell, S.M., Galinet, B.J., Renzi, A.J., and Marone, P.J. (1988): Normal and abnormal mechanics of the glenohumeral joint in the horizontal plane. J. Bone Joint Surg. Am., 70:227–232.
16. Poppen, N.K., and Walker, P.S. (1976): Normal and abnormal motion of the shoulder. J. Bone Joint Surg. Am., 58:195–201.
17. Poppen, N.K., and Walker, P.S. (1978): Forces at the glenohumeral joint in adduction. Clin. Orthop. Relat. Res., 135:165–170.
18. Warner, J.J.P., Deng, X.P., Warren, R.F., and Torzilli, P.A. (1992): Static capsular ligamentous constraints to superior-inferior translation of the glenohumeral joint. Am. J. Sports Med., 20:675–685.
19. Matsen, F.A., III (1980): Compartmental Syndromes. San Francisco, Grune & Stratton.
20. Pagnani, M.J., and Warren, R.F. (1994): Stabilizers of the glenohumeral joint. J. Shoulder Elbow Surg., 3:173–190.
21. Soslowsky, L.J., Flatow, E.L., Bigliani, L.U., et al. (1992): Quantitation of in situ contact areas and the glenohumeral joint: A biomechanical study. J. Orthop. Res., 10:524–535.
22. Bost, F.C., and Inman, V.T. (1942): The pathological changes in recurrent dislocation of the shoulder; a report of Bankart's operative procedure. J. Bone Joint Surg. Am., 24:595–613.
23. Codman, E.A. (1934): The Shoulder. Boston, Thomas Todd.
24. Steindler, A. (1955): Kinesiology of Human Body Under Normal and Pathological Conditions. Springfield, IL, Charles C Thomas.
25. Clemente, C.A. (ed.) (1985): Gray's Anatomy of the Human Body, 30th ed. Philadelphia, Lea & Febiger.
26. Basmajian, J.V., and Bazant, F.J. (1959): Factors preventing downward dislocation of the adducted shoulder joint. J. Bone Joint Surg. Am., 41:1182–1186.
27. Saha, A.K. (1971): Dynamic stability of the glenohumeral joint. Acta Orthop. Scand., 42:491–505.
28. Brewer, B.J., Wubben, R.G., and Carrera, G.F. (1986): Excessive retroversion of the glenoid cavity. J. Bone Joint Surg. Am., 68:724–726.
29. Harryman, D.T., II, Sidles, J.A., Clark, J.M., et al. (1990): Translation of the humeral head on the glenoid with passive glenohumeral motion. J. Bone Joint Surg. Am., 72:1334–1338.
30. Howell, S.M., and Galinet, S.J. (1989): The glenoid labral socket: A constrained articular surface. Clin. Orthop. Relat. Res., 243:122–129.
31. Bowen, M.K., Deng, X.H., Hannafin, J.A., et al. (1992): 1992): An analysis of the patterns of glenohumeral joint contact and their relationship of the glenoid "bare area" (Abstract). Trans. Orthop. Res. Soc., 17:496, 1992.
32. Sarrafian, S. (1983): Gross and functional anatomy of the shoulder. Clin., Orthop. Relat. Res., 173:11–19.
33. Hill, H.A., and Sachs, M.D. (1940): The grooved defect of the humeral head. A frequently unrecognized complication of dislocations of the shoulder joint. Radiology, 35:690–700.
34. Pavlov, H., Warren, R.F., Weiss, C.B., and Dines, D.M. (1985): The roentgenographic evaluation of anterior shoulder instability. Clin. Orthop. Relat. Res., 194:153–158.

35. Rowe, C.R. (1956): Prognosis in dislocation of the shoulder. J. Bone Joint Surg. Am., 38:957–977.
36. Rowe, C.R., Patel, D., and Southmayd, W.W. (1978): The Bankart procedure: A long term end-result study. J. Bone Joint Surg. Am., 60:1–16.
37. O'Brien, S.J. (1994): Glenoid labral lesions. Presented at Advances of the Knee and Shoulder, Hilton Head, SC.
38. Lippett, F.G. (1982): A modification of the gravity method of reducing anterior shoulder dislocations. Clin. Orthop. Relat. Res., 165:259–260.
39. Podromos, C.C., Perry, J.A., and Schiller, J.A. (1990): Histological studies of the glenoid labrum from fetal life to old age. J. Bone Joint Surg. Am., 72:1344–1352.
40. Andrews, J.R., Carson, W.G., and McLeod, W.D. (1985): Glenoid labrum tears related to the long head of the biceps. Am. J. Sports Med., 13:337–341.
41. Cooper, D.E., Arnoczky, S.P., O'Brien, S.J., et al. (1992): Anatomy, histology, and vascularity of the glenoid labrum. J. Bone Joint Surg. Am., 74:46–52.
42. Colachis, S.C., Strohm, B.R., and Brechner, V.L. (1969): Effects of axillary nerve block on muscle force in the upper extremity. Arch. Phys. Med. Rehabil., 50:647–654.
43. Tyler, T.F., Nicholas, S.J., Roy, T., and Gleim, G.W. (2000): Quantification of posterior capsule tightness and motion loss in patients with shoulder impingement. Am. J Sports Med., 28:668–673.
44. Basmajian, J.V. (1963): The surgical anatomy and function of the arm-trunk mechanism. Surg. Clin. North Am., 43:1475–1479.
45. Gohlke, F., Essigkrug, B., and Schmitz, F. (1994): The pattern of the collagen fiber bundles of the capsule of the glenohumeral joint. J. Shoulder Elbow Surg., 3:111–128.
46. DePalma, A.F., Callery, G., and Bennett, G.A. (1949): Variational anatomy and degenerative lesions of the shoulder joint. Instr. Course Lect., 6:255–281.
47. Moseley, H.F., and Overgaard, B. (1962): The anterior capsular mechanism in recurrent dislocation of the shoulder: Morphological and clinical studies with special reference to the glenoid labrum and glenohumeral ligaments. J. Bone Joint Surg. Br., 44:13–27.
48. O'Brien, S.J., Neves, M.C., and Arnoczky, S.J. (1990): The anatomy and histology of the inferior glenohumeral ligament complex of the shoulder. Am. J. Sports Med., 18:449–456.
49. Turkel, S., Panio, M., Marshall, J., and Girgis, F. (1981): Stabilization mechanism preventing anterior dislocation of the glenohumeral joint. J. Bone Joint Surg. Am., 63:1208–1217.
50. Ferrari, D.A. (1990): Capsular ligaments of the shoulder: Anatomical and functional study of the anterior superior capsule. Am. J. Sports Med., 18:20–24.
51. O'Brien, S.J., Schwartz, R.E., Warren, R.F., and Torzilli, P.A. (1988): Capsular restraints to anterior/posterior motion of the shoulder (Abstract). Orthop. Trans., 12:143.
52. Schwartz, R.E., O'Brien, S.J., and Warren, R.F. (1988): Capsular restraints to anterior-posterior motion of the abducted shoulder: A biomechanical study (Abstract). Orthop. Trans., 12:727.
53. Bowen, M.K., and Warren, R.F. (1991): Ligamentous control of shoulder stability based on selective cutting and static translation experiments. Clin. Sports Med., 10:757–782.
54. Braly, G., and Tullos, H.S. (1985): A modification of the Bristow procedure for recurrent anterior shoulder dislocation and subluxation. Am. J. Sports Med., 13:81–86.
55. Oveson, J., and Nielson, S. (1986): Anterior and posterior instability of the shoulder: A cadaver study. Acta Orthop. Scand., 57:324–327.
56. O'Brien, S.J., Neves, M.C., Arnoczky, S.P., et al. (1990): The anatomy and histology of the inferior glenohumeral ligament complex of the shoulder. Am. J. Sports Med., 18:449–456.
57. Schaefer, S.L., Ciarelli, M.J., Arnoczky, S.T., and Ross, H.E. (1997): Tissue shrinkage with the holmium:yttrium:aluminum:garnet laser: A postoperative assessment of tissue length, stiffness, and viscosity. Am. J. Sports Med., 25:841–848.
58. Bankart, A.S.B. (1923): The pathology and treatment of recurrent dislocation of the shoulder joint. Br. Med. J., 2:1132–1133.
59. Bankart, A.S.B. (1948): Discussion on recurrent dislocation of the shoulder. J. Bone Joint Surg. Br., 30:46–47.
60. Kaltsas, D.S. (1983): Comparative study of the properties of the shoulder joint capsule with those of other joint capsules. Clin. Orthop. Relat. Res., 173:20–26.
61. Baker, C.L., Uribe, J.W., and Whitman, C. (1990): Arthroscopic evaluation of acute initial anterior shoulder dislocations. Am. J. Sports Med., 18:25–28.
62. Matsen, F.A., Thomas, S.C., and Rockwood, C.A. (1985): Anterior glenohumeral instability. In Rockwood, C. A., and Matsen, F. A. (eds.): The Shoulder. Philadelphia, Saunders.
63. Browne, A.O., Hoffmeyer, P., An, K.N., and Morrey, B.F. (1990): The influence of atmospheric pressure on shoulder stability. Orthop. Trans., 14:259–263.
64. Gibb, T.D., Sidles, J.A., Harryman, D.T., et al. (1991): The effect of capsular venting on glenohumeral laxity. Clin. Orthop. Relat. Res., 268:120–127.
65. Kumar, V.P., and Balasubramianium, P. (1985): The role of atmospheric pressure in stabilizing the shoulder. An experimental study. J. Bone Joint Surg. Br., 67:719–721.
66. Habermeyer, P., Schuller, U., and Wiedemann, E. (1992): The intra-articular pressure of the shoulder: An experimental study on the role of the glenoid labrum in stabilizing the joint. Arthroscopy, 8:166–172.
67. Perry, J. (1988): Muscle control of the shoulder. In Rowe C.R. (ed.): The Shoulder. New York, Churchill Livingstone, pp. 17–34.
68. Wuelker, N., Wirth, C.J., Plitz, W., and Roetman, B. (1995): A dynamic shoulder model: Reliability testing and muscle force study. J. Biomech., 28:489–499.
69. Wilk, K.E., and Arrigo, C.A. (1992): An integrated approach to upper extremity exercises. Orthop. Phys. Ther. Clin. North Am., 9:337–360.

70. Wilk, K.E., and Arrigo, C.A. (1993): Current concepts in the rehabilitation of the athletic shoulder. J. Orthop. Sports Phys. Ther., 18:365–378.

71. Blackburn, T.A., McLeod, W.D., White, B.W., and Wofford, L. (1990): EMG analysis of posterior rotator cuff exercises. Athl. Train., 25:40–45.

72. Steindler, A. (1955): Kinesiology of the Human Body. Springfield IL, Charles C Thomas.

73. Kessel, L., and Watson, M. (1977): The painful arc syndrome. J. Bone Joint Surg. Br., 59:166–172.

74. Neer, C.S. (1983): Impingement lesions. Clin. Orthop. Relat. Res., 173:70–77.

75. Hollingshead, W.H. (1982): Anatomy for Surgeons, Vol. III. The Back and Limbs. New York, Hoeber & Harper.

76. DeDuca, C.J., and Forrest, W.J. (1973): Force analysis of individual muscles acting simultaneously on the shoulder joint during isometric abduction. J. Biomech., 6:385–393.

77. Rowe, C.R. (ed.). (1988): The Shoulder. New York, Churchill Livingstone.

78. Hughston, J.C. (1985): Functional anatomy of the shoulder. In Zarins B., Andrews J.R., and Carson W.G. (eds.): Injuries to the Throwing Arm. Philadelphia, Saunders.

79. Jobe, F.W., and Jobe, C.M. (1983): Painful athletic injuries of the shoulder. Clin. Orthop. Relat. Res., 173:117–124.

80. Jobe, F.W., Moynes, D.R., and Tibone, J.E. (1984): An EMG analysis of the shoulder in pitching: A second report. Am. J. Sports Med., 12:218–220.

81. Codman, E.A. (1934): Rupture of the supraspinatus tendon and other lesions in or about the subacromial bursa. In Codman E.A. (ed.): The Shoulder. Boston, Thomas Todd.

82. Kent, B. (1971): Functional anatomy of the shoulder complex: A review. Phys. Ther., 51:867–887.

83. Lucas, D.B. (1973): Biomechanics of the shoulder joint. Arch Surg. 107:425–432.

84. Saha, A. (1961): Theory of Shoulder Mechanism: Descriptive and Applied. Springfield IL, Charles C Thomas.

85. Inman, V., Saunders, M., and Abbott, L. (1944): Observations of the function of the shoulder joint. J. Bone Joint Surg. Am., 26:1–30.

86. Inman, V., and Saunders, J.B. (1946): Observations of the function of the clavicle. Calif. Med., 65:158–166.

87. Colachis, S.C., and Strohm, B.R. (1971): The effect of suprascapular and axillary nerve blocks and muscle force in the upper extremity. Arch. Phys. Med. Rehabil., 52:22–29.

88. Bechtol, C. (1980): Biomechanics of the shoulder. Clin. Orthop. Relat. Res., 146:37–41.

89. Fleisig, G.S., Dillman, C.J., and Andrews, J.R. (1997): Biomechanics of the shoulder during throwing. In Andrews J.R., and Wilk K.E. (eds.): The Athlete's Shoulder. New York, Churchill Livingstone, pp. 355–368.

90. Walsh, D.A. (1989): Shoulder evaluation of the throwing athlete. Sports Med. Update, 4:524–527.

91. Bratatz, J.H., and Gogia, P.P. (1987): The mechanics of pitching. J. Orthop. Sports Phys. Ther., 9:56–69.

92. Perry, J., and Glousman, R.E. (1990): Biomechanics of throwing. In Nicholas J.A., and Hershman E.B. (eds.): The Upper Extremity in Sports Medicine. St. Louis, Mosby, pp. 727–751.

93. McLeod, W.D., and Andrews, J.R. (1986): Mechanisms of shoulder injuries. Phys. Ther., 66:1901–1904.

94. Pappas, A.M., Zawacki, R.M., and Sullivan, T.J. (1985): Biomechanics of baseball pitching: A preliminary report. Am. J. Sports Med., 13:216–222.

95. DiGiovine, N.M., Jobe, F.W., Pink, M., et al. (1992): An electromyographic analysis of the upper extremity in pitcher. J. Shoulder Elbow Surg., 1:15–25.

96. Jobe, F.W., Tibone, J.E., Perry, J., et al. (1983): An EMG analysis of the shoulder in throwing and pitching: A preliminary report. Am. J. Sports Med., 11:3–5.

97. Blackburn, T.A. (1987): Throwing injuries to the shoulder. In Donatelli R. (ed.): Physical Therapy of the Shoulder. New York, Churchill Livingstone.

98. Fukuda, H., Mikasa, M., Ogawa, K., et al. (1983): The partial-thickness tear of the rotator cuff. Orthop. Trans., 55:137.

99. Glousman, R., Jobe, F., Tibone, J., et al. (1988): Dynamic electromyographic analysis of the throwing shoulder with glenohumeral instability. J. Bone Joint Surg. Am., 70:220–226.

100. Wick, H.J., Dillman, C.J., Wisleder, D., et al. (1991): A kinematic comparison between baseball pitching and football passing. Sports Med. Update, 6:13–16.

101. Reinold, M.M., Wilk, K.E., Fleisig, G.S., et al. (2004): Electromyographic analysis of the rotator cuff and deltoid musculature during common shoulder external rotation exercises. J. Orthop. Sports Phys. Ther., 34:385–394.

102. Jobe, F.W., and Moynes, D.R. (1982): Delineation of diagnostic criteria and a rehabilitation program for rotator cuff injuries. Am. J. Sports Med., 10:336–339.

103. Malanga, G.A., Jenp, Y.N., Growney, E.C., and An, K.N. (1996): EMG analysis of shoulder positioning in testing and strengthening the supraspinatus. Med. Sci. Sports Exerc., 28:661–664.

104. Kelly, B.T., Kadrmas, W.R., and Speer, K.P. (1996): The manual muscle examination for rotator cuff strength. An electromyographic investigation. Am. J. Sports Med., 24:581–588.

105. Townsend, H., Jobe, F.W., Pink, M., et al. (1992): EMG analysis of the glenohumeral muscles during a baseball rehabilitation program. Am. J. Sports Med., 19:264–269.

106. Harryman, D.T., II, Sidles, J.A., Clark, J.A., et al. (1990): Translation of the humeral head on the glenoid with passive glenohumeral motion. J. Bone Joint Surg. Am., 72:1334–1343.

107. Berger, R.A. (1982): Applied Exercise Physiology. Philadelphia, Lea & Febiger, p. 267.

108. Wilk, K.E., Voight, M., Keirns, M.A., et al. (2001): Preventive and Rehabilitative Exercises for the Shoulder and Elbow, 6th ed. Birmingham, AL, American Sports Medicine Institute.

109. Wilk, K.E. (1996): Conditioning and training techniques. In Hawkins R.J., and Misamore G.W. (eds.): Shoulder Injuries in the Athlete. New York, Churchill Livingstone, pp. 339–364.

110. Wilk, K.E., Voight, M., Keirns, M.A., et al. (1993): Stretch shortening drills for the upper extremity: Theory and clinical application. J. Orthop. Sports Phys. Ther., 17:225–239.

111. Chu, D. (1989): Plyometric Exercises with a Medicine Ball. Livermore, CA, Bittersweet Publishing.

112. Gambetta, V., and Odgers, S. (1991): The Complete Guide to Medicine Ball Training. Sarasota, FL, Optimum Sports Training.

113. Bigliani, L.U., Codd, T.P., Connor, P.M., et al. (1997): Shoulder motion and laxity in the professional baseball player. Am. J. Sports Med., 25:609–612.

114. Brown, L.P., Niehues, S.L., Harrah, A., et al. (1988): Upper extremity range of motion and isokinetic strength of the internal and external shoulder rotators in major league baseball players. Am. J. Sports Med., 16:577–585.

115. Johnson, L. (1992): Patterns of shoulder flexibility among college baseball players. J. Athl. Train., 27:44–49.

116. Wilk, K.E., Meister, K., and Andrews, J.R. (2002): Current concepts in the rehabilitation of the overhead athlete. Am. J. Sports Med., 30:136–151.

117. Burkhart, S.S., Morgan, C.D., and Kibler, W.B. (2003): The disabled throwing shoulder: Spectrum of pathology. Part I: Pathoanatomy and biomechanics. Arthroscopy, 19:404–420.

118. Burkhart, S.S., Morgan, C.D., and Kibler, W.B. (2003): The disabled throwing shoulder: Spectrum of pathology. Part II: Evaluation and treatment of SLAP lesions in throwers. Arthroscopy, 19:531–539.

119. Dines, J.S., Frank, J.B., Akerman, M., and Yocum, L.A. (2009): Glenohumeral internal rotation deficits in baseball players with ulnar collateral ligament insufficiency. Am. J. Sports Med., 37:566–570.

120. Ellenbecker, T.S., Roetert, E.P., Bailie, D.S., et al. (2002): Glenohumeral joint total rotation range of motion in elite tennis players and baseball pitchers. Med. Sci. Sports Exerc., 34:2052–2056.

121. Torres, R.R., and Gomes, J.L. (2009): Measurement of glenohumeral internal rotation in asymptomatic tennis players and swimmers. Am. J. Sports Med., 37:1017–1023.

122. Burkhart, S.S., Morgan, C.D., and Kibler, W.B. (2003): The disabled throwing shoulder: Spectrum of pathology. Part III: The SICK scapula, scapular dyskinesis, the kinetic chain, and rehabilitation. Arthroscopy, 19:641–661.

123. Borsa, P.A., Wilk, K.E., Jacobson, J.A., et al. (2005): Correlation of range of motion and glenohumeral translation in professional baseball pitchers. Am. J. Sports Med., 33:1392–1399.

124. Crockett, H.C., Gross, L.B., Wilk, K.E., et al. (2002): Osseous adaptation and range of motion at the glenohumeral joint in professional baseball pitchers. Am. J. Sports Med., 30:20–26.

125. Meister, K. (2000): Injuries to the shoulder in the throwing athlete. Part one: Biomechanics/pathophysiology/classification of injury. Am. J. Sports Med., 28:265–275.

126. Borsa, P.A., Dover, G.C., Wilk, K.E., and Reinold, M.M. (2006): Glenohumeral range of motion and stiffness in professional baseball pitchers. Med. Sci. Sports Exerc., 38:21–26.

127. Meister, K., Day, T., Horodyski, M., et al. (2005): Rotational motion changes in the glenohumeral joint of the adolescent/Little League baseball player. Am. J. Sports Med., 33:693–698.

128. Pieper, H.G. (1998): Humeral torsion in the throwing arm of handball players. Am. J. Sports Med., 26:247–253.

129. Reagan, K.M., Meister, K., Horodyski, M.B., et al. (2002): Humeral retroversion and its relationship to glenohumeral rotation in the shoulder of college baseball players. Am. J. Sports Med., 30:354–360.

130. Osbahr, D.C., Cannon, D.L., and Speer, K.P. (2002): Retroversion of the humerus in the throwing shoulder of college baseball pitchers. Am. J. Sports Med., 30:347–353.

131. Reinold, M.M., Wilk, K.E., Macrina, L.C., et al. (2008): Changes in shoulder and elbow passive range of motion after pitching in professional baseball players. Am. J. Sports Med., 36:523–527.

132. Wilk, K.E., Macrina, L.C., Fleisig, G.F., et al. (2011): The correlation of glenohumeral joint internal rotation deficit (GIRD) and total rotational motion to shoulder injuries in professional baseball pitchers. Am. J. Sports Med., 39:329–335.

133. Jobe, C.M. (1996): Superior glenoid impingement: Current concepts. Clin. Orthop. Relat. Res., 330:98–107.

134. Andrews, J.R. (1996): The pathomechanics of injury in the throwers' shoulder. Presented at the American Sports Medicine Institute Injuries in Baseball Course, Birmingham, AL, January 19.

135. Alderink, G.J., and Kuck, D.J. (1986): Isokinetic shoulder strength of high school and college aged pitchers. J. Orthop. Sports Phys., 7:163–172.

136. Bartlett, L.R., Storey, M.D., and Simons, D.B. (1989): Measurement of upper extremity torque production and its relationship to throwing speed in the competitive athlete. Am. J. Sports Med., 17:89–91.

137. Cook, E.E., Gray, U.L., Savinar-Nogue, E., et al. (1987): Shoulder antagonistic strength ratios: A comparison between college level baseball pitchers and non-pitchers. J. Orthop. Sports Phys. Ther., 8:451–461.

138. Hinton, R.Y. (1988): Isokinetic evaluation of shoulder rotational strength in high school baseball pitchers. Am. J. Sports Med., 16:274–279.

139. Wilk, K.E., Andrews, J.R., Arrigo, C.A., et al. (1993): The strength characteristics of internal and external rotator muscles in professional baseball pitchers. Am. J. Sports Med., 21:61–69.

140. Wilk, K.E., Andrews, J.R., and Arrigo, C.A. (1995): The abductor and adductor strength characteristics of professional baseball pitchers. Am. J. Sports Med., 23:307–311.

141. Magnusson, S.P., Gleim, G.W., and Nicholas, J.A. (1994): Shoulder weakness in professional baseball pitchers. Med. Sci. Sports Exerc., 26:5–9.

142. Kibler, W.B. (1991): Role of the scapular in the overhead throwing motion. Contemp. Orthop., 22:525–532.

143. Kibler, W.B. (1998): The role of the athletic shoulder function. Am. J. Sports Med., 26:325–337.

144. Cools, A.M., Dewitte, V., Lanszweert, F., et al. (2007): Rehabilitation of scapular muscle balance: Which exercises to prescribe? Am. J. Sports Med., 35:1744–1751.

145. McCabe, R.A., Orishimo, K.F., McHugh, M.P., and Nicholas, S.J. (2007): Surface electromyographic analysis of the lower trapezius muscle during exercises performed below ninety degrees of shoulder elevation in healthy subjects. North Am. J. Sports Phys. Ther., 2:34–43.

146. Ekstrom, R.A., Donatelli, R.A., and Soderberg, G.L. (2003): Surface electromyographic analysis of exercises for the trapezius and serratus anterior muscles. J. Orthop. Sports Phys. Ther., 33:247–258.

147. Meyers, J.B., Pasquale, M.R., Laudner, K.G., et al. (2005): On-the-field resistance-tubing exercises for throwers: An electromyographic analysis. J. Athl. Train., 40:15–22.

148. Moseley, J.B., Jr., Jobe, F.W., Pink, M., et al. (1992): EMG analysis of the scapular muscles during a shoulder rehabilitation program. Am. J. Sports Med., 20:128–134.

149. Smith, J., Dahm, D.L., Kaufman, K.R., et al. (2006): Electromyographic activity in the immobilized shoulder girdle musculature during scapulothoracic exercises. Arch. Phys. Med. Rehabil., 87:923–927.

150. Bagg, S.D., and Forrest, W.J. (1986): Electromyographic study of the scapular rotators during arm abduction in the scapular plane. Am. J. Phys. Med., 65:111–124.

151. Hardwick, D.H., Beebe, J.A., McDonnell, M.K., and Lang, C.E. (2006): A comparison of serratus anterior muscle activation during a wall slide exercise and other traditional exercises. J. Orthop. Sports Phys. Ther., 36:903–910.

152. Wiedenbauer, M.M., and Mortensen, O.A. (1952): An electromyographic study of the trapezius muscle. Am. J. Phys. Med., 31:363–372.

153. Ballantyne, B.T., O'Hare, S.J., Paschall, J.L., et al. (1993): Electromyographic activity of selected shoulder muscles in commonly used therapeutic exercises. Phys. Ther., 73:668–677; discussion 677–682.

154. Ludewig, P.M., Cook, T.M., and Nawoczenski, D.A. (1996): Three-dimensional scapular orientation and muscle activity at selected positions of humeral elevation. J. Orthop. Sports Phys. Ther., 24:57–65.

155. McClure, P.W., Michener, L.A., Sennett, B.J., and Karduna, A.R. (2001): Direct 3-dimensional measurement of scapular kinematics during dynamic movements in vivo. J. Shoulder Elbow Surg., 10:269–277.

156. Decker, M.J., Hintermeister, R.A., Faber, K.J., and Hawkins, R.J. (1999): Serratus anterior muscle activity during selected rehabilitation exercises. Am. J. Sports Med., 27:784–791.

157. Hintermeister, R.A., Lange, G.W., Schultheis, J.M., et al. (1998): Electromyographic activity and applied load during shoulder rehabilitation exercises using elastic resistance. Am. J. Sports Med., 26:210–220.

158. De Wilde, L., Plasschaert, F., Berghs, B., et al. (2003): Quantified measurement of subacromial impingement. J. Shoulder Elbow Surg., 12:346–349.

159. Roberts, C.S., Davila, J.N., Hushek, S.G., et al. (2002): Magnetic resonance imaging analysis of the subacromial space in the impingement sign positions. J. Shoulder Elbow Surg., 11:595–599.

160. Ludewig, P.M., Hoff, M.S., Osowski, E.E., et al. (2004): Relative balance of serratus anterior and upper trapezius muscle activity during push-up exercises. Am. J. Sports Med., 32:484–493.

161. Lear, L.J., and Gross, M.T. (1998): An electromyographical analysis of the scapular stabilizing synergists during a push-up progression. J. Orthop. Sports Phys. Ther., 28:146–157.

162. Davies, G.J., and Gould, J.A. (1985): Orthopaedic and Sports Physical Therapy. St. Louis, Mosby.

163. Allegrucci, M., Whitney, S.L., Lephart, S.M., et al. (1995): Shoulder kinesthesia in healthy unilateral athletes participating in upper extremity sports. J. Orthop. Sports Phys. Ther., 21:220–226.

164. Blasier, R.B., Carpenter, J.E., and Huston, L.J. (1994): Shoulder proprioception: Effects of joint laxity, joint position, and direction of motion. Orthop. Rev., 23:45–50.

165. Dempster, W.T. (1965): Mechanisms of shoulder movement. Arch. Phys. Med. Rehabil., 46A:49.

166. Bigliani, L.U., Morrison, D., and April, E.W. (1986): The morphology of the acromion and its relationship to rotator cuff tears. Orthop. Trans., 10:228.

167. Travell, J.G., and Simons, D.G. (1983): Myofascial Pain and Dysfunction: The Trigger Point Manual. Baltimore, Williams & Wilkins.

168. Andrews, J.R., and Meister, K. (1993): Classification and treatment of rotator cuff injuries in the overhead athlete. J. Orthop. Sports Phys. Ther., 18:413–421.

169. Neer, C.S. (1972): Anterior acromioplasty for the chronic impingement syndrome in the shoulder: A preliminary report. J. Bone Joint Surg. Am., 54:41–50.

170. Matsen, F.A., III, and Arntz, C.T. (1990): Subacromial impingement. In Rockwood C.A., Jr., Matsen F.A., III (eds.): The Shoulder, Vol. II. Philadelphia, Saunders pp. 623–646.

171. Flatow, E.L., Soslowsky, L.J., Ticker, J.B., et al. (1994): Excursion of the rotator cuff under the acromion: Patterns of subacromial contact. Am. J. Sports Med., 22:779–788.

172. Hawkins, R., and Kennedy, J. (1980): Impingement syndrome in athletes. Am. J. Sports Med., 8:151–158.

173. Kibler, W.B., and McMullen, J. (2003): Scapular dyskinesis and its relation to shoulder pain. J. Am. Acad. Orthop. Surg., 11:142–151.

174. Paine, R.M. (1994): The role of the scapula in the shoulder. In Andrews J.R., and Wilk K.E. (eds.): The Athlete's Shoulder. New York, Churchill Livingstone pp. 495–512.

175. Lindblom, K. (1939): On pathogenesis of ruptures of the tendon aponeurosis of the shoulder joint. Acta Radiol., 20:563–577.

176. Moseley, H.F., and Goldie, I. (1963): The arterial pattern of rotator cuff of the shoulder. J. Bone Joint Surg. Br., 45:780–789.

177. Iannotti, J.P., Swiontkowski, M., Esterhafi, J., and Boulas, H.F. (1989): Intraoperative assessment of rotator cuff vascularity using laser Doppler flowmetry (Abstract). Presented at the Meeting of the American Academy of Orthopaedic Surgeons, Las Vegas.

178. Rathbun, J.B., and Macnab, I. (1970): The microvascular pattern of the rotator cuff. J. Bone Joint Surg. Br., 52:540–553.

179. Sigholm, G., Styf, J., Korner, L., and Herberts, P. (1988): Pressure recording in the subacromial bursa. J. Orthop. Res., 6:123–128.

180. Brewer, B.J. (1979): Aging of the rotator cuff. Am. J. Sports Med., 7:102–110.

181. Morrison, D.S., and Bigliani, L.U. (1987): The clinical significance of variation in acromial morphology. Presented at the Third Open Meeting of the American Shoulder and Elbow Surgeons, San Francisco.

182. MacConnail, M., and Basmajian, J. (1969): Muscles and Movement: A Basis for Human Kinesiology. Baltimore, Williams & Wilkins.

183. Garth, W.P., Allman, F.L., and Armstrong, W.S. (1987): Occult anterior subluxations of the shoulder in non-contact sports. Am. J. Sports Med., 15:579–585.

184. Matsen, F.A., III, and Arntz, C.T. (1990): Rotator cuff tendon failure. In Rockwood C.A., Jr., Matsen F.A., III (eds.): The Shoulder, Vol. II. Philadelphia, Saunders pp. 647–677.

185. Kennedy, J.C., and Willis, R.B. (1976): The effects of local steroid injections on tendons: A biomechanical and microscopic correlative study. Am. J. Sports Med., 4:11–21.

186. Wilk, K.E., and Andrews, J.R. (1993): Rehabilitation following arthroscopic subacromial decompression. Orthopedics, 16:349–358.

187. Walch, G., Boileau, P., Noel, E., and Donell, T. (1992): Impingement of the deep surface of the supraspinatus tendon on the glenoid rim. J. Shoulder Elbow Surg., 1:239–245.

188. Andrews, J.R., and Carson, W.G. (1984): The arthroscopic treatment of glenoid labrum tears in the throwing athlete. Orthop. Trans., 8:44–49.

189. Andrews, J.R., Kupferman, S.P., and Dillman, C.J. (1991): Labral tears in throwing and racquet sports. Clin. Sports Med., 10:901–907.

190. Jobe, C.M. (1995): Posterior superior glenoid impingement. J. Shoulder Elbow Surg., 11:530–556.

191. Jobe, C.M. (1997): Superior glenoid impingement. Orthop. Clin. North Am., 28:137–143.

192. Clark, J.C., and Harryman, D.T. (1992): Tendons, ligaments, and capsule of the rotator cuff. J. Bone Joint Surg. Am., 74:713–719.

193. Howell, S.M., Imobersteg, A.M., Segar, D.H., and Marone, P.J. (1986): Clarification of the role of the supraspinatus muscle in shoulder function. J. Bone Joint Surg. Am., 68:398–404.

194. Yamanaka, K., Fukuda, H., and Mikasa, M. (1987): Incomplete thickness tears of the rotator cuff. Clin. Orthop. Relat. Res., 223:51–58.

195. DePalma, A.F. (1973): Surgery of the Shoulder, 2nd ed. Philadelphia, Lippincott.

196. Wilson, C.F., and Duff, G.L. (1943): Pathologic study of degeneration and rupture of the supraspinatus tendon. Arch. Surg., 47:121–135.

197. Boissonnault, W.G., and Janos, S.C. (1989): Dysfunction, evaluation, and treatment of the shoulder. In Donatelli R., and Wooden, M.J. (eds.): Orthopaedic Physical Therapy. New York, Churchill Livingstone.

198. Reinold, M.M., Macrina, L.C., Wilk, K.E., et al. (2008): The effect of neuromuscular electrical stimulation of the infraspinatus on shoulder external rotation force production after rotator cuff repair surgery. Am. J. Sports Med., 36:2317–2321.

199. Protzman, R.R. (1980): Anterior instability of the shoulder. J. Bone Joint Surg. Am., 62:909–918.

200. Arnheim, D. (1985): Modern Principles of Athletic Training. St. Louis, Mosby.

201. Davis, G.J., and Dickoff-Hoffman, S.D. (1993): Neuromuscular training and rehabilitation of the shoulder. J. Orthop. Sports Phys. Ther., 18:449–454.

202. Jobe, F.W., Tibone, J.E., Jobe, C.M., Kvitne, R.S., Jr. (1990): The shoulder in sports. In Rockwood C. A., Matsen F. A., III (eds.): The Shoulder. Philadelphia, Saunders.

203. Rowe, C.R. (1988): Tendinitis, bursitis, impingement, "snapping scapula" and calcific tendinitis. In Rowe C.R. (ed.): The Shoulder. New York, Churchill Livingstone pp. 105–129.

204. Aronen, J.G. (1986): Anterior shoulder dislocation in sports. Sports Med., 3:224–234.

205. Aronen, J.G., and Regan, K. (1984): Decreasing the incidence of recurrence of first-time anterior shoulder dislocations with rehabilitation. Am. J. Sports Med., 12:283–291.

206. Hovelius, L. (1987): Anterior dislocation of the shoulder in teenagers and young adults. Five-year prognosis. J. Bone Joint Surg. Am., 69:393–399.

207. Itoi, E., Hatakeyama, Y., Sato, T., et al. (2007): Immobilization in external rotation after shoulder dislocation reduced the risk of recurrence. A randomized controlled trial. J. Bone Joint Surg. Am., 89:2124–2131.

208. Cain, P.R., Mutschler, T.A., Fu, F.A., et al. (1987): Anterior stability of the glenohumeral joint: A dynamic model. Am. J. Sports Med., 15:144–148.

209. Ahmadain, A.M. (1987): The Magnuson-Stack operation for recurrent anterior dislocation of the shoulder. J. Bone Joint Surg. Br., 69:111–114.

210. Altchek, D.W., Skybar, M.J., and Warren, R.F. (1989): Shoulder arthroscopy for shoulder instability. Instr. Course Lect., 37:187–198.

211. Bland, J. (1977): The painful shoulder. Semin. Arthritis Rheum., 7:21–47.

212. Collins, K.A., Capito, C., and Cross, M. (1986): The use of the Putti-Platt procedure in the treatment of recurrent anterior dislocation. Am. J. Sports Med., 14:380–382.
213. Kuland, D. (1982): The Injured Athlete. Philadelphia, Lippincott.
214. Lilleby, H. (1984): Shoulder arthroscopy. Acta Orthop. Scand., 55:561–566.
215. Miller, L.S., Donahue, J.R., Good, R.P., and Staerk, A.J. (1984): The Magnuson-Stack procedure for treatment of recurrent glenohumeral dislocations. Am. J. Sports Med., 12:133–137.
216. Norwood, L.A. (1985): Posterior shoulder instability. In Zarins B., Andrews J.R., and Carson W.G. (eds.): Injuries to the Throwing Arm. Philadelphia, Saunders pp. 153–159.
217. Engle, R.P., and Canner, G.C. (1989): Posterior shoulder instability approach to rehabilitation. J. Orthop. Sports Phys. Ther., 10:488–494.
218. Bottoni, C.R., Franks, B.R., Moore, J.H., et al. (2005): Operative stabilization of posterior shoulder instability. Am. J. Sports Med., 33:996–1002.
219. Bradley, J.P., Baker, C.L., 3rd, Kline, A.J., et al. (2006): Arthroscopic capsulolabral reconstruction for posterior instability of the shoulder: A prospective study of 100 shoulders. Am. J. Sports Med., 34:1061–1071.
220. Hawkins, R.J., Kippert, G., and Johnston, G. (1984): Recurrent posterior instability (subluxation) of the shoulder. J. Bone Joint Surg. Am., 66:169–174.
221. Kim, S.H., Ha, K.I., Park, J.H., et al. (2003): Arthroscopic posterior labral repair and capsular shift for traumatic unidirectional recurrent posterior subluxation of the shoulder. J. Bone Joint Surg. Am., 85:1479–1487.
222. Mair, S.D., Zarzour, R.H., and Speer, K.P. (1998): Posterior labral injury in contact athletes. Am. J. Sports Med., 26:753–758.
223. Radkowski, C.A., Chhabra, A., Baker, C.L., 3rd, et al. (2008): Arthroscopic capsulolabral repair for posterior shoulder instability in throwing athletes compared with nonthrowing athletes. Am. J. Sports Med., 36:693–699.
224. Rowe, C., and Zarins, B. (1981): Recurrent transient subluxation of the shoulder. J. Bone Joint Surg. Am., 63:863–871.
225. Savoie, F.H., 3rd, Holt, M.S., Field, L.D., and Ramsey, J.R. (2008): Arthroscopic management of posterior instability: evolution of technique and results. Arthroscopy, 24:389–396.
226. Zarins, B., and Rowe, C.R. (1984): Current concepts in the diagnosis and treatment of shoulder instability in athletes. Med. Sci. Sports Exerc., 16:444–448.
227. Bigliani, L.U. (1990): Multidirectional instability. In Advances on the Knee and Shoulder. Cincinnati, Cincinnati Sports Medicine.
228. Snyder, S.J., Karzel, R.P., DelPizzo, W., et al. (1990): SLAP lesions of the shoulder. Arthroscopy, 6:274–276.
229. Rockwood, C.A., and Young, D.C. (1990): Disorders of the acromioclavicular joint. In Rockwood C.A., and Matsen F.A. (eds.): The Shoulder. Philadelphia, Saunders, pp. 413–468.
230. Neviaser, R.J. (1987): Injuries to the clavicle and acromioclavicular joint. Orthop. Clin. North Am., 18:433–438.
231. Fukuda, K., Craig, E.V., and An, K. (1986): Biomechanical study of the ligamentous system of the acromioclavicular joint. J. Bone Joint Surg. Am., 68:434–440.
232. Dehre, E., and Tory, R. (1971): Treatment of joint injuries by immediate mobilization based upon the spinal adaption concept. Clin. Orthop. Relat. Res., 77:218–232.
233. Haggmark, T., Eriksson, E., and Jansson, E. (1986): Muscle fiber type changes in human muscles after injuries and immobilization. Orthopaedics, 9:181–189.
234. Salter, R.B., Hamilton, H.W., and Wedge, J.H. (1984): Clinical application of basic science research on continuous passive motion for disorders of injures and synovial joints. J. Orthop. Res., 1:325–333.
235. Tipton, C.M., Mattes, R.D., and Maynard, J.A. (1975): The influence of physical activity on ligaments and tendons. Med. Sci. Sports Exerc., 7:165–175.
236. Wickiewicz, T.L., Pagnani, M.J., and Kennedy, K. (1993): Rehabilitation of the unstable shoulder. Sports Med. Arthrosc. Rev., 1:227–235.
237. Hawkins, R.J., and Angelo, R.L. (1990): Glenohumeral osteoarthrosis: A late complication of the Putti-Platt procedure. J. Bone Joint Surg. Am., 72:1193–1197.
238. Wilk, K.E., Reinold, M.M., Dugas, J.R., and Andrews, J.R. (2002): Rehabilitation following thermal capsular shrinkage of the glenohumeral joint. J. Orthop. Sports Phys. Ther., 32:268–292.
239. Wickiewicz, T.L., Chen, S.K., Otis, J.C., and Warren, R.F. (1995): Glenohumeral kinematics in a muscle fatigue model: A radiographic study. Orthop. Trans., 18:126.
240. Wilk, K.E. (2000): Restoration of functional motor patterns and functional testing in the throwing athlete. In Lephart S. M., and Fu, F. H. (eds.): Proprioception and Neuromuscular Control in Joint Stability. Champaign IL, Human Kinetics, pp. 415–438.
241. Warner, J.J.P., and Warren, R.F. (1991): Arthroscopic Bankart repair using a cannulated absorbable fixation device. Oper. Tech. Orthop. Surg., 1:192–198.
242. Shall, L.W., and Crowley, P.W. (1994): Soft tissue reconstruction in the shoulder: Comparison of suture anchors, absorbable staples and absorbable tacks. Am. J. Sports Med., 22:715–718.
243. Acerio, R.A., Wheeler, J.H., and Ryan, J.B. (1994): Arthroscopic Bankart repair vs. non-operative treatment for acute, initial anterior shoulder dislocations. Am. J. Sports Med., 22:589–594.
244. Grana, W., Buckley, P., and Yates, C. (1993): Arthroscopic Bankart suture repair. Am. J. Sports Med., 21:348–353.
245. Morgan, C.D. (1991): Arthroscopic transglenoid suture repair. Oper. Tech. Orthop. Surg., 1:171–179.
246. Morgan, C.D., and Bodenstab, A.B. (1987): Arthroscopic Bankart suture repair: Technique and early results. Arthroscopy, 3:111–122.
247. Hayes, K., Callanan, M., Walton, J., et al. (2002): Shoulder instability: Management and rehabilitation. J. Orthop. Sports Phys. Ther., 32:497–509.
248. Altchek, D.W., Warren, R.F., Skybar, M.J., and Ortiz, G. (1991): T-plasty modification of the Bankart procedure for multi-directional instability of the anterior and inferior types. J. Bone Joint Surg. Am., 73:105–112.
249. Caspari, R.B., and Savoie, F. (1991): Arthroscopic reconstruction of the shoulder: The Bankart repair. In McGinty J. (ed.): Operative Arthroscopy. New York, Raven Press, pp. 507–515.
250. Bigliani, L.U., Kurzweil, P.R., Schwartzback, C.C., et al. (1994): Inferior capsular shift procedure for anterior-inferior shoulder instability in athletes. Am. J. Sports Med., 22:578–584.
251. Kvitne, R.S., Jobe, F.W., and Jobe, C.M. (1995): Shoulder instability in the overhead or throwing athlete. Clin. Sports Med., 14:917–935.
252. Fleisig, G.S. (1977): Ten years in twenty minutes: Conclusions from ASMI's research. Presented at 15th Annual Injuries in Baseball Course, American Sports Medicine Institute, Birmingham, AL, January 24.

13

Rehabilitation of Elbow Injuries

Kevin E. Wilk, PT, DPT, Christopher Arrigo, PT, MS, ATC,
A.J. Yenchak, PT, DPT, CSCS, and James R. Andrews, MD

CHAPTER OBJECTIVES

- Associate anatomic structures of the elbow with particular injuries based on the function of the structures during specific athletic endeavors.

- Correlate the findings from a clinical examination to specific elbow injuries.

- Incorporate biomechanical principles as they relate to the elbow for the prevention and rehabilitation of specific injuries.

- Develop a rehabilitation program for specific pathologic elbow conditions that takes into account the biomechanical function and healing parameters of the anatomic structures involved.

- Advance an athlete through phases of rehabilitation based on specific criteria for progression.

Participation in sports can lead to numerous injuries to the elbow. Injuries involving the elbow joint complex are common occurrences, and rehabilitation after these injuries is often challenging because of the unique anatomy and significant stress applied to this complex during sport-specific movements. The most common mechanisms of injuries are repetitive microtraumatic overuse and macrotraumatic overload forces.[1,2] Complex injury patterns of the elbow are typically sport specific because of the unique demands placed on the elbow during the sport or activity. Overhead throwing athletes such as pitchers and tennis players typically exhibit chronic stress overload or repetitive traumatic stress injuries.[3] Conversely, athletes participating in collision sports such as football, ice hockey, wrestling, and gymnastics are more susceptible to traumatic elbow injuries that include fractures and dislocations.

The ultimate goal of any rehabilitation program is to gradually restore function and return the athlete to symptom-free competition as quickly and safely as possible. Functionally, the elbow plays an integral role in the interplay between the shoulder, wrist/forearm, and hand. Successful rehabilitation of the elbow joint must address this kinetic linkage to complement the usefulness of the elbow in sports. Rehabilitation requires thorough knowledge of the anatomy, biomechanics, and pathomechanics of the elbow during participation in athletics. Each patient's rehabilitation program should be progressed individually and be driven by the patient's symptoms and continuous assessment by the clinician during the rehabilitation process. A team approach

that includes the family, physician, therapist, trainer, coach, and biomechanist should be used to enhance compliance and promote proper education and management related to the rehabilitation process. Continuous feedback/communication is a necessary step to achieve a successful outcome after elbow injury.

This chapter provides an overview of the anatomy and biomechanics of the elbow during sports, along with a detailed description of common clinical examination techniques for injured athletes. Several nonoperative and postoperative rehabilitation programs for specific sports injuries based on a multiphase, progressive approach derived from current scientific research and clinical experience to ensure safe and timely return to sport are discussed.

ANATOMY

Sport-specific applied anatomy of the elbow joint complex can be broken down and divided into osseous, capsuloligamentous, musculotendinous, and neurologic components. The interplay between osseous, neurovascular, and soft tissue structures is integral in promoting static and dynamic stability of the elbow complex as it relates to function, especially in sports. Injury to any specific structure can create overwhelming complications for the athlete, such as limitations in range of motion (ROM), stability, and overall function. The following sections provide a comprehensive overview of anatomy as it relates to the elbow complex.

Osseous Structures

The elbow joint complex includes the humerus, radius, and ulna articulating together in concert to form four joints: the humeroulnar joint, the humeroradial joint, the proximal radioulnar joint, and the distal radioulnar joint (Fig. 13-1).

The humeroulnar joint is generally considered a uniaxial, diarthrodial joint with 1° of freedom. It allows flexion and extension in the sagittal plane around a coronal axis. Morrey[4] described the humeroulnar joint as a modified hinge joint because of the small amounts of internal and external rotation that occur in the extreme end ranges of both flexion and extension. The anterior aspect of the distal end of the humerus is composed of the convex trochlea. It is an hourglass-shaped surface covered with articular cartilage. The trochlear groove is located centrally within the trochlea and runs obliquely in an anterior to posterior direction. The distal end of the humerus is typically rotated 30° anteriorly with respect to the long axis of the humerus. Correspondingly, the proximal end of the ulna is normally rotated 30° posteriorly with respect to the shaft of the ulna. This paired anatomic rotation of the humerus and ulna ensures the availability of end-range elbow flexion to approximately 145° to 150°. It also serves to enhance the static stability of the elbow complex in full extension.[5]

The proximal end of the ulna contains a central ridge that runs between two bony prominences, the coronoid process anteriorly and the olecranon posteriorly. Two fossas are located on each side of the corresponding articular surfaces of the humerus. Anteriorly, the coronoid fossa articulates with the coronoid process of the ulna during flexion. Posteriorly, the olecranon fossa receives the olecranon process of the ulna, which serves to limit extension.

The congruency achieved via these articulations makes the humeroulnar joint one of the most stable joints in the human body.[6]

The medial epicondyle of the humerus also contributes significantly to the humeroulnar joint. Located proximal and medial to the trochlea, it serves as the site of origin for the flexor-pronator muscle group and the ulnar collateral ligament (UCL). Hoppenfeld[7] noted that both the size and prominence of the medial epicondyle provide an important mechanical advantage for the medial stabilizing structures of the elbow joint. The cubital tunnel is located posterior to the medial epicondyle and functions to protect the ulnar nerve as it traverses distally across the elbow joint complex.

Similarly, the humeroradial joint is a diarthrodial, uniaxial joint that allows elbow flexion and extension along with the humeroulnar joint. The humeroradial joint also pivots around a longitudinal axis to allow rotational movements in association with the proximal radioulnar joint, thus making the joint a combination hinge and pivot joint.[8]

The articular surfaces of the humeroradial joint include the concave radial head and the spherical convex capitellum at the distal end of the humerus.[9] The capitellum and trochlea are separated by a groove within the humerus, the capitulotrochlear groove. This groove guides the radial head as the elbow flexes and extends.

Immediately proximal to the capitellum on the anterior aspect of the humerus is the radial fossa. It receives the anterior aspect of the radial head when the elbow is in a maximally flexed position. The lateral epicondyle of the humerus lies just lateral to the radial fossa. It serves as the site of origin for the wrist extensor muscle group. The radial tuberosity is located on the radius just distal to the radial head. It is the attachment site for the distal biceps brachii tendon.

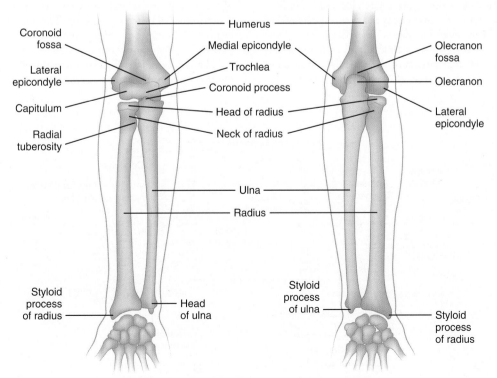

FIGURE 13-1 Osseous structures of the elbow.

The proximal and distal radioulnar joints are intimately related from a functional standpoint. Together they allow 1° of freedom in the transverse plane around a longitudinal axis, which facilitates forearm supination and pronation. During these motions the head of the radius rotates within a ring formed by the annular ligament and the radial notch of the ulna. Little motion actually occurs in the ulna. The radius and ulna lie parallel to each other when the forearm is in a pronated position. As the forearm rotates into supination, the radius crosses over the ulna. The radius and ulna are connected midway between the two bony shafts by an interosseous membrane, which serves as an additional attachment site for the forearm musculature.

Functionally, the bony articulation of the elbow joint forms the carrying angle of the elbow. This is defined as the angle formed by the long axis of the humerus and the ulna. It normally results in an abducted position of the forearm in relation to the humerus. The carrying angle is measured in the frontal plane with the elbow extended and averages 11° to 14° in males and 13° to 16° in females.[10,11] The carrying angle changes linearly as the elbow joint is flexed and extended, diminishing in flexion and increasing with extension.[4]

Capsuloligamentous Structures

The joint capsule is a relatively thin but strong structure that derives significant strength from its transverse and obliquely oriented fibrous bands. The posterior portion of the capsule is a thin transparent structure that allows visualization of the bony prominences when the elbow is fully extended. The posterior capsule originates just above the olecranon fossa and inserts distally along the medial and lateral margins of the trochlea. The anterior capsule originates proximally above the coronoid and radial fossas and attaches distally at the anterior margin of the coronoid medially and into the annular ligament laterally. The anterior capsule is taut as the elbow is extended and lax in flexion. The greatest capsular laxity occurs at approximately 80° of elbow flexion.[12] A synovial membrane lines the joint capsule and is attached anteriorly above the radial and coronoid fossas to the medial and lateral margins of the articular surface and posteriorly to the superior margin of the olecranon fossa.

The ligaments of the elbow consist of thickened parts of the medial and lateral portions of the capsule. The UCL is located on the medial aspect of the elbow. This ligamentous complex can be divided into three distinct components: the anterior, posterior, and transverse bundles (Fig. 13-2, A). The anterior bundle originates from the inferior surface of the medial epicondyle and inserts at the medial aspect of the coronoid process. Because of the posterior orientation of this portion of the ligament in relation to the center of rotation of the elbow joint, the anterior bundle is taut throughout elbow ROM. The anterior bundle can be further divided into two bands: the anterior band, which is taut in extension, and the posterior band, which tightens in flexion.[4,13] The anterior bundle of the UCL provides the main ligamentous support to resist valgus strain at the elbow.

The posterior bundle originates from the posteroinferior medial epicondyle and fans out to attach onto the posteromedial aspect of the olecranon. The transverse bundle of the UCL originates from the medial olecranon and inserts into the coronoid process. Several authors have reported that these two bundles provide minimal amounts of medial elbow stability.[6,13,14]

Laterally, the ligamentous complex helps stabilize the elbow against varus stress. It is made up of several components, including the radial collateral ligament, the annular ligament, the accessory lateral collateral ligament, and the lateral ulnar collateral ligament.[4]

The characteristics of the radial collateral ligament are not as well defined as those of the UCL. Originating from the lateral epicondyle, the radial collateral ligament fans out and inserts into the annular ligament (Fig. 13-2, B). The origin of the radial collateral ligament is in line with the axis of elbow joint rotation, which allows little change in length as the elbow moves through its full ROM.

The annular ligament is a strong fibroosseous ring that encircles and stabilizes the radial head within the radial notch of the ulna. Its origin and insertion occur along the anterior and posterior radial notch of the ulna. The anterior portion of this ligament becomes taut with supination, whereas the posterior portion becomes taut with pronation.[15]

The accessory lateral collateral ligament originates from the inferior margin of the annular ligament and inserts discretely

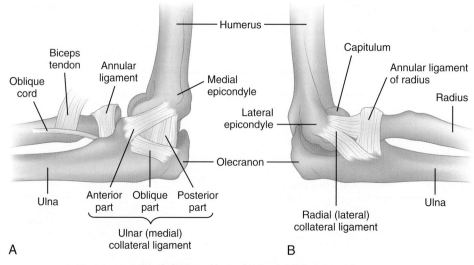

FIGURE 13-2 Medial (**A**) and lateral (**B**) capsuloligamentous structures.

into the tubercle of the supinator crest of the ulna. The accessory lateral collateral ligament further assists the annular ligament in varus stabilization of the elbow joint complex.[16]

The lateral ulnar collateral ligament originates from the lateral epicondyle and inserts into the tubercle of the crest of the supinator. This ligament provides posterolateral stability for the humeroulnar joint.[17]

The elbow joint is one of the most congruent joints in the human body and therefore is also one of its most stable. Stability is provided by the interaction of soft tissue and articular constraints. The static soft tissue stabilizers include the capsular and ligamentous structures. Table 13-1 summarizes the stabilizing influences of the ligamentous and articular components of the elbow joint.[6] When the elbow is in full extension, the anterior capsule provides approximately 70% of the restraint to joint distraction, whereas the UCL provides approximately 78% of the resistance to distractive forces at 90° of elbow flexion. The restraint to valgus displacement varies significantly, depending on the angle of elbow flexion. When the elbow is in full extension, the capsule provides 38% of the valgus restraint, the UCL provides 31%, and the osseous articulations provide the remaining 31%. Conversely, at 90° of elbow flexion, the primary restraint to valgus force is the UCL, which provides 54% of the restraint, followed by the osseous articulation (33%) and the capsule (13%). Varus stress is controlled in extension by the joint articulation (54%), lateral collateral ligament (14%), and joint capsule (32%). As the elbow flexes, the lateral collateral ligament and capsule contribute 9% and 13%, respectively, and the joint articulation provides 75% of the stabilizing force against varus stress.[6]

Musculotendinous Structures

The elbow joint musculature can be divided into six groups based on their functions: the elbow flexors, extensors, flexor-pronators, extensor-supinators, primary pronators, and primary supinators.

The three primary flexor muscles of the elbow are the biceps brachii, the brachioradialis, and the brachialis. The biceps brachii typically consists of a long and short head. The long head of the biceps brachii originates on the superior glenoid and glenoid labrum. It passes directly through the glenohumeral joint capsule and the intertubercular groove of the humerus until it joins with the short head of the biceps brachii. The short head of the biceps originates from the coracoid process of the scapula. The two heads join to form a common attachment onto the posterior portion of the radial tuberosity and via the bicipital aponeurosis, which attaches to the anterior capsule of the elbow joint. The biceps is responsible for the vast majority of elbow flexion strength when the forearm is supinated and generates its highest torque values when the elbow is positioned between 80° and 100° of flexion.[8] The biceps also acts secondarily as a supinator of the forearm, principally when the elbow is in a flexed position.

The brachialis muscle originates from the lower half of the anterior surface of the humerus. It extends distally to cross the anterior aspect of the elbow joint and inserts into both the ulnar tuberosity and the coronoid process. The brachialis muscle is active in flexing the elbow in all positions of forearm rotation.[18]

The brachioradialis muscle originates from the proximal two thirds of the lateral supracondylar ridge of the humerus and along the lateral intermuscular septum just distal to the spiral groove. It inserts into the lateral aspect of the base of the styloid process of the radius. The muscular insertion of the brachioradialis is at a significant distance from the joint axis and therefore exhibits a substantial mechanical advantage as an elbow flexor.[8]

The triceps brachii and anconeus muscles serve as the primary extensors of the elbow. The triceps brachii is a large three-headed (long, lateral, and medial) muscle that encompasses almost the entire posterior portion of the brachium. The long head of the triceps originates from the infraglenoid tubercle, whereas the lateral and medial heads originate from the posterior and lateral aspects of the humerus. At the distal end of the humerus, the three heads converge to form a common muscle that inserts into the posterior surface of the olecranon.

The small anconeus muscle originates from a broad area on the posterior aspect of the lateral epicondyle and inserts into the olecranon. The anconeus muscle covers the lateral portion of the annular ligament, the radial head, and the posterior surface of the proximal end of the ulna. Electromyographic (EMG) activity of the anconeus muscle during the early phases of elbow extension has been noted, and this muscle appears to play a stabilizing role during both pronation and supination movements.[19]

Table 13-1 Forces Contributing to Displacement of the Elbow

Elbow Position	Stabilizing Structure	Distraction (%)	Varus (%)	Valgus (%)
Elbow extended (0°)	UCL	12	–	31
	LCL	10	14	–
	Capsule	70	32	38
	Articulation	–	54	31
Elbow flexed (90°)	UCL	78	–	54
	LCL	10	9	–
	Capsule	8	13	13
	Articulation	–	75	33

LCL, Lateral collateral ligament; *UCL,* ulnar collateral ligament.

The flexor-pronator muscles include the pronator teres, flexor carpi radialis, palmaris longus, flexor carpi ulnaris, and flexor digitorum superficialis. All these muscles originate completely or in part from the medial epicondyle and serve secondary roles as elbow flexors. Their primary roles are associated with movements of the wrist and hand. This muscle group may provide a limited amount of dynamic stability to the medial aspect of the elbow in resisting valgus stress.[20]

The extensor-supinator muscles include the brachioradialis, extensor carpi radialis brevis and longus, supinator, extensor digitorum, extensor carpi ulnaris, and extensor digiti minimi muscles. Each muscle originates near or directly from the lateral epicondyle of the humerus. Like the flexor-pronators, the primary functions of the extensor-supinator muscles involve the wrist and hand. They also provide dynamic support over the lateral aspect of the elbow. Both this muscle group and the flexor-pronator musculature are susceptible to various overuse conditions and muscular strains.

The pronator quadratus and pronator teres muscles act on the radioulnar joints to produce pronation. The pronator quadratus originates from the anterior surface of the lower part of the ulna and inserts at the distal and lateral border of the radius. The pronator quadratus acts as a significant pronator in all elbow and forearm positions. The pronator teres, which possesses both humeral and ulnar heads, originates from the medial epicondyle and coronoid process of the ulna. The two heads join together and insert along the middle of the lateral surface of the radius. The pronator teres is a strong forearm pronator. It generates its highest contractile force during rapid or resisted pronation.[21] However, the contribution of the pronator teres to pronation strength diminishes when the elbow is positioned in full extension.[8] The flexor carpi radialis and brachioradialis also act as secondary pronators.

The biceps brachii and the supinator muscles are the primary supinators of the forearm, whereas the brachioradialis acts as an accessory supinator. The supinator muscle originates from three separate locations: (1) the lateral epicondyle, (2) the proximal anterior crest and depression of the ulna distal to the radial notch, and (3) the radial collateral and annular ligaments. The supinator muscle then winds around the radius and insert into the dorsal and lateral surfaces of the proximal end of the radius. The supinator, though a significant supinator of the forearm, generally appears to be weaker than the biceps.[4] The supinator acts alone during unresisted slow supination in all elbow and forearm positions and during unresisted fast supination with the elbow extended.[9] The effectiveness of the supinator is not altered by elbow position; however, elbow position does significantly affect the biceps. Because the supinator originates at the radial collateral and annular ligaments, it may also act as a supportive or stabilizing muscle for the lateral aspect of the elbow.

Neurologic Structures

The four nerves that play significant roles in normal elbow function are the median, ulnar, radial, and musculocutaneous nerves. Table 13-2 shows the effect of injury to each of these peripheral nerves.

The median nerve arises from branches of the lateral and medial cords of the brachial plexus. Nerve root levels include C5 to C8 and T1. This nerve proceeds distally over the anterior brachium and continues to the medial aspect of the antecubital fossa. From the fossa, the nerve continues its course under the bicipital aponeurosis and passes most often between the two heads of the pronator teres. The median nerve can be compressed between these two heads or by the bicipital aponeurosis, which results in either pronator or anterior interosseous syndrome. Although relatively uncommon, highly repetitive and strenuous pronation movements of the forearm can also lead to entrapment of the median nerve.[22]

The ulnar nerve emanates from the C8 and T1 nerve root levels and descends into the proximal aspect of the upper extremity from the medial cord of the brachial plexus. The ulnar nerve passes from the anterior to the posterior compartments of the brachium through the arcade of Struthers. This arcade represents a fascial bridging between the medial head of the triceps and the medial intermuscular septum. The nerve continues distally, passing behind the medial epicondyle and through the cubital tunnel. At the cubital tunnel, the bony anatomy provides little protection for the nerve (Fig. 13-3). Ulnar nerve injury, which can be caused by compression or stretching, takes place most often in the cubital tunnel. The cubital tunnel retinaculum flattens with elbow flexion, thus decreasing the overall capacity within the cubital tunnel. This can be noted clinically when nerve symptoms are reproduced during elbow flexion, which typically occurs when osteophytes are present on the ulna or medial epicondyle.[23] Injury to the medial capsular ligaments can result in increased traction forces on the medial portion of the elbow and cause a change in length of the ulnar nerve. This change in length may result in neuropathy or ulnar nerve subluxation. The nerve enters the forearm by passing between the two heads of the flexor carpi ulnaris and continues distally between the flexor digitorum profundus and flexor carpi ulnaris.

The radial nerve originates from the posterior cord of the brachial plexus and derives its nerve supply from the C6, C7, and C8 nerve root levels, with variable contributions from the C5 and T11 nerve root levels. At the midpoint of the brachium, the radial nerve descends laterally through the radial groove of the humerus and continues its course in a lateral and distal direction. The nerve descends anteriorly behind the brachioradialis and brachialis muscles to the level of the elbow, where it divides into its posterior interosseous and superficial radial branches.

The musculocutaneous nerve originates from the lateral cord of the brachial plexus at nerve root levels C5 to C7. The nerve passes between the biceps and brachialis muscles and pierces the brachial fascia lateral to the biceps tendon. The nerve continues distally and terminates as the lateral antebrachial cutaneous nerve, which provides sensation over the anterolateral aspect of the forearm. Compression between the biceps tendon and the brachialis fascia can cause entrapment of the musculocutaneous nerve.

Sensory nerves innervate the elbow cutaneously and are derived from specific nerve root levels. The lateral aspect of the arm is innervated by branches of the axillary nerve of the C5 nerve root level, whereas the lateral aspect of the forearm is innervated by the musculocutaneous nerve of the C6 nerve root level.[24] The medial aspect of the arm is innervated by the brachial cutaneous nerve from the T1 nerve root level, and the medial aspect of the forearm is innervated by branches of the antebrachial cutaneous nerve from the C8 nerve root level.[24] The T2 dermatome extends from the axilla to the posteromedial portion of the elbow.[22] The extent of innervation provided by each nerve root is variable, and overlap between dermatome distributions does occur.

Table 13-2 Effects of Injury to Specific Peripheral Nerves

Musculocutaneous Nerve (C5)	
Sensory supply	Lateral half of the anterior surface of the forearm from the elbow to the thenar eminence
Effect of injury	Severe elbow flexion weakness Weakness during supination Loss of the biceps deep tendon reflex Loss of sensation, cutaneous distribution
Radial Nerve (C5, C6, C7, C8, and T1)	
Sensory supply	Back of the arm, forearm, and wrist; radial half of the dorsum of the hand; and back of the thumb, index finger, and part of the middle finger
Effect of injury	Loss of the triceps deep tendon reflex Elbow flexion weakness Loss of supination (when the elbow is extended) Loss of wrist extension Weakness during ulnar and radial deviation Loss of extension at the MCP joints Loss of extension and abduction of the thumb
Median Nerve (C5, C6, C7, C8, and T1)	
Sensory supply	Radial half of the palm; palmar surface of the thumb, index, middle, and radial half of the ring finger; and dorsal surface of the same fingers
Effect of injury	Loss of complete pronation (the brachioradialis can bring the forearm to midpronation but not beyond) Weakness with flexion and radial deviation (ulnar deviation with wrist flexion) Loss of flexion at the MCP joints Loss of thumb opposition or abduction, loss of flexion at the IP and MCP joints
Ulnar Nerve (C7, C8, and T1)	
Sensory supply	Dorsal and palmar surfaces of the ulnar side of the hand, including the little finger and ulnar half of the ring finger
Effect of injury	Weakness in wrist flexion and ulnar deviation (radial deviation with wrist flexion) Loss of flexion of the DIP joints or ring and little fingers Inability to abduct or adduct the fingers Inability to adduct the thumb Loss of flexion of the fingers, especially the ring and little fingers at the MCP joints Loss of extension of the fingers, especially the ring and little fingers at the joint

DIP, Distal interphalangeal; *IP,* interphalangeal; *MCP,* metacarpophalangeal.

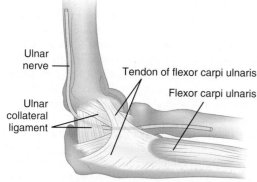

FIGURE 13-3 Ulnar nerve.

BIOMECHANICS IN SPORTS

Biomechanics of Baseball Pitching

The biomechanics of the elbow during overhead baseball pitching can be broken down into six phases: windup, stride, arm cocking, arm acceleration, arm deceleration, and follow-through.

During the windup and stride phases, minimal elbow kinetics and muscle activity are present. As the foot contacts the ground, the elbow is flexed to approximately 85°.[25]

The arm-cocking phase begins as the foot comes into contact with the ground and continues until the point of maximum shoulder external rotation. As the arm moves into external rotation, a varus torque is produced at the elbow to prevent valgus stress.[15] Shortly before maximum external rotation, the elbow is flexed to 95° and a varus torque of approximately 85 Nm is produced.[26-28] At this critical instant, excessive valgus strain may cause injury to the medial stabilizing structures of the elbow, particularly the UCL. As discussed previously, Morrey and An[14] reported that at this instant the UCL is contributing approximately 54% of the resistance to this valgus strain moment. Assuming that the UCL absorbs 54% of the 85 Nm of valgus strain observed during the arm-cocking phase, 45 Nm of strain would be applied to the UCL in this position, which approaches the maximum load capacity before failure of the UCL ensues.[3,29]

In addition, as the elbow joint sustains this valgus strain, lateral compression is applied. This may lead to compressive injuries involving the lateral compartment of the elbow as the radial head and humeral capitellum are approximated. Such compression may lead to avascular necrosis, osteochondritis dissecans, osteochondral chip fractures, or any combination of these injuries.

As the arm accelerates from maximal external rotation to ball release, elbow extension velocity peaks at approximately 2500°/sec.[3,26,27,29-31] As the elbow extends and resists valgus strain simultaneously, the olecranon can impinge against the medial aspect of the trochlear groove and olecranon fossa,[3,32] which may lead to the formation of a posteromedial osteophyte and loose bodies. This type of compression under valgus stress was described by Wilson et al[33] as valgus extension overload.

As the arm decelerates and continues into the follow-through phase, eccentric contraction of the elbow flexors must control the distractive forces at the elbow joint. Moderate activity of the biceps brachii and brachioradialis has been reported at this time.[25] Muscular activity of the elbow flexors may assist in preventing impingement of the olecranon as the elbow is rapidly extended. The elbow remains in a flexed position of approximately 20° as the arm continues into follow-through. Minimal kinetic and muscular activity at the elbow occurs during this final phase of throwing.

Biomechanics of the Elbow During Tennis

The kinematic and kinetic data during tennis vary depending on the type of stroke; therefore, the biomechanics of the serve and groundstroke will be discussed separately. The overhead serve has been compared with the mechanics of overhead throwing.[3] The elbow has been reported to extend at 1500°/sec and pronate at 347°/sec during the acceleration and deceleration phases of the tennis serve.[28,34,35] Morris et al[36] reported that the activity of the triceps and pronator teres during the tennis serve must be high to produce significant racket velocity. Because of this excessive angular velocity, eccentric contraction of the elbow flexors and supinators is critical for prevention of injuries to the elbow during an overhead tennis serve.

During a groundstroke, both the forehand and the backhand—the wrist extensors—are predominantly active as the athlete prepares the racquet for impact.[36] The extensor carpi radialis longus and brevis and the extensor communis muscles are active during both strokes, with the forehand showing additional muscular activity of the biceps brachii and brachioradialis.[36-38] As the racquet comes into contact with the ball and begins the follow-through, continued activity of the extensor carpi radialis brevis occurs. The backhand produces additional activity of the biceps brachii as the elbow decelerates into extension.[36-38]

Kelley and Weiland[37] compared the muscular activity of the elbow during the backhand stroke in subjects with and without lateral epicondylitis. The results indicated that the group of subjects exhibiting lateral epicondylitis had a significant increase in EMG activity in the extensor carpi radialis longus and brevis, pronator teres, and flexor carpi radialis. These retrospective findings may have an impact on the explanation of the etiology of lateral epicondylitis.

Biomechanics of the Golf Swing

The biomechanics of the golf swing that pertain to elbow and wrist injuries can be broken down into five phases: backswing, transition, downswing, impact, and follow-through.[39,40] As the athlete swings the club, both the lead arm and the back arm are susceptible to injuries at various moments during the swing.

The backswing phase produces few injuries in the elbow. As the backswing progresses, the lead wrist pronates, flexes, and deviates radially. The back arm flexes at the elbow and the wrist supinates, extends, and deviates radially. The wrist flexors exhibit minimal EMG activity, whereas the wrist extensors exhibit 33% of the maximum voluntary isometric contraction (MVIC).[41] As the clubhead approaches the top of the backswing, the musculature of the elbow must contract eccentrically to control the clubhead and transition from the backswing to the downswing. This motion places a great deal of stress on the stretched flexor-pronator mass of the back arm.[42]

As the downswing progresses, the wrists must uncoil to produce clubhead speed. The wrists and elbows uncoil and return to the neutral position initially observed at setup to prepare for impact. The downswing is characterized by increased muscular activity of both the wrist extensors and flexors. The wrist extensors exhibit 45% MVIC and the wrist flexors 35% MVIC during the downswing. During impact, the wrist and hands decelerate because of the force of impact.[41] McCarroll and Gioe[43] reported that more than twice as many injuries occur during downswing as during backswing because the elbows and wrists move approximately three times faster during downswing. This deceleration of force places a great deal of strain on the forearm muscles as they attempt to maintain control of the club.[42] The majority of elbow injuries take place during impact as the lateral epicondyle of the lead arm and the medial epicondyle of the back arm are placed under significant strain. The lead elbow extensor mass has been reported to be under even greater stress at impact because of the compressive force of ball impact and divots.[44] At ball contact, wrist flexor activity increases significantly to 91% MVIC. Additionally, the wrist extensors exhibit EMG activity of approximately 58% MVIC.[41]

After impact, the arm continues into follow-through. Minimal injuries occur during this phase. The wrists and hands follow a reverse pattern as that seen during the backswing. The lead arm flexes at the elbow, supinates, extends, and deviates radially at the wrist, whereas the back arm pronates, flexes, and deviates radially at the wrist. During follow-through, the EMG activity of the wrist extensors is approximately 60% to 70% MVIC. The repetitive nature of elbow and wrist motion observed may be responsible for the golfing overuse injuries commonly seen in the forearm musculature.

When the muscular activity patterns of golfers with medial epicondylitis and golfers without injuries are compared, golfers with medial epicondylitis exhibit significantly greater wrist flexor muscle activity during the backswing, transition, and downswing.[41]

CLINICAL EXAMINATION

Clinical evaluation of the elbow of an athlete requires a thorough history, extensive knowledge of the anatomy and biomechanics of the joint, and a well-organized physical examination. The goal of the examination is to identify areas of dysfunction and determine an appropriate course of intervention.

History

Before the examination begins, a complete history is imperative.[45] The location, intensity, and duration of pain should be clearly identified. The date and mechanism of injury should be explained thoroughly because this will assist in determining the structures involved. Other subjective information, such as aggravating factors, previous injuries, and primary complaints, should also be recorded to assist in assessment and development of patient-specific treatment and goals.[45]

Observation

The trunk and arms should be completely exposed to provide a full view of the neck, shoulder, and elbow for a comprehensive evaluation. The skin should be evaluated for areas of contusion, ecchymosis, swelling, burns, surgical scars, redness, blanching, petechiae, and venous congestion. The carrying angle of the elbow should also be assessed during this portion of the examination.

Palpation

Palpation of the elbow begins with the identification of specific bony landmarks. The clinician should palpate each to determine whether tenderness or deformity is present.

The medial epicondyle may exhibit tenderness for various reasons, including epicondylitis, muscle strain, and UCL injury. The medial supracondylar ridge should be examined for osteophytes, which may be entrapping the median nerve. The olecranon is easily palpated and is covered by the insertion of the triceps and the olecranon bursa, both of which may be tender in athletes with a pathologic condition. Osseous changes in the posteromedial olecranon may be associated with valgus extension overload in overhead athletes. The ulnar border should also be palpated for stress fractures, which are sometimes present in throwing athletes. The lateral epicondyle is often irritable when palpated if epicondylitis is present. Finally, the radial head lies approximately 2 cm distally from the lateral epicondyle and should be palpated during passive supination and pronation.

When one palpates the soft tissues of the elbow, it is helpful to divide the elbow into four distinct regions: the medial, posterior, lateral, and anterior aspects.

The major structures of the medial aspect of the elbow include the ulnar nerve, the flexor-pronator muscle group, the UCL, and the supracondylar lymph nodes. The clinician should manually determine whether the ulnar nerve is capable of being dislocated from within its bony sulcus. This is done by abducting and externally rotating the shoulder with the athlete in a supine position and the elbow flexed between 20° and 70°.[45] The medial epicondyle should also be palpated to determine tenderness in the flexor-pronator muscle mass or the UCL.

The posterior aspect of the elbow contains the olecranon, which should be palpated for the presence of an inflamed, swollen bursa. The triceps insertion points should also be palpated for tenderness.

Laterally, the wrist extensor group is palpated. The brachioradialis is made prominent by having the patient close the fist, place the forearm in a neutral position, and resist elbow flexion. Resisted wrist flexion allows easy palpation of the extensor carpi radialis longus and brevis.

The anterior structures of the elbow pass through the cubital fossa. From medial to lateral, these structures are the median nerve, brachial artery, and biceps tendon. The biceps can be made prominent by resisted elbow flexion.

Range of Motion

The normal ROM of the elbow is 0° of extension, 140° to 150° of flexion, 80° of pronation, and 80° of supination.[46] Passive ROM is assessed in each direction and is always compared with that on the contralateral side. In addition, the end-feel of movement should be assessed. Normal end-feel of the elbow is different for each movement: elbow extension exhibits a bony end-feel, flexion has a soft tissue approximation, and forearm pronation and supination both have a capsular end-feel.[47]

Muscle Testing

Muscle testing of the elbow musculature begins with the patient seated.[48] The brachialis is tested with the elbow flexed and the forearm pronated. The biceps is tested with the forearm supinated and the shoulder flexed to 45° to 50°. The brachioradialis is tested with the elbow flexed and the wrist in neutral rotation. Triceps extension is performed with the shoulder flexed 90° and the elbow flexed 45° to 90°. Pronation and supination of the elbow are performed with the arm by the side, the elbow flexed 90°, and the wrist in neutral rotation. Resistance is applied at the distal end of the forearm as the patient attempts to rotate in either direction. Wrist extension and flexion are performed with the elbow flexed 30° and the elbow fully extended. Isokinetic testing may also be performed to determine specific objective data on muscular strength, power, and endurance.

Special Tests

Special tests for the elbow joint are used in an attempt to elicit specific pathologic signs or symptoms. Laxity is assessed to evaluate the integrity of the medial and lateral stabilizing structures. Varus and valgus testing may be performed by stabilizing the arm with one hand and applying a fulcrum at the elbow joint with the other. The clinician imparts a varus or valgus stress and notes the amount of gapping and the end-feel of motion. The tests are conducted bilaterally and may be performed at 0° of extension and 30° of flexion. Pain, excessive gapping, or a soft end-feel may all indicate a pathologic condition of the stabilizing structures.

Several clinical tests are used to test the integrity of the UCL. The two most common techniques are the supine and prone valgus stress tests. In the first, the athlete is positioned supine while the clinician holds the elbow, externally rotates the shoulder, and blocks the upper extremity from further rotation (Fig. 13-4). The UCL is easily palpated in this position. The elbow is tested at 5° and at 25° to 30° of flexion by applying a valgus stress to determine the integrity of the ligament. The amount of opening, or gapping, is assessed, as well as the end-feel of motion. Excessive gapping, a soft end-feel, or localized medial pain may all indicate a UCL injury.[45]

Next, the athlete is placed in the prone position with the involved arm hanging over the edge of the table. The clinician internally rotates the shoulder and stabilizes the elbow and forearm in pronation before placing a valgus stress on the elbow at 5° and at 25° to 30° of flexion (Fig. 13-5). Again, the amount of opening and

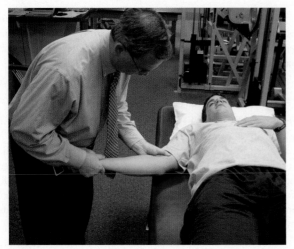

FIGURE 13-4 Clinical test for instability of the ulnar collateral ligament in the supine position.

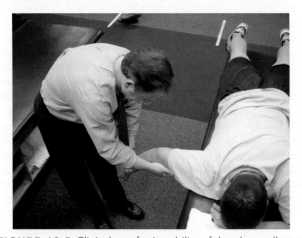

FIGURE 13-5 Clinical test for instability of the ulnar collateral ligament in the prone position.

end-feel are evaluated during the examination. The prone test is preferred by the authors because of its greater capacity for isolating the UCL and minimizing humeral rotation.

The clinical test for valgus extension overload is performed by the clinician grasping the elbow in a flexed position. As the clinician forces the elbow into extension, a valgus stress is simultaneously applied to the elbow. The clinician palpates the posteromedial aspect of the joint for tenderness and crepitation. Pain over the posteromedial portion of the olecranon process signifies a positive test result.[33]

A lateral pivot shift test is used to assess posterolateral rotatory instability of the elbow.[17] Patients who have sustained an elbow dislocation often report a posterolateral rotatory mechanism of injury that is replicated during this test. With the patient supine, the clinician holds the arm over the head with the shoulder in 90° of flexion and maximal external rotation.

The clinician applies a valgus and supination moment while flexing the elbow, which results in the semilunar notch of the ulna being displaced from the trochlea of the humerus. During this maneuver maximal displacement occurs at approximately 40°.[17] This test is often not tolerated by the patient without general anesthesia; however, signs of apprehension during testing indicate a positive clinical test result in an awake athlete.[49]

Neurologic Testing

The deep tendon reflexes that are significant during examination of the elbow are the biceps reflex, brachioradialis reflex, and triceps reflex, which are controlled by the spinal levels C5, C6, and C7, respectively. A slight response is normal, whereas an increased response could signify an upper motor neuron lesion and a decreased response may indicate the presence of a lower motor neuron lesion.

The biceps tendon reflex can be elicited with the elbow relaxed and in a flexed position; the clinician places the thumb over the biceps tendon in the cubital fossa and gently taps the thumb with a reflex hammer. The brachioradialis reflex is elicited by tapping the tendon at the lateral distal end of the radius with the flat edge of a reflex hammer. The triceps tendon reflex is elicited by tapping over the triceps tendon with a reflex hammer.

Sensory perception is assessed by pinprick and light touch of the skin. The contralateral extremity is always used for comparison. The lateral aspect of the arm is innervated by the axillary nerve (C5), and the lateral aspect of the forearm is innervated by branches of the musculocutaneous nerve (C6). The medial aspect of the arm is innervated by the brachial cutaneous nerve (C8), and the medial aspect of the forearm is innervated by the antebrachial cutaneous (T1) nerve.

Plain View Radiographs

Plain view radiographs may be a useful adjunct to the clinical examination. The views routinely taken of an elbow include both an anteroposterior and a lateral view. These views allow the clinician to identify the presence of fractures or loose bodies. Internal and external oblique views may also provide further diagnostic information and are the best views to detect the presence of posterior olecranon osteophytes.

Computed Tomographic Arthrography

A diagnostic arthrogram is extremely useful when a UCL tear is suspected. Contrast dye is injected into the elbow, and radiographs are obtained to determine whether the dye has escaped the capsule through a tear. Complete tears of the UCL will result in a positive arthrogram. A computed tomographic scan, performed immediately after the arthrogram, can enhance visualization of a capsuloligamentous injury.

Magnetic Resonance Imaging

Magnetic resonance imaging (MRI) may prove to be beneficial in the differential diagnosis of various pathologic elbow conditions. MRI of the elbow is helpful in diagnosing complete UCL tears, particularly when the elbow is injected with saline before testing. A UCL tear is indicated by leakage of dye along the medial side of the elbow both proximally and distally along the medial olecranon. Timmerman and Andrews[50] referred to this finding as a T-sign.

OVERVIEW OF ELBOW REHABILITATION

Rehabilitation after elbow injury or elbow surgery follows a sequential and progressive multiphase approach. The ultimate goal of elbow rehabilitation is to return athletes to their previous functional level as quickly and safely as possible. Several key principles must be addressed when an athlete's elbow is rehabilitated: (1) the effects of immobilization must

---

Box 13-1

General Elbow Rehabilitation Guidelines

PHASE I: IMMEDIATE-MOTION PHASE (WEEK 1)

Goals:
- Improve pain-free range of motion
- Retard muscular atrophy
- Minimize pain and inflammation

Exercises:
- Active and passive range of motion for wrist, elbow, and shoulder motions
- Grades I and II joint mobilization techniques
- Submaximal isometrics for the wrist, elbow, and shoulder complexes
- Local modalities as appropriate

PHASE II: INTERMEDIATE PHASE (WEEKS 2–4)

Goals:
- Normalize motion (particularly elbow extension)
- Improve muscular strength, power, and endurance

Exercises

A. Week 2:
- Isotonic strengthening program for the wrist and elbow musculature
- Elastic tubing exercises for the shoulder musculature
- Local modalities as necessary

B. Week 3:
- Advance the isotonic strengthening program for the upper extremity
- Initiate upper extremity rhythmic stabilization drills
- Initiate isokinetic strengthening exercises for elbow flexion/extension, forearm pronation/supination, and shoulder internal/external rotation

C. Week 4:
- Emphasize eccentric biceps and flexor pronation and concentric triceps activities
- Initiate the Thrower's Ten Exercise Program
- Increase endurance training activities
- Initiate light plyometric drills
- Begin swinging and/or hitting drills

PHASE III: ADVANCED STRENGTHENING (WEEKS 4–8)

Goals:
- Return to functional/athletic participation

Criteria to enter the advanced phase:
- Full nonpainful range of motion
- No pain or tenderness on clinical examination
- Satisfactory clinical examination
- Satisfactory isokinetic test

A. Weeks 4–5:
- Continue strengthening exercises, endurance drills, and flexibility activities
- Thrower's Ten Exercise Program
- Increase plyometric drills
- Increase swinging (hitting) drills

B. Weeks 6–8:
- Initiate phase I of the interval sport program
- Emphasize a pathologic condition–specific maintenance program

PHASE IV: RETURN TO SPORT (WEEKS 6–9)
- Continue the Thrower's Ten Exercise Program
- Continue the flexibility program
- Increase functional drills to unrestricted activity

---

be minimized, (2) healing tissue must not be overstressed, (3) the patient must fulfill certain criteria to advance through each phase of rehabilitation, (4) the program must be based on current scientific and clinical research, (5) the process must be adaptable to each patient and the patient's specific goals, and (6) the rehabilitation program must be a team effort involving the physician, physical therapist, athletic trainer, and patient. Communication between each team member is essential for a successful outcome. The following sections provide an overview of the rehabilitation process after elbow injury (Box 13-1) and surgery (Box 13-2). Discussion of rehabilitation protocols for specific pathologic conditions follows this general overview. In Box 13-3 the rehabilitation goals and criteria for entering each phase of rehabilitation are summarized.

Phase I: Immediate-Motion Phase

The first phase of elbow rehabilitation is the immediate-motion phase. The goals of this phase are to minimize the effects of immobilization, reestablish nonpainful ROM, decrease pain and inflammation, and retard muscular atrophy. The rehabilitation specialist must not overstress healing tissues during this phase.

Early ROM activities are performed to nourish articular cartilage and assist in the synthesis, alignment, and organization of collagen tissue.[51-58] ROM activities are performed in all planes of elbow and wrist motion to prevent the formation of scar tissue and adhesions.[59,60] Reestablishing full elbow extension is the primary goal of early ROM activities. These interventions are designed to minimize the development of elbow flexion contractures.[61-63] The elbow is predisposed to flexion contractures because of the intimate congruency of the joint articulations, the tightness of the joint capsule, and the tendency of adhesions to develop in the anterior capsule after injury. The brachialis muscle also attaches to the capsule and crosses the elbow joint before becoming a tendinous structure. Injury to the elbow may cause excessive scar tissue formation in the brachialis muscle, as well as functional splinting of the elbow.

Grades I and II joint mobilizations may be performed as tolerated during this early phase of rehabilitation. These grades I and II mobilization techniques are used to neuromodulate pain by stimulating type I and type II articular receptors.[64,65] Posterior glides with oscillations are performed in the midrange of elbow motion to assist in regaining full extension. Aggressive mobilization techniques are not used until the later stages of rehabilitation when the pain has subsided.

Box 13-2

Postoperative Elbow Rehabilitation

PHASE I: IMMEDIATE-MOTION PHASE (WEEK 1)

Goals:

- Improve pain-free range of motion
- Decrease pain and swelling
- Retard muscular atrophy

A. Day of surgery: Initiate elbow range of motion gently in a bulky dressing

B. Postoperative days 1 and 2:

- Remove the bulky dressing and replace with an elastic bandage
- Begin hand, wrist, and elbow exercises:
  - Putty/grip strengthening
  - Wrist flexor stretching
  - Wrist extensor stretching
  - Wrist curls
  - Reverse wrist curls
  - Neutral wrist curls
  - Pronation/supination
  - Active/active assisted elbow flexion/extension range of motion

C. Postoperative days 3–7:

- Passive range of motion elbow extension/flexion (to tolerance)
- Grades I/II joint mobilizations
- Begin 1-lb progressive resistance exercises:
  - Wrist curls
  - Reverse wrist curls
  - Neutral curls
  - Pronation/supination

PHASE II: INTERMEDIATE PHASE (WEEKS 2–4)

Goals:

- Improve muscular strength and endurance
- Normalize elbow joint arthrokinematics (particularly elbow extension)

A. Week 2:

- Range of motion exercises (overpressure into extension)
- Add biceps curl and triceps extension
- Continue advancing progressive resistance exercise weight and repetitions as tolerated

B. Week 3:

- Initiate biceps and triceps eccentric exercise program
- Initiate shoulder exercise program:
  - External rotators
  - Internal rotators
  - Deltoid
  - Supraspinatus
  - Scapulothoracic strengthening

PHASE III: ADVANCED STRENGTHENING PHASE (WEEKS 4–8)

Goal:

- Preparation for return to functional activities

Criteria to progress to the advanced phase:

- Full nonpainful range of motion
- No pain or tenderness on clinical examination
- Satisfactory clinical examination
- Satisfactory isokinetic test

Weeks 4–8:

- Thrower's Ten Exercise Program
- Initiate plyometric exercise drills
- Advance drills to emphasize eccentric control, muscular strength, and endurance
- Initiate phase I of the interval throwing program

If the patient continues to have difficulty achieving full extension during ROM and mobilization techniques, a low-load, long-duration stretch may be performed to produce creep of collagen tissue, which will result in tissue elongation.[66-69] The authors find this intervention to be extremely beneficial in regaining full elbow extension.[60,68,69] The athlete lies supine with a towel roll placed under the brachium to act as a cushion and fulcrum. Light-resistance exercise tubing is applied to the wrist of the patient and secured to the table or to a dumbbell on the ground (Fig. 13-6). The patient is instructed to relax as much as possible for 10 to 12 minutes. The amount of resistance applied should be of low magnitude to enable the athlete to tolerate the stretch for the entire duration without pain or muscle spasm.

The aggressiveness of stretching and mobilization techniques is dictated by the healing constraints of the involved tissues, as well as the amount of motion and end-feel of the joint complex. If the patient exhibits a decrease in motion and hard end-feel without pain, aggressive stretching and mobilization techniques may be used. Conversely, a patient exhibiting pain before resistance or an empty end-feel should be progressed slowly with gentle stretching.

Cryotherapy and high-voltage pulsed galvanic stimulation may be performed as required to assist in reducing pain and inflammation. When the acute inflammatory phase has passed, moist heat, warm whirlpool, ultrasound, or any combination of these modalities may be used at the onset of treatment to prepare the tissue for stretching and improve the extensibility of the capsule and musculotendinous structures.

The early phases of rehabilitation must also focus on retarding muscular atrophy. Subpainful and submaximal isometric exercises are performed initially for the elbow flexors and extensors and for the wrist flexor, extensor, pronator, and supinator muscle groups. Isometrics should be performed at multiple angles for two to three sets of 10 repetitions, with each contraction being held for 6 to 8 seconds. Shoulder isometrics may also be performed during this phase but with caution during internal and external rotation exercises if painful. Alternating rhythmic stabilization drills for shoulder flexion/extension/horizontal abduction/adduction and shoulder internal/external rotation are performed to begin reestablishing proprioception and neuromuscular control of the upper extremity.

Box 13-3

Rehabilitation Goals for Each Phase of Elbow Rehabilitation

PHASE I: IMMEDIATE MOTION

Goals:

- Minimize effects of immobilization
- Reestablish nonpainful range of motion
- Decrease pain and inflammation
- Retard muscular atrophy

The rehabilitation specialist must not overstress healing tissues during this phase

PHASE II: INTERMEDIATE PHASE

Criteria for entering this phase:

- Patient exhibits full range of motion
- Minimal pain and tenderness
- Good (4/5) manual muscle test of the elbow flexor and extensor musculature

Goals:

- Enhance elbow and upper extremity mobility
- Improve muscular strength and endurance
- Reestablish neuromuscular control of the elbow complex

PHASE III: ADVANCED STRENGTHENING

Criteria for entering this phase:

- Full nonpainful range of motion
- No pain or tenderness
- Strength that is 70% of the contralateral extremity

Goals:

- Involves progression of activities to prepare the athlete for sport participation
- Gradually increase strength, power, endurance, and neuromuscular control to prepare for gradual return to sport

PHASE IV: RETURN TO SPORT

Criteria for entering this phase:

- Full range of motion
- No pain or tenderness on clinical examination
- Satisfactory isokinetic test
- Satisfactory clinical examination

Goals:

- Allow the athlete to progressively return to full competition using an interval return to the sport program
- Sport-specific functional drills performed to prepare the athlete for the stresses involved in each particular sport

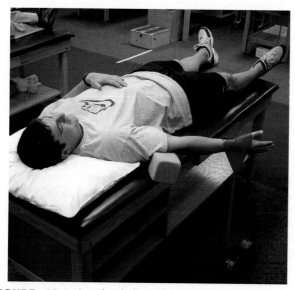

FIGURE 13-6 Low-load, long-duration stretch into elbow extension.

Phase II: Intermediate Phase

Phase II, the intermediate phase, is initiated when the patient exhibits full ROM, minimal pain and tenderness, and a good result (4/5) on the manual muscle test of the elbow flexor and extensor musculature. The emphasis in this phase includes enhancing elbow and upper extremity mobility, improving muscular strength and endurance, and reestablishing neuromuscular control of the elbow complex.

Stretching exercises are continued to maintain full elbow flexion and extension. Mobilization may be progressed to more aggressive grade III techniques as needed to apply stretch to the capsular tissue in the end range. Flexibility activities are progressed during this phase to focus on wrist flexion, extension, pronation, and supination excursion. Shoulder flexibility is also maintained in athletes with an emphasis on flexion, external and internal rotation, and horizontal adduction.

Strengthening exercises are advanced during this phase to include isotonic movements. Emphasis is placed on elbow flexion and extension, wrist flexion and extension, and forearm pronation and supination. The weight of the arm is initially used before progressing to a 1-lb dumbbell. Resistance is then advanced in a controlled progressive resistance fashion by 1 lb/wk to gradually stress the involved tissues. The shoulder and scapular muscles are also included in a progressive resistance program during the later stages of this phase. Emphasis is placed on strengthening the shoulder external rotators and scapular muscles and training eccentric control of the elbow flexors. Shoulder internal and external rotation is performed with exercise tubing at 0° of abduction; standing scaption with external rotation (full can), standing abduction, prone horizontal abduction, and prone rowing are all included in this phase.

Muscular endurance activities are also incorporated during this phase of the rehabilitation program. High-repetition, low-resistance dumbbell exercises and an upper body ergometer may be used to accomplish these goals.

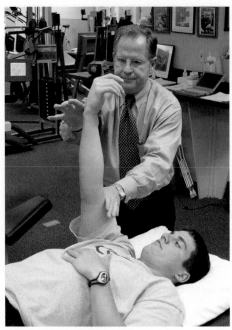

FIGURE 13-7 Manual proprioceptive neuromuscular facilitation D2 pattern with rhythmic stabilization.

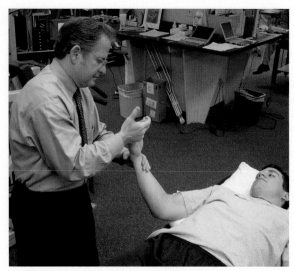

FIGURE 13-8 Manual resisted elbow and wrist flexion using both concentric and eccentric contractions of the elbow flexors.

Neuromuscular control exercises are initiated in this phase to enhance the ability of the muscle to control the elbow joint during athletic activities. These exercises include proprioceptive neuromuscular facilitation with rhythmic stabilization (Fig. 13-7) and slow-reversal, manual resistance elbow/wrist flexion drills (Fig. 13-8).

Phase III: Advanced Strengthening Phase

The third phase involves a progression of activities to prepare the athlete for participation in sports. The goals of this phase are to gradually increase strength, power, endurance, and neuromuscular control to prepare the athlete for a gradual return to sport. Specific criteria that must be met before the athlete enters this phase include full nonpainful ROM, no pain or tenderness, and strength that is 70% of that on the contralateral extremity.

Advanced strengthening activities during this phase include aggressive strengthening exercises emphasizing high-speed and eccentric contractions, as well as plyometric activities. Strengthening exercises are progressed to include the Thrower's Ten Exercise Program (see Figures A-1 through A-10 [in Appendix A] on Expert Consult @ www.ExpertConsult.com). These exercises were designed with findings from numerous EMG studies to strengthen all the shoulder, scapular, elbow, and wrist muscles that are used during upper extremity athletic activities.[70-73] Internal and external rotation exercises with exercise tubing are progressed to a functional position of 90° of shoulder abduction and 90° of elbow flexion. Exercises should be performed at both slow and fast speeds. Scapulothoracic exercises are progressed to include prone horizontal abduction at 100° and full external rotation, as well as prone rows into external rotation.

Elbow flexion exercises are advanced to emphasize eccentric control of elbow extension. The biceps muscle is an important stabilizer during the follow-through phase of overhead throwing; it eccentrically controls deceleration of the elbow and prevents pathologic abutting of the olecranon within the fossa.[70,74] Elbow flexion can be performed with elastic tubing to emphasize slow and fast concentric and eccentric contractions.

Aggressive strengthening exercises with weight machines are also incorporated during this phase. These exercises most commonly begin with bench presses, seated rowing, and front latissimus dorsi pull-downs.

Exercises to achieve neuromuscular control are progressed to include side-lying external rotation with manual resistance. Concentric and eccentric external rotation is performed against the clinician's resistance with the addition of rhythmic stabilization (Fig. 13-9). This manual resistance exercise may be progressed to standing external rotation with exercise tubing at 0° (Fig. 13-10) and finally at 90° of shoulder abduction.

Plyometric drills are an extremely beneficial form of exercise for training the upper extremity musculature.[2,59] The physiologic principles of plyometric exercise involve eccentric prestretching of the muscle tissue, thereby stimulating the muscle spindle to produce a more forceful concentric contraction. Plyometric exercises are performed with a weighted medicine ball during the later stages of this phase to train the upper extremity musculature to develop and withstand high levels of stress. Plyometric exercises initially involve two-handed chest passing, side-to-side throwing, and overhead soccer throwing. These exercises may be progressed to include one-handed activities such as 90/90 throws (Fig. 13-11), external and internal rotation throws at 0° of abduction (Fig. 13-12), and wall dribbles. Specific plyometric drills for the forearm musculature include wrist flexion flips (Fig. 13-13) and extension grips.

Phase IV: Return-to-Sport Phase

The final phase of elbow rehabilitation, the return-to-sport phase, allows the athlete to progressively return to full competition with use of an interval sport program. Sport-specific

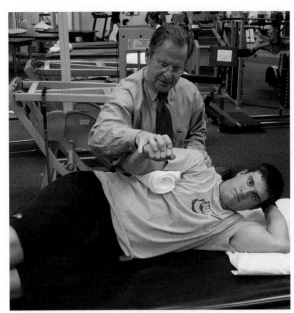

FIGURE 13-9 Manual resisted side-lying external resistance using both concentric and eccentric contractions of the external rotators.

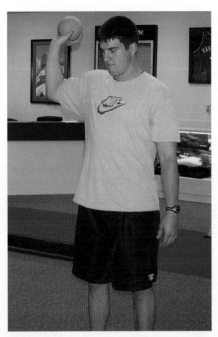

FIGURE 13-11 One-handed plyometric throws at 90° of shoulder abduction and 90° of elbow flexion using a 2-lb weighted ball.

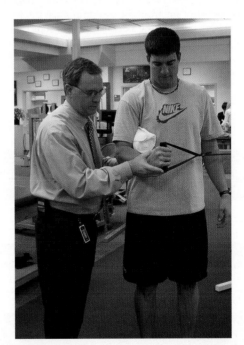

FIGURE 13-10 External rotation at 0° of shoulder abduction performed with tubing and manual resistance.

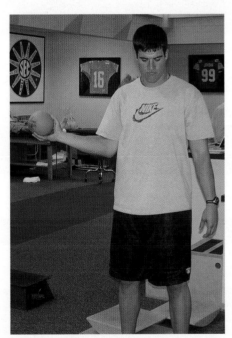

FIGURE 13-12 One-handed plyometric throws at 0° of abduction using a 2-lb weighted ball.

functional drills are performed to prepare the athlete for the stresses involved in each particular sport.

Before an athlete is allowed to begin the return-to-sport phase of rehabilitation, full ROM, no pain or tenderness on clinical examination, a satisfactory isokinetic test, and a satisfactory clinical examination must be exhibited by the athlete. Isokinetic testing is commonly used to determine the readiness of the athlete to begin an interval sport program. Athletes are routinely tested in elbow flexion/extension, shoulder internal/external rotation, and shoulder abduction/adduction at 180 and 300°/sec. Satisfactory isokinetic testing parameters are outlined in Table 13-3.

On achieving the criteria that have been outlined, a formal interval sport program should be initiated. An overhead thrower begins with a long-toss interval throwing program (see Appendix B on Expert Consult @ www.ExpertConsult.com).

The athlete throws three times per week with a day off from throwing in between. Each step must be performed at least two times on separate days without symptoms before the athlete is allowed to advance to the next step. Throwing should be performed without pain or any significant increase in symptoms. If symptoms are experienced at a particular step in the program, the athlete is instructed to regress to the previous step until the symptoms subside. It is important for the overhead athlete to perform stretching and an abbreviated strengthening program before and after performing the interval sport program. Typically, overhead throwers should warm up, stretch, and perform one set of their exercise program before throwing, followed by two additional sets of exercises after throwing. This provides an adequate warm-up but also ensures maintenance of the ROM and flexibility needed by the shoulder joint.

After completion of a long-toss program, pitchers will progress to phase II of the throwing program: throwing off a mound (see Appendix B [online]). In phase II the number of throws, their intensity, and the type of pitches are progressed to gradually increase functional stress on the upper extremity.

Interval sport programs for tennis and golf follow the same guidelines as those for the baseball program. A specific interval program for tennis is outlined in Appendix B (online). As the athlete progresses through the program, the number of forehand and backhand shots is gradually increased. Overhead serving is typically initiated during the third week of the program, and games are allowed during the fourth week if the symptoms have not been exacerbated.

Appendix B (online) outlines an interval golf program. The program begins with simple putting and chipping and progresses to include short iron swings by the end of week 1, medium iron swings by week 2, and long iron swings by week 3. Medium and long iron shots are hit from a tee to minimize the force at the elbow observed when taking a divot. Use of woods is initiated at the end of week 3 and progressed to include drives by the fourth week. The athlete can play nine holes at the end of the fourth week if asymptomatic.

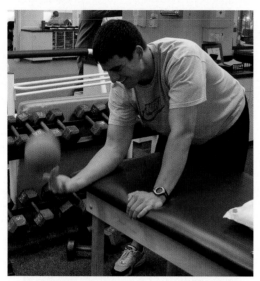

FIGURE 13-13 Plyometric wrist flips.

Table 13-3 Satisfactory Isokinetic Test Results

Bilateral Comparisons		
Velocity (°/sec)	Elbow (Flex)	Elbow (Ext)
180	110-120%	105-115%
300	105-115%	100-110%

Velocity (°/sec)	Shoulder (ER)	Shoulder (IR)	Shoulder (Abd)	Shoulder (Add)
180	98-105%	110-120%	98-105%	110-128%
300	85-95%	105-115%	96-102%	111-129%

Unilateral Muscle Ratios				
Velocity (°/sec)	Elbow (Flex/Ext)	Shoulder (ER/IR)	Shoulder (Abd/Add)	Shoulder (ER/Abd)
180	70-80%	66-76%	78-84%	67-75%
300	63-69%	61-71%	88-94%	67-75%

Peak Torque-to–Body Weight Ratios				
Velocity (°/sec)	Shoulder (ER)	Shoulder (IR)	Shoulder (Abd)	Shoulder (Add)
180	18-23%	28-33%	26-33%	32-38%
300	12-20%	25-30%	20-25%	28-34%

Abd, Abduction; *Add*, adduction; *ER*, external rotation; *Ext*, extension; *Flex*, flexion; *IR*, internal rotation.

COMMON SPORT-RELATED INJURIES

Medial and Lateral Epicondylitis

Medial and lateral epicondylitis may result from numerous factors, many of which have been discussed previously. The majority of causes are related to repetitive sport-specific microtrauma and poor biomechanics. Medially, overhead throwers most often exhibit pronator tendonitis and golfers exhibit wrist flexor tendonitis, whereas lateral epicondylitis most often occurs in tennis players. Athletes are most often seen with tenderness near the epicondyle and along the flexor-pronator or extensor-supinator muscle masses, which may be exacerbated by contraction or stretching of the musculature.

During the clinical examination an attempt should be made to distinguish the involved structures. For medial epicondylitis, wrist flexion against manual resistance should be performed, as well as pronation, to determine whether a pronation strain has occurred. For lateral epicondylitis, testing of the extensor carpi radialis longus is performed with the elbow flexed 30° and resistance applied to the second metacarpal bone.[48] The extensor carpi radialis brevis is tested with the elbow fully flexed and resistance applied to the third metacarpal bone.[48] In addition, the extensor carpi ulnaris can be differentiated by resisting ulnar deviation.[48]

The nonoperative approach for the treatment of epicondylitis is outlined in Box 13-4. The program focuses on diminishing pain and gradually improving muscular strength. The primary goals of rehabilitation are to control the applied loads and create an environment for healing. The initial treatment consists of the use of a warm whirlpool, laser, transverse friction massage, stretching exercises, and light strengthening exercises to stimulate a healing response. The authors recommend focusing on eccentric training for chronic tendinopathies, such as tendinosis. Conversely, if the condition is acute and is causing symptoms of tendinitis, an antiinflammatory program consisting of the application of ice, iontophoresis, stretching, and light concentric strengthening is used. High-voltage pulsed galvanic stimulation and cryotherapy are used after treatment to decrease pain and postexercise inflammation. The athlete should be cautioned against excessive gripping activities. When the athlete's symptoms have subsided, an aggressive stretching and strengthening program with emphasis on eccentric contractions can be initiated. Wrist flexion and extension activities should be performed initially with the elbow flexed 30° to 45° to decrease tissue stress. When the athlete can perform these isotonic exercises with a 3-lb weight, they can be done with the elbow fully extended. A gradual progression through plyometric activities precedes the initiation of an interval sport program. Because poor mechanics is often a cause of this condition, analysis of sport mechanics and proper supervision through the interval sport program are critical for successful return to symptom-free athletic participation.

Box 13-4

Epicondylitis Rehabilitation Program

PHASE I: ACUTE PHASE

Goals:
- Decrease inflammation
- Promote tissue healing
- Retard muscular atrophy

Cryotherapy
Whirlpool
Stretching to increase flexibility, wrist extension/flexion, elbow extension/flexion, forearm supination/pronation
Isometrics to increase wrist extension/flexion, elbow extension/flexion, forearm supination/pronation
High-voltage galvanic stimulation
Phonophoresis
Friction massage
Iontophoresis (with antiinflammatory agent, e.g., dexamethasone)
Avoidance of painful movements (e.g., gripping)

PHASE II: SUBACUTE PHASE

Goals:
- Improve flexibility
- Increase muscular strength/endurance
- Increase functional activities/return to function

Exercises:
- Emphasize concentric/eccentric strengthening
- Concentration on involved muscle group
- Wrist extension/flexion
- Forearm pronation/supination
- Elbow flexion/extension
- Initiate shoulder strengthening (if deficiencies noted)
- Continue flexibility exercises
- May use counterforce brace
- Continue use of cryotherapy after exercise/function
- Gradual return to stressful activities
- Gradually reinitiate once painful movements

PHASE III: CHRONIC PHASE

Goals:
- Improve muscular strength and endurance
- Maintain/enhance flexibility
- Gradual return-to-sport/high-level activities

Exercises:
- Continue strengthening exercises (emphasize eccentric/concentric)
- Continue to emphasize deficiencies in shoulder and elbow strength
- Continue flexibility exercises
- Gradually decrease use of counterforce brace
- Use of cryotherapy as needed
- Gradual return to sport activity

Equipment modification (grip size, string tension, playing surface)
Emphasize maintenance program

Ulnar Neuropathy

Numerous theories about the cause of ulnar neuropathy of the elbow in athletes have been proposed.[75] Ulnar nerve changes can result from tensile forces, compressive forces, or nerve instability. Any one or a combination of these mechanisms may be responsible for producing ulnar nerve symptoms.

A leading mechanism for tensile force on the ulnar nerve is valgus stress. This may also be coupled with an external rotation–supination stress overload mechanism. The traction forces are further magnified when underlying valgus instability from a UCL injury is present. Ulnar neuropathy is often a secondary pathologic consequence of UCL insufficiency.

Compression of the ulnar nerve is frequently due to hypertrophy of the surrounding soft tissues or the presence of scar tissue. The nerve may also be trapped between the two heads of the flexor carpi ulnaris.

Repetitive flexion and extension of the elbow with an unstable nerve can irritate or inflame the nerve. The nerve may sublux or rest on the medial epicondyle, thereby rendering it vulnerable to direct trauma. Complete dislocation of the nerve may occur anteriorly and lead to friction neuritis.

Three stages of ulnar neuropathy are recognized.[76] The first stage includes an acute onset of radicular symptoms. The second stage is characterized by recurrence of the symptoms as the athlete attempts to return to competition. The third stage is associated with persistent motor weakness and sensory changes. When the athlete is seen in the third stage of injury, conservative management may not be effective.

Clinical examination often reveals tenderness along the cubital tunnel. Additionally, the clinician may perform a Tinel test by tapping on the cubital tunnel. A positive Tinel test result consists of paresthesia or tingling over the ulnar nerve distribution.

Nonoperative treatment of ulnar neuropathy focuses on diminishing ulnar nerve irritation, enhancing dynamic medial joint stability, and gradually returning the athlete to competition.

After the diagnosis of ulnar neuropathy, throwing athletes are instructed to discontinue throwing activities for at least 4 weeks. The athlete progresses through the immediate-motion and intermediate phases of rehabilitation over the course of 4 to 6 weeks with emphasis placed on eccentric control and dynamic stabilization drills. Plyometric exercises are performed to facilitate dynamic stabilization of the medial side of the elbow. The athlete is allowed to begin an interval throwing program when the following criteria have been fulfilled: (1) full pain-free ROM, (2) satisfactory findings on clinical examination, (3) no neurologic symptoms, (4) adequate medial stability, and (5) satisfactory muscular performance. The athlete may gradually return to sport if progression through an interval sport program does not reproduce further neurologic symptoms.

Ulnar Nerve Transposition

Surgical transposition of the ulnar nerve entails stabilizing the nerve with fascial slings. Caution is taken to not overstress the soft tissue structures involved when relocating the nerve. The rehabilitation process after ulnar nerve transposition is outlined in Box 13-5. A posterior splint at 90° of elbow flexion is used for the first 2 weeks postoperatively to prevent excessive ROM and tension on the nerve while the fascial slings heal. Use of the splint is discontinued at week 2, and light ROM activities are initiated. Full ROM is usually restored by weeks 3 to 4. Gentle isotonic strengthening is begun during week 4 and progressed to the full Thrower's Ten Exercise Program (see Appendix A [online]) by 6 weeks after surgery. Aggressive strengthening, including eccentric and plyometric training, can typically be incorporated by weeks 7 to 8 and an interval sport program at weeks 8 to 9 if all previously outlined criteria have been met. Return to sport can usually take place between postoperative weeks 12 and 16.

Valgus Extension Overload

Valgus extension overload occurs in repetitive sport activities such as throwing, tennis serving, and javelin throwing. Injury generally occurs during the acceleration or deceleration phase as the olecranon wedges up against the medial olecranon fossa during elbow extension.[33] This mechanism may result in osteophyte formation and can potentially produce loose bodies. Repetitive extension stress from the triceps may further contribute to this injury. A certain degree of underlying valgus elbow laxity is often seen in these athletes and further facilitates osteophyte formation through compression of the radiocapitellar joint and the posteromedial aspect of the elbow.[77]

Athletes typically have pain along the posteromedial region of the elbow that is exacerbated by forced extension and valgus stress. The clinical test for valgus extension overload involves the clinician grasping the elbow in a flexed position. As the clinician forces the elbow into extension, a valgus stress is simultaneously applied to the elbow (Fig. 13-14). The clinician palpates the posteromedial region of the joint for tenderness and crepitation. Pain over the posteromedial olecranon process signifies a positive test result.[33]

A conservative treatment approach is often attempted before surgical intervention is considered. Initial treatment involves relieving the posterior aspect of the elbow of pain and inflammation. As symptoms subside and ROM normalizes, strengthening exercises are initiated. Emphasis is placed on improving eccentric strength of the elbow flexors in an attempt to control the rapid extension that occurs at the elbow during athletic activities. Manual resistance exercises consisting of concentric and eccentric elbow flexion, as well as elbow flexion, are performed with exercise tubing to accentuate the functional control required. Another key goal of the nonoperative program is to improve dynamic stabilization of the medial aspect of the elbow. Exercises should focus on the flexor pronator muscle group.

Excision of Posterior Olecranon Osteophytes

Surgical excision of posterior olecranon osteophytes is performed with an osteotome or motorized bur. Approximately 5 to 10 mm of the olecranon tip is typically removed concomitantly, and a motorized bur is used to contour the coronoid, olecranon tip, and fossa to prevent further impingement with extreme flexion and extension.[78,79]

The rehabilitation program after arthroscopic excision of posterior olecranon osteophytes is slightly more conservative in restoring full elbow extension because of postsurgical pain. ROM is progressed within the athlete's tolerance. Normally, by the tenth postoperative day the athlete should exhibit at least

Box 13-5

Rehabilitation After Ulnar Nerve Transposition

PHASE I: IMMEDIATE POSTOPERATIVE PHASE (WEEKS 1–2)

Goals:
- Allow soft tissue healing of the relocated nerve
- Decrease pain and inflammation
- Retard muscular atrophy

A. Week 1:
- Posterior splint at 90° of elbow flexion with the wrist free for motion (sling for comfort)
- Compression dressing
- Exercises such as gripping exercises, wrist ROM, and shoulder isometrics

B. Week 2:
- Discontinue the posterior splint
- Progress to greater elbow ROM (PROM of 15° to 120°)
- Initiate elbow and wrist isometrics
- Continue shoulder isometrics

PHASE II: INTERMEDIATE PHASE (WEEKS 3–7)

Goals:
- Restore full pain-free ROM
- Improve strength, power, and endurance of the upper extremity musculature
- Gradually increase functional demands

A. Week 3:
- Advance elbow ROM with emphasis on full extension

- Initiate flexibility exercise for wrist extension/flexion, forearm supination/pronation, and elbow extension/flexion
- Initiate strengthening exercises for wrist extension/flexion, forearm supination/pronation, and elbow extension/flexion, as well as a shoulder program

B. Week 6:
- Continue all exercises listed above
- Initiate light sport activities

PHASE III: ADVANCED STRENGTHENING PHASE (WEEKS 8–12)

Goals:
- Increase strength, power, and endurance
- Gradually initiate sporting activities

A. Week 8:
- Initiate eccentric exercise program
- Initiate plyometric exercise drills
- Continue shoulder and elbow strengthening and flexibility exercises
- Initiate interval throwing program

PHASE IV: RETURN-TO-SPORT PHASE (WEEKS 12–16)

Goals:
- Gradually return to sporting activities

A. Week 12:
- Return to competitive throwing
- Continue Throwers' Ten Exercise Program

PROM, Passive ROM; *ROM*, range of motion.

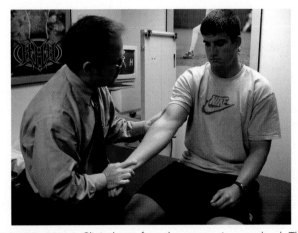

FIGURE 13-14 Clinical test for valgus extension overload. The clinician forcefully extends the elbow while applying a valgus stress.

15° to 100° of ROM and 10° to 110° by day 14. Full ROM is typically restored by days 20 to 25 after surgery. The rate of progression of ROM is most often limited by pain from osseous structures and synovial joint inflammation.

The strengthening program is progressed in a similar fashion to that discussed previously. Isometric exercises are performed

for the first 10 to 14 days. Isotonic strengthening is incorporated from weeks 2 to 6. The full Thrower's Ten Exercise Program is initiated by week 6. An interval sport program can typically be started by weeks 10 to 12. The rehabilitation focus is similar to that for nonoperative treatment of valgus extension overload, with an emphasis on eccentric control of the elbow flexors and dynamic stabilization of the medial aspect of the elbow.

Andrews and Timmerman[80] reported on the outcome of elbow surgery in 72 professional baseball players. Sixty-five percent of these athletes exhibited a posterior olecranon osteophyte and 25% of the athletes who underwent isolated olecranon excision later required UCL reconstruction.[80] These results may suggest that subtle medial instability may accelerate osteophyte formation.

Conversely, the effects of excising the posterior olecranon on medial elbow stability should elicit a certain amount of concern. Because such excision alters the static stability of the humeroulnar articulation, medial elbow stability may be compromised. Andrews et al[78] examined the amount of stress applied to the anterior bundle of the UCL after varying degrees of excision of the posterior olecranon. UCL strain was measured with an intact olecranon and after 2-mm incremental resections of the medial olecranon up to 8 mm. Further resection of 13 mm was also performed. The UCL was then strained to failure during an applied valgus stress at degrees of elbow flexion varying from

50° to 100°. The results indicated no significant differences in strain on the UCL with changes in the extent of the osteotomy performed with a given applied load and angle of elbow flexion. Thus, it appears that UCL strain is not significantly increased after posterior olecranon resection.

Ulnar Collateral Ligament Injury

Injuries to the UCL are becoming increasingly more common in overhead throwing athletes, although the higher incidence of injury may be due to an improved ability to accurately diagnose these injuries. As described briefly in the section on biomechanics, the elbow experiences a tremendous amount of valgus stress during overhead throwing. These stresses approach the ultimate failure load of the ligament with each throw. The repetitive nature of overhead sports activities such as baseball pitching, football passing, tennis serving, and javelin throwing further increases susceptibility for UCL injury by exposing the ligament to repetitive microtraumatic forces.

An athlete with an injury to the UCL usually complains of pain and tenderness in the medial aspect of the elbow. Generalized joint effusion may also be present. The athlete's subjective history typically reveals either recurring medial elbow symptoms or a single traumatic incident of medial elbow pain while throwing. The athlete recalls a sudden, sharp, medial elbow pain, often with a popping sensation. As described earlier, the physical examination and isolated analysis of UCL laxity via prone and supine valgus stress testing are critical for accurate assessment. Additionally, MRI enhanced by the intraarticular injection of dye may be useful in evaluating an athlete with a suspected UCL injury. A UCL tear is indicated by a T-sign as discussed previously.[50]

Various opinions exist about the efficacy of nonoperative treatment of UCL strains or partial tears in throwing athletes. If an injury to the UCL is suspected, the rehabilitation program outlined in Box 13-6 is initiated. ROM is initially permitted in a nonpainful arc of motion, usually 10° to 100°, to allow a decrease in inflammation and alignment of collagen tissue. A brace may be used to restrict motion and prevent valgus strain. Isometric exercises are performed for the shoulder, elbow, and wrist to deter muscular atrophy. Ice and antiinflammatory medications are prescribed to control pain and inflammation.

ROM of both flexion and extension are gradually increased during the second phase of treatment as tolerated. Full ROM should be achieved by at least 3 to 4 weeks after surgery. Rhythmic stabilization exercises are initiated to develop dynamic stabilization and neuromuscular control of the upper extremity. As dynamic stability is advanced, isotonic exercises are incorporated for the entire upper extremity.

The advanced strengthening phase is usually initiated at 6 to 7 weeks after injury. During this phase the athlete is progressed to the isotonic strengthening program and plyometric exercises in the Thrower's Ten Exercise Program (see Appenidx A [online]). After performing the Thrower's Ten Exercise Program for 3 to 4 weeks, the athlete is progressed to the Advanced Thrower's Ten Program (see Figures D-1 through D-21 [in Appendix D] on Expert Consult @ www. ExpertConsult.com). An interval sport program is initiated

when the athlete regains full motion, adequate strength, and dynamic stability of the elbow. The athlete is allowed to return to sport after asymptomatic completion of an appropriate interval sport program. If symptoms continue to persist, the athlete's condition is reassessed, and surgical intervention is considered.

Box 13-6

Nonoperative Rehabilitation of the Ulnar Collateral Ligament

ACUTE PHASE

Goals:
- Diminish ulnar nerve inflammation
- Restore normal motion
- Maintain/improve muscular strength

1. Brace (optional)
2. Range of motion: restore full nonpainful range of motion as soon as possible. Initiate stretching exercises for the wrist, forearm, and elbow musculature
3. Strengthening exercises: If the elbow is extremely painful and/or inflamed, use isometrics for approximately 1 week. Initiate isotonic strengthening:
- Wrist flexion/extension
- Forearm supination/pronation
- Elbow flexion/extension
- Shoulder program

4. Pain control/inflammation control:
- Warm whirlpool
- Cryotherapy
- High-voltage galvanic stimulation

ADVANCED STRENGTHENING PHASE (WEEKS 3–6)

Goals:
- Improve strength, power, and endurance
- Enhance Dyonics joint stability
- Initiate high-speed training

1. Exercise—Thrower's Ten Exercise Program:
- Eccentric exercises for the wrist/forearm muscles
- Rhythmic stabilization drills for the elbow joint
- Isokinetics for the elbow flexor/extensor
- Plyometric exercise drills

2. Continue stretching exercises

RETURN-TO-SPORT PHASE (WEEKS 4–6)

Goals:
- Gradual return to functional activities
- Enhanced muscular performance

Criteria to begin throwing:
- Full nonpainful range of motion
- Satisfactory clinical examination
- Satisfactory muscular performance

1. Initiate interval sport program
2. Continue Thrower's Ten Exercise Program
3. Continue all stretching exercise

Reconstruction of the Ulnar Collateral Ligament

The goal of surgical reconstruction of the UCL is to restore the stabilizing functions of the anterior bundle of the UCL.[24,81] The palmaris longus or an alternative graft source is harvested and passed in a figure-of-eight pattern through drill holes in the sublime tubercle of the ulna and the medial epicondyle.[82] If the palmaris longus tendon is not available, a gracilis graft can be used. At our center the contralateral gracilis tendon is frequently used. An ulnar nerve transposition is often performed at the time of UCL reconstruction.[24,82]

The docking procedure is another surgical technique used to reconstruct the UCL. This procedure has been thoroughly described by Dodson et al[83] and Bowers et al.[84] The docking proce-dure involves the use of a muscle-splitting technique for visualiza-tion and a single humeral tunnel for surgical fixation of the graft.

The rehabilitation program after UCL reconstruction varies according to the surgical technique, the method of transposition of the ulnar nerve, and the overall extent of injury to the elbow. The rehabilitation programs currently used by the authors after UCL reconstruction is outlined in Boxes 13-7 and 13-8.[60,85] The athlete is placed in a posterior splint with the elbow immobi-lized at 90° of flexion for the first 7 days postoperatively. This allows adequate healing of the UCL graft and soft tissue slings involved in the nerve transposition. The athlete is allowed to perform wrist ROM, gripping, and submaximal isometrics for the wrist and elbow. The athlete is progressed from the poste-rior splint to an elbow ROM brace, which is adjusted to allow

---

Box 13-7

Accelerated Postoperative Rehabilitation After Ulnar Collateral Ligament Injury (Gracilis Graft)

PHASE I. IMMEDIATE POSTOPERATIVE PHASE (WEEKS 1–3)

Goals:
- Protect healing tissue
- Decrease pain/inflammation
- Retard muscular atrophy
- Protect the graft site—allow healing

A. Postoperative Week 1

Brace: Posterior splint at 90° of elbow flexion
Range of motion:
- Wrist AROM extension/flexion immediately postoperatively
- Knee ROM on day 1

Compression dressings:
- Elbow postoperative compression dressing (5-7 days)
- Calf (graft site) compression dressing in 7-10 days

Exercises:
- Gripping exercises
- Wrist ROM
- Shoulder isometrics (no shoulder ER)
- Biceps isometrics
- No involved leg exercises in the first week

Cryotherapy: Elbow joint and graft site below the knee
Crutch: Use one crutch as needed for 3-5 days

B. Postoperative Week 2

Brace: Elbow ROM of 15° to 105° (gradually increase ROM—5° of extension/10° of flexion per week)

Exercises:
- Continue all exercises listed above
- Elbow ROM in a brace (30° to 105°)
- Initiate elbow extension isometrics
- Continue knee ROM exercises

Initiate light scar mobilization over the distal incision (graft)
Cryotherapy: Continue applying ice to the elbow and graft site

C. Postoperative Week 3

Brace: Elbow ROM of 5°/10° to 115°/120°
Exercises:
- Continue all exercises listed above
- Elbow ROM in a brace
- Initiate AROM of the wrist and elbow (no resistance)
- Initiate light hamstring stretching
- Initiate AROM of the shoulder:
  - Full can
  - Lateral raises
  - ER/IR tubing
  - Elbow flexion/extension
- Initiate light scapular-strengthening exercises
- Initiate bicycle for lower extremity ROM and strength
- May initiate light hamstring isometrics

PHASE II. INTERMEDIATE PHASE (WEEKS 4–7)

Goals:
- Gradual increase to full ROM
- Promote healing of repaired tissue
- Regain and improve muscular strength
- Restore full function of the graft site

A. Week 4

Brace: Elbow ROM at 0° to 135°
Exercises:
- Begin light resistance exercises for the arm (1 lb):
  - Wrist curls, extensions, pronation, supination
  - Elbow extension/flexion
- Advance the shoulder program with emphasis on rotator cuff and scapular strengthening
- Initiate shoulder strengthening with light dumbbells
- Isometrics for the hamstrings and calf muscles

B. Week 5

ROM: Elbow ROM at 0° to 135°
Discontinue the brace
Continue all exercises: Advance all shoulder and upper extremity exercises (advance weight 1 lb)

(Continued)

Box 13-7

Accelerated Postoperative Rehabilitation After Ulnar Collateral Ligament Injury (Gracilis Graft)—cont'd

C. Week 6

AROM: 0° to 145° without a brace or full ROM

Exercises:

- Initiate Thrower's Ten Exercise Program
- Increase elbow-strengthening exercises
- Initiate shoulder ER strengthening
- Advance the shoulder program
- Initiate isotonic strengthening for the graft site hamstrings/calf

D. Week 7

Progress to more advanced phases of the Thrower's Ten Exercise
    Program (increase weights)

Initiate PNF diagonal patterns (light)

**PHASE III. ADVANCED STRENGTHENING PHASE
(WEEKS 8–14)**

Goals:

- Increase strength, power, and endurance
- Maintain full elbow ROM
- Gradually initiate sporting activities

A. Week 8

Exercises:

- Initiate eccentric elbow flexion/extension
- Continue isotonic program: forearm and wrist
- Continue shoulder program—Thrower's Ten Exercise Program
- Manual resistance diagonal patterns
- Initiate plyometric exercise program (two-handed plyometrics
  close to the body only):
  - Chest pass
  - Side throw close to the body
- Continue stretching the calf and hamstrings

B. Week 10

Exercises:

- Continue all exercises listed above
- Program plyometrics to two-handed drills away from the body:
  - Side-to-side throws
  - Soccer throws
  - Side throws

C. Weeks 12–14

Continue all exercises

Initiate isotonic machine strengthening exercises (if desired):

- Bench press (seated)
- Latissimus pull-down

Initiate golf, swimming

Initiate interval hitting program

**PHASE IV. RETURN-TO-SPORT PHASE
(WEEKS 14–32)**

Goals:

- Continue to increase strength, power, and endurance of the
  upper extremity musculature
- Gradual return to sport activities

A. Week 14

Exercises:

- Continue strengthening program
- Emphasis on elbow and wrist strengthening and flexibility
  exercises
- Maintain full elbow ROM
- Initiate one-handed plyometric throwing (stationary throws)
- Initiate one-handed wall dribble
- Initiate one-handed baseball throws into a wall

B. Week 16

Exercises:

- Initiate interval throwing program (phase I; long-toss
  program)
- Continue Thrower's Ten Exercise Program and plyometrics
- Continue to stretch before and after throwing

C. Weeks 22–24

Exercises: Progress to phase II throwing (once phase I is
    successfully completed)

D. Weeks 30–32

Exercises: Gradually progress to competitive throwing/sports

AROM, Active ROM; *ER,* external rotation; *IR,* internal rotation; *PNF,* proprioceptive neuromuscular facilitation; *ROM,* range of motion.

ROM from 30° to 100° of flexion. Motion is increased by 5° of extension and 10° of flexion thereafter to restore full ROM (0° to 145°) by the end of week 6. Use of the brace is discontinued by weeks 5 to 6 after surgery. A recent change in our rehabilitation is to allow earlier return of full elbow ROM. We prefer full elbow extension to occur by weeks 4 to 5. Bernas et al[86] reported minimal to no strain on the UCL from 0° to approximately 50° to 60° of flexion. Thus, it appears safe to obtain full extension soon after surgery.

Isometric exercises are progressed to include light-resistance isotonic exercises at week 4 and the full Thrower's Ten Exercise Program by week 6.[87] Sport-specific exercises are incorporated at weeks 8 to 9. Focus is again placed on developing dynamic stabilization of the medial aspect of the elbow. Because of the anatomic orientation of the flexor carpi ulnaris and flexor digitorum

superficialis overlaying the UCL, isotonic and stabilization activities for these muscles may assist the UCL in stabilizing valgus stress at the medial aspect of the elbow.

Aggressive exercises involving eccentric and plyometric contractions are included in the advanced phase, usual during weeks 9 through 14. We initiate a program called the Advanced Thrower's Ten Program (see Appendix D [online]) at approximately 3 months after surgery.[88] An interval sport program is typically allowed 16 weeks postoperatively. In most cases, throwing from a mound is initiated within 6 to 8 weeks after starting an interval throwing program, and competitive throwing is resumed approximately 6 to 9 months after surgery.[89] Azar et al[89] and later Cain et al[90] reported 85% to 88% success rates (return to sport after UCL reconstruction in athletes).

Box 13-8

Accelerated Postoperative Rehabilitation After Ulnar Collateral Ligament Injury (Palmaris Longus Graft)

PHASE I. IMMEDIATE POSTOPERATIVE PHASE (WEEKS 1–3)
Goals:
- Protect healing tissue
- Decrease pain/inflammation
- Retard muscular atrophy
- Protect the graft site—allow healing

A. Postoperative Week 1
Brace: Posterior splint at 90° of elbow flexion
AROM: Wrist extension/flexion immediately postoperatively
Compression dressing:
- Elbow postoperative compression dressing (5–7 days)
- Wrist (graft site) compression dressing in 7–10 days as needed

Exercises:
- Gripping exercises
- Wrist ROM
- Shoulder isometrics (no shoulder ER)
- Biceps isometrics
Cryotherapy: To elbow joint and to graft site at the wrist

B. Postoperative Week 2
Brace: Elbow ROM of 25° to 100° (gradually increase ROM by 5° of extension/10° of flexion per week)
Exercises:
- Continue all exercises listed above
- Elbow ROM in a brace (30° to 105°)
- Initiate elbow extension isometrics
- Continue wrist ROM exercises
- Initiate light scar mobilization over the distal incision (graft)

Cryotherapy: Continue application of ice to elbow and graft site

C. Postoperative Week 3
Brace: Elbow ROM of 10° to 120°
Exercises:
- Continue all exercises listed above
- Elbow ROM in a brace
- Initiate AROM of the wrist and elbow (no resistance)
- Initiate light wrist flexion stretching
- Initiate AROM of the shoulder:
  - Full can
  - Lateral raises
  - ER/IR tubing
- Elbow flexion/extension
- Initiate light scapular-strengthening exercises
- May incorporate bicycle for lower extremity strength and endurance

PHASE II. INTERMEDIATE PHASE (WEEKS 4–7)
Goals:
- Gradual increase to full ROM
- Promote healing of repaired tissue
- Regain and improve muscular strength
- Restore full function of the graft site

A. Week 4
Brace: Elbow ROM of 0° to 125°

Exercises:
- Begin light resistance exercises for the arm (1 lb):
  - Wrist curls, extensions, pronation, supination
  - Elbow extension/flexion
- Advance the shoulder program with an emphasis on rotator cuff and scapular strengthening
- Initiate shoulder strengthening with light dumbbells

B. Week 5
ROM: Elbow ROM of 0° to 135°
Discontinue brace
Maintain full ROM
Continue all exercises: Advance all shoulder and upper extremity exercises (increase weight 1 lb)

C. Week 6
AROM: 0° to 145° without a brace or full ROM
Exercises:
- Initiate the Thrower's Ten Exercise Program
- Advance elbow-strengthening exercises
- Initiate shoulder ER strengthening
- Advance the shoulder program

D. Week 7
Advance the Thrower's Ten Exercise Program (increase weights)
Initiate PNF diagonal patterns (light)

PHASE III. ADVANCED STRENGTHENING PHASE (WEEKS 8–14)
Goals:
- Increase strength, power, and endurance
- Maintain full elbow ROM
- Gradually initiate sporting activities

A. Week 8
Exercises:
- Initiate eccentric elbow flexion/extension
- Continue isotonic program: forearm and wrist
- Continue shoulder program—Thrower's Ten Exercise Program
- Manual resistance diagonal patterns
- Initiate plyometric exercise program (two-handed plyometrics close to the body only):
  - Chest pass
  - Side throw close to the body
- Continue stretching the calf and hamstrings

B. Week 10
Exercises:
- Continue all exercises listed above
- Advance plyometrics to two-handed drills away from the body:
  - Side-to-side throws
  - Soccer throws
  - Side throws

C. Weeks 12–14
Continue all exercises
Initiate isotonic machine strengthening exercises (if desired)
- Bench press (seated)
- Latissimus pull-down

(Continued)

Box 13-8

Accelerated Postoperative Rehabilitation After Ulnar Collateral Ligament Injury (Palmaris Longus Graft)—cont'd

Initiate golf, swimming
Initiate interval hitting program

PHASE IV. RETURN-TO-SPORT PHASE (WEEKS 14–32)

Goals:
- Continue to increase strength, power, and endurance of the upper extremity musculature
- Gradual return to sport activities

A. Week 14

Exercises:
- Continue strengthening program
- Emphasis on elbow and wrist strengthening and flexibility exercises
- Maintain full elbow ROM
- Initiate one-handed plyometric throwing (stationary throws)

- Initiate one-handed wall dribble
- Initiate one-handed baseball throws into a wall

B. Week 16

Exercises:
- Initiate interval throwing program (phase I; long-toss program)
- Continue Thrower's Ten Exercise Program and plyometrics
- Continue to stretch before and after throwing

C. Weeks 22–24

Exercises: Progress to phase II throwing (once phase is successfully completed I)

D. Weeks 30–32

Exercises: Gradually progress to competitive throwing/sports

AROM, Active ROM; *ER,* external rotation; *IR,* internal rotation; *PNF,* proprioceptive neuromuscular facilitation; *ROM,* range of motion.

ADOLESCENT ELBOW INJURIES

Skeletal immaturity in adolescents alters the typical pathomechanics such that a very different set of lesions are seen at the elbow than in adult athletes. The elbow is the most common area of symptoms in young baseball players, and the vast majority of the osseous changes seen as a result of pitching occur at the radiohumeral joint.[91-93] The two most common injuries occurring at the adolescent elbow are osteochondritis dissecans and Little Leaguer's elbow.

Osteochondritis Dissecans

Osteochondritis dissecans of the elbow is a compression lesion of the radiocapitellar joint that results in damage to bone and articular cartilage on the anterolateral surface of the capitellum.[81] Though most often seen in throwers, osteochondritis dissecans of the elbow has been reported as a result of participation in various athletic activities.[94-96] It is considered the leading cause of permanent elbow disability in young pitching athletes.[97,98] Unlike lesions occurring on the medial side of the elbow, lateral lesions can result in permanent elbow damage and often shorten or terminate a throwing athlete's career.[91]

Although the exact cause of osteochondritis dissecans is unknown, it is believed that repeated traumatic impact of the radial head against the capitellum during the cocking and acceleration phases of throwing can result in a circulatory disturbance in the radiocapitellar joint. This disturbance produces primary changes in the bone and secondary changes in the articular cartilage.[17] Osteochondritis dissecans of the adolescent elbow is seen as aseptic necrosis of the radial head. It can result in the progressive formation of loose bodies, overgrowth of the radial head, and early arthritic changes.

Osteochondritis dissecans represents a major threat to the elbow joint, and it is important that it be diagnosed early. The athlete typically complains of anterolateral elbow tenderness along with decreased pronation and supination, findings suggestive of radiocapitellar incongruity or radial head fracture.[99] The most common finding is loss of full elbow extension that can involve as much as a 20° loss of full extension.[98,100,101]

Conservative treatment consists of a period of active rest during which the athlete avoids all throwing and other exacerbating activities, along with the use of local modalities to decrease pain and inflammation. When the athlete can tolerate it, an elbow rehabilitation program may be started; however, an overly aggressive approach can result in progressive loss of motion. If avascular changes are noted on the lateral side of the elbow in a young thrower, abstinence from throwing should be maintained until revascularization of the affected area has occurred.

Most authors recommend surgical removal of symptomatic loose bodies and avoidance of other surgical procedures unless changes have occurred that could compromise architectural support of the capitellum.[101,102] The prognosis of individuals with osteochondritis dissecans after simple loose body removal is good if the diagnosis is made early and no associated degenerative changes are present. Recovery to normal function is slow, however, and some limitation of full extension is likely to remain. Tivnon et al[98] reported an average preoperative elbow ROM of 30° to 134° that improved to 11° to 136° after surgery. If ROM is to be reestablished or increased after loose body extraction in individuals with this condition, appropriate early mobilization is paramount.

Degenerative changes in the radiocapitellar joint have a poor prognosis for an athlete returning to pitching.[97] Although the osteophytes and loose bodies can be removed surgically, ankylosis of the elbow complex may result and leave the young athlete unable to throw effectively.[103]

Little Leaguer's Elbow

Brogdon and Crow[104] first used the term *Little Leaguer's elbow* to describe an avulsion of the ossification center of the medial epicondyle in an adolescent athlete caused by pitching. Little

Leaguer's elbow is now a catchall term used to describe several pathologic conditions that occur at the elbow, including strain of the flexor-pronator muscle group, ulnar neuropathy, and osteochondritis dissecans.

The forces associated with this condition injure the epiphyseal plate because it is the weakest link in the adolescent kinetic chain. The injury is associated with repetitive throwing, which produces medial traction forces during the acceleration phase of the activity. Hypertrophy of the medial epicondyle develops as a physiologic response to throwing. A widened growth line or displacement of the epicondyle is evidence of a fracture.

Little Leaguer's elbow is commonly manifested by a history of medial elbow pain progressing over the course of a few weeks. These symptoms typically worsen with pitching and are relieved by rest. Additional signs and symptoms include limitation of complete extension, tenderness over the medial epicondyle, and pain with passive extension of the wrist and fingers. Radiographic changes include accelerated growth, separation, and fragmentation of the medial epicondylar epiphysis. Less commonly, the athlete may have dramatic symptoms, including the report of a popping sensation followed by medial elbow pain, an inability to throw because of pain, and swelling accompanied by medial elbow ecchymosis.

Prevention remains the best treatment of Little Leaguer's elbow. It is important that coaches and parents be educated about proper warm-up, conditioning, and off-season training of an adolescent pitcher. Moreover, the throwing of curve balls and other breaking pitches by pitchers in the 9- to 14-year-old age group should be prohibited because the stress associated with these pitches considerably increases the forces placed on wrist flexion and pronation.[102,105] Pitchers should be taught proper pitching mechanics, and appropriate pitching limits or maximum should be established. Currently, Little League International pitching rules advise six innings per week, with 3 days of rest between pitching outings.[106] However, there are no rules or recommendations that govern the intensity and frequency of pitching practice that an athlete can engage in.

Treatment in the early stages of Little Leaguer's elbow includes rest from noxious stimuli, local modalities to decrease pain and inflammation, and possibly immobilization. If radiography reveals osteochondritis dissecans of the capitellum, it is recommended that the player stop pitching for the remainder of the baseball season. After initial conservative treatment, if the athlete returns to throwing and any of the symptoms recur, the athlete should abstain completely from throwing until the next season.

A medial epicondylar fracture that is displaced by more than 1 cm may occur in a small percentage of athletes. These injuries should be opened and fixed internally with a screw. After open reduction and internal fixation, the elbow is immobilized for approximately 3 to 4 weeks, and the athlete should not engage in any throwing activity until the following season. Criteria for return to competition include no pain, normal elbow ROM, and no weakness in muscle strength or endurance in all planes of wrist and elbow ROM. Return to throwing should be gradual and follow the Little League interval throwing program (see Appendix B [online]). Fortunately, most elbow injuries in an adolescent thrower are treated adequately by rest and cause no permanent disability.

ATYPICAL SPORT-RELATED INJURIES

Osteochondritis Dissecans

Osteochondritis dissecans of the elbow may develop as a result of valgus strain on the elbow joint, which produces not only medial tension but also lateral compressive forces. This is observed as the capitellum of the humerus compresses with the radial head. Patients often complain of lateral elbow pain on palpation and valgus stress. Morrey[107] described a three-stage classification of pathologic progression. Stage 1 includes patients without evidence of subchondral displacement or fracture, whereas stage 2 refers to lesions showing evidence of subchondral detachment or articular cartilage fracture. Stage 3 lesions involve detached osteochondral fragments and resultant intraarticular loose bodies. Nonsurgical treatment is attempted for patients with stage 1 lesions only and consists of relative rest and immobilization until the elbow symptoms have resolved.

Nonoperative treatment includes 3 to 6 weeks of immobilization at 90° of elbow flexion. ROM activities for the shoulder, elbow, and wrist are performed three to four times per day. As the symptoms resolve, a strengthening program consisting of isometric exercises is initiated. Isotonic exercises are included after approximately 1 week of isometric exercise. Aggressive high-speed, eccentric, and plyometric exercises are progressively included to prepare the athlete for the start of an interval sport program.

If nonoperative treatment fails or evidence of loose bodies exist, surgical intervention, including arthroscopic abrading and drilling of the lesion with fixation or removal of the loose body, is indicated.[8] Long-term follow-up studies on the outcome of patients undergoing surgery to drill or reattach the lesions have not shown favorable results, thus suggesting that prevention and early detection of symptoms may be the best form of treatment.[108]

Degenerative Joint Disease

Degenerative joint disease of the elbow may occur prematurely in certain athletes who participate in sport activities that repetitively load the articular surfaces of the elbow joint. Acceleration of joint degeneration and osteophyte formation may occur. Pain and joint effusion may be observed during examination, as well as tenderness to palpation over the joint lines. Although this particular pathologic condition may not restrict normal function and activities of daily living, the pain and loss of motion associated with degenerative joint disease may restrict further participation in sports.

Conservative treatment is thus focused on first diminishing pain and inflammation and then improving ROM and soft tissue flexibility. Warm whirlpool treatment before stretching and gentle joint mobilization techniques may be beneficial to enhance soft tissue extensibility. As the pain is relieved and ROM normalizes, overall enhancement of upper extremity strength and endurance is emphasized. If conservative treatment does not produce favorable results, open or arthroscopic débridement may be indicated to alleviate the symptoms.

Synovitis

Generalized joint synovitis may occur as a result of the repetitive nature of throwing or other overhead sports. Athletes often complain of diffuse joint pain not specific to one area, and a flexion contracture is apparent on examination. Initial treatment includes antiinflammatory medications and modifications in activity to allow a period of rest and recovery.

A rehabilitation program focused on restoring elbow extension is initiated. ROM, stretching, and mobilization exercises are performed as necessary to restore and maintain full ROM. The clinician must be cautioned against overaggressive stretching and mobilization during the acute phases of recovery to avoid contributing to the inflammatory synovial reaction. Tepid to warm whirlpool treatment may be used before ROM exercises. Contrast treatment (cold to warm) may also be beneficial. Submaximal isometric exercises are performed until the inflammatory response has diminished, followed by the initiation of an isotonic strengthening program. Return to sport–specific drills and an interval sport program are instituted once the athlete has achieved proper strength and has satisfactory results on clinical examination.

Dislocations

Dislocations of the elbow joint most commonly occur in collision sports such as football and wrestling or in noncontact sports when an athlete lands onto an outstretched hand. A hyperextension injury occurs as the olecranon is forced into the olecranon fossa and the trochlea translates posteriorly or posterolaterally over the coronoid process.[24] Disruption of the UCL and possibly the lateral collateral ligament may occur during this type of severe injury. Concomitant fractures of the radial head or capitellum may also be produced.[24]

A lateral pivot shift test may be used to assess posterolateral stability of the elbow.[17] Initial reduction of the injury may be achieved by applying traction to the forearm and humerus with the elbow in 30° of flexion.[24] Neurovascular integrity should be assessed immediately, and surgical intervention may be necessary to repair concomitant ligament instability and osseous fractures.

Treatment depends greatly on the severity of the injury and any associated injuries that are present. An initial period of rest and immobilization may be warranted to allow soft tissue healing and a decrease in pain and inflammation. Early motion should be initiated within the first week after injury to minimize the chance for loss of motion, which is one of the primary complications after elbow dislocation.[109] Rehabilitation follows a progressive sequence similar to that described earlier for regaining motion and strength of the entire elbow and forearm complex.

Fractures

Various fractures of the elbow may occur in the athletic population, including extraarticular and intraarticular distal humeral fractures, radial head fractures, and olecranon fractures.[109] Stress fractures of the olecranon have been reported in overhead throwers and can occur in any part of the olecranon, especially in the midarticular area.[110] The most likely cause of injury involves repetitive stress applied to the olecranon as the elbow extends from triceps contraction during the acceleration, deceleration, and follow-through phases of throwing. Patients often subjectively report an insidious onset of pain in the posterolateral region of the elbow while throwing. The symptoms appear similar to those of triceps tendinitis; however, tenderness over the involved site of the olecranon is often detected on palpation. Plain radiographs are typically taken, and the diagnosis may be further enhanced with the aid of a bone scan or MRI (or both).

Aggressive stretching and strengthening exercises are restricted for the first 6 to 8 weeks to allow adequate healing of the fracture site. The athlete should maintain motion with light ROM exercises. Heavy lifting, plyometrics, and sport-specific drills are not allowed until bony healing is seen on radiographic evaluation, typically by 8 to 12 weeks. When adequate healing has been documented, an interval sport program may be allowed. Complete recovery occurs in approximately 3 to 6 months after injury. Open reduction and internal fixation may be indicated if conservative management fails.

Arthrolysis

Many of the pathologic conditions that have been discussed earlier involve loss of motion as a primary complication. The elbow is one of the joints in which functional loss of motion most commonly develops as a result of injury or after surgery.[50,62] After injury, the elbow flexes in response to pain and hemarthrosis. The periarticular soft tissue and joint capsule become shortened and fibrotic, and loss of motion develops. Arthroscopic arthrolysis may be necessary for patients whose injury does not respond to conservative treatment.

During the first postoperative week, the athlete is instructed to perform elbow and wrist ROM exercises hourly. Treatment to regain ROM at this time is cautiously aggressive.[111] Full motion should be obtained quickly; however, a pace that does not cause additional inflammation of the joint capsule is necessary to avoid further pain and reflexive splinting. Low-load, long-duration stretching has been an extremely beneficial clinical treatment technique in these instances. Full passive ROM is usually restored by 10 to 14 days after surgery.

Isometric strengthening is begun during week 2 and progressed to isotonic dumbbell exercises during weeks 3 to 4. Strengthening exercises are progressed as tolerated by the athlete. During the later phases of rehabilitation the emphasis on maintaining full motion is continued. Athletes are educated to continue a motion maintenance program several times per day and before and after sport activities for at least 2 to 3 months after surgery.

CONCLUSION

- The elbow joint is a common site of injury in the athletic population.
- Injuries vary widely from repetitive microtraumatic injuries to gross macrotraumatic dislocations.
- Thorough understanding of the functional anatomy and biomechanics of the elbow joint is necessary for successful clinical examination, assessment, and rehabilitation prescription.
- Rehabilitation of the elbow, whether after injury or surgery, must follow a progressive and sequential order to ensure that the healing tissues are not overstressed.
- An elbow rehabilitation program that limits immobilization, achieves full ROM early, progressively restores strength and neuromuscular control, and gradually incorporates sport-specific activities is essential to successfully return athletes to their previous level of competition as quickly and safely as possible.
- The elbow can potentially become an unyielding joint when injured, and lengthy periods of immobilization often result in elbow stiffness, impaired function, and pain; rehabilitation programs should therefore focus on immediate or early motion to prevent these complications from occurring.

REFERENCES

1. Wilk, K.E., Arrigo, C., and Andrews, J.R. (1993): Rehabilitation of the elbow in the throwing athlete. J. Orthop. Sports Phys. Ther., 17:305–317.
2. Wilk, K.E., and Levinson, M. (2001): Rehabilitation of the athlete's elbow. In Altchek, D.W., and Andrews, J.R. (eds.): The Athlete's Elbow. Philadelphia, Lippincott Williams & Wilkins, pp. 249–273.
3. Fleisig, G.S., and Barrentine, S.W. (1995): Biomechanical aspects of the elbow in sports. Sports Med. Arthrosc. Rev., 3:149–159.
4. Morrey, B.F. (1985): Anatomy of the elbow. In Morrey, B.F. (ed.): The Elbow and Its Disorders. Philadelphia, Saunders, pp. 7–40.
5. Lehmkuhl, D.L., and Smith, L.R. (1983): Brunnstrom's Clinical Kinesiology. Philadelphia Davis, pp. 149–170.
6. Morrey, B.F., An, K.N., and Dobyns, J. (1985): Functional anatomy of the elbow ligaments. Clin. Orthop. Relat. Res., 201:84.
7. Hoppenfeld, S. (1976): Physical Examination of the Spine and Extremities. New York, Appleton-Century-Crofts, pp. 35–55.
8. Norkin, C., and Levangie, P. (1985): Joint Structure and Function: A Comprehensive Analysis. Philadelphia, Davis, pp. 191–210.
9. Kapandji, I.A. (1970): The Physiology of the Joints, Vol. 1. London, E & S Livingston, pp. 82–83. 112-117.
10. Atkinson, W.B., and Elftman, H. (1945): The carrying angle of the human arm as a secondary sex character. Anat. Rec., 91:49–54.
11. Keats, T.E., Teeslink, R., Diamond, A.E., and Williams, J.H. (1966): Normal axial relationships of the major joints. Radiology, 87:904.
12. Johansson, O. (1962): Capsular and ligament injuries of the elbow joint. A clinical and arthrographic study. Acta Chir. Scand. Suppl., 287:1–159.
13. Schwab, G.H., Bennett, J.B., Woods, G.W. (as quoted by Lanz), and Tullos, H.S. (1980): The biomechanics of elbow stability: The role of the medial collateral ligament. Clin. Orthop. Relat. Res, 146:42.
14. Morrey, B.F., and An, K.N. (1983): Articular and ligamentous contributions to the static stability of the elbow joint. Am. J. Sports Med., 11:315–319.
15. Spinner, M., and Kaplan, E.B. (1970): The quadrate ligament of the elbow—Its relationship to the stability of the proximal radioulnar joint. Acta Orthop. Scand., 41:632.
16. Martin, B.F. (1958): The annular ligament of the superior radioulnar joint. J. Anat., 52:473.
17. O'Driscoll, S.W., Bell, D.F., and Morrey, B.F. (1991): Posterolateral rotatory instability of the elbow. J. Bone Joint Surg. Am., 73:440–446.
18. Basmajian, J.V., and DeLuca, C.J. (1985): Muscles Alive: Their Function Revealed by Electromyography. Baltimore, Williams & Wilkins, pp. 279–280.
19. Pavly, J.E., Rushing, J.L., and Scheving, L.E. (1967): Electromyographic study of some muscles crossing the elbow joint. J. Anat., 159:47–53.
20. Jobe, F.W., Moynes, D.R., Tibone, J.E., and Perry, J. (1984): An EMG analysis of the shoulder in pitching. Am. J. Sports Med., 12:218–220.
21. Soderberg, G.L. (1981): Kinesiology Application to Pathological Motion. Baltimore, Williams & Wilkins, pp. 131–136.
22. Magee, D.J. (1987): Orthopaedic Physical Assessment. Philadelphia, Saunders.
23. St. John, J.N., and Palmaz, J.C. (1986): The cubital tunnel in ulnar entrapment neuropathy. Musculoskel. Radiol., 158:119.
24. Andrews, J.R., and Whiteside, J.A. (1993): Common elbow problems in the athlete. J. Orthop. Sports Phys. Ther., 17:289–295.
25. Werner, S., Fleisig, G.S., Dillman, C.J., et al. (1993): Biomechanics of the elbow during baseball pitching. J. Orthop. Sports Phys. Ther., 17:274–278.
26. Dun, S., Kingsley, D., Fleisig, G.S., et al. (2008): Biomechanical comparison of the fastball from wind-up and the fastball from stretch in professional baseball pitchers. Am. J. Sports Med., 36:137–141.
27. Fleisig, G.S., Loftice, J., and Andrews, J.R. (2006): Elbow biomechanics during sports: 21st century research. Tech. Orthop., 21:228–238.
28. Fleisig, G.S., Nicholls, R.L., Elliott, B.C., and Escamilla, R.F. (2003): Kinematics used by world class tennis players to produce high-velocity serves. Sports Biomech., 2:17–30.
29. Fleisig, G.S., Weber, A., Hassell, N., and Andrews, J.R. (2009): Prevention of elbow injuries in youth baseball pitchers. Curr. Sports Med. Rep., 8:250–25409.
30. Escamilla, R.F., Barrentine, S.W., Fleisig, G.S., et al. (2007): Pitching biomechanics as a pitcher approaches muscular fatigue during a simulated baseball game. Am. J. Sports Med., 35:23–33.
31. Chu, Y., Fleisig, G.S., Simpson, K.J., and Andrews, J.R. (2009): Biomechanical comparison between elite female and male baseball pitchers. J. Appl. Biomech., 25:22–31.
32. Fleisig, G.S., Andrews, J.R., Dillman, C.J., and Escamilla, R.F. (1995): Kinetics of baseball pitching with implications about injury mechanisms. Am. J. Sports Med., 23:233–239.
33. Wilson, F.D., Andrews, J.R., Blackburn, T.A., and McClusky, G. (1983): Valgus extension overload in the pitching elbow. Am. J. Sports Med., 11:83–88.
34. Kibler, W.B. (1994): Clinical biomechanics of the elbow in tennis: implications for evaluation and diagnosis. Med. Sci. Sports Exerc., 26:1203–1206.
35. Elliott, B., Fleisig, G., Nicholls, R., and Escamilla, R. (2003): Technique effects on upper limb loading in the tennis serve. J. Sci. Med. Sport, 6:76–87.
36. Morris, M., Jobe, F.W., Perry, J., et al. (1989): EMG analysis of elbow function in tennis players. Am. J. Sports Med., 17:241–247.
37. Kelley, B.T., and Weiland, A.J. (2001): Posterolateral rotatory instability of the elbow. In Altchek, D.W., and Andrews J.R. (eds.): The Athlete's Elbow. Philadelphia, Lippincott Williams & Wilkins, pp. 175–189.
38. Rhu, K.N., McCormick, J., Jobe, F.W., et al. (1988): An electromyographic analysis of shoulder function in tennis players. Am. J. Sports Med., 16:481.
39. Zheng, N., Barrentine, S.W., Fleisig, G.S., and Andrews, J.R. (2008): Swing kinematics for male and female pro golfers. Int. J. Sports Med., 29:965–970.
40. Zheng, N., Barrentine, S.W., Fleisig, G.S., and Andrews, J.R. (2008): Kinematic analysis of swing in pro and amateur golfers. Int. J. Sports Med., 29:487–493.
41. Glazebrook, M.A., Curwin, S., Islam, M.N., et al. (1994): Medial epicondylitis. An electromyographic analysis and an investigation of intervention strategies. Am. J. Sports Med., 22:674–679.
42. Stanish, W.D., Loebenberg, M.I., and Kozey, J.W. (1994): The elbow. In Stover C. N., McCarroll, J.R., and Mallon W.J. (eds.): Feeling Up to Par: Medicine From Tee to Green. Philadelphia, Davis, pp. 143–149.
43. McCarroll, J.R., and Gioe, T.J. (1982): Professional golfers and the price they pay. Physician Sports Med., 10:64–70.
44. McCarroll, J.R. (1985): Golf. In Schneider, R.C., et al. (eds.): Sports Injuries: Mechanisms, Prevention, and Treatment. Baltimore, Williams & Wilkins, pp. 290–294.
45. Andrews, J.R., Wilk, K.E., Satterwhite, Y.E., and Tedder, J.L. (1993): Physical examination of the thrower's elbow. J. Orthop. Sports Phys. Ther., 17:296–304.
46. Norkin, C.C., and White, D.J. (1995): Measurement of Joint Motion: A Guide to Goniometry, 2nd ed. Philadelphia, Davis.
47. Cyriax, J. (1982): Textbook of Orthopedic Medicine, Vol. 1, Diagnosis of Soft Tissue Lesions, 8th ed. London, Bailliere Tindall, pp. 52–54.
48. Kendall, F.P., and McCreary, E.K. (1983): Muscles, Testing, and Function, 3rd ed. Baltimore, Williams & Wilkins, pp. 86–87.
49. Kelley, J.D., Lombardo, S.J., Pink, M., et al. (1994): EMG and cinematographic analysis of elbow function in tennis players with lateral epicondylitis. Am. J. Sports Med., 22:359–363.
50. Timmerman, L.A., and Andrews, J.R. (1994): Undersurface tears of the ulnar collateral ligament in baseball players. A newly recognized lesion. Am. J. Sports Med., 22:33–36.
51. Coutts, R., Rothe, C., and Kaita, J. (1981): The role of continuous passive motion in the rehabilitation of the total knee patient. Clin. Orthop. Relat. Res., 159:126–132.
52. Dehne, E., and Tory, R. (1971): Treatment of joint injuries by immediate mobilization based upon the spiral adaptation concept. Clin. Orthop. Relat. Res., 77:218–232.
53. Haggmark, T., and Eriksson, E. (1979): Cylinder or mobile cast brace after knee ligament surgery: A clinical analysis and morphologic and enzymatic studies of changes of the quadriceps muscle. Am. J. Sports Med., 7:48–56.
54. Noyes, F.R., Mangine, R.E., and Barber, S.E. (1987): Early knee motion after open and arthroscopic anterior cruciate ligament reconstruction. Am. J. Sports Med., 15:149–160.
55. Perkins, G. (1954): Rest and motion. J. Bone Joint Surg. Br., 35:521–539.
56. Salter, R.B., Hamilton, H.W., and Wedge, J.H. (1984): Clinical application of basic research on continuous passive motion for disorders and injuries of synovial joints. A preliminary report of a feasibility study. J. Orthop. Res., 1:325–342.
57. Salter, R.B., Simmonds, D.F., Malcolm, B.W., et al. (1980): The effects of continuous passive motion on healing of full thickness defects in articular cartilage. J. Bone Joint Surg. Am., 62:1232–1251.
58. Tipton, C.M., Mathies, R.D., and Martin, R.F. (1978): Influence of age and sex on strength of bone-ligament junctions in knee joints in rats. J. Bone Joint Surg. Am., 60:230–236.
59. Wilk, K.E. (2000): Elbow injuries. In Schenck R.C. (ed.): Athletic Training and Sports Medicine. Rosemont, IL, American Academy of Orthopaedic Surgeons, pp. 293–334.
60. Wilk, K.E., Arrigo, C.A., Andrews, J.R., and Azar, F.M. (1996): Rehabilitation following elbow surgery in the throwing athlete. Oper. Tech. Sports Med., 4:114–132.
61. Akeson, W.H., Amiel, D., and Woo, S.L.Y. (1980): Immobilization effects on synovial joints. The pathomechanics of joint contracture. Biorheology, 17:95–107.
62. Green, D.P., and McCoy, H. (1979): Turnbuckle orthotic correction of elbow flexion contractures. J. Bone Joint Surg. Am., 61:1092.
63. Nirschl, R.P., and Morrey, B.F. (1985): Rehabilitation. In Morrey, B.F. (ed.): The Elbow and Its Disorders, Philadelphia, Saunders, pp. 147–152.
64. Maitland, G.D. (1977): Vertebral Manipulation. London, Butterworths, pp. 84–105.
65. Wyke, B.D. (1966): The neurology of joints. Ann. R. Coll. Surg. (Lond.), 41:25–29.
66. Kottke, F.J., Pauley, D.L., and Ptak, R.A. (1966): The rationale for prolonged stretching for connective tissue. Arch. Phys. Med. Rehabil., 47:345–352.
67. Sapega, A.A., Quedenfeld, T.C., Moyer, R.A., and Butler, R.A. (1976): Biophysical factors in range of motion exercise. Arch. Phys. Med. Rehabil., 57:122–126.
68. Warren, C.G., Lehmann, J.F., and Koblanski, J.N. (1971): Elongation of rat tail tendon: Effect of load and temperature. Arch. Phys. Med. Rehabil., 52:465–474.
69. Warren, C.G., Lehmann, J.F., and Koblanski, J.N. (1976): Heat and stretch procedures: An evaluation using rat tail tendon. Arch. Phys. Med. Rehabil., 57:122–126.
70. Fleisig, G.S., and Escamilla, R.F. (1996): Biomechanics of the elbow in the throwing athlete. Oper. Tech. Sports Med., 4:62–68.
71. Moseley, V.B., Jobe, F.W., and Pink, M. (1992): EMG analysis of the scapular muscles during a shoulder rehabilitation program. Am. J. Sports Med., 20:128–134.
72. Townsend, H., Jobe, F.W., Pink, M., and Perry, J. (1991): Electromyographic analysis of the glenohumeral muscles during a baseball rehabilitation program. Am. J. Sports Med., 19:264–272.
73. Blackburn, T.A., McCleod, W.D., and White, B. (1990): EMG analysis of posterior rotator cuff exercises. J. Athl. Train., 25:40–45.
74. Andrews, J.R., and Frank, W. (1985): Valgus extension overload in the pitching elbow. In Andrews J.R., Zarins B., and Carson W.B. (eds.): Injuries to the Throwing Arm. Philadelphia, Saunders, pp. 250–257.

75. Glousman, R.E. (1990): Ulnar nerve problems in the athlete's elbow. Clin. Sports Med., 9:365–377.

76. Alley, R.M., and Pappas, A.M. (1995): Acute and performance-related injuries of the elbow. In Pappas, A.M. (ed.): Upper Extremity Injuries in the Athlete. New York, Churchill Livingstone, pp. 339–364.

77. Anderson, K. (2001): Elbow arthritis and removal of loose bodies and spurs, and techniques for restoration of motion. In Altchek D.W., and Andrews, J.R. (eds.): The Athlete's Elbow. Philadelphia, Lippincott Williams & Wilkins, pp. 219–230.

78. Andrews, J.R., Heggland, E.J., Fleisig, G.S., and Zheng, N. (2001): Relationship of UCL strain to amount of medial olecranon osteotomy. Am. J. Sports Med., 29:716–726.

79. Martin, S.D., and Baumgarten, T.E. (1996): Elbow injuries in the throwing athlete: Diagnosis and arthroscopic treatment. Oper. Tech. Sports Med., 4:100–108.

80. Andrews, J.R., and Timmerman, L. (1995): Outcome of elbow surgery in professional baseball players. Am. J. Sports Med., 23:245–250.

81. Jobe, F.W., and Nuber, G. (1986): Throwing injuries of the elbow. Clin. Sports Med., 5:621–636.

82. Andrews, J.R., Jelsma, R.D., Joyse, M.E., and Timmerman, L.A. (1996): Open surgical procedures for injuries to the elbow in throwers. Oper. Tech. Sports Med., 4:109–113.

83. Dodson, C.C., Thomas, A., Dines, J.S., et al. (2006): Medial ulnar collateral ligament reconstruction in throwing athletes. Am. J. Sports Med., 34:1926–1932.

84. Bowers, A.L., Dines, J.S., Dines, D.M., and Altchek, D.W. (2010): Elbow medial ulnar collateral ligament reconstruction: Clinical & the docking technique. J. Shoulder Elbow Surg., 19:110–117.

85. Wilk, K.E., Voight, M., Keirns, M.D., et al. (1993): Plyometrics for the upper extremities: Theory and clinical application. J. Orthop. Sports Phys. Ther., 17:225–239.

86. Bernas, G.A., Thiele, R.A., Kinnaman, K.A., et al. (2009): Defining safe rehabilitation for ulnar collateral ligament reconstruction of the elbow. Am. J. Sports Med., 37:2392–2400.

87. Wilk, K.E., Azar, F.M., and Andrews, J.R. (1995): Conservative and operative rehabilitation of the elbow in sports. Sports Med. Arthrosc. Rev., 3:237–258.

88. Wilk, K.E., Arrigo, C.A., Macrina, L., and Yenchak, A.J. (2011): The Advanced Throwers Ten Program. Physician Sports Med. Submitted for publication.

89. Azar, F.M., Andrews, J.R., Wilk, K.E., and Groh, D. (2000): Operative treatment of ulnar collateral ligament injuries of the elbow. Am. J. Sports Med., 28:16–23.

90. Cain, E.L., Andrews, J.R., Dugas, J.R., et al. (2010): Outcome of ulnar collateral ligament reconstruction of the elbow in 1281 athletes. Am. J. Sports Med., 38:2426–2434.

91. Tullos, H.S., and King, J.W. (1972): Lesion of the pitching arm in adolescents. JAMA, 220:264–271.

92. Olsen, S.J., Fleisig, G.S., Dun, S., et al. (2006): Risk factors for shoulder and elbow injuries in adolescent baseball pitchers. Am. J. Sports Med., 34:905–912.

93. Roberts, W., and Hughes, R. (1950): Osteochondritis dissecans of the elbow joint: A clinical study. J. Bone Joint Surg. Br., 32:348–360.

94. Inoue, G. (1991): Bilateral osteochondritis dissecans of the elbow treated with Herbert screw fixation. Br. J. Sports Med., 25:142–144.

95. Pintore, E., and Maffulli, N. (1991): Osteochondritis dissecans of the lateral humeral epicondyle in a table tennis player. Med. Sci. Sports Exerc., 23:889–891.

96. Singer, K.M., and Roy, S.P. (1984): Osteochondrosis of the humeral capitellum. Am. J. Sports Med., 12:351–360.

97. Indelicato, P.A., Jobe, F.W., Kerlan, R.K., et al. (1979): Correctable elbow lesions in professional baseball players: A review of 25 cases. Am. J. Sports Med., 7:72–75.

98. Tivnon, M.C., Anzel, S.H., and Waugh, T.R. (1976): Surgical management of osteochondritis dissecans of the capitellum. Am. J. Sports Med., 4:121–128.

99. Tullos, H.S., and Bryan, W.J. (1985): Examination of the throwing elbow. In Zarins, B., Andrews J.R., and Carson, W.G. (eds.): Injuries to the Throwing Athlete. Philadelphia, Saunders, pp. 201–210.

100. Brown, R., Blazina, M.E., Kerlan, R.K., et al. (1974): Osteochondritis of the capitellum. J. Sports Med., 2:27–46.

101. Woodward, A.H., and Bianco, A.J., Jr. (1975): Osteochondritis dissecans of the elbow. Clin. Orthop. Relat. Res., 110:35–41.

102. Pappas, A.M. (1982): Elbow problems associated with baseball during childhood and adolescence. Clin. Orthop. Relat. Res., 164:30–41.

103. Hunter, S.C. (1985): Little Leaguer's elbow. In Zarins, B., Andrews, J.R., and Carson W.G. (eds.): Injuries to the Throwing Arm. Philadelphia, Saunders, pp. 228–234.

104. Brogdon, B.S., and Crow, M.D. (1960): Little Leaguer's elbow. Am. J. Roentgenol., 85:671–677.

105. DeHaven, K.E., and Evarts, C.M. (1973): Throwing injuries of the elbow in athletes. Orthop. Clin. North Am., 4:801–808.

106. Little League International (1996): Youth Baseball Handbook. Williamsport, PA, Little League International.

107. Morrey, B.F. (1994): Osteochondritis desiccans. In DeLee J.C., and Drez D. (eds.): Orthopedic Sports Medicine. Philadelphia, Saunders, pp. 908–912.

108. Baur, M., Jonsson, K., Josefson, P.O., et al. (1992): Osteochondritis dissecans of the elbow: A long-term follow-up study. Clin. Orthop. Relat. Res., 284:156–160.

109. Richardson, J.K., and Iglarsh, Z.A. (1994): Clinical Orthopaedic Physical Therapy. Philadelphia, Saunders, pp. 227–230.

110. Bennett, G.E. (1941): Shoulder and elbow lesions of the professional baseball player. JAMA, 117:510–514.

111. Wilk, K.E. (1994): Rehabilitation of the elbow following arthroscopic surgery. In Andrews J.R., and Soffer, S.R. (eds.): Elbow Arthroscopy. St. Louis, Mosby, pp. 109–116.

Rehabilitation of Wrist and Hand Injuries

Greg Pitts, MS, OTR/L, CHT, Jason Willoughby, MS, OTR/L, CHT,
Bradley Cummings, PT, CHT, and Tim L. Uhl, PT, PhD, ATC, FNATA

CHAPTER OBJECTIVES

- Apply rehabilitation guidelines to sports-related wrist and hand injuries.
- Describe the mechanism of injury and clinical picture with common hand injuries.
- Identify treatment pitfalls to help avoid poor functional outcomes.
- Apply rehabilitation principles for common wrist and hand injuries to advance an athlete from an acute phase of healing to return to sport.
- Choose appropriate splint types for specific wrist and hand injuries.

The purpose of this chapter is to provide a practical approach to the treatment of athletes with injuries involving their wrists and hands. Upper extremity injuries are often not given the full attention that they deserve because athletes resume participation after minimal care. However, left untreated, these injuries can result in permanent disability.[1] Complete recovery to maximize function in performing daily tasks is the primary goal in the treatment of hand and wrist injuries. Fortunately, progress in surgical techniques, rehabilitation techniques, and custom splinting has allowed athletes to realize good functional outcomes.

The primary goal after a sports injury is to return the athlete to full participation as soon as possible without risking further injury or permanent disability.[2] However, formal informed discussion about the potential long-term outcome of an undertreated hand or wrist injury should be a primary goal of the initial evaluation. The primary emphasis in this chapter is on the management of common wrist, hand, and finger injuries to minimize time until return to sport and prevent permanent disability or deformity.

In this chapter, common mechanisms of injury, pathologic characteristics of the involved structures, and clinical assessment of the injury are discussed. Practical management of the injury is presented with regard to evaluation, protective splinting, and initiation of rehabilitation. A summary of rehabilitation recommendations for each injury can be found in Table 14-10. Exercises are described to help the clinician return the athlete to participation and maximize full functional performance of the injured structure. Consideration should always be given to the importance of evaluation and providing appropriate treatment of the entire upper extremity kinetic chain, as well as the body's core, when rehabilitating an injured athlete. Whether a throwing athlete or not, a solid foundation in treating the upper extremity is essential to achieve normal mechanics for performing functional or sports activities after a hand or wrist injury. Failure to address weak trunk musculature, scapulothoracic dyskinesia, poor posture, neural tension or compression issues, and thoracic mobilization can result in further injury when return to sport is achieved.

MALLET FINGER (DISTAL INTERPHALANGEAL TENDON INJURY)

Mallet finger injury often occurs in ball-catching sports such as football, basketball, baseball, and softball. Typically, a ball or some object strikes the distal phalanx and forces it into hyperflexion while the extensor mechanism is active.[3-6] A mallet finger deformity is readily observed because the athlete is unable to actively extend the distal phalanx. Additional clinical signs of this injury are listed in Box 14-1. McCue[7] classified mallet finger into five types (Table 14-1). Indications for physician referral include the following:

- Extensor lag of the distal interphalangeal (DIP) joint
- Passive range of motion (ROM) greater than active ROM (AROM) extension of the DIP joint
- Pain and swelling focal to the DIP joint

Box 14-1

Signs of a Mallet Finger Injury

The athlete is unable to actively extend the distal phalanx.
Radiographs must be obtained to rule out the presence of a fracture, but it is not generally necessary to acquire radiographs immediately.
Crepitus and point tenderness in the distal phalanx are classic signs of a fracture.
Along with the fracture, the digit may have a subungual hematoma.

Table 14-1 Classification of Mallet Finger Injury

Type	Injury
I	Tendon stretch
II	Tendon rupture
III	Tendon rupture with avulsion of the distal phalanx
IV	Distal phalanx fracture involving the articular surface
V	Epiphyseal fracture

Data from McCue, F.C. (1982): The elbow, wrist, and hand. In Kulund, D.N. (ed.): The Injured Athlete. Philadelphia, Lippincott, pp. 295-329.

- Ligamentous instability
- Painful passive compression of the finger; radiographs must be obtained to rule out fractures
- Absence of hyperextension of the proximal interphalangeal (PIP) joint
- Need for surgical treatment for type IV and V injuries

Open mallet injuries may require surgical débridement to prevent infection and surgical repair of the damaged soft tissues to restore the biomechanics of the joint.[8] Table 14-2 lists considerations for splint use and pitfalls in the treatment of a mallet finger.

Treatment of mallet finger depends on the type of injury that the DIP joint and extensor mechanism have sustained. If an open dislocation has occurred, care is taken to prevent wound infection.[12] Initial swelling can be managed with the use of a Coban wrap*, application of ice, elevation, and motion of the unaffected joints and digits while wearing a protective splint (Fig. 14-1). The athlete must be supervised and instructed to keep the DIP joint in full extension at all times during the 8-week course of treatment.

Clinical Pearl #1

Regular splint removal after a mallet finger injury is necessary to keep the area under the splint clean and dry and to ensure skin integrity. It is imperative that the athlete maintain joint extension during this cleaning process. The splint must be worn continuously for 6 to 8 weeks to achieve a good functional outcome.

---

*Available from 3M, St. Paul, MN.

Table 14-2 Splint Considerations and Treatment Pitfalls for Mallet Finger

Joint Position	Conservative Treatment by Splinting the DIP Joint in Full Slight Hyperextension[9]
Duration of splint wear	6 to 8 weeks of constant splinting, acute injury
Splinting for competition	3 additional weeks monitored by a physician
Splint type	DIP dysfunction tendon injury: a variety of splints, including commercially available dorsal or volar aluminum and custom-made thermoplastic (preferred) (see Fig. 14-1)[10]
Pitfalls of treatment	Poor understanding and poor healing rate of the distal extensor mechanism, which has a negative impact on compliance with the treatment protocol Flexion occurring at any time during the immobilization phase: the 8-week immobilization period starts again from that day and may need to be longer Fracture malunion as a result of poor compliance DIP joint splinted into extreme hyperextension, which may cause an impairment of the blood supply to the skin and result in skin sloughing over the DIP joint[11] Heavy scar tissue formation The splint and skin must be kept dry to prevent maceration Infection or skin irritation because of poor splint fit
Goals of treatment	Protect the distal extensor mechanism, fracture, or joint dislocation Avoid deformity Preserve dexterity and strength Maintain independence in ADL tasks

Data from McCue, F.C., and Garroway, R.Y. (1985): Sport injuries to the hand and wrist. In Schneider, R.C. (ed.): Sport Injuries: Mechanism, Prevention, and Treatment. Baltimore, Lippincott Williams & Wilkins, pp. 743–764.
ADL, Activity of daily living; *DIP,* distal interphalangeal.

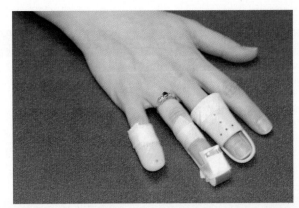

FIGURE 14-1 Three types of splints for mallet finger.

After the initial 8 weeks of continuous splinting, the athlete is advised to continue wearing the splint during athletic activities for 6 to 8 more weeks with assurance that return to sport has been authorized by the physician.[11,13] Athletes participating in a formal rehabilitation program may not realize full ROM of the DIP joint with an intraarticular fracture. Consult Tables 14-9 and 14-10 for an expected time line for return to sport.

JERSEY FINGER (FLEXOR DIGITORUM PROFUNDUS RUPTURE)

An athlete may sustain this injury when attempting to tackle an opponent if a digit is caught in the opponent's jersey while the opponent is breaking away. The flexor digitorum profundus (FDP) tendon undergoes eccentric loading at the distal phalanx with the force exceeding the tendon's tensile strength. This can create an avulsion of the FDP tendon at the insertion of the distal phalanx.[14-16] The injury can occur at any finger, but most commonly the ring finger is involved because of the longer length of the digit when grasping objects.[15,17]

Physical examination of this injury requires isolating the function of the flexor tendons.[18] The FDP is isolated by blocking PIP joint motion while actively flexing the DIP joint. Inability to isolate and actively flex the DIP joint should raise suspicion for FDP injury.[8,19] Palpating for the retracted tendon along the flexor sheath is important for identifying the level of retraction. Jersey finger is classified by Leddy and Packer[15] into three levels of retraction (Table 14-3), with type I injury being most severe.

Management of a jersey finger injury depends on the level of tendon retraction (available blood supply from an intact vinculum), delay in repairing the injury, future sports career plans, philosophy of the treating physician, and the athlete's commitment to participate in the rehabilitation protocol after surgery. Common pitfalls that can occur in the management of this injury are described in Table 14-4.

Table 14-3 **Classification of Jersey Finger Injury**

Type	Amount of Retraction	Time to Repair
I	Retracted to the palm	7 days
II	Retracted to the PIP joint	10 days
III	Avulsion of the distal phalanx	2 weeks

Data from Leddy, J.P., and Packer, J.W. (1977): Avulsion of the profundus tendon insertion in athletes. J. Hand Surg., 2:66-69.
PIP, Proximal interphalangeal.

Flexor tendon injuries should be monitored by a physician and a trained certified hand therapist (CHT) for the first 8 to 10 weeks to maximize the athlete's functional outcome. The Kleinert method of dynamic digital flexion can be used to assist in the rehabilitation process (Fig. 14-2). A dorsal block splint

Table 14-4 **Common Pitfalls in the Treatment of Jersey Finger**

Consideration	Pitfall
Human and anatomic factors	Compliance is poor. Adhesions of digital tendons impede flexion and extension of the fingers. Quadriplegia (diminished ability to create movement because of adverse effect of the pathologic condition on common muscle belly performance) may occur. Intrinsic tightness will result in loss of dexterity and grip strength. Extrinsic tightness will result in loss of gross motor dexterity of the wrist and strength of the hand.
Splinting	Awareness of flexion contractures of the PIP joint is inadequate, and it is often untreated.
Treatment	Injury is often missed because of soft tissue trauma. Postsurgically, the athlete must have the capacity to passively flex all fingers to the palm and actively extend the fingers to the dorsal block splint before leaving the first treatment session. Extreme edema may impede early tendon gliding and should be an early primary treatment goal.[4] The athlete must be cautioned to not allow the fingers or wrists to actively flex or extend outside the protected dorsal block splint.

PIP, Proximal interphalangeal.

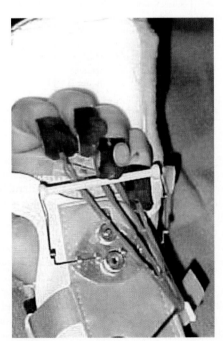

FIGURE 14-2 Dorsal blocking splint via a palmar pulley for flexor tendon repairs. This technique diminishes stress on the flexor tendon repair through reciprocal inhibition of the flexors while extending against resistance.

Table 14-5 Modified Kleinert-Duran Protocol

	3 Days–3 Weeks	4½–6 Weeks	6 Weeks	8–10 Weeks	10–12 Weeks
Splint	Wrist placed in a dorsal block splint Wrist placed in 20° of flexion MCP joints placed in 60° of flexion IP joints placed in maximum extension Dynamic traction via a daytime palmar pulley with nighttime resting strap	Dorsal block splint can be worn at night Postoperative flexor tendon splint can be worn during the day. This splint provides finger pulley flexion to palm all digits and allows wrist flexion and extension	Dorsal block splint and postoperative flexor tendon splint can be discontinued	Protective DIP joint splint at 30° of flexion to be used with gross motor strengthening activities and athletic activities	Buddy tape for functional activities that exceed a medium demand level (25 lb) with one hand Use protective DIP joint splint when performing competitive activities At 12 weeks all splints can be discontinued

Levels of Care	0 3 Days–3 Weeks	I 4½–6 Weeks	I and II 6 Weeks	II 8–10 Weeks	III 10–12 Weeks
Exercise	Active extension of IP joints to the hood of the splint, 8 repetitions every hour without traction through the palmar pulley Passive flexion of the digits, working toward a full fist and isolated MCP, PIP, and DIP flexion; 10 repetitions 4–6 times per day in the splint	Emphasize tendon gliding with basic four hand postures: dorsal compartment ROM (elbow extended, pronated; full fist; actively flexed wrist) Volar compartment ROM (elbow extended, supinated; fingers extended; actively extended wrist)	Continue intrinsic and extrinsic compartment stretching Passive overpressure exercise can be used in a protected posture (flexed wrist to stretch the lumbricals)	Start isometric and isotonic strengthening: Thera-Putty Functional passive ROM to restore intrinsic and extrinsic motion without protective posture Start pushing activities (push-ups and bench press) and general conditioning tasks but avoid pulling exercises	Continue progressive strengthening exercises Continue stretching exercises to regain full motion Start sport-specific training activities, including pulling exercises, in preparation for return to full sport participation
Precautions	No lifting, carrying, pushing, or pulling done with the repaired hand	No lifting, carrying, pushing, or pulling done with the repaired hand	Self-care activities at a sedentary physical level (not to exceed 5 lb)	Activity progressed to a light physical demand level (not to exceed 10 lb)	Ballistic pulling tasks with force greater than 20 lb
Special considerations	Use a Coban wrap to control edema At 2 weeks postoperative, the fingers can be placed in a fist-like posture and AROM of wrist flexion and extension initiated (with the therapist) Avoid the pain reflex with aggressive rehabilitation	Biofeedback training for fine motor and gross motor self-care tasks; need physician's clearance before starting AROM	Neuromotor reeducation Light resisted activities for increasing motor output of the flexor tendons	Explore correction of joint flexion deformity if present with physician's consent Scapular stabilization is key to focal movement of flexor tendons	Pushing tasks for conditioning can exceed pulling tasks

AROM, Active ROM; *DIP*, distal interphalangeal; *IP*, interphalangeal; *MCP*, metacarpophalangeal; *PIP*, proximal interphalangeal; *ROM*, range of motion.

is custom-fabricated by a CHT to protect the repaired tendon from excessive stress associated with wrist and digital extension. The fingertips are passively flexed to the palm with rubber bands attached to the fingernails via hooks and adhesive. This passive flexion ROM pushes the repaired tendon proximally, reduces stress on the repair, and promotes tendon glide. The exercise program consists of passive ROM with dynamic flexion to the palm followed by active extension. Active extension against the dynamic flexion creates reciprocal inhibition and thus reduces stress on the repair and relaxes the repaired flexor tendon. The athlete exercises with the dorsal block splint in place at all times for the first 6 weeks. Joints with excessive edema require a graded and slower approach to realize full passive flexion. These athletes should be seen more often to ensure that full active extension and passive flexion motion is achieved early in rehabilitation. A modified Klienert and Duran postoperative rehabilitation protocol after repair of a torn FDP is described in

Table 14-5.[20,21] The presurgical and postsurgical rehabilitation programs include a focus on control of edema with compression, elevation, and protected movement based on the selected protocol (Fig. 14-3), as well as education of the athlete with regard to long-term disabilities, precautions, and appropriate compliance with the rehabilitation protocol.

Clinical Pearl #2

Stress on the FDP tendon repair at 6 to 8 weeks should occur slowly with a focus on AROM, avoidance of joint stiffness, and management of scar pain and adhesions (Fig. 14-4). The tendon repair will be at half strength 12 weeks after surgery.

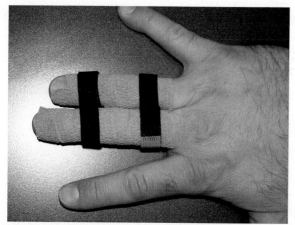

FIGURE 14-3 Coban wrap for swelling of the ring finger and a double-digit sleeve on the index and middle fingers. Buddy straps help initiate normal grasp, protect the volar plates, and promote tendon gliding.

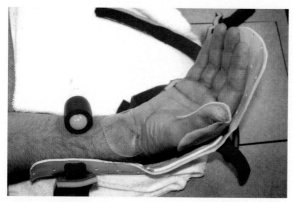

FIGURE 14-4 Flexor tendon treatment options to avoid scar pain and web space contractures.

BOUTONNIÈRE INJURIES (EXTENSOR TENDON INJURY OF THE PROXIMAL INTERPHALANGEAL JOINT)

A boutonnière deformity is a flexion deformity of the PIP joint with a hyperextension deformity of the DIP joint. Common mechanisms of injury include a direct blow to the dorsum of the PIP joint or forced flexion of the PIP joint while the extensor mechanism is actively extending the joint (e.g., opening the hand to catch a pass and being struck on the dorsum of the hand at the same time). This deformity can occur as a result of lengthening or complete rupture of the central slip at the PIP joint.[22] Swelling from the traumatic injury can displace the lateral bands volarly and further retract the ruptured extensor mechanism.

Anatomically, the central slip of the extensor mechanism is ruptured at the base of the middle phalanx.[22] The extensor mechanism may glide volar to the axis of the PIP joint. The injury can change the mechanical function of the extensor mechanism to a flexor of the PIP joint. This change coupled with unopposed action of the flexor digitorum superficialis (FDS) results in the boutonnière deformity.[23]

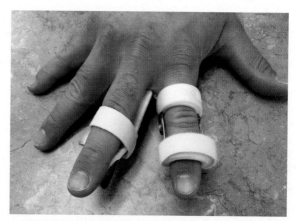

FIGURE 14-5 Splints for boutonnière deformities.

In acute injuries, it is difficult to differentiate a PIP joint sprain from a boutonnière injury. With either injury, swelling, pain, and an inability to actively extend the PIP joint can be noted. A digital block performed by a physician can limit the inhibiting effect of the pain and assist in detection of a ruptured extensor mechanism.[24] An extension lag at the PIP joint of greater than 15° after injury as a result of joint or contractile tissue problems is an indication for referral to a specialist. Surgical repair is rarely an option because the results are less predictable than with conservative management.[25] If this injury goes untreated or is managed as a PIP joint sprain by splinting the finger in slight flexion, a boutonnière deformity can occur. Other complications that may develop if this injury is not diagnosed appropriately include volar plate tightness, oblique retinacular tightness, and adhesions of the lateral bands. PIP joint dysfunction can result in loss of dexterity and long-term stiffness. A variety of splinting techniques are used to treat a PIP joint contracture. If a soft end-feel is present and contracture of the PIP joint is less than 35°, a custom static progressive splint may be used. If a firm end-feel contracture of greater than 25° is present, serial casting is recommended to stress the dense connective tissue contracture and correct the extension lag.[26] Splints that correct dense connective tissue should be provided by a CHT to maximize extension and avoid skin breakdown (Fig. 14-5). When full extension is achieved, the PIP joint is splinted continuously in full extension for 4 more weeks, and AROM exercises for the DIP and metacarpophalangeal (MCP) joints are then started.[19]

During the period of immobilization, the athlete is encouraged to perform AROM and passive ROM exercises for the DIP and MCP joints to prevent joint contracture and assist in healing of the extensor mechanism.[16] Short-arc AROM exercises for the PIP joint are initiated after the initial immobilization period. Splinting should continue until full pain-free motion is restored.[27]

Clinical Pearl #3

Extension lag as a result of volar plate stiffness of the PIP joint should be eliminated and healing of the extensor mechanism realized before implementation of ROM. Early recognition and priority treatment of these problems are essential in the first 2 to 4 weeks following injury to ensure a good functional outcome.

If loss of active extension develops, exercises are discontinued and splinting restarted for a minimum of 2 weeks.[28] Strengthening exercises can commence once active extension is ensured 8 weeks after injury. See Tables 14-9 and 14-10 for an approximate time line for return to sport. Injuries that do not respond to rehabilitation, have full passive extension of the PIP joint, and exhibit unacceptable extension lag are considered for surgery.

PROXIMAL INTERPHALANGEAL JOINT SPRAINS AND DISLOCATIONS

Painful stiff PIP joints can develop without appropriate follow-up and are commonly called coach's finger.[9] PIP joint sprains and dislocations are very common, so much so that they are often overlooked and undertreated. The mechanism of injury varies, and they are generally poorly reported by the athlete other than "I jammed my finger." Frequently, PIP joint dislocations are reduced on the field and the player then allowed to return to the game with buddy taping.[25] The problem with this approach is that the athlete may not have a simple dislocation but instead a fracture or other soft tissue trauma such as a volar plate injury. If the dislocation is reduced on the field, follow-up radiographs are required. Sotereanos et al[26] advise that reduction be delayed until radiographic evaluation is performed.

Joint stability must be assessed with the PIP joint in extension and flexion. [29] Anatomically, the collateral ligaments of the PIP joint are under the greatest tension when the joint is in full extension and the accessory ligaments in maximum flexion.

Three types of dislocations can occur: dorsal, lateral, and volar. Dorsal dislocations of the middle phalanx are the most common type and often cause the volar plate to be torn from its insertion on the middle phalanx. A lateral dislocation injures the collateral ligaments and volar plate, whereas a volar dislocation can cause an avulsion of the central slip of the extensor mechanism.[30] The dislocated PIP joint is typically treated by closed reduction. However, surgical intervention may be necessary if the joint is unstable after reduction or if the dislocation cannot be reduced.

Treatment of dislocations and sprains can be successful with simple finger-based splints. Dorsal blocking PIP joint splinting at 30° of flexion is often used for dorsal dislocations and side-by-side stabilization with buddy taping for lateral dislocations. Protective taping (see Fig. 14-3) or splinting must be continued during off-field activities for 3 to 6 weeks to prevent small aggravations of the injured joint, which can prolong recovery. Active exercises are begun as soon as possible, and continued splinting or taping is recommended for 8 to 12 weeks during participation in sports.

Clinical Pearl #4

Stability of the PIP joint must be supported for at least 6 weeks during daily activities and for 10 to 12 weeks during sporting tasks. Paraffin bathes and application of gentle flexion stress to the PIP joint can diminish joint stiffness and improve outcomes.

Box 14-2

Splint Considerations for Proximal Interphalangeal Joint Sprains and Dislocations After Reduction

DORSAL DISLOCATION

The finger is blocked with a dorsal extension gutter and the PIP joint in 25° to 30° of flexion.[26]
Edema should be controlled with a 1-inch Coban wrap (see Fig. 14-3).
The athlete is instructed to not extend the PIP joint beyond the limits of the splint for 2 weeks to protect the volar plate and prevent hyperextension.

VOLAR DISLOCATION

Splint the PIP joint in full extension with the DIP joint allowed full motion.
Protect against extensor lag for 6 weeks.

TREATMENT

After the protected phase, the athlete is instructed to progress to full AROM exercises.
Strengthening exercises are initiated at 6 to 8 weeks after injury if no PIP lag is present.
Protective splinting with buddy straps (see Fig. 14-3) is continued during athletic events until complete, pain-free motion is achieved.

AROM, Active range-of-motion; *DIP*, distal interphalangeal; *PIP*, proximal interphalangeal.

Flexor tendon adhesions commonly develop as a result of this injury. It is important for the athlete to receive follow-up evaluations and corrective splinting for 2 to 3 months after injury to avoid a painful, stiff, or deformed finger. Without this simple but appropriate care, these sprains can affect the athlete throughout the entire season. Splinting guidelines are listed in Box 14-2, and Tables 14-9 and 14-10 address an approximate time line for return to sport.

PSEUDOBOUTONNIÈRE DEFORMITY (VOLAR PLATE INJURY OF THE PROXIMAL INTERPHALANGEAL JOINT)

Pseudoboutonnière deformity occurs after a forceful hyperextension injury to the PIP joint that involves the volar plate.[31] Its clinical manifestations are very similar to that of a boutonnière deformity, with flexion deformity of the PIP joint. The slight difference occurs in the DIP joint: in a boutonnière deformity the DIP joint is in hyperextension, whereas a pseudoboutonnière deformity allows normal DIP joint motion.[31] If a flexion contracture of greater than 45° is present, surgical intervention is usually necessary. If the athlete has a flexion contracture of less than 45°, a static progressive extension splint applied by a CHT may be used to correct the deformity. Stiff PIP joints that do not respond to splints can be treated with serial casts applied by a CHT.

Table 14-6 Splinting Summary

	Boutonnière Injuries	PIP Sprains and Dislocations	Pseudoboutonnière Deformity
Splint type	Static custom finger-based splint	Custom dorsal block splint	Static progressive or dynamic splint to defeat flexor contracture
Joint position	PIP joint in extension while allowing MCP and DIP flexion	PIP joint in 15°-30° of flexion	Maintain PIP joint at end range of extension
Duration of splint wear	Continuous splinting for 6-8 weeks and participation in sports allowed[31]*	Dorsal block splint for 3-6 weeks*	6-8 weeks*
Splinting for competition	Static finger- or hand-based splint at 10-12 weeks*	Static finger- or hand-based splint at 10-12 weeks*	Static finger- or hand-based splint at 10-12 weeks*

DIP, Distal interphalangeal; *MCP*, metacarpophalangeal; *PIP*, proximal interphalangeal.
*Clearance from physician.

Rehabilitation includes initiation of AROM exercises during splinting to facilitate active gliding of the flexor and extensor tendons. Splints can be removed to perform exercises during the day.[30] Care must be taken to avoid injury to the volar plate as a result of the use of excessive force during exercise and daily tasks (buddy taping/straps, see Fig. 14-3). A strength program can be initiated at 6 to 8 weeks after injury, provided that the PIP joint is stable and no pain reflex is present.[29] Tables 14-9 and 14-10 provide an approximate time line for return to sport. Additionally, Table 14-6 presents a summary of splinting for boutonnière injuries, PIP joint sprains and dislocations, and pseudoboutonnière deformities.

METACARPAL FRACTURES

Metacarpal fractures can be the result of direct trauma, compression, or excessive rotational force on the hand.[6,32] Metacarpal fractures are generally associated with point tenderness at the fracture site and swelling within the hand. Careful inspection of rotation is done by having the athlete attempt to make a flat fist (MCP and PIP joint flexion and DIP joint extension) and observing whether all fingers have proper convergence. Before selecting the type of stabilization, radiographs are necessary to confirm the severity, location, and angulation of the fracture.

Stabilizing the fracture without bulky immobilization is critical to reduce edema and return the hand to normal ROM.[33] Ulnar or radial gutter thermoplastic splints have the advantage of being able to be remolded as needed for changes in edema to ensure fracture stability (Fig. 14-6). Table 14-7 provides an outline of splinting guidelines for metacarpal fractures.[35]

Clinical Pearl #5

When a metacarpal fracture is splinted, caution must be taken to avoid malalignment or abnormal rotation, which can result in long-term dysfunction. Splints should focus on maximum flexion of the MCP joints and maximum extension of the interphalangeal (IP) joints to maintain the closed-pack safe position and keep the joints from contracture (see Fig. 14-6).

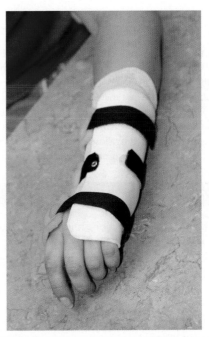

FIGURE 14-6 A metacarpal splint is designed to protect the healing facture and keep the ligaments in a closed-pack position.

Inadequate stabilization, insufficient control of edema, and poor adhesion prevention may lead to complications and delay return to sport. Edema is managed with the application of ice (dorsum of the hand only), elevation, and compression during and after the splinting phase. AROM is initiated with physician clearance to facilitate tendon glide and minimize the potential for tendon adhesions. Rehabilitation of metacarpal fractures that are managed by closed reduction and casting involves AROM of the unaffected joints during the initial immobilization period of 3 to 6 weeks.[19] Passive motion can be initiated after clinical healing, at approximately 6 weeks.[19,36] An approximate time line for return to sport can be found in Tables 14-9 and 14-10.

Table 14-7 Guidelines for Splinting Metacarpal Fractures

Clinical Reasoning	Splinting
Joint position	Wrist in 20° to 30° of extension MCP joint in 60° to 70° of flexion PIP and DIP joints in full extension Allows the MCP collateral ligaments to maintain proper length and avoid joint contracture The closed-pack position helps stabilize the fracture[34]
Duration of splint wear	4-8 weeks, depending on the severity of the fracture and the healing rate of the bone
Splinting for competition	Forearm-based custom splint in the same position as described earlier
Goals of splinting	Protect the healing fracture by placing the hand in a safe position and maintain the length of supporting structures

DIP, Distal interphalangeal; *MCP,* metacarpophalangeal; *PIP,* proximal interphalangeal.

BENNETT FRACTURE

A Bennett fracture is a small intraarticular fracture of the carpo-metacarpal (CMC) joint of the thumb caused by axial compression. Focal swelling at the CMC joint of the thumb and pain with movement or palpation of the first metacarpal are clinical indications of the presence of this injury. Every athlete in whom this injury is suspected should be referred to a hand specialist. This small-fragment fracture is generally treated by closed reduction and percutaneous pin fixation.[25] Splint considerations are presented in Table 14-8.

Clinical Pearl #6

Thumb supination, abduction, and extension must be maintained and retrained to ensure proper opposition and good dexterity. Stabilization of the CMC joint and early active ROM of the MCP and IP joints are key to a good outcome after a Bennett fracture.

If the fracture is treated by rigid internal fixation, the player may return to sport earlier, with external stability provided by a protective forearm-based thumb spica cast or splint and physician clearance.[37] Protective splinting (Fig. 14-7) is continued during competition until full strength and pain-free ROM have been reestablished.[25] This injury can have a major and long-standing impact on function. Restoration of joint biomechanics and healing of the fracture are keys to a good functional outcome. Consult Tables 14-9 and 14-10 for an expected time line for return to sport.

INJURY TO THE ULNAR COLLATERAL LIGAMENT OF THE THUMB

Commonly referred as gamekeeper's thumb or skier's thumb, this injury is caused by forceful hyperabduction or hyperextension of the thumb or a combination of the two. Injury to the ulnar collateral ligament (UCL) is common in skiers who fall on a ski pole and in football players and wrestlers who are attempting

Table 14-8 Splint Considerations for Bennett Fractures

Clinical Reasoning	Splinting
Joint position	Thumb spica cast or splint applied and worn for 3-4 weeks continuously Thumb placed in midposition of abduction and extension
Duration of splint wear	Forearm-based thumb spica split for 4-8 weeks, depending on severity index and clinical healing
Splinting for competition	Hand-based thumb spica for an additional 4 weeks with competition
Goals of splint	Protect healing structures at the base of the first metacarpal
Rehabilitation	At approximately 4 weeks, intraarticular pin removed and active motion of the thumb and wrist begins After 6-8 weeks, rehabilitation progresses to passive and resistance exercises[30] Protective splint for ADLs for 4 weeks and for sports for 8 weeks

ADLs, Activities of daily living.

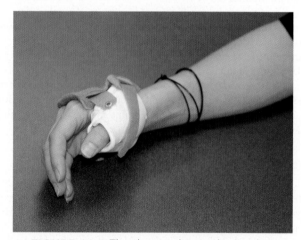

FIGURE 14-7 Thumb spica thermoplastic splint.

to grab their opponents.[4,34] The UCL is dense connective tissue that requires 8 to 12 weeks of healing before initiation of full functional stress. A combination of many structures can be involved with this lesion: UCL proper, UCL accessory, adductor pollicis, and the volar plate. Complete avulsion of the UCL at the first proximal phalanx is referred to as a Stener lesion and requires surgical intervention to achieve full recovery.

Athletes with UCL injuries have pain and swelling on the ulnar side of the MCP joint of the thumb.[38] Clinical examination of the UCL requires stressing the MCP joint in full flexion to evaluate the accessory ligament and in full extension to assess the proper ligament.[38,39] Hyperextension laxity of the MCP joint is indicative of volar plate involvement. Stress radiographs are indicated for documenting abduction instability and identifying involvement of bone.[40]

Surgical treatment and specialty care of these injuries are indicated for acute trauma with gross clinical instability (Fig. 14-8). These injuries cannot be reduced because of significant fragmentation of the articular surface, displacement of bone, or a rotation fracture fragment. Surgical management of chronic UCL

Table 14-9 Hierarchic Plan for Functional Return: Levels of Care*[7,12]

Level	Activity	Load	Pace	Goal
Level I: Restoration and balance phase (inflammatory and proliferation phase of healing)	Rest with a custom splint ADL fine motor dexterity training (lacing, buttoning, pegboard) Tendon glides (see Fig. 14-13) Nerve glides (avoid increase in pain or symptoms) Scapular and posture awareness (to increase proximal stability) Resume cardiovascular training if no open wounds	No load to avoid increasing the inflammatory phase of healing Sedentary functional tasks conducted below shoulder level	Therapist directed Self-paced	Athlete education on potential loss of function and need for compliance Establish a balance of hand function to minimize potential for deformity Maximize tendon excursion Treat edema Desensitize scar tissue Maintain neuromotor control Independence in self-care activities Postural control
Level II: Load and correction phase (maturation phase of healing)	Focus on strengthening linear motion patterns of the wrist and arm below shoulder level Thera-Putty Isometric grip and hold Isotonic wrist flexion and extension Core stability of proximal stabilizers critical to establish during this rehabilitation phase Closed kinetic chain exercises Continue level I tasks	Increase in physical demand level load from sedentary to light, light medium Increase in duration of rehabilitation activity from 1-2 hours total	Self-paced	Increase motor control Increase work capacity of injured structures in preparation for strength and conditioning program Start measures to correct joint deformities Eliminate compensatory movement patterns Master postural control
Level III (return-to-sport phase); level considered to be the highest level of function	Use of dynamic functional sport simulation tool Exposure to dynamic open kinetic chain strengthening tasks Overhead weight lifting Ulnar and radial deviation Pronation and supination	Increase in physical demand level load from medium to heavy	Sport pace	Maximize motor control Safe return to sport

Data from Lindsay, M., Lindsay, L., and Pitts, D.G. (1992): Levels of functional return. Personal communication; and Pitts, D.G., Hall, L.D., and Murray, P.M. (1999): Rehabilitation aspects of external fixation for distal radius fractures. Tech. Hand Upper Extremity Surg., 3:210–220.

ADL, Activity of daily living.

*Based on healing rates of involved tissues. The levels of care can provide clear communication on the hierarchic plan for functional return between clinicians and physicians during the rehabilitation process. This communication will help minimize the chance of overloading the recovering tissue, thereby producing a setback, which occurs easily in hand rehabilitation. Consultation with the team physician should be considered before a change in level.

instability is determined by MCP joint instability, loss of pinch strength, and loss of the ability to use a large grasp pattern.[25]

Clinical Pearl # 7

Good functional outcomes following a UCL injury depend on avoiding excessive stress on the UCL during early rehabilitation and everyday tasks. Athlete's who are non-compliant with splinting and engage in sports or strengthening activities too early can have a poor outcome.

UCL sprains are generally treated with a forearm-based thumb spica splint or cast with the thumb in slight adduction, approximately 40° from the palm, continuously for 4 to 6 weeks. UCL healing will progress slowly. AROM exercises can be initiated at 4 weeks and slowly progressed to avoid excessive stress on healing tissue. Protective splinting is recommended for at least another 10 weeks to ensure complete healing.[40,41] The time frame for return to sport is outlined in Tables 14-9 and 14-10.

SCAPHOID FRACTURE

Of all the carpal bones, the scaphoid is the most commonly fractured. Falling on an outstretched hand with the wrist in extension is the usual mechanism of injury.[28,42,43] Scaphoid fractures should be suspected in any athlete who has tenderness over the anatomic snuffbox, palmar side of the scaphoid, or radial side of the wrist. Pain with weight bearing, such as an inability to do push-ups with an open hand, may indicate a previously missed fracture. Diagnostic radiographic series should include anteroposterior, lateral, right and left oblique, and clenched-fist views in maximal radial and ulnar deviation.[44] If the radiographic findings are normal but the athlete remains symptomatic, a bone scan may be indicated to evaluate the status of the scaphoid.[44]

A large number of scaphoid fractures result in nonunion or avascular necrosis.[6,29,45] Avascular necrosis develops in 30% of waist (middle region) fractures and 90% of proximal fractures because the blood supply flows distal to proximal in the scaphoid and is carried by a single artery arising from the dorsal branch of the radial artery. Today, many scaphoid fractures are repaired immediately when the lesion is located at the proximal pole or

Table 14-10 Treatment Guidelines Summary

Injury and Location	Key Anatomic Structures	Splint Description	Splint Wear Schedule	Start Level I: AROM	Start Level I: PROM	Start Level II: Strength Program	Level III: Return to Sport
Mallet finger, fingertip	Terminal extensor mechanism	Custom Stax splint with DIP joint in full extension	24 hr/day, 7 days/week for 8 weeks	8 weeks	10 weeks	10 weeks	S/P injury with physician consent with 80% strength
Jersey finger with FDP repair, fingertip	Rupture of FDP tendon	Dorsal block splint with wrist at 20°-30° of flexion and dynamic finger flexion	24 hr/day, 7 days/week for 4.5-6 weeks	6 weeks	8-10 weeks with physician consent	8 weeks	8-10 weeks with protective splinting and physician consent with 80% strength
Boutonnière, deformity of the PIP joint	Rupture of central slip	Finger-based splint for PIP joint only in full extension and disallowing movement	24 hr/day, 7 days/week for 2-4 weeks*	4 weeks	6-8 weeks only with physician consent	8-10 weeks with physician consent	S/P injury with physician consent with 80% strength
Pseudoboutonnière, PIP joint sprains and dislocations	Volar plate, collateral ligaments	Dorsal block splint with PIP joint in 30° of flexion	24 hr/day, 7 days/week for 4-6 weeks*	1-4 weeks	6-10 weeks	10-12 weeks	S/P injury with physician consent and protective splinting with 80% strength
Metacarpal fracture	Most common on the fourth or fifth metacarpal	Forearm-based ulnar gutter splint with the MCP joints in maximum flexion and the IP joints in maximum extension	24 hr/day, 7 days/week for 4-6 weeks*	4-6 weeks	8-10 weeks	8-10 weeks	10-12 weeks with 80% strength
UCL sprain of the thumb	Sprain or rupture of UCL of the MCP joint of the thumb	Hand-based thumb spica splint with the thumb in midabduction and extension to protect the web space	24 hr/day, 7 days/week for 4-6 weeks*	6-8 weeks	10-12 weeks	10-12 weeks	12 weeks with 80% strength

Condition	Description	Splint	Immobilization				
Bennett fracture	Fracture at the base of the thumb	Hand-based thumb spica splint with the thumb in midabduction and extension to protect the web space	24 hr/day, 7 days/week for 6-8 weeks* Start rehabilitation if cleared by physician	8-10 weeks AROM ADL therapy splint with sports	10-12 weeks corrective splinting	10-12 weeks start strengthening level II	12 weeks Full sport if no pain and 80% strength
Scaphoid fracture	Fracture of the scaphoid located just distal to the radius	Forearm-based thumb spica splint with the thumb in midabduction and extension to protect the web space	24 hr/day, 7 days/week for 12-16 weeks*	8-12 weeks Splint to protect tender glide of digits	12-16 weeks AROM of wrist if healed Cleared by physician	14-16 weeks Advance strength tasks	S/P injury with physician consent with 80% strength
Ganglion cyst	Fluid-filled cyst normally appearing on the dorsal radial surface of the wrist	Forearm-based wrist cock-up splint with the wrist in neutral to 10° of extension	24 hr/day, 7 days/week for 2 weeks*	0-2 weeks AROM	3-6 weeks Strength	7-10 weeks Full sports and splint	Return to sport with splint in 1 week with physician consent with 80% strength
Wrist sprain, TFCC injury	Located at the distal end of the ulna	Wrist gauntlet with the wrist in neutral to 10° of extension	24 hr/day, 7 days/week for 8-12 weeks*	4-6 weeks AROM of digit 3	8-12 weeks AROM of the digits	12 weeks Slow progression in strength training if cleared by physician	12+ weeks with 80% strength
de Quervain tenosynovitis	Tendonitis of the first extensor compartment	Forearm-based thumb spica splint with the thumb in midabduction and extension to rest the first extensor compartment	24 hr/day, 7 days/week for 4-6 weeks*	2-3 weeks Nest with splint	4-6 weeks Tendon glides Grip strength	6-8 weeks Work simulation	6-8 weeks with 80% strength

ADL, Activities of daily living; *AROM*, active range of motion; *DIP*, distal interphalangeal; *FDP*, flexor digitorum profundus; *IP*, interphalangeal; *MCP*, metacarpophalangeal; *PIP*, proximal interphalangeal; *PROM*, passive range of motion; *S/P*, status post; *TFCC*, triangular fibrocartilage complex; *UCL*, ulnar collateral ligament.

*Physician's approval should be obtained before progression by all.

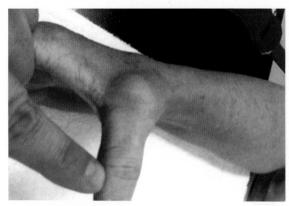

FIGURE 14-8 Laxity of the ulnar collateral ligament— "gamekeepers thumb."

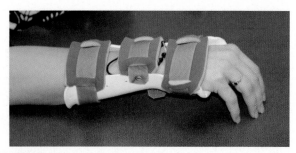

FIGURE 14-9 A wrist gauntlet splint is used to stabilize, protect, and allow use of the hand without stressing injured tissue.

waist (middle) region. Distal pole fractures are repaired if no evidence of healing is seen on radiographs at 4 weeks. Scaphoid fractures are classified (and seen clinically) in the following anatomic distributions[45]:

- 20% involving the proximal pole
- 70% involving the waist (middle region)
- 10% involving the distal pole

Clinical Pearl #8

Rehabilitation of scaphoid fractures should focus first on AROM, grip strength, and wrist flexion and extension to 80% of that on the unaffected side before weight-bearing tasks. Torquing tasks of pronation-supination, radial-ulnar deviation, and overhead activities must be progressed slowly.

Continuous long arm casting for stable nondisplaced fractures of the distal pole for up to 3 months is a common treatment. Radiographs and refitting of a cast every 3 to 4 weeks is necessary to ensure that stability of the healing scaphoid is maintained.[25] Removal of the cast for showering and wearing one cast for practice and another for daily tasks can have a negative impact during the early healing period. Some physicians choose early fixation and a thumb spica cast or splint (see Fig. 14-7) for wrist and proximal pole scaphoid fractures. Casts or splints must be worn at all times until healing is evident on radiographs. With all scaphoid fractures, treatment compliance is critical because of their poor healing rates. An approximate time frame for return to sport is presented in Tables 14-9 and 14-10. Progression of treatment must be slow to avoid reinjury.

GANGLION CYSTS

Ganglion cysts generally arise from ligamentous structures around the wrist. They are most common on the dorsal, radial side of the wrist. Ganglion cysts can arise from the synovial lining of a tendon sheath or from the joint capsule.[46] Ligamentous injuries involving the wrist should be ruled out before return to sport. The athlete will complain of wrist pain with motion and tenderness on palpation. Physician referral is needed to differentiate between a cyst and a tumor.

The conservative treatment of choice is rest with a wrist cock-up splint (Fig. 14-9) and modification of activity, along with nonsteroidal antiinflammatory medications. Aspiration and surgical intervention are alternative treatments if conservative methods fail. See Tables 14-9 and 14-10 for an approximate time line for return to sport.

Clinical Pearl #9

Postsurgical treatment of a ganglion cyst focuses on wrist flexion with the fingers flexed to maximize extrinsic extensor distal glide and scar management. Wrist extension with weight bearing should be progressed slowly.

INJURY TO THE TRIANGULAR FIBROCARTILAGE COMPLEX

The main function of the triangular fibrocartilage complex (TFCC) is to act as a strut and stabilize the distal radioulnar joint during functional pronation and supination activities, and it is critical for support of the ulnar carpus.[8,47] The TFCC supports approximately 20% of axial loading through the wrist below shoulder level and 80% above shoulder level. Injury to the TFCC commonly results from a fall on the outstretched hand and the carpus in ulnar deviation. Therefore, this structure is commonly injured with distal radius fractures and wrist sprains.[48] The TFCC can sustain injuries in both the medial meniscus disk area and the outer support structures.

Palmer's[47] classification divides TFCC injuries into two types: type 1 is traumatic injury, which results from an acute injury, and type 2 is degenerative injury, which is attributed to degenerative processes such as arthritis. TFCC meniscus disk perforations increase with age, with an estimated 7% incidence rate by the age of 30 and a 53% incidence by the age of 60.

Athletes with a TFCC tear will have pain and discomfort with palpation directly over the ulnar side of the wrist. They will complain of painful catching and snapping of the wrist during rotational tasks. Weight-bearing and ulnar-deviated tasks with the forearm pronated place a high level of stress on the TFCC. Such activities include but are not limited to strengthening exercises such as dips, bench press, overhead press, and dumbbell exercises.

Nonoperative treatment consisting of rest and avoidance of painful activities should be the first treatment option.[30] Immobilization with the forearm in a neutral position is maintained with a custom-fitted long arm or Munster splint (Fig. 14-10). The wrist is placed in 10° to 20° of extension and included in the splint.[5] A wrist gauntlet splint (see Fig. 14-9) (10° to 20° of wrist extension) is a second choice to support the wrist against ulnar and radial deviation for 4 to 6 weeks. The athlete should limit pronation, supination, and joint-loading activities

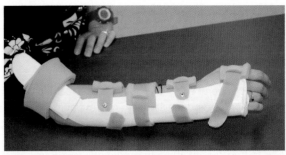

FIGURE 14-10 A Munster splint disallows forearm pronation and supination while allowing elbow flexion and extension. This splint allows the distal radioulnar joint to rest.

and avoid heavy lifting/carrying and pushing/pulling activities. Overhead and torquing tasks that incorporate radial/ulnar deviation and pronation/supination activities are also contraindicated. Consult Tables 14-9 and 14-10 for an approximate time line for return to sport.

Clinical Pearl #10

Improper wearing of splints and inappropriate torque stress are the main reasons for poor functional outcomes after TFCC injures. Aggressive use of pronation/supination and radial/ulnar deviation exercises without an appropriate healing time (10 to 12 weeks) can result in reinjury. Athletes must first regain adequate AROM, strength of wrist flexion/extension, and weight-bearing tolerance before torque to achieve a good functional outcome.

DE QUERVAIN TENOSYNOVITIS

de Quervain tenosynovitis involves irritation of the extensor pollicis brevis and abductor pollicis longus tendons in the first dorsal extensor compartment of the wrist. It is usually caused by overuse, although it may result from a direct blow to the first dorsal compartment. It is seen most often in players of racquet sports, gymnasts, and golfers.[10,49,50] The athlete complains of pain on the radial side of the wrist localized over the radial styloid area. A positive Finkelstein test result indicates a strong possibility of de Quervain tenosynovitis. The test is performed by the athlete flexing the thumb into the palm and making a full fist; the wrist is then passively deviated with gentle force in an ulnar direction. The test is positive if the athlete feels excruciating pain over the first dorsal wrist compartment.[51] Evaluation of the thumb includes assessing for muscular tightness of the flexor pollicis longus (FPL) and tenderness on palpation of the first CMC joint.

Clinical Pearl #11

FPL tightness, inappropriate work/rest cycles, and initiation of a strengthening and torquing program before pain-free full AROM is mastered can have a detrimental impact on recovery from de Quervain tenosynovitis.

Conservative treatment consists of therapeutic modalities to decrease the pain and inflammation and splinting with a forearm-based thumb spica (see Fig. 14-7) to rest the first dorsal wrist compartment. The forearm-based thumb spica splint should place the wrist in approximately 15° of extension and the thumb in 40° of abduction and 10° of metacarpal flexion with the IP joint free. The splint is worn all the time for 3 weeks and then 6 weeks for heavy tasks.[19] Nonsteroidal antiinflammatory medications may be prescribed, and steroid injections may also be considered.[44] If symptoms persist, surgery may be necessary to release the tendon sheath.[6] Tables 14-9 and 14-10 contain an approximate time line for return to sport.

CONCLUSION

Hand injuries are very common in athletes and pose many challenges to the health care professional. Because of pressure for early return to sport, a good long-term functional outcome can be difficult to achieve. Advancements in hand surgery techniques, evidence-based rehabilitation programs, and improvements in splinting material and methods have resulted in enhanced outcomes. The following points have proved to provide safe, reliable, and excellent functional outcomes.

- "Do no harm"—the hand is a complex system designed to produce power and dexterity. If mismanaged, dysfunction and a poor outcome will occur.
- Advanced upper extremity evaluation skills will enhance the quality of care. These skills require knowledge of surface anatomy, postural analysis, joint function, and nerve function and the ability to distinguish between contractile and noncontractile tissue dysfunction.
- "Don't feed a pain reflex"—excessive passive ROM can increase muscle guarding and decrease function.
- Advance treatment according to the stages of wound healing. Always consider the type of tissue injured and its location, function, and adjacent structures when setting rehabilitation and functional goals.
- Seek to restore balance of function.
- Treat pitfalls before development of the following problems:
  - Scar adhesions
  - Intrinsic and extrinsic muscle tightness
  - Joint stiffness
  - Pain reflexes: joint, nerve, muscle, and skin
- Strive for core stability/postural alignment. "Edema is scar in evolution"—use assertive edema management to prevent tendon adhesions, joint stiffness, and painful scars. Techniques include the following:
  - Elevation
  - Compression
  - Rest
  - Movement
  - Pressure on scars with silicon
- Use the hierarchy of hand rehabilitation to guide treatment. This approach will help prevent pitfalls and restore function. Treat the whole body. Performance of functional and sport-specific activities requires a mobile thoracic spine, stable shoulder, proper postural alignment, and strong core musculature to reduce the mechanical load on the hand, wrist, or elbow.
- Advance the treatment of postsurgical athletes only with prior communication and consent of the physician.

Level I (Inflammatory and Proliferation Phase of Healing)

ACTIVE MOTION EXERCISES FOR THE DIGITS AND UPPER EXTREMITY

Individual AROM exercises for the fingers are described in this section and can be used for all injuries after clearance for AROM exercises. These exercises establish a balance by maximizing excursion of tendons and eliminating imbalance of the intrinsic and extrinsic muscle systems. If these exercises are performed while compensatory movements are eliminated, the formation of adhesions will be minimized. Each exercise is performed within the pain tolerance of the injured athlete. Sets and repetitions depend on the clinician's preference; generally one to two sets of 10 to 15 repetitions four to six times per day are used with these active exercises. Additionally, the injured athlete is educated in all appropriate exercises so that proper exercise technique is used. The athlete is encouraged to take responsibility for performing the exercises several times a day independently.

Compensatory movement patterns are common with hand and wrist injuries. These learned abnormal movement patterns occur because of joint stiffness, tendon adhesions, pain, edema, or focal weakness. Such patterns include scapular destabilization with protraction, elevation, and internal rotation. Compensatory hand patterns include thumb adduction and wrist flexion with grasp. These abnormal movement patterns are best addressed with rote functional tasks. These tasks defeat the pain reflex and restore the natural motor patterns of the hand and upper extremities.

INTRINSIC HAND EXERCISES

Dorsal and Palmar Interossei Muscle Exercises

Interossei Stretch. To stretch the interossei muscles, the MCP joint is placed in slight hyperextension and the athlete's PIP joint is only slowly and passively moved into flexion. This stretch will improve flexibility around the MCP and PIP joints and help restore the athlete's natural grasp. Care should be taken to not overstretch the extensor mechanism with aggressive passive flexion exercises (Fig. 14-11).

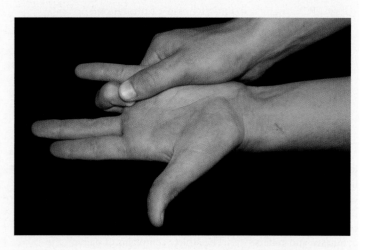

FIGURE 14-11 To stretch the interosseous muscles, the metacarpophalangeal (MCP) joint is put into slight hyperextension and the athlete's proximal interphalangeal (PIP) joint receives only slow passive range of motion (ROM) into flexion. This stretch will improve flexibility around the MCP and PIP joints and help restore the natural grasp. This exercise should be done before AROM of the lumbricals. Level I.

Finger Abduction and Adduction. The athlete spreads the fingers apart and then places them together. This facilitates fluid shift in the palm and decreases edema when working the interossei musculature of the hand.

Lumbrical Exercises

The athlete flexes the MCP joint to 90° and then alternately flexes and extends the IP joints into full flexion and full extension to facilitate stretching of the interossei and lumbricals (Fig. 14-12).[52] To stretch the lumbrical, the MCP is positioned in slight hyperextension, and the athlete is asked to flex the DIP and PIP joints. This stretch will restore normal length to the lumbrical and allow the FDP to achieve full excursion and restore the natural grasp reflex.

Opposition

The athlete touches every fingertip with the thumb starting with the index finger and progressing by sliding the thumb down the small finger into the palm of the hand to facilitate full flexion of the thumb.

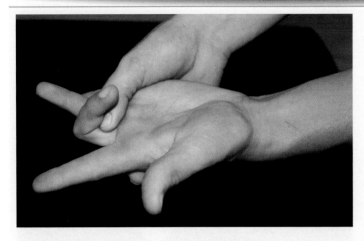

FIGURE 14-12 To stretch the lumbrical, the metacarpophalangeal joint is put into slight hyperextension, and the athlete is asked to flex the distal interphalangeal and proximal interphalangeal joints. This stretch will improve flexor digitorum profundus function and help restore the natural grasp pattern. Level I.

EXTRINSIC HAND EXERCISES

Tendon-Gliding Exercises or Staged Fisting

This exercise involves making various types of fists with the digits in a progression that starts with full extension followed by a tabletop (intrinsic-plus) position, a flat fist, a full fist without thumb, and finally a hook (intrinsic-minus) position (Fig. 14-13). These exercises are designed to facilitate gliding of the FDS and FDP tendons through zone II and restore balance between the intrinsic and extrinsic muscles.

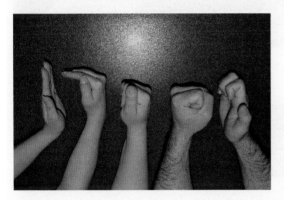

FIGURE 14-13 Tendon-gliding exercises. From left to right: beginning position in full extension, a tabletop position (intrinsic-plus position), flat fist (flexor digitorum superficialis [FDS]), full fist (flexor digitorum profundus [FDP]), and a hook position (intrinsic-minus position for maximum differential tendon glide of the FPD versus the FDS and to detect tightness of the lumbricals). Level I.

Isolated Tendon Excursions or Joint-Blocking Exercises

These exercises are designed to isolate the FDS, FDP, and FPL tendons to increase AROM of a specific joint (Fig. 14-14). The athlete holds the MCP joints of all fingers in extension. To isolate FDP tendon excursion, the athlete holds the finger below the DIP joint crease and then flexes and extends the DIP joint (see Fig. 14-14). To isolate the FDS tendon, the athlete places the fingers beside the tested finger and then flexes and extends the PIP joint (Fig. 14-15). To isolate the FPL tendon, the athlete holds the finger below the crease of the thumb IP joint and then flexes and extends the IP joint. It is critical that the joints be properly stabilized during these exercises to prevent substitution.

EXTRINSIC FOREARM MUSCLE STRETCH

Extrinsic extensor stretch is conducted with the elbow extended, the forearm pronated, a full fist, and wrist flexion stretching in conjunction with passive overpressure from the opposite hand. This exercise stretches the extrinsic extensor muscles and improves grip strength and endurance (Fig. 14-16). Extrinsic flexor stretch is conducted with the elbow in extension, the forearm supinated, the wrist in extension, and the digits fully extended. This exercise will stretch the extrinsic flexor muscles and improve grip strength and endurance (Fig. 14-17).

(Continued)

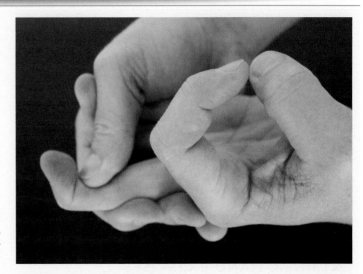

FIGURE 14-14 Joint-blocking exercise for distal interphalangeal joint flexion of the index finger. This is focal tendon glide and motor reeducation for the flexor digitorum profundus. Level I.

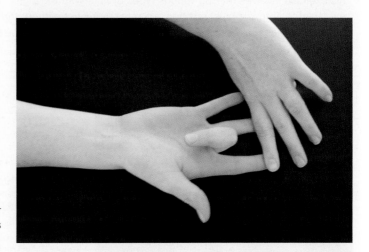

FIGURE 14-15 Isolation motor function test for the flexor digitorum superficialis of the ring finger. This exercise helps avoid tendon adhesions and improves dexterity. Level I.

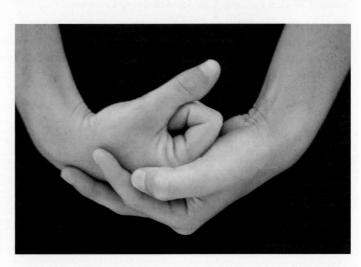

FIGURE 14-16 Passive wrist flexion to stretch the extrinsic extensors. This will improve motor control, endurance, and minimize pain. Level I. (Stay below the pain reflex.)

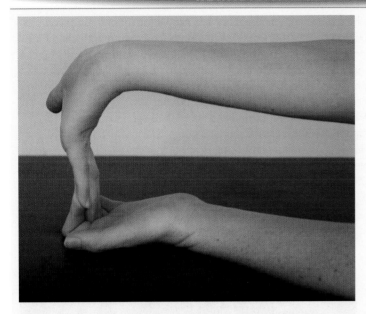

FIGURE 14-17 Passive wrist extension to stretch the extrinsic flexors. This will improve motor control and endurance and minimize pain. Level I.

PASSIVE MOTION EXERCISES FOR THE DIGITS

The goal of rehabilitation for digits is to obtain full flexion without losing extension. Pushing the joint beyond the pain threshold should be avoided because this can cause an inflammatory reaction and slow progression. Do not feed a pain reflex! Passive ROM exercises should be gentle and not be performed if extension of the digit is being compromised. Passive exercises are often combined with the active exercises described earlier and are performed with gentle overpressure by either the athlete or treating clinician. Stretches should be held for 5 to 10 seconds and repeated 5 to 10 times as needed. Passive ROM exercises are generally initiated after 2 weeks of AROM activities.

Treatment of Edema and Scarring

Edema is a scar in evolution. All hand injuries should be treated for edema and scar formation. Several techniques can be used to accomplish this. Overhead fisting should be performed at 5 to 10 repetitions per hour, which opens the lymphatic chain and allows the edema to be pumped out of the hand. Overhead fisting also incorporates elevation and mobility to diminish the edema. The injured hand should be elevated above heart level at all times, which allows gravity to have a positive impact on edema. Compression is obtained with a Coban wrap and edema glove to decrease edema in the digits and hand.

The use of thin silicone sheets or elastomer over a nonopen incision site for several hours per day will assist in scar management. Soft tissue massage is commonly prescribed to loosen a stiff joint or facilitate scar mobility. Minivibrators are also often used in the maturation phase to enhance this technique.

Level II (Maturation Phase of Healing)

STRENGTHENING EXERCISES

Rehabilitation should focus on gradual ramping of load while maintaining focal excursion and differential glide of affected structures. Care must be taken to not regress to the inflammatory stage by overloading tissue. The athlete must be made aware of compensatory movement patterns and avoid them to have a complete and speedy recovery. Rehabilitation exercises should be conducted below shoulder level. Wrist and forearm strengthening should be conducted with linear motion planes. Core stability exercises are initiated to establish proximal strength and avoid compensation.

All AROM exercises described earlier can be used for strengthening exercises with the use of manual resistance or light resistive elastic bands. Gripping exercises are commonly performed to strengthen the flexor tendons. Various devices can be used for strengthening the intrinsic and extrinsic muscles of the hand and wrist.

(Continued)

Soft Thera-Putty is ideal for early rehabilitation because it provides light biofeedback and allows full tendon excursion. Start with light resistance 3 to 5 times per day for 5 to 10 minute at a time. Focus should be placed on strengthening the extrinsic flexors. This is accomplished by making a hook posture while using Thera-Putty. The athlete's strength will improve with a decrease in intrinsic tightness. Isometric grip and hold tasks help restore a natural grasp reflex with controlled exposure to work without repetition. Start with a 30-second hold and build up to 1 minute and then a 1-minute rest period for 10 repetitions 3 times per day with a 10-lb gripper. If no flare-up from the putty and gripper occurs, resistance can be increased to 30% of maximum grip and 3 to 4 sets of 15 repetitions performed and held for 10 seconds (Fig. 14-18). The use of wrist flexion and extension with resistance is a great way to restore a natural grasp. Start with 2 sets of 10 repetitions 3 times per day at 20% to 30% of maximum force (Figs. 14-19 and 14-20). Postural stability exercises are an effective way to enhance upper extremity function and include closed kinetic chain scapular stabilization exercises (Fig. 14-21). Progression should be guided by pain, maintenance of active excursion, and healing restraints of the particular injury.

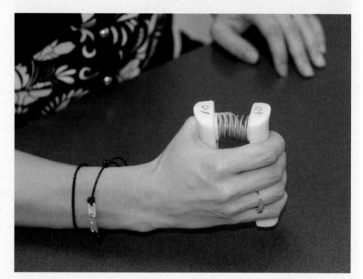

FIGURE 14-18 Grip and hold exercise. This exercise is used to improve grasp endurance and strength. Start slow at 10 lb of resistance and hold 1 minute on and 1 minute off. If no pain is felt after the exercise, 30% of grip strength can be a safe starting point. The duration of grasp is decreased to 10 seconds, and repetitions and sets can be progressed as tolerated. Level II.

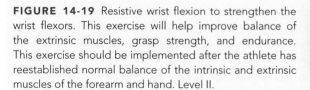
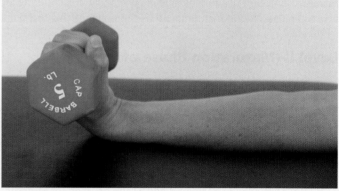

FIGURE 14-19 Resistive wrist flexion to strengthen the wrist flexors. This exercise will help improve balance of the extrinsic muscles, grasp strength, and endurance. This exercise should be implemented after the athlete has reestablished normal balance of the intrinsic and extrinsic muscles of the forearm and hand. Level II.

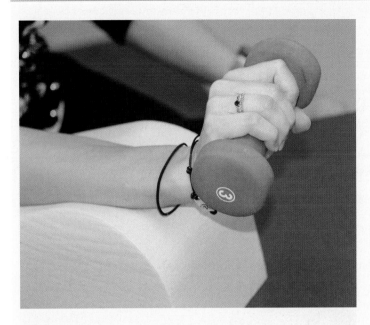

FIGURE 14-20 Resistive wrist extension to strengthen the wrist extensors. This exercise will help improve balance of the extrinsic muscles, grasp strength, and endurance. This exercise should be implemented after the athlete has reestablished normal balance of the intrinsic and extrinsic muscles of the forearm and hand. Level II.

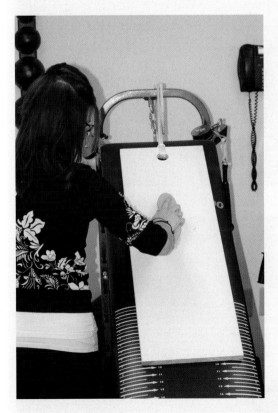

FIGURE 14-21 Stress-loading exercise with the Dystrophile can restore scapular stabilization with closed kinetic chain strengthening and diminish hypersensitivity of the hand and wrist. Level II.

(Continued)

Level III (Return-to-Sport Phase)

DYNAMIC STRENGTHENING EXERCISES FOR THE WRIST AND FOREARM

These exercises are performed to facilitate the highest level of return to functional activities. This group of exercises facilitates synergetic muscle recruitment to maximize motor control and coordination for return to sport. Exposure to forearm- and wrist-torquing exercises, overhead weight-bearing tasks, and kinetic chain exercises is the cornerstone of this phase of rehabilitation. These types of exercises should be attempted only after the athlete has mastered level I and level II tasks.

- Fast grip exercise is started with a 10-lb gripper for up to a set of 100 repetitions or the development of fatigue (which ever occurs first), 1 per second followed by a 1-minute rest period between sets. This exercise can be progressed to 25% of maximum grip to improve grip strength and endurance.
- Resistive radial deviation, ulnar deviation, supination, and pronation are considered to be high-level movement patterns and strengthening techniques (Figs. 14-22 through 14-25).
- Open kinetic chain tasks include but are not limited to weight lifting and Thera-Band tasks.
- Closed kinetic chain tasks include but are not limited to stress loading and push-ups.

Note: All these exercises are recommended for all wrist and hand injuries with physician consent.

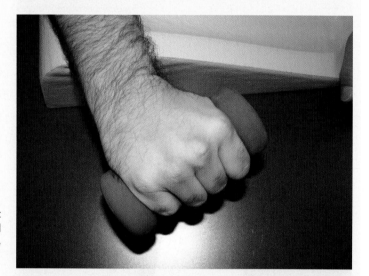

FIGURE 14-22 Resistive radial deviation. This movement is considered to be a high-level movement pattern and strengthening technique for all wrist pathologies. Incorporate this exercise after successful completion of level II tasks. Level III.

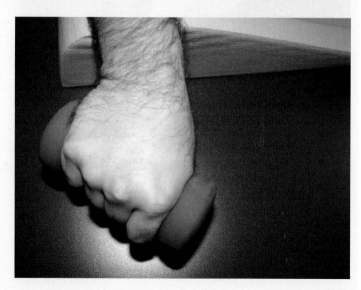

FIGURE 14-23 Resistive ulnar deviation. This movement is considered to be a high-level movement pattern and strengthening technique for all wrist pathologies. Incorporate this exercise after successful completion of level II tasks. Level III.

REHABILITATIVE EXERCISES—cont'd

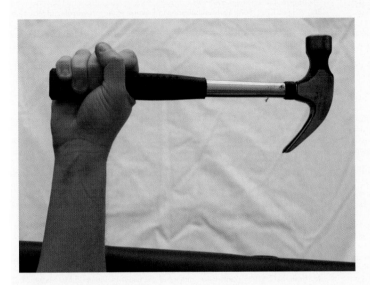

FIGURE 14-24 Resistive supination. This movement is considered to be a high-level movement pattern and strengthening technique for all wrist pathologies. Incorporate this exercise after successful completion of level II tasks. Level III.

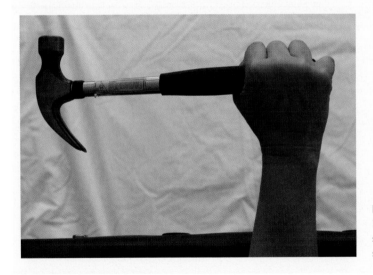

FIGURE 14-25 Resistive pronation. This movement is considered to be a high-level movement pattern and strengthening technique. Incorporate this exercise after successful completion of level II tasks. Level III.

REFERENCES

1. Foreman, S., and Gieck, J.H. (1992): Rehabilitative management of injuries to the hand. Clin. Sports Med., 11:239–252.
2. Leadbeter, W.B., Buckwalter, J.A., and Gordon, S.L. (1990): Sport-Induced Inflammation: Clinical and Basic Science Concepts. Park Ridge, IL, American Academy of Orthopaedic Surgeons.
3. Abouna, J.M., and Brown, H. (1968): The treatment of mallet finger. The results in a series of 148 consecutive cases and a review of the literature. Br. J. Surg., 55:653–667.
4. Kulund, D.N. (1982): The Injured Athlete. Philadelphia, Lippincott, pp. 295–329.
5. McCue, F.C., Hakala, M.H., Andrews, J.R., and Gieck, J.H. (1974): Ulnar collateral ligament injuries of the thumb in athletes. J. Sports Med., 2:70–80.
6. Posner, M.A. (1990): Hand injuries. In Nicholas, J. A., and Hershman, E.B. (eds.): The Upper Extremity in Sports Medicine. St. Louis, Mosby, pp. 495–594.
7. McCue, F.C. (1982): The elbow, wrist, and hand. In Kulund, D.N. (ed.): The Injured Athlete. Philadelphia, Lippincott, pp. 295–329.
8. Werner, F.M., Glisson, R.R., Murphy, D.J., and Palmer, A.K. (1986): Force transmission through the distal radioulnar carpal joint: Effect of ulnar lengthening and shortening. Handchir. Mikrochir. Plast. Chir., 18:304–308.
9. McCue, F.C., Honner, R., Gieck, J.H., et al. (1975): A pseudo-boutonniere deformity. Hand, 7:166–170.
10. Weiker, G.G. (1992): Hand and wrist problems in the gymnast. In Culzer, J.E. (ed.): Clinical Sports Medicine: Injuries of the Hand and Wrist. Philadelphia: Saunders, pp. 189–202.
11. McCue, F.C., and Cabrera, J.N. (1992): Common athletic digital joint injuries of the hand. In Strickland, J.W., and Rettig, A.C. (eds.): Hand Injuries in Athletes. Philadelphia, Saunders, pp. 49–94.
12. Redler, M. (1989): Dislocation of the interphalangeal joints and metacarpophalangeal joints. Sport Injury Manage., 2:59–66.
13. Leddy, J.F., and Dennis, T.R. (1992): Tendon injuries. In Stricklan, J.W., and Rettig, A.C. (eds.): Hand Injuries in Athletes. Philadelphia, Saunders, pp. 175–207.
14. Carroll, R.E., and Match, R.M. (1970): Avulsion of the profundus tendon insertion. J. Trauma, 10:1109.
15. Leddy, J.P., and Packer, J.W. (1977): Avulsion of the profundus tendon insertion in athletes. J. Hand Surg., 2:66–69.
16. Schneider, L.H. (1990): Tendon injuries of the hand. In Nicholas, J.A., and Hershman, E.B. (eds.): The Upper Extremity in Sports Medicine. St. Louis, Mosby, pp. 595–618.
17. Lester, B. (1999): Sport Injuries. In The Acute Hand. Stamford, CT, Appleton Lange, pp. 361–390.

18. Russe, O. (1960): Fracture of the carpal navicular: Diagnosis, non-operative and operative treatment. J. Bone Joint Surg. Am., 42:759–768.

19. Sadler, J.A., and Koepfer, J.M. (1992): Rehabilitation and the splinting of the injured hand. In Strickland, J.W., and Rettig, A.C. (eds.): Hand Injuries in Athletes. Philadelphia, Saunders, pp. 235–276.

20. Duran, R., and Houser, R. (1975): Controlled passive motion following flexor tendon repair in zone 2 and 3. AAOS Symposium on Tendon Surgery in the Hand. St. Louis, Mosby.

21. Kleinert, H.E., Kutz, J.E., and Cohen, M.J. (1975): Primary repair of zone 2 flexor tendon lacerations. AAOS Symposium on Tendon Surgery in the Hand. St. Louis: Mosby.

22. Rettig, A.C. (1992): Closed tendon injuries of the hand and wrist in the athlete. Clin. Sports Med., 11:77–99.

23. Rosenthal, E.A. (1995): The extensor tendons: Anatomy and management. In Hunter, J.M., Macken, E.J., and Callhan, A.B. (eds.): Rehabilitation of the Hand: Surgery and Therapy. St. Louis, Mosby–Year Book, pp. 519–564.

24. Burton, R.I., and Eaton, R.G. (1973): Common hand injuries in the athlete. Orthop. Clin. North Am., 4:809–838.

25. McCue, F.C., and Wooten, S.L. (1986): Closed tendon injuries of the hand in athletics. Clin. Sports Med., 5:741–755.

26. Sotereanos, D.G., Levy, J.A., and Herndon, J.H. (1994): Hand and wrist injuries. In Fu, F.H., and Stone, D.A. (eds.): Sport Injuries: Mechanisms, Prevention, Treatment. Baltimore, Williams & Wilkins, pp. 937–947.

27. McCue, F.C., Hussamy, O.D., and Gieck, J.H. (1996): Hand and wrist injuries. In Zachazewski, J.E., Magee, D.J., and Quillen, W.S. (eds.): Athletic Injuries and Rehabilitation. Philadelphia, Saunders, pp. 585–597.

28. Wilson, R.L., and Hazen, J. (1995): Management of joint injuries and intraarticular fractures of the hand. In Hunter, J.M., Macken, E.J., and Callhan, A.B. (eds.): Rehabilitation of the Hand: Surgery and Therapy. St. Louis, Mosby–Year Book, pp. 377–394.

29. Kapandji, I.A. (1982): The Physiology of Joints, Vol. I, Upper Limb. New York, Churchill Livingstone, pp. 1860–1891.

30. McCue, F.C., and Garroway, R.Y. (1985): Sport injuries to the hand and wrist. In Schneider, R.C. (ed.): Sport Injuries: Mechanism, Prevention, and Treatment. Baltimore, Williams & Wilkins, pp. 743–764.

31. McCue, F.C., and Redler, M.R. (1990): Coach's finger. In Torg, J.S., Welsh, P.R., and Shepard, R.J. (eds.): Current Therapy in Sports Medicine. Toronto, Decker, pp. 438–443.

32. Hastings, H. (1992): Management of extraarticular fractures of the phalanges and metacarpals. In Strickland, J.W., and Rettig, A.C. (eds.): Hand Injuries in Athletes. Philadelphia, Saunders, pp. 129–153.

33. Wright, S.C. (1990): Fracture and dislocation in the hand and wrist. In Torg, J.S., Welsh, P.R., and Shepard, R.J. (eds.): Current Therapy in Sports Medicine. Toronto, Decker, pp. 443–446.

34. Lane, L.B. (1995): Acute ulnar collateral ligament rupture of the metacarpophalangeal joint of the thumb. In Torg, J.S., and Shepard, R.J. (eds.): Current Therapy in Sports Medicine. St. Louis, Mosby, pp. 151–161.

35. Colditz, J.C. (1995): Functional fracture bracing. In Hunter, J.M., Macken, E.J., and Callhan, A.B. (eds.): Rehabilitation of the Hand: Surgery and Therapy. St. Louis, Mosby–Year Book, pp. 395–406.

36. Wright, T.A. (1968): Early mobilization in fractures of the metacarpals and phalanges. Can. J. Surg., 11:491–498.

37. Rettig, A.C., and Rowdon, G.A. (1995): Metacarpal fractures. In Torg, J.S., and Shepard, R.J. (eds.): Current Therapy in Sports Medicine. St. Louis, Mosby, pp. 152–156.

38. Melone, C.P. (1990): Fracture of the wrist. In Nicholas, J.A., and Hershman, E.B. (eds.): The Upper Extremity in Sports Medicine. St. Louis, Mosby, pp. 419–456.

39. Adams, B.D., and Muller, D.L. (1996): Assessment of thumb positioning in the treatment of ulnar collateral ligament injuries. A laboratory study. Am. J. Sports Med., 24:672–675.

40. Pitts, D.G., Hall, L.D., and Murray, P.M. (1999): Rehabilitation aspects of external fixation for distal radius fractures. Tech. Hand Upper Extremity Surg., 3:210–220.

41. McCue, F.C., and Bruce, J.F. (1994): Hand and wrist. In DeLee, J.C., and Drez, D., Jr. (eds.): Orthopaedic Sports Medicine Principles and Practice, Vol. I. Philadelphia, Saunders, pp. 913–944.

42. Cooney, W.P., Linscheid, R.L., and Dobyns, J.H. (1996): Fracture and dislocation of the wrist. In Rockwood, C.A., Green, D.P., and Bucholz, R.W. (eds.): Fracture in Adults. Philadelphia, Lippincott, pp. 745–867.

43. Weber, E.R., and Chao, E.Y. (1978): An experimental approach to the mechanism of scaphoid wrist fractures. J. Hand Surg., 3:142–148.

44. Shaw Wilgis, E.F., and Yates, A.Y. (1990): Wrist pain. In Nicholas, J.A., and Hershman, E.B. (eds.): The Upper Extremity in Sports Medicine. St. Louis, Mosby, pp. 483–494.

45. Gelberman, R.H., Panagis, J.S., Taleisnk, J., and Baumgaertner, M. (1983): The arterial anatomy of the human carpus. Part I. The extraosseous vascularity. J. Hand Surg., 8:367–375.

46. Bush, D.C. (1995): Soft-tissue tumors of the hand. In Hunter, J.M., Macken, E.J., and Callhan, A.B. (eds.): Rehabilitation of the Hand: Surgery and Therapy. St. Louis, Mosby–Year Book. pp. 1017–1033.

47. Palmer, A.K. (1987): The distal radial ulnar joint. Anatomy, biomechanics, and triangular fibrocartilage complex abnormalities. Hand Clin, 3:31–40.

48. Redler, M. (1989): Phalangeal and metacarpal fractures. Sport Injury Manage., 2:53–58.

49. Manske, P.R., and Lesker, P.A. (1978): Avulsion of the ring finger digitorum profundus tendon: An experimental study. Hand, 10:52–55.

50. Wright, H.H., and Rettig, A.C. (1995): Management of common sports injuries. In Hunter, J.M., Macken, E.J., and Callhan, A.B. (eds.): Rehabilitation of the Hand: Surgery and Therapy. St. Louis, Mosby–Year Book, pp. 1809–1838.

51. Finkelstein, H. (1930): Stenosing tendovaginitis at the radial styloid process. J. Bone Joint Surg., 12:509–540.

52. Evans, R.B. (1995): An update on extensor tendon management. In Hunter, J.M., Macken, E.J., and Callhan, A.B. (eds.): Rehabilitation of the Hand: Surgery and Therapy. St. Louis, Mosby–Year Book, pp. 565–606.

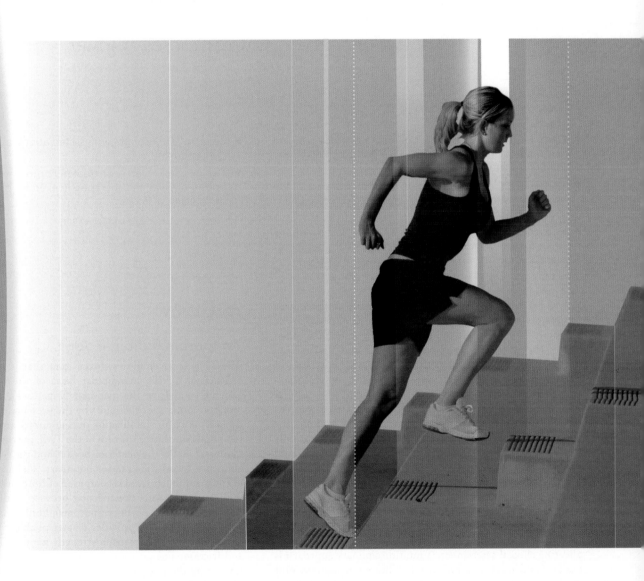

Section III

Spine

15

Temporomandibular Joint

Todd R. Hooks, PT, SCS, ATC, MOMT, MTC, CSCS, FAAOMPT

CHAPTER OBJECTIVES

- Describe the bony anatomy, ligamentous structures, and surrounding musculature of the temporomandibular joint, including their functions.

- Understand the arthrokinematics and biomechanics of the temporomandibular joint that occur during osteokinematic movements of the mandible.

- Recognize the relationship and causative factors of the cervical spine as it relates to pathology of the temporomandibular joint.

- Perform a thorough and systematic evaluation of the temporomandibular joint.

- Design and implement a treatment program that includes both a manual and therapeutic exercise program based on the clinical findings.

Sports rehabilitation specialists often manage athletes with complaints of head, neck, or maxillofacial pain in which the etiologic factors of their complaints can be difficult to diagnose. Disorders and complaints of pain and dysfunction can be difficult to care for because of the wide spectrum of pathology of dental, infectious, metaplastic, musculoskeletal, neurologic, otolaryngologic, psychologic, and vascular origin.[1-3] The temporomandibular joint (TMJ) is a complex synovial joint with a capsule and meniscus that connects the mandible with the cranium. This joint is connected not only to the cranium but also to the spine and shoulder girdle via soft tissue attachments.[4] Therefore, when evaluating and treating athletes with possible TMJ disorders, the clinician should assess the cranium, cervical and thoracic spine, and TMJ as one functional unit because of the interdependency and functional relationship of these joint systems.[4] The TMJ can both refer pain and be a referral site of pain, thus complicating clinical assessment. A multidisciplinary approach is used that includes conservative rehabilitation to address joint mechanics, postural adaptations, and muscular function and control, as well as dental care and possibly the use of oral appliances.

ANATOMY

Temporomandibular Joint

The TMJ is a complex synovial joint that is formed by the articulation of the mandibular fossa of the temporal bone and the condyle of the mandible (Fig. 15-1). The TMJ differs from other synovial joints by the presence of teeth, which can offer anterior stabilization during surface articulation. The temporal bone forms the roof of the TMJ, the concave mandibular fossa marks the posterior border, and the convex articular eminence forms the anterior boundary. The articular surface of the mandibular fossa is composed of fibrocartilage, not hyaline cartilage, and is nonarticular because of the presence of the posterior band of the temporomandibular disk. This fibrocartilaginous surface provides greater pliability during translation and increased tensile strength for prolonged pressure and friction. The posterior border of the mandibular fossa is formed by the postglenoid spine or process. The postglenoid spine is a downward extension of the squamosal portion of the temporal bone that is located anterior to the external auditory meatus.[5] The postglenoid spine serves as an attachment site for

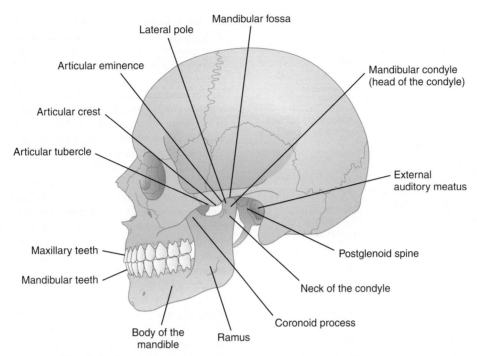

FIGURE 15-1 Lateral view of the skeletal anatomy. *(Adapted from Kraus, S.L. [1993]: Temporomandibular disorders. In Saunders, H.D., and Saunders, R. [eds.]: Evaluation, Treatment, and Prevention of Musculoskeletal Disorders, Vol. 1, The Spine, 3rd ed. Philadelphia, Saunders, pp. 173–210.)*

the capsule.[6] The articular tubercle, which is the most anterior portion of the roof of the TMJ, is separated from the articular eminence by the articular crest. The articular eminence is convex anteroposteriorly and concave mediolaterally. With mandibular opening, the condyle translates along the eminence. However, with full mouth opening, the mandible may translate onto the articular tubercle, a condition indicative of TMJ hypermobility.[2,7]

The condyle of the mandible forms the floor of the TMJ. This condyle is biconvex and has an elliptical shape measuring approximately 20 mm mediolaterally and 10 mm anteroposteriorly (Fig. 15-2).[8] This elliptical shape is oriented approximately 15° to the frontal plane, which places the lateral pole of the condyle anterior to the transverse axis of the condyle and the medial pole posterior to the frontal plane. The coronoid process is a projection located at the superior border between the neck and the ramus (of the mandible) that serves as the attachment for the temporalis muscle. Inferior to the head of the condyle is the neck, which continues as the ramus before becoming the body of the mandible. The maxillary teeth are contained in the maxillary bone. The position, form, and relationship of the teeth are important to function of the TMJ in that they can affect positioning during occlusion, with deviations or irregularities creating malocclusion.[9] Centric occlusion or maximum intercuspation has been defined as the "relationship of the mandible to the maxilla when the teeth are in maximum occlusal contact, irrespective of the position or alignment of the condyle-disc assemblies."[10]

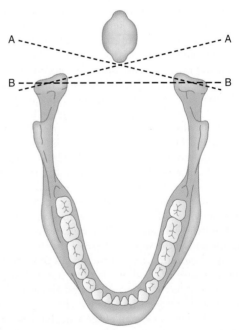

FIGURE 15-2 A line drawn from the medial to the lateral pole of each condyle crosses anterior to the foramen magnum. The lateral pole of the condyle is noted to lie anterior to the transverse axis of the condyle, whereas the medial pole lies posterior to the axis. *(Adapted from Kraus, S.L. [1993]: Temporomandibular disorders. In Saunders, H.D., and Saunders, R. [eds.]: Evaluation, Treatment, and Prevention of Musculoskeletal Disorders, Vol. 1, The Spine, 3rd ed. Philadelphia, Saunders, pp. 173–210.)*

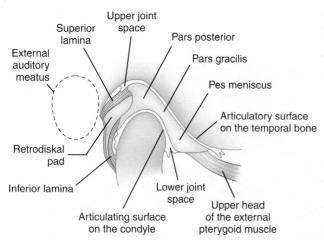

FIGURE 15-3 Sagittal view of the temporomandibular joint, including the articular disk. *(Adapted from Kraus, S.L. [1993]: Temporomandibular disorders. In Saunders, H.D., and Saunders, R. [eds.]: Evaluation, Treatment, and Prevention of Musculoskeletal Disorders, Vol. 1, The Spine, 3rd ed. Philadelphia, Saunders, pp. 173–210.)*

The articular disk is a firm yet flexible biconcave fibrocartilage structure consisting of dense bundles of collagenous fibers, which allows it to conform to the incongruence of the TMJ (Fig. 15-3).[6,11,12] The TMJ is divided into two compartments or spaces by the disk. The superior compartment is formed by the articulation of the superior surface of the meniscus and the glenoid fossa, whereas the inferior compartment is located between the inferior surface of the meniscus and the condylar head. The superior joint space is larger, with a volume of 1.2 mL, than the inferior compartment, which has a volume of 0.9 mL.[13]

The articular disk can be divided into three bands based on thickness: anterior (pes meniscus), intermediate (pars gracilis), and posterior (pars posterior).[14] The peripheral portions of the disk are non–load-bearing regions that are vascularized and innervated, whereas the intermediate band of the disk, located between the temporal bone and the head of the condyle, is avascular and aneural and is the portion of the disk where load bearing occurs.[15,16] The anterior band is anterior to the condyle on the articular eminence and serves as an attachment site for the superior division of the lateral pterygoid muscle. The anterior disk attaches to the anterior joint capsule and to the superior head of the lateral pterygoid muscle. The thinnest portion of the disk is the intermediate band. Its biconcave shape allows it to be positioned over the anterosuperior aspect of the condyle and along the articular eminence and conform to the condyle. No capsular attachments are located in this region of the articular disk; however, the medial and lateral collateral ligaments do originate from this region. The intermediate band, along with the medial and lateral collateral ligaments, allows the disk to rotate anteriorly and posteriorly on the condyle without being displaced anterior to the condyle.[17-19] The posterior band is the thickest portion of the articular disk; it is positioned superior on the condyle and in the mandibular fossa during centric occlusion. The posterior superior portion of the disk attaches to the postglenoid spine via the superior stratum, and the posterior inferior aspect of the disk attaches onto the neck of the mandibular condyle via the inferior stratum. The superior stratum is composed primarily of elastic fibers, whereas the inferior

stratum is mainly collagenous fibers. Posteriorly, the superior stratum attaches to the tympanic plate, which is stretched with forward translation of the condyle and the disk. The inferior stratum is attached to the condyle posteriorly, which serves to limit further forward displacement of the disk during forward translation. Between these layers of strata is the highly vascular retrodiscal pad. During forward translation of the condyle, the volume of the retrodiscal tissue expands and fills the mandibular fossa and then returns to its original shape and size during closure.[16,20]

The TMJ is surrounded by a capsule composed of fibrous connective tissue. The capsule has attachments superiorly to the temporal bone and inferiorly to the neck of the condyle and blends mediolaterally with a thickening in the capsule that forms the medial and lateral collateral ligaments.[21] Superiorly, the capsule does not have a medial or lateral attachment to the disk; posteriorly, it attaches to the postglenoid spine; and anteriorly, it blends with the upper and lower heads of the lateral pterygoid muscle and to the disk.[21] The synovial capsule provides nutrients to the avascular regions of the joint. The capsule, lateral collateral ligaments, and posterior attachment are highly innervated with mechanoreceptors and nociceptors that provide kinesthetic and perceptional joint sense, but the disk and synovial tissue are void of receptors. Although all four types of mechanoreceptors are present, type II is the most prominent, followed by type I receptor in the joint capsule (see Table 24-2 for a summary of mechanoreceptor classification). Cranial nerve V supplies innervation to this region via the deep temporal, masseteric, and auriculotemporal nerves, which are branches of the mandibular division.[22]

Temporomandibular Ligaments

Four main ligamentous structures support the TMJ: the lateral ligament (TMJ ligament), internal ligament (sphenomandibular ligament), stylomandibular ligament, and anterior malleolar ligament. The TMJ ligament is a fan-shaped ligament that strengthens the lateral capsule; it originates from the lateral surface of the zygomatic arch and articular eminence and inserts onto the posterolateral portion of the neck of the mandible (Fig. 15-4). This ligament resists excessive retrusion of the mandible and compression of the posterior tissues of the joint; prevents separation of the condyle, disk, and temporal fossa; and assists in the transition from condylar rotation to condylar translation.[23] The ligament is believed to work in synchrony with the surrounding musculature during arthrokinematic transition from condylar rotation to the translation that occurs during mandibular opening. Translation is achieved by tension placed on the oblique portion of the TMJ ligament at approximately 10 mm of opening as the condyle rotates posteriorly and the neck of the condyle moves posteriorly. Therefore, for additional opening to take place, the condyle must translate anteriorly, which decreases tension on the TMJ ligament.[23]

The sphenomandibular and stylomandibular ligaments are extracapsular ligaments (Fig. 15-5). The sphenomandibular ligament runs from the spine of the sphenoid, blends with the medial capsule, and inserts into the lingual aspect of the mandible at the mandibular foramen. The stylomandibular ligament originates from the styloid process of the temporal bone and inserts into the posterior medial angle of the ramus. The exact roles of these ligaments are uncertain, but they may help protect the TMJ during wide excursion. Individually, it is thought

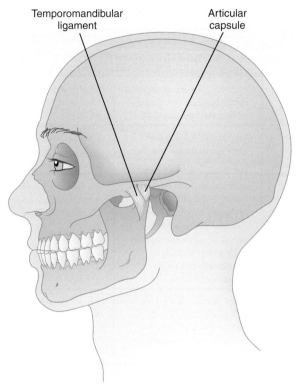

FIGURE 15-4 Lateral view displaying the temporomandibular ligament and its relationship to the articular capsule. *(Adapted from Kraus, S.L. [1993]: Temporomandibular disorders. In Saunders, H.D., and Saunders, R. [eds.]: Evaluation, Treatment, and Prevention of Musculoskeletal Disorders, Vol. 1, The Spine, 3rd ed. Philadelphia, Saunders, pp. 173–210.)*

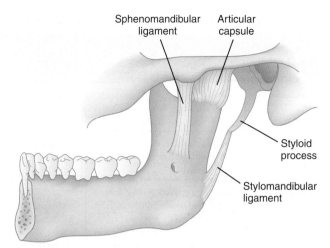

FIGURE 15-5 Medial view of the right mandible illustrating the sphenomandibular and stylomandibular ligaments. *(Adapted from Kraus, S.L. [1993]: Temporomandibular disorders. In Saunders, H.D., and Saunders, R. [eds.]: Evaluation, Treatment, and Prevention of Musculoskeletal Disorders, Vol. 1, The Spine, 3rd ed. Philadelphia, Saunders, pp. 173–210.)*

Temporomandibular Joint Musculature

The cervical spine plays an important role in the biomechanics and function of the TMJ; therefore, it is important for the rehabilitation specialist to have a through understanding of its function and relationship to the TMJ. The focus in this section of the chapter is on the skeletal muscles involved in mandibular movement and function. Table 15-1 lists these muscles, including the origin, insertion, action, and innervation of each muscle.

BIOMECHANICS

The TMJ is a synovial ginglymoarthrodial joint with osteokinematic motions that are described as depression, elevation, protrusion, retrusion, and lateral excursion. The arthrokinematic movements can be divided into active accessory and passive accessory movements. Active accessory movements are a result of muscle contraction and include translation, rotation, compression, and spin. Passive accessory movements (joint play) include distraction and lateral glide. In addition to these accessory motions, rotary movements occur between the head of the condyle and the disk during mandibular opening and closing. During mandibular opening, rotation occurs between the disk and condylar head with concomitant translation occurring between the disk and temporal bone (Fig. 15-6).

Mandibular depression occurs as a result of condylar rotation during the first 10 mm of opening; the neck of the condyle moves posteriorly and places tension on the TMJ ligament. As the TMJ ligament checks rotatory motion, additional movement occurs as the inferior belly of the lateral pterygoid induces anterior translation of the condylar head for approximately 10 mm, after which rotation and translation occur together until functional opening takes place.[23] Mandibular protrusion occurs as a result of condylar translation, whereas mandibular lateral deviation is produced by condylar translation contralaterally and condylar spin ipsilaterally.

Although the disk is firmly attached to the head of the condyle, they rotate independently of one another with mandibular movement. During the initial 10 mm of mandibular opening the

that the sphenomandibular ligament may help maintain congruency of the condyle, disk, and temporal bone whereas the stylomandibular ligament may restrict anterior translation of the mandibular condyle.

The anterior malleolar ligament extends from the neck of the malleus and inserts into the medial-posterior-superior aspect of the capsule or the meniscus of the TMJ. Because of its close approximation to the sphenomandibular ligament, tension on this ligament or the medial capsule causes movement of the chain of ossicles and the tympanic membrane.[24] Tension on the anterior malleolar ligament can be caused by either tension from the sphenomandibular ligament at the end range of jaw movement or tension on the medial capsule as a result of disk displacement. This tension on the anterior malleolar ligament is thought to give rise to middle ear symptoms.

Innervation

The TMJ receives innervation from both primary specific articular nerves and multiple accessory articular nerves from the adjoining musculature. The mandibular nerve, which is a division of the trigeminal nerve, has two branches that provide the primary innervation to the TMJ. The posterior attachment and the posterior and lateral joint capsule are supplied by the auriculotemporal nerve, the anterior and anterolateral capsule is innervated by the masseteric nerve, and the posterior deep temporal nerve innervates the anteromedial and medial aspect of the capsule, as well as the deep and superficial temporalis muscle.

Table 15-1 Origin, Insertion, Action, and Innervation of the Temporomandibular Joint Musculature

	TMJ Musculature			
Muscle	**Origin**	**Insertion**	**Action**	**Innervation**
Buccinator	Alveolar processes of the maxilla, buccinator ridge of the mandible, and pterygomandibular ligament	Orbicularis oris at the angle of the mouth	Compresses the cheeks against the teeth, aids in whistling and smiling, assists in mastication	Buccal branch of the facial nerve (cranial nerve VII)
Orbicularis oris	Strata of the muscular fibers surrounding the orifice of the mouth	Skin and mucous membrane of the lips; blends with the surrounding muscles	Compresses the lips against the teeth; brings the lips together	Buccal and mandibular branches of the facial nerve (cranial nerve VII)
Masseter	*Superficial:* Zygomatic process of the maxilla and anterior two thirds of the lower border of the zygomatic arch *Middle:* Anterior two thirds of the deep surface of the zygomatic arch and lower border of the zygomatic arch *Deep:* Deep surface of the zygomatic arch	*Superficial:* Angle and lower, lateral surface of the ramus of the mandible *Middle:* Middle of the ramus of the mandible *Deep:* Upper ramus of the mandible and coronoid process	Initiates elevation of the mandible and adds force to closure; contributes to clenching during emotional stress and nocturnal clenching and bruxing; assists in protraction and lateral deviation	Masseteric nerve from the mandibular division of the trigeminal nerve
Temporalis	Temporal fossa, deep surface of the temporal fascia	Coronoid process of the mandible and anterior border of the ramus of the mandible; some fibers insert into the skeletal orbit of the eye	Elevates the mandible; unilaterally deviates to the ipsilateral side; retracts the mandible from a protracted position	Deep temporal branch of the mandibular nerve
Lateral pterygoid	*Superior head:* Greater wing of the sphenoid bone *Inferior head:* Lateral surface of the lateral pterygoid plate	Anterior head of the mandibular head, articular capsule, and TMJ disk	Opens and protrudes the mandible, pulls the disk forward, and assists in the rotary motion of chewing; acts with the medial pterygoid to move the jaw side to side *Superior head:* Eccentrically controls the disk with a backward glide during closure *Inferior head:* Translates the mandibular head downward with opening	Lateral pterygoid branch of the mandibular nerve
Medial pterygoid	Palatine bone and tuberosity of the maxilla	Medial surface of the ramus and mandibular angle	Elevates the mandible; protrudes the jaw; unilaterally deviates the mandible contralaterally	Medial pterygoid branch of the mandibular division of the trigeminal nerve
Digastric	*Posterior belly:* Mastoid notch of the temporal bone *Anterior belly:* Digastric fossa of the mandible	Greater cornu and body of the hyoid bone by a fibrous loop midway along the body of the mandible	Depresses the mandible; elevates the hyoid	*Posterior:* Facial nerve *Anterior:* Mylohyoid branch of the mandibular division of the trigeminal nerve
Stylohyoid	Posterior surface of the styloid process	Body of the hyoid bone at the juncture with the greater cornu	Elevates and draws the hyoid back to elongate the floor of the mouth; fixes the hyoid for the tongue muscles	Mylohyoid branch of the inferior alveolar division of the mandibular nerve
Mylohyoid	Mylohyoid line of the mandible	Hyoid bone and median fibrous raphe	Elevates the floor of the mouth; elevates the hyoid bone; depresses the mandible	Mylohyoid branch of the inferior alveolar division of the mandibular nerve
Geniohyoid	Inferior mental spine on the back of the symphysis menti	Anterior surface of the hyoid bone	Elevates the hyoid; with the hyoid fixed, depresses the mandible	C1 via the hypoglossal nerve
Sternohyoid	Posterior medial surface of the clavicle, posterior sternoclavicular ligament, upper and posterior manubrium sterni	Inferior body of the hyoid	Depresses the hyoid, assists in speech and mastication	Ansa cervicalis (C1-C3)

Table 15-1 Origin, Insertion, Action, and Innervation of the Temporomandibular Joint Musculature—cont'd

TMJ Musculature				
Muscle	Origin	Insertion	Action	Innervation
Sternothyroid	Posterior surface of the manubrium sterni and cartilage of the first rib	Oblique line, lamina of the thyroid cartilage	Draws the larynx down after it has been elevated	Ansa cervicalis (C1-C3)
Thyrohyoid	Oblique line, lamina of the thyroid cartilage	Lower border of the greater cornu and adjacent body of the hyoid	Depresses the hyoid; elevates the larynx	C1, C2 fibers from the hypoglossal nerve
Omohyoid	Upper border of the scapula near the scapular notch	*Inferior belly:* Intermediate tendon *Superior belly:* Lower border of the hyoid	Depresses and elevates the hyoid; may assist in inspiration	*Inferior belly:* Ansa cervicalis (C2-C3) *Superior belly:* Superior root of the ansa cervicalis (C1)

TMJ, Temporomandibular joint.

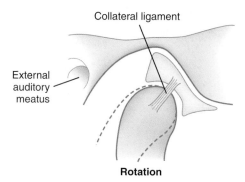

Rotation

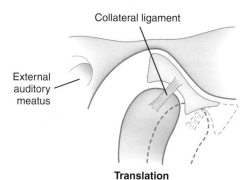

Translation

FIGURE 15-6 Normal arthrokinematic movement during mandibular opening of the lower joint surface. Rotation occurs between the inferior surface of the disk and the condyle, and translation occurs in the upper joint space between the superior disk surface and the temporal bone. *(Adapted from Kraus, S.L. [1993]: Temporomandibular disorders. In Saunders, H.D., and Saunders, R. [eds.]: Evaluation, Treatment, and Prevention of Musculoskeletal Disorders, Vol. 1, The Spine, 3rd ed. Philadelphia, Saunders, pp. 173–210.)*

condyle rotates on a relatively stationary disk, followed by anterior translation of both the condyle and disk. However, because of the "self-seating" disk-to-condyle relationship and the tension that develops at the posterior attachment, a relative posterior rotation occurs between the disk and the condyle after the initial 10 mm of opening. Conversely, during mandibular closing, although both the condylar head and disk translate posteriorly, the disk rotates relatively anteriorly on the condyle because of the conforming "self-seating" disk-to-condyle articulation and tension in the lateral pterygoid[25] (Fig. 15-7). During normal movement, the disk and condyle move forward approximately 7 and 14 mm, respectively.[26]

Clinical Pearl #1

"The interdependency of the cranium, cervical and thoracic spine, and TMJ requires that the interaction between these components be considered as one functional, intricately-balanced unit"—Ola Grimsby, PT, DMT, FFAAOMPT.

EVALUATION

Evaluation of the TMJ is warranted in patients with complaints of headache or maxillofacial, cervicogenic, or shoulder girdle pain because of the common referral patterns of the TMJ. When pathology in the TMJ is suspected, the sports rehabilitation specialist should assess the cervical and thoracic spine and the shoulder girdle because of the attachment of the surrounding musculature, as well as the biomechanical relationship of these joint systems. This can be illustrated with the common head forward/rounded shoulder posture, which as a result of increased tension placed on the hyoid muscles and a relative posterior position of the mandible, gives rise to retracted malocclusion in the sagittal plane. In addition, a dysfunction such as scoliosis causes the upper cervical spine to compensate and "right" the cranium in the horizontal plane. This corrected compensation is achieved by upper cervical side bending with concomitant contralateral rotation, which results in the frontal plane occlusion of a crossbite.

Box 15-1 outlines the sequence of examination. A systematic approach to the evaluation process is helpful to ensure that the clinician does not overlook any step in the assessment and that the examination flows smoothly. By performing all the elements of the evaluation listed in Box 15-1, the sports rehabilitation specialist will be able to determine which tissues are involved from their response to the tests imposed. Each tissue is suspected as being a potential source of the pain (Fig. 15-8) until the tissue has been cleared by careful examination. To clear a tissue, the

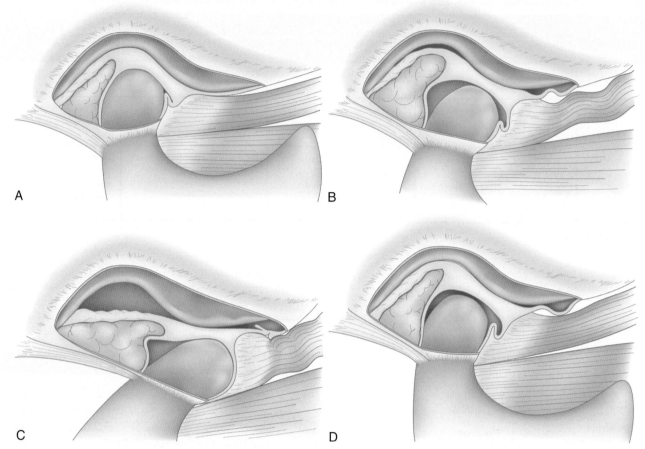

A

B

C

D

FIGURE 15-7 Normal disk movement during mandibular depression and elevation. **A,** Normal positioning with mandibular occlusion. **B,** At 10 mm of mandibular opening, the disk rotates posteriorly in relation to the condyle as condylar rotation and anterior translation occur. **C,** At full opening, the disk has translated anteriorly on the temporal bone and is rotated posteriorly relative to the condyle. **D,** During condylar closing, the disk rotates anteriorly relative to the condyle as the condyle undergoes rotation and posterior translation. *(Adapted from Kraus, S.L. [1993]: Temporomandibular disorders. In Saunders, H.D., and Saunders, R. [eds.]: Evaluation, Treatment, and Prevention of Musculoskeletal Disorders, Vol. 1, The Spine, 3rd ed. Philadelphia, Saunders, pp. 173–210.)*

Box 15-1

Sequence of Examination of the Temporomandibular Joint

Initial observation
- Posture of the head and cervical spine
- Mouth movement with speaking
- Personality and attitude of the athlete

Patient's subjective history
Structural inspection
- Anterior/posterior/lateral
- Standing/sitting position
- Assessment of the vertical and horizontal alignment of head position
- Oral inspection
- Respiration pattern
- Quick tests of the cervical spine to rule out pathology

Active motion (assess range, speed, quality, aberrations in movement, clicking)
- Mandibular opening (40 mm)
- Lateral deviation (1 tooth wide, 8 mm)

- Mandibular protrusion
- Mandibular retrusion
- Teeth clinching
- Bilateral molar biting on a cotton roll (joint distraction)
- Unilateral molar biting on a cotton roll (ipsilateral distraction, contralateral compression)

Passive motion
- Vertical opening
- Lateral movements
- Retraction
- Protraction

Resisted motion (each motion tested in a neutral position)
- Mandibular depression
- Mandibular elevation
- Lateral deviation
- Retrusion
- Protrusion

Box 15-1

Sequence of Examination of the Temporomandibular Joint—cont'd

Palpation (note variations in temperature, atrophy, swelling, tenderness, thickness, dryness, moisture, abnormalities, crepitus, and pain)
- Crepitation, grinding, clicking with mandibular movement
- Temporomandibular ligament
- Posterior glenoid spine
- Medial/lateral pterygoid muscle
- Temporalis muscle
- Anterior and posterior digastric muscle
- Occipital nerve

Neurologic tests
- Sensation tests
- Reflexes
  - Mandibular
  - Biceps/triceps/brachioradialis/abductor digiti minimi

- Myotomes
- Cranial nerve testing (I to XII)

Special tests
- Chvostek

Mobility tests
- Distraction
- Anterior glide
- Lateral glide

Diagnostic tests
- Radiographs, magnetic resonance imaging, computed tomography, myelography, electromyography, laboratory tests

Adapted from The Ola Grimsby Institute (2004): Temporomandibular Joint: Residency Course Notes; Systems Course, pp. 44–46.

Δ The Diagnostic Pyramid Δ

Facility: Date:
Patient: Therapist:
Medical Diagnosis:

Summation of Tissue(s) in Lesion	SKIN	SUB-CUTANEOUS	LIGAMENT FASCIA	MUSCLE TENDON	JOINT CAPSULE	BURSA	JOINT CARTL	JOINT ENTRAP	NERVE	DISC	BONE	VASCULAR	META-BOLISM
X-RAY/LAB MR/CAT/EMG	144	145	146	147	148	149	150	151	152	153	154	155	156
SEGMENTAL PLAY	131	132	133	134	135	136	137	138	139	140	141	142	143
JOINT PLAY	118	119	120	121	122 - extremity	123	124	125 - blocked	126	127	128	129	130
SPECIAL TESTS	105	106	107	108	109	110	111	112	113	114	115	116	117
NEURO TESTS	92	93	94	95	96	97	98	99	100	101	102	103	104
PALPATION	79	80	81	82	83	84	85	86	87	88	89	90	91
RESISTED MOTION	66	67	68	69	70 - Spine	71	72	73	74	75	76	77	78
PASSIVE MOTION	53	54	55	56	57	58	59	60	61	62	63	64	65
ACTIVE MOTION	40	41	42	43	44	45	46	47	48	49	50	51	52
STRUCTURAL INSPECTION	27	28	29	30	31	32	33	34	35	36	37	38	39
HISTORY INTERVIEW	14	15	16	17	18	19	20	21	22	23	24	25	26
INITIAL OBSERVATION	1	2	3	4	5	6	7	8	9	10	11	12	13
	SKIN	SUB-CUTANEOUS	LIGAMENT FASCIA	MUSCLE TENDON	JOINT CAPSULE	BURSA	JOINT CARTL	JOINT ENTRAP	NERVE	DISC	BONE	VASCULAR	META-BOLISM

KEY

+	Positive means indicative of the tissue
×	Eliminated
0	More testing (or clarifying tests) required

?	Test (information) does not determine the tissue
-	It is not indicative of the tissue
(shaded)	Test does not apply to the ELIMINATION of tissue
(bold box)	Tissue eliminated or confirmed by this block

FIGURE 15-8 The Ola Grimsby Institute Pyramid. *(From The Ola Grimsby Institute [2004]: Evaluation: Residency Course Notes; Science Course, p. 7.)*

examiner must perform tests that create stress or tension on that tissue. If a positive response does not occur, the tissue can be excluded as a source of the pain.

Initial Observation

The examination process begins with initial observation of the athlete. The clinician watches the athlete walk into the room and observes the position of the head, neck, and shoulder girdle. The sports rehabilitation specialist should observe the way the athlete speaks and develop an understanding of how the dysfunction is affecting the athlete's functional ability.

History

The athlete's subjective history is a crucial part of the evaluation process. A complete and thorough history allows the sports rehabilitation specialist to determine the causative factors locally, regionally, or globally, as well the direction and goal of treatment. In addition to a general history, Box 15-2 contains some specific information the clinician should obtain.

Structural Inspection

A structural inspection can be performed with the athlete in both standing and sitting positions as warranted by the history and should consist of a full examination that includes an anterior, posterior, and lateral view of the entire body to note any postural problems and possible compensations. The face

should be observed to ascertain facial symmetry in the vertical plane, which can be assessed via the bipupillary, otic, and occlusive lines (Fig. 15-9), as well as by dividing the face into normal vertical dimensions (Fig. 15-10). The examiner should note any malposition of the jaw if present, such as a crossbite (lateral positioning of the mandible), underbite (mandibular teeth lying anterior to the maxillary teeth), or overbite (maxillary incisors extending anterior beyond the normal position of 2 to 3 mm). The athlete should be asked to swallow and chew to allow observation of any deviations or abnormal movements. The lips should be observed to determine whether their positioning is normal, with the upper lip covering the maxillary teeth and the lower lip reaching the lower quarter of the superior incisors. If proper lip closure is not present, the activity of the mentalis and masticatory muscles could be increased. The examiner should also note the available mobility of the tongue, as well as any habitual movement patterns of the tongue such as thrusting.

The sports rehabilitation specialist should also perform quick tests to rule out involvement of the cervical spine. Such tests can include active, passive, and resisted motion

---

Box 15-2

Questions Specific to the Temporomandibular Joint That Should Be Asked During the Evaluation

Does the athlete have any pain with activities such as chewing, talking, yawning, biting, swallowing, or shouting?

Was any injury associated with this condition?

Does the athlete have any pain with the mouth fully opened or during biting?

Does the athlete have any complaints of clicking when opening the jaw, or does the jaw ever lock in place?

Does the athlete grind the teeth, clench the jaw, have any painful or sensitive teeth, or have any difficulty swallowing?

Does the athlete awaken in the morning with pain or soreness in the TMJ or surrounding musculature?

Has the athlete had any ear problems such as ringing, earaches, dizziness, or feeling faint?

Does the athlete have a history of headaches and if so in what location?

Does the athlete have any habitual or postural habits that can add stress to the TMJ, such as nail biting, chewing gum, smoking, leaning on the chin, or holding a telephone between the shoulder and ear?

Has the athlete ever undergone any previous treatment of this condition and what was the outcome of this treatment?

Has any diagnostic tests such as radiography or magnetic resonance imaging been performed?

TMJ, Temporomandibular joint.

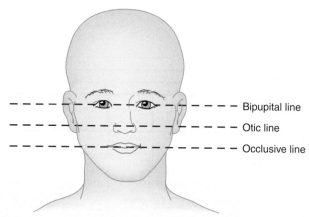

FIGURE 15-9 The bipupillary, otic, and occlusive lines, which are normally parallel. *(Adapted from Magee, D.J. [1997]: Temporomandibular joint. In Magee, D.J. [ed.]: Orthopedic Physical Assessment, 3rd ed. Philadelphia, Saunders.)*

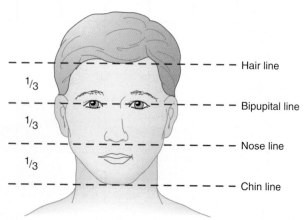

FIGURE 15-10 Vertical dimensions of the face divided into equal thirds. *(Adapted from Magee, D.J. [1997]: Temporomandibular joint. In Magee, D.J. [ed.]: Orthopedic Physical Assessment, 3rd ed. Philadelphia, Saunders.)*

and special tests of the cervical spine (see Chapter 16). Adjunctive motion of the mandible, such as the normal anterior-superior movement that occurs with cervical flexion and the inferior-posterior movement that occurs during cervical extension, should be assessed. The athlete may have soft tissue or muscular dysfunction in the cervical region that is creating altered tension on the mandible during cervical movements. The examiner should evaluate both available movement and quality of motion and note whether the athlete's tissue mobility allows movements to be performed with the mouth closed.

Active Movements

Clinical Pearl #2

Hyperactivity or a trigger point can interfere with eccentric contraction of the lateral pterygoid muscle as it guides the disk to its resting position during mandibular closing.

When assessing osteokinematic movements it is important for the clinician to understand that the spectrum of normal values is wide because of variables such as age and gender. Each movement is commonly assessed during two to three repetitions; in addition to available range of motion (ROM), the speed and quality of motion, any abnormal deviation in movement, and the presence of clicking should be noted. Because a patient can have significant intracapsular dysfunction and be able to achieve full mandibular motion as a result of pathologic adaptations, it is important for the examiner to understand that the athlete's ability to obtain full motion is not the most important aspect of the examination. As the athlete performs active movements, the examiner should palpate just below the zygomatic arch, 1 to 2 cm anterior to the tragus (Fig. 15-11). The posterior aspect of the joint can be palpated through the external auditory canal (Fig. 15-12). The examiner should observe the mandible during active movements for

any asymmetric patterns that may be described as an "S" or "C" curve. An altered movement pattern may result from TMJ dysfunction (intracapsular or extracapsular), abnormal muscle activity or imbalance, abnormal bone growth or development, or derangement of an oral structure. Functional mandibular depression is reported to be 40 mm; however, normal values for maximal opening range from 33 to 72 mm in healthy subjects (Fig. 15-13).[27,28]

The mandible should move in a symmetric straight line during mandibular depression; if any deviation is present, the examiner should note the dysfunctional arc of motion and type of curve. Two types of curves are commonly described: a C-type curve occurs when the jaw deviates unilaterally during opening, which could possibly indicate hypomobility on the side toward the deviation, whereas an S-type curve could result from muscle spasm or imbalance, capsulitis, joint hypermobility, decreased coordination, or medial displacement of the condylar head. The first phase of opening, which is rotation, can be assessed by asking the athlete to open the mouth as wide as possible while

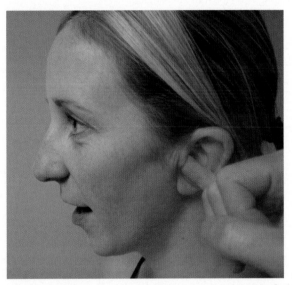

FIGURE 15-12 Palpation of the posterior aspect of the temporomandibular joint via the external auditory meatus.

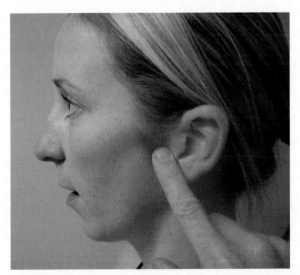

FIGURE 15-11 Palpation performed over the lateral aspect of the temporomandibular joint (TMJ) to detect any crepitus or clicking, as well as provoke signs from the joint capsule and TMJ ligament.

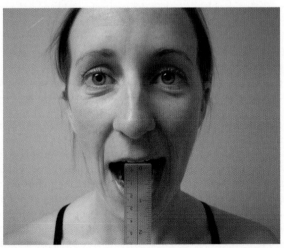

FIGURE 15-13 Objective assessment of mandibular opening measured in millimeters.

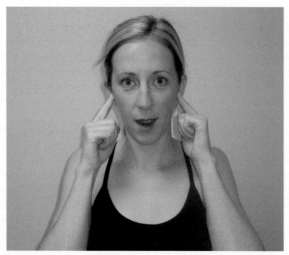

FIGURE 15-14 Active mandibular opening limited to the first phase of opening (condylar rotation) by having the athlete maintain the tongue on the roof of the mouth.

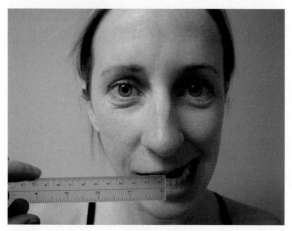

FIGURE 15-15 Lateral deviation as measured by picking a point on the upper teeth that is parallel to a point on the lower teeth at rest and then having the athlete perform lateral deviation.

maintaining the tongue on the roof of the mouth (Fig. 15-14). Translation then begins when the tongue is unable to make contact with the roof of the mouth.

The athlete is asked to perform protrusion and retrusion of the mandible while the examiner assesses the quality and quantity of movement; normal ROM can vary between 3 and 6 mm of protrusion and 3 and 4 mm of retrusion. When evaluating the athlete for protrusion and retrusion, the examiner should assess for any altered movements such as lateral deviation. If a restriction in the TMJ is present, the mandible will deviate to the side with restriction.

Lateral deviation is determined bilaterally by measuring the distance that the lower teeth move in relation to the upper teeth (Fig. 15-15). This can be measured by selecting points on the upper and lower teeth that are vertical to each other at rest and having the athlete laterally deviate from that position, with normal lateral deviation being 10 to 15 mm (or approximately one tooth in width). In addition, the relationship of lateral deviation should be proportional to the amount of mandibular opening, with a normal ratio being 1:4. Therefore, for every 1 mm of

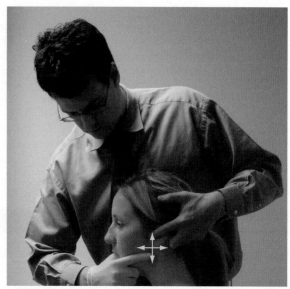

FIGURE 15-16 Passive assessment of the temporomandibular joint performed while concomitantly palpating the joint. Passive movements can be performed either intraorally or extraorally.

lateral deviation, the athlete should demonstrate approximately 4 mm of mandibular opening. When evaluating lateral deviation of the mandible, the examiner is actually assessing lateral excursion of the TMJ on the opposite side. Rotation and translation should occur at approximately a 1:1 ratio; if a dysfunction such as an anteromedially displaced disk is present, lateral excursion will be restricted as a result of diminished medial translation of the mandibular head.

Passive Movements

Passive ROM is performed to allow the sports rehabilitation specialist to appreciate the end-feel for each motion. The examiner can perform all TMJ planar motions: mandibular opening and closing, lateral excursion, retraction, and protraction (Fig. 15-16). As the passive movements are performed, the clinician palpates the TMJ to check for the presence of any joint crepitus while also assessing the end-feel of motion. Crepitus noted when palpating the joint may be indicative of cartilage damage. Depending on the direction of movement, patient comfort, and other variables, the examiner may provide resistance with either the hand on the outside of the mouth or the fingers or thumb on the teeth while wearing gloves.

Resisted Movements

Resisted isometrics are performed with the mandible in the resting position and instructing the athlete, "Don't let me move you." Isometric testing is performed for all movement patterns: vertical opening, vertical closing, protraction, retraction, and lateral deviation (Fig. 15-17). During testing the examiner should provide proper stabilization of the head, neck, or both while providing isometric resistance to the mandible. Depending on the direction of movement, patient comfort, and other variables; the examiner may provide resistance with either the hand on the outside of the mouth or the fingers or thumb on the teeth while wearing gloves.

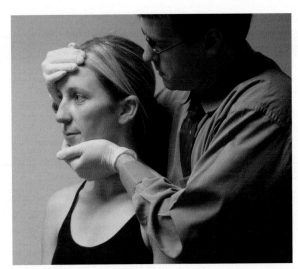

FIGURE 15-17 Resisted isometrics performed with the mandible in the resting position.

Palpation

Clinical Pearl #3

Joint clicking is indicative of sliding anterior or posterior to the disk, whereas crepitus is a result of degenerative joint disease or a perforation in the disk.

Proper assessment and screening of the cervical spine should be included in a complete TMJ evaluation. Therefore, the sports rehabilitation specialist should also palpate the cervical spine as part of the evaluation. Box 15-3 lists some of the more commonly palpated structures in the cervical spine.

Palpation of the TMJ is performed by placing a finger with the pad facing anteriorly into the external auditory meatus as the athlete actively opens and closes the mouth. The clinician applies light pressure anteriorly to palpate the posterior attachment of the disk. In addition, the capsule and lateral aspect of the joint, including the ligamentous structures, are palpated by placing the finger slightly posterior to the lateral pole and anterior to the tragus. The examiner notes any pain, provocation of symptoms, clicking, or crepitus during palpation.

The examiner also palpates the ligamentous, muscular, lymphatic, fascial, and skeletal structures in the maxillofacial region. Although most structures are palpated extraorally, some require intraoral examination. If an intraoral examination is indicated, it is important for the clinician to ask the patient about any latex allergies if latex gloves are worn by the examiner. The examiner should identify any local or radiating muscle pain, myositis, fibrosis, trigger points, variations in muscle volume or tone, and edema.[29] The practitioner should have thorough knowledge of maxillofacial anatomy to allow proper identification of structures and apply both parallel and perpendicular pressure during the assessment. Box 15-4 lists some of the common structures palpated during evaluation of the TMJ; a few of these structures are discussed in the following sections.

Box 15-3

Commonly Palpated Structures During Assessment of the Cervical Spine

POSTERIORLY

External occipital protuberance
Superior nuchal line
Mastoid process
Ligamentum nuchae
Upper trapezius
Levator scapulae
Spinous processes
Transverse processes
Facet joints

ANTERIORLY

Sternum
Clavicle
Supraclavicular fossa
First rib
Sternocleidomastoid muscle
Scalene muscles
Hyoid bone
Thyroid cartilage
Thyroid gland
First cricoid ring
Lymph nodes
Carotid pulse
Temporomandibular joints
Mandible
Parotid gland

Hyoid Bone

This bone serves as an important structure in the stomatognathic system by influencing mandibular movements, swallowing, and sound formation during speech. The hyoid is situated superior to the thyroid cartilage at the level of the C2-C3 vertebrae. The lateral masses of the hyoid bone are palpated as the athlete swallows, and the examiner notes any complaints such as difficulty or tightness when swallowing. The mobility of the hyoid is assessed to determine its available movement and the presence of normal crepitus as the hyoid bone is translated laterally. If crepitus is absent with lateral translation, muscle spasm of either the longus colli or infrahyoid muscle or swelling in the bursa may be present. Soft tissue such as the anterior longitudinal ligament can also exhibit swelling following trauma to the cervical spine.

Temporalis Muscle

This muscle can be palpated extraorally at the temporal fossa to assess the anterior, middle, and posterior muscle fibers. The insertion of the temporalis at the coronoid process can be palpated extraorally, inferior to the zygomatic arch, while the patient opens the mouth or intraorally by following the ramus of the mandible posteriorly to the tip of the mandible.

Masseter Muscle

The masseter muscle is palpated below the zygomatic arch to the inferior angle of the mandible. This muscle can display hypertrophy as a result of parafunctional activity. The deep portion of

Box 15-4

Commonly Palpated Structures During Assessment of the Temporomandibular Joint

TEMPOROMANDIBULAR JOINT

Presence of clicking

Condyle translating past the eminence (false clicking)

Grinding and/or crepitation

BONY ANATOMY

Posterior glenoid spine

Articular tubercle

Lateral pole of the mandibular condyle

SOFT TISSUE/LIGAMENTS/MUSCULAR TISSUE

Retrodiscal pad (mouth open, posterior to the condyle)

Articular capsule

Temporomandibular ligament

Occipital nerve

Temporalis muscle

Masseter

Medial pterygoid

Lateral pterygoid

Buccinator

Orbicularis oris (internus and externus)

Anterior and posterior digastric muscle belly

Mylohyoid

Sternocleidomastoid

Upper trapezius

Levator scapularis

Rhomboids

Table 15-2 Cranial Nerve Testing

Nerve	Test
Cranial nerve I (olfactory)	Smell coffee or familiar substance
Cranial nerve II (optic)	Visual acuity (eye chart); peripheral visual field
Cranial nerve III (oculomotor)	Assess for drooping of the eyelid; ability to move the eyes up, down, and medially; light reflex
Cranial nerve IV (trochlear)	Assess ability of the eye to adduct and look downward
Cranial nerve V (trigeminal)	Sensation in the forehead, maxillary portion of the cheek, and mandible Motor testing of the masseter and temporalis Corneal reflex by touching the cornea (positive if the athlete does not blink)
Cranial nerve VI (abducens)	Assess the ability to look laterally
Cranial nerve VII (facial)	Test the athlete's ability to smile and frown, move the eyebrows, purse the lips, show teeth, whistle
Cranial nerve VIII (vestibulocochlear)	Assess the athlete's hearing Equilibrium testing: balance, nystagmus, vestibular ocular reflexes
Cranial nerve IX (glossopharyngeal)	Gag reflex; taste in the posterior third of the tongue
Cranial nerve X (vagus)	Assess the uvula's ability to rise as the athlete says "ah"
Cranial nerve XI (spinal accessory)	Assess the sternocleidomastoid and trapezius muscles
Cranial nerve XII (hypoglossal)	Assess the athlete's ability to protrude and move the tongue left and right

this muscle can be palpated intraorally between the index finger and thumb near the athlete's posterior molars.

Lateral Pterygoid Muscle

This muscle is palpated intraorally by placing the finger posterior to the third maxillary molar in a posterior, superior, and medial direction. Only the inferior head can be palpated, and the examiner should use light pressure because this is a region of pain and is often very tender.

Medial Pterygoid Muscle

The clinician intraorally palpates along the body of the mandible at its angle while placing the other index finger on the external portion of the angle of the mandible. This allows examination of the inferior portion of the medial pterygoid insertion.

Greater Occipital Nerve

This nerve arises from the first and second cervical vertebrae and emerges from the suboccipital triangle between the inferior oblique and semispinalis capitis muscle. It innervates the scalp along the top of the head, the area above the ears, and region over the salivary glands. Because pathology affecting this nerve can mimic temporomandibular disorders, it is important to palpate this structure for reproduction of symptoms. A disorder affecting the greater occipital nerve often causes headaches that are frequently on the side of the head, neck pain, pain behind the eyes, and sensitivity to light.

Neurologic Tests

It is important that a complete and thorough neurologic evaluation of the cervical region be performed, including sensation, myotomes, and deep tendon reflexes. The cranial nerves (I to XII), with particular emphasis on cranial nerves V, VII, and XII, should also be assessed to rule out any pathologic conditions that may mimic or contribute to temporomandibular disorders (Table 15-2). To assess the jaw reflex (cranial nerve V), the examiner places a thumb on the athlete's chin and then taps the thumbnail with a reflex hammer as the athlete's mouth is opened and relaxed. If a sensory deficit is noted during the sensory evaluation, the sports rehabilitation specialist should determine whether this loss of sensation is in a dermatomal (Fig. 15-18) or cutaneous sensory nerve pattern (Fig. 15-19).

Special Tests

Special tests for the TMJ consist of assessing for cranial nerve pathology. The Chvostek test (Fig. 15-20) is performed to assess for pathology of cranial nerve VII (facial). This test is performed by tapping the parotid gland overlying the masseter muscle. A positive sign is twitching of the facial muscles.

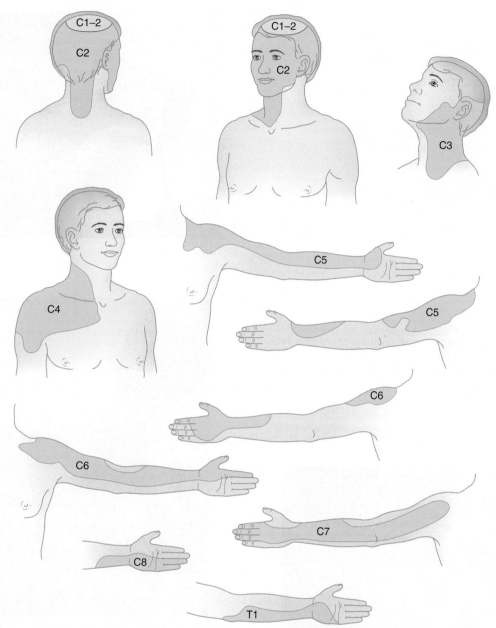

FIGURE 15-18 Dermatomal nerve pattern of the upper extremity. *(Adapted from Magee, D.J. [1997]: Temporomandibular joint. In Magee, D.J. [ed.]: Orthopedic Physical Assessment, 3rd ed. Philadelphia, Saunders.)*

The sports rehabilitation specialist can also listen to the TMJ during active movements with a stethoscope. Normally, sound is detected only on occlusion, and reciprocal clicking can be detected when the mouth opens and closes. The first click occurs when the condyle slides under the posterior aspect of the disk (reduces) or anterior to the disk (subluxates) with opening. The second click occurs when the condyle translates posterior to the disk (subluxates) or into its correct position and is reduced. A single click may be heard if the condyle gets caught behind the TMJ disk during opening or translates posteriorly on the disk during closing. Crepitus can be indicative of degenerative joint disease or perforation of the disk. If painful crepitus is noted, it could be indicative of loss of fibrocartilage causing the condyle and temporal bone to wear as a result of the disk being degenerated.

The athlete's swallowing and lingual functions should be evaluated. A normal adult swallows with the tip of the tongue pressed against the rugae, the teeth together in centric occlusion, the lips sealed without suction or perioral muscle activity, the food or liquid held above the tongue and sealed against the maxillary arch, and peristaltic propulsion of food as the hyoid bone ascends during swallowing.[29,30] During altered swallowing habits, such as a tongue thrust, the tip of the tongue presses against the front incisors and acts like a fulcrum pressing the tongue backward. The tongue can fall into the oral pharynx and either occlude or make swallowing difficult without adequate styloglossus activity. Altered posture such as a forward head position can affect lingual function because of the tongue's attachment to the hyoid bone, mandible, and cranium.[30] A forward head posture increases the distance between the hyoid

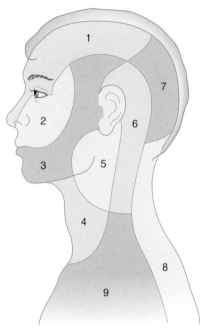

FIGURE 15-19 Cutaneous nerve distribution of the face, head, and neck. *1*, Ophthalmic nerve; *2*, maxillary nerve; *3*, mandibular nerve; *4*, transverse cutaneous nerve of the neck (C2-C3); *5*, greater auricular nerve (C2-C3); *6*, lesser auricular nerve; *7*, greater occipital nerve (C2-C3); *8*, cervical dorsal rami (C3-C5); *9*, suprascapular nerve (C5-C6). *(Adapted from Magee, D.J. [1997]: Temporomandibular joint. In Magee, D.J. [ed.]: Orthopedic Physical Assessment, 3rd ed. Philadelphia, Saunders.)*

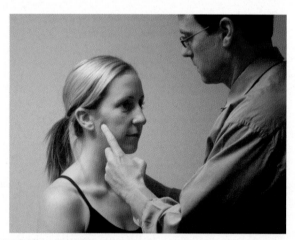

FIGURE 15-20 Chvostek test. This test is performed to determine whether pathology involving the seventh cranial nerve is present.

bone and the mandible, thus changing the length-tension relationship of the hyoglossus muscle and causing an inferior force on the tongue.[30] These forces can be amplified when the head is brought forward or when the cranium is rotated posteriorly.

Mobility Testing

TMJ mobility is assessed to determine the available passive joint mobility, as well as to detect any joint dysfunction. The examiner can perform these techniques either intraorally or extraorally, depending on variables such as test direction, patient comfort, and whether the athlete's mouth opens sufficiently to

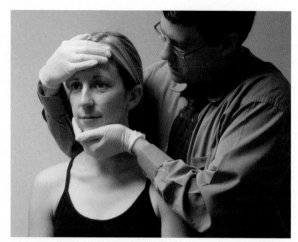

FIGURE 15-21 Medial/lateral glide assessment performed extraorally.

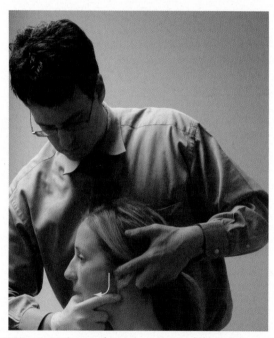

FIGURE 15-22 Intraoral passive anterior glide mobility testing.

allow intraoral examination. The sports rehabilitation specialist examines lateral and medial glide of the mandibular condyles with the athlete in the supine or sitting position and the athlete's head supported against the examiner's body, as seen in Figure 15-21. If this examination is performed intraorally, the examiner places a gloved thumb on top of the molars with the hand molded around the athlete's chin as the middle finger palpates the TMJ and the athlete's head stabilized against the examiner's body with the opposite hand. The clinician performs a lateral and medial glide of the condyle while the mouth is opened and in a relaxed position. Anterior glide of the mandibular condyle is performed with the same hand placement; the clinician translates the mandible caudally and slightly posteriorly to produce joint distraction, followed by anterior mobilization (Fig. 15-22). In addition, cervical and thoracic mobility (see Chapter 16) should also be assessed to allow the clinician to effectively treat the entire joint system.

REHABILITATION TECHNIQUES FOR THE TEMPOMANDIBULAR JOINT

Clinical Pearl #4

Restoration of myokinematic control is important in the rehabilitation process because of the joint's dependency on musculature support for stability.

The sports rehabilitation specialist should have a good understanding of the causative effects and the tissues involved following a complete evaluation. This allows the clinician to develop a specific program for treating the condition because TMJ dysfunction or pain (or both) may be a result of cervical spine dysfunction. The athlete's rehabilitation program might consist of modalities to reduce pain, muscle tone and spasticity, and edema. The clinician can also incorporate manual techniques in conjunction with fundamental exercises with the ultimate goal of providing the optimal stimulus for regeneration of the tissues involved in the pathologic process.

Soft Tissue Mobilization

During evaluation the clinician should appreciate the status of the soft tissues of the maxillofacial region, including any edema, change in temperature, moisture, decreased skin mobility (direction and relative restrictions), muscle properties (mobility, tone, and pliability), trigger points, and provocation of symptoms. Depending on the findings, the clinician implements soft tissue mobilization techniques to address the pain, muscle guarding and tension, collagen extensibility, decreased circulation, lymphatic congestion, scar adhesions, decreased fluid dynamics, altered muscle recruitment and coordination, and joint stiffness. Numerous mobilization techniques can be used by the clinician, depending on the findings on evaluation, to specifically address the involved tissue. Petrofsky et al demonstrated that muscle blood flow begins diminishing at 10% of maximum voluntary contraction; therefore, soft tissue mobilization techniques to diminish muscle guarding can be used.[31,32] In addition, passive or active muscle pump techniques (or both) can be used to create an arterial-venous pressure gradient to help restore normal circulation.

Joint Mobilization Techniques

The sports rehabilitation specialist should reassess joint mobility following soft tissue mobilization to determine whether previous restrictions were a result of muscle guarding and tone. The clinician can perform oscillatory techniques at the beginning and midrange of collagen tension to influence type II mechanoreceptors or a sustained hold at the beginning or end range of collagen tension for type I mechanoreceptors. Joint mobilization techniques can be used to reestablish the TMJ capsule's functional range of tension bound by adhesions or scaring, facilitate type I and II mechanoreceptors, normalize joint biomechanics, relieve excessive joint compression, promote joint lubrication through production of synovial fluid, and release any entrapment.[4] Figure 15-23 demonstrates the use of manual distraction to restore normal joint mobility caused by displacement of the intraarticular disk. In addition, the previously described mobility maneuvers can be used to increase joint mobility by performing

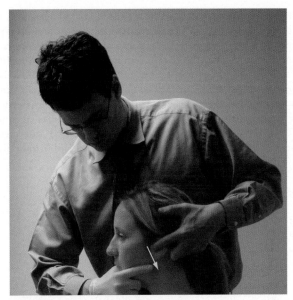

FIGURE 15-23 Joint distraction mobilization technique performed in a caudal and slightly posterior direction to restore normal joint mobility.

sustained holds (10 to 15 seconds) at the end range of joint mobility. Mobilizations of the cervical spine, as indicated, may also be warranted to address any postural faults.

THERAPEUTIC TREATMENT

The rehabilitation specialist should incorporate a complete program that includes education on oral habits such as gum chewing, biting on pens or fingernails, smoking, or activities in which the mouth is opened widely. Pain and dysfunction can cause tonic reflexogenic muscle guarding, which can affect normal arthrokinematic motion, reduce osteokinematic range, and cause secondary myositis.[4] Fundamental exercises should be performed first to address the functional quality of coordination before endurance and strength training is initiated to restore normal movement patterns. The functional qualities of exercise training can be individualized by adjusting repetitions, range, speed, concentric or eccentric muscle activity, direction of movement, and other variables. Therefore, the clinician should be able to individualize each treatment to address pain, edema, mobility, coordination, motor recruitment and coordination, vascularity, and endurance.

Self-Mobilization Exercises

The athlete may be instructed in self-mobilization exercises as determined by the findings on manual joint assessment. These exercises can be prescribed on the basis of direction (distraction, anterior or lateral), mobilization intent (collagen plasticity, joint lubrication, or neuromodulation of pain), and muscle status (tonic guarding or tightness). Normal arthrokinematic motion for mandibular opening consists of posterior rolling initially, followed by anterior gliding along with rotation, and finally a roll at the end of ROM. If the initial rolling component (first 6 to 10 mm of opening) of this arthrokinematic sequence is diminished, an increase in compensatory anterior translation will occur. Therefore, in this common clinical example the patient should be instructed in self-distraction to increase capsular mobility and improve rolling (Fig. 15-24). Mobilization exercises can be performed with tongue depressors or dental cotton rolls. If mandibular opening is limited to less than 30 mm, loss of anterior translation is typically present. In addition to the clinician performing mobilization treatment, the athlete can be prescribed self-mobilization exercises for anterior translation (Fig. 15-25, *A* and *B*). Active protrusion can also be performed to help improve mobility and coordination for the arthrokinematic anterior translation needed for movement of the component during mandibular opening (Fig. 15-26).[4] To ensure a proper relationship and movement pattern (1 mm of lateral deviation for every 5 mm of mandibular

opening), when 30 mm of opening is obtained, lateral deviation exercises are emphasized over protrusion exercises. Limited lateral deviation can be detected by noting a "C" curve during mandibular opening, with deviation toward the affected side because of capsular restriction. If normal opening is achieved with lateral deviation, excessive anterior translation may be present. This excessive translation can place deleterious stress and tension on the capsule and posterior stratum. If limited arthrokinematic lateral deviation is noted, the athlete is instructed to perform unilateral biting on the ipsilateral side (Fig. 15-27),

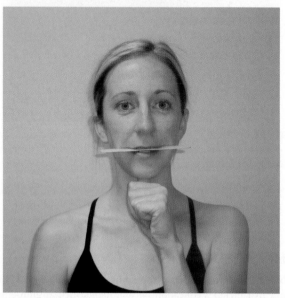

FIGURE 15-24 Distraction self-mobilization performed with a tongue depressor placed behind the incisors. The athlete is instructed to create a light external force with the thumb pressing under the chin in a cranial direction. The mandible will fulcrum around the tongue depressor to create a distraction force at the temporomandibular joint. This technique can be also be performed with a pencil or cotton roll.

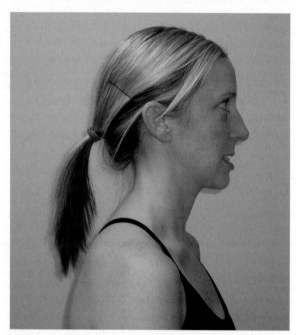

FIGURE 15-26 Active protrusion performed to improve anterior translation. Cotton rolls can be placed between the teeth to place the temporomandibular joint in a more open-packed position that will reduce the amount of compressive and shear force at the joint.

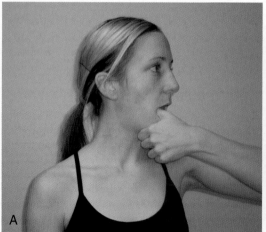

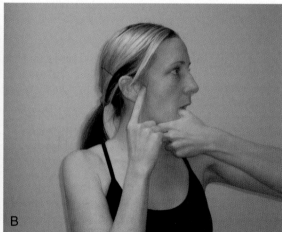

FIGURE 15-25 A, Self-mobilization treatment of anterior translation. The athlete slightly rotates the neck toward the hand used for mobilization. The thumb is placed on the molars and a slight distraction force is created in a caudal and posterior direction, followed by anterior translation of the mandible. **B,** Alternative hand position for self-mobilization treatment of anterior translation. The athlete performs the self-mobilization treatment as described previously and assists by using the contralateral hand to provide a gentle anterior translation force on the posterior aspect of the mandible.

which has been shown to reduce ipsilateral joint compression and produce lateral glide,[33] or to perform lateral glide mobilizations with dental cotton rolls (Fig. 15-28).

Fundamental Exercises

Stage 1

The proper sequence of muscle activity, as well as adequate capsular mobility, is critical in the restorative process to regain normal function. As arthrokinematic and osteokinematic mobility is restored, the athlete can continue with exercise training to improve dynamic control of the TMJ. The athlete can perform the exercises within all planes of movement by performing active movements with the assistance of gravity (Fig. 15-29), with resistance to gravity, and with movements resisted with a tongue depressor, manual resistance, or weighted resistance. It is advisable, at least initially, to have the athlete perform the exercises in front of a mirror. This will give valuable visual input as the athlete performs these activities because proprioception is greatly affected when joint mechanoreceptors are damaged during capsular and musculoskeletal trauma.

LATERAL DEVIATION

Lateral deviation can be performed in the initial phases of treatment, particularly if the athlete is symptomatic during mandibular opening.[30] Left lateral deviation is performed by the right pterygoids and initially includes high repetitions in a pain-free range of movement for coordination training (Fig. 15-30). If anteromedial disk subluxation is suspected, this exercise can be performed with a dental cotton roll to increase joint space and prevent compression of the disk (see Fig. 15-28).

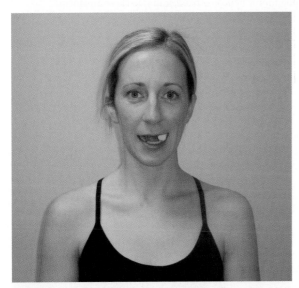

FIGURE 15-27 Unilateral biting performed on the involved side to create joint distraction and slight lateral deviation of the mandible.

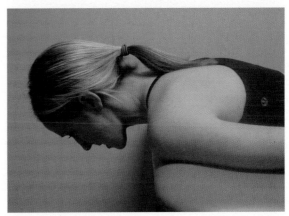

FIGURE 15-29 Mandibular protrusion performed in the prone position. Gravity assistance may reduce the amount of muscle activity and allow reduced symptoms with exercise. The prone position requires increased posterior cervical activity, which can provide reciprocal inhibition of the suprahyoid and infrahyoid during this exercise.

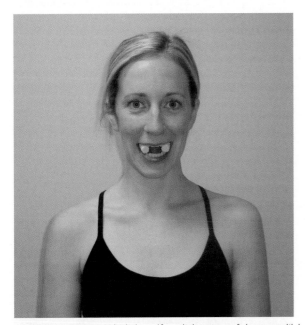

FIGURE 15-28 Lateral glide self-mobilization of the mandible. A dental cotton roll is placed bilaterally between the front teeth to place the joint in a neutral position. The athlete deviates the mandible to the ipsilateral side to perform a lateral glide.

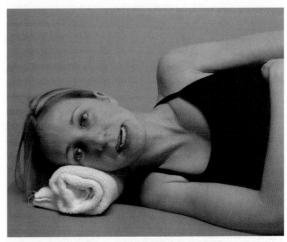

FIGURE 15-30 Left lateral deviation against gravity to coordinate muscular activity of the right pterygoids performed in a side-lying position.

PROTRUSION/RETRUSION

Protrusion and retrusion are not normal functional movements; however, they are an effective means of training the pterygoid muscles (Fig. 15-31). A weak or neurologically inhibited pterygoid may have difficulty coordinating bilateral protrusion. The clinician may have the athlete provide facilitatory cueing by applying a lateral force to the chin with a finger to increase recruitment (Fig. 15-32).

MANDIBULAR OPENING

Mandibular opening can be performed to provide proprioceptive input, coordination of training, and normal tissue stress and strain on the healing tissues. If emphasis is on the initial rolling component of opening, the athlete can be instructed to perform this activity with the tongue maintained on the roof of

the mouth (Fig. 15-33).[34] This will limit arthrokinematic movement to the condylar rolling phase of mandibular opening.

Stage 2

As an athlete progresses to stage 2 training, isometric training can be added to the exercise regimen. Isometrics are performed to improve strength in the ROM gained and to sensitize the muscle spindle to stretch (Fig. 15-34).[30] Sensitization training is important because mechanoreceptor input can become diminished following trauma, which reduces the afferent reflex response. Therefore, as the muscle is lengthened into the hypermobile range, sensory input from the spindle will cause increased recruitment of alpha motor neurons to assist in muscle recruitment.

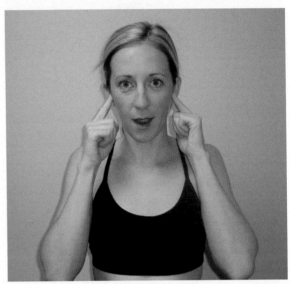

FIGURE 15-33 Mandibular opening isolated to the rotation phase by having the athlete maintain the tongue on the roof of the mouth. The athlete can additionally palpate the temporomandibular joint to limit any protrusion motion with this exercise, as well as limit the exercise to ranges that are void of any clicking or pain.

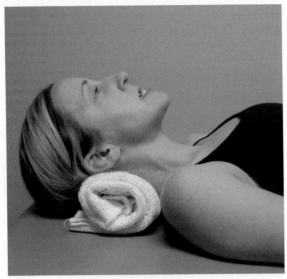

FIGURE 15-31 Mandibular protrusion performed supine against gravity. Dental cotton rolls can be used to maintain the joint in a more neutral position. Resistance can be added as symptoms and movement quality improve.

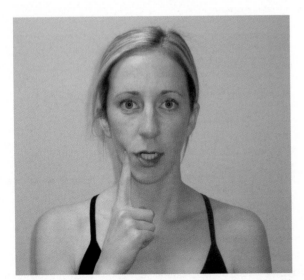

FIGURE 15-32 Mandibular protrusion performed with a concomitant lateral deviation force to facilitate lateral pterygoid activity.

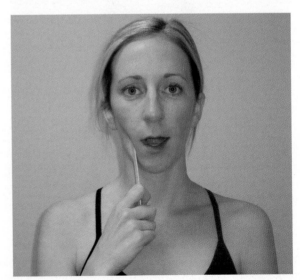

FIGURE 15-34 Isometric lateral deviation performed to achieve strength in a pain-free range and sensitize the muscle spindles to stretch in a hypermobile joint.

Stage 3

As the athlete progresses to stage 3 training, a progressive strengthening program is added to the dynamic stabilization exercises. The clinician may have the athlete continue to perform the exercises in a limited ROM because of joint clicking or dysfunction, as well as continue cervical stabilization, respiration, and postural reeducation training.

ECCENTRIC TRAINING

Eccentric muscle activity plays a critical role in the TMJ because the lateral pterygoid muscle assists in controlling movement of the articular disk as the mandible is elevated. Because the initial phases of treatment have focused on decreasing tone, relieving pain, and restoring joint mobility, the clinician can now instruct the athlete in eccentric training to restore/retrain normal motor function to assist in TMJ arthrokinematic motion (Fig. 15-35).

Stage 4

STRENGTH TRAINING

As the athlete progresses into stage 4, the function of the TMJ should be normalized. The athlete can continue with the cervical stabilization and postural reeducation exercises. Further strengthening exercises can be incorporated as deemed necessary by the sports rehabilitation specialist and may include chewing exercises. Although chewing activities (such as gum chewing) are generally avoided when an athlete has an unstable joint, it can be used as a form of resistance training in a stable joint. Brekhaus et al reported that patients increased their maximum bite force from 527 to 634 N following 50 days of chewing paraffin for 1 hour per day.[35]

POSTURAL INFLUENCE

The cervical spine has a direct relationship to the function of the TMJ and should therefore be assessed and treated as necessary. Assessment and treatment of the cervicothoracic spine is important because dysfunction in this region can both mimic and cause TMJ pain. Cervical pain can be perceived in the face, head, and mandibular region through transmission of nociceptive input via the trigeminocervical nucleus.[36] Cervical pain and dysfunction have been reported to be present in 70% of patients with TMJ dysfunction.[37] The incidence of bruxism has also been reported to be higher in patients with cervical spine pain.[38] Although TMJ dysfunction is multifactorial, the correlation between cervical spine pain/dysfunction and TMJ disorders warrants assessment of this region (see Chapter 16). Cervical spine pain may have a neurophysiologic basis, or postural adaptations may create abnormal tension.

A common clinical finding is a head forward, rounded shoulder posture, which has been shown to have a direct relationship with malocclusion, masticatory myofascial pain, and the resting position of the mandible and its movements, as listed in Table 15-3.[39,40] A forward head posture places the upper cervical spine in an extended position and the lower cervical spine in flexion because of the gravitational line being posterior to the atlantooccipital joint. This position creates weight bearing on the posterior facets of the mid and upper cervical spine, which can cause irritation of the posterior suboccipital nerves, dorsal root ganglia of C2, and blood vessels and, consequently, headaches and tonic reflexogenic guarding of muscles innervated by the trigeminal-cervical nucleus.[30] Because the soft tissues of the TMJ extend into the cervical region, both the available mobility and posture of the cervical spine can affect the tension and tone of the soft tissues of the TMJ. In addition, premature occlusion of the TMJ will occur and cause excessive compression and resultant joint irritation.[4] A malaligned forward head posture can cause irritation of the joint cartilage of both the TMJ and upper cervical and midcervical facets, collagen adaptations (capsular adhesions, elongation of the posterior-superior collagen stratum, and deformation of the intraarticular disk), muscle guarding, and diminished coordination of the surrounding musculature.[4] The athlete's rehabilitation program therefore consists of exercises and manual treatment to address any postural adaptations or abnormalities. The athlete can be instructed to perform cervical retraining exercises with the tongue placed on the roof of the mouth, the lips closed, and the teeth slightly apart to inhibit activity of the mandibular depressor muscles.[41]

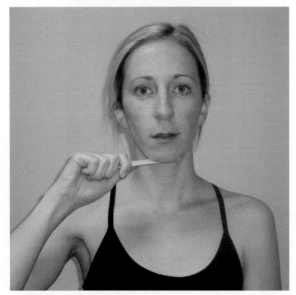

FIGURE 15-35 Eccentric muscle training for mandibular opening. This exercise can be performed with a tongue depressor or the fingers for resistance. It begins with the mandible in an open position and resistance applied under the mandible, and the athlete is instructed to slowly allow the mandible to elevate.

Table 15-3 Resultant Mandibular and TMJ Positioning With Altered Head and Cervical Posture

Altered Postural Position	Resultant TMJ Malocclusion
Forward head posture	Retrusion of the mandible
Retracted head	Protrusion of the mandible
Cranial right side bended	Right lateral glide of the mandible
Cranial right side bended/ left rotated	Right lateral glide of the mandible, retrusion of the right TMJ (posterior translation), and protrusion of the left TMJ (anterior translation)

TMJ, Temporomandibular joint.

SWALLOWING AND LINGUAL FUNCTION

Posture and breathing patterns affect lingual function and occlusion patterns. Normally, an individual is able to swallow with the chin tucked and the head in a neutral or retracted position; however, if normal lingual strategies are not present, the athlete may require the head to be in a forward position. Similarly, normal breathing patterns may be influenced by muscle weakness or reflexive inhibition of the tongue in which it is prevented from elevating on the maxillary arch. If such inhibition occurs, an individual will assume a forward head position to increase pharyngeal airway space because of positioning of the tongue in the pharynx. The tongue attaches via soft tissues to the hyoid bone, so a forward head posture creates a biomechanical increase in the muscle length relationship; this results in an increase in muscle activity to elevate the mandible, which promotes a depressed tongue and static hyoid position.

Coordination and sensory awareness training for lingual function can be done effectively with a mirror for biofeedback. The athlete is instructed to watch for subcranial movement and excessive perioral activity during tongue retraining exercises, as illustrated in Figure 15-36. When the athlete has developed a proper movement and swallowing pattern, these exercises can be performed with the use of water or a tongue depressor for added coordination and functional training (Fig. 15-37). In addition, water can be used to retrain the athlete's maxillary seal by cupping water above the tongue while the tongue is held against the rugae with the mouth opened. This exercise can be progressed to having the athlete maintain this position followed by swallowing the water while the mouth is maintained in an open position.

REDUCTION OF DISK DISPLACEMENT

Manual reduction of a displaced disk may be necessary. Various techniques can be used, and an understanding of the biomechanics and pathologic factors contributing to the disorder will aid the clinician in reducing the disk (Fig. 15-38).[29,42] If clicking in the

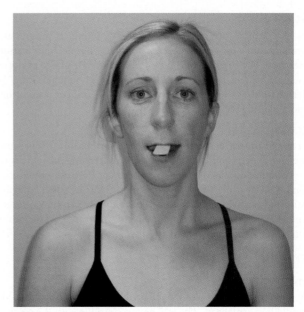

FIGURE 15-37 Resisted tongue elevation. A tongue depressor or finger can be used to apply external resistance to elevation. The depressor is placed as posterior as comfortably allowed to incorporate this posterior region of the tongue because of it more commonly being weaker.

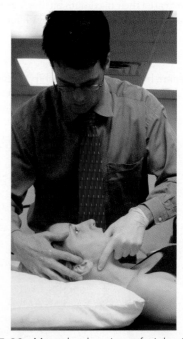

FIGURE 15-38 Manual relocation of right-sided anterior temporomandibular subluxation as described by Grimsby.[4] The clinician palpates the temporomandibular joint with the stabilizing hand. The clinician places the gloved left thumb on top of the bottom molars as the hand is molded around the mandible and chin. The mobilization technique is performed by first depressing the right mandible caudally, and then while maintaining joint distraction, the mandible is pulled anteriorly as far as tolerated. While still maintaining distraction, the mandible is moved posteriorly into mandibular retrusion, and the clinician then releases the joint distraction.

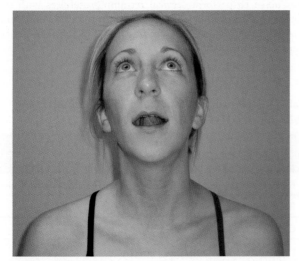

FIGURE 15-36 Tongue tip clucking. The athlete is instructed to place the tongue behind the incisors and make a clucking sound. This exercise is performed to coordinate placement of the tip of the tongue against the rugae.

TMJ is a result of displacement of the intraarticular disk, a relocation exercise can be performed (Fig. 15-39, *A* to *D*).[30] The athlete is instructed to open the mouth maximally with the opening click, and slight lateral deviation is performed away from the involved side. The jaw is then closed while maintaining the protrusion and lateral deviation. As the teeth make contact, the athlete deviates laterally to the neutral position and retrudes the mandible to the position just before the click is perceived to occur. The mouth is then opened again to the point just before the opening click.[4]

ORAL APPLIANCE

Despite a wide range of opinions regarding the effectiveness and mechanism of oral appliances, they are commonly used in the treatment of TMJ disorders. Some of the more common theories are the occlusal disengagement theory, the restored vertical dimension theory, the maxillomandibular realignment theory, the TMJ repositioning theory, and the cognitive awareness theory.[43] It is beneficial for the clinician to become knowledgeable in appliance design and theory and the prescribing dentist's aim

and goal with this device. It is equally important for the clinician to understand and recognize that although oral appliances can be effective in the treatment of TMJ dysfunction, they can sometimes worsen or aggravate the symptoms.

PROPHYLAXIS

The athlete should be educated about avoidance of certain activity, corrections in posture, and behavior modifications to diminish the stress placed on the TMJ. This will help prevent overuse of the masticatory muscles and stress on the TMJ. Box 15-5 summarizes prophylactic education for the TMJ.

CONCLUSION

General Principles

- Evaluation and diagnosis are multifaceted and frequently involve the cervical spine.
- Assessment of respiratory and lingual function is included in a complete evaluation of the TMJ.

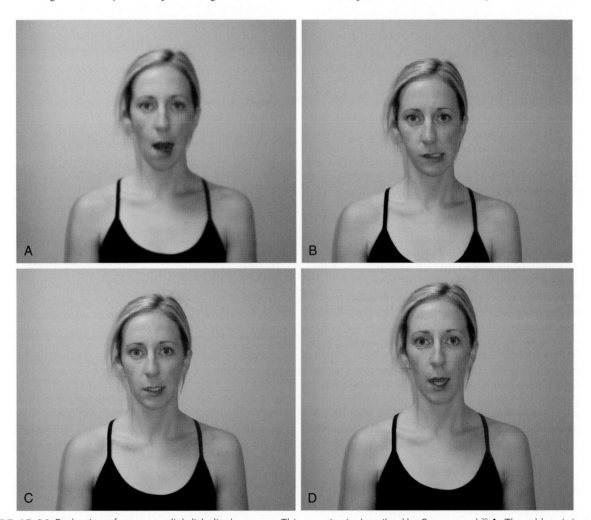

FIGURE 15-39 Reduction of anteromedial disk displacement. This exercise is described by Sayson et al.[30] **A,** The athlete is instructed to open the mouth maximally with an opening click while slight lateral deviation is performed toward the contralateral side. **B,** The mandible is elevated while maintaining a position of protrusion and lateral deviation. **C,** When the upper and lower teeth make contact, the athlete performs lateral deviation to neutral and retrusion as allowed without a click occurring. **D,** The athlete then opens the mouth to a point before the opening click.

Box 15-5

Prophylactic Education for the Treatment of Temporomandibular Joint Disorders

Avoid isometric parafunctional muscle activities such as clenching and chewing on pencils, pens, and fingernails.

Avoid wide mouth opening greater than three finger widths

Avoid hard food, and cut hard and tough food into smaller pieces.

Chew evenly on both sides with the back molars.

Unilateral chewing on the involved side may be less painful because of less joint compression ipsilaterally than contralaterally.

Maintain a neutral posture of the head and neck to promote a neutral position of the mandible when chewing.

Avoid a side-lying sleeping position if lateral shear of the TMJ is problematic.

Hold the mandible in the resting zone to reduce activity of the masticator muscles.

Avoid a forward head posture.

Avoid ranges and movements that produce clicking or locking of the TMJ.

Address malocclusion with dental intervention.

Avoid the rest position of the tongue thrust forward, which causes protrusion of the mandible.

TMJ, Temporomandibular joint.

- The TMJ is more dependent on muscular tissues than on ligamentous and bony tissues for joint stability.
- The sports rehabilitation specialist should determine whether joint hypomobility or hypermobility is present to design an effective treatment strategy.

Evaluation

- Patients with complaints of headaches or maxillofacial, cervicogenic, or shoulder girdle pain warrant evaluation of the TMJ because of common referral patterns.
- Altered posture such as a forward head position or cervical side bending will produce malocclusion of the mandible and altered muscle tension.
- A systematic and thorough evaluation is helpful to ensure that all aspects of the examination are performed.
- Posture, including the athlete's habitual posture, should be assessed for possible abnormalities and compensatory positions.
- Cervical screening should be performed when assessing the TMJ to rule out pathology.

Rehabilitation

- The clinician should base the rehabilitation program on the pathologic tissue involved, with treatment, such as education on posture and respiration and lingual training, included as necessary.
- The therapeutic program should consist of soft tissue mobilization to address altered muscle status and prepare tissue for exercise.

- The clinician can include joint mobilization treatment to improve joint mobility and diminish pain and muscle guarding as needed.
- The athlete should be properly educated regarding avoidance of certain activity and modifications in posture to expedite the rehabilitation program and avoid the deleterious effects that can occur at the TMJ.

REFERENCES

1. Mohl, N.D., and Dixon, D.C. (1994): Current status of diagnostic procedures for temporomandibular disorders. J. Am. Dent. Assoc., 125:56–64.
2. Kraus, S.L. (2004): Temporomandibular disorders. In Saunders, H.D., and Saunders Ryan, R. (eds.): Evaluation, Treatment, and Prevention of Musculoskeletal Disorders, Vol. 1, The Spine, 3rd ed. Philadelphia, Saunders, pp. 173–210.
3. Marbach, J.J. (1992): The "temporomandibular pain dysfunction syndrome" personality: Fact or fiction? J. Oral Rehabil., 19:545–560.
4. The Ola Grimsby Institute (2005): Temporomandibular Joint: Residency Course Notes; Systems Course, p. 685.
5. Eggleton, T.M., and Langton, D.P. (1994): Clinical anatomy of the TMJ complex. In Kraus, S.L. (ed.): Clinics in Physical Therapy; Temporomandibular Disorders, 2nd ed. New York, Churchill Livingstone.
6. Mohl, N.D. (1982): Functional anatomy of the temporomandibular joint. In Laskin, D.M., Greenfield, W., and Gale, E., et al. (eds.): The President's Conference on the Examination, Diagnosis and Management of Temporomandibular Disorders. Chicago, American Dental Association.
7. Dijkstra, P.U., de Bont, L.G.M., Leeuw, R., et al. (1993): Temporomandibular joint osteoarthrosis and temporomandibular joint hypermobility. J. Craniomandibular Pract., 11:268–275.
8. Yale, S.H., Allison, B.D., and Hauptfuehrer, J.D. (1966): An epidemiological assessment of mandibular condyle morphology. Oral Surg., 21:169.
9. Abdel-Fattah, R.A. (1997): An introduction to occlusal biomechanics in temporomandibular disorders. Cranio, 15:349–350.
10. Dawson, P. (1989): Evaluation, Diagnosis, and Treatment of Occlusal Problems, 2nd ed. St. Louis, Mosby.
11. Mills, D., Fiandaca, D., and Scapino, R. (1994): Morphologic, microscopic, and immunohistochemical investigations into the function of the primate TMJ disc. J. Orofac. Pain, 8:136–154.
12. Minarelli, A., Del Santo, M., and Liberti, E. (1997): The structure of the human temporomandibular joint disc: A scanning electron microscopy study. J. Orofac. Pain, 11:95–100.
13. Bays R.A. (2000): Surgery for internal derangement. In Fonseca, R.J., Bays, R.A., and Quin, P.D. (eds.): Oral and Maxillofacial Surgery. Vol. 4, Philadelphia, Saunders.
14. Rees, L.A. (1954): The structure and function of the mandibular joint. Br. Dent. J., 96:125.
15. Wong, G.V., Weinberg, S., and Symingen, J.M. (1985): Morphology of the developing articular disc of the human temporomandibular joint. J. Oral Maxillofac. Surg., 43:565–569.
16. Turell, J., and Ruiz, G. (1987): Normal and abnormal findings in temporomandibular joints in autopsy specimens. J. Orofac. Pain, 1:257–275.
17. Bell, W.E. (1982): Temporomandibular Disorders; Classification, Diagnosis and Management, 3rd ed. Chicago, Year Book.
18. Mahan, P.E. (1980): The temporomandibular joint in function and pathofunction. In Solberg, W.K., and Clark, G.T. (eds.): Temporomandibular Joint Problems. Lombard, IL, Quintessence.
19. Okeson, J.P. (1993): The Management of Temporomandibular Disorders and Occlusion, 3rd ed. St. Louis, Mosby.
20. Scapino, R. (1991): The posterior attachment: Its structure, function and appearance in TMJ imaging studies. Part 1. J. Orofac. Pain, 5:83–94.
21. Ide, Y., and Nakazawa, K. (1991): Anatomical Atlas of the Temporomandibular Joint. Tokyo, Quintessence.
22. Klineberg, I.J., Greenfield, B.E., and Wyke, B.D. (1970): Contributions to the reflex control of mastication from mechanoreceptors in the temporomandibular joint capsule. Dent. Pract., 21:73–83.
23. Hesse, J.R., and Hansson, T. (1988): Factors influencing joint mobility in general and in particular respect of the craniomandibular articulation: A literature review. J. Orofac. Pain, 2:19–28.
24. Pinto, O.F. (1962): A new structure and function of the mandibular joint. J. Prosthet. Dent., 12:95–103.
25. Pertes, R., and Attanasio, R. (1991): Internal derangements. In Kaplan, A.S., and Assael, L.A. (eds.): Temporomandibular Disorders, Diagnosis and Treatment. Philadelphia, Saunders.
26. Friedman, M.H., and Weisberg, J. (1990): The temporomandibular joint. In Gould, J.A. (ed.): Orthopedic and Sports Physical Therapy. St. Louis, Mosby.
27. Hochstedler, J.L., Allen, B.A., and Follmar, M.A. (1996): Temporomandibular joint range of motion: A ratio of interincisal opening to excursive movement in a healthy population. J. Craniomandibular Pract., 14:296–300.
28. Szentpetery, A. (1993): Clinical utility of mandibular movement ranges. J. Orofac. Pain, 7:163–168.

29. Rocabado, M., and Iglarsh, Z.A. (1991): Neuromuscular evaluation of the maxillofacial region. In Rocabado, M., and Iglarsh, Z.A. (eds.): Musculoskeletal Evaluation of the Maxillofacial Region. Philadelphia, Lippincott.

30. Sayson, J., Rivard, J., Grimsby, O., and Wong, W. (2008): Exercise rehabilitation of the TMJ. In Rivard, J., and Grimsby, O. (eds.): Science, Theory and Clinical Application in Orthopaedic Manual Physical Therapy. Taylorsville, UT, Academy of Graduate Physical Therapy.

31. Petrofsky, J.S., and Hendershot, D.M. (1984): The interrelationship between blood pressure, intramuscular pressure, and isometric endurance in fast and slow twitch skeletal muscle in the cat. Eur. J. Appl. Physiol. Occup. Physiol., 53:106–111.

32. Petrofsky, J.S., Phillips, C.A., Sawka, M.N., et al. (1981): Blood flow and metabolism during isometric contractions in cat skeletal muscle. J. Appl. Physiol., 50:493–502.

33. Naeije, M., and Hofman, N. (2003): Biomechanics of the human temporomandibular joint during chewing. J. Dent. Res., 82:528–531.

34. Gelb., H. (1977): Clinical management of head, neck, and TMJ pain and dysfunction. In Gelb, H. (ed.): A Multi-Disciplinary Approach to Diagnosis and Treatment, 1st ed. Philadelphia, Saunders, pp. 73–117.

35. Brekhaus, P.J., Armstrong, W.D., and Simon, W.G. (1941): Stimulation of the muscles of mastication. J. Dent. Res., 20:87.

36. Bogduk, N. (1986): Cervical causes of headache and dizziness. In Grieve G. (ed.): Modern Manual Therapy. Edinburgh, Churchill Livingstone, pp. 289–302.

37. Padamsee, M., Mehtan, N., Forgione, A., et al. (1994): Incidence of cervical disorders in a TMD population [IADR; abstract No. 680]. J. Dent. Res., p. 73.

38. Isaccsson, G., Linde, C., and Isberg, A. (1989): Subjective symptoms in patients with temporomandibular joint disc displacement versus patients with myogenic craniomandibular disorders. J. Prosthet. Dent., 61:70–77.

39. Mohl, N.D. (1976): Head posture and its role in occlusion. N.Y. State Dent. J., 42:17–23.

40. Fricton, J.R., Kroening, R., Haley, D., and Siegert, R. (1985): Myofascial pain syndrome of the head and neck: A review of clinical characteristics of 164 patients. Oral Surg. Oral Med. Oral Pathol., 60:615–623.

41. Chiu, T.T., Law, E.Y., and Chiu, T.H. (2005): Performance of the craniocervical flexion test in subjects with and without chronic neck pain. J. Orthop. Sports Phys. Ther., 35:567–571.

42. Yoda, T., Sakamoto, I., Imai, H., et al. (2003): A randomized controlled trial of therapeutic exercise for clicking due to disk anterior displacement with reduction in the temporomandibular joint. Cranio, 21:10–16.

43. Clark, G.T. (1984): A critical evaluation of orthopedic interocclusal appliance therapy: Design, theory, and overall effectiveness. J. Am. Dent. Assoc., 108:359–368.

16

Cervical Spine Rehabilitation

Todd R. Hooks, PT, SCS, ATC, MOMT, MTC, CSCS, FAAOMPT

CHAPTER OBJECTIVES

- Describe the orientation and function of the anatomic structures in the cervical spine.
- Explain the arthrokinematics and biomechanics of the cervical spine during active range of motion and joint mobilizations.
- Perform special tests for the cervical spine and be able to explain the technique and differentiate positive and negative test findings.

- Appreciate the clinical thought process involved during the evaluation.
- Design and implement a therapeutic program on the basis of clinical findings noted during the evaluation.
- Describe common pathologic conditions in the cervical spine and the therapeutic considerations needed to address the pathology.

The cervical spine is one of the most commonly injured areas in the human body, with pathologies ranging from chronic in nature because of poor postural habits to those occurring as a result of acute, traumatic injuries. Rehabilitation techniques have changed in recent years because of a more thorough understanding of this region. Such understanding has allowed rehabilitation to evolve from structured protocols that have relied solely on static, isometric exercises to programs that address the need for normalization of the tissue's tolerance of functional loading (forces causing stretching or compression) so that dynamic, isotonic exercises can be instituted to restore postural deficits and regain neuromuscular control, strength, and endurance. This chapter addresses the anatomic, arthrokinematic, and biomechanical considerations needed during the evaluation and treatment process. Differential assessment of the tissues related to the cervical spine and evaluation of joint play and mobility will allow the clinician to determine whether tissue lesions and pathologic hypermobility or hypomobility are present and to address these pathologies with manual techniques and the application of an exercise regimen to expedite the healing process. Various special tests are presented that allow the clinician to determine the specific cause of pain and loss of function. By performing a complete evaluation procedure, the sports rehabilitation specialist will develop a better understanding of the exact tissues involved in the pathology. This will allow the clinician to provide the optimal stimulus to facilitate healing of that tissue.

ANATOMY

It is imperative that the clinician be competent in locating and identifying the anatomic structures of the cervical spine and have proficient understanding of their biomechanical functions to allow a thorough evaluation and institute a proper rehabilitation program. Therefore, this section addresses the cervical vertebral column and its surrounding ligaments, muscles, and neurovascular structures. Because various pathologic conditions can affect one or more of these systems, it is important that the rehabilitation specialist have a thorough functional understanding of these structures.

Bony Configuration

The cervical spine consists of seven vertebrae. The anatomic structure of the midcervical spine (C3-C6) is similar to that of the thoracic and lumbar spine in that each vertebra has a vertebral body, pedicle, lamina, and spinous process. However, the midcervical spine also has a number of anatomic structures that are unique to this region (Fig. 16-1). Each midcervical vertebra has an uncinate process and a foramen transversarium, and their spinous processes are bifid. The foramen transversarium accommodates the vertebral artery and vein and is found in all cervical vertebrae except C7, although variations do exist. The spinous processes are bifid to allow greater range of motion (ROM) into extension and to provide a mechanical advantage for muscular attachments.

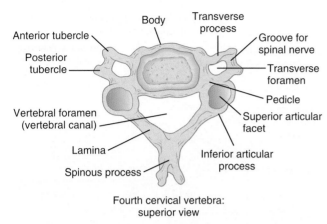

FIGURE 16-1 Superior view of the midcervical vertebrae.

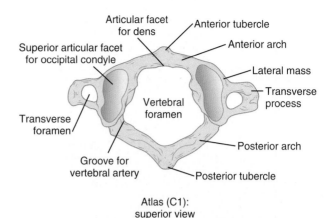

Atlas (C1):
superior view

FIGURE 16-3 Superior view of the atlas (C1).

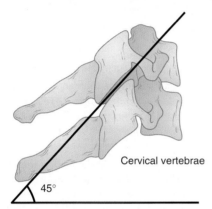

FIGURE 16-2 Lateral view of the midcervical vertebrae depicting the plane of the facet joints. *(From Iglarsh, Z.A., and Snyder-Mackler, L. [1994]: Temporomandibular joint and the cervical spine. In Richardson, J.K., and Iglarsh, Z.A. (eds.): Clinical Orthopedic Physical Therapy. Philadelphia, Saunders, p. 12.)*

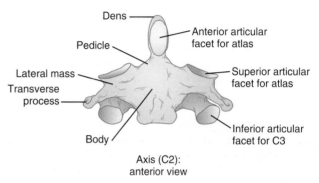

Axis (C2):
anterior view

FIGURE 16-4 Anterior view of the axis (C2).

The superior surface of the vertebral bodies in the midcervical spine is concave in the frontal plane and convex in the sagittal plane, and the opposite is true for the inferior surfaces. These cervical vertebrae have two superior and two inferior facets that are located on the pedicles. The superior facets are oriented in a posterior direction, whereas the inferior facets are oriented in an anterior direction. The biplanar orientation of these joints requires that rotation and lateral flexion be coupled movements. These facets articulate with the adjacent vertebrae to form facet joints (zygapophyseal joints). They have an approximate angle of 45° from the horizontal plane in the midcervical region (C3-C6) that decreases to approximately 30° in the lower cervical region (C7-T3) (Fig. 16-2). The facet joints are planar synovial joints with articular cartilage on the surfaces that is enclosed in a fibrosis joint capsule. Found within the joint capsule is meniscoid, adipose, and connective tissue.[1] The medial branch of the dorsal primary ramus innervates the facet joints.

The first cervical vertebra (C1), the atlas, articulates with the occiput superiorly and the axis (C2) inferiorly. The atlas does not have a spinous process or a real vertebral body; however, the odontoid process (dens) of the axis functions as the body of C1 (see Fig. 16-4). The atlas consists of two lateral masses connected by anterior and posterior arches and transverse processes

that provide for acceptance of weight through the articular processes. The posterior surface of the anterior arch has a facet lined with hyaline cartilage that articulates with the odontoid process of C2 (Fig. 16-3). The superior articular processes are biconcave and articulate with the biconvex occipital condyles, and the inferior articular processes are biconvex and articulate with the biconvex superior facets of the axis.

The axis (C2) contains a superior projection, the odontoid process, that articulates with the posterior aspect of the anterior arch of the atlas. The axis, like the atlas, has small transverse processes and a posterior arch instead of pedicles (Fig. 16-4). In the upper cervical spine (C1-C2), the foramen transversarium is located more laterally than in the midcervical spine, thus requiring the vertebral artery to ascend in a lateral direction in this region. Weight bearing is absorbed superiorly as the axis articulates with the inferior facets located on the lateral masses of the atlas and is transmitted inferiorly through the inferior facet joints, which are located more posteriorly on the axis, similar to those in the midcervical region.

Uncovertebral joints (joints of Luschka), first described by von Luschka, are believed to develop because of degenerative changes in the annulus fibrosus (Fig. 16-5). They are located on the lateral aspect of the midcervical vertebra and on the posterolateral aspect of C7-T1.[2] Uncovertebral joints function to deepen the articular surface and provide stability as they articulate with the adjacent vertebral body. However, because of their close proximity to the spinal nerves, osteophyte formation in this region can encroach on these structures. They also limit motion, especially lateral flexion, and serve to prevent lateral disk herniation.

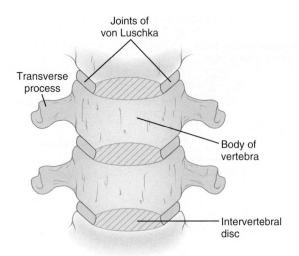

FIGURE 16-5 Anterior view of the midcervical vertebrae displaying uncovertebral joints (joints of Luschka). *(From Iglarsh, Z.A., and Snyder-Mackler, L. [1994]: Temporomandibular joint and the cervical spine. In Richardson, J.K., and Iglarsh, Z.A. (eds.): Clinical Orthopedic Physical Therapy. Philadelphia, Saunders, p. 12.)*

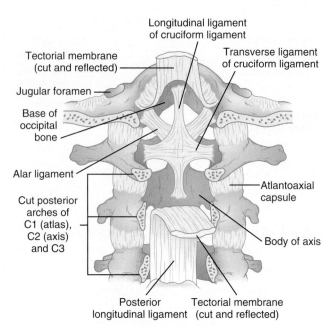

FIGURE 16-6 Posterior view of ligaments in the upper cervical spine. *(From Iglarsh, Z.A., and Snyder-Mackler, L. [1994]: Temporomandibular joint and the cervical spine. In Richardson, J.K., and Iglarsh, Z.A. (eds.): Clinical Orthopedic Physical Therapy. Philadelphia, Saunders, p. 12.)*

Intervertebral Disk

An intervertebral disk (IVD) is present between each cervical vertebra except for the occiput and atlas (C0-C1) and the atlas and axis (C1-C2). The disks in the cervical spine are relatively thicker than those in the thoracic and lumbar spine, which allows greater ROM. The cervical disks are slightly higher anteriorly and thereby contribute to the lordotic curve in the cervical spine. The IVD is divided into a central region, the nucleus pulposus, and a peripheral ring, the annulus fibrosus. No true demarcation is found between the nucleus and the annulus, but rather a gradual change in tissue structure is seen from the inner layer to the outer ring. Because of the collagenous properties of the nucleus pulposus, which contains primarily type II collagen, it functions to resist axial compression and distributes these forces. The annulus fibrosus is composed of primarily type I collagen and functions to resist tensile forces within the disk. As a person ages, the amount of proteoglycan and therefore the amount of water begin to diminish.[3] The IVDs are avascular and depend on diffusion from the vertebral end plates for their nutrition. The disk is innervated along the periphery of the annulus fibrosus through the sinuvertebral nerve.[4]

Nerve Roots

Although there are seven cervical vertebrae, there are eight pairs of nerve roots in the cervical spine. This discrepancy is due to the fact that the first nerve root (C1) exits between the occiput and the atlas and nerves 2 through 7 also exit above the vertebrae for which they are named. The transition of the nerve root exiting below the vertebra for which it derives its name occurs at C8, and this continues throughout the thoracic and lumbar spine. Therefore, because the C5 nerve root exists above the C5 vertebra, protrusion of the C4-C5 IVD would most likely affect this nerve. The cervical nerves differ from the lumbar nerves in that the ventral (motor) and dorsal (sensory) roots do not unite to form a mixed spinal nerve until it is in the intervertebral foramen. Because of this anatomic relationship, cervical

disk herniations would be more likely to affect the spinal cord or the ventral root, whereas nerve irritation from the facet or uncovertebral joint could encroach on either the nerve roots or the spinal nerve. The nerve roots then exit the vertebral column in the intervertebral foramen and divide into the anterior (ventral) and posterior (dorsal) primary rami. The posterior primary rami innervate the deep erector spinae muscles and the facet joints. The anterior primary rami of C5-T1 combine to form the brachial plexus supplying the upper part of the arms.[5]

Ligamentous Support

Because the upper cervical spine has sacrificed osteokinematic stability for greater arthrokinematic mobility, it is dependent on ligamentous support to allow basic function and avoid injury. Because of the unique and complex articulations present in the upper cervical region, specialized ligaments provide the needed stability. The dens is connected to the anterior rim of the foramen magnum by the apical ligament and the two obliquely oriented alar ligaments. The alar ligaments limit the amount of contralateral rotation that occurs at the atlantoaxial joint.[6] The cruciform (cruciate) ligament consists of three bands of fibers oriented in superior, inferior, and transverse directions (Fig. 16-6). The transverse band is approximately 7 to 8 mm in thickness,[2] which makes it the largest and strongest of all the atlantoaxial ligaments. The cruciform ligament functions to stabilize the dens against the posterior aspect of the anterior arch of the atlas and to prevent subluxation into the spinal canal. Posterior to the cruciform ligaments is the tectorial membrane. It originates at the basilar occipital bone and forms the continuation of the posterior longitudinal ligament (PLL). The PLL attaches to the IVD of adjacent vertebrae and their vertebral margins and functions to prevent cervical disk herniation and excessive flexion of the vertebral bodies.[7] In the cervical spine the PLL is broader and thicker than in the lumbar spine. The anterior longitudinal ligament

Table 16-1 Origin, Insertion, Action, and Innervation of the Anterior Cervical Spine Musculature

Muscle	Origin	Insertion	Action	Innervation
Sternocleidomastoid	Sternal head: anterior sternum	Mastoid process	Bilaterally: flexes the head	C2
	Clavicular head: medial third of the clavicle	Mastoid process	Unilaterally: side-bends the head toward and rotates the head to the opposite side	Spinal accessory nerve (cranial nerve XI)
Scalene anterior	Anterior tubercles of the transverse processes of C3-C6	Scalene tubercle of the first rib	Elevates the first rib Unilaterally: side-bends the neck toward and rotates the neck to the opposite side Bilaterally: flexes the neck	C5-C8
Scalene medius	Posterior tubercles of the transverse processes of C2-C7	Superior surface of the first rib behind the subclavian groove	Elevates the first rib Unilaterally: side-bends the neck toward and rotates the neck to the opposite side Bilaterally: flexes the neck	C3-C4
Scalene posterior	Posterior tubercles of the transverse processes of C4-C6	Second rib posterior to the attachment of the serratus anterior	Elevates the second rib Unilaterally: side-bends the neck toward and rotates the neck to the opposite side Bilaterally: flexes the neck	C4-C8
Longus capitis	Anterior tubercles of the transverse processes of C3-C6	Basilar part of the occipital bone	Flexes the head and neck and assists in rotation	C1-C4
Longus colli	Vertebral bodies of C5-T3 and anterior tubercles of the transverse processes of C3-C5	Vertebral bodies of C2-C4 Anterior tubercle of the atlas Anterior tubercles of the transverse processes of C5-C6	Flexes the head and neck and assists in rotation Unilaterally: side-bends the neck	C2-C8
Rectus capitis anterior	Lateral mass of the atlas	Basilar part of the occipital bone	Bilaterally: flexes the head Unilaterally: side-bends and rotates the head ipsilaterally	C1-C2
Rectus capitis lateralis	Anterior tubercle of the transverse process of the atlas	Jugular process of the occiput	Bilaterally: flexes the head Unilaterally: side-bends the head	C1-C2

(ALL) originates from inferior surface of the basilar occiput bone and extends to the sacrum. It attaches to the vertebral bodies and IVD, but not to the bony rims.[8] This ligament functions in preventing hyperextension of the vertebral bodies.

The posterior vertebral elements have specialized ligaments to provide stability. The ligamentum flavum connects adjoining laminae, and because of its attachment to the anterior aspect of the facet joint, it serves to prevent entrapment of the facet capsule and meniscus in the facet joints. The ligamentum nuchae is posterior to the ligamentum flavum and is a fibroelastic membrane that functions to limit cervical flexion. The posterior cervical ligament originates at the occiput and inserts into the spinous processes of the cervical spine before terminating at C7. It functions to resist excessive flexion and divides the posterior cervical muscles into right and left sides.

Muscular Arrangement

The cervical spine has numerous muscles that have an influence on proprioceptive input and postural control and provide active movements for the occiput, cervical spine, and upper part of the trunk. These muscles can be divided into anterior and posterior groups according to their attachment in relation to the transverse processes. Tables 16-1 and 16-2 list these muscles, including their origin, insertion, action, and innervation.

BIOMECHANICS

Clinical Pearl #1

The forces and stresses that are controlled and generated by the body ensure the proper histologic, biomechanical, and physiologic properties of each tissue.

"Structure governs function and function dictates structure."
—Rob Tillman, PT, MOMT

Osteokinematic motion in the cervical spine is a result of interaction of the cervical vertebrae, IVDs, ligaments, joint capsules, and the orientation of the facet joints working together to control and dictate the movements that occur in

Table 16-2 Origin, Insertion, Action, and Innervation of the Posterior Cervical Spine Musculature

Muscle	Origin	Insertion	Action	Innervation
Upper trapezius	Medial third of the superior nuchal line, external occipital protuberance, and ligamentum nuchae	Lateral third of the clavicle	Extends, side-bends, and rotates the head to the opposite side Elevates the scapula	Spinal accessory nerve (cranial nerve XI) C3-C4
Levator scapulae	Transverse processes of the upper 3-4 cervical vertebrae	Medial border of the scapula above the spine	Extends, side-bends, and rotates the neck to the ipsilateral side Elevates and downwardly rotates the scapula	Dorsal scapular nerve (C5) C3-C4
Splenius capitis	Ligamentum nuchae, spinous processes of C7 and upper 4-5 thoracic vertebrae	Mastoid process and superior nuchal line	Extends, side-bends, and rotates the head and neck to the ipsilateral side	C4-C6
Splenius cervicis	Spinous processes of T3-T6	Posterior tubercles of the transverse processes of the upper 3–4 cervical vertebrae	Extends, side-bends, and rotates the neck to the ipsilateral side	C4-C6
Longissimus capitis	Transverse processes of the upper 4-5 thoracic vertebrae	Mastoid process	Extends, side-bends, and rotates the head to the ipsilateral side	C6-C8
Longissimus cervicis	Transverse processes of the upper 4-5 thoracic vertebrae	Posterior tubercles of the transverse processes of C2-C6	Side-bends and rotates the neck to the ipsilateral side	C6-C8
Semispinalis capitis	Transverse processes of C7 and upper 6-7 thoracic vertebrae, C4-C6 articular processes	Between the superior and inferior nuchal lines	Extends, side-bends, and rotates the head to the ipsilateral side	C1-C8
Semispinalis cervicis	Transverse processes of the upper 5-6 thoracic vertebrae	Spinous processes of C2-C5	Extends, side-bends, and rotates the neck to the ipsilateral side	C1-C8
Obliquus capitis inferior	Spinous process of the axis	Transverse process of the atlas	Extends, side-bends, and rotates the head to the ipsilateral side Side-bends and rotates the neck to the ipsilateral side	C1-C2
Obliquus capitis superior	Transverse process of the atlas	Above the inferior nuchal line	Extends and side-bends the head	C1
Rectus capitis posterior major	Spinous process of the axis	Lateral aspect of the inferior nuchal line	Extends, side-bends, and rotates the head to the ipsilateral side	C1
Rectus capitis posterior minor	Posterior tubercle of the atlas	Medial third of the inferior nuchal line	Extends and side-bends the head	C1

this region. Active ROM is a result of the interaction of the entire cervical spine to produce a desired movement. However, because of anatomic differences between the upper cervical and midcervical spine, the upper cervical spine is able to perform motions independent of those of the midcervical region. This allows the cervical spine to correctly position the head for optimal orientation of the visual, auditory, and olfactory nervous systems.

The arthrokinematic motions of the upper cervical spine are discussed in detail because of the complex articulations in this region. Notably, the desired motion occurs as a result of these actions occurring in unison. The following processes described are a teaching tool that is meant to promote biomechanical understanding of what occurs, although functionally these

movements are occurring together and in synchrony. Because normal variations occur in osseous and connective tissue properties and orientation, structural discrepancies can exist and produce altered arthrokinematic movements.

During flexion of the upper cervical spine (Fig. 16-7), (1) the convex condyles of the occiput glide in a posterior direction on the concave facets of the atlas, which produces (2) an anterior tilt of the occiput. (3) The atlas is pushed approximately 2 to 3 mm in an anterior direction because of the force created in the facet joints. This translation creates approximation between the dens and the transverse ligament, which restricts further motion. (4) The atlas tilts 15° to 20° anteriorly, (5) thus causing its anterior arch to move inferiorly 2 to 4 mm as the posterior arch is elevated. (6) The superior tilt of the posterior

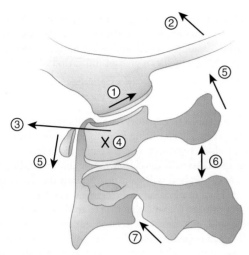

FIGURE 16-7 Biomechanics of the upper cervical spine during flexion. *(From The Ola Grimsby Institute [1998]: Cervical Biomechanics. Residency Course Notes; Systems Course, 680:33.)*

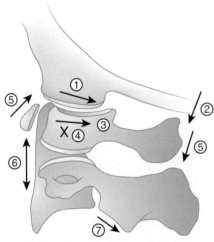

FIGURE 16-8 Biomechanics of the upper cervical spine during extension. *(From The Ola Grimsby Institute [1998]: Cervical Biomechanics. Residency Course Notes; Systems Course, 680:33.)*

Right   Left

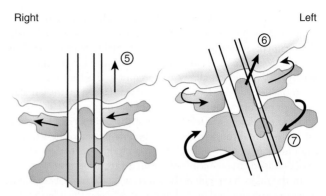

FIGURE 16-9 Biomechanics of the upper cervical spine during lateral flexion. *(From The Ola Grimsby Institute [1998]: Cervical Biomechanics. Residency Course Notes; Systems Course, 680:33.)*

Right   Left

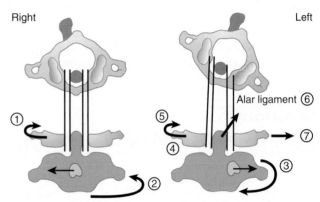

FIGURE 16-10 Biomechanics of the upper cervical spine during rotation. *(From The Ola Grimsby Institute [1998]: Cervical Biomechanics. Residency Course Notes; Systems Course, 680:33.)*

arch increases tension on the posterior ligamentous structures between C1 and C2. (7) The increased tension causes movement between C2 and C3.[9]

Extension of the upper cervical spine (Fig. 16-8) occurs as a result of (1) the convex occipital condyles gliding forward on the concave facet joints of the atlas, which produces (2) a posterior tilt of the occiput. (3) The compressive forces cause the atlas to translate 2 to 3 mm posteriorly, and such translation is restrained by the anterior arch of the atlas approximating against the odontoid process. (4) The atlas tilts posteriorly approximately 12°, which causes (5) its anterior arch to translate 2 to 4 mm superiorly on the dens as the posterior arch moves inferiorly. (6) As the anterior ligamentous structures become taut, (7) the axis glides posteriorly on C3.[9]

Right lateral flexion of the upper cervical spine (Fig. 16-9) is produced as the convex condyles of the occiput glide 3° to 5° to the left, which causes a relative right translation of the atlas.

This translation is prevented as the dens approximates against the lateral mass of the atlas. Lateral flexion between C1 and C2 does not occur because of the approximation between the odontoid process and the atlas and their biconvex articulating surfaces. Because of the lateral forces exerted by the occiput and atlas, the axis side-bends 5° to the right on C3 as a result of the inability of C1 to glide laterally on C2. The atlas will then rotate immediately to the left on the axis to maintain an anterior orientation of the face. (5) The left occipital condyle elevates as a result of the wedge-shaped lateral masses of the atlas gliding to the right. This elevation causes tension in the left alar ligament, which (6) produces compression between C2 and C1 as the axis is elevated. (7) The joint compression between the biconvex surfaces of both the atlas and the axis produces a right rotation of the axis. As lateral flexion is increased, the occiput and atlas will rotate to the left on the axis to allow anterior orientation of the face.[9]

Rotation of the upper cervical spine (Fig. 16-10) to the right begins with (1) the occiput rotating on the atlas a minute amount (approximately 1°). As joint approximation occurs, the atlas is pulled into right rotation, thereby bringing the left lateral mass of C1 closer to the dens. (2) The compressive forces that occur between the atlas and the axis produce 2° to 3° of left rotation of

C2 as a result of the biconvex surfaces. (3) The occiput and atlas rotate to the right approximately 40° and apply tension on the left alar ligament, which brings the axis into right rotation. (4) The axis will continue to rotate and side-bend to the right approximately 10°, (5) which allows the occiput and atlas to rotate to the available end ROM. (6) The increased tension on the left alar ligament produces left side bending of the occiput. (7) The atlas is forced to glide to the left because of the compressive forces of the left occipital condyle. As the atlas side glides to the left, the amount of left side bending of the occiput is increased as the wedge-shaped lateral masses of the atlas tilt the occiput.[9]

In the midcervical spine, the superior facets are oriented in a superior, posterior, and medial direction, whereas the inferior facets are oriented in an anterior, inferior, and lateral direction. As a result, during cervical rotation the contralateral inferior facet glides in a superior and medial direction, which produces lateral flexion in the same direction. Therefore, in the cervical region, rotation and lateral flexion always occur together in the same direction.

During flexion, the superior vertebral body slides and tilts anteriorly on the inferior vertebra, which causes separation of the facet joints. During extension, the superior vertebral body slides and tilts posteriorly. This motion is limited because of joint approximation and tension in the ALL. The facet joints are oriented to allow an increase in the amount of flexion and extension.

EVALUATION

Clinical Pearl #2

"The least reliable way to diagnose in soft tissue lesions is to palpate immediately for tenderness in the area outlined by the patient."
—James Cyriax, M.D.

During evaluation of the cervical spine it is important to perform a screening examination of the thoracic spine, temporomandibular joint, and upper extremities to ensure that the pathology is cervical in nature. Box 16-1 outlines an examination flow. It is helpful to take a systemic approach to the evaluation process to ensure that no step in the assessment is overlooked and to allow a smooth, systematic flow of the examination. By performing all the aspects of the examination listed in Box 16-1, the sports rehabilitation specialist will be able to determine which tissue or tissues are affected as a result of the tissue's response to the test imposed. Each tissue is suspected as being a potential source of pain until that tissue has been cleared by careful examination. To clear a tissue, the clinician must perform tests that create stress or tension on that tissue. If a positive response does not occur, the tissue can be excluded as a source of pain.

Visual Observation

The examination process begins with visual observation of the athlete. The clinician watches the athlete walk into the room and observes the positioning of the athlete's head, neck, and shoulder girdle. The sports rehabilitation specialist may be able to detect any defects or abnormalities that are present

and develop an understanding of how the pain is affecting the patient's functional ability. The clinician may be able to ascertain the athlete's ability, speed, and willingness to move the head and upper limbs, which can give an indication of the degree of injury present.

History

The athlete's subjective history is an important aspect of the evaluation process. By eliciting a complete history, the clinician can obtain clues regarding the patient's diagnosis. The rehabilitation specialist will develop a better understanding of the athlete's condition and will gain insight into the direction and intensity of the examination and treatment needed.

It is important to allow the athlete to describe the current complaint and any previous related conditions. The athlete should be encouraged to describe the symptoms, including the location and nature of the pain, as well as any conditions that increase or relieve these symptoms. A visual analog pain-rating scale is commonly used to allow the athlete to indicate the severity of the pain. Although many different types of analog scales are available for use, it is important to use the same scale for consistency.[10] The clinician should be aware of the athlete's goals and the time frame for achieving these goals. This will ensure that both the clinician and the athlete clearly understand one another and will allow insight into the athlete's motivation.

Structural Inspection

The clinician begins an inspection of the athlete in a standing position after the athlete has undressed. The visual inspection can include the patient standing in a normal, habitual stance and in the anatomic position. The clinician should briefly perform a full examination of the entire body of the patient in anterior, lateral, and posterior views while observing body contours and looking for any structural abnormalities or postural faults that may be present. The clinician can observe the athlete's respiratory pattern to assess rate and rhythm and determine whether inspiration originates from the diaphragm or from the upper thoracic region. The clinician may also choose to perform an inspection while the patient is in both habitual and upright sitting postures. Because postural abnormalities (i.e., forward head, rounded shoulders) profoundly amplify any decreased ROM and function, the clinician should make note of such abnormalities because of their potential contribution to tissue irritation.

Active Movements

The first motions performed by the athlete are active movements. This allows the clinician to observe not only the patient's available ROM but also the quality of motion, pain elicited, and the speed and willingness to move. The athlete begins by performing cardinal plane motions. As the patient performs the active movements, the clinician should observe for segmental areas that have either an abrupt or reduced angulation. This may indicate areas where segmental motion is altered with respect to the rest of the cervical spine.

Movements that are most painful should be performed last to ensure that the pain is not carried over during the remaining motions.[11] If an athlete complains of pain with repetitive

---

Box 16-1

Examination Flow

INITIAL OBSERVATION

Posture and position of the head and cervical sprain

General demeanor of the athlete

ATHLETE'S SUBJECTIVE HISTORY

STRUCTURAL INSPECTION

Observe from the anterior/posterior/lateral views for alignment and position

May perform both in seated/standing postures

Observe in both habitual/corrected postures

ACTIVE MOTION

The examiner notes the speed, willingness to move, range, quality of movement, and availability of segmental movement:

- Flexion
- Extension
- Lateral flexion
- Rotation
- Combined motions
- Repetitive motions

PASSIVE MOTION

The examiner notes the end-feel, availability of movement, and restrictions:

- Flexion
- Extension
- Lateral flexion
- Rotation
- Prolonged positions
- Overpressure

RESISTED MOTION

Each motion is tested in three positions (mid, inner range, outer range):

- Flexion
- Extension
- Lateral flexion
- Rotation

PALPATION

Note temperature variations, atrophy, muscle bulk, tone, swelling, tenderness, thickness, dryness, moisture, abnormalities, crepitus, and pain

NEUROLOGIC TESTS

Sensation tests

Reflexes

Myotomes

SPECIAL TESTS

Vascular tests:

- DeKleyn test (vertebral artery test)
- Hautant test
- Underburg test

Neurologic tests:

- Distraction
- Compression
- Shoulder abduction test
- Valsalva maneuver

Upper limb tension tests (ULTTs):

- ULTT1
- ULTT2
- ULTT3
- ULTT4

Instability tests:

- Odontoid fracture
- Transverse ligament

Thoracic outlet syndrome tests:

- Roos test
- Adson test
- Allen test
- Costoclavicular compression maneuver
- Pectoralis minor test
- Wright hyperabduction test

MOBILITY TESTS

Lower and midcervical spine:

- Flexion
- Extension
- Lateral flexion
- Rotation

Upper cervical spine:

- Atlantooccipital:
  - Flexion
  - Extension
  - Lateral flexion
  - Rotation
- Atlantoaxial:
  - Rotation

DIAGNOSTIC TESTS

Radiographs, magnetic resonance imaging, computed tomography, myelography, electromyography, laboratory tests

---

movements, prolonged positions (i.e., cervical flexion, extension, sitting, standing), or a combined motion, the clinician should instruct the patient to perform these actions last. In such cases it may be necessary to have the athlete repeat a movement (5 to 10 times), maintain a position (15 to 20 seconds), or perform combined movements in an attempt to reproduce the symptoms.

Passive Movements

The rehabilitation specialist performs passive ROM to assess the cervical spine for possible restrictions and to determine each motion's end-feel. In the cervical spine, the normal end-feel for all cardinal plane movements is a tissue stretch. If ROM is restricted in multiple directions, the clinician should determine whether the limitation is in a capsular or noncapsular pattern.

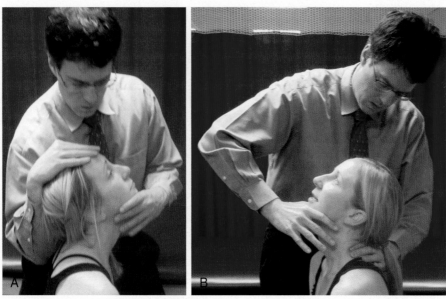

FIGURE 16-11 **A,** Overpressure bias applied to the upper cervical spine. **B,** Overpressure bias applied to the lower cervical spine.

The capsular pattern of the cervical spine is side flexion and rotation equally limited, slight limitation of extension, and full flexion.[11] A noncapsular pattern will have limitations in ROM, but these limitations do not resemble those in the capsular pattern. Noncapsular restriction may result from pain, adhesions, or internal derangement.[11] During assessment of passive ROM it is important to remember that greater ROM will occur if the passive movements are assessed while the athlete is supine as opposed to when the patient is seated. This is a result of the increased muscular tone present in the seated position to maintain an erect head.

The clinician may choose to hold a movement for a sustained period or to apply overpressure at the end range. The clinician may also opt to bias the amount of overpressure on the upper or lower cervical spine to evoke symptoms.[12] For example, overpressure into extension for the upper cervical spine (Fig. 16-11, *A*) can be performed by passively flexing the midcervical and cervicothoracic spine followed by extending the upper cervical segments. Extension overpressure on the lower cervical spine (see Fig. 16-11, *B*) can be induced by flexing the upper cervical spine and then introducing extension into the lower segments. The clinician must be careful to not generally overstress the system without an appropriate differential assessment, which may require radiologic testing.

Resisted Motion

During resisted motion testing, the athlete is asked to repeat the same movements as performed during the active and passive parts of the examination (flexion, extension, side bending, and rotation) and instructed to maintain a static, isometric position during the test. Each movement is tested in three positions of the patient's available ROM. The athlete is first tested with the cervical spine in a midrange position, then in the beginning of

the available ROM, and followed by the outer limits of the available ROM. Each movement is tested in similar fashion with the athlete's head placed in three different positions. By testing each motion in three positions, various amounts of joint compressive force and tensile force are generated in the contractile and noncontractile tissues.

The purpose of this part of the examination is not to determine muscular strength but to give the clinician insight on feedback of the affected tissues' response when tensile force and joint compression/decompression occur as a result of muscle activation. If, however, muscle weakness is noted, the clinician must determine whether it is a result of pain inhibition, injury to contractile tissues, or the presence of neurologic pathology. It may be necessary to perform more muscle-specific manual muscle testing to allow appropriate muscle differentiation.[13,14] In addition, a neurologic examination should be conducted to rule out any possible upper or lower motor neuron lesion.

Clinical Pearl #3

The clinician can determine whether the affected tissue is inert or contractile tissue after performing the active, passive, and resisted motions. If active and passive motions are painful in the same direction and no pain is reported with resistive isometric movements, an inert tissue is suspected.[11] If active and passive motions are painful in the opposite direction and pain occurs with resisted isometrics in the same direction as active motion, it is indicative of a contractile tissue lesion.[11]

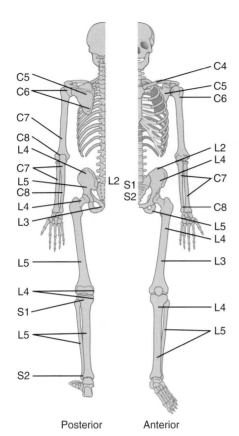

Posterior   Anterior

FIGURE 16-12 Skeletal representation of the sclerotomes of the body. *(From Magee, D.J. [1997]: Principles and concepts. In: Magee, D.J. (ed.), Orthopedic Physical Assessment, 3rd ed. Philadelphia, Saunders, p. 14.)*

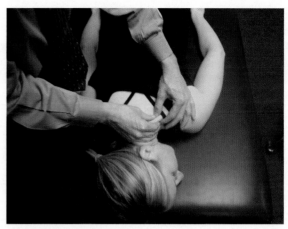

FIGURE 16-13 Skin-rolling technique used during evaluation of the mobility of the skin and underlying fascia.

Box 16-2
Commonly Palpated Structures During Assessment of the Cervical Spine

POSTERIORLY
External occipital protuberance
Superior nuchal line
Mastoid process
Ligamentum nuchae
Upper trapezius
Levator scapulae
Spinous processes
Transverse processes
Facet joints

ANTERIORLY
Sternum
Clavicle
Supraclavicular fossa
First rib
Sternocleidomastoid muscle
Scalene muscles
Hyoid bone
Thyroid cartilage
Thyroid gland
First cricoid ring
Lymph nodes
Carotid pulse
Temporomandibular joints
Mandible
Parotid gland

Palpation

Palpation allows the clinician to assess the status of the athlete's tissues. Although the clinician will make note of any tenderness occurring during palpation, because of the possibility of referred symptoms, the clinician must rely on manual skills while palpating the athlete. Irritation of a spinal nerve or a structure innervated by that spinal nerve can cause referred pain in a dermatomal, myotomal, or sclerotomal pattern (Fig. 16-12).[11] Therefore, to rely solely on patient feedback for identification of lesions can be misleading.

Palpation begins superficially on the skin and progresses to deeper underlying structures. The rehabilitation specialist can identify any variations in skin temperature that may be present in the cervical spine area by using the back of the hand. A histamine reaction can be observed and compared bilaterally by making a light scratch on the skin in the cervical spine area with the dorsum of the thumb. To assess the skin and subcutaneous tissues the clinician can roll the skin in multiple directions. Skin rolling is performed by grasping the dermis and superficial fascia between the fingers and thumb and then lifting and rolling the skin (Fig. 16-13). The clinician may notice restrictions or abnormalities in the consistency of the tissues that may indicate fibrosis.

During palpation, the clinician should make note of tenderness, altered muscular tone, crepitus, bony abnormalities or defects, or any other indication of pathologic conditions. Box 16-2 contains a list of commonly palpated anterior and posterior structures. Proper orientation to bony landmarks and surrounding soft tissue is imperative during the evaluation process.[15]

Neurologic Tests

A neurologic evaluation should be performed on every athlete to assess the status of the neurologic system and to verify that the athlete does not have a previously undetected neurologic dysfunction. The clinician examines the reflexes and the sensory and motor functions of the athlete to determine whether an upper or lower motor neuron lesion is present (Table 16-3). Because of the motor and sensory fibers remaining split in the foramina of the cervical spine, it is

Table 16-3 Comparison of an Upper and Lower Motor Neuron Lesion

Upper Motor Neuron Lesion	Lower Motor Neuron Lesion
Spasticity	Flaccidity
Hyperreflexia	Hyporeflexia
Hypertonicity	Hypotonicity
Muscle weakness distal to the lesion	Weakness of innervated muscles
Pathologic reflexes positive bilaterally	Pathologic reflexes absent

possible that an anterior pathology (disk, uncovertebral joint) will cause only motor changes whereas pathology in the facet can create sensory changes. The clinician should also determine the state or stage of the nerve injury: irritated, mixed, or compressed. When a nerve is in a state of compression, the motor and sensory levels will be in a compressed state. A nerve that is in a mixed state will create the potential for some tests to show that the nerve is compressed, some normal, and some demonstrating signs of nerve irritation. This stage of nerve root pathology is a transition between the irritated and compressed state. A nerve that is irritated will display increased excitability with an increase in sensation and deep tendon reflexes, complaints of pain will be most severe, and muscle spasms will be noted in the muscles innervated by the spinal nerve.

To prevent any visual cues during testing of sensation, the athlete's eyes should be closed as the clinician lightly runs the hands in a dermatomal pattern on the patient. The clinician notes any areas of hyposensitivity or hypersensitivity. Although only light touch sensation is frequently performed, other sensory components should also be assessed, such as sharp touch, temperature, vibration, and two-point discrimination. This is important because there are different tracts or pathways for sensory input. Consequently, it is possible to have loss in one or more sensory components without affecting the others, and to limit testing to just one area of sensation could produce a false-negative result. The rehabilitation specialist then determines whether the altered sensation is in a dermatomal pattern (Fig. 16-14) or follows the distribution of a peripheral nerve (Fig. 16-15).

The deep tendon reflexes of the biceps (C5-C6), brachioradialis (C5-C6), triceps (C7-C8), and abductor digiti minimi (C8-T1) are tested and graded bilaterally. If the clinician is having difficulty obtaining a reflexive response, the athlete can be instructed to perform a Jendrassik maneuver[16] by pressing the legs together, thereby facilitating the nervous system. The deep tendon reflexes of the athlete are compared bilaterally to determine whether any hyporeflexive or hyperreflexive responses are present.

Because reflexes can vary from person to person, the clinician should not be alarmed if the athlete has a weakened or heightened reflexive response bilaterally, although an altered unilateral response should be noted. A hyporeflexive response indicates a lower motor neuron lesion, whereas a hyperreflexive response is indicative of an upper motor neuron lesion.

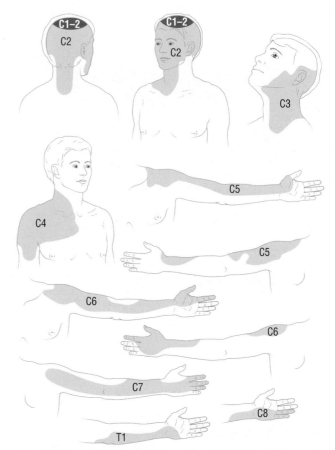

FIGURE 16-14 Dermatomal pattern of the upper extremity. *(From Magee, D.J. [1997]: Principles and concepts. In Magee, D.J. (ed.): Orthopedic Physical Assessment, 3rd ed. Philadelphia, Saunders, p. 135.)*

If signs of an upper motor neuron lesion are present, pathologic reflex testing is indicated. The Babinski sign (see online appendix Fig. A16-1 on Expert Consult @ www.expertconsult.com) for the lower extremity and the Hoffmann sign (see online appendix Fig. A16-2 on Expert Consult @ www.expertconsult.com) for the upper extremity are two examples of pathologic reflex tests that are commonly used. The pathologic reflexes should be examined bilaterally to note a difference on either side.

The rehabilitation specialist also assesses the motor responses of the cervical myotomes (Table 16-4) to determine whether neurologic weakness is present. The athlete is instructed to maintain an isometric contraction while the joint being tested is held in a neutral position. Because most muscles receive innervation from more than one neurologic level, a lesion involving a single nerve root may not result in complete paralysis of a muscle. It can result in only mild muscle weakness in the early stages of injury, which can make it difficult for the clinician to detect a difference. The clinician should therefore require the athlete to maintain an isometric contraction for a minimum of 5 seconds to allow any subtle weakness to be manifested.

Although the pathologic cause of the patient's symptoms may not yet be determined, the clinician will at this point be able to conclude whether the neurologic tests are indicating an upper or lower motor neuron lesion, as well as the state of nerve root pathology. Table 16-5 provides the clinical findings to help differentiate a nerve root lesion from a peripheral nerve injury.

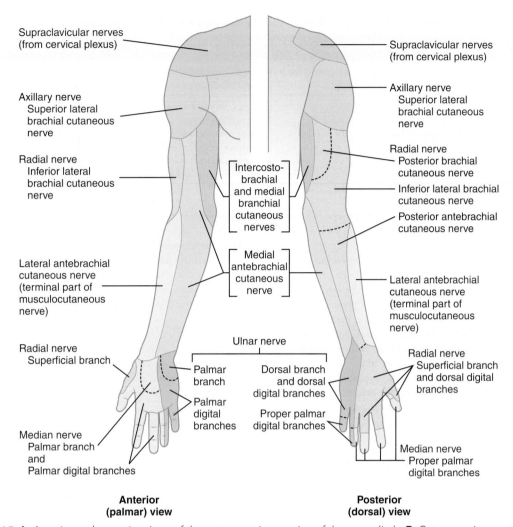

FIGURE 16-15 A, Anterior and posterior views of the cutaneous innervation of the upper limb. **B,** Cutaneous innervation of the face, head, and neck.

Table 16-4 Cervical Myotomes

Action	Nerve Root	Muscles
Chin tuck	C1-C2	Rectus capitis anterior Rectus capitis lateralis
Head side flexion	C3	Longus capitis Longus cervicis Scalene
Shoulder elevation	C4	Trapezius Levator scapulae
Shoulder abduction	C5	Deltoid
Elbow flexion Wrist extension	C6	Biceps Extensor carpi radialis brevis Extensor carpi radialis longus
Elbow extension Wrist flexion	C7	Triceps Flexor carpi radialis Flexor digitorum superficialis
Thumb extension	C8	Extensor pollicis longus Extensor pollicis brevis
Finger abduction/ adduction	T1	Intrinsic muscles of the hand

SPECIAL TESTS

A variety of special tests can assist the clinician in determining the status of the osseous, neurovascular, and ligamentous structures. Although many tests are available for evaluating the cervical spine, the rehabilitation specialist must use clinical judgment to determine which tests are clinically relevant in accordance with the athlete's subjective history and objective findings. The rehabilitation specialist should also use the subjective history and objective information for determining whether to perform a test in a unilateral or bilateral manner. This will ensure a more efficient and streamlined evaluation for the clinician. The special tests include vascular, neurologic, and instability tests (for descriptions, see online Figs. A16-3 through A16-16 [in Appendix 16] on Expert Consult @ www.expertconsult.com).

THORACIC OUTLET SYNDROME

In thoracic outlet syndrome, the brachial plexus or the subclavian artery or vein in the neck or upper extremity is compromised by surrounding anatomic structures. In 95% of all cases the brachial plexus is involved, the arterial system is involved in 5%, and the venous system is involved in 2%.[17,18] Although the condition most often affects middle-aged women with respiratory dysfunction and a forward head posture, the condition should not be

Table 16-5 **Differential Diagnosis Between a C6 Nerve Root Lesion and a Radial Nerve Lesion**

Lesion	Altered Sensation	Muscle Deficits	Abnormal Reflexes
C6 nerve root	Lateral arm and forearm, radial side of the wrist, thumb, and index finger	Biceps, brachioradialis, supinator, extensor carpi radialis longus	Biceps Brachioradialis
Radial nerves C5-C8, T1	Posterior lateral aspect of the arm; posterior forearm; hand into the thumb, index, middle, and radial side of the ring fingers, excluding the fingertips	Triceps, anconeus, brachioradialis, extensor carpi radialis longus, supinator, extensor carpi radialis brevis, extensor carpi ulnaris, extensor digitorum, extensor digiti minimi, extensor indicis, abductor pollicis longus, extensor pollicis brevis	None

dismissed in individuals not meeting this stereotype. Thoracic outlet syndrome can result from congenital anomalies, postural faults, or environmental or traumatic stress.

An athlete will have different symptoms depending on the structures that are being compressed. Athletes with irritation of the nerves will describe pain radiating down the arm in a segmental distribution and hypersensitivity or hyposensitivity in these regions. Patients with obstruction of the vascular system will describe ischemic pain in the entire hand. Common patient complaints include pain, weakness of grip, and numbness and tingling that are frequently present in the ulnar nerve distribution. Athletes may also report vascular symptoms, including changes in the temperature of the upper extremity and hand, feelings of heaviness, swelling, and quick fatigue that is relieved with rest.

The neurologic and vascular structures of the upper extremity pass through four possible anatomic spaces that serve as potential pathologic sites for thoracic outlet syndrome: the sternocostovertebral space, the scalene triangle, the costoclavicular space, and the pectoralis minor space.

Sternocostovertebral Space

The sternocostovertebral space is formed by the sternum anteriorly, the spine posteriorly, and the first rib laterally. The subclavian artery and vein and the brachial plexus travel through this space. Though unusual, compression can occur in this region from a tumor of the thyroid, lymph nodes, or a Pancoast tumor of the lung.

Scalene Triangle

The scalene triangle is formed by the anterior scalene anteriorly, the middle scalene posteriorly, and the first rib inferiorly. Muscle tightness is commonly found in the scalenes in patients exhibiting a forward head postural dysfunction. Athletes with respiratory problems may recruit the scalenes to assist in inspiration. Conditions that cause muscle tightness or hyperactivity of the scalene muscles can produce neurovascular compression between the anterior and middle scalene muscles or can elevate the first rib, which causes a reduction in the dimensions of the scalene triangle.

Costoclavicular Space

The costoclavicular space is formed by the medial third of the clavicle anteriorly, the first rib posteriorly, and the scapula posterolaterally. Costoclavicular syndrome occurs as a result of depression of the shoulder girdle and fixation of the clavicle onto the first rib.[19,20] When the shoulder is in a depressed and retracted position, the clavicle is approximated on the neurovascular structures as traction is placed on these structures. The first rib may become elevated in someone with an abnormal breathing pattern that originates from the accessory respiratory muscles (scalenes) or because of tightness in this muscle group. Elevation of the first rib can create a reduced volume in this space and compress the neurovascular structures.

Pectoralis Minor Space

The pectoralis minor space is formed by the pectoralis minor tendon anteriorly and the ribs posteriorly. Compression can occur in this region when the arm is placed in an abducted position, which causes the neurovascular structures to curve around the coracoid process and become compressed as the pectoralis minor and subclavius muscles are stretched. Hyperactivity of the pectoralis minor muscle can also cause compression in this region and can be seen with conditions that cause the muscle to be used as an accessory muscle for respiration. Other conditions that can create compression of neurovascular structures in this region include postural kyphosis or trauma to the pectoralis minor or upper rib.

Thoracic Outlet Testing

Several special tests can be performed to aid in determining the presence of thoracic outlet syndrome. For descriptions of these tests, see Figures A16-12 through A16-17 (in Appendix 16) on Expert Consult @ www.expertconsult.com.

MOBILITY TESTING

The rehabilitation specialist can apply passive joint movements to the cervical vertebrae to assess intervertebral mobility and determine the presence of hypomobility or hypermobility. Because normal joint mobility is relative from person to person, it is important for the clinician to examine the surrounding joints for comparison. In addition, it is possible for a joint to be hypomobile with certain movements and have normal mobility or be hypermobile during other movements. Because an athlete may have sufficient neuromuscular control of a joint's translational movements, it is important to remember that the presence of hypomobility or hypermobility is not necessarily indicative of a pathologic condition.

The clinician may inspect the mobility of the entire cervical spine or a particular joint or region. Passive intervertebral movement is assessed with the same movements used during the active and passive ROM parts of the examination—that is, flexion, extension, rotation, and lateral flexion.

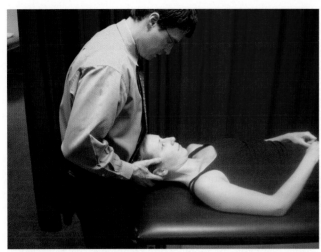

FIGURE 16-16 Testing flexion mobility of the occiput on the atlas. The clinician detects for the amount of motion occurring as the head is flexed.

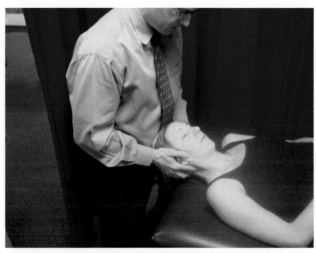

FIGURE 16-17 Right lateral flexion mobility testing of C4-C5. The athlete's head is flexed laterally while the clinician palpates C4 translating posteriorly and inferiorly onto C5 on the right side.

The upper cervical spine can be assessed with the athlete in the seated or supine position. To test flexion of the occiput on C1 (Fig. 16-16), the clinician holds the athlete's head in a neutral position and places the index fingers on the lateral aspect of the patient's neck between the transverse processes of the atlas and the mastoid processes of the occiput.[9] The clinician introduces flexion into the upper cervical spine by passively nodding the athlete's head and then detects the motion occurring as a separation between the mastoid and transverse processes of the atlas. The clinician can assess extension, lateral flexion, and rotation of the occiput and atlas in a similar manner performed during flexion.

Rotation of the atlas on the axis is examined with the athlete in a seated position. The clinician's right hand is positioned on top of the athlete's head and the left hand is placed in the midline of the spine with the index finger over the spinous process of the axis. The clinician rotates the head to the right while palpating to detect the C2 spinous process rotating to the left. The axis will begin to rotate to the left as the C1-C2 joint is taken to end range, which occurs at approximately 40°. A comparison is made between right and left rotation to assess for possible hypomobility or hypermobility. The sports rehabilitation specialist may also inspect lateral flexion of C1-C2 in a similar fashion to determine the motion available during this movement.

The clinician can assess flexion, extension, and rotational mobility of the midcervical spine with the athlete supine. To examine passive intervertebral right lateral flexion of C4-C5, the clinician places fingers over these facet joints while supporting the patient's head (Fig. 16-17). The clinician laterally flexes the cervical spine while palpating the right inferior facet of C4 as it translates inferiorly and posteriorly onto the C5 right superior facet. This is repeated on the other side for bilateral comparison. This process can be repeated in the remaining vertebral segments in this region.

The lower cervical and upper thoracic spine (which is frequently included in the cervical evaluation) can be tested in a seated position. The clinician can assess flexion, extension, lateral flexion, and rotation to determine passive intervertebral mobility.

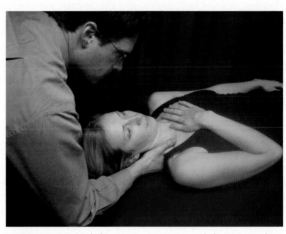

FIGURE 16-18 Mobility testing or joint mobilization technique for the first rib. The clinician uses the web space between the thumb and index finger and directs a force in an anterior and caudal direction.

Mobility of the first rib is often included in assessment of the cervical spine. The first rib serves as an attachment site for the anterior and middle scalenes. Tightness or neurologic facilitation of this musculature or other conditions could cause decreased mobility in this region. The athlete is examined in a supine position as the clinician uses the web space between the thumb and index finger to apply a force directed in an anterior and caudal direction to the first rib (Fig. 16-18). The clinician compares the available motion and end-feel of the first rib bilaterally.

DIAGNOSTIC TESTS

After clinical examination of the athlete, the clinician should review any diagnostic testing that the athlete has undergone to verify the clinical findings obtained from the evaluation. Plain film radiographs are commonly taken for musculoskeletal injuries. These films allow determination of possible vertebral fractures, dislocations, developmental vertebral abnormalities, metabolic bone diseases, and tumors. Anteroposterior, lateral, and oblique views are routinely obtained to allow complete examination of the entire cervical spine.

In addition, the athlete may have had further studies performed, such as magnetic resonance imaging, computed tomography, or myelography. If a nerve injury is suspected, electromyographic studies can be used to determine the grade of nerve injury present. Laboratory tests can assist in determining whether an infection or disease is present, such as osteoporosis, osteomalacia, rheumatoid arthritis, hyperthyroidism, and hypothyroidism.

REHABILITATION TECHNIQUES FOR THE CERVICAL SPINE

After completing a thorough evaluation, the sports rehabilitation specialist should be able to determine the pathologic tissue or tissues that are contributing to the athlete's condition. The athlete can have a wide variety of symptoms and limitations that will determine and dictate the intensity and direction of treatment. The athlete's injury can be treated with various modalities, manual techniques, and therapeutic exercise programs. It is important that the rehabilitation program chosen address the athlete's individual injuries and deficiencies. This allows a therapeutic program that is both patient and tissue specific. It is also important that the sports rehabilitation specialist continuously monitor the athlete's current conditions and symptoms to ensure an optimal therapeutic program at all times and allow adjustments as needed and dictated by the athlete's condition.

Numerous rehabilitation techniques, treatment strategies, and exercises have been described. Much has been written and studies have been performed to determine the best forms of treatment. The most effective treatment in patients with cervical pathology is a combination of manual therapy and exercise.[21,22] This form of treatment has been shown to be highly effective in patients with whiplash-associated disorders and acute and chronic mechanical neck pain with or without headaches.[23] Although the basic principles of exercise (histology, neurophysiology, and tissue healing) are the same as for other body segments, the sympathetic nervous system, vestibular system, ocular reflexes, and potential side effects of cervical instabilities warrant specialized treatment of the cervical spine.[23] Injuries involving the cervical spine can cause reorganization of normal muscle activation to possibly minimize the activity of painful muscles on the cervical spine and shoulder. The decrease in muscle recruitment, whether from pain inhibition or the reduced gamma motor loop,[24] and altered sensory input from the muscular and articular tissue can contribute to the diminished proprioceptive deficits that occur after injury. Because loss of proprioception can cause difficulty in proper head positioning for activities of daily living, the rehabilitation program should consist of coordination activities, proprioceptive drills, and postural training.[23]

Loss of coordinated movement and muscle firing patterns is common after injury, and the clinician should therefore design a program that targets the appropriate muscles and movement patterns to effectively train the motor patterns. In general, coordination training involves high repetitions per set; however, because of the complex interactions of the cervical afferent and vestibular and ocular systems, as well as the vascular supply to the brain, the initial rehabilitation exercises are limited to 10 repetitions.[23] After the initial few visits, if the athlete shows no

adverse signs or symptoms, repetition volume can be increased. Mechanoreceptors that give proprioceptive input can be found in the joint capsules of the cervical spine and the muscle spindles, and they can become damaged following injury or immobilization. Proprioceptive loss can affect cervicocephalic kinesthesia, which is the ability to accurately reposition the head on the trunk, and can cause significant motor incoordination because of the diminished dorsal root activity. Therefore, proprioceptive training should also be included in the rehabilitation program of the athlete.

The clinician should base the rehabilitation program on the goal of treatment, the tissues involved, and the current status of the tissue or tissues. Exercise prescription will vary in speed, range, use of concentric/eccentric activity, and repetition, depending on whether the treatment goal is to improve mobility, vascularity, or muscle fiber atrophy; repair tissue; or reduce edema. Similarly, the mobilization techniques can be varied to modify the intent of treatment, such as to neuromodulate pain, decrease muscle tone, impede synovial fluid, and improve joint mobility.

Modalities

During the acute phase of treatment, therapeutic modalities are commonly used to reduce pain and muscle tone and spasticity, decrease stiffness, increase blood flow and the metabolic rate, and reduce edema. The modality chosen should be determined by the target tissue and the desired therapeutic benefit. It is also important that the modality chosen not be contraindicated by the athlete's current condition (e.g., application of ultrasound to a hypermobile joint).

Soft Tissue Mobilization

After a sports-induced cervical injury it is common for musculoskeletal dysfunction to develop in an athlete. Sports rehabilitation specialists commonly perform various soft tissue mobilization techniques to decrease muscle soreness, stiffness, spasm, hypertonicity, and edema; improve joint lubrication; and prepare the tissues for therapeutic activities. The clinician should also be aware of conditions that may be a contraindication to soft tissue mobilization at that time, such as infections or a fracture.

Before implementing a soft tissue mobilization program, the clinician must decide on the desired treatment goals and outcomes to determine which specific technique to use. Dysfunctions of the neuromusculoskeletal system often require an approach that involves multiple techniques. Effleurage and kneading techniques are useful in increasing circulation and neuromodulating pain. Decreased mobility is often found in the muscle, fascia, and skin surrounding postural muscles after trauma and chronically habitual postures. After evaluation the clinician should have a good understanding of the state of the soft tissues, the target tissue, and the aim of treatment when initiating soft tissue mobilization techniques. The direction, depth of force, and technique used will dictate which tissue will be affected. Myofascial mobilization techniques can be used to restore decreased mobility and reduce the associated pain. Soft tissue techniques can be performed with and without the addition of joint motion; the addition of joint motion will allow additional tension to be applied to the soft tissues, as well as promote mechanoreceptor input to the joint and permit absorption of synovial fluid.

In addition, muscle pump techniques performed either actively or passively can be used to help increase local circulation (Fig. 16-19). These techniques are used to increase local circulation. During the contraction phase of soft tissue mobilization, arteriovenous flow is decreased, whereas during the relaxation phase of treatment, the gradient is reduced and fluid exchange improves.

Flexibility Exercises

Stretching exercises can be performed for the treatment of muscle spasms, hypertonicity, and adaptive shortening. Before beginning a stretching program it is important for the rehabilitation specialist to determine whether the muscle tightness or increased tone is being caused by cervical hypermobility or a facilitated segment (reactive innervated level) that is producing a protective muscle splint. Although a light stretching program to relax the muscles can be implemented, a therapeutic program aimed at addressing the causative factor is needed to provide long-term relief of symptoms. Pain and muscle guarding are common during both the acute and chronic stages of injury. The decreased muscular mobility is typically related to the increased tone and decreased extensibility of collagen. Therefore, in athletes with increased neurologic tone and guarding, dynamic movements can be used to increase circulation and remove the metabolic waste products that create secondary pain and facilitate tonic reflexogenic activity in the muscle. This repetitive activity will also improve tensile properties and elasticity in the collagenous tissues.[23]

The clinician can use various flexibility exercise programs. A vapor coolant spray, such as Fluori-Methane (Gebauer Chemical Co., Cleveland, OH), can be used to stimulate the sensory receptors of the skin and allow an increase in passive stretching without causing pain. The spray-and-stretch technique is performed with the patient sitting upright and the head supported to allow relaxation of the cervical musculature. The Fluori-Methane bottle is held approximately 18 inches away and at an angle from the targeted muscle, and the spray is applied in a unidirectional motion parallel to the muscle fibers. The clinician simultaneously stretches the muscle while the Fluori-Methane spray is being applied. Work by Travell and Simons[25] describes patient positioning and the direction of stretching and vapor coolant spraying. (See Chapters 6 and 8 for additional information regarding the spray-and-stretch technique.)

Contract-relax or contract-relax contract-antagonist techniques can also be used to stretch tight musculature. A contract-relax stretch is performed by taking the muscle to a position of mild stretch and instructing the patient to match the resistance applied by the therapist by mildly contracting the target muscle. This contraction is maintained for 3 to 5 seconds, followed by the clinician applying a further stretch for 5 to 10 seconds as the patient exhales and relaxes. This process is repeated throughout a full ROM. The contract-relax contract-antagonist stretch is performed in a similar manner, except that after contraction of the agonist muscle, contraction of the antagonist muscle provides a reciprocal inhibition as a stretch is applied (see Chapter 6).

Joint Mobilization

Joint mobilization techniques can be performed not only to restore motion but also to provide a neurophysiologic effect that reduces pain and muscle spasms. The sports rehabilitation specialist must evaluate intervertebral mobility and the possible presence of pain originating from a cervical segment or surrounding tissue to determine whether the application of joint mobilizations is justified. It is important for the clinician to understand the role and application of joint mobilization techniques to allow optimal use in a rehabilitation setting. When performing a joint mobilization technique, the practitioner should maintain close approximation to the joint being mobilized and also use the legs and body to transfer weight and provide the force needed for the mobilization. This technique allows the clinician to produce the needed movement while generating a minimal amount of force and allowing greater palpatory sense. A few examples of mobilization techniques are described in Figures 16-20 through 16-25. The cervical

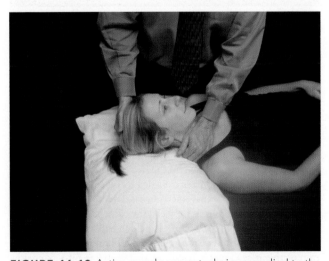

FIGURE 16-19 Active muscle pump technique applied to the sternocleidomastoid to increase local circulation. The clinician side-bends the head to place slight tension on the muscle, and the athlete is instructed to slightly contract the muscle while minimum resistance is applied to the movement and manual compression is placed on the muscle. As tension develops in the involved muscle, the compression force is removed to allow reflux of fluid. This movement will be repeated throughout a pain-free range of motion.

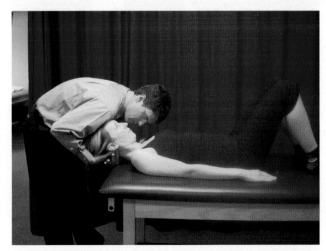

FIGURE 16-20 The clinician performs a flexion mobilization of the occiput on the atlas by stabilizing the atlas as the head is moved into a flexed position.

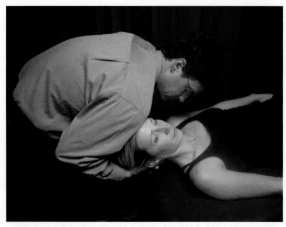

FIGURE 16-21 Mobilizing the atlas on the axis into left rotation. The left transverse process of the axis is stabilized as the clinician rotates the athlete's head into left rotation.

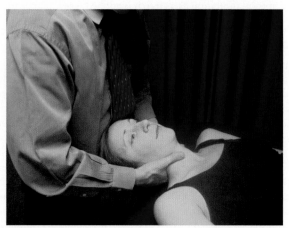

FIGURE 16-22 Left lateral flexion mobilization of C4-C5. The left transverse process of C5 is stabilized while mobilizing C4 into a left side-bending position.

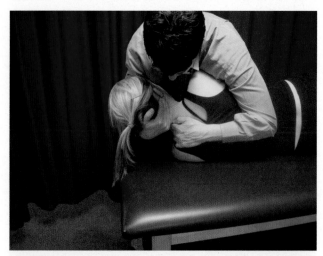

FIGURE 16-23 Side-lying extension mobilization of C5-C6. The clinician stabilizes the C6 spinous process while imposing extension mobilization onto C5-C6 parallel to the articular surfaces.

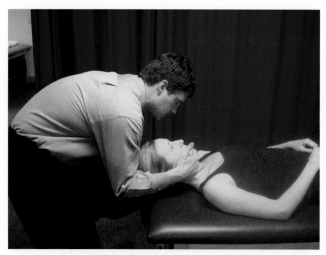

FIGURE 16-24 Manual cervical traction.

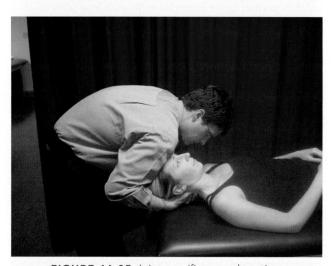

FIGURE 16-25 Joint-specific manual traction.

spine can be mobilized with motions other than those described earlier by applying arthrokinematic principles to the cervical joints. Other techniques can also be used, depending on the joint mobilization school of thought adhered to by the rehabilitation specialist.

Joint mobilization techniques for the upper cervical spine can be applied with the athlete in a supine or seated position. Flexion mobilization of the occiput on the atlas is performed with the athlete in a supine position and the head placed in a neutral position. The clinician stabilizes the atlas by placing the thumb and index finger on its transverse processes (see Fig. 16-20). The athlete's head is supported between the clinician's opposing forearm and shoulder as the occiput is held in the hand. The occiput is moved into a flexed position while maintaining a fixated position of the atlas. The clinician can also mobilize into extension, side bending, and rotation, as needed, by using the same hand placements and altering the direction of mobilization.[9]

Mobilization of the atlas on the axis into left rotation in a supine position is illustrated in Figure 16-21. The athlete is supine with the head held in a neutral position. The left hand of the rehabilitation specialist is used to stabilize the axis by placing the thumb over the right transverse process. As the athlete's head is held between the clinician's right hand and chest, the body of the clinician is rotated to the left. Because of the motion of the axis being restricted, this rotation will cause mobilization between the atlas and the axis. The rehabilitation specialist can mobilize C2-C3 with the same technique.[9]

Mobilization of the midcervical vertebrae is more efficiently performed with the patient in the supine position because of the otherwise longer arm movement that occurs when the clinician generates motion through the occiput with the athlete in a seated position. Mobilization of C4-C5 into a left side-bending position is illustrated in Figure 16-22. The clinician supports the athlete's head in a neutral position, identifies the superior articular process of C5, and uses the left index finger to fixate the transverse process of C5 while the right index finger is placed on inferior articular process of C4. The clinician stabilizes C5 as C4 is bent to the left side by using the right hand and forearm to induce motion of the head and upper segments of the cervical spine. The rehabilitation specialist can mobilize the midcervical spine into flexion, extension, and rotation by applying the same principles of stabilizing the inferior spinal segment and mobilizing the superior spinal segment.

An extension mobilization of C5-C6 can be performed with the athlete in a side-lying position (see Fig. 16-23). The athlete's head is supported and cradled between the clinician's hand and the anterior aspect of the arm as the clinician grasps the spinous and transverse processes with the web space of the left hand. The clinician positions the web space of the right hand to stabilize the spinous and transverse processes of C4. By shifting body weight, the rehabilitation specialist introduces motion.[9]

Cervical traction is often performed as a generalized technique when initiating joint mobilizations. The athlete is placed in a supine position and the clinician supports the athlete's head with one hand cupping the occiput. The other hand is placed under the athlete's chin to provide positioning so that no force is translated to the chin (see Fig. 16-24). By shifting body weight back the clinician introduces a traction force. This technique can also be modified to allow the traction force to be specific to an intervertebral joint. The clinician performs joint-specific traction mobilization by stabilizing the spinous process of the inferior vertebrae with one hand as motion is introduced to that intervertebral level by the other hand applying a distractive force to the superior vertebrae (see Fig. 16-25). During both traction techniques, the clinician should mobilize the cervical spine in a superior and anterior direction to allow motion to occur along the longitudinal axes.[9]

Cervical Manipulation

The clinician may include manipulation as part of the rehabilitation program as determined during the evaluation process. Manipulations can potentially be of benefit by relieving symptoms, releasing adhesions, restoring joint mobility, reducing positional faults, normalizing muscle tension, promoting neurologic and sympathetic function, and improving posture. The clinician should also determine whether any contraindications are present, and specific segmental mobility testing should be performed before any high-velocity thrust is applied. Cervical manipulations can be performed for the upper, mid, and lower cervical spine in a weight-bearing (seated) or non–weight-bearing (lying) position. Figure 16-26 demonstrates traction manipulation of

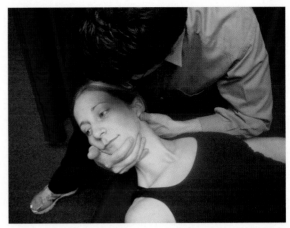

FIGURE16-26 Occipitoaxial traction manipulation on the left side. The clinician side-bends the cervical spine to the left and rotates it to right below C2 to lock the inferior segments. The occiput is extended to decrease tension on the alar ligament. The clinician then imparts a distraction manipulation.

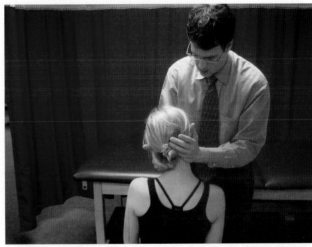

FIGURE 16-27 The clinician conforms the right hand around the left side of the athlete's spine at the facet joints of C3. The left hand is supporting the right side of the head and neck. The cervical spine is flexed and side-bent to C2 while C3 and C4 are maintained in a neutral position. The clinician performs a high-speed thrust with the right hand.

the left occipitoaxial joint. This technique is performed with left side bending and right rotation to lock the mid and upper cervical spine. A manipulation thrust of the occipitoaxial joint is performed in the direction of the long axis of the cervical spine with the left hand. A midcervical manipulation ("Mitnehmer Griff") can be performed by placing the right hand around the patient's cervical spine with the fingers along the facet joints of C3 and the left hand on the side of the patient's head to offer support. The cervical spine is flexed and bent to side of the affected joint to lock the superior joints. A manipulative thrust is applied to the C3-C4 joint (see Fig. 16-27). Manipulation of the lower cervical spine can be performed by fixating the indicated spinous process as the cervical spine is flexed, side-bent, and rotated toward the affected joint. A unilateral distraction manipulation is then performed as illustrated in Figure 16-28.

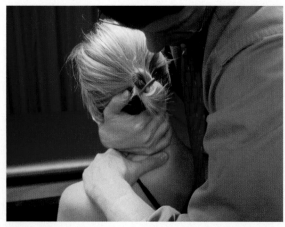

FIGURE 16-28 Right C6-C7 manipulation. The sports rehabilitation specialist places the right hand around the athlete's head and grasps C6 as the left hand stabilizes the spinous process of C7. The cervical spine is then flexed, side-bent, and rotated down to C6. The clinician then performs a rotation manipulation of C6-C7.

Fundamental Exercises

Clinical Pearl #4

To provide the optimal stimulus for tissue repair, regeneration, and growth, the clinician should include adequate stress and force (resistance) in the athlete's rehabilitation program while avoiding stress that can create deleterious effects in pathologic tissue. The tissues must be able to tolerate functional loads to adequately prepare an athlete for return to sports.

"Challenge the tissue."

—Rob Tillman, PT, MOMT.

Pathologic conditions can be extremely variable in symptoms and can affect the athlete's ability to voluntarily move and control movement in the cervical spine. Therefore, the rehabilitation specialist's therapeutic exercise program must be sufficiently specific to address the athlete's symptoms and causative pathology. Cervical isometrics or isotonics can be performed in a ROM near midline to promote stabilization. The clinician can address postural concerns by having the patient perform exercises at high repetitions while in a corrected posture. The athlete's neuromuscular system can be challenged by adding a proprioceptive component to the rehabilitation. If the athlete reports pain and is unable to perform exercises in a seated (weight-bearing) position, the athlete is assessed for the ability to begin exercises in a non–weight-bearing (supine) position. The clinician therefore can not only alter the rehabilitation program just by changing the exercises that the athlete performs, but also by adjusting the athlete's position, repetition, level of proprioceptive difficulty, and ROM of the exercises. This allows a program to be prescribed that addresses the athlete's individual needs.

If the athlete has pain originating from a weight-bearing structure (facet joints, disk), exercises may not be able to be performed in an upright posture during the early phases of rehabilitation because of an increase in pain. Accordingly, it may be

necessary to have the athlete perform ROM activities while in a supine, non–weight-bearing position. The athlete is encouraged to perform active movements within a pain-free ROM while in a gravity-eliminated (supine or semisupine) position (Fig. 16-29, A and B). The athlete may also be able to tolerate external resistance such as with a Thera-Band (Akron, OH), pulley system, or manual resistance sooner than in an upright position (Fig. 16-30). This allows earlier initiation of exercises to avoid the deleterious effects associated with immobilization.

Cervical isometric exercises in which the athlete exercises against self-administered manual resistance are commonly performed to allow early initiation of the rehabilitation program. As the athlete's condition improves, the sports rehabilitation specialist can further challenge the athlete's ability to stabilize and control the cervical spine by adding external resistance to the exercise. This can be achieved with a pulley system or Thera-Band. The plane of resistance (angle of the pulley), as well as the anterior or posterior attachment of the pulley resistance, can be altered to allow targeting of different muscle groups. These slight alterations will allow the clinician to emphasize or train specific muscle groups with the exercise. A posterior attachment will create less torque because it is closer to the joint axis, whereas an anterior attachment will have an increased torque moment, so depending on the athlete's symptoms and stage of recovery, the clinician can alter this attachment. The athlete can perform cervical rotation exercises with the posterior attachment of the pulley set below the horizontal to facilitate a slight extension moment to assist the deep cervical flexors in achieving stabilization; if the anterior attachment of the pulley is set below the horizontal, a slight flexion moment will be produced that will require the athlete to stabilize or counter this moment with resistance from the cervical extensors (Figs. 16-31 and 16-32). The athlete may also be instructed to perform upper extremity resistance exercises while maintaining a static, isometric position of the cervical spine (Fig. 16-33, A to C).

Postural faults that may cause or contribute to the pathologic condition of the athlete must be addressed. A typical posture identified is a forward-head, rounded-shoulder posture. This posture can elevate the inferior angle of the scapula and depress the acromion as the scapula fulcrums at its ventral midpoint on the resultant increased thoracic kyphosis.[26] This can result in adaptive shortening of the pectoralis minor and stretch the lower trapezius. This excessive stretching is referred to as stretch weakness because of the resultant weakness that occurs after prolonged elongation.[14] The athlete can perform self-mobilization exercises to correct the increased thoracic kyphosis, flexibility exercises for the anterior musculature, and strengthening exercises for the posterior musculature. Extension mobilization exercises as illustrated in Figure 16-34 can be performed by the patient to assist in restoring normal thoracic and cervicothoracic mobility. To increase the mobilization moment, the athlete can be instructed to perform the exercise with the elbows extended or with either pulleys or dumbbells to provide a further increase in extensor moment. Seated rows can be performed to target the scapula retractors and the thoracic and cervical extensors. The athlete is instructed to retract the scapula as the thoracic spine is extended and the cervical spine retracted. The clinician may provide tactile cueing so that the athlete can maintain proper form during the exercise. In similar fashion, the athlete can perform prone dumbbell flies. A hinged bench can be used to allow the athlete to simultaneously extend the thoracic spine

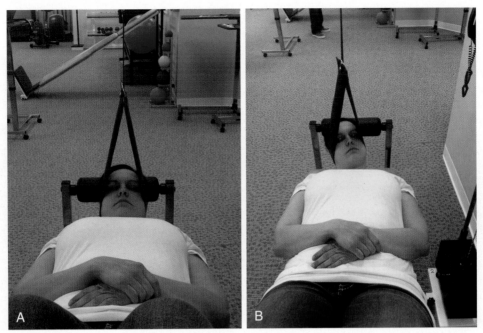

FIGURE 16-29 Cervical lateral flexion performed in a pulley sling to allow movement without resistance within a pain-free range of motion. This resistance-free motion allows an athlete who is unable to perform weight-bearing exercises because of pain the ability to initiate therapeutic activities at high repetitions to facilitate coordination, reduce pain, and normalize local vascularity to expedite the healing process. **A,** Starting position. **B,** Ending position.

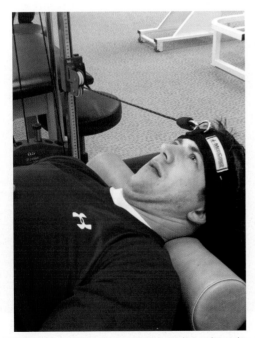

FIGURE 16-30 Supine isotonic resistance with combined isometric stabilization. The athlete is placed in the supine position with a bolster under the neck to support normal cervical lordosis; depending on the aim of treatment, the isometric/isotonic component of the exercise can be switched. The athlete can be instructed to perform a chin tuck while maintaining isometric cervical rotation against the pulley, or the athlete can maintain an isometric chin tuck while performing active cervical rotation.

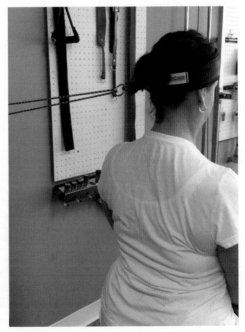

FIGURE 16-31 Cervical rotation performed with a posterior resistance attachment on the pulley. The posterior attachment provides less torque than an anterior attachment because of its close approximation to the cervical axis of rotation. The resistive moment can be adjusted to impart a secondary force moment. The clinician can place the resistance below the axis of rotation to create an extension moment that will assist the deep cervical flexors in countering this movement.

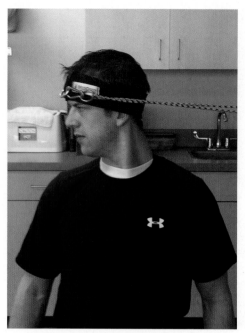

FIGURE 16-32 Cervical rotation performed with an anterior resistance attachment on the pulley. An anterior attachment allows greater torque production than a posterior attachment does. The angle of resistance can be adjusted to provide a secondary resistance moment, with resistance above the horizontal imparting a secondary extensor moment that will require increased cervical flexor stabilization; resistance below the horizontal produces a secondary flexor moment that will result in facilitation of the cervical extensors.

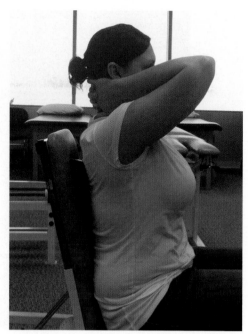

FIGURE 16-34 Cervicothoracic self-mobilization extension performed over a mobilization wedge. The clinician places the wedge inferior to the segment to be mobilized to provide stabilization. The athlete is instructed to support the cervical spine with both hands behind the neck while performing an extension moment of the upper part of the trunk and maintaining a gentle chin tuck.

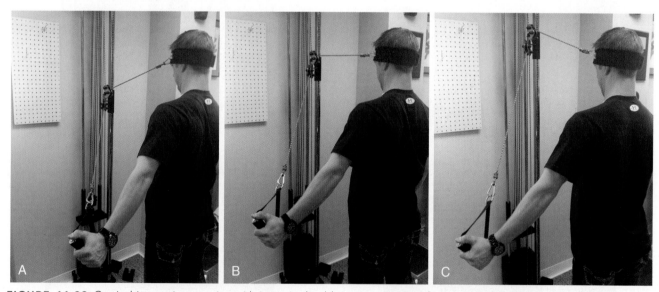

FIGURE 16-33 Cervical isometric extension with isotonic shoulder extension. **A,** Inferior isometric resistance increases the upper cervical extension moment. **B,** Horizontal isometric resistance requires upper and lower cervical extensor stability. **C,** Superior isometric resistance creates a smaller upper cervical extension moment, thus requiring greater lower cervical stabilization.

and retract the cervical spine and scapula. The athlete can perform wall-bar push-ups in a dynamic movement to elongate the pectoralis musculature (Fig. 16-35). Having the athlete perform low-resistance, repetitive exercises will improve local circulation, reduce tone, and improve tissue elasticity.

A proprioceptive component can be added to the exercise regimen. This is achieved by having the athlete lie, sit, or stand on an unstable surface. The athlete performs stabilization, postural reeducation, and strengthening exercises in a fashion similar to those performed with a stable base of support.

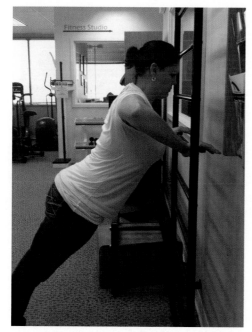

FIGURE 16-35 Wall-bar push-up.

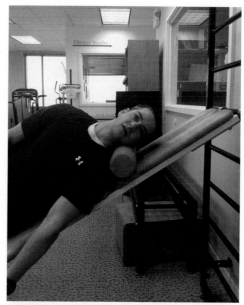

FIGURE 16-36 Midcervical locking with upper cervical active movement. With the athlete in a side-lying position, the clinician can place a bolster under the cervical spine to maintain the midcervical spine in a left side-bending and rotated position that will prevent right side bending and rotation. The athlete can then perform active upper cervical rotation or side bending to improve joint mobility.

Because of the high physical demands associated with athletics, the rehabilitation program should also include exercises that strengthen the upper extremities, improve core stability, and increase cardiovascular endurance.

Therapeutic Exercise Principles

Clinical Pearl # 5

"If we could give every individual the right amount of nourishment and exercise, not too little or too much, we would have found the safest way to health."
—Hippocrates

The therapeutic rehabilitation program can be divided into stages of treatment, with each stage emphasizing various functional qualities. Accordingly, the clinician can alter the dosage, speed, direction of movement, use of concentric/eccentric/isometric work, and other parameters to specially train for such variables as edema reduction, coordination, vascularity, joint mobility, local muscle endurance, and strength.[23]

If the athlete is determined to have hypomobility, exercises can be performed in the outer ranges of available normal physiologic motion, whereas for hypermobility, exercises would be performed that emphasize mid to inner ROM. If needed, the clinician may opt to perform locking techniques of the cervical spine when treating hypomobility in the early stages of rehabilitation because of the frequency of neighboring hypermobility (Fig. 16-36). Following trauma or in the presence of acute pain, to minimize the use of painful muscles, reorganization of normal muscle activation may have taken place.[23] In this case, the clinician should incorporate exercises to improve coordination and diminish pain. To avoid compensatory muscle activity, the athlete may need to perform an exercise in an alternative position. This compensatory pattern is commonly seen

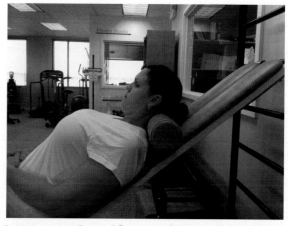

FIGURE 16-37 Cervical flexion performed on a slant board to facilitate activation of the deep cervical flexors. The athlete can perform cervical flexion in an inclined position to reduce weight and allow decreased participation of the sternocleidomastoid.

during cervical flexion; when training the deep neck flexors in the supine position, the sternocleidomastoid and the anterior scalene muscles will compensate. This compensation can be minimized by performing cervical flexion with a concomitant chin tuck, which will allow the sternocleidomastoid to relax or eccentrically lengthen[23] (Fig. 16-37). The sports rehabilitation specialist can facilitate a flexion pattern by incorporating upper extremity resistive movements to augment deep cervical flexion training (Fig. 16-38). In addition, to minimize recruitment of the mandibular depressors during cervical flexion activities, the athlete can place the tongue on the roof of the mouth with the lips closed and the teeth slightly apart.

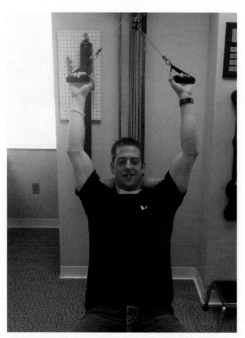

FIGURE 16-38 Neutral cervical spine stabilization. The athlete maintains a neutral cervical position and resists cervical extension as the upper extremity performs shoulder extension from a starting elevated position. As symptoms improve, the athlete can incorporate active cervical flexion as the upper extremities are extended.

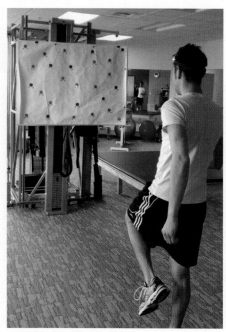

FIGURE 16-39 This activity can be performed while either jogging in place and maintaining level gaze fixation or jogging in place and separating cervical and eye movement by maintaining the laser at one fixation point as the eye searches for other points marked on the board. When the eyes locate a marked area, the laser is guided to that point as the eyes now search for the next identified location.

Isometrics can be added to fixate strength as it relates to neurologic adaptation and to sensitize the muscle spindle for stabilization of pathologic ROM. Isometric holds can be performed in any plane of movement and at any point in the cervical ROM as dictated by the athlete's symptoms and tolerance. Resistance can be increased 20% to 40% for isometric contraction and be maintained for 10 to 30 seconds. The increased weight and long duration of hold will help achieve greater muscle facilitation and recruit an increased number of motor units to augment the neurologic adaptation.

Because of the relationship of the ocular and vestibular systems to function of the cervical spine, the sports rehabilitation specialist should include training of these systems with cervical rehabilitation. It is very helpful for the clinician to have an understanding of the functional relationship of the oculomotor and vestibular system to the cervical spine. These systems combine afferent information (proprioceptive, visual, and vestibular end-organs) with efferent output to allow movements and activities to be performed without retinal slipping/visual bobbing or altered movement patterns. The vestibuloocular reflex functions to stabilize the eyes while the head is moving, both independently and dependently of each other. The vestibular nucleus receives information from the ocular system via the pontine reticular formation and from the vestibular end-organs that facilitates coordinated activity with other sensory systems to orient the body, head, and eyes. It allows postural adjustments to maintain equilibrium, calculate linear and angular movements, stimulate the ocular reflexes, and work with the brain to perform tasks such as ambulation, athletics, or subcortical activities.[23,27]

Cervical-oculomotor-vestibular training is performed to normalize the function and integration of these systems and thereby correct biomechanical, proprioceptive, and oculomotor dysfunction. This dysfunction may be the result of diminished cervical ROM, reduced coordination, loss of proprioception, disequilibrium, pain, integrated ocular and cervical motion, or any combination of these causes.[23] The clinician performs testing and individualizes the treatment based on these findings (Figs. 16-39 and 16-40, *A* and *B*).

Pathologic Rehabilitation Considerations

Cervical Spondylosis

Cervical spondylosis can develop as a result of many different conditions and can have a wide array of signs and symptoms. Depending on its severity and location, the neurovascular system of the athlete may be compromised. Spondylosis can result from numerous factors, including a genetically small diameter of the intervertebral foramen or spinal canal or enlargement of a nerve root secondary to a tumor, hematoma, or cyst. Osteophytes can develop at the facet or uncovertebral joint as a result of excessive tensile force and joint motion. Ligaments, such as the PLL or the ligamentum flavum, can become thickened and calcified because of excessive traction force or trauma. The clinician should be aware of the anatomic structure that is causing encroachment on the neurovascular system and whether the athlete has any genetically predisposing factors that are possibly contributing to this condition.

Treatment of athletes with cervical spondylosis consists of restoring mobility in the hypomobile vertebral segments secondary to spurring and calcifications through active and passive movements. Frequently, the athlete will also display

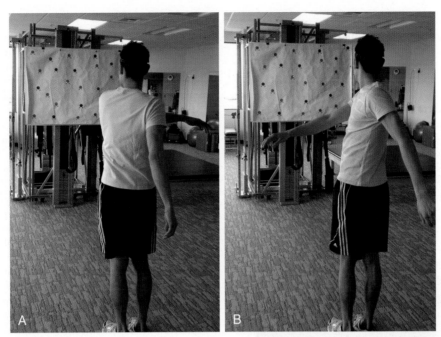

FIGURE 16-40 The athlete maintains fixation of the laser while performing various upper extremity/body movements. **A,** Trunk rotation to the right. **B,** Trunk rotation to the left.

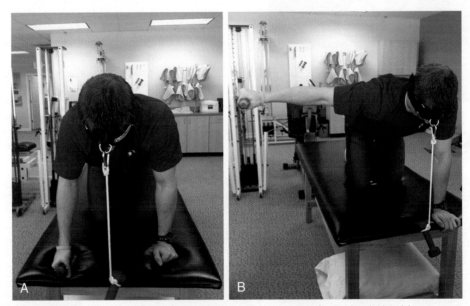

FIGURE 16-41 Quadruped cervical extension isometrics. This exercise can be performed with shoulder movement while maintaining a neutral isometric position and can be progressed by incorporating active cervical rotation with arm elevation. **A,** Starting position. **B,** Ending position.

hypermobility in adjacent segments to compensate for the lack of mobility. The athlete needs to perform stabilization exercises (i.e., cervical isometrics, midline ROM exercises) to control this excessive motion. The surrounding cervical soft tissue commonly has signs of tightness and spasm caused by neuromuscular facilitation, so the sports rehabilitation specialist will need to perform soft tissue mobilization techniques to restore mobility and decrease spasms. If the athlete has any associated postural adaptations, such as a forward-head, rounded-shoulder posture, the clinician should address this problem with flexibility, strengthening, and postural exercises (Fig. 16-41, *A* and *B*).

Facet Joint Lock

Facet joint impingement occurs as a result of the facet joint capsule or a meniscoid body becoming entrapped between a facet joint in the cervical spine. This can result from a rapid approximation of the joint surfaces, such as extension, side bending, and rotation or holding the head in an awkward position for an extended period (e.g., sleeping in an uncomfortable position). The head will be in a side-bent and rotated position, and the athlete will complain of a "locked" neck and unilateral neck pain. Assessment will reveal pain and decreased motion with contralateral side bending and rotation. Tenderness will be elicited on palpation of the affected facet joint, and muscle guarding will be detected in the surrounding musculature.

Because of the presence of pain and muscle guarding, the clinician may provide inhibition through modalities, soft tissue mobilization techniques, or both. The rehabilitation specialist can administer manual traction while simultaneously passively side-bending and rotating the athlete's head. This is initially performed in the pain-free direction and is gradually progressed into the restricted direction. The clinician can also provide manual resistance against ipsilateral cervical rotation throughout a full available ROM while also applying manual traction to help reduce muscle guarding and neuromodulate the athlete's pain (Fig. 16-42).

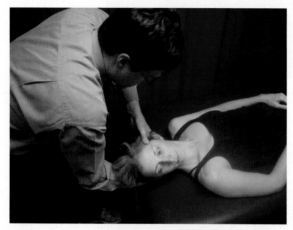

FIGURE 16-42 Manual cervical traction combined with contract-relax cervical rotation and passive range of motion can release an entrapped meniscoid and restore range of motion.

Cervical Sprain

A cervical sprain is a common injury because of the strenuous nature of athletics. It can be a result of a traumatic injury such as a fall or tackle that causes excessive motion or tension in the cervical spine. Because a cervical sprain can cause injury to muscular and ligamentous structures, the sports rehabilitation specialist should determine the status of the cervical ligaments through palpation and provocation tests (see online Figs. A16-9 through A16-11 [in Appendix 16] on Expert Consult @ www.expertconsult.com).

Initially after the injury, the athlete may require modalities to help control pain and inflammation. The clinician initiates pain-free passive and active ROM exercises and soft tissue mobilization to help neuromodulate the athlete's pain and facilitate soft tissue repair and regeneration. If the athlete does not have gross ligamentous instability, light stretches can be performed to help reduce muscle spasms. As soon as it can be tolerated, the athlete should begin performing an isotonic program to increase strength and stabilization of the cervical spine, diminish pain, and reduce metabolic exudates. This program should be progressed to a functional rehabilitation program as dictated by the condition of each athlete (Fig. 16-43, *A* and *B*).

Thoracic Outlet Syndrome

Treatment of thoracic outlet syndrome, along with any other pathologic condition, is dependent on the clinician's findings during the examination. Compression of neurovascular structures can result from altered kinematics related to posture or from decreased mobility in the surrounding joints or soft tissue (or both). The athlete typically performs exercises that address postural concerns, such as flexibility and strengthening exercises with special attention to the posterior rotator cuff, scapular retractors, and cervical and thoracic extensors.

The athlete may display signs of decreased joint mobility in the cervical and thoracic regions because of an increase in

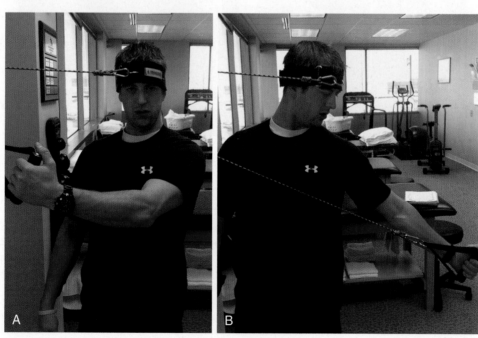

FIGURE 16-43 Combined resisted cervical rotation with upper extremity movement. This exercise allows training and coordination of cervical and upper extremity movements. **A,** Starting position. **B,** Ending position.

cervical lordosis and thoracic kyphosis. Although thoracic function has not been addressed in this chapter, the clinician can perform soft tissue and joint mobilization techniques to correct both these conditions. Compression of neurovascular structures can be caused by an elevated and hypomobile first rib, which can be due to overuse of the upper respiratory muscles—the sternocleidomastoid and scalenes—during inspiration. Normal mobility in this case will need to be restored through joint mobilizations of the first rib (see Fig. 16-18). If the athlete does not breathe from the diaphragm but rather from the upper thoracic region, the clinician should instruct the athlete in a diaphragmatic breathing pattern (Fig. 16-44). The clinician should also rule out any pathology involving the C3-C6 spinal levels that could cause irritation of the phrenic nerve.[9] The athlete will also perform flexibility and strengthening exercises to restore normal mobility and regain normal postural alignment.

CONCLUSION

Principles

- Because of the complexity of the cervical region, pain in this area has many possible origins.
- The osseous and connective tissues in the cervical spine interact to allow balance between functional mobility and stability.
- The facet joint planes, ligamentous tension, and muscle actions act together to provide the necessary arthrokinematic movements.

Evaluation

- The clinician should be cautious in assuming the source of pain without performing a thorough evaluation to determine which tissue is at fault.
- A quick screening of the temporomandibular joint, thoracic spine, and shoulder should be performed during a cervical evaluation because of common pain referral.

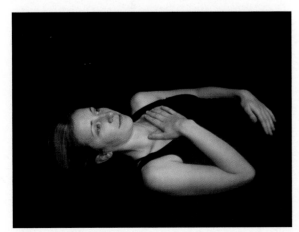

FIGURE 16-44 Diaphragmatic breathing technique. The clinician can assess the athlete's breathing pattern in this manner and instruct the athlete as needed. If treatment is warranted, the athlete is instructed to place one hand on the upper part of the chest and one hand over the stomach and is given verbal and tactical cueing to breathe with the diaphragm.

- Special tests, including neurologic, vascular, and ligamentous tests, should be performed to assist the clinician in the evaluation process.
- The clinician should perform mobility testing of the cervical spine to evaluate for any hypomobility or hypermobility and the relative mobility of the surrounding vertebral segments.
- In the event of traumatic injury to the head and neck with resultant paresthesia or vertebral insufficiency (or both), upper cervical instability can be ruled out with radiologic and instability tests.
- The clinician can determine whether hypermobilities or hypomobilities are present by mobility testing of the cervical region.

Rehabilitation

- The clinician should base the treatment program on addressing the cause of the pain and providing return to function.
- Soft tissue mobilization techniques can be used to provide relaxation and allow the performance of joint mobilizations and therapeutic exercises.
- The rehabilitation specialist can perform joint mobilization techniques to neuromodulate pain and address any hypomobilities.
- The clinician can ensure that the athlete receives a customized rehabilitation program by altering the fundamental exercises through the use of isometrics, isotonics, adjustment of the range of motion of the exercise, and addition of a proprioceptive component.
- The therapeutic program should be individualized based on the athlete's clinical findings and tolerance, as well as the tissue or tissues affected, with specific treatment aimed at healing the tissue involved.
- Rehabilitation programs that combine manual therapy and exercise have been shown to be most effective for patients with cervical pathology.
- The rehabilitation specialist should include soft tissue mobilization and manual mobilization to decrease muscle spasm, hypertonicity, and edema; improve joint lubrication; diminish pain; and prepare the tissues for exercise.
- Therapeutic exercises should be prescribed to achieve the treatment outcome desired while concomitantly refraining from movements, speed, and range that could create a deleterious response from the cervical-ocular-vestibular system.
- Oculomotor-vestibular assessment and training should be included in the treatment of an athlete with cervical pathology.

REFERENCES

1. Calliet, R. (1996): Soft Tissue Pain and Disability. Philadelphia, Davis.
2. Panjabi, M.M., and White, A.A. (1978): Clinical Biomechanics of the Spine. Philadelphia, Lippincott.
3. Gower, W.E., and Pedrini, V. (1969): Age-related variations in protein polysaccharides from human nucleus pulposus, annulus fibrosus and costal cartilage. J. Bone Joint Surg. Am., 51:1154–1162.
4. Mednel, T., Wink, C.S., and Zimny, M.L. (1992): Neural elements in human cervical intervertebral discs. Spine, 17:132–135.
5. Williams, P.L., and Warwick, R. (1983): Gray's Anatomy, 36th British ed. Baltimore, Williams & Wilkins.
6. Greenberg, A.D. (1968): Atlanto-axial dislocations. Brain, 91:655–684.
7. Bland, J.H. (1994): Disorders of the Cervical Spine. Philadelphia, Saunders.
8. Kapandji, I.A. (1974): The Physiology of Joints, Vol 3: The Trunk and the Vertebral Column. New York, Churchill Livingstone.

9. Ola Grimsby Institute (1998): Cervical Biomechanics: Residency Course Notes; Systems Course, San Diego, 680:33.

10. Magee, D.J. (1997): Orthopedic Physical Assessment, 3rd ed. Philadelphia, Saunders.

11. Cyriax, J.C. (1982): Textbook of Orthopaedic Medicine, Vol 1: Diagnosis of Soft Tissue Lesions, 8th ed. London, Bailliere Tindall.

12. Elvey, R.L. (1994): The investigation of arm pain. In Boyling, J.D., and Palastanga, N. (eds.): Grieve's Modern Manual Therapy: The Vertebral Column. Edinburgh, Churchill Livingstone.

13. Hislop, H.J., and Montgomery, J. (2002): Daniels and Worthington's Muscle Testing: Techniques of Manual Examination, 7th ed. Philadelphia, Saunders.

14. Kendall, F.P., and McCreary, E.K. (1993): Muscles Testing and Function, 4th ed. Baltimore, Lippincott Williams & Wilkins.

15. Hoppenfeld, S. (1976): Physical Examination of the Spine and Extremities. New York, Appleton-Century-Crofts.

16. Evans, R.C. (1994): Illustrated Essentials in Orthopedic Physical Assessment. St. Louis, Mosby–Year Book.

17. Cuetter, A.C., and Bartoszek, D.M. (1989): The thoracic outlet syndrome: Controversies, overdiagnosis, overtreatment and recommendations for management. Muscle Nerve, 12:410–419.

18. Roos, D.B., and Wilbourn, A.J. (1990): The thoracic outlet syndrome is underrated. Arch. Neurol., 47:327–328.

19. Stanton, P.E., Wo, N.M., Haley, T., et al. (1988): Thoracic outlet syndrome: A comprehensive evaluation. Am. Surg., 54:129–133.

20. Turek, S. (1967): Orthopaedics: Principles and Their Applications. Philadelphia, Saunders.

21. Bronfort, G., Evan, R., Nelson, B., et al. (2001): A randomized clinical trial of exercise and spinal manipulation for patients with chronic neck pain. Spine, 26:788–797.

22. Evans, R.C. (1992): Some observations on whiplash injuries. Neurol. Trauma, 10: 975–997.

23. Rivard, J., Kring, R., Gramont, D., and Grimsby, O. (2008): Exercise rehabilitation of the cervical spine. In Rivard, J., and Grimsby, O. (eds.): Science, Theory and Clinical Application in Orthopedic Manual Physical Therapy. Taylorsville, UT, Academy of Graduate Physical Therapy.

24. Mense, S., and Skeppar, P. (1991): Discharge behavior of feline gamma-motoneurones following induction of an artificial myositis. Pain, 46:201–210.

25. Travell, J.G., and Simons, D.G. (1983): Myofascial Pain and Dysfunction: The Trigger Point Manual. Baltimore, Williams & Wilkins.

26. Kaltenborn, F.M. (1980): Mobilization of the Extremity Joints: Examination and Basic Treatment Techniques. Oslo, Olaf Norlis Bokhandel.

27. Baloh, R., and Honrubia, V. (2001): Clinical Neurophysiology of the Vestibular System, 3rd ed. Oxford, Oxford University Press.

Low Back Rehabilitation

Julie Fritz, PT, PhD, ATC

CHAPTER OBJECTIVES

- Explain the need for classification methods designed to direct the treatment of patients with low back pain.
- Recognize red flags indicating the potential for a serious underlying condition.
- Explain the importance of yellow flags to the management of patients with low back pain.
- Determine the stage of a patient with low back pain.

- Identify key signs and symptoms and determine the classification of the patient and the treatments associated with a patient classified to be in stage I.
- Identify key impairments and the treatments designed to eliminate these impairments in patients determined to be in a stage II classification.

Low back pain (LBP) is a nearly universal experience in the adult population. Studies have documented the lifetime prevalence rate of LBP to be as high as 80%.[1] Although most cases are self-limited and recover with little intervention, those who recover are prone to recurrences at a rate of up to 60%.[2] The past few decades has witnessed numerous advances in the medical community's understanding of the lumbar spine. The functional anatomy of the lumbar spine has been investigated in detail, the biomechanics of the lumbar motion segments has been studied, and new technology has allowed more precise diagnostic imaging of the spine. Despite these advances, the prevalence of LBP and its associated costs has been growing at an alarming rate in recent decades, which has led to the characterization of back pain as an epidemic.[3]

LBP is also a prevalent and problematic condition in athletes. Up to 20% of all sports-related injuries are reported to involve the spine.[4] Athletes in certain sports appear to be particularly susceptible to LBP. For example, high rates of LBP in athletes participating in the following sports have been reported: gymnastics, swimming, tennis, volleyball, and football, as well as others.[5-9] Rehabilitation of individuals with LBP, including athletes, remains largely enigmatic. Numerous approaches to rehabilitation have been advocated, yet for any given individual with LBP, selection of a treatment method from among the many competing approaches has been said to take on the characteristics of a lottery,[10] with the rehabilitation specialist often being left uncertain of the best course of action to undertake with any particular patient. This chapter presents a classification-based approach to the evaluation and treatment of patients with LBP. This approach seeks to classify patients with LBP on the basis

of clusters of signs and symptoms. The patient's classification is then matched to a treatment strategy believed to be most effective for that individual patient.

EVALUATION AND TREATMENT: THE IMPORTANCE OF CLASSIFICATION

Identifying the anatomic structure responsible for LBP is often difficult, and in up to 90% of patients, a precise diagnosis cannot be made on the basis of pathology.[11] In this large group of patients a nominal diagnosis such as "lumbar strain" or "back pain" is typically made, and it has been considered a homogeneous entity. Although it is generally agreed that most of these patients should be treated conservatively, the search for effective conservative treatment measures has been elusive. It has been suggested that undiagnosed LBP is not actually a homogeneous entity but instead consists of subtypes or classifications of patients who can be identified on the basis of specific signs and symptoms noted during examination.[12] The classification in turn directs the clinician to a specific treatment intervention. An effective classification system for LBP should improve the clinician's decision making and may be necessary before the therapeutic benefit of specific conservative treatment interventions can be documented in research studies.

Delitto et al[12,13] have proposed a treatment-based classification system for use in the evaluation and treatment of individuals with LBP. This system uses information gathered from the physical examination and from patient self-reports to guide patient management. Three basic levels of decision making or classification are required: (1) the athlete must be screened for red flags and yellow flags to ascertain suitability for rehabilitation, (2) the acuity (or stage) of the low back condition must be determined, and finally (3) a treatment approach is selected.

Assessing for Red and Yellow Flags: First-Level Classification

Red Flags

Even though a specific pathoanatomic source cannot be identified in most individuals with LBP, the cause in most cases can be attributed to mechanical factors. In a much smaller percentage of patients, the cause may be something more serious such as a fracture, cauda equina syndrome, neoplastic condition, or inflammatory disease.[14] Red flags are signs or symptoms that suggest a more serious underlying pathology and may necessitate referral for medical or surgical intervention.

Several findings from the patient's history should alert the clinician to the potential for a serious underlying pathology. Spinal fractures can occur as a result of major trauma or falls. Compression fractures most commonly occur in postmenopausal women or in individuals with other bone-weakening conditions such as chronic corticosteroid use. Stress fractures are also not uncommon in athletes with persistent LBP. Stress fractures of the sacrum have been reported as a cause of LBP in athletes.[15] The pars interarticularis of the vertebral arch is the most common site of stress fractures in the spine, particularly in athletes involved in sports activities that involve repeated extension and rotation movements. The term *spondylolysis* describes a bony defect in the pars interarticularis region.[16] Rates of spondylolysis are particularly high in gymnasts, weight lifters, throwing athletes in track and field, divers, and rowers.[17,18] Spondylolysis may progress to spondylolisthesis, or forward slippage of one vertebra in relation to the vertebra below (Fig. 17-1).[19] Red flags that

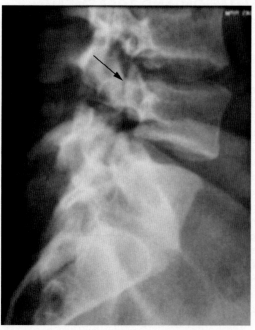

FIGURE 17-1 Grade 1 spondylolisthesis of the L4 vertebra in a 17-year-old football offensive lineman with low back pain.

may indicate the presence of spondylolysis or spondylolisthesis include teenage athletes with LBP, participation in sports involving repetitive hyperextension of the spine, and pain with extension activities. If a spondylolytic lesion is suspected, referral for further diagnostic imaging should be considered. Early identification of these conditions may prevent a nonunion fracture or progression of the slippage.[20] Treatment may involve bracing and limitation of activity. Rehabilitation typically focuses on stabilization exercises.

LBP caused by a spinal neoplasm is rare and occurs in less than 1% of individuals with LBP.[21] A missed or delayed diagnosis is possible if an awareness of red flags for the condition is lacking. Deyo and Diehl[21] identified several red flags that should raise suspicion for spinal tumors, including older than 50 years of age, unexplained weight loss, and no relief with bed rest. The most significant red flag is a previous history of cancer. The most common cancers that may result in metastases to the spine involve the breast, lung, and prostate.[22] LBP caused by infectious conditions such as osteomyelitis or septic discitis are also rare; red flags include fever, chills, a recent history of an infectious condition such as a urinary tract infection, or intravenous drug use.[23] The medical history may also provide the first clues for detecting ankylosing spondylitis, a rheumatic inflammatory disorder more common in male individuals and characterized by fibrosis and ossification of ligaments and joint capsules. Most affected individuals are younger than 35 years of age when they first experience symptoms and will describe morning stiffness. The finding of relief with exercise and the need to get out of bed at night are also important in raising suspicion for ankylosing spondylitis.[24,25]

Cauda equina syndrome occurs when a large midline disk herniation causes compression of the cauda equina nerve roots. The condition is rare, with estimates of it occurring in less than 0.01% of patients with LBP,[14] but when present it represents a surgical emergency that requires immediate referral. Red flags for cauda equina syndrome are sensory deficits in the perineal (i.e., "saddle") region, urinary retention, or loss of sphincter control.[26] Box 17-1 provides a contrasting view of red flags that could potentially be a serious condition causing LBP.

Yellow Flags

LBP is a common experience, and most affected individuals are able to recover and resume normal activities within a few weeks.[27] Research has shown that psychosocial variables are far more important than findings on physical examination for predicting which patients are at risk for not making a rapid recovery.[28,29] Yellow flags are findings that indicate an increased risk for prolonged pain and disability because of psychosocial factors.[30] Research suggests that fear-avoidance beliefs may be the most important psychosocial yellow flag indicating increased risk for prolonged LBP.[31,32]

The Fear-Avoidance Model was developed to help explain why some individuals with acute painful conditions progress to chronic pain whereas others are able to recover.[33] The model proposes that pain perception has both a sensory component and an emotional reaction component. During normal conditions these two components have a proportional relationship. In some instances, however, the relationship between the sensory component and the emotional reaction component can become dissociated and result in pain experience or behavior, or both, that is out of proportion to the demonstrable pathology.[34] The most important determinant of the relationship between the sensory and emotional components of pain perception is proposed to be an individual's fear of pain and subsequent avoidance behavior.[33,34]

The response of an individual to a painful experience may fall somewhere along a continuum between two extremes: avoidance and confrontation.[35] Confrontation is seen as an adaptive response in which the individual resumes activities in a graded manner and eventually returns to a normal level of activity. Conversely, avoidance is viewed as a maladaptive response in

which activities anticipated to cause pain are avoided. Avoidance may result in decreased activity levels, continued disability, and adverse psychologic consequences.

Clinical Pearl #1

Fear-avoidance beliefs may be the most important psychosocial factor that increases the risk for prolonged disability caused by LBP. Patients with high levels of fear-avoidance beliefs need to be managed with an active rehabilitation approach that includes ample positive reinforcement when functional goals are achieved.

The presence of an avoidance response to LBP has been associated with increased risk for prolonged disability and work loss.[28,32,36,37] Yellow flags indicating increased risk for prolonged disability caused by heightened fear-avoidance beliefs can be assessed by clinical evaluation or by questionnaire. Several attitudes and behaviors may represent yellow flags.[38] Waddell et al[32] developed the Fear-Avoidance Beliefs Questionnaire (FABQ) to quantify fear-avoidance beliefs in patients with LBP (Fig. 17-2). The questionnaire is designed to assess the impact of fear-avoidance beliefs on two aspects of function: physical activity and work.

When yellow flags are identified, the rehabilitation approach used with the patient may need to be modified. An emphasis on active rehabilitation and positive reinforcement of functional accomplishments is recommended for patients with increased fear-avoidance beliefs.[39] Graded exercise programs that direct attention toward attaining certain functional goals and away from the symptom of pain have also been recommended.[40] Finally, graduated exposure to specific activities that a patient fears as being potentially painful or difficult to perform may be helpful.[41] Box 17-2 summarizes the attitudes and types of behavior that may be associated with yellow flags.

Staging the Patient: Second-Level Classification

Determining the acuity of the patient's LBP is an important consideration for rehabilitation. Acuity is not based strictly on the duration of symptoms but also includes the nature of the patient's examination and the goals for rehabilitation. Patients who have difficulty performing basic daily activities such as sitting, standing, or walking are considered to be in stage I (i.e., acute). Patients in stage I tend to have increased levels of pain and disability, and the goals for rehabilitation are directed toward reducing the patient's symptoms and permitting progression to stage II of treatment. Patients who are able to perform basic daily activities but experience difficulty with more demanding activities such as running, lifting, and sporting activities are considered to be in stage II. Patients in stage II will generally have less severe symptoms, but they tend to have had their symptoms for a longer duration, and the symptoms possibly limit their ability to work or engage in sports activities. The goals of rehabilitation for patients in stage II focus on reducing impairments in strength, flexibility, endurance, and neuromuscular control and returning to full participation in work or sports activities.

Box 17-1

Red Flags for Potentially Serious Conditions Causing Low Back Pain

FRACTURES

Spinal fracture:

- Major trauma such as a motor vehicle accident, a fall from a height, or a direct blow to the lumbar spine

Compression fracture:

- Minor trauma or strenuous lifting in older or potentially osteoporotic individuals; prolonged corticosteroid use

Pars interarticularis stress fracture:

- Persistent back pain in younger individuals involved in repetitive hyperextension activities

CAUDA EQUINA SYNDROME

Saddle anesthesia

Recent onset of bladder dysfunction, such as urinary retention, increased frequency, or overflow incontinence

Serious or progressive neurologic deficit in the lower extremity

NEOPLASTIC CONDITIONS

Older than 50 years of age

Previous history of cancer

Unexplained weight loss

No relief with bed rest

ANKYLOSING SPONDYLITIS

Getting out of bed at night

Morning stiffness

Male gender

At onset, younger than 35 years of age

No relief when lying down

Relief with exercise and activity

SPINAL INFECTION

Recent fever and chills

Recent bacterial infection, intravenous drug abuse, or immunosuppression (from steroids, organ transplantation, or human immunodeficiency virus infection)

Data from Bigos S., Bowyer, O., Braen, G., et al. (1994): Acute low back problems in adults. AHCPR Publication 95–0642. Rockville, MD, Agency for Health Care Policy and Research, Public Health Service, US Department of Health and Human Services; and Deyo, R.A., and Diehl, A.K. (1988): Cancer as a cause of back pain: Frequency, clinical presentation, and diagnostic strategies. J. Gen. Intern. Med., 3:230–238.

FEAR-AVOIDANCE BELIEFS QUESTIONNAIRE

Here are some of the things other patients have told us about their pain. For each statement please mark the number from 0 to 6 to indicate how much physical activities such as bending, lifting, walking or driving affect or would affect your back pain.

	Completely disagree			Unsure			Completely agree
1. My pain was caused by physical activity	0	1	2	3	4	5	6
2. Physical activity makes my pain worse	0	1	2	3	4	5	6
3. Physical activity might harm my back	0	1	2	3	4	5	6
4. I should not do physical activities which (might) make my pain worse	0	1	2	3	4	5	6
5. I cannot do physical activities which (might) make my pain worse	0	1	2	3	4	5	6

The following statements are about how your normal work affects or would affect your back pain.

	Completely disagree			Unsure			Completely agree
6. My pain was caused by my work or by an accident at work	0	1	2	3	4	5	6
7. My work aggravated my pain	0	1	2	3	4	5	6
8. I have a claim for compensation for my pain	0	1	2	3	4	5	6
9. My work is too heavy for me	0	1	2	3	4	5	6
10. My work makes or would make my pain worse	0	1	2	3	4	5	6
11. My work might harm my back	0	1	2	3	4	5	6
12. I should not do my regular work with my present pain	0	1	2	3	4	5	6
13. I cannot do my normal work with my present pain	0	1	2	3	4	5	6
14. I cannot do my normal work until my pain is treated	0	1	2	3	4	5	6
15. I do not think that I will be back to my normal work within 3 months	0	1	2	3	4	5	6
16. I do not think that I will ever be able to go back to that work	0	1	2	3	4	5	6

FIGURE 17-2 Fear-Avoidance Beliefs Questionnaire.[32] The physical activity subscale is computed as the sum of questions 2 through 5. The work subscale is computed as the sum of questions 6, 7, 9 to 12, and 15. *(From Waddell, G., Newton, M., Henderson, I., et al. [1993]: A Fear-Avoidance Beliefs Questionnaire [FABQ] and the role of fear-avoidance beliefs in chronic low back pain and disability. Pain, 52:157–168.)*

Box 17-2

Attitudes and Types of Behavior That May Represent Yellow Flags

ATTITUDES AND BELIEFS

Belief that pain is harmful or disabling and resulting in guarding and fear of movement

Belief that all pain must be abolished before returning to activity

Expectation of increased pain with activity or work, lack of ability to predict capabilities

Catastrophe focused, expecting the worst

Belief that pain is uncontrollable

Passive attitude to rehabilitation

BEHAVIOR

Use of extended rest

Reduced activity level with significant withdrawal from daily activities

Avoidance of normal activity and progressive substitution of lifestyle away from productive activity

Reports of extremely high pain intensity

Excessive reliance on aids (braces, crutches, and other aids)

Sleep quality reduced after the onset of back pain

High intake of alcohol or other substances with an increase since the onset of back pain

Smoking

Determining the Best Treatment Approach: Third-Level Classification

When the patient has been screened for red and yellow flags and the stage of the condition has been judged, the next decision is determining which treatment approach is most likely to benefit the patient. Instead of focusing on a pathoanatomic diagnosis, the clinician should seek to classify the patient's condition on the basis of clusters of signs and symptoms. The classification assignment should in turn assist in determination of the most appropriate treatment approach. The treatment-based classification system used in this chapter was originally described by Delitto et al[12] in 1995 and has been updated and modified based on research developments since that time.[13,42-45] The system uses information gathered from the patient's medical history and physical examination to place the patient into a classification, which in turn guides treatment of the patient. Four basic classifications are used for patients in stage I: manipulation/mobilization, specific exercise (flexion, extension, and lateral shift patterns), stabilization, and traction. Each of these classifications is associated with several key examination findings and a unique treatment approach. Components of the examination are assessed through patient self-report measures, neurologic evaluation, the patient's medical history, and findings on physical examination. Table 17-1 summarizes the key examination findings and treatments for patients with a stage I classification.

Table 17-1 Key Examination Findings and Treatments for Stage I Classifications

Classification	Key Examination Findings	Treatments
Stabilization	Frequent previous episodes of low back pain Increasing frequency of episodes of low back pain "Instability catch" or painful arcs during lumbar flexion/extension ROM Hypermobility of the lumbar spine Positive prone segmental instability test	Trunk-strengthening stabilization exercises
Manipulation/mobilization	No symptoms distal to the knee Recent onset of symptoms Low levels of fear-avoidance beliefs Hypomobility of the lumbar spine Increased hip internal rotation (>35°) or discrepancy in hip internal rotation ROM between the right and left hip	Manipulation or mobilization techniques targeted to the sacroiliac or lumbar region. ROM exercises
Specific Exercise		
Extension pattern	Symptoms distal to the knee Signs and symptoms of nerve root compression Symptoms centralize with lumbar extension Symptoms peripheralize with lumbar flexion	Extension exercises Mobilization to promote extension Avoidance of flexion activities
Flexion pattern	Older age (>55 years) Symptoms distal to the knee Signs and symptoms of nerve root compression and/or neurogenic claudication Symptoms peripheralize with lumbar extension Symptoms centralize with lumbar flexion	Flexion exercises Mobilization to promote flexion Deweighted ambulation Avoidance of extension activities
Lateral shift pattern	Visible frontal plane deviation of the shoulders relative to the pelvis Asymmetric side-bending active ROM Painful and restricted extension active ROM	Pelvic translocation exercises Autotraction
Traction	Signs and symptoms of nerve root compression No movements centralize symptoms	Mechanical or autotraction

ROM, Range of motion.

Self-Report Measures

Several self-report measures provide useful information for the classification process and may also serve as useful indicators of the effectiveness of treatment. Three self-report measures are recommended: a pain diagram and pain rating scale, the FABQ, and a disability measure.

PAIN DIAGRAM AND RATING SCALE

A pain body diagram is used to determine the nature and distribution of the patient's symptoms. The patient is asked to indicate the location and nature (e.g., aching, burning, numbness) of symptoms on the body diagram. If symptoms are noted to extend distal to the knee, a classification of manipulation/mobilization becomes less likely.[42] The presence of symptoms distal to the knee or symptoms of numbness and tingling increases the likelihood of a specific exercise or traction classification. A pain diagram may also serve as an additional yellow flag screening tool. A nondermatomal or widespread distribution of symptoms may indicate that psychosocial factors are affecting the patient's perception of pain.[46] A pain rating scale asks the patient to rate the level of pain on a 0 to 10 scale, with 0 indicating no pain and 10 the worst imaginable pain. Ratings of pain may serve as a useful outcome measure to document treatment success or failure.

FEAR-AVOIDANCE BELIEFS QUESTIONNAIRE

The FABQ is a helpful screening tool for yellow flags. It has both work and physical activity subscales (see Fig. 17-2). The work subscale of the FABQ may be particularly helpful for classifying patients. It contains seven items, each scored 0 to 6, with higher numbers indicating greater levels of fear-avoidance beliefs. Research has found that total scores greater than 34 should raise concern about prolonged disability.[31] Total scores higher than 18 have been associated with a reduced likelihood of success with a manipulation treatment approach,[42] and these patients may need a more active rehabilitation program.

MODIFIED OSWESTRY DISABILITY QUESTIONNAIRE

The two most commonly used self-report disability scales are the Modified Oswestry Disability Questionnaire and the Roland Morris Questionnaire.[47] We have used the Oswestry questionnaire for the purposes of staging patients and assessing the outcomes of treatment. The Oswestry questionnaire has 10 sections: 1 section for pain severity and the other 9 representing various functional activities (Fig. 17-3). The patient indicates the degree of limitation in that activity because of LBP. Each section contains six responses, scored from 0 to 5. Each section score is summed to obtain the final score. The final score is then multiplied by 2, and the degree

---

MODIFIED OSWESTRY LOW BACK PAIN DISABILITY QUESTIONNAIRE

This questionnaire has been designed to give your therapist information as to how your back pain has affected your ability to manage in every day life. Please answer every question by placing a mark in the **one** box that best describes your condition today. We realize you may feel that two of the statements may describe your condition, but **please mark only the box which most closely describes your current condition**.

Pain intensity
- ☐ I can tolerate the pain I have without having to use pain medication.
- ☐ The pain is bad but I can manage without having to take pain medication.
- ☐ Pain medication provides me complete relief from pain.
- ☐ Pain medication provides me with moderate relief from pain.
- ☐ Pain medication provides me with little relief from pain.
- ☐ Pain medication has no effect on my pain.

Lifting
- ☐ I can lift heavy weights without increased pain.
- ☐ I can lift heavy weights but it causes increased pain.
- ☐ Pain prevents me from lifting heavy weights off the floor, but I can manage if weights are conveniently positioned (ex. on a table).
- ☐ Pain prevents me from lifting heavy weights, but I can manage light to medium weights if they are conveniently positioned.
- ☐ I can lift only very light weights.
- ☐ I cannot lift or carry anything at all.

Walking
- ☐ Pain does not prevent me from walking any distance.
- ☐ Pain prevents me from walking more than 1 mile.
- ☐ Pain prevents me from walking more than $1/2$ mile.
- ☐ Pain prevents me from walking more than $1/4$ mile.
- ☐ I can only walk with crutches or a cane.
- ☐ I am in bed most of the time and have to crawl to the toilet.

Standing
- ☐ I can stand as long as I want without increased pain.
- ☐ I can stand as long as I want but it increases my pain.
- ☐ Pain prevents me from standing more than 1 hour.
- ☐ Pain prevents me from standing more than $1/2$ hour.
- ☐ Pain prevents me from standing more than 10 minutes.
- ☐ Pain prevents me from standing at all.

Social life
- ☐ My social life is normal and does not increase my pain.
- ☐ My social life is normal, but it increases my level of pain.
- ☐ Pain prevents me from participating in more energetic activities (ex. sports, dancing, etc.).
- ☐ Pain prevents me from going out very often.
- ☐ Pain has restricted my social life to my home.
- ☐ I have hardly any social life because of my pain.

Employment/homemaking
- ☐ My normal homemaking/job activities do not cause pain.
- ☐ My normal homemaking/job activities increase my pain, but I can still perform all that is required of me.
- ☐ I can perform most of my homemaking/job duties, but pain prevents me from performing more physically stressful activities (ex. lifting, vacuuming).
- ☐ Pain prevents me from doing anything but light duties.
- ☐ Pain prevents me from doing even light duties.
- ☐ Pain prevents me from performing any job/homemaking chores.

Personal care (washing, dressing, etc.)
- ☐ I can take care of myself normally without causing increased pain.
- ☐ I can take care of myself normally but it increases my pain.
- ☐ It is painful to take care of myself and I am slow and careful.
- ☐ I need help but I am able to manage most of my personal care.
- ☐ I need help every day in most aspects of my care.
- ☐ I do not get dressed, wash with difficulty and stay in bed.

Sitting
- ☐ I can sit in any chair as long as I like.
- ☐ I can only sit in my favorite chair as long as I like.
- ☐ Pain prevents me from sitting for more than 1 hour.
- ☐ Pain prevents me from sitting for more than $1/2$ hour.
- ☐ Pain prevents me from sitting for more than 10 minutes.
- ☐ Pain prevents me from sitting at all.

Sleeping
- ☐ Pain does not prevent me from sleeping well.
- ☐ I can sleep well only by using pain medication.
- ☐ Even when I take pain medication, I sleep less than 6 hours.
- ☐ Even when I take pain medication, I sleep less than 4 hours.
- ☐ Even when I take pain medication, I sleep less than 2 hours.
- ☐ Pain prevents me from sleeping at all.

Traveling
- ☐ I can travel anywhere without increased pain.
- ☐ I can travel anywhere but it increases my pain.
- ☐ Pain restricts travel over 2 hours.
- ☐ Pain restricts my travel over 1 hour.
- ☐ Pain restricts my travel to short necessary journeys under $1/2$ hour.
- ☐ Pain prevents all travel except for visits to the doctor/therapist or hospital.

FIGURE 17-3 The Modified Oswestry Disability Questionnaire. *(Reprinted with permission from Fritz, J.M., and Irrgang, J.J. [2001]: A comparison of a Modified Owestry Low Back Pain Disability Questionnaire and the Quebec Back Pain Disability Scale. Phys. Ther., 81:776–788.)*

of disability is expressed as a percentage. Higher scores on the Oswestry questionnaire indicate greater levels of perceived disability.[48] The Oswestry score can assist in staging the patient. Generally, patients in stage I will have Oswestry scores at or greater than 30%, and patients in stage II will have scores lower than 30%.

Neurologic Assessment

Neurologic evaluation is required for any patient who has symptoms that extend below the buttock. The neurologic examination consists of four components: (1) strength of key muscles for each lumbar and sacral myotome, (2) sensation within dermatomes of the lower quarter, (3) deep tendon reflexes of the

lower quarter, and (4) signs of neural tension. Results of the neurologic examination will determine whether signs of nerve root compression are present and need to be monitored throughout treatment. Results of the neurologic assessment may also provide prognostic information. Individuals with positive findings on the neurologic examination may be more likely to experience long-term pain and disability.[49]

STRENGTH ASSESSMENT

Evaluation of key muscles in each lumbar and sacral myotome is performed. Myotomal weakness may be indicative of lower motor neuron lesions, most commonly nerve root compression

Table 17-2 Key Muscles to Be Tested and Corresponding Myotomes

Muscles	How to Test
Hip flexion (L1-L2)	The hip is flexed to near end range and pressure is applied to the anterior aspect of the thigh into hip extension.
Knee extension (L3-L4)	The knee is placed in a position slightly less than full extension. One hand stabilizes the patient's thigh while the other applies pressure on the anterior aspect of the tibia into knee flexion.
Dorsiflexion (L4-L5)	Dorsiflexion is best tested by having the patient walk on the heels. Non–weight-bearing assessment of dorsiflexion strength can be performed but may be less sensitive to subtle deficits in strength. For non–weight-bearing assessment, the foot is placed in full dorsiflexion with some inversion. One hand stabilizes the distal end of the tibia while the other hand applies pressure on the dorsum of the foot into plantar flexion with some eversion.
Great toe extension (L5)	With the shoes off, the great toe is placed in extension. One hand stabilizes the foot while the other hand applies pressure on the dorsum of the distal phalanx of the great toe into flexion.
Ankle plantar flexion (S1-S2)	Plantar flexion is best tested by having the patient walk on the toes. Non–weight-bearing assessment of plantar flexion strength can be performed but may be less sensitive to subtle deficits. For non–weight-bearing assessment, the foot is placed in full plantar flexion. One hand stabilizes the distal end of the tibia while the other applies pressure on the plantar aspect of the foot into plantar flexion. (With the knee flexed the soleus muscle is the primary plantar flexor.)

caused by intervertebral disk herniation. More generalized weakness may indicate more serious pathology or simply generalized disuse atrophy of the lower limb. The key muscles to be tested and corresponding myotomes are listed in Table 17-2.

SENSORY ASSESSMENT

Evaluation for sensory loss is performed by lightly brushing the hand over key dermatomal areas. Any region of diminished or absent sensation should be tested further with the use of a pin to clearly map the area of sensory deficit. Box 17-3 contains the key areas used to assess specific dermatomes. Considerable overlap and individual variations in dermatomal patterns are known to exist. The results of sensory testing should be collaborated with the results of other components of the neurologic assessment to determine the presence and extent of nerve root compression.

DEEP TENDON REFLEX ASSESSMENT

Diminished deep tendon reflexes may represent nerve root compression. Hyperactive reflexes can be another area of concern related to upper motor neuron disturbances (e.g., myelopathy). At the same time, hyperactive reflexes can be a normal variant. If encountered, the clinician should at least suspect a myelopathic process or upper motor neuron pathology. Confirming evidence for these conditions would be clonus or the presence of a Babinski response. If these findings exist, referral for further diagnostic work-up is probably required. Table 17-3 describes two lower extremity reflexes that are assessed.

NEURAL TENSION TESTS

These tests are procedures designed to place tension on neural structures to assist in the diagnosis of nerve root compression that is typically caused by lumbar intervertebral disk herniation. Two different neural tension tests are used (Fig. 17-4, A and B).

Straight Leg Raise A straight leg raise is used to place tension on the sciatic nerve to aid in diagnosis of the presence of nerve root compression of the lower lumbar nerve roots (L4-S1) (see Fig. 17-4, A). The patient is prone and the lower extremity is raised by the clinician to the maximum tolerable

---

Box 17-3

Key Areas Used to Assess Specific Dermatomes

Inguinal area (L1)
Anterior aspect of the midthigh region (L2)
Distal anterior aspect of the thigh and medial part
    of the knee (L3)
Medial aspect of lower part of the leg and foot (L4)
Lateral aspect of the lower part of the leg and foot (L5)
Posterior of the calf (S1)

Table 17-3 Lower Extremity Reflex Tests

Reflex	Test Integrity of Nerve Roots	Technique
Patellar tendon reflex	L3-L4 nerve roots	The patient is seated with the knee flexed to approximately 90°. The patellar tendon is struck with the reflex hammer and reflexive knee extension is observed.
Achilles tendon reflex	S1-S2 nerve roots	The patient is seated and the ankle is supported at approximately neutral dorsiflexion. The ankle dorsiflexor muscles must be relaxed. The Achilles tendon is struck with the reflex hammer and reflexive plantar flexion is observed and felt with the supporting hand.

level of hip flexion range of motion (ROM). The test must be performed passively and the patient's knee maintained in full extension and the hip in neutral rotation. The opposite leg is kept in extension. For each test, the clinician notes any symptoms produced during the test and also the degree of hip flexion at which the symptoms are produced. A positive test result requires reproduction of the patient's familiar leg symptoms between 30° and 70° of hip flexion. It is important to distinguish between reproduction of familiar symptoms and hamstring tightness.

Both the symptomatic and contralateral lower extremities are examined. A positive contralateral straight leg raise test result occurs when a straight leg raise of the asymptomatic lower extremity reproduces the symptoms in the symptomatic extremity. A positive contralateral straight leg raise test result is highly specific for lower lumbar disk herniation.[50]

Femoral Nerve Stretch Femoral nerve stretch is a neural tension test used to place tension on the femoral nerve to diagnose nerve root compression of the midlumbar nerve roots (L2-L4) (see Fig. 17-4, *B*). The femoral nerve stretch is performed with the patient prone. The clinician first passively extends the patient's hip and then passively flexes the knee. If the patient's familiar anterior thigh symptoms are reproduced or intensified with these maneuvers, the test is considered positive. It is important to distinguish between reproduction of the patient's familiar symptoms caused by tension on the femoral nerve and stretching of the rectus femoris muscle.

STAGE I MANAGEMENT

Manipulation/Mobilization Classification

Spinal manipulation is an intervention with at least some supporting evidence of its effectiveness. Several randomized trials have found spinal manipulation to be more effective than placebo or other interventions for patients with LBP.[51-54] Manipulation/mobilization techniques may be directed at either the sacroiliac (SI) region or the lumbar spine. Many theoretic approaches to identifying patients likely to benefit from spinal manipulation have been proposed; however, little to no evidence support their use and reliability. These approaches are frequently based on pathoanatomic and biomechanical theories that use various examination procedures to identify a pathologic motion segment or a biomechanical dysfunction toward which a manipulative intervention is then directed.

An alternative to the traditional tests used to classify patients is the development of a clinical prediction rule. A clinical prediction rule is a tool designed to assist in the classification process and improve decision making for clinicians.[55] Flynn et al[42] developed a clinical prediction rule consisting of multiple factors from the medical history and physical examination to predict a priori which patients will most likely benefit from spinal manipulation. The results of this study identified a set of five criteria that accurately identified patients who would benefit from a manipulative intervention. The five criteria are listed in Box 17-4. The presence of at least four of five of these findings was strongly predictive of a dramatic response to a manipulative intervention, and the presence of three findings was moderately predictive of success.[42] Therefore, a classification of manipulation/mobilization should be strongly considered when at least three of these findings are present.

Examination for the Manipulation/Mobilization Classification

Patients who are most likely to respond to a manipulation/mobilization intervention are generally those with a more recent onset of symptoms and localization of the symptoms to the low back region, to the buttock, and possibly into the thigh. Patients with signs of nerve root compression (i.e., positive straight leg raise and strength tests, reflex, or sensory deficits) are likely to respond more favorably to an alternative treatment approach. Traditionally, classifying a patient for a manipulation/mobilization intervention has relied predominately on mobility assessments and special tests. Many of these diagnostic tests have been found to have poor reliability and questionable validity,[42,56,57] and therefore clinicians should be cautious about basing classification decisions on any one of these findings in isolation. Confirmatory findings from the physical examination are outlined later in this chapter.

FURTHER EXAMINATION OF THE SACROILIAC REGION

Tests of Bony Landmark Symmetry The clinician assesses the symmetry of the pelvic landmarks, including the posterior superior iliac spines (PSISs), anterior superior iliac spines

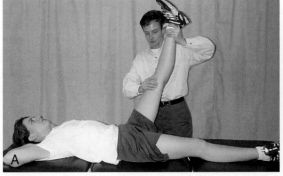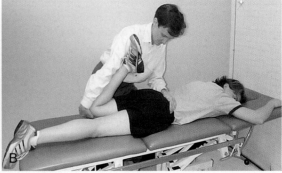

FIGURE 17-4 A, Straight leg raise. The hip is passively flexed with the knee maintained in extension. The test is positive if the patient's familiar leg symptoms are reproduced between 30° and 70° of hip flexion. **B,** Femoral nerve stretch. The knee and hip are passively flexed. The test is positive if the patient's familiar anterior thigh symptoms are reproduced or intensified with these maneuvers.

(ASISs), and the iliac crests with the patient standing. The iliac crests are evaluated from the posterior aspect of the patient with the clinician's hands at the pelvic level. The clinician judges the symmetry of the heights of the iliac crests. A difference between the right and left sides can indicate a leg length discrepancy, iliac rotation, or both. Asymmetry of the iliac crests must be correlated with the positional findings of the PSISs and ASISs. PSIS levels are determined by placing the tips of the index fingers directly beneath the inferior aspect of the PSIS on each side and visually comparing the height. The same procedure is used in comparing ASIS heights.

After each of the landmarks has been palpated, the results are compiled to arrive at one of three possible determinations:

- Long leg: symmetrically increased height of the ASIS, PSIS, and iliac crest on one side
- Innominate rotation: asymmetric heights of the ASISs, PSISs, and iliac crests (e.g., low PSIS on the right, high iliac crest on the right, and high ASIS on the right)
- Normal: even pelvic landmarks while standing

PSIS levels are palpated in a similar manner with the patient sitting. Palpation of the ASISs is difficult with the patient seated and is not performed. Interpretation of the position of the PSISs with the patient sitting is correlated with the results of palpation in the standing position. Asymmetry that was present while standing and remains while sitting may indicate dysfunction in the SI region. If the asymmetry is eliminated by sitting, a leg length discrepancy should be suspected.

The Standing and Seated Flexion Tests The clinician places the tips of the index fingers directly beneath the PSISs on both sides. The fingers are directed against the inferior margin of the PSISs with maintenance of upward pressure. The patient is instructed to bend forward as far as possible while the clinician continues to monitor the position of the PSISs and observes for symmetry of cranial movement of these bony landmarks (Fig. 17-5, *A*). Normally, the superior movement of each PSIS should be equal. A positive finding occurs when the cranial

excursion of one PSIS is judged to be greater than the other. The side that moves further in a cranial direction is presumed to be the hypomobile side that requires manipulation/mobilization.

The seated flexion test is performed and interpreted in an identical manner, except that the patient is seated. The clinician palpates the PSISs on both sides and the patient is then asked to flex forward while the clinician continues to monitor the position of the PSISs. If one PSIS is found to move further in a cranial direction than the other, the test is considered to be positive. The side that moves further in a cranial direction is presumed to be the hypomobile side.

Gillet Test With the patient standing, the clinician places one thumb under the PSIS on the side being tested. The other thumb is placed in the midline over the S2 spinous process. The patient is instructed to stand on one leg and flex the hip and knee on the side being testing while bringing the leg toward the chest. The clinician continues to palpate the PSIS on the tested side. The test is considered to be positive if the PSIS fails to move posterior and inferior with respect to the S2 spinous process (see Fig. 17-5, *B*).

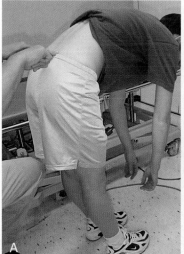
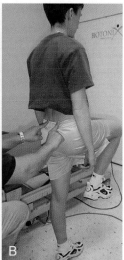
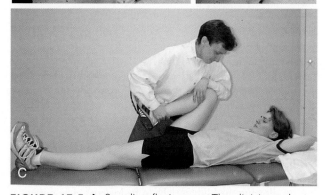

FIGURE 17-5 A, Standing flexion test. The clinician palpates the posterior superior iliac spines (PSISs) while the patient flexes forward. The test is positive if one PSIS moves further in a cranial direction. **B,** Gillet test. The clinician palpates the PSIS while the patient flexes the hip and knee. The test is positive if the PSIS does not move in a caudal direction. **C,** Gaenslen test. The clinician flexes the knee and hip and then applies overpressure. The test is positive if the patient's familiar symptoms are reproduced.

Box 17-4

Key Examination Findings Leading to a Classification of Manipulation/Mobilization*

- Low Fear-Avoidance Beliefs Questionnaire work subscale score (<19 points)
- Short duration of current symptoms (<16 days)
- No symptoms extending distal to the knee
- At least one hypomobile lumbar spine segment (judged from lumbar spring testing)
- At least one hip with more than 35° of internal rotation ROM

No increasing frequency of low back pain episodes noted by the patient

No signs of nerve root compression

No peripheralization during lumbar active movement testing

From Flynn, T., Fritz, J., Whitman, J., et al. (2002): A clinical prediction rule for classifying patients with low back pain who demonstrate short-term improvement with spinal manipulation. Spine, 27:2835–2843.

*The five findings prefaced by bullets make up the clinical prediction rule.

Gaenslen Test The Gaenslen test is a provocation test for dysfunction of the SI region. The patient is supine with both legs extended. The leg being tested is passively brought into full hip and knee flexion while the opposite hip is maintained in an extended position. Overpressure is applied by the clinician to the flexed extremity (see Fig. 17-5, *C*). A positive test result occurs when the patient's familiar symptoms are reproduced in either SI region with the application of the overpressure.

FURTHER EXAMINATION OF THE LUMBAR REGION
Lumbar Active Motion Assessment: The Movement Diagram
Active ROM is performed with the patient standing. In performing these procedures, the clinician needs to determine the ROM present in each direction, as well as the behavior of the patient's symptoms during and immediately after the movement in question. The patient is asked to perform the following movements:

● Side bending to the right and left
● Extension
● Forward bending

Reliable methods of measurement with a single inclinometer have been described for quantification of forward bending and extension.[58] For ease of recording the ROM present and the location of symptoms, we have developed a movement diagram and a shorthand system to denote the effect of movements on the patient's symptoms and to record the pattern of motion restriction present (Fig. 17-6).

For the classification of manipulation/mobilization, the focus of active movement testing is on identification of a noncapsular pattern of movement restriction that may indicate the need for manipulation or mobilization of the lumbar spine. Noncapsular patterns in the lumbar region were characterized by Cyriax[59] as occurring when a gross limitation in side bending is present in only one direction. Noncapsular patterns may be further distinguished as either opening or closing restrictions.[12] A closing restriction theoretically occurs when side bending is limited toward the side of pain and extension is also limited. The movement diagram of a left closing restriction is shown in Figure 17-7. An opening restriction is proposed to occur when the restricted motions are side bending away from the painful side and flexion. The movement diagram of a left opening restriction is shown in Figure 17-8.

Passive Segmental Motion Testing Passive segmental motion tests include both provocation and tests of mobility of the lumbar motion segments. The patient lies prone and the clinician places the hypothenar eminence over the spinous process of the vertebra to be tested. The contact point of the hand is just distal to the pisiform. When the clinician's hand is positioned appropriately, the wrist and elbow are extended and gentle but firm anteriorly directed pressure is applied to the spinous process. The force is applied not by pushing with the arms but by allowing the body weight to be lowered. The patient is instructed to report any change in symptoms during performance of the test. The clinician also judges the mobility as normal, hypomobile, or hypermobile. The presence of hypomobile lumbar motion segments is an indication for a manipulation/mobilization classification.

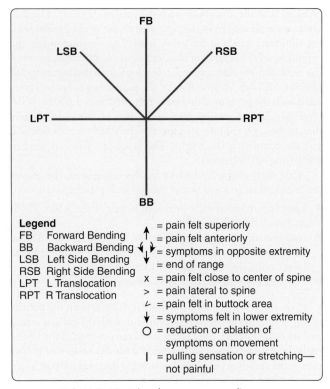

FIGURE 17-6 Lumbar movement diagram.

Treatment for the Manipulation/Mobilization Classification
Although it has not been studied extensively, a few studies have found greater benefit from manipulative techniques than from mobilization of the lumbosacral region.[60,61] Patients in whom spondylolisthesis, lumbar instability, or osteoporosis has been diagnosed or with any concern for a stress fracture should be approached with caution, and manipulative techniques are generally contraindicated in these individuals. Many different manipulation and mobilization techniques have been described, but currently no evidence has shown the superiority of one approach over another. Correct identification of a patient who actually needs manipulation/mobilization interventions is probably more important than the particular technique chosen by the clinician. Several manipulation/mobilization techniques are described in Figure 17-9, *A* to *D*. After these interventions are applied, the patient should be instructed in non–weight-bearing active ROM exercises. They may be performed in the supine or quadruped positions. In the supine position, the patient is instructed to actively tilt the pelvis anteriorly and posteriorly to create motion in the lumbar spine. In the quadruped position, the patient can be asked to rock backward over the heels and forward over the hands to create lumbar flexion and extension, respectively.

TREATMENT OF THE LUMBAR REGION
For lumbar region techniques, the lumbar motion segment to be manipulated or mobilized is determined from the accessory motion testing. The segment that seems to be the most hypomobile or painful should be treated first. After performing the

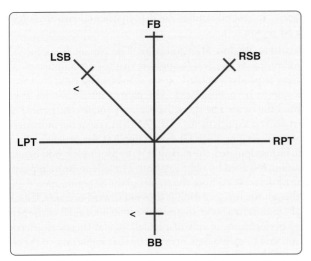

FIGURE 17-7 Movement diagram depicting a left closing pattern. (See Figure 17-6 for definitions.)

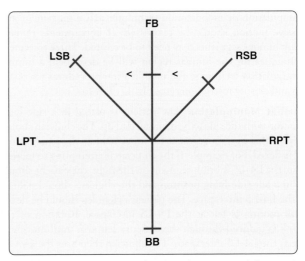

FIGURE 17-8 Movement diagram depicting a left opening restriction. (See Figure 17-6 for definitions.)

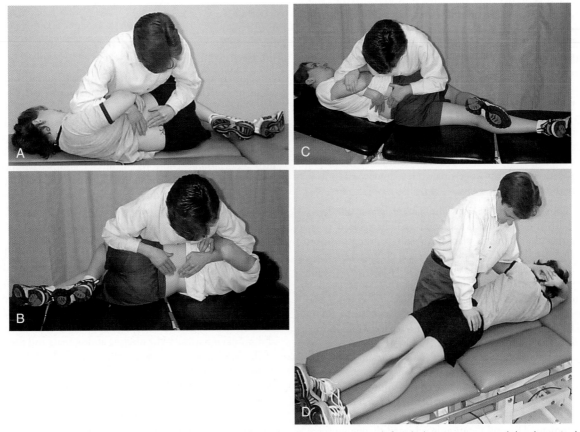

FIGURE 17-9 A, Manipulation of the L4-L5 segment on the right. The patient is in a left side-lying position and the thrust is delivered through the clinician's left arm. **B,** Mobilization of L4-L5 for a left opening restriction. The patient is in a right side-lying position. Mobilization is delivered through the clinician's hands and forearms. **C,** Mobilization of L4-L5 for a right closing restriction. The patient is in a left side-lying position. Mobilization is delivered through the clinician's right hand and forearm. **D,** Manipulation of the left sacroiliac region. The patient is in a left side-bending position with right rotation. Manipulation is delivered through the patient's left anterior superior iliac spine.

manipulation or mobilization technique, active movement and passive motion should be reassessed. If impairments remain, other lumbar segments may need to be treated. Three treatment techniques for the lumbar region will be described: a lumbar manipulation technique and mobilization procedures for opening and closing restrictions (see Fig. 17-9, A to C).

Lumbar Manipulation The patient is placed in a side-lying position with the side to be manipulated up. The clinician should palpate this motion segment for movement as the patient's top leg is flexed. For example, if the clinician is attempting to manipulate the L4-L5 motion segment on the right, the patient should be in a left side-lying position and the clinician should palpate in the L4-L5 interspace. The patient's right leg should be flexed until motion is felt at the L4-L5 interspace. Rotation of the trunk is induced through the patient's left arm until motion is felt at the L4-L5 interspace. The clinician then uses the arm on the patient's pelvis to induce a thrust in the anterior direction (see Fig. 17-9, A)

Lumbar Opening Mobilization The patient is in a side-lying position with the side to be mobilized up. If possible, the table is positioned to side-bend the patient away from the painful side. For example, with a left opening restriction at L4-L5, the patient would be in the right side-lying position with the table positioned in the right side-bending configuration. The clinician should palpate the L4-L5 interspace while flexing the patient's hips and knees until motion is felt at that segment. The upper part of the patient's leg is flexed further to allow the foot to rest behind the opposite knee. The clinician next palpates the L4-L5 interspace and induces flexion and rotation of the trunk to that level by pulling the patient's right arm parallel to the table. The clinician places one arm against the patient's trunk and the other arm over the pelvis. The fingertips of both hands are placed at the segment with pressure directed against the lower side of the spinous processes. Mobilization is performed by lifting the spinous processes with the fingertips while a downward force is created by the forearms (see Fig. 17-9, B).

Lumbar Closing Mobilization The patient is in a side-lying position with the side to be mobilized up. The table is positioned so that the patient is placed in a side-bending position toward the top side. For example, for a right closing restriction at L4-L5, the patient would be in a left side-lying position with the table positioned into the right side-bending configuration. The clinician palpates the L4-L5 interspace and extends the part lower of the patient's hip until motion is felt at the interspace. The clinician next palpates the interspace while inducing trunk rotation and extension by pulling the lower part of the patient's arm toward the ceiling. The clinician places the right arm against the patient's trunk. The hand is positioned with the thumb on the superior side of the spinous process of L4. The opposite arm blocks the patient's pelvis. The fingertips are placed on the inferior side of the lower vertebra in the motion segment. The mobilization is achieved through a force against the superior spinous process in a caudal and downward direction (see Fig. 17-9, C). The force can be accentuated by the superior arm pushing into further extension and side bending.

TREATMENT OF THE SACROILIAC REGION

Many manipulation and mobilization techniques have been described for the SI region.[62,63] The manipulation technique described in this section has been demonstrated to be effective in several studies for many patients with findings in the SI region.[52,53]

Sacroiliac Region Manipulation The patient is supine. The clinician stands on the side opposite that to be manipulated. The patient is passively moved into a side-bending position toward the side to be manipulated. The patient interlocks the fingers behind the head. The therapist passively rotates the patient and then delivers a quick thrust to the ASIS in a posterior and inferior direction (see Fig. 17-9, D). For example, if the patient's left side is to be manipulated, the patient is moved into a left side-bending position, followed by right rotation. The side to be manipulated may be determined from the results of the SI region special tests. Although the manipulation is directed toward one side, Cibulka et al[64] found changes in innominate tilt on both sides of the pelvis after performance of this manipulation, and therefore selection of the side to manipulate may not be that important to the outcome of the technique.

Clinical Pearl #2

Although the SI manipulation technique is described as targeting the SI region, it is often helpful for patients with pain and hypomobility in the lumbar spine as well.

Stabilization Classification

Strengthening the muscles of the lumbar spine is often the focus of exercise programs for patients with LBP. Although a link between LBP and lumbar muscle weakness may appear intuitive, research has produced some conflicting results. Some researchers report differences in strength between asymptomatic subjects and those with back pain,[65] whereas others report little association.[66] More recent investigations have focused on aspects of muscle performance other than maximal force output. These studies indicate that the properties of muscular endurance,[67] muscle balance,[68] and neuromuscular control[69] may be more important than maximum muscle strength in preventing and rehabilitating patients with LBP.

A lumbar spine devoid of any muscle activity is highly unstable, even under very low loads.[70] Muscle activity is therefore important for maintaining spinal stability. Stability during lifting and rotational movements has been studied most extensively. The erector spinae muscles provide most of the extensor force needed for lifting.[71] Rotation is produced mostly by the oblique abdominal muscles.[72] The oblique abdominals and the majority of the lumbar erector spinae muscle fibers lack direct attachment to the lumbar spinal motion segments and are therefore unable to stabilize individual motion segments. The multifidus muscle is better suited for the purpose of segmental stabilization. The multifidus originates from the spinous processes of the lumbar vertebrae and forms a series of repeating fascicles attaching to the inferior lumbar transverse processes, the ilium, and the sacrum. The multifidus is proposed to function as a stabilizer during lifting and rotational movements of the lumbar spine.[73] The quadratus lumborum has been proposed to be the primary stabilizer for side-bending movements.[74]

The oblique abdominals and transversus abdominis also contribute to spinal stabilization. These muscles have a more horizontal orientation and have been proposed to contribute to spinal stability by creating a rigid cylinder and increasing the stiffness of the lumbar spine.[75,76] This hypothesis is supported by studies demonstrating continuous activity of the transversus abdominis muscle throughout flexion and extension movements of the lumbar spine.[77]

Examination for the Stabilization Classification

Many of the findings leading to a stabilization classification are derived from the patient's medical history and include frequent recurrent episodes of LBP precipitated by minimal perturbations, deformity (e.g., lateral shift) with previous episodes, short-term relief from manipulation, a history of trauma, use of oral contraceptives, or improvement in symptoms with the use of a brace.[12] Other authors recommend palpatory techniques to detect the presence of a "step-off" between the spinous processes of adjacent vertebrae or passive intervertebral motion testing to detect hypermobility.[78,79] The reliability of these techniques, however, has been questioned, and their validity has not been demonstrated.[80] Others emphasize aberrant motions such as the "instability catch" occurring during active ROM testing of the motion.[79,81] The instability catch has been described by numerous authors as a sign of segmental instability[66,81,82]; however, its presence has never been related to symptoms or abnormal movements on diagnostic imaging studies.

Hicks[83] investigated a clinical prediction rule for predicting which patients with LBP are likely to benefit from a stabilization treatment approach. The most important factors were numerous previous episodes of LBP, particularly if the patient reports that the frequency of episodes is increasing (Box 17-5). From the physical examination, the most important factors were aberrant motions during active ROM, hypermobility detected during passive accessory motion testing, and a positive prone segmental instability test result. These examination findings are detailed in the following sections.

ABERRANT MOTIONS

While standing, the patient is asked to perform flexion and extension ROM. Several different aberrations may occur that are considered to be signs of a stabilization classification. Most aberrations will occur during flexion or on return from a forward flexed position. An "instability catch" is a sudden movement that occurs out of the plane of the intended motion.[70] For example, the patient may suddenly rotate, side-bend, or both

---

Box 17-5

Key Examination Findings Leading to a Classification of Stabilization

Increasing frequency of episodes of low back pain
More than three previous episodes of low back pain
At least one hypermobile lumbar spine segment
   (judged from lumbar spring testing)
Aberrant movements during lumbar flexion/extension
   active range of motion
Positive prone segmental instability test

From Hicks, G.E. (2002): Predictive Validity of Clinical Variables Used in the Determination of Patient Prognosis Following a Lumbar Stabilization Program [doctoral dissertation]. University of Pittsburgh.

---

while performing flexion. "Thigh climbing" occurs when the patient is attempting to return from a flexed position and uses an external support to assist in extending the spine.[12] Frequently, the patient will be observed to assist spinal extension by pushing on the thighs. A "painful arc" is defined as symptoms occurring during the midrange of a motion that are not present at the beginning or end of the motion.[59] A painful arc may occur in flexion or on return from flexion. Any of these aberrations (instability catch, thigh climbing, or a painful arc) are considered signs of a stabilization classification.

PASSIVE ACCESSORY MOTION TESTING

Passive accessory motion testing was described previously. For the stabilization classification, the clinician is looking for hypermobility at any level of the lumbar spine. The presence of hypermobility is an indication for a classification of stabilization.

PRONE INSTABILITY TEST

The patient lies prone with the trunk on the examining table, legs over the edge, and feet resting on the floor (Fig. 17-10, A and B). While the patient rests in this position, the clinician performs passive accessory motion testing on each level of the lumbar spine. The patient is asked to report any provocation of pain during the motion testing. Next, the patient is asked to lift the legs off the floor (hands holding the table may be used to maintain this position). With the patient holding this position, the motion testing is repeated. The test is positive if a lumbar segment was painful in the resting position but is not painful or the pain is markedly reduced in the leg-lifting position. Lifting the legs causes the spinal extensor muscles to activate, which assists in spinal stabilization. If the prone instability test is positive, a stabilization classification is indicated.[83]

Treatment for the Stabilization Classification

Treatment of patients in the stabilization classification begins with patient education. Education should focus on abstaining from end-range movements of the lumbar spine to avoid positions that may overload the passive stabilizing structures of the spine. Lifting even light loads from a position of near end-range spinal flexion should be avoided because of the potentially damaging forces created in the ligaments and intervertebral disks of the spine by such movements.[84] Though important for anyone with LBP, patients in the stabilization classification need to be educated regarding the importance of maintaining trunk strength and overall endurance. Fatigue can have an adverse impact on the ability of the spinal musculature to respond to imposed loads, which may further compromise the stabilizing structures.[85]

Many exercise programs have been advocated for spinal stabilization. Although the literature supports the usefulness of active strengthening exercise programs, studies comparing different stabilization-strengthening routines have not generally found any differences.[86,87] One approach is to identify exercises that optimally challenge important stabilizing muscles without imposing any potentially dangerous loads on the spine.[52,74] Important stabilizing muscles of the lumbar spine include the abdominal muscles, erector spinae and multifidus, and quadratus lumborum. Basic exercises can be identified to address each of these muscle groups (Fig. 17-11, A to E).

ABDOMINAL MUSCLES AND TRANSVERSUS ABDOMINIS

The muscles of the abdominal wall include the rectus abdominis, external and internal obliques, and transversus abdominis. The primary function of these muscles is flexion and rotation of the trunk.[72] The oblique abdominals have a somewhat horizontal orientation and contribute to spinal stability by increasing the stiffness of the lumbar spine. The oblique abdominals have been shown to cocontract with the spinal extensors during side-bending or extension movements, thereby increasing the stiffness and stability of the torso.[75] The rectus abdominis, because of its midline orientation, is primarily a trunk flexor and is not emphasized during the rehabilitation of patients

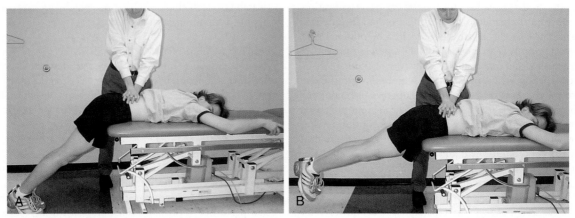

FIGURE 17-10 Prone instability test. **A,** Step 1. With the patient's feet on the floor, the clinician identifies any lumbar segments that are painful with passive motion testing. **B,** Step 2. The patient lifts the legs off the floor and the clinician retests any lumbar segments that were painful in step 1. A positive test result occurs when the pain is substantially reduced or eliminated in step 2.

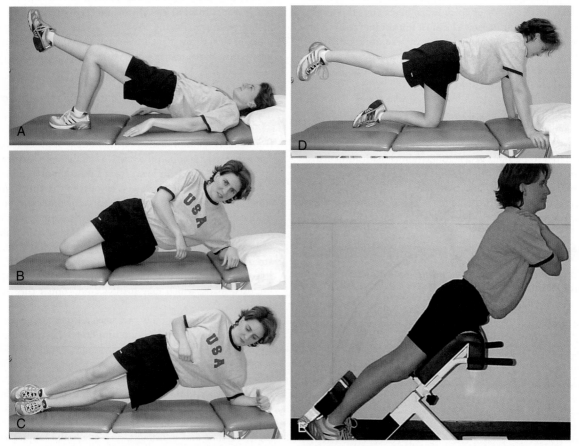

FIGURE 17-11 Stabilization exercise treatment program. **A,** Hollowing while bridging. **B,** Side support with the knees flexed. **C,** Side support with the knees extended. **D,** Quadruped single-leg lift. **E,** Roman chair extension exercise.

with LBP. The transversus abdominis is a deep abdominal muscle with a horizontal orientation that helps stabilize the spine by forming a rigid cylinder. Studies have demonstrated that a feed-forward postural response occurs with transversus abdominis contraction and limb movement.[76,88] In subjects without LBP, the transversus abdominis contracts before extremity movement, theoretically to stabilize the spine in preparation for movement. However, in patients with back pain, the onset of transversus abdominis contraction is delayed.[89] This has led to the hypothesis that the transversus abdominis plays an important role in spinal stabilization.

Training the transversus abdominis may be initiated by teaching the patient the abdominal hollowing maneuver.[90] The patient is instructed to draw the navel up toward the head and in toward the spine so that the stomach flattens but the spine remains in its neutral position. Patients with LBP may have difficulty performing this seemingly simple maneuver. The key to the exercise is to isolate the deep abdominals and avoid substitution with the rectus abdominis. Palpation for muscle contraction by the patient just medial to the ASIS will often provide helpful feedback for proper performance of the exercise. The quadruped position is also useful for learning the hollowing maneuver because substitution with the rectus abdominis may be more difficult in this position.

When the patient can perform the abdominal hollowing maneuver properly, more challenging activities can be added. From the supine position, leg movements (i.e., marching or leg raises) can be incorporated while maintaining the hollowing. Performing bridging exercises while maintaining the hollowing is also a challenge to both the transversus abdominis and gluteus maximus (see Fig. 17-11, *A*). It is recommended that hollowing be combined with other aspects of the stabilization exercise program and eventually be incorporated into more functional positions and postures that would challenge each individual patient in everyday activities. For example, if the patient complains of pain while sitting at work, the hollowing maneuver should be used in that position to control symptoms.

The oblique abdominal muscles can be exercised effectively with the horizontal side support exercise. This exercise produces high levels of activity in the oblique abdominals (50% maximum voluntary contraction [MVC]) with low compressive force.[91] To perform the horizontal side support, the patient is a side-lying position with the knees bent and upper part of the body supported on the lower portion of the elbow. The patient then lifts the pelvis from the table (see Fig. 17-11, *B* and *C*). The side support should be performed on both sides to achieve balance of strength. If a patient has unilateral low back symptoms, it may be more difficult for the patient to perform the exercise on the symptomatic side. The patient should perform the side support exercise for progressively longer sustained periods and with more repetitions. If asymmetry exists, the goal should be to achieve equality in strength and endurance between the left and right sides. The side support exercise can also be progressed by extending the knees and using the ankles as the distal contact instead of the knees.

Performing curl-ups with rotation of the torso has also been found to target the oblique abdominals while imposing relatively low compressive loads.[91] Performing curl-ups without any trunk rotation will target mostly the rectus abdominis muscle and is therefore less useful in the rehabilitation process. The position

of the legs during the curl-up does not appear to affect muscle activity or compression on the spine.[91] A more challenging exercise for the oblique abdominals is a hanging straight leg raise. To perform this exercise, the patient is hanging with body weight supported by the upper extremities. The legs are lifted to the horizontal position (90° of hip flexion). This exercise provides high levels of oblique abdominal activity (nearly 100% MVC) while producing low levels of compressive force on the spine.[91]

ERECTOR SPINAE AND MULTIFIDUS

Strengthening of the erector spinae muscles may be important because they are the primary source of extension torque for lifting tasks.[71] The lumbar extensors can be divided into two groups: the multisegmental erector spinae muscles that attach to the thoracic spine and the pelvis, with most fibers spanning the lumbar region without any attachment, and the segmental extensors, which attach to individual lumbar vertebrae.[92,93] The erector spinae muscles produce the extensor force needed for lifting, whereas the segmental extensors, primarily the multifidus muscle, provide stabilization of individual lumbar motion segments.[73,94] The multifidi originate from the spinous processes of the lumbar vertebrae and form a series of repeating fascicles attaching to the lumbar transverse processes below, as well as to the ilium and sacrum. The multifidus is proposed to function as a segmental stabilizer during both lifting and rotational movements. Current evidence suggests that decreased endurance of the multifidus and erector spinae muscles may be a risk factor for recurrence of LBP.[95] Research has also shown that the multifidi do not automatically recover full strength and endurance after the first episode of LBP unless specific exercises are performed.[96] These findings emphasize the need for clinicians to focus attention on rehabilitation of the extensor musculature, with a particular focus on regaining endurance.

The erector spinae and multifidus muscles can be trained by performing extension exercises. Caution must be exercised, however, because extension exercises also tend to produce high levels of compression on the lumbar spine, which may not be tolerated by all patients.[97] The safest position to begin an extension exercise program is a quadruped one. While in the quadruped position, the patient is asked to extend one leg or one arm to a horizontal position while maintaining the abdominal hollowing (see Fig. 17-11, *D*). Raising the opposite arm and leg simultaneously offers more efficient training of the multifidus and erector spinae with muscle activity levels in the realm of 30% MVC while maintaining safe levels of lumbar compression.[98] Abdominal hollowing should be maintained while performing quadruped extension exercises to stabilize the spine in a neutral position, with avoidance of flexion or extension.

Extension exercises can be progressed to the prone position and performed dynamically instead of statically when a greater challenge to the extensor muscles is desired, which is often true for athletes. From a prone lying position, the patient is asked to raise the trunk and legs off the table while keeping the pelvis in contact. Alternatively, the patient may perform active extension using a Roman chair to vary the angle of extension (see Fig. 17-11, *E*).[99] For these exercises the patient's legs are fixed and the trunk is unsupported. The patient flexes the trunk forward and then extends against gravity to return to the starting position. These exercises produce high levels of activity in the erector spinae and multifidus muscles (40% to 60% MVC); however, compressive loads on the lumbar spine are greater than when the quadruped position is used and may not be tolerated early in rehabilitation.[52] The use of prone extension exercises as described should be limited to patients who are hopeful of returning to athletic competition or demanding work activities and who can tolerate the compressive force produced by such exercises. Quadruped exercises will be sufficient for the majority of patients, for whom the emphasis of retraining will be on endurance and high levels of MVC are not required.

QUADRATUS LUMBORUM

The quadratus lumborum appears to play a key role in stabilization of the spine during side-bending movements in the frontal plane or during compression of the spine. When compression is applied to the spine in an upright position, the activity of the quadratus lumborum most closely correlates with the increased need for stability because of compressive loads.[74] The horizontal side support exercise described previously produces the greatest muscle activity in the quadratus lumborum (54% MVC) with low compressive loads. The horizontal side support exercise effectively targets both the oblique abdominals and the quadratus lumborum and is a key component in a stabilization exercise program.

Clinical Pearl #3

The horizontal side support exercise promotes high levels of activity in the oblique abdominal and quadratus lumborum muscles while placing low compressive loads on the spine. This exercise is quite useful for patients in the stabilization classification and for those who have progressed to stage II management.

Specific Exercise Classifications

The important clinical characteristic of patients in stage I likely to benefit from specific exercise routines is the presence of the centralization phenomenon. Centralization was originally described by McKenzie[100] as a phenomenon occurring during lumbar movement testing when the patient reports that the pain moves from an area more distal or lateral to a location more central or near the midline position in the lumbar spine. Peripheralization occurs when the patient reports movement of pain from an area more proximal in the lumbar spine to an area more distal or lateral. Movements that do not produce centralization or peripheralization are judged to be status quo.[43,100]

The centralization phenomenon is an important finding in patients with LBP. Patients with LBP, particularly those with radiation to the buttock, thigh, or calf, who do not exhibit centralization are less likely to have a successful treatment outcome.[101,102] Long[103] studied patients with chronic LBP entering a work-hardening program and found that the presence of centralization during the initial evaluation was associated with greater reductions in pain and higher percentages of return to work after completion of the program. Karas et al[104] found that an inability to centralize symptoms during the initial evaluation decreased the likelihood of return to work within 6 months.

The presence of centralization has also been proposed to be an important finding for classifying patients into treatment-based subgroups.[12,100] When patients are found to centralize during

the examination, the movements producing centralization are then used as treatment techniques. Three different movements are typically found to centralize symptoms: extension, flexion, or pelvic translocations for a patient with a lateral shift. The three subgroups of patients in the specific exercise classification are defined by which movement is found to produce centralization.

Other examination factors are also used to make a classification of specific exercise. Patients who centralize with extension and fit an extension classification often have signs and symptoms consistent with intervertebral disk herniation. These patients will probably report that standing or walking is preferable to sitting and that sitting tolerance may be limited to less than a few minutes. These patients are also likely to report symptoms that extend into the buttock or lower extremity, or both, and may have signs of nerve root compression.

Patients fitting a flexion classification frequently report a clear preference for sitting versus standing or walking, and they may not have any symptoms at all when sitting.[105,106] Patients who centralize with flexion tend to be somewhat older and often have degenerative or stenotic spinal conditions.[13] Spinal stenosis causes narrowing of the spinal canal. This narrowing is exacerbated with spinal extension and is relieved with spinal flexion.[107] Patients with spinal stenosis will therefore often be found to centralize with flexion movements and peripheralize with extension movements. Neurogenic claudication, defined as poorly localized pain, paresthesias, and cramping of one or both lower extremities of a neurologic origin that is brought on by walking and relieved when sitting,[108] frequently occurs with lumbar spinal stenosis.[2] Signs of nerve root compression may also be present on examination.

Patients fitting a lateral shift classification usually have a visible lateral shift deformity. A lateral shift deformity can be defined as shifting of the patient's trunk and shoulders relative to the pelvis in the frontal plane.[109] Patients with a lateral shift will most often have symptoms in the lower extremity and signs of nerve root compression.[12] Lumbar intervertebral disk pathology is also common in patients fitting a lateral shift classification.[110] On examination, patients fitting a lateral shift classification will typically have substantially asymmetric side-bending ROM, with gross limitation of side-bending ROM in the direction opposite the lateral shift.[111]

Examination for the Specific Exercise Classifications

The portion of the physical examination most central to the specific exercise classifications is the active motion assessment. The focus of active movement testing is not ROM, but rather the response of symptoms to movement (i.e., centralization or peripheralization). In addition, neurologic assessment for signs of nerve root compression is often required for patients fitting specific exercise classifications because distal symptoms are common.

LUMBAR ACTIVE MOTION ASSESSMENT: CENTRALIZATION/PERIPHERALIZATION

Lumbar motion assessment begins with testing side bending, flexion, and extension with the patient standing. For the purpose of detecting centralization/peripheralization, it is important to establish the baseline symptoms of the patient before any movements. The patient is asked to explain the symptoms experienced before motion testing in terms of both location and intensity and instructed to report any change in these factors that occurs with testing. The patient is then asked to side-bend to the left and right, extend backward, and flex forward. After each movement the patient is asked about the effect of the movement on the symptoms. If the symptoms are abolished or move centrally, centralization has occurred. If the symptoms fluctuate in intensity but do not centralize, the patient is judged to be status quo with respect to that movement. If the symptoms move peripherally, away from the spine, the patient is judged to have peripheralized with the movement. Any movement producing centralization is noted. This movement will be used as the basis for the patient's specific exercise program. Any movement causing peripheralization is also noted, and these movements are avoided in further motion assessment and treatment procedures.

For patients with a visible lateral shift deformity, pelvic translocation movements are also assessed with the patient standing. The clinician stands at the patient's side, on the same side toward which the patient has shifted. The clinician then stabilizes the patient's shoulders and trunk with his or her body and translates the pelvis in the frontal plane in the direction that corrects the shift. For example, if the patient had a right lateral shift deformity, the clinician would stand on the patient's right side and translate the patient's pelvis to the right (i.e., right pelvic translocation). The status of the patient's symptoms with this movement is judged to be either centralized, peripheralized, or status quo.

If single movements produce centralization, these movements will form the basis for the patient's classification and treatment. If single movements cause peripheralization, these movements are avoided. However, many patients will remain status quo with single-movement testing performed with the patient standing. If the patient's history suggests a specific exercise classification but single movements while standing are judged to be status quo, further movement testing may be performed. The clinical decision-making scheme for movement testing is pictured in Figure 17-12. Further movement testing may be accomplished by changing the patient's position, performing repeated movements, or sustaining the end-range movement position. Spinal flexion or extension, or both, may be assessed in the seated, supine, prone, or quadruped positions, as well as in the standing position. The quadruped position is particularly useful for evaluation because both flexion and extension can be assessed by having the patient rock back and forth and the position decreases weight-bearing stress on the spine. The movement tests in any position can be repeated 5 to 10 times consecutively or can be sustained for 20 to 30 seconds. After each test the patient is questioned regarding its impact on symptoms, and the same judgments are made: centralization, peripheralization, or status quo. If centralization occurs with flexion, extension, or lateral shifts with any movement testing, the patient is assigned to the corresponding specific exercise classification. Box 17-6 summarizes the key examination findings leading to a classification of specific exercises.

Treatment for the Specific Exercise Classifications

The basic principle for treating patients with a specific exercise classification is to use the motions that were found to produce centralization on examination as interventions. The overall goal of interventions is to produce lasting centralization of symptoms and permit the patient to progress to later stages of treatment.

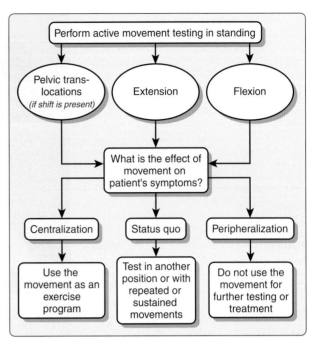

FIGURE 17-12 Decision making with lumbar active movement testing.

Box 17-6

Key Examination Findings Leading to a Classification of Specific Exercise

Centralization during active lumbar movement assessment
Symptoms distal to the knee
Signs of nerve root compression
Clear preference for flexed or extended postures (sitting vs. standing/walking)
Visible lateral shift deformity

TREATMENT FOR THE FLEXION CLASSIFICATION

Exercises to Promote Flexion Flexion exercises are usually easiest to perform in the supine or quadruped position. Patients fitting a flexion classification will frequently find the position of supine with the hips and knees flexed (i.e., the "hook-lying position") to be a comfortable position from which to exercise and therefore a good place to begin a program. From this position, the patient may bring a single knee or both knees to the chest to create further flexion of the lumbar spine. The knee-to-chest position can be sustained for 20 to 30 seconds and repeated. Another simple flexion exercise to perform from this position is a posterior pelvic tilt. The patient is instructed to flatten the back against the support surface to reduce lumbar lordosis and increase lumbar flexion. The quadruped position is also a useful position for performing flexion exercises. From the quadruped position, the patient can move from the neutral position back onto the heels to promote lumbar flexion (Fig. 17-13, A). This motion can be repeated as a gentle rocking movement from neutral into lumbar flexion.

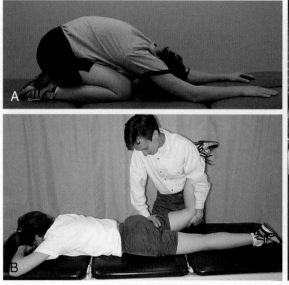
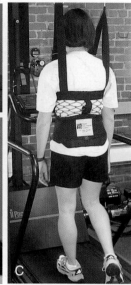

FIGURE 17-13 Treatment for the flexion-specific exercise classification. **A,** Quadruped flexion exercise. **B,** Hip extension mobilization. **C,** Deweighted ambulation.

Mobilizations to Promote Flexion Joint mobilization can serve as a useful adjunctive treatment for patients fitting a flexion classification. Because patients in this classification tend to be older with degenerative changes, stiffness of the lumbar spine and hip joints is not uncommon. If stiffness is detected in the lumbar spine with passive accessory mobility testing, mobilizations may be performed. Several techniques may be used. Prone posterior-to-anterior mobilization is useful for many patients. The patient is prone and then positioned with the lumbar spine in flexion. This may be accomplished either by positioning the table into flexion or by using pillows under the patient's abdomen. The clinician contacts the lumbar spinous process to be mobilized with the hypothenar eminence of the hand. An oscillatory mobilization force is produced through the clinician's trunk while the elbows are maintained in extension[112].

Mobilization or flexibility exercises, or both, for the hip joints are often indicated for patients fitting a flexion classification. If hip joint mobility is limited, particularly hip joint extension, an increased demand for extension ROM in the lumbar spine may be created. Patients fitting a flexion classification often cannot tolerate lumbar extension; therefore, improving mobility of the hip joints may help reduce stress on the lumbar spine. Stretching techniques for the hip joint flexor muscles (i.e., iliopsoas, rectus femoris, and tensor fasciae latae) may be used. Mobilization of the hip joint to improve extension ROM is indicated when hypomobility of the joint is detected. Mobilization to improve hip joint extension is performed with the patient prone. A posterior-to-anterior mobilization force is directed to the proximal end of the femur. The angle of hip extension can be increased for further progression of the mobilization technique (see Fig. 17-13, *B*).

Deweighted Treadmill Ambulation Patients fitting a flexion classification often have substantial limitations in walking tolerance[110]; therefore, addressing this functional limitation is an important goal of treatment. The limitation in walking in these patients is at least partly caused by the narrowing of the spinal canal that results from the axial loading and extension that occur during walking.[113] Deweighted treadmill ambulation uses harness support to provide a vertical traction force and thereby reduce axial loading during walking (see Fig. 17-13, *C*). Flynn et al[114] found an average 24% reduction in vertical ground reaction forces during walking with 20% of the body's weight supported. Training with deweighted treadmill ambulation is begun with sufficient traction force to reduce or abolish the patient's lower extremity symptoms while walking. Usually, a traction force equal to 20% to 40% of the patient's body weight is sufficient to accomplish this goal.[45] Over the course of treatment, the amount of walking time is gradually increased while the amount of traction force is gradually diminished.

TREATMENT FOR THE EXTENSION CLASSIFICATION

Exercises to Promote Extension Extension exercises can be performed in a variety of ways. Quadruped is usually a comfortable position for beginning an extension exercise program. Extension is achieved by having the patient rock forward over the arms and then returning to the starting position. This gentle rocking motion is repeated 10 to 20 times. The patient should not rock back into flexion at this stage of treatment. Another basic activity that may be useful early in treatment is having the patient lie prone. Lying prone promotes extension of the lumbar spine. The prone position is sustained for 30 seconds up to a few minutes. With all exercises the response of the patient's symptoms is the key to determining their effectiveness. Exercises that help centralize the patient's pain are continued; those that do not are modified or discarded. A transient increase in central LBP may initially occur with extension exercises. An exercise should not be discontinued if centralization is being achieved but central LBP is increased.

After the patient is comfortable with the basic extension activities, the treatment program may be progressed to include having the patient prop onto the elbows while lying prone. This position is held for 15 to 30 seconds and repeated several times. The patient will need to be able to keep the extensor musculature relaxed in this position and maintain the pelvis in contact with the support surface. Propping on elbows can be progressed to prone press-ups, in which the patient extends the elbows to lift the upper part of the body while the pelvis remains in contact with the support surface. This exercise is repeated 10 to 20 times, depending on the patient's upper body strength

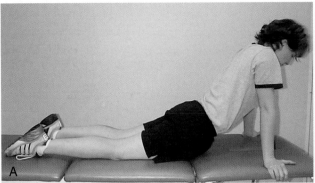
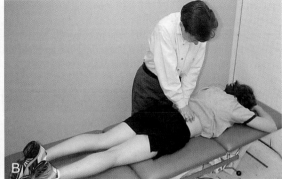

FIGURE 17-14 Treatment for the extension-specific exercise classification. **A,** Prone press-up. **B,** Lumbar mobilization in the prone lying position.

(Fig. 17-14, *A*). It is important to realize that prone press-ups are a more aggressive form of extension exercises that have been shown to require substantial amounts of spinal extensor muscle activity.[115] This muscle activity may not be tolerated by all patients, particularly early in the course of treatment.

Motions that produce peripheralization of symptoms should be avoided during the initial stage of treatment. The motion most often of concern is lumbar flexion. The lumbar flexion exercises described in the previous section should be avoided until the patient has progressed with treatment. Patients whose status worsens rapidly with spinal flexion may need to wear a brace to prevent flexion during the initial stages of treatment.

Mobilization to Promote Extension Patients in an extension classification may also benefit from mobilization procedures that are designed to promote lumbar extension. Although these procedures are passive, they may help the patient gain more benefit from active extension activities and are therefore often a useful adjunct to an extension exercise program. Mobilization is performed with the patient prone. The clinician contacts the lumbar spinous process to be mobilized with the hypothenar eminence of the hand. An oscillatory mobilization force is produced through the clinician's trunk while the elbows are maintained in extension (see Fig. 17-14, *B*). The patient may be progressively positioned into more extension by having the patient prop onto the elbows or perform a prone press-up while the mobilization is delivered.

TREATMENT FOR THE LATERAL SHIFT CLASSIFICATION

Patients with a lateral shift who are able to centralize their symptoms on pelvic translocation movement testing while standing are treated with weight-bearing shift correction exercises. The patient is taught to perform the pelvic translocation movement in the direction that produced the centralization. It is important that the patient be taught to translate the pelvis in the frontal plane and not to simply side-bend the trunk. This instruction can be facilitated by having the patient stand in a door frame and use the forearms to stabilize the trunk (Fig. 17-15, *A*). The patient is then instructed to perform the pelvic translocation in the appropriate direction. When the patient's lateral shift is diminished, the next goal is frequently to restore extension ROM. The doorway shift correction exercises can be progressed by having the patient perform lumbar extension along with the pelvic translocation, as long as this combination does not create

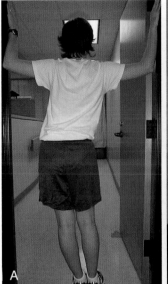
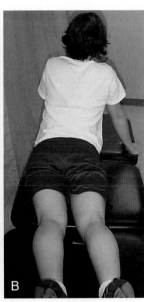

FIGURE 17-15 A, Standing shift correction exercises. The patient stands in a door frame to brace the trunk and prevent lumbar side bending. The pelvis is shifted in the direction that corrects the lateral shift and centralizes the symptoms. **B,** Prone shift correction exercises. The patient is prone and the pelvis is positioned to correct the lateral shift. The patient may perform prone on elbows or prone press-up exercises while maintaining the pelvis in the corrected position.

any peripheralization of symptoms. The exercises to promote extension described earlier may also be helpful once the visible shift has been reduced.

If the patient is unable to achieve centralization of symptoms with standing pelvic translocation movements, two options exist. One would be to treat a patient in the traction classification via autotraction (see the discussion of traction classification later in this chapter). The second option would be to position the patient prone and then gradually work to restore lumbar extension. The magnitude of a patient's lateral shift is typically reduced substantially when not bearing weight; therefore, the patient may be able to effectively centralize symptoms with a prone progression of extension exercises. It may begin by merely lying prone with the pelvis passively moved into translocation to correct the lateral shift (see Fig. 17-15, B). This may be progressed to prone on elbows and prone press-ups as tolerated by the patient. Although these exercises may be effective in centralizing symptoms while the patient is prone, when a weight-bearing position is assumed, the symptoms often return rapidly.

Clinical Pearl #4

A patient with a visible lateral shift who is unable to centralize symptoms with standing pelvic translocations will often benefit from treatment in the traction classification with autotraction. After two to three autotraction treatments, it is likely that the patient will be able to centralize symptoms with standing pelvic translocations.

Traction Classification

The use of traction has not been supported by research, and it is not generally recommended for patients with LBP.[51,116] Studies that have shown no benefit in using traction have not sought to identify patients who are most likely to benefit from the intervention but instead have used nonspecific inclusion criteria that essentially include all patients fitting a broad definition of "acute" or "chronic."[117,118] The results of these studies should be interpreted to indicate that traction should not be a widely used intervention for patients with LBP. There does, however, appear to be a small subgroup of patients with LBP who may benefit from traction.[13]

Examination for the Traction Classification

Patients fitting a traction classification will most likely have symptoms that extend into the lower extremity, often distal to the knee. Signs of nerve root compression are frequently present, and the patient may have diagnostic imaging that shows herniation of a disk. The key examination finding that indicates a traction classification is an inability to centralize symptoms with any active movement testing, including repeated, sustained movements, or with movements in an alternative posture. Because of the evidence against the use of traction, clinicians should exhaust all movement-testing options before placing a patient in a traction classification. A trial of specific exercise interventions may even be attempted before using a traction intervention.

Treatment for the Traction Classification

Traction treatment can be delivered by using pelvic traction devices or autotraction. In general, autotraction devices are preferred when available because the intervention is more active, and they can be made more specific to the patient because the table can be positioned. Mechanical traction may be performed with the patient either prone or supine. If the patient is supine, flexing the hips and knees will tend to place the lumbar spine in more flexion and may be better tolerated by older patients with imaging findings suggesting lumbar spinal stenosis. The goal of treatment with mechanical traction is to centralize the patient's symptoms and permit the patient to progress to another classification, such as specific exercise. Patients in the traction classification should be monitored closely. If reassessment shows that the patient is able to centralize symptoms with active movements, progression to a specific exercise classification would be indicated. If the patient's symptoms and signs of nerve root

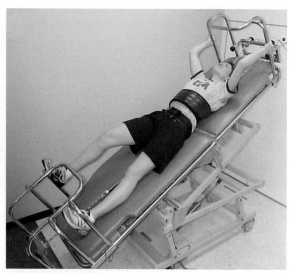

FIGURE 17-16 Autotraction treatment for the traction classification. The patient produces the traction force by pulling with the arms and pushing with the legs.

compression continue to worsen, referral for surgery, injections, or other treatment options is warranted.

Treatment with autotraction may be preferred over mechanical traction for patients in the traction classification. Autotraction is particularly indicated for patients with a lateral shift deformity who are unable to centralize symptoms or who actually experience peripheralization of symptoms with pelvic translocation. Autotraction involves the use of a specially designed table that allows the patient to be positioned in a variety of ways. The patient is initially positioned in a manner that centralizes symptoms to the greatest extent possible. For patients with a lateral shift, this is most often accomplished by having the patient lie supine with lumbar flexion or lie on the side opposite the direction of the shift. After positioning the patient, the table can be elevated and the patient asked to produce the traction force by pulling with the arms and pushing with one or both feet (Fig. 17-16). As the patient is producing the traction force, the table can gradually be repositioned to move the patient away from the accommodated position into a more neutral posture.

STAGE II MANAGEMENT

The goal of stage I management, regardless of the classification, is to reduce pain and disability and advance the patient to stage II treatment. The goals for management of patients with LBP in stage II are more focused on improving functional abilities and addressing any impairments in strength or flexibility that can be identified. Another goal of stage II management is to reduce the likelihood of the patient experiencing a recurrence of LBP. Rates of recurrence are reported to be as high as 60% to 80%.[119,120] The stage II treatment approach has three basic components: specific trunk strengthening, general strength and flexibility exercises, and aerobic conditioning.

Specific Trunk Strengthening

Some evidence suggests that failure to regain strength of the important trunk-stabilizing muscles may increase the risk for poor recovery from LBP or for recurrence of an episode of LBP.[121,122]

Hides et al[96] have shown that a program of trunk-strengthening and stabilization exercises can reduce the likelihood of recurrence after an episode of LBP. If patients did not receive specific trunk-strengthening exercises as part of stage I treatment, those exercises should be initiated once the patient moves into stage II. Strengthening exercises for the abdominal muscles, erector spinae and multifidus, and quadratus lumborum should be used as previously described (see Fig. 17-11, *A* to *E*).

Clinical Pearl #5

Adequate strength of the trunk-stabilizing muscles may be an important factor in preventing the recurrence of LBP. When a patient reaches stage II, specific stabilizing exercises should be initiated if not done already.

General Strength and Flexibility Exercises

In addition to training the stabilizing muscles of the trunk, the clinician may also need to focus a portion of the stage II rehabilitation program on some of the large muscle groups of the lower extremities. This is particularly important when a patient is having difficulty performing lifting tasks. Current theory suggests that the proper way to perform a lifting task is to lift from a squatted position and flex the hips and knees while minimizing flexion of the lumbar spine.[98] When lumbar flexion predominates in a lifting task, the risk for injury is increased. To lift from a squatted position, an individual must have adequate strength and endurance of the gluteus maximus and quadriceps muscle groups in particular. If the gluteus maximus and quadriceps are deconditioned, correct lifting may not be performed and the risk for recurrence of LBP may be increased. The gluteus maximus in particular is often weak in individuals with chronic LBP and has been found to be more fatigable than those in healthy individuals.[123] Strengthening of the gluteus maximus can be achieved with bridging exercises or quadruped single-leg extension exercises with the knee flexed to reduce the contribution of the hamstring muscles. It has also been reported that performance of balance exercises in the standing position may improve the strength and timing of gluteus maximus contractions.[124] Performance of squatting exercises will incorporate both the quadriceps and gluteus maximus muscles.[125]

Although a link between lower extremity flexibility and LBP is often assumed, research has not shown this to be the case.[126] A few studies have suggested a relationship between flexibility of the hamstring and hip flexor muscles and LBP, particularly in adolescents.[127,128] Stretching of these muscle groups may be important for some patients during stage II treatment. Flexibility of the hamstring muscles can be assessed with the straight leg raise test described earlier. Hip flexor flexibility is best evaluated by using the Thomas test (see Greenman,[63] pp. 462–464). Caution may need to be exercised when instructing a patient with LBP in proper stretching techniques. When stretching the hamstrings, the patient should be instructed to avoid excessive lumbar flexion. This may be accomplished by instructing the patient to maintain a neutral to slightly lordotic lumbar spine while stretching or by using the supine position for stretching. The best position for stretching the hip flexors while avoiding undue stress on the lumbar spine is often a kneeling position.

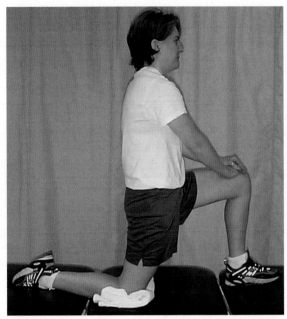

FIGURE 17-17 Kneeling hip flexor stretch for stage II. To stretch the right hip flexor, the patient is instructed to kneel on the right knee and then perform a posterior pelvic tilt to produce hip extension. Extension of the lumbar spine should be avoided.

The patient kneels on the side to be stretched and is taught to perform a posterior tilt of the pelvis to stretch the hip flexors, particularly the iliopsoas (Fig. 17-17). Careful instruction may be required to ensure that the patient is able to achieve the stretch with a posterior tilt of the pelvis and not by extending the lumbar spine. Placing the hip in slight adduction will place greater emphasis on the iliotibial band.

Aerobic Exercises

Increased levels of aerobic fitness have been linked to a decreased incidence of low back injury and may help avoid recurrence.[129] Evidence also suggests that low-stress aerobic exercise may be effective in the treatment of patients with acute or chronic LBP.[51,116] An aerobic exercise component should be incorporated into all stage II treatment programs. The particular aerobic activity used depends on the preferences and tolerance of the individual patient. Walking results in low levels of compression on the lumbar spine and is well tolerated by most patients in stage II. Because walking also requires constant, submaximal effort from the stabilizing muscles of the trunk while placing low compressive loads on the spine,[52] it is an effective aerobic exercise for patient with LBP who have progressed to stage II treatment. Progressive walking programs can generally be initiated early in the rehabilitation process and can be progressed as the patient's tolerance of activity increases.

Not all patients with LBP, even those in stage II treatment, will be able to tolerate walking as an aerobic activity. Walking places the lumbar spine in a more extended position, and this position may not be tolerated for prolonged periods by all patients. These patients may be better suited to stationary cycling as an aerobic exercise. Another option for aerobic activity in patients who experience an increase in symptoms while walking is the use of aquatic exercise. Having the patient walk while in a pool permits the buoyancy of the water to reduce the compressive force of gravity (see Chapter 11). This usually allows a patient to walk without any increase in symptoms. The depth of the water will correspond to the amount of reduction in compression. Exercise progression can therefore be achieved by having the patient walk in progressively shallower water until the patient can tolerate walking out of the water without any increase in symptoms.

Deweighted treadmill ambulation may also be an option for patients who do not tolerate regular walking because of increased symptoms. As described earlier, deweighted treadmill walking uses a traction harness system to decrease the weight that the body must support during walking, thereby reducing compressive force on the lumbar spine and probably reducing the symptoms experienced when walking. When beginning an aerobic exercise program consisting of deweighted treadmill ambulation, the clinician should use sufficient traction force to permit the patient to walk without any increase in symptoms. The amount of traction force can then be gradually reduced over the course of treatment until the patient is able to walk without any external support or increase in symptoms.

Another popular and effective aerobic exercise is jogging or running. Running has not been associated with an increased risk for the development of LBP, and running has actually been found to place participants at lower risk for degenerative changes in the lumbar intervertebral disks than has participation in other activities such as soccer or weight lifting.[130] Running has been found to create increased compressive load on the lumbar spine[112] and may therefore not be tolerated by some patients in stage II rehabilitation after an episode of LBP. If return to running is a goal of a patient, caution should be exercised and gradual return emphasized. If a patient experiences difficulty returning, use of a deweighting device to reduce compression along with running on a treadmill may be helpful.

CONCLUSION

Background

- LBP is a common occurrence that results in substantial pain and disability.
- It is frequently not possible to identify the underlying cause of LBP.
- Classification systems seek to group patients on the basis of clusters of signs and symptoms found on examination instead of seeking to identify the underlying cause.
- Each classification category has a specific treatment approach associated with it that is believed to be most effective for patients in that category.

Assessing for Red and Yellow Flags: First-Level Classification

- Red flags are findings that may indicate a serious underlying pathology.
- Clinicians should be aware of red flags for conditions such as fracture, cancer, cauda equina syndrome, and others that would warrant referral to a physician.
- Yellow flags are findings indicating that the patient may be at risk for prolonged disability because of psychosocial factors.

- The most important psychosocial factor for patients with LBP is fear-avoidance beliefs.
- Patients with high levels of fear-avoidance beliefs should be treated with active interventions with an emphasis on functional ability rather than pain.

Staging the Patient: Second-Level Classification

- Staging is not based strictly on acuity but also on the signs and symptoms of the patient and the goals for rehabilitation.
- Patients in stage I have high levels of disability and difficulty performing basic daily activities. The goals for rehabilitation are to reduce symptoms and progress to stage II.
- Patients in stage II have lower levels of disability but difficulty performing more complex tasks. The goals for rehabilitation are to resume full functioning and prevent recurrence.

Determining the Best Treatment Approach: Third-Level Classification

- Information from the medical history and physical examination is used to classify the patient.
- For patients in stage I, four classifications exist: manipulation/mobilization, specific exercise, stabilization, and traction.
- Patients in the manipulation/mobilization classification tend to have a more recent onset of symptoms, stiffness in the spine, and no symptoms distal to the knee. Interventions include manipulation and mobilization techniques and ROM exercises.
- Patients in the stabilization classification tend to have frequent previous episodes that are increasing in frequency, hypermobility in the spine, and a positive prone instability test result. Interventions include strengthening exercises for the trunk-stabilizing muscles.
- Patients in the specific exercise classification are characterized by the presence of centralization during lumbar ROM testing. Interventions involve repeated end-range exercises in the direction that produces the centralization (flexion, extension, or lateral shift).
- Patients in the traction classification tend to have signs of nerve root compression and do not centralize with lumbar ROM testing. Interventions include mechanical traction and autotraction.
- Interventions for patients in stage II focus on eliminating impairments in trunk strength, lower extremity strength, and flexibility and on achieving aerobic conditioning.

REFERENCES

1. Nachemson, A.L. (1985): Advances in low back pain. Clin. Orthop. Relat. Res., 200:266–278.
2. Turner, J.A., Ersek, M., Herron, L., and Deyo, R. (1992): Surgery for lumbar spinal stenosis. Attempted meta-analysis of the literature. Spine, 17:1–8.
3. Waddell, G. (1987): A new clinical model for the treatment of low back pain. Spine, 12:632–639.
4. Cypress, B.K. (1983): Characteristics of physician visits for back symptoms: A national perspective. Am. J. Public Health, 73:389.
5. Goldstein, J.D., Berger, P.E., Windler, G.E., and Jackson, J.W. (1991): Spine injuries in gymnasts and swimmers. An epidemiologic investigation. Am. J. Sports Med., 19:463–468.
6. Hutchinson, M.R., Laprade, R.F., Burnett, Q.M., et al. (1995): Injury surveillance at the USTA Boys' Tennis Championships: A 6-yr study. Med. Sci. Sports Exerc., 27:826–830.

7. NCAA. (1998): NCAA Injury Surveillance System (1997–1998). Overland Park, KS, National Collegiate Athletic Association.

8. Sands, W.A., Shultz, B.B., and Newman, A.P. (1993): Women's gymnastics injuries. A 5-year study. Am. J. Sports Med., 21:271–276.

9. Thompson, N., Halpern, B., Curl, W.W., et al. (1987): High school football injuries: Evaluation. Am. J. Sports Med., 15:117–124.

10. Sikorski, J.M. (1985): A rationalized approach to physiotherapy for low back pain. Spine, 10:571–578.

11. Valkenburg, H.A., and Haanen, H.C.M. (1982): The epidemiology of low back pain. In White, A.A., and Gordon, S. (eds.): American Academy of Orthopedic Surgeons Symposium on Low Back Pain. St. Louis, Mosby, pp. 9–22.

12. Delitto, A., Erhard, R.E., and Bowling, R.W. (1995): A treatment-based classification approach to low back syndrome: Identifying and staging patients for conservative treatment. Phys. Ther., 75:470–489.

13. Fritz, J.M., and George, S. (2000): The use of a classification approach to identify subgroups of patients with acute low back pain: Inter-rater reliability and short-term treatment outcomes. Spine, 25:106–114.

14. Jarvik, J.G., and Deyo, R.A. (2002): Diagnostic evaluation of low back pain with emphasis on imaging. Ann. Intern. Med., 137:586–597.

15. Shah, M.K., and Stewart, G.W. (2002): Sacral stress fractures: An unusual cause of low back pain in an athlete. Spine, 27:E104–E108.

16. Wiltse, L.L., Newman, P.H., and Macnab, I. (1976): Classification of spondylolysis and spondylolisthesis. Clin. Orthop. Relat. Res., 117:23–29.

17. Soler, T., and Calderon, C. (2000): The prevalence of spondylolysis in the Spanish elite athlete. Am. J. Sports Med., 28:57–62.

18. Standaert, C.J., and Herring, S.A. (2000): Spondylolysis: A critical review. Br. J. Sports Med., 34:415–422.

19. Fredrickson, B.E., Baker, D., McHolick, W.J., et al. (1984): The natural history of spondylolysis and spondylolisthesis. J. Bone Joint Surg. Am., 66:699–707.

20. Micheli, L.J., and Wood, R. (1995): Back pain in young athletes: Significant differences from adults in causes and patterns. Arch. Pediatr. Adolesc. Med., 149:15–18.

21. Deyo, R.A., and Diehl, A.K. (1988): Cancer as a cause of back pain: Frequency, clinical presentation, and diagnostic strategies. J. Gen. Intern. Med., 3:230–238.

22. van Tulder, M.W., Assendelft, W.J., Koes, B.W., and Bouter, L.M. (1997): Spinal radiographic findings and nonspecific low back pain. A systematic review of observational studies. Spine, 22:427–434.

23. Waldvogel, F.A., and Papageorgiou, P.S. (1980): Osteomyelitis: The past decade. N. Engl. J. Med., 303:360–370.

24. Calin, A., Porta, J., Fries, J.F., and Schurman, D.J. (1977): Clinical history as a screening tool for ankylosing spondylitis. JAMA, 237:2613–2614.

25. Gran, J.T. (1985): An epidemiological survey of the signs and symptoms of ankylosing spondylitis. Clin. Rheumatol., 4:161–169.

26. Deyo, R.A., Rainville, J., and Kent, D. (1992): What can the history and physical examination tell us about low back pain? JAMA, 268:760–765.

27. Thomas, E., Silman, A.J., Croft, P.R., et al. (1999): Predicting who develops chronic low back pain in primary care: A prospective study. BMJ, 318:1662–1667.

28. Fritz, J.M., George, S.Z., and Delitto, A. (2001): The role of fear avoidance beliefs in acute low back pain: Relationships with current and future disability and work status. Pain, 94:7–15.

29. Macfarlane, G.J., Thomas, E., Croft, P.R., et al. (1999): Predictors of early improvement in low back pain amongst consulters to general practice: The influence of pre-morbid and episode-related factors. Pain, 80:113–119.

30. Pincus, T., Vlaeyen, J.W., Kendall, N.A., et al. (2002): Cognitive-behavioral therapy and psychosocial factors in low back pain. Spine, 27:E133–E138.

31. Fritz, J.M., and George, S.Z. (2002): Identifying specific psychosocial factors in patients with acute, work-related low back pain: The importance of fear-avoidance beliefs. Phys. Ther., 82:973–983.

32. Waddell, G., Newton, M., Henderson, I., et al. (1993): A Fear-Avoidance Beliefs Questionnaire (FABQ) and the role of fear-avoidance beliefs in chronic low back pain and disability. Pain, 52:157–168.

33. Lethem, J., Slade, P.D., Troup, J.D.G., and Bentley, G. (1983): Outline of a fear avoidance model of exaggerated pain perception—I. Behav. Res. Ther., 21:401–408.

34. Slade, P.D., Troup, J.D.G., Lethem, J., and Bentley, G. (1983): The fear-avoidance model of exaggerated pain perception—II. Behav. Res. Ther., 21:409–416.

35. Phillips, H.C. (1987): Avoidance behaviour and its role in sustaining chronic pain. Behav. Res. Ther., 25:273–279.

36. Crombez, G., Vlaeyen, J.W., Heuts, P.H., and Lysens, R. (1999): Pain-related fear is more disabling than pain itself: Evidence on the role of pain-related fear in chronic back pain disability. Pain, 80:329–339.

37. Klenerman, L., Plade, P.D., Stanley, M., et al. (1995): The prediction of chronicity in patients with an acute attack of low back pain in a general practice setting. Spine, 20:478–484.

38. Kendall, N.A., Linton, S.J., and Main, C.J. (1997): Guide to Assessing Psychosocial Yellow Flags in Acute Low Back Pain: Risk Factors for long-Term Disability and Work Loss. Wellington. New Zealand: Accident Rehabilitation and Compensation Insurance Corporation of New Zealand and the National Health Committee.

39. Moore, J.E., Von Korff, M., Cherkin, D., et al. (2000): A randomized trial of a cognitive-behavioral program for enhancing back pain self-care in primary care setting. Pain, 88:145–153.

40. Linton, S.J., and Andersson, T. (2000): Can chronic disability be prevented? A randomized trial of a cognitive-behavioral intervention for spinal pain patients. Spine, 25:2585–2591.

41. Vlaeyen, J.W., de Jong, J., Geilen, M., et al. (2001): Graded exposure in vivo in the treatment of pain-related fear: A replicated single-case experimental design in four patients with chronic low back pain. Behav. Res. Ther., 39:151–166.

42. Flynn, T., Fritz, J., Whitman, J., et al. (2002): A clinical prediction rule for classifying patients with low back pain who demonstrate short-term improvement with spinal manipulation. Spine, 27:2835–2843.

43. Fritz, J.M., Delitto, A., Vignovic, M., and Busse, R.G. (2000): Inter-rater reliability of judgments of the centralization phenomenon and status change during movement testing in patients with low back pain. Arch. Phys. Med. Rehabil., 81:57–61.

44. Fritz, J.M., Erhard, R.E., and Hagen, B.F. (1998): Update: Segmental instability of the lumbar spine. Phys. Ther., 78:889–896.

45. Fritz, J.M., Erhard, R.E., and Vignovic, M. (1997): A nonsurgical treatment approach for patients with lumbar spinal stenosis. A case report. Phys. Ther., 77:962–973.

46. Chan, C.W., Goldman, S., Ilstrup, D.M., et al. (1993): The pain drawing and Waddell's nonorganic physical signs in chronic low back pain. Spine, 18:1717–1722.

47. Bombardier, C. (2000): Outcome assessment in the evaluation of treatment of spinal disorders: Summary and general recommendations. Spine, 25:3100–3103.

48. Fritz, J.M., and Irrgang, J.J. (2001): A comparison of a Modified Oswestry Disability Questionnaire and the Quebec Back Pain Disability Scale. Phys. Ther., 81:776–788.

49. Balagué, F., Nordin, M., Sheikhzadeh, A., et al. (1999): Recovery of severe sciatica. Spine, 24:2516–2524.

50. Supik, L.F., and Broom, M.J. (1994): Sciatic tension signs and lumbar disc herniation. Spine, 19:1066–1069.

51. Bigos, S., Bowyer, O., Braen, G., et al. (1994): Acute low back problems in adults, AHCPR Publication 95–0642. Agency for Health Care Policy and Research, Public Health Service. Rockville, MD: US Department of Health and Human Services.

52. Delitto, A., Cibulka, M.T., Erhard, R.E., et al. (1993): Evidence for use of an extension-mobilization category in acute low back syndrome: A prescriptive validation pilot study. Phys. Ther., 73:216–222.

53. Erhard, R.E., Delitto, A., and Cibulka, M.T. (1994): Relative effectiveness of an extension program and a combined program of manipulation and flexion and extension exercises in patients with acute low back syndrome. Phys. Ther., 74:1093–1100.

54. Koes, B.W., Bouter, L.M., van Mameren, H., et al. (1992): The effectiveness of manual therapy, physiotherapy, and treatment by the general practitioner for nonspecific back and neck complaints. A randomized clinical trial. Spine, 17:28–35.

55. Laupacis, A., Sekar, N., and Stiell, I. G. (1997): Clinical prediction rules. A review and suggested modifications of methodological standards. JAMA, 277:488–494.

56. Dreyfuss, P., Michaelsen, M., Pauza, K., et al. (1996): The value of medical history and physical examination in diagnosing sacroiliac joint pain. Spine, 21:2594–2602.

57. Riddle, D.L., and Freburger, J.K. (2002): Evaluation of the presence of sacroiliac joint region dysfunction using a combination of tests: A multicenter intertester reliability study. Phys. Ther., 82:772–781.

58. Waddell, G., Somerville, D., Henderson, I., and Newton, M. (1992): Objective clinical evaluation of physical impairment in chronic low back pain. Spine, 17:617–628.

59. Cyriax, J. (1982): Textbook of Orthopaedic Medicine, Vol 1: Diagnosis of Soft Tissue Lesions, 6th ed. London, Bailliere Tindall.

60. Hadler, N.M., Curtis, P., Gillings, D.B., and Stinnett, S. (1987): A benefit of spinal manipulation as an adjunctive therapy for acute low-back pain: A stratified controlled study. Spine, 12:703–706.

61. Meade, T.W., Dyer, S., Browne, W., et al. (1990): Low back pain of mechanical origin: Randomised comparison of chiropractic and hospital outpatient treatment. BMJ, 300:1431–1437.

62. Boyling, J.D., Palastanga, N., and Grieve, G.P. (1994): Grieve's Modern Manual Therapy: The Vertebral Column, 2nd ed. St. Louis, Churchill Livingstone.

63. Greenman, P.E. (1996): Principles of Manual Medicine, 2nd ed. Philadelphia: Lippincott Williams and Wilkins.

64. Cibulka, M.T., Delitto, A., and Koldehoff, R.M. (1988): Changes in innominate tilt after manipulation of the sacroiliac joint in patients with low back pain. An experimental study. Phys. Ther., 68:1359–1363.

65. Mayer, T.G., Smith, S.S., Keeley, J., et al. (1985): Quantification of lumbar function. Part 2. Sagittal plane trunk strength in chronic low back pain patients. Spine, 10:765–770.

66. Ogon, M., Bender, B.R., Hooper, D.M., et al. (1997): A dynamic approach to spinal instability. Part II. Hesitation and giving-way during interspinal motion. Spine, 22:2859–2866.

67. Hultman, G., Nordin, M., Saraste, H., et al. (1993): Body composition, endurance, strength, cross-sectional area, and density of erector spinae in men with and without low back pain. J. Spinal Dis., 6:114–120.

68. Lee, J.H., Hoshino, Y., Nakamura, K., et al. (1999): Trunk muscle weakness as a risk factor for low back pain: A 5-year prospective study. Spine, 24:54–61.

69. Luoto, S., Taimela, S., Hurri, H., et al. (1996): Psychomotor speed and postural control in chronic low back pain patients: A controlled follow-up study. Spine, 21:2621–2629.

70. Panjabi, M.M. (1992): The stabilizing system of the spine. Part II. Neutral zone and instability hypothesis. J. Spinal Disord., 5:390–398.

71. Bogduk, N., Macintosh, J.E., and Pearcy, M.J. (1992): A universal model of the lumbar back muscles in the upright position. Spine, 17:897–913.

72. MacIntosh, J.E., Pearcy, M.J., and Bogduk, N. (1993): The axial torque of the lumbar back muscles: Torsion strength of the back muscles. Aust. N. Z. J. Surg., 63:205–212.

73. Macintosh, J.E., and Bogduk, N. (1986): The biomechanics of the lumbar multifidus. Clin Biomech., 1:205–213.

74. McGill, S.M. (1997): Distribution of tissue loads in the low back during a variety of daily and rehabilitation tasks. J. Rehabil. Res. Dev., 34:448–458.

75. Gardner-Morse, M.G., and Stokes, I.A.F. (1998): The effects of abdominal muscle coactivation on lumbar spine stability. Spine, 23:86–92.

76. Hodges, P.W., and Richardson, C.A. (1996): Inefficient muscular stabilization of the lumbar spine associated with low back pain. Spine, 21:2640–2649.

77. Cresswell, A.G., Grundstrom, H., and Thorstensson, A. (1992): Observations on intra-abdominal pressure and patterns of abdominal intra-muscular activity in man. Acta Physiol. Scand., 144:409–418.

78. Maitland, G.D. (1986): Vertebral Manipulation, 5th ed. Oxford: Butterworth Heinemann, pp. 74–76.

79. Paris, S.V. (1985): Physical signs of instability. Spine, 10:277–279.

80. Maher, C., and Adams, R. (1994): Reliability of pain and stiffness assessments in clinical manual lumbar spine examination. Phys. Ther., 74:801–811.

81. Kirkaldy-Willis, W.H., and Farfan, H.F. (1982): Instability of the lumbar spine. Clin. Orthop. Relat. Resl, 165:110–123.

82. Nachemson, A. (1985): Lumbar spine instability: A critical update and symposium summary. Spine, 10:290–291.

83. Hicks, G.E. (2002): Predictive Validity of Clinical Variables Used in the Determination of Patient Prognosis Following a Lumbar Stabilization Program [doctoral dissertation]. University of Pittsburgh.

84. McGill, S.M. (1988): Estimation of force and extensor moment contributions of the disc and ligaments at L4-L5. Spine, 13:1395–1402.

85. Wilder, D.G., Aleksiev, A.R., Magnusson, M.L., et al. (1996): Muscular response to sudden load: A tool to evaluate fatigue and rehabilitation. Spine, 21:2628–2637.

86. Danneels, L., Vanderstraeten, G., Cambier, D., et al. (2001): Effects of three different training modalities on cross-sectional area of the lumbar multifidus muscle in patients with chronic low back pain. Br. J. Sports Med., 35:186–192.

87. Mannion, A., Taimela, S., Montener, M., and Dvorak, J. (2001): Active therapy for chronic low back pain. Part 1. Effects on back muscle activation, fatigability, and strength. Spine, 26:897–908.

88. Hodges, P.W., and Richardson, C.A. (1998): Delayed postural contraction of transversus abdominis in low back pain associated with movement of the lower limb. J. Spinal Dis., 11:46–52.

89. Hodges, P.W., and Richardson, C.A. (1997): Contraction of the abdominal muscles associated with movement of the lower limb. Phys. Ther, 77:132–141.

90. Richardson, C.A., and Jull, G.A. (1995): Muscle control–pain control: What exercises would you prescribe? Manual Ther., 1:2–11.

91. Axler, C.T., and McGill, S.M. (1997): Low back loads over a variety of abdominal exercises: Searching for the safest abdominal challenge. Med. Sci. Sports Exerc., 29:804–811.

92. Kippers, V., and Parker, A.W. (1984): Posture related to myoelectric silence of erectores spinae during trunk flexion. Spine, 7:740–745.

93. MacIntosh, J.E., and Bogduk, N. (1987): The morphology of the lumbar erector spinae. Spine, 12:658–668.

94. MacIntosh, J.E., and Bogduk, N. (1996): The anatomy and function of the lumbar back muscles. In Boyling, J.D., and Palastanga, N. (eds.): Grieve's Modern Manual Therapy. The Vertebral Column, 2nd ed. New York, Churchill Livingstone, pp. 189–209.

95. Sihvonen, T., Lindgren, K.A., Airaksinen, O., et al. (1997): Movement disturbances of the lumbar spine and abnormal back muscle electromyographic findings in recurrent low back pain. Spine, 22:289–297.

96. Hides, J.A., Jull, G.A., and Richardson, C.A. (2001): Long-term effects of specific stabilizing exercises for first-episode low back pain. Spine, 26:E243–E248.

97. Callaghan, J.P., Gunning, J.L., and McGill, S.M. (1998): The relationship between lumbar spine load and muscle activity during extensor exercises. Phys. Ther., 78:8–18.

98. McGill, S.M. (1998): Low back exercises: Evidence for improving exercise regimens. Phys. Ther., 78:754–766.

99. Verna, J.L., Mayer, J.M., Mooney, V., et al. (2002): Back extension endurance and strength: The effect of variable-angle Roman chair exercise training. Spine, 27:1772–1777.

100. McKenzie, R.A. (1989): The Lumbar Spine: Mechanical Diagnosis and Therapy. Waikanae, New Zealand, Spinal Publications.

101. Donelson, R., Silva, G., and Murphy, K. (1990): Centralization phenomenon: Its usefulness in evaluating and treating referred pain. Spine, 15:211–213.

102. Werneke, M., and Hart, D.L. (2001): Centralization phenomenon as a prognostic factor for chronic low back pain and disability. Spine, 26:758–764.

103. Long, A.L. (1995): The centralization phenomenon: Its usefulness as a predictor of outcome in conservative treatment of low back pain (a pilot study). Spine, 20:2513–2521.

104. Karas, R., McIntosh, G., Hall, H., et al. (1997): The relationship between nonorganic signs and centralization of symptoms in the prediction of return to work for patients with low back pain. Phys. Ther., 77:354–360.

105. Fritz, J.M., Erhard, R.E., Delitto, A., et al. (1997): Preliminary results of the use of a two-stage treadmill test as a clinical diagnostic tool in the differential diagnosis of lumbar spinal stenosis. J. Spinal Dis., 10:410–416.

106. Katz, J.N., Dalgas, M., Stucki, G., and Lipson, S.G. (1995): Degenerative lumbar spinal stenosis. Diagnostic value of the history and physical examination. Arthritis Rheum., 38:1236–1241.

107. Penning, L. (1992): Functional pathology of lumbar spinal stenosis. Clin. Biomech., 7:3–15.

108. Porter, R.W. (1996): Spinal stenosis and neurogenic claudication. Spine, 21:2046–2052.

109. Kilpikoski, S., Airaksinen, O., Kankaanpaa, M., et al. (2002): Interexaminer reliability of low back pain assessment using the McKenzie method. Spine, 27:E207–E214.

110. Porter, R.W., and Miller, C.G. (1986): Back pain and trunk list. Spine, 11:596–600.

111. Donahue, M.S., Riddle, D.L., and Sullivan, M.S. (1996): Intertester reliability of a modified version of McKenzie's lateral shift assessments obtained on patients with low back pain. Phys. Ther., 79:412–418.

112. Whitman, J.M., Flynn, T.W., and Fritz, J.M. (2003): Nonsurgical management of patients with lumbar spinal stenosis: A literature review and a case series of three patients managed with physical therapy. Phys. Med. Rehabil. Clin. N. Am., 14:1–23.

113. Willen, J., Danielson, B., Gaulitz, A., et al. (1997): Dynamic effects on the lumbar spinal canal. Axially loaded CT-myelography and MRI in patients with sciatica and/or neurogenic claudication. Spine, 22:2968–2976.

114. Flynn, T.W., Canavan, P.K., Cavanagh, P.R., et al. (1997): Plantar pressure reduction in an incremental weight-bearing system. Phys Ther., 77:410–419.

115. Fiebert, I., and Keller, C. D. (1994): Are "passive" extension exercises really passive? J. Orthop. Sports Phys. Ther., 19:111–117.

116. van Tulder, M.W., Koes, B.W., and Bouter, L.M. (1997): Conservative treatment of acute and chronic nonspecific low back pain. A systematic review of randomized controlled trials of the most common interventions. Spine, 22:2128–2156.

117. Beursken, A.J., de Vet, H.C., Köke, A.J., et al. (1997): Efficacy of traction for nonspecific low back pain. 12-week and 6-month results of a randomized clinical trial. Spine, 22:2756–2762.

118. van der Heijden, G.J., Beurskens, A.J., Dirx, M.J., et al. (1995): Efficacy of lumbar traction: A randomized clinical trial. Physiotherapy, 81:29–35.

119. Bergquist-Ulman, M., and Larsson, U. (1970): Acute low back pain in industry: A controlled prospective study with special reference to therapy and confounding factors. Acta Orthop. Scand., 170:S1–S117.

120. Von Korff, M., Deyo, R.A., Cherkin, D., et al. (1993): Back pain in primary care: Outcomes at one year. Spine, 18:855–862.

121. Cholewicki, J., and McGill, S.M. (1996): Mechanical stability of the in vivo lumbar spine: Implications for injury and low back pain. Clin. Biomech., 11:1–15.

122. Rantenen, J., Hurme, M., Ralck, B., et al. (1993): The lumbar multifidus muscle five years after surgery for a lumbar intervertebral disc herniation. Spine, 18:568–574.

123. Kankaanpaa, M., Taimela, S., Laaksonen, D., et al. (1998): Back and hip extensor muscle fatigability in chronic low back pain patients and controls. Arch. Phys. Med. Rehabil., 79:412–418.

124. Bullock-Saxton, J. E., Janda, V., and Bullock, M.I. (1993): Reflex activation of gluteal muscles during walking. An approach to restoration of muscle function for patients with low-back pain. Spine, 18:704–709.

125. Vakos, J.P., Nitz, A.J., Threlkeld, A.J., et al. (1994): Electromyographic activity of selected trunk and hip muscles during a squat lift. Effect of varying the lumbar posture. Spine, 19:687–694.

126. Nadler, S.F., Wu, K.D., Galski, T., and Feinberg, J.H. (1998): Low back pain in college athletes. A prospective study correlating lower extremity overuse or acquired ligamentous laxity with low back pain. Spine, 23:828–833.

127. Feldman, D.E., Shrier, I., Rossignol, M., and Abenhaim, L. (2001): Risk factors for the development of low back pain in adolescence. Am. J. Epidemiol., 154:30–36.

128. Kujala, U.M., Salminen, J.J., Taimela, S., et al. (1992): Subject characteristics and low back pain in young athletes and nonathletes. Med. Sci. Sports Exer., 24:627–632.

129. Cady, L.D., Bischoff, D.P., and O'Connell, E.R. (1979): Strength and fitness and subsequent back injuries in firefighters. J. Occup. Med., 21:269–279.

130. Videman, T., Sarna, S., and Battie, M.C. (1995): The long-term effects of physical loading and exercise lifestyles on back-related symptoms, disability and spinal pathology among men. Spine, 20:700–705.

Lower Extremity

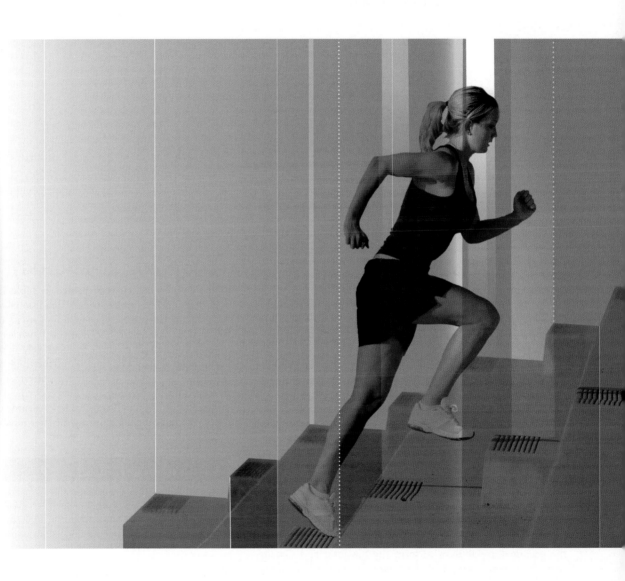

18

Rehabilitation of Thigh Injuries

Jason Brumitt, PT, PhD, SCS, ATC, CSCS

CHAPTER OBJECTIVES

- Identify common muscular injuries involving the quadriceps, hamstring, and groin areas.
- Recall typical sports-related injuries to the thigh and apply appropriate treatment and rehabilitation strategies.
- Apply different rehabilitation strategies based on stages of healing for soft tissue injuries of the thigh.

- Recognize appropriate activities to increase muscular strength and endurance for the hamstring, quadriceps, and groin muscle groups.
- Identify appropriate functional activities for rehabilitation of thigh injuries.

Sports-related injuries involving the thigh are frequently sustained by athletes during practice and competition.[1-6] The pathomechanics associated with a sports-related thigh injury can be the result of repetitive overuse, degeneration (age-related changes), or trauma. The nature and severity of a thigh injury will dictate how quickly an athlete is able to resume play. In some cases an athlete may miss little, if any, time from sports. In other situations an athlete may need to complete a lengthy rehabilitation program before returning to activities. For others, additional medical interventions, including surgery, may be required for the athlete to have a successful outcome.[7-11] The purpose of this chapter is to identify common sports-related injuries involving the thigh and to present evidence-based or evidence-supported rehabilitation strategies for each type of injury.

FUNCTIONAL ANATOMY

The thigh is the anatomic region of the human body located between the proximal end of the pelvis and the distal knee joint. The femur, the only bone in the thigh, articulates with the proximal acetabulum to form the hip joint and distally with the superior aspect of the tibia to form the knee joint. The thigh consists of 18 muscles housed in one of three fascial compartments (Figs. 18-1 to 18-3). The muscles of the thigh allow flexion, extension, rotation, abduction, and adduction of the hip and flexion, extension, and rotation at the knee (Table 18-1). Primary vascularization of the thigh is provided by the femoral artery and vein, obturator artery, and popliteal vein. The femoral, obturator, tibial sciatic, and common peroneal nerves innervate the muscles of the thigh.

FUNCTIONAL KINESIOLOGY

The muscular functions presented in Table 18-1 describe how a muscle contracts concentrically. Traditional open kinetic chain exercises, performed with or without gym equipment, can effectively train concentric movements. However, rarely does one muscle (or muscle group) contract solely in a concentric fashion during sports. The muscles of the thigh are synergistically activated to perform concentric, isometric, and eccentric contractions during functional athletic movements such as running, jumping, cutting, and lifting. Functional and sport-specific exercises should be included during the later rehabilitation stages to optimize an athlete's return to sport.

Clinical Pearl #1

Closed kinetic chain exercises should be included in an athlete's rehabilitation program. Prescribe exercises that reproduce an athlete's functional movement patterns.

MUSCLE AND TENDON INJURIES OF THE THIGH

An athletic injury occurs when forces experienced by the body, during training or competition, exceed the strength of a tissue (or tissues). Muscle injuries are classified by how they occurred: either by a direct (or external) mechanism or by an indirect (or internal) mechanism. Direct injury occurs when an external force applied to the body results in trauma. For example,

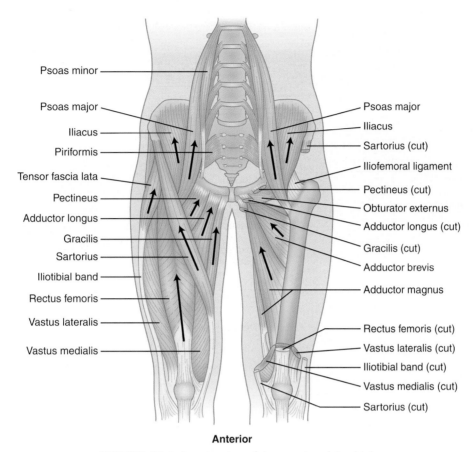

Anterior

FIGURE 18-1 Anterior view of the muscles of the thigh.

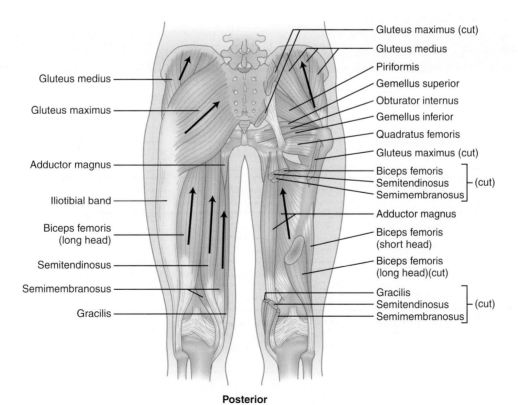

Posterior

FIGURE 18-2 Posterior view of the muscles of the thigh.

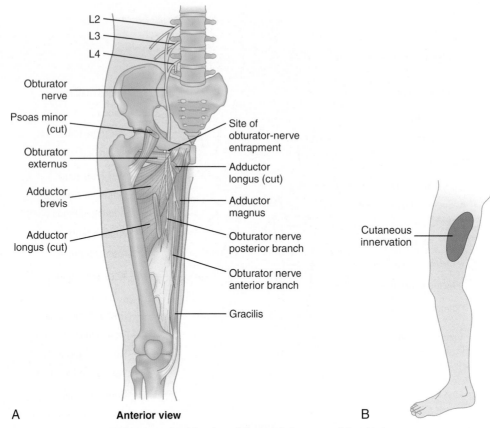

A **Anterior view**   B

FIGURE 18-3 Muscles of the medial aspect of the thigh.

Table 18-1 Functional Anatomy of the Thigh

Muscle	Function	General Origins (O) and Insertions (I)	Nerve Innervation	Fascial Compartment
Rectus femoris	Hip flexion, knee extension	O: Anterior inferior iliac spine I: Tibial tuberosity	Femoral nerve	Anterior
Vastus medialis	Knee extension	O: Intertrochanteric line and linea aspera I: Tibial tuberosity via patellar tendon	Femoral nerve	Anterior
Vastus intermedius	Knee extension	O: Anterior and lateral femur I: Tibial tuberosity via patellar tendon	Femoral nerve	Anterior
Vastus lateralis	Knee extension	O: Greater trochanter and linea aspera I: Tibial tuberosity via patellar tendon	Femoral nerve	Anterior
Psoas major	Hip flexion, stabilization	O: T12-L5 vertebrae laterally, transverse processes, and intervertebral disks I: Lesser trochanter	Ventral rami of L1-L3	Anterior
Psoas minor	Hip flexion, stabilization	O: T12-L1 vertebrae and intervertebral disks I: Pectineal line, iliopectineal eminence	Ventral rami of L1-L2	Anterior
Iliacus	Hip flexion, stabilization	O: Iliac crest, iliac fossa, anterior sacroiliac ligaments, ala of sacrum I: Psoas major tendon, iliopectineal eminence	Femoral nerve	Anterior
Tensor fasciae latae	Hip abduction, internal rotation, flexion	O: Anterior superior iliac spine, anterior portion of iliac crest I: Lateral tibial condyle via iliotibial tract	Superior gluteal nerve	Anterior

Table 18-1 Functional Anatomy of the Thigh—cont'd

Muscle	Function	General Origins (O) and Insertions (I)	Nerve Innervation	Fascial Compartment
Sartorius	Hip flexion, abduction, external rotation; knee flexion	O: Superior to anterior superior iliac spine I: Pes anserine	Femoral	Anterior
Biceps femoris	Hip extension; knee flexion, external rotation	O: Ischial tuberosity (posterior), sacrotuberous ligament, linea aspera I: Head of fibula	Tibial and common fibular portions of sciatic nerve	Posterior
Semimembranous	Hip extension; knee flexion, internal rotation	O: Ischial tuberosity I: Superior-medial tibia	Tibial division of sciatic nerve	Posterior
Semitendinosus	Hip extension; knee flexion, internal rotation	O: Ischial tuberosity I: Posterior portion of medial condyle (tibia)	Tibial division of sciatic nerve	Posterior
Pectineus	Hip adduction, flexion, external rotation	O: Superior pubic ramus I: Posterior surface of femur	Femoral nerve, branch of obturator nerve	Medial
Adductor longus	Hip adduction	O: Pubis (anterior) I: Linea aspera (proximal third)	Obturator	Medial
Adductor brevis	Hip adduction	O: Inferior pubic ramus I: Linea aspera (middle third)	Obturator	Medial
Adductor magnus	Hip adduction	O: Ischial ramus, ischial tuberosity I: Linea aspera, adductor tubercle	Obturator, tibial portion of sciatic nerve	Medial
Gracilis	Hip adduction, flexion, internal rotation	O: Pubis (anterior), inferior ramus of pubis I: Superior-medial tibia	Obturator	Medial
Obturator externus	Hip external rotation	O: Obturator foramen and membrane I: Trochanteric fossa (femur)	Obturator	Medial

a muscle contusion may be caused by a direct blow to the thigh during a football tackle. An indirect injury takes place independent of an external force. An example of an indirect injury is a strain that transpires when a muscle experiences excessive stretching or a violent, eccentric muscle contraction.[5,12,13] A classic example of this type of injury is a running-related hamstring strain.[5] Additional soft tissue injuries may arise when tissue is stressed repeatedly or constantly over time.

The majority of sports-related thigh injuries are muscular strains or contusions.[14,15] Clinicians should also be cognizant of potential complications associated with a thigh injury or other medical conditions that would require immediate referral to a physician. Table 18-2 addresses common musculoskeletal injuries to the anterior, lateral, and medial aspects of the thigh and their differential diagnoses.[1,16-22]

Tendon injuries are classified by the tissue's pathologic state (Table 18-3). The most common primary tendon injuries are either tendinitis (an acute inflammatory condition) or tendinosis (a chronic degenerative condition). Symptoms associated with tendinitis include pain, loss of function (strength, range of motion [ROM]), and the other inflammatory signs (warmth, swelling, redness). An athlete who has been diagnosed with tendinitis may be describe having performed either a novel or intense workout or an excessive amount of repetitive activity within the past 1 to 7 days. If an athlete, however, has tendon pain without inflammatory signs, it is likely that tendinosis is present. The degenerative tendon changes associated with tendinosis are the result of strain levels that over time damage the tendon's microstructure. A patient in whom tendinosis is diagnosed frequently reports that the pain has been present for prolonged periods (months to years) before seeking medical attention.

GENERAL SOFT TISSUE TREATMENT

Selection of treatment or treatments for an injured athlete should be based on the findings from musculoskeletal evaluation and the current healing stage (time frame after injury). Soft tissue healing progresses through three stages: acute, subacute, and chronic (Table 18-4). Prescription of inappropriate therapeutic measures can delay healing or exacerbate the injured athlete's condition (or both).

During the acute healing stage, treatments are directed toward controlling or reducing the effects of inflammation, modulating pain, initiating controlled (gentle) movement to restore ROM, and reducing loss of muscular strength with isometric exercises.[23]

In the course of the subacute healing phase, immature (functionally weak) collagen fibers are deposited in the injured region. The clinician should prescribe exercises that stress the newly formed tissue. The orientation and tensile strength of collagen are influenced by the therapeutic exercise program prescribed. Pain, however, should be avoided during exercise and, if incurred, may be an indication that the exercise is damaging the newly deposited collagen.

Table 18-2 Sports-Related Musculoskeletal Injuries to the Thigh and Their Differential Diagnosis

Region of the Thigh	Primary Soft Tissue Injuries	Secondary Soft Tissue Injuries	Differential Diagnosis
Anterior	Quadriceps strain Quadriceps contusion Coxa saltans Iliopsoas strain Iliotibial band syndrome Patella tendinitis Patella tendinosis	Sartorius strain Gracilis strain Trochanteric bursitis Iliopsoas bursitis Iliopsoas tendinitis Lacerations Muscular avulsions Greater trochanteric pain syndrome Compartment syndrome	Myositis ossificans Legg-Calvé-Perthes disease Osteomyelitis Osteitis pubis Femoral stress fracture Femoral nerve entrapment Obturator nerve entrapment Tumors Labral tears Arthritis Infection Avascular necrosis of the hip
Posterior	Hamstring strains Hamstring tendinitis	Proximal hamstring avulsion Distal hamstring avulsion	Myositis ossificans Lumbar radiculopathy Sacroiliac dysfunction Piriformis syndrome Infection Tumors
Medial	Adductor muscle, group strain	Hip bursitis	Sports hernia Stress fracture Osteitis pubis Obturator nerve entrapment Ilioinguinal neuralgia Genitourinary disorders Intraabdominal disorders

Table 18-3 Tendon Injury Classifications

Pathology	Definition
Tendinitis	Acute tendon injury with associated inflammatory response
Tendinosis	Degeneration of the tendon not associated with an inflammatory process and caused by one or more factors (e.g., microtrauma, age-related changes)
Tenosynovitis	Inflammation of the tendon's synovial membrane
Tenovaginitis	Inflamed, thickened tendon sheath
Peritenonitis	Inflammation of only the peritenon

In the subacute stage of healing the athlete initially performs exercises with the goal of improving muscular endurance (performing each set with high repetitions and low weights). This allows the athlete to gradually increase strength while protecting tissues from potentially injurious loads. In addition to the prescription of therapeutic exercises, electrical stimulation may further assist in restoration of muscular strength.[24]

Clinical Pearl #2

Strengthening exercises prescribed during the subacute phase should be performed with low loads and high repetitions. The risk of reinjuring tissue is reduced by performing high repetitions (15 or more per set). The level of resistance may be gradually increased when the athlete is able to perform the desired number of repetitions per set.

Finally, during the chronic stage of healing, collagen alignment is influenced by the stress applied to the body while the tissue is maturing and remodeling. Exercise prescription can now include multijoint, closed kinetic chain exercises using strength-training variables (sets of 8 to 12 repetitions). If, however, the athlete experiences discomfort with increasing loads, continue with previous exercises that address muscular endurance. Advance the athlete to closed kinetic chain exercises, plyometrics, power training, and sport-specific training when pain-free full active ROM is restored. A more detailed description of tissue healing and its associated stages can be found in Chapters 2 and 7.

ANTERIOR THIGH INJURIES

The quadriceps is at risk for overuse, traumatic, and degenerative injury. The majority of sports-related injuries involving the anterior aspect of the thigh are muscular strains and contusions.[14,25,26] Other common injuries that an athlete may experience in this area include iliopsoas strain, coxa saltans, abrasions, and lacerations.[21]

Quadriceps Strains

An athlete will experience a range of physical loads and stress during practice or competition. A muscular strain can occur in response to a one-time supraphysiologic load that is greater than the tissue's tolerance or in response to repeated subfailure loads experienced during the course of a game or practice.[27] Potential risk factors associated with a quadriceps strain include muscular fatigue, lack of flexibility, previous history of strains, muscular weakness, muscular imbalance, or inadequate warm-up routine.[13,28,29]

Table 18-4 General Rehabilitation Strategies for Soft Tissue Injuries

Stages of Healing	Time Frame (Approximate)	Treatment Goals	Treatment
Acute (inflammatory response)	1-3 days	Modulate pain	Modalities PRN
		Decrease swelling	Modalities PRN
		Maintain or improve ROM	Gentle ROM: PROM, AAROM, passive stretching
		Limit muscle atrophy	Isometric strengthening
Subacute (repair and healing phase)	3-27 days	Modulate pain	Modalities PRN Joint mobilizations: grades I-II
		Increase ROM	Joint mobilization grades III-V Soft tissue mobilization Increase ROM: PROM → AROM, stretching
		Increase strength	Strengthening exercises: endurance (15-25 repetitions per set) and strength-training parameters
		Restore cardiovascular fitness	Stationary bicycling, stairmaster
Chronic (maturation and remodeling phase)	27 days-1 year	Increase strength, functional strengthening	Stretching and eccentric exercises Strengthening: strength training (sets of 8-12 repetitions) Functional training
		Plyometrics, sport-specific conditioning	Plyometrics Sport-specific training

AAROM, Active assisted range of motion; *PRN,* as needed; *PROM,* passive range of motion; *ROM,* range of motion.

Table 18-5 Signs and Symptoms of First-, Second-, and Third-Degree Strains

Injury Charcteristic	First Degree	Second Degree	Third Degree
Extent of muscle damage	Tear of a few muscle fibers	Tear of approximately half of the muscle fibers	Rupture of the entire muscle
Functional loss	None to minor	Moderate	Major
Pain	Minor	Moderate to severe	None
Motor weakness	Minor	Moderate	Major
Swelling	Minimal to none	Noticeable degree of swelling	Significant degree of swelling

A strain may occur anywhere along the length of the quadriceps muscle or tendon, or both; however, the majority of strains occur at the myotendinous junction.[2,30] Strains are clinically described by the degree of muscle damage. Table 18-5 presents the characteristics of first-, second-, and third-degree strains.

Treatment of a strain begins as soon as possible after the onset of injury. Immediate management will take place either on the sideline or in the athletic training facility/clinic (Table 18-6). Immediate treatment of an athlete suffering a strain is rest, ice, compression, and elevation (RICE).[30]

Cross et al[27] reported success using a specific rehabilitation protocol to return injured Australian Rules football players back to sport after suffering a sport-related quadriceps strain. Athletes who completed the two-phase rehabilitation program were able to return to sport without reoccurrence of injury.[27]

Treatments performed during the first phase of recovery ("acute management period"—the first 48 hours after injury) include RICE.[27] The second phase, the remodeling phase, is a four-stage program involving a return to running and kicking (Table 18-7) combined with a progressive therapeutic exercise routine and "soft tissue therapy."[27] The injured athlete is allowed to begin the running program once full pain-free ROM and the ability to hop on the involved leg for three sets of 10 repetitions are demonstrated.[27] The athlete is allowed to progress from one stage to the next when the previous stage's goal has been completed (see Table 18-7).[27]

Quadriceps Contusions

A muscular contusion is caused by a traumatic force that damages the injured region's musculature.[1,31] The damage to the region's capillaries leads to a collection of blood that, depending on its severity, may cause pain. In addition to the muscular pain or soreness associated with the contusion, the athlete may have a palpable mass and swelling, experience pain with movement, and have loss of motion at the adjacent joint or joints.[1,2,14,31]

Table 18-6 **Quadriceps Strain Rehabilitation Progression**

Phase	Time Frame	Treatment Goals	Treatment
Immediate management	First 24 hours	Decrease swelling and pain	Protection, rest, cryotherapy (ice), compression, elevation
		Protect injured region	Crutches if injury severe
Acute stage (inflammatory response)	1-3 days	Decrease swelling and pain	Cryotherapy Electrical stimulation
		Restore ROM	Gentle ROM exercises (e.g., passive hip and knee ROM, kneeling hip flexor stretch [Fig. 18-4], standing quadriceps stretch [Fig. 18-5])
		Restore neuromuscular function	Isometric exercises: quadriceps and hamstring sets (Fig. 18-6)
Subacute stage (repair and healing phase)	3-27 days	Continue ROM activities; improve muscular flexibility	ROM and flexibility exercises
		Increase strength	Progressive resistance exercises: Four-way SLR exercises (hip flexion, extension, abduction, and adduction) Short-arc quads Large-arc quads Leg press, shuttle, or Total Gym (double and single leg) Total body strengthening: address lower kinetic chain muscular weakness
		Improve cardiovascular fitness	Stationary bicycle Elliptical machine
Chronic stage (maturation and remodeling phase)	27 days and on	Increase strength, progress to functional training Improve cardiovascular fitness Increase power	Cardiovascular fitness: stationary bicycle, Elliptical machine, Stairmaster Return to running program Endurance training: continue progressive resistance exercises as necessary Strength training: squats, lunges, step-downs, knee extensions (machine) Total body strengthening: address lower kinetic chain muscular weakness Plyometrics Agility drills Sport-specific training

ROM, Range of motion; *SLR*, straight leg raise.

Table 18-7 **Four-Stage Program for Return to Running and Kicking**

Stage	Goal
1	Able to jog 2 sets for 10 minutes each.
2	80-m striding intervals (3 sets of 5 repetitions) performed at 40%-60% of maximum ability. Stretch and rest between sets.
3	80-m sprints while sprinting at 90%-100% of ability during the middle 30-m of the run. This must be performed for 3 sets of 5 repetitions. Stretch and rest between sets. Begin a kicking program by progressing from a small ball and kicking for short distances.
4	80-m sprints while sprinting at 90%-100% of ability for 60-80 m. Sport-specific drills include shuttle runs, figure-of-eights, and kicking the ball. Perform 3 sets of 5 repetitions each. Kick a normal-sized ball for all distances. Stretch and rest between sets.

From Cross, T.M., Gibbs, N., Houang, M.T., and Cameron, M. (2004): Acute quadriceps muscle strains: Magnetic resonance imaging features and prognosis. Am. J. Sports Med., 32:710–719.

Anterior thigh contusions have been reported in soccer, football, rugby, and the martial arts; however, any athlete is at risk for a quadriceps contusion when participating in contact or collision sports.[1,14,6,32] Although many contusions may go unreported or cause minimal dysfunction, some athletes can experience significant loss of time from sports after sustaining a moderate to severe contusion. In 1973 Jackson and Feagin[33] reported that the average time lost from sports was 45 days (range, 2 to 180 days). Since then, intervention strategies have evolved to allow athletes to return to sports sooner.[3]

Typical conservative management of a thigh contusion includes RICE and therapeutic exercises.[3,14] Aronen et al[3] were able to return injured midshipmen back to sports with no limitations in an average of 3.5 days (range, 2 to 5 days) by following the treatment plan presented in Table 18-8. Furthermore, within 24 hours, all injured individuals had maintained pain-free active ROM to 120° of knee flexion, and more than 75% could perform a pain-free quad set and a straight leg raise without a lag. Within 3 days, all individuals demonstrated full pain-free active ROM equal to that on the uninvolved side. On return to sports, each midshipman was required to wear a thigh pad.[3]

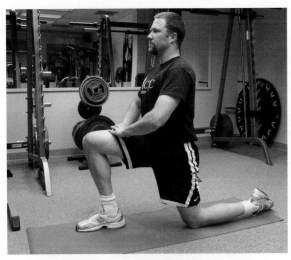

FIGURE 18-4 Kneeling hip flexor stretch.

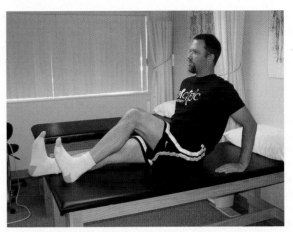

FIGURE 18-6 Isometric hamstring set.

Table 18-8 Quadriceps Contusion Treatment Protocol

Injury Time Line	Intervention
Immediate management: sideline management	Immobilize the knee in 120° of knee flexion with an elastic wrap technique. Transfer the injured individual to the clinic.
Immediate management: in the clinic	Remove the elastic wrap. Replace with a knee brace and immobilize the knee at 120°. Provide crutches and instruct the patient to wear the brace for next 24 hours.
Twenty-fours hours after injury	Remove the brace. Initiate pain-free active quadriceps stretching and quad sets. The patient performs the prescribed exercises and continues crutch ambulation until able to demonstrate full pain-free active range of motion and restoration of quad function equal to that on the ipsilateral side.

From Aronen, J.G., Garrick, J.G., Chronister, R.D., and McDevitt, E.R. (2006): Quadriceps contusions: Clinical results of immediate immobilization in 120 degrees of knee flexion. Clin. J. Sports Med., 16:383–387.

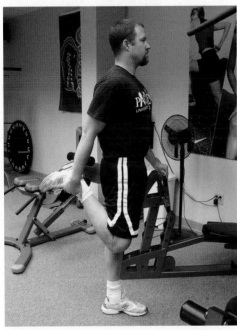

FIGURE 18-5 Standing quadriceps stretch.

Myositis Ossificans

Athletes risk significant impact trauma to their joints and soft tissues when competing in high-impact or collision sports such as football, martial arts, soccer, and rugby. An athlete who sustains a muscle contusion after a football tackle or other direct blow may require rehabilitation and time off from the sport.[3,14,34] A potential complication associated with muscle trauma is myositis ossificans (MO).[34] An athlete must be assessed for MO if conservative treatment fails to alleviate the symptoms and restore function.[15,34,35,36]

MO is a condition marked by abnormal bone formation at the site of muscle trauma (see Fig. 7-5). Three types of MO have been reported.[14,15,34] Two forms, a "thin stalk" and the "periosteal" type, develop in response to the availability of progenitor cells from the bone's damaged periosteum.[15,34] Ossification of bone is the third type, often seen as bone development within the muscle belly, and has a different pathophysiology from the first two types. In some individuals (who may have a predisposition

for the development of MO in the presence of a proper stimulus), calcification of a hematoma will occur and be followed by ossification of bone within the muscle.

MO will usually occur in the injured quadriceps muscle of teen-aged to young adult male athletes.[15,34,35] MO should be suspected in an individual who has a history of muscle trauma (or repeated trauma to the same site) and muscle pain, swelling, loss of ROM, and a palpable mass.[14,34,36] If MO is suspected, the athlete should be referred to a physician for assessment, and active or manual therapy (or both) should be discontinued immediately.

As mentioned previously, initial treatment of an athlete with muscle trauma is focused on alleviating the symptoms associated with the primary injury and reducing risk for the development of MO. It has been suggested that localized tenderness and swelling combined with loss of flexion may indicate an imminent case of MO.[34] In addition, contusions that are considered moderate to severe have a greater likelihood of MO developing.[2] An athlete with signs and symptoms consistent with muscle trauma or MO is treated first with RICE.[14,34,36] The treatment protocol of Aronen et al[3] following a muscle contusion successfully returned 100% ($N = 47$) of midshipmen back to full, pain-free activity within 2 to 5 days after injury (see Table 18-8). Radiographic follow-up of 23 subjects at 3 and 6 months revealed only 1 individual with MO. The 4% incidence of MO after quadriceps contusion found by Aronen et al[3] is below the 9% to 17% previously reported in the literature.[32-38]

King[34] suggested that it might not be possible to immobilize the individual's leg in 120° of knee flexion for the first 24 hours; rather, the use of RICE and avoidance of aggressive treatment are appropriate in the acute stage. Application of heat, manual treatments such as massage and instrument-assisted soft tissue mobilization, or prescription of therapeutic exercise may exacerbate the condition. Despite the success demonstrated by Aronen et al,[3] some athletes may lack access to immediate medical services or may continue to compete despite pain. In the aforementioned examples, it may be too late to reduce the risk for MO.

If MO is suspected, the athlete should be referred to a physician for assessment. Imaging studies will help reveal the location and size of the MO, as well as monitor its progression.[14,37] Initial medical management of an athlete in whom MO is diagnosed includes immobilization of the extremity and ambulation with crutches. Antiinflammatory medication may also be prescribed to reduce symptoms.[14,35] Rehabilitation is resumed when ROM is restored to 90° of flexion.[35]

Coxa Saltans

Coxa saltans, also known as a snapping hip, is a condition marked by an audible snapping sound that may be associated with hip pain during activity. Coxa saltans may be of either intraarticular or extraarticular origin.[9,39] An intraarticular snapping hip is associated with some form of intraarticular pathology. An extraarticular snapping hip will have either an "external" or an "internal" cause.

External coxa saltans occurs when the iliotibial band (ITB) pathologically moves over the greater trochanter as the hip flexes from an extended position.[9] This condition is frequently marked by an audible snapping sound at the hip and may be associated with pseudosubluxation (a term coined by Byrd[40] to describe the patient's perception that the hip is dislocating). Internal coxa saltans is associated with pain and snapping of the iliopsoas tendon.[40] It is theorized that "snapping" of the iliopsoas tendon may be due to movement either across the femoral head or over the lesser trochanter.[40]

Internal coxa saltans occurs when an individual extends and internally rotates the hip from a flexed, abducted, and externally rotated position. During this specific movement pattern the involved iliopsoas tendon or the iliacus muscle is believed to sublux across the anterior portion of the femoral head or the iliopectineal eminence.[41-43]

Repetitive overuse (specifically hip flexion greater than 90°), trauma, and anatomic factors may contribute to the onset of an extraarticular snapping hip.[8,39,44] Physical therapy interventions should address asymmetries in flexibility and core dysfunction. Standard treatments include rest, modalities, lower extremity flexibility exercises (specifically for the hip flexors and the tensor fasciae latae [TFL]/ITB), and strengthening exercises for the lower quadrant.[41,45-50]

Iliotibial Band Syndrome

The ITB is a tendinous-like structure (a thick band of fibrous tissue) originating proximally from the TFL and the gluteus maximus muscles and inserting distally on the fibular head, the Gerdy

tubercle, and the lateral retinaculum of the knee. Iliotibial band syndrome (ITBS) is an overuse injury marked by pain at either the lateral aspect of the knee or the lateral hip area. Frequently experienced by distance runners, ITBS is often the result of poor training, poor footwear, anatomic factors, muscular inflexibility, muscle weakness, or any combination of these factors.[51,52]

It has been reported that specific stretching and strengthening exercises help reduce the symptoms associated with ITBS. Fredericson et al[53] assessed the effectiveness of three ITB stretches for their ability to improve flexibility (Figs. 18-7 to 18-9). They found that the stretch depicted in Figure 18-8 was the most

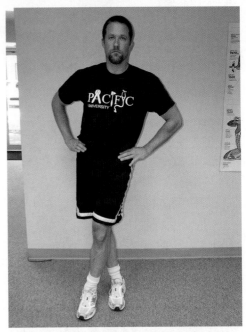

FIGURE 18-7 Iliotibial band stretch.

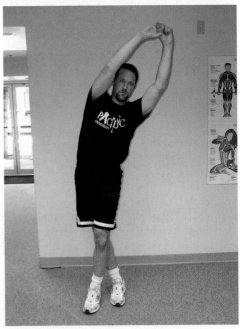

FIGURE 18-8 Iliotibial band stretch with the arms extended overhead.

effective technique of the three; however, each position may help improve ITB flexibility. Stretching exercises for the TFL, the ITB, and other muscles should be performed throughout the rehabilitation period. In addition to stretching exercises for the ITB, some individuals have reported experiencing decreased pain both during and after performing the ITB foam roll exercise (Fig. 18-10). The effectiveness of foam roll exercise in increasing muscular flexibility is unknown. The reduction in pain that some report may be due to the pressure applied to trigger points in the TFL or ITB.

Fredericson et al[51] proposed a therapeutic exercise progression designed to address muscular weakness patterns associated with ITBS. Their program starts with side-lying hip abduction and progresses "to single-leg balance, step downs, and single-leg balance, pelvic drop exercise."[51,54] Some athletes may need to improve core endurance before initiating weight-bearing exercises. A core progression program is presented in Table 18-9. The athlete performs either several sets of multiple repetitions (15 or more repetitions) of exercises involving active movement of the lower extremity or several repetitions of plank exercises while holding each pose for a minimum of 10 seconds. Hold times are increased as tolerated by the athlete.

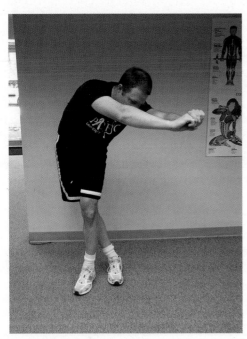

FIGURE 18-9 Iliotibial band stretch with lateral trunk flexion.

Clinical Pearl #3

Core stabilization exercises should be prescribed for athletes who have sustained a sports-related thigh injury.

The program promoted by Fredericson et al[51] has evolved to now include eccentric, multiplanar exercises (Table 18-10). They recommend that these exercises be performed bilaterally for two to three sets of 5 to 8 repetitions initially, with the number of repetitions gradually increased to 15.

MEDIAL THIGH INJURIES

Adductor Strains

The adductors are a collection of six muscles that form the medial aspect of the thigh (see Fig. 18-3). In a non–weight-bearing position the primary function of the adductors is to adduct the thigh (see Table 18-1). During weight bearing (i.e., during functional movements), the adductors will eccentrically decelerate and stabilize the thigh. The incidence of adductor strains is high in sports such as ice hockey, soccer, swimming, American football, and Australian Rules football.[47,49,50,55,56]

Strain injuries at the hip are the most likely cause of groin pain in athletes.[41] Poor flexibility, dysfunctional hip strength, and a previous history of an adductor strain have been reported as potential risk factors for athletes who sustain a hip adductor

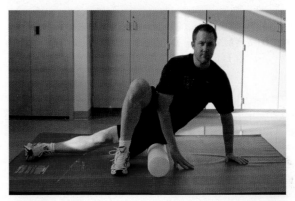

FIGURE 18-10 Foam roll exercise for the iliotibial band.

Table 18-9 Core Exercise Progression for Athletes With Iliotibial Band Syndrome

Position	Basic Exercise	Intermediate Exercise	Advanced Exercise
Side lying	Clamshells	Side plank	Side plank with the feet on a BOSU (with or without hip abduction) (Figs. 18-11 and 18-12)
		Side-lying hip abduction	Side plank with hip abduction (Fig. 18-13)
Prone	Prone abdominal isometric	Front planks	Front plank with lower extremity extension (Fig. 18-14)
		Prone hip extension	Front plank with the feet on a BOSU (with or without hip extension)
Supine	Supine abdominal isometric	Bridges Crunches	Bridging with lower extremity extension

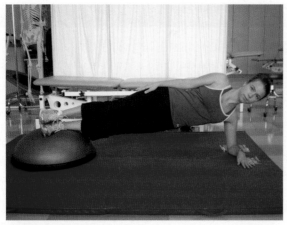

FIGURE 18-11 Side plank with the feet on a BOSU.

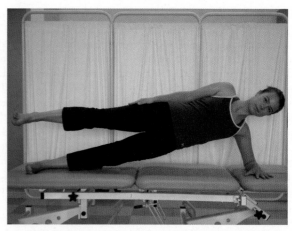

FIGURE 18-13 Side plank with hip abduction.

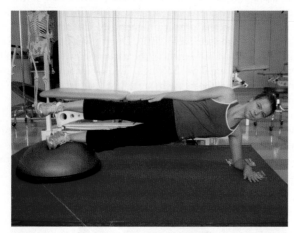

FIGURE 18-12 Side plank with hip abduction on a BOSU.

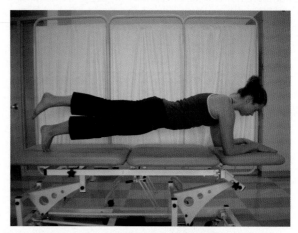

FIGURE 18-14 Front plank with lower extremity extension.

Table 18-10 **Descriptions of Eccentric Exercises for Iliotibial Band Syndrome**

Eccentric Exercise	Description
Modified matrix exercise	Stand as shown in Figure 18-15, *A*, with the involved leg back. The athlete performs an abdominal bracing contraction. Next, the athlete rotates the hips anteriorly and transfers weight to the front leg; at the same time the upper extremity of the involved side reaches toward the contralateral hip. While reaching forward and across the body, the athlete lowers the involved hip (Fig. 18-15, *B*). The action is repeated for the desired number of repetitions.
Wall-bangers	Stand approximately 6-12 inches from a wall as shown in Figure 18-16, *A*. The involved extremity is closest to the wall. Instruct the athlete to reach away from the wall and rotate the hips in the same direction while flexing and lowering the involved hip toward the wall (Fig. 18-16, *B*). The action is repeated for the desired number of repetitions.
Frontal plane lunges	Start in a standing pose. Three lunges can be performed with this exercise. The first is a lunge with the leg reaching out to the side (Fig. 18-17, *A*). The second involves a leg reach with a medial reach of the upper extremities (Fig. 18-17, *B*). The third exercise is similar to the previous exercise; however, the athlete now reaches to the opposite side.

From Fredericson, M., and Wolf, C. (2005): Iliotibial band syndrome in runners: Innovations in treatment. Sports Med., 35:451–459.

strain (Table 18-11).[48,49,56,57] Soccer players who started their sport season with decreased hip abduction ROM experienced a higher rate of adductor strain than did their counterparts who possessed optimal hip ROM.[49] Tyler et al[57] reported that professional hockey players who were found to have muscular imbalance between the abductors and adductors in the preseason were more likely to experience an adductor strain than were uninjured hockey players. In addition, adduction strength in injured hockey players was found to be less than that in their uninjured counterparts.[57] However, other reports have found no correlation between experiencing an adductor strain and either lack of flexibility or muscular strength imbalance at the hip.[48,57,60] Additional prospective investigations are warranted to improve our appreciation of these and other potential risk factors.

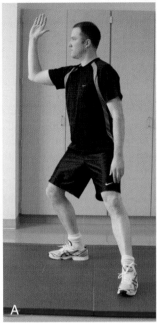
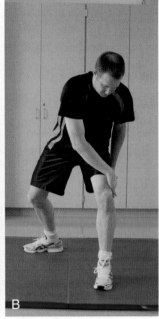

FIGURE 18-15 **A,** Modified matrix exercise starting position. **B,** Modified matrix exercise end position.

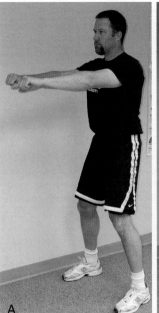
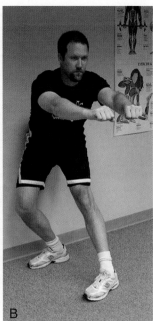

FIGURE 18-16 **A,** Wall-banger starting position. **B,** Wall-banger end position.

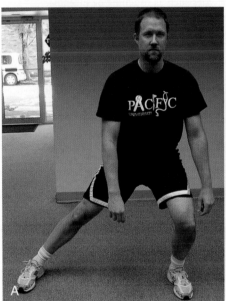
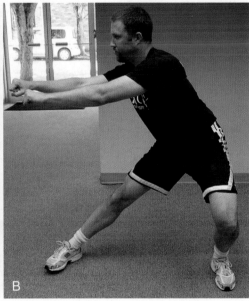

FIGURE 18-17 **A,** Lunge in the frontal plane with the leg to the side. **B,** Lunge with lateral reach.

In at-risk athletes, the primary mechanism of injury on land occurs when eccentric loads generated by the adductors exceed the tissue's failure tolerance. This frequently occurs when an athlete attempts to decelerate the leg in response to powerful hip abduction and external rotation.[58] The primary mechanism of injury in swimmers appears to be associated with the repetitive adduction that occurs during the terminal portion of the breaststroke leg kick.[55,59]

Of the six adductor muscles, the adductor longus is the most frequently strained.[1,50,61] Key findings associated with an adductor strain include pain with adduction (against manual resistance) and pain during palpation of the adductor muscles, tendons, or the tendon insertion sites.[1,45,41,50,62]

Tyler et al[63] developed an injury prevention program designed to strengthen the hip adductors in professional ice hockey players who had been identified in the preseason as being at risk for an adductor strain.[62] After implementing their injury prevention program (Box 18-1), a decrease in hip adductor strains from 3.2 to 0.71 per 1000 player game exposures was realized.[63]

Clinical reports suggest that a progressive strengthening program should be prescribed to an injured athlete whether a primary, acute adductor injury has occurred or whether a chronic adductor strain is present and continuing to cause pain.[62,64] Initial rehabilitation in an athlete who has sustained an acute injury should address decreasing pain, restoring ROM, and initiating non–weight-bearing strengthening exercises.[62,64] Strengthening exercises are progressed as tolerated from concentric, open chain positions to functional eccentric weight-bearing exercises (Box 18-2).[62,64] To be able to return to a high level of play, exercises that mimic sport-specific situations are prescribed, such as plyometric drills, drills on the Fitter (Fitterfirst International; Calgary, Alberta, Canada) (Fig. 18-18, *A* and *B*), and lunges in all directions.

Osteitis Pubis

Osteitis pubis is a chronic groin pain that has been reported in runners and soccer players.[65] It is caused by either shearing forces on the pubic symphysis or supraphysiologic traction forces created locally by the pelvic muscles.[65,66] Conservative treatment includes resting from sports, addressing lower extremity asymmetries (leg length), and stretching of the hip adductor muscles (Fig. 18-19).[65]

Athletic Pubalgia

Athletic pubalgia, also known as a *sports hernia*, is an enigmatic, controversial medical diagnosis. Physicians disagree regarding the existence of this "condition."[45] The pain

associated with a *sports hernia* is thought to result from attenuation or tearing of the transversalis fascia or the conjoined tendon.[1] The pain may also be caused by entrapment of the genital branches of the ilioinguinal or genitofemoral nerves as a result of inflammation or scarring (or both) at the injury site.[1]

Athletic pubalgia is most prevalent in high-performance male athletes whose sport requires high-velocity twisting, cutting, and striding, such as ice hockey, lacrosse, soccer, football, and tennis.[1,67] Several injury mechanisms have been proposed: abnormal hip adductor–to–lower abdominal musculature strength ratio and lack of hip internal rotation.[1,46-48] An abnormal hip adductor–to–lower abdominal musculature strength ratio results in an inability of the abdominal muscles to reduce the shear forces created during hip adduction moments. This imbalance increases risk for injury to the transversalis fascia. Adequate hip internal rotation is critical because powerful adduction creates shear forces across the pubic symphysis that ultimately strain the abdominal musculature along the inguinal wall.[1] Frequently, an individual with athletic pubalgia will be seen by the clinician after having failed initial medical or self-management for a groin strain. The injured athlete, typically a male, will often complain of having had unilateral groin pain for several months without any known trauma.[1,46-48] He will report that his pain is exacerbated during high-intensity exercise and may complain of pain during lower-intensity activities such as coughing or sneezing.[1,46-48]

Typically, traditional ROM and special testing performed during the physical examination will be negative or fail to identify asymmetries. Palpation of the inguinal region will probably fail to reveal a palpable bulge or "hernia."[1,46-48] Frequently reported physical examination findings associated with this diagnosis include pain on palpation of the pubic tubercle, inguinal region, or superficial inguinal ring; a dilated superficial inguinal ring; pain with resisted hip adduction; and pain when manually resisting a sit-up.[1,46-48] It has been noted that assessment of this area requires significant experience and that diagnosis of a hernia should not rely solely on palpation findings. Imaging studies are performed to rule out other potential conditions and to identify potential abnormalities.[1] In some cases, arthroscopy is required to confirm the diagnosis.[1]

Table 18-11 Reported Risk Factors for Hip Adductor Strain per Sport

Sport	Injury Risk Factors
Soccer	Decreased hip abduction range of motion (preseason)
Ice hockey	Decreased hip adduction strength (preseason) Muscular imbalance between the hip adductors and abductors Previous hip adductor injury Athletes who did not practice during the off season
Australian Rules football	Previous history of groin strain
Swimming	Those who compete in the breaststroke

Data from references 47, 48, 55-59.

Box 18-1

Adductor Strain Prevention Program*

WARM-UP
Bike
Adductor stretching
Sumo squats (Fig. 18-20)
Side lunges
Kneeling pelvic tilts

STRENGTHENING PROGRAM
Ball squeezes (legs bent to legs straight) with different ball sizes
Concentric adduction with weight against gravity
Adduction while standing on a cable column or with elastic resistance
Seated adduction machine
Standing with the involved foot on a sliding board moving in the sagittal plane

Bilateral adduction on a sliding board moving in the frontal plane (i.e., bilateral adduction simultaneously)
Unilateral lunges with reciprocal arm movements

SPORT-SPECIFIC TRAINING
On-ice kneeling adductor pull-together exercises
Standing resisted stride lengths on a cable column to simulate skating
Slide skating
Cable column crossover pulls

CLINICAL GOAL
Adduction strength at least 80% of abduction strength

From Tyler, T.F., and Nicholas, S.J. (2007): Rehabilitation of extra-articular sources of hip pain. N. Am. J. Sports Phys. Ther., 2:207–216.
*Designed for professional ice hockey players.

Box 18-2

Adductor Strain Postinjury Protocol*

PHASE I (ACUTE)

RICE (rest, ice, compression, and elevation) for approximately the first 48 hours after injury

Nonsteroidal antiinflammatory drugs

Massage

Transcutaneous electrical nerve stimulation

Ultrasound

Submaximal isometric adduction with the knees bent and knees straight progressing to maximal isometric adduction, pain free

Hip passive range of motion in the pain-free range

Non–weight-bearing hip progressive resistive exercises without weight in an antigravity position (all except abduction).

Pain-free, low-load, high-repetition exercise

Upper body and trunk strengthening

Contralateral lower extremity strengthening

Flexibility program for noninvolved muscles

Bilateral balance board

Clinical Milestone: Concentric adduction against gravity without pain

PHASE II (SUBACUTE)

Bicycling/swimming

Sumo squats (Fig. 18-20)

Single-limb stance

Concentric adduction with weight against gravity

Standing with the involved foot on a sliding board moving in the frontal plane

Adduction while standing on a cable column or elastic tubing

Seated adduction machine

Bilateral adduction on a sliding board moving in the frontal plane (i.e., bilateral adduction simultaneously)

Unilateral lunges (sagittal) with reciprocal arm movements

Multiplane trunk tilting

Balance board squats with throwbacks

General flexibility program

Clinical Milestone: Involved lower extremity passive range of motion equal to that on the uninvolved side and involved adductor strength at least 75% that of the ipsilateral abductors

PHASE III (SPORT-SPECIFIC TRAINING)

Phase II exercises with an increase in load, intensity, speed, and volume

Standing resisted stride lengths on a cable column to simulate skating

Slide board

On-ice kneeling adductor pull-together exercises

Lunges (in all planes)

Correct or modify ice-skating technique

Clinical Milestone: Adduction strength at least 90% to 100% of the abduction strength and involved muscle strength on the contralateral side

From Tyler, T.F., and Nicholas, S.J. (2007): Rehabilitation of extra-articular sources of hip pain. N. Am. J. Sports Phys. Ther., 2:207–216.

*Designed for professional ice hockey players.

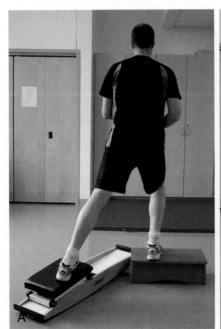
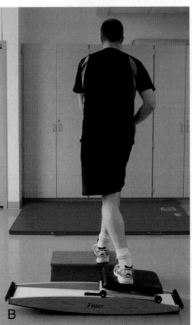

FIGURE 18-18 A, Functional hockey exercise on the Fitter. **B,** Functional hockey exercise for hip adduction.

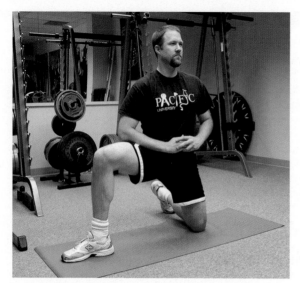

FIGURE 18-19 Stretching of the left adductors.

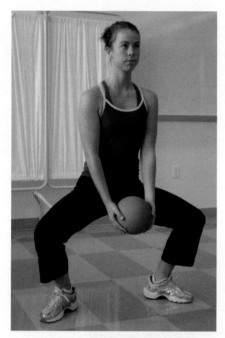

FIGURE 18-20 Sumo squats.

Nonoperative treatment of suspected sports hernias may be effective; however, several reports suggest that the majority of patients will require surgical repair.[1,46–48,67] Nonoperative and postoperative rehabilitation should address the following: weak abdominal musculature, tight or overdeveloped hip adductors, and poor neuromuscular control of the trunk, hip, and pelvis.[1,46–48]

Surgical repair is necessary if conservative treatment fails. It is frequently performed laparoscopically, and the damaged posterior abdominal wall is repaired with a mesh insert.[1] With a mesh repair the athlete should be able to return to sports in 6 to 12 weeks.[1] Therapeutic exercise progression should address any initial deficits in ROM or strength. As asymmetries in flexibility and muscular weakness are corrected, the athlete progresses from functional strengthening exercises (e.g., squats, lunges) to sport-specific drills and plyometrics.

POSTERIOR THIGH INJURIES

Hamstring Strains

Hamstring strains can cause athletes significant pain and loss of function.[4,68] An eccentric hamstring muscle contraction while the knee is extending during the terminal portion of the swing phase of gait is the primary injury mechanism. Another common injury mechanism is concentric contraction of the hamstring during a hip extension movement. Askling et al[68] reported that the mean time frame for return to sports after a hamstring strain was 31 weeks (range, 9 to 104 weeks). In addition, return to sports is influenced by the type of injury. Individuals sustaining a hamstring strain while stretching required a significantly longer recovery period (median, 50 weeks; range, 30 to 76 weeks) than did those who sustained a strain while sprinting (median, 16 weeks; range, 6 to 50 weeks).[4]

Several risk factors for injury can predispose an athlete to a hamstring strain (Box 18-3). At-risk athletes (sprinters and field sport athletes) should be assessed in the preseason and be prescribed exercises to correct asymmetries or muscular imbalances.

As mentioned previously, a hamstring strain may require an athlete to participate in a lengthy rehabilitation program (mean length, 31 weeks; range, 9 to 104 weeks) before returning to sports (Table 18-12).[5,68] To reduce the risk for sustaining a hamstring strain, at-risk athletes should participate in a preseason training program.

A recent trend is to address hamstring deficits by having the athlete perform eccentric exercises. Hamstring injuries tend to occur during eccentric lengthening of the muscle. The inclusion of eccentric exercises is postulated to address an athlete's strength deficits in a functional manner. In addition, eccentric exercises may help improve an athlete's muscular inflexibility.[75,76] Table 18-13 presents a list of exercises that train the hamstrings eccentrically.

RETURNING TO SPORT

Returning an athlete back to sport too quickly may affect performance or increase the risk for reinjury (or both). Administering tests and measures throughout the course of the athlete's rehabilitation will help guide progression of treatment and identify when the athlete is ready to return to sport. Several functional tests have been used to assess an athlete's ability to return to sport after a lower extremity injury.[77-80]

Three tests—a double-legged jump for distance, a single-leg jump for distance, and the lower extremity functional test (LEFT)—when performed together have been reported to assess functional strength and power, agility, and lower extremity anaerobic power.[6,14,76] Davies and Zillmer[77] included these three tests in the "functional testing algorithm," a rehabilitation strategy originally created to assist clinicians' decision-making process when advancing a patient through the anterior cruciate ligament reconstruction program. The algorithm is designed to test and advance an individual from the acute stage of therapy through functional tests that assess sport-specific movements. These three functional tests may be administered to any patient with a lower extremity injury.

The first test to administer in the testing sequence is the double-legged jump for distance. This test is designed to measure bilateral lower extremity power.[77,78] The athlete stands with both feet situated behind a line (or a piece of tape) on the floor. Before jumping, the athlete clasps both hands behind the back. Clasping the hands behind the back is necessary to reduce potential contributions from the upper extremities. For a test to count, the athlete must land on both legs, under control, and hold this position for 5 seconds.[77,78] Davies and Zillmer[77] suggest that when an athlete is able to meet the distance goal (for males, at least 90% of one's height; for females, at least 80% of one's height), the athlete may progress to the next test. If the athlete is unable to achieve this goal, the focus of rehabilitation is on improving bilateral lower extremity power.

The single-leg jump for distance assesses the athlete's ability to hop for distance and to land on the involved leg. The testing procedure is similar to that of the double-legged jump for distance. The athlete assumes the same starting position as described previously, except for standing on one leg. For a test to count, the athlete must land under control on the test leg and hold the landing for 5 seconds.[77,78] The length of each jump is measured from the back of the tape (starting point) to the heel of the foot. Males should be able to jump at least 80% of their height, with less than a 15% difference between

---

Box 18-3

Injury Risk Factors Associated With a Hamstring Strain

Hamstring weakness (eccentric)[69]
Muscular imbalances[70,71]
Previous history of a hamstring injury[29,70-74]
Muscular inflexibility[70,71,74]
Muscular fatigue[13]
Failure to properly warm up before a sport[70,71]
Athlete's age[70-73]
Athlete's position in a sport[72]

Table 18-12 Hamstring Strain Rehabilitation Protocol

Phase	Time Frame	Treatment Goals	Treatment
Immediate management	First 24 hours	Decrease swelling and pain	Protection, rest, cryotherapy (ice), compression, elevation
		Protect the injured region	Crutches if injury severe
Acute stage (inflammatory response)	1-3 days	Decrease swelling and pain	Cryotherapy Electrical stimulation
		Restore ROM	Gentle ROM exercises (e.g., passive hip and knee ROM, hamstring stretch [long sitting] [Fig. 18-21], hamstring stretch [supine], standing quadriceps stretch)
		Restore neuromuscular function	Isometric exercises
Subacute stage (repair and healing phase)	3-27 days	Continue ROM activities; improve muscular flexibility	ROM and flexibility exercises
		Increase strength	Progressive resistance exercises: Hamstring curls (Fig. 18-22) Prone straight leg raise Leg press, shuttle, or Total Gym (double and single leg) Total body strengthening: address lower kinetic chain muscular weakness
		Improve cardiovascular fitness	Stationary bicycle Elliptical machine
Chronic stage (maturation and remodeling phase)	27 days and on	Increase strength, progress to functional training Improve cardiovascular fitness Increase power	Cardiovascular fitness: stationary bicycle, Elliptical machine, Stairmaster Return to running program Endurance training: continue progressive resistance exercises as necessary Strength training: eccentric hamstring exercises (e.g., good mornings, dead lifts, squats, lunges, step-downs, knee extensions [machine]) Total body strengthening: address lower kinetic chain muscular weakness Plyometrics Agility drills Sport-specific training

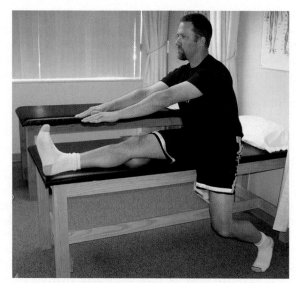

FIGURE 18-21 Hamstring stretch.

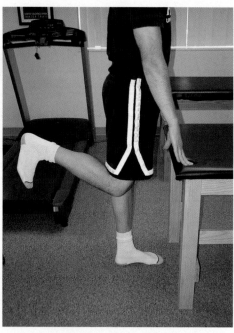

FIGURE 18-22 Hamstring curl.

Table 18-13 Eccentric Exercises for the Hamstrings

Exercise	Technique
Inverted hamstring	Start by balancing on one leg with the knee in full extension. Next, the athlete bends from the hip, not the back, while maintaining a neutral spine. Stretch the arms to the side to assist with balance (Fig. 18-23). Hold each repetition for up to 30 seconds.
Romanian dead lift	Stand with the feet shoulder width apart and the knees slightly bent. Have the athlete grasp a pair of dumbbells or place a weighted bar along the upper trapezius muscles (Fig. 18-24). Instruct the athlete to shift the hips posteriorly to lower the weights toward the ground.
Nordic (also called Russian) hamstring curl	Assume a high kneeling pose on a padded surface. The clinician is positioned behind the athlete and provides support/assistance by grasping the ankles. Instruct the athlete to lower the upper part of the body as far as possible toward the floor, followed by performing a hamstring curl at the knees to bring oneself back to a vertical position (Fig. 18-25 [also see Fig. 7-9])

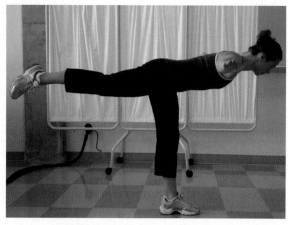

FIGURE 18-23 Inverted hamstring.

each leg.[77] Females should be able to jump at least 70% of their height, with less than a 15% difference between the legs.[77] If the test is passed successfully, the athlete may progress to the LEFT. If the athlete fails to pass this test, rehabilitation is directed at improving strength and power in the involved lower extremity.

The LEFT is a reliable, timed test that incorporates several multidirectional movement patterns.[77,78,80] The LEFT is performed on a gym floor, and four cones are placed in a diamond shape.[77,78,80] The cones are oriented 30 feet apart in the north-south direction and 10 feet apart in the east-west direction. The LEFT has 10 components (Box 18-4).[77,78,80] A complete description of the components of the LEFT and how

to administer it is beyond the scope of this chapter, and it is described in detail in other sources.[77,78]

Davies and Zillmer[77] state that the average male should be able to complete the course in 100 seconds (range, 90 to 120 seconds) and females should be able to finish in 135 seconds (range, 120 to 150 seconds). If the athlete fails to pass the test, rehabilitation is directed at improving speed and agility.

When these three functional tests are completed successfully, the athlete can advance to sport-specific training with integration to full practice and competition. The athlete should be observed over the next few weeks during practice and competition for hesitation or apprehension during drills, inability to perform power movements, or fatigue because further assessment and exercise prescription may be indicated.

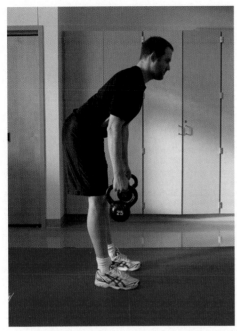

FIGURE 18-24 Romanian dead lift.

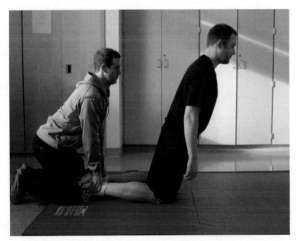

FIGURE 18-25 Nordic (also called Russian) hamstring curl.

Box 18-4
Components of the Lower Extremity Functional Test

1. Forward run
2. Backward run
3. Side shuffles (both ways)
4. Cariocas (both ways)
5. Figure-of-eight run (both ways)
6. 45° angle cuts (outside foot, both ways)
7. 90° angle cuts (outside foot, both ways)
8. 90° crossover cuts (both ways)
9. Forward run
10. Backward run

CONCLUSION

- Several sports-related injuries of the thigh are common. The majority of injuries are either strains or contusions; however, some thigh injuries may be severe and require significant time off from sports.
- Rehabilitation of thigh injuries should begin as soon as possible after injury, with initial treatments directed toward modulating pain and reducing signs of inflammation.
- During the subacute and chronic stages of healing, the clinician should begin an athlete's rehabilitation program with exercises that address deficits and advance the routine to exercises that reproduce functional, sport-specific movements.
- Quadriceps strains and contusions, myositis ossificans, coxa saltans, and iliotibial band syndrome are examples of anterior thigh injuries experienced by athletes.
- Sports-related injuries involving the medial aspect of the thigh include adductor strains, athletic pubalgia, and osteitis pubis.
- A hamstring strain (posterior aspect of the thigh) may be a debilitating injury requiring extensive rehabilitation before returning to sports.
- Athletes at risk for hamstring strains should perform eccentric exercises as part of a training program.
- Before returning to a sport, the athlete should undergo functional assessment. In one testing strategy, the athlete progresses from a double-legged jump, to a single-leg jump for distance, to the lower extremity functional test. The athlete must meet a minimum test score before advancing to the next test.

REFERENCES

1. Anderson, K., Strickland, S.M., and Warren, R. (2001): Hip and groin injuries in athletes. Am. J. Sports Med., 29:521–533.
2. Armfield, D.R., Kim, D.H., Towers, J.D., et al. (2006): Sports-related muscle injury in the lower extremity. Clin. Sports Med., 25:803–842.
3. Aronen, J.G., Garrick, J.G., Chronister, R.D., and McDevitt, E.R. (2006): Quadriceps contusions: Clinical results of immediate immobilization in 120 degrees of knee flexion. Clin. J. Sports Med., 16:383–387.
4. Askling, C., Saartok, T., and Thorstensson, A. (2006): Type of acute hamstring strain affects flexibility, strength, and time to return to pre-injury level. Br. J. Sports Med., 40:40–44.
5. Askling, C.M., Tengvar, M., Saartok, T., and Thorstensson, A. (2007): Acute first-time hamstring strains during high-speed running: A longitudinal study including clinical and magnetic resonance imaging findings. Am. J. Sports Med., 35:197–206.
6. Chomiak, J., Junge, A., Peterson, L., and Dvorak, J. (2000): Severe injuries in football players. Influencing factors. Am. J. Sports Med., 28(5 Suppl.):S58–S68.
7. Gidwani, S., and Bircher, M.D. (2007): Avulsion injuries of the hamstring origin—a series of 12 patients and management algorithm. Ann. R. Coll. Surg. Engl., 89:394–399.
8. Gruen, G.S., Scioscia, T.N., and Lowenstein, J.E. (2002): The surgical treatment of internal snapping hip. Am. J. Sports Med., 30:607–613.
9. Hoskins, J.S., Burd, T.A., and Allen, W.C. (2004): Surgical correction of internal coxa saltans. A 20-year consecutive study. Am. J. Sports Med, 32:998–1001.
10. Konan, S., and Haddad, F. (2010): Successful return to high level sports following early surgical repair of complete tears of the proximal hamstring tendons. Int. Orthop., 34:119–123.
11. Lempainen, L., Sarimo, J., Mattila, K., et al. (2007): Distal tears of the hamstring muscles: Review of the literature and our results of surgical treatment. Br. J. Sports Med., 41:80–83.
12. Askling, C.M., Tengvar, M., Saartok, T., and Thorstensson, A. (2007): Acute first-time hamstring strains during slow-speed stretching: Clinical, magnetic resonance imaging, and recovery characteristics. Am. J. Sports Med., 35:1716–1724.
13. Garrett, W.E. (1996): Muscle strain injuries. Am. J. Sports Med, 24(Suppl.):S2–S8.
14. Beiner, J.M., and Joki, P. (2001): Muscle contusion injuries: Current treatment options. J. Am. Acad. Orthop. Surg., 9:227–237.
15. Beiner, J.M., and Joki, P. (2002): Muscle contusion injury and myositis ossificans traumatica. Clin. Orthop. Relat. Res. 403(Suppl.):S110–S119.
16. Bonsell, S., Freudigman, P.T., and Moore, H.A. (2001): Quadriceps muscle contusion resulting in osteomyelitis of the femur in a high school player. A case report. Am. J. Sports Med., 29:818–820.
17. Johnston, C.A.M., Wiley, J.P., Lindsay, D.M., and Wiseman, D.A. (1998): Iliopsoas bursitis and tendinitis. A review. Sports Med., 25:271–283.

18. Miller, A.E., Davis, B.A., and Beckley, O.A. (2006): Bilateral and recurrent myositis ossificans in an athlete: A case report and review of treatment options. Arch. Phys. Med. Rehabil., 87:286–290.

19. Sarimo, J., Lempainen, L., Mattila, K., and Orava, S. (2008): Complete proximal hamstring avulsions: A series of 41 patients with operative treatment. Am. J. Sports Med., 36:1110–1115.

20. Vazquez, M.T., Murillo, J., Maranillo, E., et al. (2007): Femoral nerve entrapment: A new insight. Clin. Anat., 20:175–179.

21. Viegas, S.F., Rimoldi, R., Scarborough, M., and Ballantyne, G.M. (1988): Acute compartment syndrome in the thigh. A case report and a review of the literature. Clin. Orthop. Relat. Res., 234:232–234.

22. Williams, B.S., and Cohen, S.P. (2009): Greater trochanteric pain syndrome: A review of anatomy, diagnosis and treatment. Anesth. Analg., 108:1662–1670.

23. Decoster, L.C., Cleland, J., Altieri, C., and Russell, P. (2005): The effects of hamstring stretching on range of motion: A systematic literature review. J. Orthop. Sports Phys. Ther., 35:377–387.

24. Meier, W., Mizner, R.L., Marcus, R.L., et al. (2008): Total knee arthroplasty: Muscle impairments, functional limitations, and recommended rehabilitation approaches. J. Orthop. Sports Phys. Ther., 38:246–256.

25. Jarvinen, M., and Lehto, M.U.K. (1993): The effects of early mobilisation and immobilisation on the healing process following muscle injuries. Sports Med., 15:78–89.

26. Jarvinen, T.A., Jarvinen, T.L., Kaariainen, M., et al. (2005): Muscle injuries: Biology and treatment. Am. J. Sports Med., 33:745–764.

27. Cross, T.M., Gibbs, N., Houang, M.T., and Cameron, M. (2004): Acute quadriceps muscle strains: Magnetic resonance imaging features and prognosis. Am. J. Sports Med., 32:710–719.

28. Mair, S.D., Seaber, A.V., Glisson, R.R., and Garrett, W.E. (1996): The role of fatigue in susceptibility to acute muscle strain injury. Am. J. Sports Med., 24:137–143.

29. Orchard, J.W. (2001): Intrinsic and extrinsic risk factors for muscle strains in Australian football. Am. J. Sports Med., 29:300–303.

30. Pescasio, M., Browning, B.B., and Pedowitz, R. A. (2008): Clinical management of muscle strains and tears. J. Musculoskelet. Med., 25:526–532.

31. Diaz, J.A., Fischer, D.A., Rettig, A.C., et al. (2003): Severe quadriceps muscle contusions in athletes. A report of three cases. Am. J. Sports Med., 31:289–293.

32. Ryan, J.B., Wheeler, J.H., Hopkinson, W.J., et al. (1991): Quadriceps contusions. West Point Update. Am. J. Sports Med., 19:299–304.

33. Jackson, D.W., and Feagin, J.A. (1973): Quadriceps contusions in young athletes. Relation of severity of injury to treatment and prognosis. J. Bone Joint Surg. Am., 55:95–105.

34. King, J.B. (1998): Post-traumatic ectopic calcification in the muscles of athletes: A review. Br. J. Sports Med., 32:287–290.

35. Nalley, J., Jay, M.S., and Durant, R.H. (1985): Myositis ossificans in an adolescent following sports injury. J. Adolesc. Health Care, 6:460–462.

36. Webner, D., Huffman, R., and Sennett, B.J. (2007): Myositis ossificans traumatica in a recreational marathon runner. Curr. Sports Med. Rep., 6:351–353.

37. Ryan, J.M. (1999): Myositis ossificans: A serious complication of a minor injury. CJEM, 1:198.

38. Rothwell, A.G. (1982): Quadriceps hematoma. A prospective clinical study. Clin. Orthop. Relat. Res., 171:97–103.

39. Lewis, C.L. (2010): Extra-articular snapping hip: A literature review. Sports Health Multidisciplinary Approach, 2:186–190.

40. Byrd, J.W. (2005): Snapping hip. Oper. Tech. Sports Med., 13:46–54.

41. Byrd, J.W.T. (2007): Evaluation of the hip: History and physical examination. N. Am. J. Sports Phys. Ther., 4:231–240.

42. Deslandes, M., Guillin, R., Cardinal, E., et al. (2008): The snapping iliopsoas tendon: New mechanisms using dynamic sonography. A.J.R. Am. J. Roentgenol., 190:576–581.

43. Winston, P., Awan, R., Cassidy, J.D., and Bleakney, R.K. (2007): Clinical examination and ultrasound of self reported snapping hip syndrome in elite ballet dancers. Am. J. Sports Med., 35:118–126.

44. Wahl, C.J., Warren, R.F., Adler, R.S., et al. (2004): Internal coxa saltans (snapping hip) as a result of overtraining: A report of 3 cases in professional athletes with a review of causes and the role of ultrasound in early diagnosis and management. Am. J. Sports Med., 32:1302–1309.

45. Braly, B.A., Beall, D.P., and Martin, H.D. (2006): Clinical examination of the athletic hip. Clin. Sports Med., 25:199–210.

46. Caudill, P., Nyland, J., Smith, C., et al. (2008): Sports hernias: A systematic literature review. Br. J. Sports Med., 42:954–964.

47. Emery, C.A., Meeuwisse, W.H., and Powell, J.W. (1999): Groin and abdominal strain injuries in the National Hockey League. Clin. J. Sports Med., 9:151–156.

48. Emery, C.A., and Meeuwisse, W.H. (2001): Risk factors for groin injuries in hockey. Med. Sci. Sports Exerc., 33:1423–1433.

49. Ekstrand, J., and Gillquist, J. (1983): The avoidability of soccer injuries. Int. J. Sports Med., 4:124–128.

50. Macintyre, J., Johnson, C., and Schroeder, E.L. (2006): Groin pain in athletes. Curr. Sports Med. Rep., 5:293–299.

51. Fredericson, M., and Wolf, C. (2005): Iliotibial band syndrome in runners: Innovations in treatment. Sports Med., 35:451–459.

52. Paluska, S.A. (2005): An overview of hip injuries in running. Sports Med., 35:991–1014.

53. Fredericson, M., White, J.J., Macmahon, J.M., and Andriacchi, T.P. (2002): Quantitative analysis of the relative effectiveness of 3 iliotibial band stretches. Arch. Phys. Med. Rehabil., 83:589–592.

54. Fredericson, M., and Weir, A. (2006): Practical management of iliotibial band friction syndrome in runners. Clin. J. Sport Med., 16:261–268.

55. Grote, K., Lincoln, T.L., and Gamble, J.G. (2004): Hip adductor injury in competitive swimmers. Am. J. Sports Med., 32:104–108.

56. Seward, H., Orchard, J., Hazard, H., and Collinson, D. (1992): Football injuries in Australia at the elite level. Med. J. Aust., 159:298–301.

57. Tyler, T.F., Nicholas, S.J., Campbell, R.J., and McHugh, M.P. (2001): The association of hip strength and flexibility with the incidence of adductor muscle strains in professional ice hockey players. Am. J. Sports Med., 29:124–128.

58. Hrysomallis, C. (2009): Hip adductors' strength, flexibility, and injury risk. J. Strength Cond. Res., 23:1514–1517.

59. Tonsoline, P.A. (1993): Chronic adductor tendinitis in a female swimmer. J. Orthop. Sports Phys. Ther., 18:629–633.

60. Witvrouw, E., Danneels, L., Asselman, P., et al. (2003): Muscle flexibility as a risk factor for developing muscle injuries in male professional soccer players. A prospective study. Am. J. Sports Med., 31:41–46.

61. Taylor, D.C., Meyers, W.C., Moylan, J.A., et al. (1991): Abdominal musculature abnormalities as a cause of groin pain in athletes. Inguinal hernias and pubalgia. Am. J. Sports Med., 19:239–242.

62. Tyler, T. F., and Nicholas, S. J. (2007): Rehabilitation of extra-articular sources of hip pain in athletes. N. Am. J. Sports Phys. Ther., 2:207–216.

63. Tyler, T.F., Nicholas, S.J., Campbell, R.J., et al. (2002): The effectiveness of a preseason exercise program to prevent adductor muscle strains in professional ice hockey players. Am. J. Sports Med., 30:680–683.

64. Nicholas, S.J., and Tyler, T.F. (2002): Adductor muscle strains in sport. Sports Med., 2:339–344.

65. Waite, B.L., and Krabak, B.J. (2008): Examination and treatment of pediatric injuries of the hip and pelvis. Phys. Med. Rehabil. Clin. N. Am., 19:305–318.

66. Fricker, P. A. (1997): Osteitis pubis. Sports Med. Arthrosc. Rev., 5:305–312.

67. Unverzagt, C.A., Schuemann, T., and Mathisen, J. (2008): Differential diagnosis of a sports hernia in a high-school athlete. J. Orthop. Sports Phys. Ther., 38:63–70.

68. Askling, C.M., Tengvar, M., Saartok, T., and Thorstensson, A. (2008): Proximal hamstring strains of stretching type in different sports: Injury situations, clinical and magnetic resonance imaging characteristics, and return to sport. Am. J. Sports Med., 36:1799–1804.

69. Sugiura, Y., Saito, T., Sakuraba, K., et al. (2008): Strength deficits identified with concentric action of the hip extensors and eccentric action of the hamstrings predispose to hamstring injury in elite sprinters. J. Orthop. Sports Phys. Ther., 38:457–464.

70. Croisier, J.L., Forthomme, B., Namurois, M.H., et al. (2006): Hamstring muscle strain recurrence and strength performance disorders. Am. J. Sports Med., 30:199–203.

71. Croisier, J.L. (2004): Factors associated with recurrent hamstring injuries. Sports Med., 34:681–695.

72. Engebretsen, A.H., Myklebust, G., Holme, I., et al. (2010): Intrinsic risk factors for hamstring injuries among male soccer players. A prospective cohort study. Am. J. Sports Med., 38:1147–1153.

73. Gabbe, B.J., Bennell, K.L., Finch, C.F., et al. (2006): Predictors of hamstring injury at the elite level of Australian football. Scand. J. Med. Sci. Sports, 16:7–13.

74. Worrell, T.W., Perrin, D.H., Gansneder, B., and Gieck, J. (1991): Comparison of isokinetic strength and flexibility measures between hamstring injured and non-injured athletes. J. Orthop. Sports Phys. Ther., 13:118–125.

75. Carlson, C. (2008): The natural history and management of hamstring injuries. Curr. Rev. Musculoskelet. Med., 1:120–123.

76. Copland, S.T., Tipton, J.S., and Fields, K.B. (2009): Evidence-based treatment of hamstring tears. Curr. Sports Med. Rep., 8:308–314.

77. Davies, G.J., and Zillmer, D.A. (2000): Functional progression of a patient through a rehabilitation program. Orthop. Phys. Ther. Clin. N. Am., 9:103–117.

78. Ellenbecker, T.S., and Davies, G.J. (2001): Closed Kinetic Chain Exercise—A Comprehensive Guide to Multiple Joint Exercises. Champaign, IL, Human Kinetics.

79. Manske, R.C., Smith, B., and Wyatt, F. (2003): Test-retest reliability of lower extremity functional tests after a closed kinetic chain isokinetic testing bout. J. Sport Rehabil., 12:119–132.

80. Tabor, M.A., Davies, G.J., Kernozek, T.W., et al. (2002): A multicenter study of the test-retest reliability of the Lower Extremity Functional Test. J. Sport Rehabil., 11:190–201.

19

Knee Rehabilitation

Mark D. Weber, PT, PhD, ATC, SCS, and William R. Woodall, PT, EdD, ATC, SCS

CHAPTER OBJECTIVES

- Identify activities that may cause detrimental stress on a healing/reconstructed anterior cruciate ligament, posterior cruciate ligament, medial collateral ligament, or lateral collateral ligament.
- Identify activities that may cause detrimental stress on the patellofemoral joint.
- Develop appropriate rehabilitation programs for athletes with a variety of knee injuries.

- Determine when to advance an athlete's rehabilitation program by using specific measurable criteria.
- Discuss the reliability, sensitivity, and specificity of arthrometry, lower extremity functional tests, and isokinetics.
- Interpret information obtained from an arthrometer, lower extremity functional tests, and measures of strength.

The knee joint is one of the most frequently injured joints in the body, especially in those engaging in athletic activity. In the functional anatomy section of this chapter some of the key information used for developing safe and effective rehabilitation programs is presented. The rehabilitation programs are goal oriented, modified by time instead of being driven by it. Also emphasized are knee rehabilitation of the entire kinetic chain, early controlled motion, return to participation along a functional progression, and restoration of lower extremity muscular strength, power, endurance, and neuromuscular control.

FUNCTIONAL ANATOMY

To make appropriate clinical decisions for rehabilitation of knee injuries, the clinician must have a thorough understanding of lower extremity anatomy and biomechanics. In the following sections some of the more important biomechanical factors related to rehabilitation of knee injuries are presented.

Ligaments

The knee is inherently unstable because of its location between the two longest bones in the body. Knee stability is maintained through static restraints (e.g., ligaments) and dynamic restraints (e.g., muscles). The role of the ligamentous restraints in controlling forces applied to the knee joint has been studied extensively. Loads produced on the knee by rehabilitation activities have been the subject of a number of investigations.

The data gained from these studies provide the clinician with the information necessary to develop safe and effective rehabilitation programs.

Anterior Cruciate Ligament

The anterior cruciate ligament (ACL) is the primary restraint to anterior translation of the tibia on the femur. Grood et al[1] reported that the ACL provides 85% of the ligamentous restraining force to an anterior drawer test at 30° and 90° of flexion. In addition to controlling anterior tibial translation, the ACL has several other functions, including the screw-home mechanism,[2] assisting in the control of varus and valgus stress,[3] control of hyperextension stress,[4-6] and a guiding function during tibiofemoral flexion-extension.[2,7] Because of its position in the femoral intercondylar notch, if a valgus stress is placed on a flexed knee, the ACL becomes a restraint to external tibial rotation.[6] The ACL also assists the medial collateral ligament (MCL) in controlling tibial internal rotation.[8]

The stresses placed on the ACL by rehabilitation exercises have been studied in a number of investigations. Henning et al[9] implanted a strain gauge in two patients with grade II ACL sprains. The patients then performed various rehabilitation activities and the strain was recorded. The strain on the ACL was reported as a percentage of the strain of an 80-lb Lachman test (Table 19-1). Although conclusions should be drawn with care from a study with only two subjects, it still provides some useful information about the relative rank of strain on the ACL during particular rehabilitation activities.

Beynnon et al[10] implanted a Hall effect transducer in the knees of 11 subjects with normal ACLs and then determined the strain on the ACL during open chain knee flexion and extension, as well as during isometric contractions. They concluded that the following open chain exercises produce either low or no strain on the ACL: isometric contractions of the hamstrings at 15°, 30°, 60°, and 90°; isometric quadriceps contractions at 60° and 90°; cocontractions of the quadriceps and hamstrings at 30°, 60°, and 90°; active knee flexion and extension between 35° and 90°; and knee flexion and extension with a 45-N (10-lb) weight between 45° and 90°. Exercises that proved to significantly increase strain on the ACL included the following: knee extension exercise with a 45-N weight (particularly at 10° and 20° of knee flexion), isometric quadriceps contractions

(at 15° and 30°), and isometric cocontractions of the quadriceps and hamstrings at 15°. During the knee extension exercise the transition from unstrained ACL to strained ACL shifted from 35° of flexion during active unweighted knee extension to 45° during the weighted knee extension condition.

Beynnon et al[11] also compared closed chain with open chain exercises for peak strain on the ACL. They reported the following peak ACL strains: open chain active knee flexion-extension with no load, 2.8%; squatting, 3.6%; open chain knee flexion-extension with a 45-N load, 3.8%; squatting with a sport cord, 4.0%; and 30-Nm isometric quadriceps contractions at 15°, 4.4%. To put these ACL strain values into clinical perspective, these authors reported the peak ACL strain to be 3.7% for a 150-N Lachman test and 1.7% for stationary bicycling.[12] The results of this study regarding the influence of open chain quadriceps activity on ACL strain are predictable from the results of other studies,[13-16] but the strain results during the closed chain activities are somewhat surprising given that Escamilla et al[13] reported no tensile load on the ACL during loaded squats or leg presses.

Kvist and Gillquist[14] measured anterior tibial translation during knee extension exercises and several types of squats. During active knee extension, as loads increased, so did tibial translation, with the ACL-deficient knee demonstrating greater anterior translation than the uninjured knee. Anterior translation was greater during the eccentric phase than during the concentric phase of the exercise. The greatest anterior translation occurred between 15° and 20° of knee flexion. This matches the range in which Escamilla et al[13] reported the greatest tensile load on the ACL during weighted open chain knee extension. Kvist and Gillquist[14] also reported that anterior translation was less under all squat conditions than during loaded open chain extension exercises in knees with deficient ACLs. Similar results were reported in two different studies by Yack et al.[15,16]

In most studies investigating anterior shear during rehabilitation activities the results have been reported as strain on the ACL or anterior translation. A few researchers have calculated their results relative to body weight. Table 19-2 contains such data.

Posterior Cruciate Ligament

The primary function of the posterior cruciate ligament (PCL) is to limit posterior translation of the tibia on the femur.[20,21] It also assists in controlling varus, valgus, and hyperextension stress on the knee.[1,22] The role of the PCL in controlling

Table 19-1 Strain on the Anterior Cruciate Ligament

Activity	Relative ACL Strain (%)*
Running downhill at 5 mph	125
Isometric quadriceps contraction at 22° of flexion against a 20-lb weight	62–121
Isometric quadriceps contraction at 0° of flexion against a 20-lb weight	87–107
Jogging on the floor	89
Lift the leg in 22° of knee flexion	12–79
Jogging 5 mph on a treadmill	62–64
Isometric quadriceps contraction at 45° of flexion against a 20-lb weight	50
Walking without an assistive device	36
Half-squat, one leg	21
Quad set	18
Walking with crutches, weight bearing at 50 lb	7
Stationary cycle	7
Isometric hamstring contraction	−7

Data compiled from Henning, C.E., Lynch, M.A., and Glick, K.R. (1985): An in vivo strain gauge study of elongation of the anterior cruciate ligament. Am. J. Sports Med., 13:22–26.
*A single recording indicates that the activity was reported for one subject only, whereas a range indicates recordings reported for both subjects.

Table 19-2 Anterior Shear Forces Across the Tibiofemoral Joint During Various Activities

Reference	Activity	Knee Position at Peak Anterior Shear(°)	Calculated Force Times Body Weight
Ericson and Nisell[17]	Cycling at 60 RPM, 120-W workload	60–70	0.05
Kaufman et al[18]	Isokinetic knee extension at 60°/sec	25	0.3
	Isokinetic knee extension at 180°/sec	25	0.2
Nisell et al[19]	Isokinetic knee extension at 30°/sec	45	1.3
	Isokinetic knee extension at 180°/sec	40	0.5

RPM, Rotations per minute.

rotational force appears to be minimal.[20,21] The importance of the PCL in normal knee arthrokinematics is indicated by the increased compression force observed in the patellofemoral joint and medial compartment in cadaveric specimens when the PCL is sectioned.[23] This correlates with the common complaints of anterior knee pain and medial compartment arthrosis in patients with a PCL-deficient knee.[23-25] Rehabilitation activities that cause large posterior shear force include isometric hamstring contractions, jogging, lunges, ascending and descending stairs, and squats involving greater than 60° of knee flexion (especially as hip flexion is increased).[24-28] In addition, during early PCL rehabilitation, the clinician may want to avoid activities that require high force from the gastrocnemius because of evidence that these activities may produce significant strain on the PCL.[28] Isokinetic testing of the hamstrings also produces significant posterior shear force on the tibiofemoral joint.[18] Box 19-1 contains a summary of exercises that may cause excessive stress during the early healing phase after ACL or PCL reconstruction. Table 19-3 contains calculated posterior shear data for several rehabilitation exercises.

Collateral Ligaments

The MCL is the primary restraint against valgus stress on the knee.[1] It has a role in control of internal rotation torsional force through the knee, but this role decreases as the knee is flexed.[30] The MCL also assists in controlling excessive external rotation.[6] The MCL is taut in extension and external rotation.[31] Consequently, as flexion is initiated, tension within the ligament assists in reversal of the screw-home mechanism.[2] Rehabilitation activities that stress the

---

Box 19-1

Exercises to Avoid During Early Anterior Cruciate Ligament (ACL) or Posterior Cruciate Ligament (PCL) Rehabilitation

ACL

Loaded open chain knee extension from 50°–5°

PCL

Open chain hamstring exercises in any part of the range of motion
Loaded open chain knee extension from 90°–50°
Closed chain activities with the knee in greater than 50° of flexion

---

MCL would include any hip adductor strengthening exercises in which resistance is placed distal to the knee. In addition, care must be taken during closed kinetic chain activities if the athlete lacks hip control because the hip has a tendency in these conditions to adduct and internally rotate, which creates valgus stress on the knee.

The lateral collateral ligament (LCL) is the primary restraint to varus stress on the knee.[1] The tendon of the biceps femoris overlaps the LCL[32] and may act as an active mechanism to bias the tension of the LCL.[1] The LCL, along with the posterolateral capsule, appears to play a large role in control of external tibial rotation.[20,30] Rehabilitation activities that stress the LCL would include any hip abductor strengthening exercises in which resistance is placed distal to the knee.

Capsular Restraints

The posterior medial and lateral "corners" of the knee joint capsule play an important role in the control of torsional force through the knee. The posteromedial capsule is supported by the semimembranosus muscle and the oblique popliteal ligament, which is an expansion of the tendon of the semimembranosus.[32] The posterior medial corner provides some restraint to valgus stress when the knee is in extension,[1] but it is primarily involved in the control of internal torsional stress.[38]

The posterolateral capsule is reinforced by the arcuate ligament and the popliteus tendon.[21] The posterolateral corner, with the LCL, is primarily involved in control of external rotation stress; however, in an ACL-deficient knee, it also plays a role in controlling internal rotation of the knee.[20,21] The posterolateral corner plays a minor role in control of varus stress on the knee when the knee is extended.[21] The posterior capsule is less prone to injury when the knee is in the flexed position because the structure is relatively slack.[1]

In vitro isolated sectioning of the ACL or PCL is not generally associated with rotational instability,[1,20,21,30,33] but when coupled with sectioning of either of the posterior corners, rotational instability becomes apparent. Clinically, this would suggest that an athlete with acute rotational instability probably does not have an isolated cruciate injury.[33]

Menisci

The meniscus serves a number of important functions, including increasing the stability and congruence of the knee joint,[34,35] load distribution and transmission,[34-37] shock absorption,[34,35]

Table 19-3 Posterior Shear Force Across the Tibiofemoral Joint During Various Activities

Reference	Activity	Knee Position at Peak Posterior Shear(°)	Calculated Force Times Body Weight
Ericson and Nisell[17]	Cycling at 60 RPM, 120-W workload	105	0.05
Kaufman et al[18]	Isokinetic knee flexion at 60°/sec	75	1.7
	Isokinetic knee flexion at 180°/sec	75	1.4
Ohkoshi et al[27]	Squat	15	<0.25
		30	<0.3
		60	0.25–0.5
		90	1.0–1.25

RPM, Rotations per minute.

joint proprioception,[34] and aiding in joint lubrication and nutrition.[34,35] Its shape, attachments, and collagen arrangement allow the meniscus to effectively transmit compressive force across the tibiofemoral joint. Removal of the meniscus reduces the contact area between the femur and tibia, which substantially increases the force per unit area between the two articular surfaces.[36] It is likely that the increase in force per unit area leads to the degenerative changes that often occur after removal of the meniscus.[37,38] The structure and attachments of the menisci also allow early controlled weight bearing after longitudinal meniscal repairs because the sutured edges are approximated by weight-bearing stress.[37]

The peripheral 10% to 30% of the meniscus has a vascular supply from the perimeniscal capillary plexus.[34] The rest of the meniscus, 70% or more, receives nutrition by passive diffusion and mechanical pumping (intermittent compression during joint loading and unloading).[34] Because of the important role that the meniscus plays in the health of the knee joint, meniscal tears in the vascular zone are usually repaired surgically.[34] By extrapolation from animal studies, the tensile strength of the meniscus 12 weeks after repair is approximately 80%.[39]

The menisci move or distort during tibiofemoral motion,[6] distorting posteriorly during flexion and anteriorly during extension. This distortion is caused by a shear from the oblique reaction force between the femur and meniscus.[6] During active flexion, contraction of the semimembranosus and popliteus muscles also assists in pulling the menisci posteriorly.[40] This is why open chain hamstring strengthening is usually avoided in the early rehabilitation phases after meniscal repairs. During internal and external rotation of the knee, the menisci distort in opposite directions. With internal rotation of the femur on the tibia, the medial meniscus distorts posteriorly, whereas the lateral meniscus distorts anteriorly.[6] The opposite occurs during external rotation of the femur on the tibia. In summary, during flexion and extension of the knee, the direction of meniscal distortion follows the direction of movement of the tibial plateau, and during rotation the distortion follows the direction of movement of the femoral condyle. This means that during combined flexion-extension and internal-external rotation movements, the distortions in the anterior and posterior portions of one meniscus are in opposite directions, whereas in the other meniscus the distortion is primarily in one direction. This is why a frequent mechanism of isolated meniscal injury is combined knee flexion and rotation.[41]

PATELLOFEMORAL BIOMECHANICS

It is important to understand patellofemoral biomechanics when one prescribes knee exercises, regardless of the diagnosis. The connection between the tibiofemoral and patellofemoral joints must not be overlooked, nor should these joints be treated independently. Ignoring important aspects of the biomechanics of the patellofemoral joint during rehabilitation of a tibiofemoral joint problem often creates patellofemoral joint problems and unnecessarily extends the rehabilitation process.

Stability of the patellofemoral joint is based on the interplay among bony geometry, ligamentous-retinacular restraints, and muscles.[42] To function optimally, the patellofemoral joint must be able to control forces in the sagittal and frontal planes. Additionally, the hip and foot must control transverse plane forces through the patellofemoral joint. Three factors play an

important role in the sagittal plane mechanics of the patellofemoral joint: the quadriceps force of contraction, the sagittal plane angle of the knee, and the contact area between the patella and femur. The interaction between the force of the quadriceps contraction and the knee angle determines the amount of compressive force that occurs between the patella and femur. The compression force is known as the patellofemoral joint reaction (PFJR) force.[42-44] Increasing the quadriceps force of contraction or increasing the knee angle increases PFJR force[42,43] (Fig. 19-1). It is important to note that at knee angles of less than 25° to 30°, even large quadriceps forces do not produce tremendous compression force because the magnitude of the posteriorly directed resultant force vector is sufficiently reduced.[42,43] During most rehabilitation activities, gravity has a profound influence on the force of the quadriceps contraction. As the torque of gravity increases during an exercise, the force of the quadriceps must increase. For typical open chain quadriceps exercises, as the knee moves toward extension, the torque of gravity increases and therefore the force of the quadriceps must increase. The opposite is true for common closed chain activities: the torque of gravity decreases as the knee moves toward extension and thus the force of the quadriceps decreases as well.

The third factor to consider in sagittal plane forces is the contact area between the patella and femur. The contact area depends on the contact points between the patella and femur, which change based on the tibiofemoral joint flexion angle (Fig. 19-2).[42,44-47] In general, the contact area between the articular surfaces of the patella and femur increases as knee flexion progresses toward 90°.[42,44,47] Because the patellofemoral contact area varies, it is important to account for it when the influence of the PFJR force is examined. This relationship, PFJR force applied per unit area of contact, is known as patellofemoral contact stress.

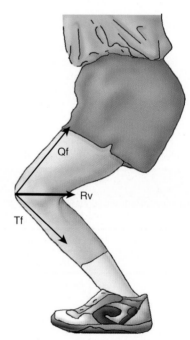

FIGURE 19-1 Resolution of quadriceps force (*Qf*) and patellar tendon force (*Tf*) produces a resultant posteriorly directed force (*Rv*).

During typical open chain quadriceps exercises, as the knee extends, patellofemoral joint contact stress increases significantly because of the increasing PFJR force and decreasing contact area.[42-44] Experimentally, it appears that during open chain quadriceps exercises, maximal contact stress peaks at approximately 35° to 40°. It then declines as extension continues because of the reduced sagittal plane angle of the knee.[42,43] During typical closed chain exercises, as the knee extends, the patellofemoral joint contact stress decreases despite the decreasing contact area. This occurs because PFJR force is decreasing rapidly as a result of the decreasing torque of gravity and decreasing sagittal plane angle of the knee. Patellofemoral contact stress is also influenced by patellar position in the frontal and transverse planes. Inappropriate alignment in these planes can produce a nonuniform pressure distribution with higher peak stress in some areas and relative unloading in others.[47]

Figure 19-3 is a graphic representation of data from several studies of patellofemoral contact stress versus knee flexion angle during both open and closed chain activities.[42-44] The lines for open and closed chain contact stress cross at approximately 50°. These data suggest that for an athlete with an extensor mechanism problem, open chain strengthening activities for the quadriceps are safest from 90° to 50° and from 10° to 0°, whereas closed chain activities are safest from 50° to 0°. These "safe" and "unsafe" ranges should be used only as a guide, with the truly detrimental ranges and loads being determined by the signs and symptoms of the athlete. Initially, athletes with extensor mechanism problems will often experience an increase in pain and symptoms if exercises are performed in the suggested unsafe ranges. However, as the athlete's condition improves, loads through greater ranges, including the suggested unsafe ranges, will typically be tolerated without symptoms. Decisions

on when to advance the exercise program should be based on the signs and symptoms of the athlete. Most athletic endeavors will require the athlete to tolerate loads through a wide range of motion (ROM) under a wide variety of situations. Therefore, in the late stages of the rehabilitation process, it is often necessary for the athlete to perform activities in the unsafe ranges if these activities are to be tolerated on return to sport.

Table 19-4 contains calculated PFJR force data for a variety of rehabilitation activities. Care must be taken when interpreting the data in this table because they do not account for the contact area through which the PFJR force is being applied. Direct comparison should be made only between activities with peak compression force at similar angles of knee flexion and therefore similar contact area. For example, a comparison between knee extension with a 9-kg weighted boot and cycling, which appear to have similar PFJR force values (1.4 and 1.3, respectively), would be misleading. Because the patellofemoral contact area is greater at 83° than at 36°, patellofemoral joint contact stress will be much greater during the knee extension exercise. Box 19-2 provides a summary of activities with high and low patellofemoral contact pressure.

The frontal plane forces that must be balanced by the extensor mechanism also originate from forces developed by the quadriceps. As with the sagittal plane forces, contraction of the vastus lateralis (VL), vastus intermedius, rectus femoris, and vastus medialis longus (VML) produces a superiorly directed force that is resisted by an inferiorly directed force from the patellar tendon. In the frontal plane these two opposing forces do not form a straight line but instead form an angle similar to the physiologic valgus angulation between the femur and tibia (Fig. 19-4).[45] Resolving these two forces provides a resultant force that is directed laterally. This resultant force is referred

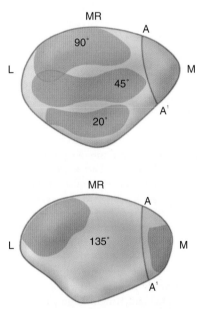

FIGURE 19-2 Patellofemoral contact pattern during knee flexion. *A-A¹*, Ridge separating the medial and odd facets, *L*, lateral; *M*, medial; *MR*, median ridge. *(From Goodfellow, J., Hungerford, D.S., and Zindel, M. [1976]: Patellofemoral joint mechanics and pathology: 1. Functional anatomy of the patello-femoral joint. J. Bone Joint Surg. Br., 58:287–290.)*

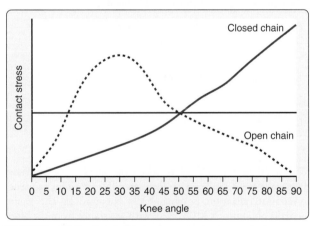

FIGURE 19-3 Patellofemoral contact stress during open and closed chain activities. The area below the *horizontal line* indicates relatively low contact stress, a potentially "safe" zone. The area above the *horizontal line* indicates relatively high contact stress and therefore a potentially "unsafe" zone. *(Graph developed from data reported by Hungerford, D.S., and Barry, M. [1979]: Biomechanics of the patellofemoral joint. Clin. Orthop. Relat. Res., 144:9-15; Reilly, D.T., and Martens, M. [1972]: Experimental analysis of the quadriceps muscle force and patellofemoral joint reaction force for various activities. Acta Orthop. Scand., 43:126-137; and Steinkamp, L.A., Dillingham, M.F., Markel, M.D., et al. [1993]: Biomechanical considerations in patellofemoral joint rehabilitation. Am. J. Sports Med., 21:438–444.)*

Table 19-4 Patellofemoral Compressive Forces During Various Activities*

Reference	Activity	Knee Position at Peak Patellofemoral Compressive Force	Calculated Force Times Body Weight
Dahlkvist et al[48]	Squat, slow ascent	45°	4.73
	Squat, slow descent	—	7.41
	Squat, fast ascent	55°–60°	5.99
	Squat, fast descent	60°	7.62
Ericson and Nisell[49]	Cycling at 60 RPM, 120-W workload	83°	1.3
Flynn and Soutas-Little[50]	Forward running	35% of stance phase	5.6
	Backward running	52% of stance phase	3.0
Huberti and Hayes[47]	Squat	90°	6.5
Kaufman et al[18]	Isokinetic knee extension at 60°/sec	70°	5.1
	Isokinetic knee extension at 180°/sec	80°	4.9
Reilly and Martens[43]	Walking	8°	0.5
	Straight leg raise	0°	0.5
	Knee extension with a 9-kg weighted boot	36°	1.4
	Ascending and descending stairs	40°–60°	3.3
	Deep squat	135°	7.6
Scott and Winter[51]	Running	Midstance	7.0–11.1

*Because of the change in patellofemoral contact area at different points in the range of motion, it is appropriate to compare activities that occur only in similar ranges

---

Box 19-2

Contact Pressure and the Patellofemoral Joint

ACTIVITIES WITH HIGH CONTACT PRESSURE
Loaded open chain knee extension from 50°–20°
Closed chain activities with the knee in greater than 50° of flexion

ACTIVITIES WITH LOW CONTACT PRESSURE
Loaded open chain knee extension from 90°–50° and from 20°–0°
Closed chain activities with the knee in less than 50° of flexion

---

to as a valgus vector.[45] Thus, when the quadriceps contracts, the patella has a tendency to shift laterally.[45,52,53] This tendency toward lateralization is dynamically balanced by the vastus medialis obliquus (VMO)[45,52,53] with assistance from the static restraints of the medial portion of the extensor retinaculum. When the patella is seated in the femoral sulcus, the lateral wall of the sulcus will also assist in resisting the laterally directed resultant force vector.[45,54]

Several factors have been suggested to influence the magnitude of this valgus vector, including hip position, extensibility of the lateral retinacular structures, competence of the medial retinacular structures, femoral and tibial alignment, foot alignment, and ineffective firing or weakness of the VMO. Excessive hip internal rotation during the loading response in walking or running causes a functional increase in physiologic valgus of the femur and tibia.[55,56] This leads to a greater valgus vector, which can decrease the efficiency of the extensor mechanism.

Several factors can contribute to excessive hip internal rotation during gait, including weakness of the gluteus medius, tightness of the tensor fasciae latae, weakness of the hip lateral rotators, and excessive foot pronation.[55,56] Tightness in the lateral retinaculum is associated with lateral compression syndrome in the patellofemoral joint.[45,55] Loss of static restraint from the medial retinacular structures can also result in an increased tendency of the patella to track laterally.[45]

Lower extremity bony malalignment can contribute to an increased valgus vector. Such malalignment includes genu valgum, anteversion of the femoral neck, and external tibial torsion.[55-57] Hughston et al[57] referred to combined femoral neck anteversion and external tibial torsion as the "treacherous extensor mechanism malalignment." Varus deformity of the foot leading to excessive pronation during gait is another lower extremity alignment problem that contributes to an increased valgus vector.[55,58] Eng and Pierrynowski[58] reported that use of a soft foot orthosis with medial posting was effective in reducing pain in patients with symptomatic patellofemoral pain syndrome and varus foot deformities.

Some evidence in the literature suggests that closed chain exercise may positively influence tracking of the patellofemoral joint.[59-61] Ingersoll and Knight[61] compared patellar tracking angles in a group of normal subjects trained in biofeedback who were in a program involving both open and closed chain activities with a group of normal individuals performing a program of entirely open chain progressive resistance exercises. The group performing the combination of open and closed chain exercises with biofeedback had improved tracking measures, whereas the open chain–only group actually had an increase in lateral glide.

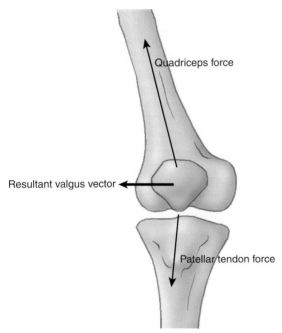

Quadriceps force

Resultant valgus vector ←

Patellar tendon force

FIGURE 19-4 Frontal plane valgus vector created by resolution of the quadriceps and patellar tendon forces.

Doucette and Child[59] investigated the patellar congruency angle with computed tomography during an open chain activity and a closed chain activity in patients with lateral compression syndrome. The patellar congruence angle was improved in the closed chain activity versus the open chain activity at knee angles of 0°, 10°, and 20°. Their results also suggested that patellar tracking during open chain activities improves with greater amounts of flexion. They concluded that open chain exercise appears to be more appropriate at angles greater than 30° of flexion, which corresponds to the safe ranges of patellofemoral joint contact stress for open chain activities.[42,44,59]

MUSCLE FUNCTION

The quadriceps femoris is the primary dynamic stabilizer of the knee and is responsible for knee extension. Functionally, it plays an important role in decelerating knee flexion and absorbing shock when one lands on the lower extremity.[62] As would be predicted based on the influence of gravity, open chain knee extension exercises with a 12–repetition maximum (RM) load produce greater quadriceps activity than do squats or leg presses with a 12-RM load as the knee extends from approximately 45° of flexion to 0°. Squats and leg presses produce more quadriceps activity from about 60° to 95° of knee flexion than does a 12-RM open chain knee extension load in the same ROM.[13]

The straight leg raise, isometric quadriceps contraction (quad set), and knee extension exercises are typical therapeutic exercises prescribed after knee injury or surgery. Total quadriceps activity is greater during a quad set than during a straight leg raise or unweighted knee extension exercise.[63,64] Soderberg and Cook[65] reported electromyographic (EMG) data for the rectus femoris and vastus medialis during a straight leg raise and quad sets. They noted an increase in rectus femoris activity with a straight leg raise and an increase in vastus medialis activity when a quad set was performed. These results were supported by a study of EMG activity from the VMO, VML, vastus lateralis, and rectus femoris by Karst and Jewett.[66]

These authors also tested whether a straight leg raise performed with the hip in external rotation or while resisting an abduction force would preferentially recruit the VMO. They found no difference in VMO recruitment under these conditions. Karst and Jewett[66] concluded was that if the goal was to address the vasti group, the quad set was a better exercise than the straight leg raise.

Currently, there is no way to test the strength of the VMO in isolation from the rest of the quadriceps musculature, so it is impossible to directly measure isolated weakness in the VMO. Consequently, researchers have used electromyography to quantify the firing patterns and behavior of the heads of the quadriceps. In particular, attention has centered around the firing patterns of the VMO and VL and VMO-to-VL ratios.[59,60,67-73] The results of these studies have not been conclusive. It has been reported that in persons without patellofemoral pain syndrome, the VMO fires significantly faster than the VL does, whereas in persons with patellofemoral pain, the VL fires first.[72] These results, however, were not supported by a more recent study.[70] The VMO-to-VL ratio in both symptomatic and asymptomatic individuals engaged in a variety of open and closed chain activities has been reported to be approximately 1:1 in two studies[67,71] and 2:1 in another.[73] The discrepancy between these results is in part due to the large individual variability in the VMO-to-VL ratio even within the normal asymptomatic population.[67] In normal individuals, Worrell et al[73] reported a range of VMO-to-VL ratios of 0.35 to 17.21. Additionally, the reliability of the measurement is also problematic, with reported intraclass correlation coefficients being as low as 0.40.[73]

Probably the most comprehensive investigation of quadriceps activity during different rehabilitation exercises was performed by Cerny.[67] In this study, EMG activity was measured from the VMO, VL, and adductor magnus during more than 20 exercises in both normal individuals and patients with patellofemoral pain. The exercises with the greatest quadriceps EMG activity in this study appeared to be quad sets and step-downs. Cerny concluded that none of the exercises studied selectively recruited the VMO in either normal individuals or patients with patellofemoral pain syndrome. The addition of resisted hip adduction to squats or leg presses does not appear to have an impact on recruitment of the VMO[74] or improve the outcome of patients with patellofemoral pain.[75] In all the studies discussed, it should be noted that the VMO never functioned independently of any other head of the quadriceps during any of the exercises evaluated. Thus, the clinical results from these exercises would, in all likelihood, be a generalized quadriceps-strengthening effect.[76]

Much debate has arisen about the different roles of the quadriceps musculature, especially the VMO, in the various ranges of motion. Historically, it was accepted that the VMO was responsible for terminal knee extension. Some of this interpretation was based on the fact that atrophy of the vastus medialis is more visible because of the normal prominence of the muscle and the thinness of its fascial covering in comparison to that over the VL.[53] This visibility misled clinicians into the belief that the quadriceps atrophy was specific rather than general. At the same time, clinicians noted that patients had difficulty performing terminal knee extension and that an extensor lag was often present.[77] In a classic series of studies, Lieb and Perry[53,78] defined the role of the VMO as a dynamic stabilizer against lateral displacement of the patella. Their studies determined that the VMO in isolation could not produce any extension of the knee. Each of the other parts of the quadriceps, in isolation, could produce knee extension. Interestingly, the first study was published in 1968, and confusion

---

Box 19-3

Vastus Medialis Obliquus (VMO) Function

Is the VMO active during terminal knee extension? Yes, but so are the other parts of the quadriceps. In fact, the VMO is active through any range of knee extension when the other parts of the quadriceps are active.

Does the VMO become more active during open chain terminal knee extension than during open chain knee extension from 90°–60°? Yes, but so do the other parts of the quadriceps. It is estimated that the terminal ranges of knee extension require twice as much quadriceps force to accomplish the last 15° of extension[79,80] because of lessening of the quadriceps mechanical advantage and an improvement in the mechanical advantage of gravity.[6]

Is the VMO strengthened with terminal knee extension exercises? Yes, but so are the other parts of the quadriceps.[76] It gets stronger through training, not because it is extending the knee, but because it is contracting against the patellar lateralizing force of the other parts of the quadriceps.

If the VMO is weak in isolation, can that weakness reduce knee extension torque? Yes, because without the function of the VMO to stabilize the patella, the extension torque created by the other parts of the quadriceps is not being applied through an efficient patellofemoral mechanism.

Box 19-4

General Principles for Developing and Implementing Any Knee Rehabilitation Program

Awareness of the process of inflammation in the joint
Level of muscle control or strength
Amount of range of motion available
Establishment of weight-bearing status
Present functional status and desired outcomes

Note: The rehabilitation specialist should always be mindful of these principles when working within the time constraints placed on the rehabilitation program by any particular protocol.

---

still lingers over the role of the VMO. Some of this confusion can be related to the subtlety of the function of the VMO in relation to the other quadriceps muscles. Box 19-3 summarizes the function of the VMO in the form of clinically relevant questions.

The hamstrings produce knee flexion, tibial rotation, and hip extension. Functionally, the hamstrings act more as hip extensors than as knee flexors because under most closed chain conditions, gravity produces the necessary knee flexion. For the knee joint, providing stability is a more important hamstring role than creating flexion. Hamstring contractions reduce loads on the ACL by creating a posterior shear force on the tibia. Cocontraction with the quadriceps also stiffens the knee joint and thus makes it more stable.[81] The semitendinosus has been found to contract against valgus loads on the knee, whereas the biceps femoris contracts against varus loads.[82] The biceps femoris rotates the tibia externally, and the semimembranosus and semitendinosus rotate the tibia internally. In the presence of anterolateral rotatory instability or anteromedial rotatory instability, facilitation of enhanced neuromuscular control of the biceps femoris (anterolateral rotatory instability) and the semimembranosus and semitendinosus (anteromedial rotatory instability) may assist in the control of abnormal tibial excursions.

AN OVERVIEW OF KNEE REHABILITATION PRINCIPLES

Before rehabilitation guidelines and protocols for specific pathologic knee conditions and surgical procedures can be addressed, an overview of general knee rehabilitation principles should be offered. Significant changes have recently occurred in the area of knee rehabilitation, with the greatest change being the speed at

which patients are progressed through the rehabilitation process. Although the process has become much more rapid, the rehabilitation specialist should not simply focus on time frames to advance a patient's rehabilitation program but should always keep in mind certain basic rehabilitation principles when evaluating the patient's condition and the appropriateness of the rehabilitation program (Box 19-4).

After trauma to the knee, whether from surgery or injury, the acute inflammatory process must be addressed. Specifically, joint effusion should be evaluated and treated and pain management techniques should be initiated. Appropriate, early treatment focused on controlling acute inflammation can significantly affect the rehabilitation program, both immediately and at the final outcome. This early antiinflammatory treatment can help minimize losses in both strength and ROM. Ice, compression, and elevation, applied in conjunction with safe, pain-free condition-appropriate exercise, can aid in progressing through the acute stage of inflammation as rapidly as possible. Care should be taken by the rehabilitation specialist to not further irritate an acutely inflamed joint. Being too aggressive with exercises, weight-bearing status, or functional activities can keep the knee acutely inflamed and significantly lengthen the time needed for rehabilitation or even lead to permanent damage within the joint.

At the knee, achieving adequate quadriceps recruitment early in the rehabilitation process is extremely important. Quadriceps recruitment can be inhibited by the effects of acute inflammation. Kennedy et al[83] determined that as little as 60 mL of saline injected into the knee decreases quadriceps recruitment by 30% to 50%. In a patient with true acute inflammation, the presence of pain could further diminish the ability to recruit the quadriceps. Biofeedback units may be used to aid the patient in developing a strong voluntary quadriceps contraction. If any voluntary contraction is difficult to perform, electrical muscle stimulation can be used to aid the patient in developing a contraction. Because Spencer et al[84] found that as little as 20 mL of knee joint effusion may selectively inhibit contraction of the vastus medialis, this head of the quadriceps should be targeted when biofeedback or electrical stimulation is used.

Early knee motion after surgery or injury is critical to help prevent joint fibrosis, provide nutrition to the articular cartilage,[7] and initiate controlled stress. This stress will help align the collagen fibers and thereby provide a flexible, strong scar and promote the return of normal joint mechanics.[85] Active ROM at the knee, within case-appropriate range limitations, can be initiated as soon as pain allows. Supine heel slides can be used to aid in regaining knee flexion. However, such slides can be painful

Table 19-5 **Pain Resistance Sequence**

Reaction to Movement*	Joint Status	Treatment Action
Pain before resistance	Acute	Red light—No attempt should be made to gain ROM.
Pain with resistance	Subacute	Yellow light—A gentle attempt can be made to regain ROM but should be done cautiously. (Vigorous attempts may cause reversion to the acute state.)
Resistance before pain	Chronic	Green light—Vigorous intervention may be necessary to restore ROM.

Data from Wallace, L.A., Mangine, R.E., and Malone, T. (1985): The knee. In: Gould, J.A. III, and Davies, G.J. (eds.), Orthopaedic and Sports Physical Therapy. St. Louis, Mosby.

ROM, Range of motion.

*Refers to passive movement through the physiologic range.

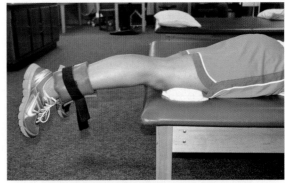

FIGURE 19-5 Prone passive knee extension with weight. To improve effectiveness, the hip should be maintained in neutral rotation.

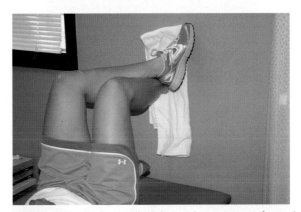

FIGURE 19-6 Supine wall slides with assistance from the uninvolved lower extremity.

at the knee because of contraction of the rectus femoris during flexion at the hip. Active knee flexion can also be done in either the seated or side-lying positions. Active assisted ROM can be very effective in regaining ROM. Techniques such as using a towel to pull the knee into more flexion or having the clinician aid the athlete in taking the knee into more flexion often allow greater gains in ROM to be achieved, as long as the patient's complaints of pain are not increased significantly. Slow pedaling on a stationary bike is another excellent way to increase knee ROM, as long as care is taken to not irritate the tibiofemoral or patellofemoral joints. If no substitution is allowed, the knee requires approximately 105° to 110° of flexion to complete a revolution on a properly fitted bike.

Mobilization of the patellofemoral joint should be initiated during the early-motion phase to help restore its normal arthrokinematics.[86] Without normal patellofemoral arthrokinematics, it is very difficult for the patient to regain normal, pain-free knee flexion and extension. The patella should be mobilized superiorly, inferiorly, medially, and laterally. A decrease in superior and inferior patellar glide can decrease knee extension and flexion ROM, respectively. Stretching of the lateral patellar retinaculum, as described by McConnell,[87] can possibly help decrease the incidence of patellofemoral pain by aiding in restoration of normal patellofemoral arthrokinematics.

As progress out of the acute stage of knee inflammation is made, more aggressive rehabilitation techniques can be initiated. However, it is imperative that the rehabilitation specialist accurately determine the status of the joint. Signs such as increased temperature, effusion, and levels of pain should be used to classify the stage of inflammation. For example, when the clinician feels soft tissue resistance to passive ROM before the athlete complains of any joint pain, more aggressive passive ROM techniques may be used (Table 19-5). Knee extension is often the most difficult ROM to regain, but normal extension ROM is required before a normal gait pattern can be achieved. Regaining extension, both passive and, when appropriate, active, should be set as a very high priority in any knee rehabilitation program. Various techniques can be used. One method involves placing the athlete prone with the thigh resting on the edge of the table, just proximal to the patella. As the athlete relaxes, the knee is pulled into extension. Weight can be added to the ankle to increase the force of the

stretch. This method provides a low-load, long-duration stretch that can lead to plastic deformation of the tissues limiting extension (Fig. 19-5). Spring-loaded splints are available commercially, such as the Dynasplint (see Fig. 6-8),* that can be used to deliver a low-load, long-duration stretch to tissues that surround the patient's knee.

Numerous techniques can be used in an attempt to regain flexion at the athlete's knee. For example, supine wall slides can be performed to regain early amounts of flexion. However, when the athlete achieves approximately 110° of flexion, wall slides may no longer be effective unless an additional outside force is applied, such as the athlete's other leg (Fig. 19-6). The final ranges of flexion can also be achieved by the athlete doing towel pulls while in a seated position. In addition, passive flexion can be achieved by the athlete using body weight while sliding forward from a seated position (Fig. 19-7). Another method to increase flexion is by using a Total Gym† setup as pictured in Figure 19-8. The stress that is applied to the knee is controlled by the angle of the slide of the board or by the range-limiting protection strap (or by both). Joint mobilization is an important adjunctive treatment that can be used to aid in regaining flexion. Both inferior glides of the patella and posterior glides of the tibiofemoral joint can be used to aid in increasing the athlete's flexion. As gains in knee flexion are made, it is important

---

*Available from Dynasplint Systems, Severna Park, MD.

†Available from Engineering Fitness International, San Diego, CA.

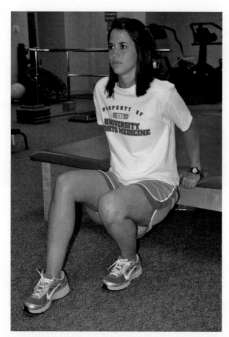

FIGURE 19-7 Passive knee flexion using body weight.

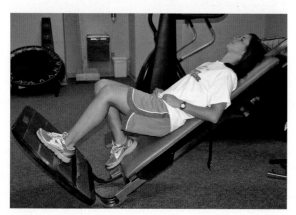

FIGURE 19-8 Total Gym. Passive flexion is controlled by the angle of the slide board or by the range-limiting protection strap.

to stretch the rectus femoris muscle. In addition to assisting in maintenance of the flexion gained, rectus femoris flexibility also reduces some of the patellofemoral joint compression force that occurs during flexion ROM activities.

Strengthening exercises should be initiated in a controlled fashion to ensure that the athlete properly executes the various strengthening exercises. These exercises should be progressed in a manner that both provides protection to healing structures and prevents abnormal muscle recruitment patterns or habits from developing. For example, additional resistance should not be added to straight leg raises or terminal knee extension exercises until the athlete can go through the full, case-appropriate ROM. If additional resistance is added too soon, the athlete might not be able to exercise throughout the full ROM and weakness in certain areas of the range might develop. For example, if too much resistance is added to an athlete's terminal knee extension exercises and full extension ROM is not achieved during the exercise, an extensor lag could develop. This extensor lag could then be manifested in a patient's functional activities as a deviation during gait.

Initially, simple exercises such as four-quadrant straight leg raises, multiple-angle isometrics, and both supine and prone terminal knee extension exercises can be started. These initial exercises are open chain exercises that allow isolation of muscles. These simple, one-plane exercises allow the rehabilitation specialist to concentrate on single muscle groups or physiologic movements that can be considered components of larger functional movements or skills. For example, four-quadrant straight leg raises can be used to strengthen the thigh and hip musculature in preparation for the athlete beginning more advanced functional activities such as single-leg squats.

Clinical Pearl #1

Verbal, physical, and visual cues should be used to assist the athlete in maintaining correct lower extremity alignment during weight-bearing activities; examples include the following:
- Verbal cues remind the athlete to keep the knee directly over the foot during closed chain activities.
- Physical cues, such as rubber tubing (or Thera-Band), can be used to apply a valgus-directed load on the knee. The athlete is then instructed to resist the pull of the tubing (while keeping the knee over the foot) as squats, leg press, and other exercises are performed.
- Visual cues, such as performing the exercises in front of a full-length mirror, allow the athlete to see when lower extremity alignment is inappropriate.

When weight bearing is allowed, the athlete can begin performing appropriate closed chain exercises. This type of exercise uses muscles that cross joints both proximally and distally to assist with motion at the desired joint. These exercises allow athletes to strengthen muscles throughout their ROM but do not provide isolated strengthening of a particular muscle, which is why both open chain and closed chain exercises should be part of the rehabilitation program. Close attention must be paid to proper performance of these exercises. During closed chain exercises, each joint depends on other joints both proximally and distally to assist in proper body alignment. If closed chain exercises are begun too early or an athlete's rehabilitation program is limited to just these types of exercise, weak muscles can be substituted for and abnormal habit patterns might develop. For example, if the hip musculature is not strong enough to control adduction and internal rotation of the thigh, the knee will assume a valgus alignment and the foot will be pronated. This alignment increases the Q angle at the knee and predisposes the athlete to the development of patellofemoral pain during the rehabilitation program. This can occur with a lateral step-up or leg press exercise (Figs. 19-9 and 19-10). If this pattern of movement then becomes ingrained into the athlete's movements during sporting activity, the athlete can become more susceptible to both overuse and traumatic injuries.

As strength and ROM levels in the lower extremity improve, proprioception exercises can be added to the rehabilitation program. Proprioception, as defined by Sherrington, refers to all neural input from joints, muscles, tendons, and associated deep tissues.[88] Proprioception, also referred to as joint position sense, seems to primarily be determined by muscle spindle receptors.

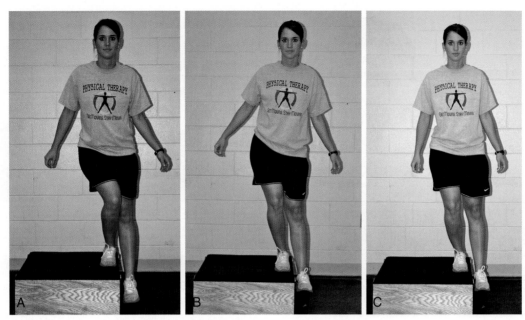

FIGURE 19-9 Lateral step-up. **A,** Performed incorrectly, with the hip being allowed to adduct and rotate internally. **B,** Performed incorrectly. The pelvis should be maintained level and not allowed to drop. **C,** Performed correctly.

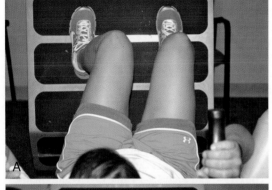

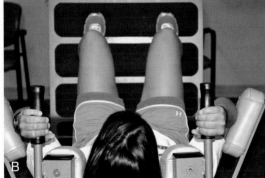

FIGURE 19-10 Leg press. **A,** Performed incorrectly. The hip is adducted and internally rotated. **B,** Performed correctly.

> **Box 19-5**
>
> **Example of Closed Chain Progression of Minisquat**
>
> Weight shifts with support
> ↓
> Weight shifts without support
> ↓
> Bilateral minisquats with support
> ↓
> Bilateral minisquats without support
> ↓
> Bilateral minisquats against a wall
> ↓
> Bilateral minisquats against a wall with weights in hands
> ↓
> One-legged minisquats with support
> ↓
> One-legged minisquats without support
> ↓
> One-legged minisquats against a wall
> ↓
> One-legged minisquats against a wall with weights in hands
> ↓
> Bilateral minisquats with tubing
> ↓
> One-legged minisquats with tubing
> ↓
> Gradual increase in tubing strength and speed of movement

These muscle receptors are assisted to a lesser degree by cutaneous and joint receptors, thereby providing the neuromuscular control required for a joint to perform efficiently. Proprioception can initially be addressed in the rehabilitation program even before the patient progresses to full weight bearing. Patients can perform partial weight-bearing activities on the Biomechanical Ankle Platform System (BAPS)*or Total Gym to begin stimulating the

proprioceptive system. As the patient progresses to full weight-bearing activities, the proprioception exercises can be advanced in difficulty in a variety of ways. A sequenced minisquat program (Box 19-5) is often a good method to begin this progression. When the minisquat program is initiated, the athlete has a tendency to excessively flex the trunk and pelvis to achieve the desired depth of motion (Fig. 19-11). This substitution pattern

*Available from Camp International, Jackson, MI.

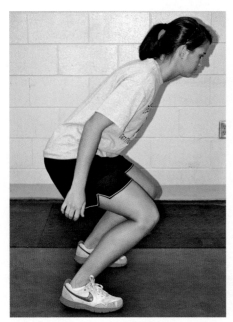

FIGURE 19-11 Squat performed incorrectly. Excessive trunk and hip flexion reduces the load on the quadriceps and knee range of motion.

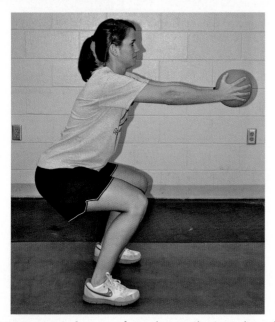

FIGURE 19-12 Squat performed correctly. A medicine ball held in this manner assists in training the proper technique.

reduces knee ROM and the load on the quadriceps. To train appropriate squat technique, especially as the depth of the squat sequence increases, it is often helpful to have the athlete hold a medicine ball or dumbbell out in front of the body (Fig. 19-12). This provides a slight forward shift in the center of gravity, which in turn allows the athlete to learn how to "sit back" when performing a squat-type activity. To assist in the transition to single-leg full weight-bearing activities, a sled-style leg press or Total Gym is useful. For example, the athlete can hop from spot to spot while on the leg press machine (Fig. 19-13). Progression of this exercise is accomplished by increasing load, increasing performance time, and changing the hop sequence.

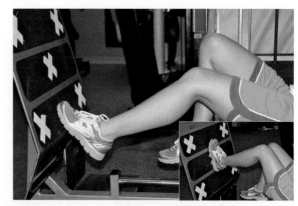

FIGURE 19-13 Leg press bounding. *Inset,* Starting position.

Box 19-6
Lunge Progression*
Balance and reach forward
Balance and reach backward
Balance and reach laterally
Forward lunge
Backward lunge
Lateral lunge
Diagonal lunge
Crossover lunge
Crossover diagonal lunge
*Lunges can be further progressed by having the athlete carry dumbbells, toss medicine balls, or work against rubber tubing resistance.

As the athlete successfully progresses through a minisquat program, further challenges can be achieved with a lunge program (Box 19-6 and Figs. 19-14 and 19-15) and finally a hop/plyometric program (Box 19-7 and Fig. 19-16). Single-leg balance activities can also be performed with a Medi-Ball Rebounder*(Fig. 19-17). This type of activity can be progressed by changing from a stable weight-bearing surface to an unstable one, such as a wobble board. If a rebounder is not available, Thera-Band[†] can be used to increase the difficulty of proprioception exercises. The athlete stands on the involved leg with the Thera-Band attached to the uninvolved leg (Fig. 19-18). Various activities can then be performed with the Thera-Band, such as flutter kicks, hip abduction/adduction, or hip flexion with knee flexion, and again the weight-bearing surface can be changed from stable to unstable as the exercises progress.

Other proprioception activities include the use of devices such as the BAPS and the slide board (Fig. 19-19). Chapter 24 contains examples of lower extremity proprioceptive exercises. Care should be taken when one adds proprioception exercises to make sure that the athlete has the strength and coordination needed to safely perform the exercises. All the proprioception activities described force the involved leg to make numerous high-speed adjustments for the athlete to maintain balance.

---

*Available from Engineering Fitness International, San Diego, CA.
[†]Available from The Hygenic Corporation, Akron, OH.

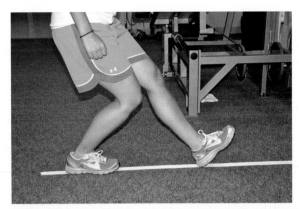

FIGURE 19-14 Forward balance and reach exercise, a low-level lunge activity.

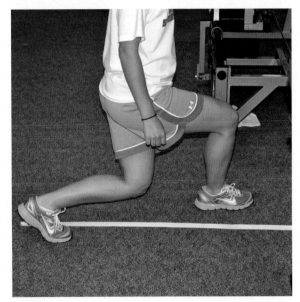

FIGURE 19-15 Crossover lunge, an advanced lunge activity.

As ROM, strength, and proprioception improve, cardiovascular and muscular endurance must be addressed in preparation for the athlete to return to full functional levels. Biking can be used to increase endurance when knee ROM is adequate. Pool exercises, including swimming, use of a kick board, or water running, can be used to increase endurance (see Chapter 11). Elliptical trainers are a good choice for a weight-bearing endurance activity. Because the elliptical motion is somewhat similar to running, but without the impact loading of running, it can be used as a precursor to a running program. Running can be used as an endurance activity, but care must be taken to not irritate the knee by advancing the program too aggressively. Table 19-6 contains an example of a running progression program. Threlkeld et al[89] determined that backward running avoids the rapid initial loading of the knee that occurs with forward running because of the absence of heel strike. This may benefit an athlete who is unable to perform forward running as a result of pain.

Isokinetic equipment may be useful for the development of muscular power and endurance near the end of the rehabilitation process. Because anterior knee pain is often a complication of knee rehabilitation programs, caution must be used

---

Box 19-7

Hop Functional Progression*

DOUBLE LEG
Hop in place
Forward hop
Backward hop
Triple hop
Side to side
Crossover
Scissors hop
Dot drills
180° hops

SINGLE LEG
Forward hop
Triple hop
Backward hop
Side to side
Crossover
Dot drills
Lateral bounds

---

*The athlete should land as quietly as possible with good knee flexion to dissipate force. Difficulty is increased by increasing speed, distance, and time and by adding cones to jump over or adding external loads (or both). Lateral bounds are performed by taking off and landing on different lower extremities.

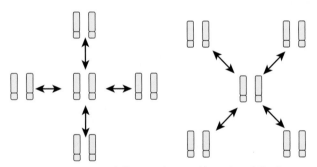

FIGURE 19-16 Dot drills are advanced hopping drills that can be increased in difficulty from two-leg hops to single-leg hops.

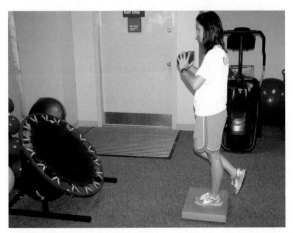

FIGURE 19-17 Medi-Ball Rebounder balance activity. The athlete stands on the involved leg.

with these types of open chain exercises because of both the potential for high patellofemoral joint compression force and the possibility of excessive tibial translatory effects. For these reasons, one may have to limit the ROM that the athlete exercises through on this equipment.

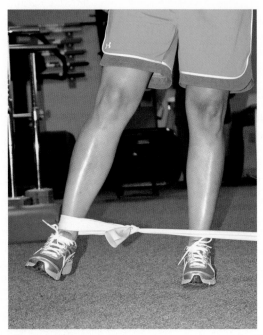

FIGURE 19-18 Proprioceptive exercise with use of a Thera-Band. The athlete stands on the involved leg and attaches the Thera-Band to the uninvolved ankle. The Thera-Band is pulled in each direction with the uninvolved leg while the involved leg attempts to maintain balance.

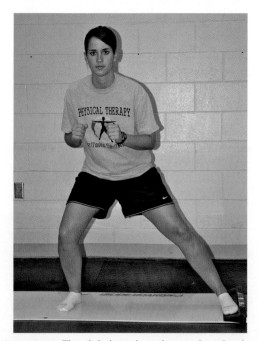

FIGURE 19-19 The slide board can be used to develop muscular strength, proprioception, eccentric firing of the hamstring muscles, and cardiovascular conditioning.

The final stage of any knee rehabilitation program should be return to normal activities through the implementation of an appropriate progression of functional exercises. No athlete should be released back to sports simply on the basis of scores from various strength and ROM measurements. Functional activities should begin with exercises as simple as jogging in a straight line and progress from there. Both the speed and the difficulty of the exercises should be increased until athletes are able to perform activities similar to those that they will be expected to perform when they return to their sport. Specific functional progressions are discussed later in the chapter. Functional testing is covered later in the chapter as well.

In rehabilitation of the knee, every possible option should be offered to help the athlete return to the preinjury level. Each athlete should be constantly reevaluated throughout rehabilitation so that the program can be adjusted appropriately to address specific conditions and requirements. No two injuries are identical because every athlete's physical, mental, and healing capabilities are different. Consequently, there are no specific "cookbook" approaches, and each rehabilitation program should be designed to maximize the athlete's potential as quickly and as safely as possible.

REHABILITATION FOR SPECIFIC KNEE INJURIES

Patellofemoral Dysfunction

Patellofemoral joint dysfunction with pain is one of the most prevalent pathologic knee conditions seen in athletes.[70] This problem can be either the primary diagnosis or a secondary complication found with other knee injuries or after surgical procedures. Even if the patellofemoral joint is not the primary site of injury or dysfunction, care must be taken to not irritate or damage the joint during other lower extremity rehabilitation programs.

Many conditions fall under the broad heading of patellofemoral dysfunction. Anterior knee pain is often the phrase used to describe any condition that leads to pain in the extensor mechanism at the knee. Because the diagnosis is frequently one of a very general nature, rehabilitation can be viewed as general in nature as well. As with other overuse injuries, rehabilitation is often done to correct or improve the biomechanics of the entire lower extremity in an attempt to decrease the patient's pain and dysfunction.

Table 19-6 Running Functional Progression

Initial Activities	Advanced Activities
Jogging in place	Jogging in figure of eights (large to small)
Jumping rope	Jog-sprint-jog (changing speeds)
Jogging	Sprinting/reversing/cutting on specified spot
Jogging forward/reversing on command	Sprinting/reversing/cutting on command
Side-to-side sliding	Sport-specific drills

The need for a comprehensive lower extremity evaluation is paramount in athletes complaining of anterior knee pain. Functioning of the patella depends on a fine balance between ligaments and muscles because of the lack of inherent bony stability at the patellofemoral joint. When this balance is disrupted by weakness, tightness, or other biomechanical problems, improper tracking of the patella can occur.[67] Lateral tracking of the patella is the most common tracking abnormality seen at the patellofemoral joint. Common causes of lateral tracking include VMO dysfunction, tight lateral soft tissues, and various biomechanical problems that increase the tendency of the patella to track laterally. VMO dysfunction can be caused by weakness of the VMO from disuse or effusion-induced neuromuscular shutdown. If the VMO is not pulling with enough force, it cannot offer the medially directed dynamic stability that is required to counteract the other heads of the quadriceps and keep the patella tracking appropriately. Tight lateral soft tissues around the knee can also increase lateral tracking of the patella. If structures such as the patellar retinaculum, iliotibial band, and tensor fasciae latae are tight, they can cause the patella to track more laterally and possibly lead to pain in the area. Biomechanical problems anywhere along the lower extremity that affect alignment of the femur on the tibia can affect tracking of the patella. Many of these malalignment problems can be bony in nature, and it is not possible for the rehabilitation specialist to change them. For example, a wide pelvis that leads to an increased genu valgum angle at the knee cannot be "corrected" by rehabilitation. However, some malalignment problems are able to be treated. For example, excessive pronation of the subtalar joint can lead to an increased Q angle at the knee and possibly increased lateral tracking at the patellofemoral joint. The rehabilitation specialist can treat this excessive pronation as described later in this chapter.

Rehabilitation of patellofemoral dysfunction, after a comprehensive evaluation, should concentrate on recruiting the VMO, normalizing patellar mobility, increasing general flexibility and muscular control of the entire lower extremity, and addressing any other biomechanical problems that can be altered by treatment (Box 19-8). The most important concept to keep in mind when the patellofemoral joint is being rehabilitated is that no exercise should cause pain at the joint. Both the patient and the rehabilitation specialist should always proceed with this guiding factor in mind.

Although various exercises have been touted to isolate the VMO, no specific exercises have been proved to isolate the VMO.

Therefore, when the rehabilitation specialist is attempting to recruit and strengthen the VMO, no specific exercise should be considered superior to all others. Any knee extension exercise that elicits contraction of the VMO and does not cause pain at the patellofemoral joint is appropriate. Use of a biofeedback unit to monitor VMO contraction is one method that is extremely helpful in ensuring that exercises are having an impact on the VMO. A biofeedback unit can be used in conjunction with a variety of open and closed chain exercises. Electrical stimulation units may also be used to obtain a strong contraction in the VMO.

Clinical Pearl #2

Lower extremity biomechanical problems frequently lead to or potentiate patellofemoral dysfunction. Key areas to evaluate and address during rehabilitation include hip abductor strength, foot alignment, and the flexibility of the rectus femoris, hamstrings, gastrocsoleus, and tensor fascia latae.

Several techniques have been reported to be helpful in normalizing patellar mobility in patients who have a laterally tracking patella because of tight lateral structures. The three most commonly reported techniques are manual patellar mobilization, patellar taping as described by McConnell, and iliotibial band/tensor fasciae latae stretching. Kramer[90] reported success with manual lateral retinaculum stretching when it was used as part of a comprehensive patellofemoral rehabilitation program. He described two manual maneuvers: (1) medial patellar glide held for 1 minute with the knee extended to stretch the lateral retinaculum and (2) patellar compression with tracking. This second technique is performed with the athlete sitting and the knee flexed to 90°. The patella is compressed against the patellofemoral articular surface and tracked medially by the clinician as the athlete extends the knee (Fig. 19-20). Neither of these techniques should cause any pain in the athlete's patellofemoral joint. Another method of stretching the lateral structures involves flexing the knee to approximately 30° to 60° of flexion and then applying a posterolateral force against the medial border of the patella. This pushes the medial border of the patella down and lifts the lateral border, thereby stretching the lateral structures.

Box 19-8

Patellofemoral Rehabilitation

After a comprehensive lower extremity evaluation:
- Facilitate recruitment of the VMO
- Normalize patellar mobility
- Increase lower extremity flexibility
- Address any alterable lower extremity biomechanical problems
- Be sure that *all* activities are pain free at the patellofemoral joint

VMO, Vastus medialis obliquus.

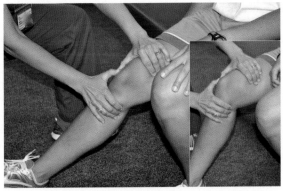

FIGURE 19-20 Patellar compression with tracking to stretch the lateral retinaculum performed as the knee is actively extended. *Inset,* Starting position.

Patellar taping as described by McConnell[87] remains somewhat controversial in patellofemoral rehabilitation, in large part because the mechanism of how it works remains to be elucidated. The results of studies examining the effects of taping on quadriceps activity, joint kinematics, and patellar positioning have been inconsistent and are generally of low study quality.[91] Derasari et al[92] also suggested that changes in these variables in the posttaped condition are very much influenced by their baseline. However, the majority of studies using pain as an outcome measure have demonstrated a reduction in pain.[91,93] Therefore, if taping techniques allow the athlete to exercise with reduced or no complaints of anterior knee pain, the techniques should be used. However, the athlete should not rely on taping techniques for prophylaxis; an appropriate rehabilitation program addressing the underlying causes of the pain should be followed.

McConnell based the application of tape on various evaluative measurements. She looked at several components of patellar orientation: (1) the medial/lateral glide component, (2) the medial/lateral tilt component, (3) the rotation component, and (4) the anterior/posterior tilt component. It has been reported that these measurements are not able to be obtained reliably, either between testers or even by the same tester at different times.[94] However, there are other methods of determining which taping techniques should be used. It is rather simple to quickly ascertain whether the taping techniques will benefit a particular patient. One activity that reliably replicates a patient's complaints of patellofemoral pain must be found before the taping techniques can be used. This activity is referred to as the *asterisk sign.* Usually, a lateral step-up or minisquat is found to be an asterisk sign for these patients. As individual pieces of tape are placed on the patient's knee, the asterisk sign is reevaluated to determine whether the tape has decreased the patient's pain. McConnell described four main types of tape application: (1) correcting lateral glide, (2) correcting lateral tilt, (3) correcting external rotation, and (4) correcting anterior-posterior tilt, in which the inferior pole of the patella is tilted posteriorly (Fig. 19-21). Although whether these pieces of tape correct the position that McConnell described is still being questioned, the tape can still be of clinical use. If pain with the patient's asterisk sign is decreased or alleviated after an individual piece of tape is applied, that piece of tape is left on. If the tape does not have an impact on pain with the asterisk sign, that piece of tape is removed. This simple procedure is used for all four of the taping techniques that are described. Although attempting to answer why these techniques might work is very difficult, one may quite simply determine whether the tape is a reasonable adjunct to the treatment regimen. The authors have anecdotally found taping techniques to be a reasonable addition that can help many patients progress through a patellofemoral rehabilitation program if they are used appropriately.

Finally, in the area of normalizing patellar mobility, specific attention should be paid to the iliotibial band and tensor fasciae latae. If, during the evaluation, these structures are found to be tight, stretching should be instituted. It is important that stretching of these structures be performed correctly (Fig. 19-22). Ultrasound applied to these structures in conjunction with stretching may aid in gaining flexibility.

The next area that should be addressed in patellofemoral rehabilitation is increasing general flexibility and muscular control of the entire lower extremity. It is especially important that the athlete have normal levels of flexibility in the rectus femoris, iliopsoas, and hamstring muscles. A tight rectus femoris can

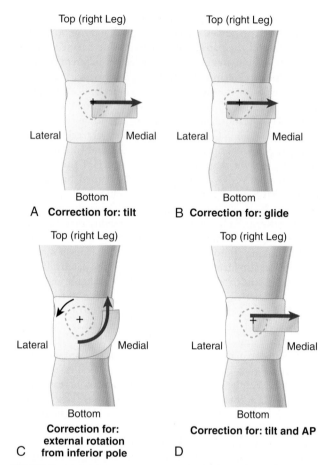

FIGURE 19-21 Tape correction. **A,** For lateral patellar tilt. **B,** For lateral patellar shift. **C,** For external rotation of the patella. **D,** For anteroposterior (AP) tilt of the patella. *(Illustration courtesy Smith & Nephew DonJoy, Inc., Carlsbad, California.).*

cause increased patellofemoral joint pressure. Tight iliopsoas and hamstrings can lead to abnormal gait patterns that increase muscular activity at the knee and patellofemoral joint pressure. Strengthening of the hip abductors to better control the hip in the transverse plane is extremely important (Fig. 19-23). It has been reported that excessive medial rotation of the femur during weight bearing has more impact on patients with patellofemoral pain than does lateral movement of the patella.[95] The athlete should not perform any closed chain exercise in which the hip cannot be controlled (Fig. 19-24; also see Figs. 19-9 and 19-10). As flexibility and strength of the lower extremity increase, the athlete must be able to show good muscle control and coordination for the entire lower extremity. This idea of appropriate control at various speeds of activity was discussed earlier in this chapter.

One final topic to be discussed is correctable biomechanical problems that affect lower extremity alignment. The most common problem in this area is excessive pronation at the subtalar joint, which can lead to an increased Q angle at the patellofemoral joint. This excessive pronation is often a compensation for a forefoot varus malalignment. Arch taping techniques, such as the Low-Dye (see Fig. 20-37) or Herzog technique, can be used to determine whether controlling pronation will affect the patient's patellofemoral pain. If taping does lessen the symptoms, orthotics can be used. In a patient with forefoot varus, the orthotic would be constructed with a medial forefoot post to control motion of

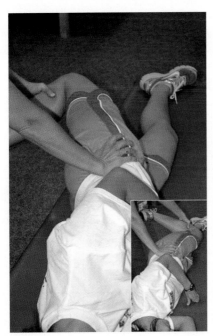

FIGURE 19-22 Method for stretching the tensor fasciae latae. The correct position maintains hip extension and external rotation as the thigh is adducted. *Inset,* Incorrect position allowing the hip to flex during adduction.

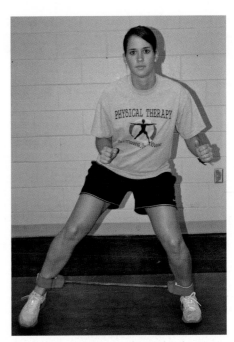

FIGURE 19-23 Lateral lunge performed with resistance tubing to increase recruitment of the hip abductors.

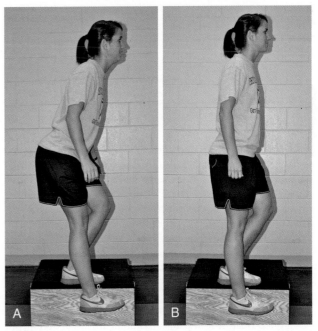

FIGURE 19-24 Lateral step-up technique. **A,** Performed incorrectly, with the hip compensating by excessively flexing the hip and trunk. **B,** Correct technique with the trunk maintained upright.

the forefoot. Appropriate shoe selection and replacement of worn shoes can also aid in control of excessive pronation.

If conservative treatment fails, surgery may be indicated. One of the most common procedures is lateral retinacular release in which the lateral retinaculum is cut to free the patella medially. Additionally, advancement of the VMO can be done in patients who have a VMO with a line of pull more vertical than normal. This is a type of proximal realignment. Table 19-7 shows a lateral release rehabilitation protocol for patients who have not undergone some sort of proximal realignment involving the VMO. The goals in this postoperative rehabilitation program are very similar to those of the conservative rehabilitation program for patellofemoral dysfunction. Emphasis should be placed on regaining patellar mobility and VMO/quadriceps control. Although this surgical procedure was quite popular in the past, it is presently performed less often and only after a course of conservative therapy has failed.

Other more involved surgical procedures, such as distal realignment, can be performed if conservative therapy fails. In a distal realignment procedure the tibial tubercle and patellar tendon are transferred to decrease the patient's Q angle. The main concern with this procedure is advancing knee flexion ROM and weight-bearing status in a fashion that does not excessively stress the tissues involved in surgery. The speed of the rehabilitation program is controlled by the quality of fixation of the realigned bone. Overaggressive flexion ROM work or weight bearing can place too much stress on the fixation site and lead to complications.

Patellar Tendinopathy

Within patellofemoral pain/dysfunction one can consider patellar tendinopathy a special subset of this type of dysfunction. Patellar tendinopathy is a common source of anterior knee pain in athletes engaged in jumping sports, hence the common name

"jumper's knee." Although the same principles discussed for patellofemoral dysfunction earlier apply to rehabilitation of patellar tendinopathy, it appears that the quadriceps-strengthening program should emphasize eccentric training.[96-101] Several specialized eccentric training programs have been recommended, with performance of single-leg squats on a decline board being one of the most common. The typical protocol used with single-leg squats on a decline board includes 3 sets of 15 repetitions performed 2 times a day. Load is increased in 5-kg increments

Table 19-7 Rehabilitation Protocol for Lateral Release

	Week 1	Weeks 2–4	Weeks 4–6	Week 6
Functional progression	Begin WB and four-quadrant lifts	Begin WB without crutches	Begin strengthening Absence of pain	Return to sport No effusion
Criteria	As pain allows	SLR with no extensor lag Full extension in gait No limp No increase in pain No increase in edema/effusion	No increase in edema/effusion Full ROM	Functional testing >85% Quadriceps strength >85%
Evaluation	Pain Incision Effusion/edema Active flexion Quadriceps recruitment Passive extension Patellar mobility Hamstring flexibility	Pain Gait Incision/scar Effusion/edema ROM/patellar mobility Quadriceps recruitment	ROM Quadriceps recruitment Patellar mobility Standing balance Self-report functional status	Functional testing Strength testing Self-report functional status
Treatment	Pain management Effusion/edema control Active flexion exercise Quadriceps recruitment exercises Passive extension Patellar mobilization Hamstring stretching IT band stretching	Pain management Effusion/edema control Scar massage Active ROM exercise Patellar mobilization Quadriceps recruitment General strengthening Flexibility exercise Minisquat progression	Strengthening Endurance exercise Proprioception exercise Hop and lunge progression Jogging progression	Strengthening Endurance exercise Sport-specific drills
Goals	75% WB Increase patellar mobility Full passive extension SLR without extensor lag	WB without crutches AROM 0°–110° Normal patellar mobility Good flexibility	Full AROM Strengthening without pain	Return to sport

AROM, Active range of motion; *IT,* iliotibial; *ROM,* range of motion; *SLR,* straight leg raise; *WB,* weight bearing.

when the athlete's pain during the exercise is less than 3 on a 0 to 10 visual analog pain scale. Load is reduced if the athlete's pain is greater than 5 on the same scale. The athlete performs the eccentric (lowering) phase of the squat with the involved lower extremity and the concentric (raising) phase with the uninvolved lower extremity. The most commonly recommended decline is 25°, but declines anywhere from 15° to 30° produce similar loads on the patellar tendon,[102] so any decline within this range can be chosen based on the athlete's comfort and control of the exercise. Because of loads on the patellofemoral joint itself during this activity, the athlete should avoid knee flexion angles greater that 60° when performing this exercise.[102]

Surgical treatment of patellar tendinopathy is an option, but the results of a randomized controlled study directly comparing surgical intervention with eccentric training demonstrated no difference in outcome between the two groups.[96] If the athlete chooses surgical treatment, the emphasis of rehabilitation for the first 6 weeks after surgery is on normalizing ROM and flexibility, controlling inflammation, and gradually introducing pain-free strengthening exercises. After 6 weeks, if the athlete has met the criteria of full ROM, normal flexibility, normal gait, no effusion, and good quadriceps control, the emphasis can shift to an eccentric training program. This can be performed similar to the conservative eccentric treatment program described earlier, with the exception that the athlete should not experience pain during the exercise and any progression should be pain free.[96]

Anterior Cruciate Ligament Injuries

Injuries involving the ACL continue to be relatively common in athletics. Although rehabilitation of this injury still varies, there is greater agreement now than there was historically, especially in the early phase of intervention. We will present an overview of commonly accepted guidelines. The time frames discussed in any protocols should be adapted to fit various situations, with progression through any protocol being defined by criteria-based guidelines instead of time alone.

Regardless of whether an athlete has decided to undergo a surgical procedure or conservative treatment, intervention immediately following an ACL injury is the same. The immediate goal is to control the hemarthrosis and general inflammatory process. The athlete should be given crutches and instructed in a pain-free partial weight-bearing gait, and the traditional anti-inflammatory program of ice, compression, and elevation should be started. A brace is not required unless other associated ligamentous injuries are present. Motion exercises should be started immediately, with concentration on passive extension to help prevent rapid scarring in the intercondylar notch. Full extension also allows greater ease of quadriceps recruitment, which is extremely important after ACL injury. Friden et al[103] stated that quadriceps strength decreases after injury because of defects in afferent inflow from the ACL-deficient knee. It is also thought that the lack of voluntary contraction of the quadriceps after

ACL injury may be due to reflex inhibition or arthrogenous muscle inhibition.[104] Weight bearing should be increased as pain decreases, joint effusion decreases, quadriceps control increases, and full active knee extension is achieved. The athlete should not be progressed to full weight bearing until these goals have been accomplished.

If the athlete has chosen conservative care, rehabilitation should progress with emphasis placed on quadriceps strengthening, as well as neuromuscular control of the hamstrings. Historically, emphasis was placed on strengthening of the hamstrings because of their role as the primary dynamic restraint in controlling anterior tibial translation.[105] The importance of the quadriceps to outcome is now better understood, and accordingly, emphasis has changed to addressing general muscle control around the knee. A study by Friden et al[103] in which 26 patients with ACL-deficient knees were tested before and after rehabilitation revealed that loss of strength in the hamstrings was minimal and that the best outcomes were obtained when both general muscular strength and coordination were addressed. The importance of the hamstrings in an ACL-deficient knee might lie more in hamstring control and proprioception. Studies indicate that athletes with complete tears of the ACL experience a decrease in proprioception at the knee.[7] The loss of proprioception may be due to the "ACL-mechanoreceptor reflex arc" to the hamstrings. Beard et al[106] found that the latency of reflex hamstring contraction in an ACL-deficient knee was twice that of the contralateral, uninjured knee. It has been suggested that improving recruitment time of the hamstrings may place less stress on the ACL during functional activities.[7] In addition, it has been reported that using active hamstring control to reduce the pivot shift found with an ACL injury might be the key to successfully avoiding reconstructive surgery. Based on all this information, the rehabilitation specialist should concentrate on facilitating control of the hamstrings, as opposed to simple strengthening in the sagittal plane. Engle and Canner[107-109] reported success in achieving this type of hamstring control in ACL-deficient knees with a program that uses proprioceptive neuromuscular facilitation (PNF) exercises for the hamstrings (Figs. 19-25 and 19-26). More advanced exercises using devices such as the BAPS board, slide board, and Medi-Ball Rebounder facilitate hamstring control and proprioception in functional positions and at higher speeds to control anterior tibial translation during more aggressive functional activities. PNF patterns and seated Thera-Band exercises can also be used to help incorporate the tibial rotation component of the function of the hamstrings. Progressive perturbation training has likewise shown promise[110] when added to standard program of strengthening, aerobic endurance training, agility, and sport-specific activities. Fitzgerald et al[110] reported that ACL-deficient subjects in their progressive perturbation plus standard rehabilitation group were almost five times more likely to return to full sports participation than were ACL-deficient subjects in the standard rehabilitation group. Studies have shown that patellofemoral arthrokinematics is altered in ACL-deficient knees. This should be kept in mind during rehabilitation of an ACL-deficient knee, and care should be taken to not irritate or damage the patellofemoral joint.[111,112]

Although surgery is the most commonly chosen treatment option for competitive athletes, surgery should be delayed until the acute inflammatory process has run its course at the knee. There is great concern that performing surgery on an acutely inflamed joint will lead to more complications during rehabilita-

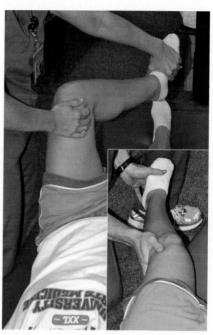

FIGURE 19-25 Proprioceptive neuromuscular facilitation pattern for D₁ flexion. *Inset,* Starting position for D₁ extension.

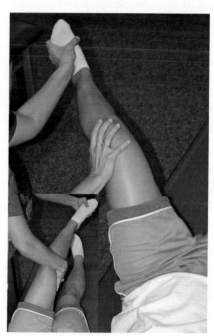

FIGURE 19-26 Proprioceptive neuromuscular facilitation pattern for D₂ flexion. *Inset,* Starting position for D₂ extension.

tion. When the period of acute inflammation has passed, the athlete, using information provided by the sports medicine team, must decide whether a reconstructive procedure is the most appropriate treatment to choose. Whether to reconstruct the ACL or treat it with just a rehabilitation program continues to be a subject of debate. Many factors should be considered when this decision is made, the most important being the ultimate level of function that the patient wishes to achieve. Noyes[113] has recommended that to have the best results, competitive or recreational athletes need surgical intervention whereas light recreational athletes and nonathletes, both of whom can limit their activities, may be able to avoid surgery. Clinically, it appears that a competitive athlete does not generally perform well with an ACL-deficient knee. We are just beginning to understand the combinations of examination measures that may identify the few athletes who might function well without surgery.[114] Noyes et al[115] used subjective and objective measurements to clinically evaluate 84 individuals with ACL-deficient knees. Their conclusion was that an ACL tear leads to functional disability in the majority of patients. They found that one third of the population compensated for the deficiency, knew their limits, and did well; one third of the population compensated for the deficiency but found the instability aggravating; and one third became worse and needed surgery to correct their instability. For the majority of patients who did not undergo surgical reconstructions, knee "giving way" episodes became a common problem.[116] These giving way episodes increase the possibility of a meniscal tear or chondral injury developing. It is well documented that ACL-deficient knees demonstrate abnormal joint kinematics during gait and functional activities, both of which increase the possibility for the development of early degenerative changes.[113,117,118]

When surgery is the chosen treatment, the ACL must be reconstructed because of the lack of success with direct repair of the ligament. The one exception to this rule might be repair of a bony avulsion. If an adolescent has an avulsion fracture without significant ligament failure, primary repair can be a viable option. Concerns that must be addressed when surgery is the treatment of choice include timing of the procedure, graft selection, and surgical technique. The timing of surgery in relation to the inflammatory condition of the joint can greatly affect rehabilitation and ultimate outcomes. It has been shown that reconstructions performed on an acutely inflamed joint are more prone to postoperative complications such as loss of ROM and deficits in function.[119,120] Allowing the patient to go through rehabilitation before surgery helps decrease the number and severity of postoperative complications.

Surgical technique is an area that includes both procedures that are chosen and how well these procedures are ultimately performed. Procedures relate mainly to intraarticular versus extraarticular reconstructions. Extraarticular reconstructions, such as the Ellison or Losee procedures, have been shown to reduce pivot shift but do not reliably limit anterior translation of the tibia or restore normal arthrokinematics through the axis of a normal ACL. Long-term control of knee instability with these extraarticular procedures is poor because of the gradual stretching that occurs in the soft tissues used in the surgical procedure, and therefore extraarticular procedures are used rarely. One remaining use for extraarticular procedures is in skeletally immature patients. Procedures that require drilling through an open physis are often avoided by surgeons because of the possibility of bone growth complications. Although reports are inconsistent, studies have shown that complications have occurred, including leg length discrepancy and physis arrest with the concomitant development of bone deformity.[121,122] For these reasons it is suggested that skeletally immature patients, especially those who are prepubescent, be treated with physis-sparing surgical procedures if surgery is the treatment of choice.

Intraarticular procedures are by far the most commonly used for reconstruction of the ACL. Both graft fixation and graft placement are extremely important surgical variables that will affect the patient's outcome. After years of refinement, the choice of fixation device is now less of a concern than the material that the surgeon is attempting to fixate. In other words, it is easier to obtain early stable fixation when the graft has a bony end as opposed to just tendon. Moreover, it is imperative that isometric graft placement be achieved at the time of surgery. If the graft placement sites are not appropriate, deficits in ROM or abnormal ligament tension might be the result.

A variety of different grafts have been examined for use in intraarticular procedures. Important factors to take into consideration when deciding on graft material are graft strength, fixation required, and comorbid conditions that might be present (including factors such as donor site complications and the possibility of disease transmission). Many types of tissue have been used for intraarticular repair of the ACL, including autografts (tissue transferred from one part of a person's body to another), allografts (human donor tissue), and prosthetics (synthetic material). The most commonly used tissue for both autografts and allografts is a bone-tendon-bone (BTB) taken from the central third of the patellar tendon and the semitendinosus tendon from the hamstrings. Other material can be used as an allograft, including fascia lata and Achilles tendon. Each type of graft has advantages and disadvantages (Table 19-8), which must be taken into consideration when planning the surgery. At one point a BTB autograft was considered the "gold standard" in ACL reconstruction, and although it remains one of the more commonly used grafts, metaanalyses[123-126] have failed to find significant differences in outcome based on the type of graft used. This suggests that according to currently available evidence, factors other than the type of graft used play larger roles in affecting outcome.

The times needed and the percentages of graft strength and revascularization achieved have engendered much debate. Noyes et al[127] reported that at the time of harvesting, 14-mm-wide patellar tendon grafts exhibited 168% of the strength of a normal

Table 19-8 Advantages and Disadvantages of Anterior Cruciate Ligament Grafts

Graft	Advantages	Disadvantages
Patellar BTB autograft	High graft strength Good fixation because of bone-to-bone healing Ease of obtaining graft material	Complications with the extensor mechanism, such as patellar fractures, patellar tendinitis, patellar tendon rupture, and anterior knee pain
Hamstring tendon autograft	Fewer complications with the extensor mechanism Comparable results to BTB autograft	Complications with fixation of graft Possible hamstring weakness More technically complicated procedure
Allograft	No complications with donor sites Increased availability of material	Higher cost Possible disease transmission Possible recipient rejection

BTB, Bone-tendon-bone.

ACL. Cooper et al[128] tested the strength of 10-mm–wide grafts. They chose 10-mm–wide grafts because they believed that most surgeons use this size of graft to minimize the possibility of impingement of the graft in the femoral intercondylar notch. They reported that at the time of harvest the 10-mm–wide graft exhibited 174% of the strength of a normal ACL. Others have reported 10-mm–wide BTB autograft strength to be less (107%) but still above normal values for the ACL. Unfortunately, because of the graft's loss of vascular supply at the time of harvest, its strength decreases significantly from the time of implantation, and it never regains its initial strength levels. The avascular necrosis that occurs after implantation causes the graft to be its weakest somewhere in the 4- to 8-week postoperative period. On the basis of data from animal models, it is generally accepted that BTB autografts undergo a "ligamentization" process that results in a graft whose vascular and histologic appearance 1 year postoperatively resembles that of a normal ACL.[129-131] Using the medial third of the patellar tendon in rhesus monkeys, Clancy et al[131] reported transplanted patellar tendon graft strength to be 53% of normal ACL strength at 3 months, 52% of normal at 6 months, 81% of normal at 9 months, and 81% of normal at 12 months. Although these values are below normal strength levels and far below the strength values at the time of harvesting and implantation, Noyes et al[127] suggested that in most strenuous activities, the ACL is seldom exposed to more than 50% of its maximal load. Allografts appear to go through the same process of avascular necrosis followed by revascularization and cellular proliferation.[132] However, it is believed that patellar tendon allografts are generally weaker throughout the rehabilitation process, which accounts for the slight differences that are often seen in rehabilitation protocols.

Although numerous rehabilitation protocols have been developed, the majority of the most commonly used protocols have certain common themes. Most protocols recommend rehabilitation before surgery. The goals for this stage of rehabilitation include regaining full ROM and neuromuscular control, as well as minimizing the inflammatory process.[125] The risk for arthrofibrosis and other postoperative complications is increased when surgery is performed on an acutely inflamed joint.[133,134] Eitzen et al[135] recommend a 5-week rehabilitation program before surgery that in addition to ROM, includes strengthening, aerobic exercise, plyometric exercises, and perturbation training.

Early Postsurgical Phase

Immediate postsurgical protocols now emphasize early motion, control of inflammation, quadriceps facilitation activities, and patellar mobility. Depending on the surgeon's preference, controlled weight bearing and initiation of low-load closed chain exercises can also begin in this stage. Even though the exact time frames vary from protocol to protocol, it has been found that achieving the early goals of full passive extension, good quadriceps control, and minimal joint effusion/inflammation leads to better ultimate outcomes for the patient (Box 19-9). In this initial period of rehabilitation, emphasis should be placed on gaining and maintaining full extension because flexion ROM will usually increase as pain and effusion decrease. Full extension is critical for gaining early quadriceps control. In this immediate postoperative phase, quadriceps facilitation activities often include quad sets, multiple-angle knee extension isometrics, neuromuscular electrical stimulation, and weight bearing in extension (if weight bearing is allowed). Because of stress on the ACL

graft, protocols often avoid multiple-angle knee isometrics in the 45° to 5° range. Straight leg raises can also be used in this stage as long as the athlete can perform the exercise without a quadriceps lag. If the surgeon is confident about graft fixation, active terminal knee extension exercises can be initiated as soon as the postoperative pain has decreased. These exercises should be done with no more resistance than simply the weight of the leg. Traditionally, any loaded open chain knee extension exercise in the 45° to 0° range has been avoided because of the stress placed on the graft. However, because the graft is strong when it is initially placed in the knee and loses strength only as it necroses and goes through its revascularization process, active terminal knee extension exercises with no added resistance can be used early in rehabilitation to aid in facilitating quadriceps recruitment. If the athlete has difficulty performing supine terminal knee extension exercises, they can be performed in the prone position, where the hip extensors can aid in achieving full knee extension (Fig. 19-27).

When a patellar tendon autograft is used as the graft material, it is important to achieve normal patellar mobility so that scarring around the harvest site does not occur and lead to infrapatellar contracture syndrome.[120] If the patella loses mobility as a result of scarring, ROM and strength can be significantly decreased. Early in the rehabilitation process, the patellar area might be too tender because of the incision at the graft harvest site to allow productive mobilization. Facilitation of early quadriceps recruitment will help in obtaining patellar movement.[136] Electrical stimulation can be extremely valuable in facilitating a quadriceps contraction great enough to result in superior mobilization of the patella. If electrical stimulation is being used in this early stage for quadriceps strengthening instead of merely facilitation, the knee should be placed in approximately 60° or greater of flexion.[137] Developing quadriceps control at full knee extension is extremely important for several reasons. Quadriceps contractions increase patellar mobility, these quadriceps contractions help maintain full extension ROM, and without good

---

Box 19-9

Goals for Early Rehabilitation After Reconstruction of the Anterior Cruciate Ligament

Decrease knee joint effusion
Achieve full passive knee extension
Develop good quadriceps control, especially in extension
Develop/maintain patellar mobility

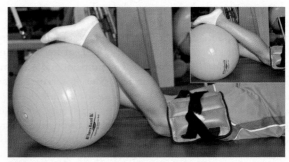

FIGURE 19-27 Prone terminal knee extension. The quadriceps is assisted in performing knee extension by the hip extensors. *Inset,* Ending position.

quadriceps control in full extension the athlete will not be able to ambulate with a normal gait pattern. When passive knee extension ROM is obtained during rehabilitation, it can be very difficult to maintain unless the patient has enough quadriceps strength to actively go into full extension.

When the patient can actively recruit the quadriceps, using biofeedback units to increase the level of recruitment can be extremely helpful. Biofeedback requires complete patient involvement because it monitors only what the patient is doing and offers no stimulation of the muscle. For patients who tolerate electrical stimulation, Snyder-Mackler et al[137] found that it helped them regain quadriceps strength at a faster rate. In a study of 110 patients, they found that high-intensity electrical stimulation performed at 65° of flexion in a closed chain position resulted in 70% recovery of quadriceps strength by 6 weeks postoperatively. This compared favorably with the 57% recovery of quadriceps strength in a group that performed only closed chain strengthening exercises. In addition, the group that received electrical stimulation showed better knee control at midstance than did the group that exercised without electrical stimulation.

Weight-bearing status varies between protocols, but most commonly at least partial weight bearing is initiated within days of surgery. It is extremely important to have patients walk with as normal a gait as possible while they are on crutches. Poor habits during gait can be developed in this early stage of rehabilitation, and once a poor gait pattern becomes ingrained, it can be very difficult to break the habit. The most common gait deviation is ambulation with the knee in flexion and never going into full extension.[137] This lack of full extension in gait may be due to lack of strength or ROM (or both), a habit pattern developed before surgery as a result of instability at the knee or a habit pattern developed after surgery. Some protocols require the patient to wear a brace at 0° immediately after surgery so that ambulating with the knee in flexion is not as common a complication. Low-load closed chain exercises can be safely performed in this early stage without creating stresses that are harmful to the graft. The decreased stress that is afforded by the use of closed chain exercises is due to the compression forces at the tibiofemoral joint and the cocontraction of other muscles to help control motion at the hip, knee, and ankle. An excellent initial closed chain exercise is terminal knee extension in the standing position with the use of a Thera-Band (Fig. 19-28).

Progressive Strengthening and Balance Training Stage

The next stage of rehabilitation shifts the focus of the program to progressive strengthening and balance activities. The athlete should advance into this phase only after demonstrating full knee extension, at least 110° of flexion, minimal or no effusion, no quadriceps lag, no pain, and a normal gait pattern without assistive devices. Muscle soreness is not uncommon in this stage, especially as loads and depth of motion are increased, but any activities that cause joint pain should be avoided. Progression of activities through this stage should be curtailed if joint soreness or effusion occurs. If the athlete has also undergone meniscus repair, the rate of progression for lunges, squats, and leg presses (in particular, the depth of motion for these activities) is often slower. If the sur-

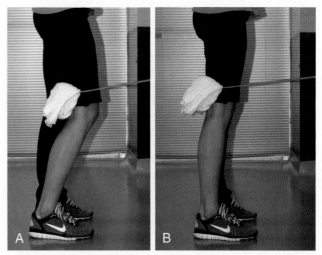

FIGURE 19-28 Closed chain terminal knee extension. **A,** Starting position. **B,** Ending position.

geon used a hamstring autograft for the reconstruction, the rate of progression of open chain hamstring strengthening is frequently slower because of symptoms from the donor site. When the athlete begins this phase, strengthening activities are usually performed with closed chain exercises. It is critical that as loads are increased in closed chain activities, the athlete maintains proper technique. Medial collapse of the lower extremity (see Figs. 19-9 and 19-10), "leaking" too far forward (see Figs. 19-11 and 19-24), and lack of symmetric loading (Fig. 19-29) are common errors in technique that occur if the athlete cannot control the load. If progressive resistance open chain quadriceps strengthening is included before postoperative week 8 to 10, it is generally still blocked from full extension. The amount of extension that is blocked varies from 30° to 60°, depending on the protocol. Full-range, open chain quadriceps strengthening is generally allowed any time from 10 to 12 weeks after surgery, depending on the specific protocol being followed. It is important to use both closed and open chain quadriceps strengthening activities during this stage because the combination has been demonstrated to produce greater quadriceps strength and earlier return to sports participation than closed chain strengthening activities alone.[138] Because the speed of protocols for rehabilitation after ACL reconstruction has increased so much in recent years, it is imperative that the exercises chosen produce a safe amount of stress on the revascularizing ACL. These exercises were presented earlier in this chapter in the section on functional anatomy of the ACL. An understanding of the exercises that place high loads on the ACL is necessary to determine safe exercises at different time frames in the rehabilitation program.

Hip strength should be addressed to decrease the excessive frontal plane motion that might occur as resistance is increased during closed chain exercises (see Figs. 19-9 and 19-23). Lack of control at the hip can contribute to lower extremity malalignment and lead to overuse problems such as patellofemoral pain. Hip-strengthening exercises can include both open and closed chain activities. Both the speed and the difficulty of these exercises can be increased as the patient works through the rehabilitation program.

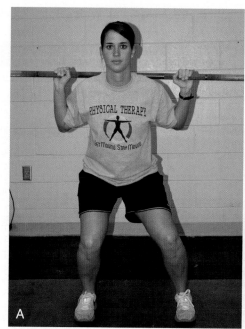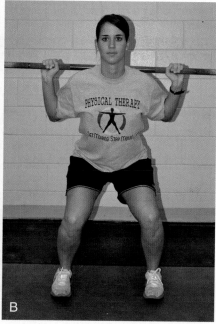

FIGURE 19-29 Squats. **A,** Performed incorrectly because of lack of symmetric loading of the lower extremities. **B,** Performed correctly.

Sport Activity Stage

The final stage of rehabilitation incorporates generic sports activities, including running (see Table 19-6), hopping (see Box 19-7), agility training, and sport-specific activities. The strengthening and balance activities continue in this stage. Most protocols allow this stage to begin somewhere between the tenth and twelfth weeks after surgery. However, to enter this stage the knee should be stable and the athlete should have full knee ROM with respect to the uninvolved side, normal lower extremity flexibility, no effusion, no pain, less than a 20% deficit in quadriceps strength in comparison to the uninvolved side, and the ability to single-leg press more than the athlete's body weight. Myer et al[139] also recommend that that athlete score at least 70 on the International Knee Documentation Committee (IKDC) Subjective Knee Form and be able to hold a single-leg squat at 60° of knee flexion for at least 5 seconds. The purpose of this phase is to gradually challenge the athlete with higher-demand and higher-risk activities in a controlled manner. Progression through this phase should be based on lack of effusion, improving subjective scores (e.g., IKDC), improving strength, and improving control and symmetry in acceleration, deceleration, and landing activities. Successful completion of this phase allows the athlete to return to sport, which usually occurs between 4 and 6 months after surgery. Table 19-9 and Box 19-10 provide examples of rehabilitation protocols for ACL reconstruction with a BTB autograft, and Box 19-11 outlines a program following ACL reconstruction with the semitendinosus.

Although the final outcome may be similar, it is not uncommon for the early rehabilitation stage after reconstruction with an allograft to be slightly slower than that with an autograft (Table 19-10). Depending on surgeon preference, weight bearing is often delayed, commonly from 4 to 6 weeks postoperatively.

When weight bearing is allowed, the order and timing of rehabilitation progression for an allograft are similar to those for an autograft. It should be stressed that regardless of the graft material used, objective criteria should be used to determine whether an athlete is ready to progress to the next stage of the rehabilitation program. Table 19-10 contains the key differences between the rehabilitation programs for a BTB autograft versus an allograft or hamstring autograft.

Functional Knee Braces

Functional braces, whether custom-made or off-the-shelf, are not able to control shear stress through the knee under physiologic loads.[140,141] Even without the ability to control such stress, some athletes report feeling more stable when they wear functional braces. Subjective improvements while an athlete wears a brace have been attributed to changes in proprioception.[142-144] Some evidence indicates that braces alter timing and recruitment of the thigh and calf musculature[145,146] and that patients with greater than a 20% quadriceps deficit perform cutting maneuvers better while wearing a brace.[135] It has also been reported that 3 weeks after ACL reconstruction, patients ambulate with a more erect gait pattern, including greater knee extension, when they wear a functional brace.[147] When braced, patients adopted a strategy that increases use of the hip and ankle joint to control forces through the lower extremity, whereas forces controlled by the knee are reduced. Risberg et al[148] reported better Cincinnati Knee scores 3 months after ACL reconstruction in patients randomly assigned to wear a functional brace. Despite this potential early benefit, no difference was seen between the braced and nonbraced groups at 1- and 2-year follow-up with respect to KT1000* scores, Cincinnati Knee scores, functional hop

*Available from Medmetric, San Diego, CA.

Table 19-9 Rehabilitation Protocol After Anterior Cruciate Ligament Reconstruction With a Bone–Patellar Tendon–Bone Autograft

	Week 1	Weeks 2–4	Weeks 5–8	3 Months	4–6 Months
Functional progression	PWB with 2 crutches	WB with 1 crutch or FWB exercises	Advance strengthening	Begin jogging	Return to sport
Criteria	As postoperative pain allows	Full knee extension during gait SLR with no extensor lag No increase in effusion	No increase in effusion AROM 0°–125° Normal patellar mobility KT1000 <2 mm increase	No increase in effusion No pain Full AROM Eccentric control with one-leg minisquat Leg press strength >70% KT1000 unchanged	No increase in effusion Functional tests >85% Isokinetic tests >85% Pain free KT1000 unchanged Self-report functional measures
Evaluation	Pain Effusion Patellar mobility AROM Passive extension Quadriceps recruitment Incision/portals	Pain Gait AROM/PROM Effusion Patellar mobility Quadriceps recruitment Incision/portals	Pain Gait AROM/PROM Effusion Patellar mobility Flexibility Standing balance KT1000	Pain AROM Effusion KT1000 Leg press strength test One-leg minisquat Lateral step-ups Self-report functional measures	Pain Effusion Functional tests Isokinetic tests KT1000 Self-report functional measures Proprioception tests
Treatment	Pain management Control effusion Patellar mobilization Passive extension and flexion Active flexion Quadriceps NMES or biofeedback	Pain management Control effusion Patellar mobilization AROM/PROM Quadriceps NMES or biofeedback Closed chain exercises Gait training General strengthening (hamstrings, hip, etc.) Scar mobility	Flexibility exercises Proprioception exercises Endurance exercises General strengthening (hamstrings, hip, etc.) Open chain quadriceps strengthening from 60°–90° Increase loads with closed chain exercises	Increase isotonic exercise Aerobic conditioning Open chain quadriceps-strengthening full ROM Begin jogging progression Begin hop progression Proprioception exercises	Increase isotonic exercise Aerobic conditioning Running progression Hop activities Sport-specific activities Proprioception exercises
Goals	PROM 0°–90° 50% WB SLR without extensor lag	AROM 0°–100° 75%–100% WB	Full AROM Normal gait Increase strength and endurance No increase in effusion with 20–30 minutes of biking or ambulating	No pain or increase in effusion with increased resistance through full ROM 85% with functional and strength tests	Return to sport

Adapted from Mangine, R.E., Noyes, F.R. and DeMaio, M. (1992): Minimal protection program: Advanced weight bearing and range of motion after ACL reconstruction: Weeks 1 to 5. Orthopedics, 15:504-515; and DeMaio, M., Mangine, R.E., and Noyes, F.R. (1992): Advanced muscle training after ACL reconstruction: Weeks 6 to 52. Orthopedics, 15:757-767.

AROM, Active range of motion; *FWB*, full weight bearing; *NMES*, neuromuscular electrical stimulation; *PROM*, passive range of motion; *PWB*, partial weight bearing; *ROM*, range of motion; *SLR*, straight leg raise; *WB*, weight bearing.

test scores, pain scores, and patient satisfaction scores. These results are further supported by a systematic review of bracing that found no benefit with the "routine" use of bracing following ACL reconstruction.[149] Additional consideration has to be given to the evidence that bracing increases energy expenditure, decreases maximal torque output from the quadriceps, and increases the rate of fatigue.[150]

Based on the evidence just presented, the use of functional bracing after ACL reconstruction should probably be reserved for athletes who are having difficulty returning to sport because of lack of confidence in the reconstructed knee. While keeping in mind that the benefit associated with the brace is probably only improved proprioceptive function and not control of physiologic

loads, the clinician and athlete must decide whether a custom-made brace is worth the extra cost to the athlete given the off-the-shelf alternatives. It has been the authors' experience that a large percentage of athletes, even those who request one, stop using a functional brace within a year.

Programs to Prevent Anterior Cruciate Ligament Injury

A substantial number of ACL injuries occur in noncontact situations,[151] especially in female athletes (see Chapter 9). A number of factors have been proposed as potential causes of noncontact ACL injuries, including lack of control of abduction/adduction forces across the knee,[152] hamstring weakness,[81,152] electromechanical

Box 19-10

Accelerated Rehabilitation After Reconstruction of the Anterior Cruciate Ligament With a Patellar Tendon Graft

PREOPERATIVE PHASE

Goals:

- Diminish inflammation, swelling, and pain
- Restore normal ROM (especially knee extension)
- Restore voluntary muscle activation
- Protect the knee from further injury—especially the meniscus
- Provide education to prepare the patient for surgery

Brace—Elastic wrap or knee sleeve to reduce swelling
Weight Bearing—As tolerated with or without crutches

Exercises:

- Ankle pumps
- Passive knee extension to 0°
- Passive knee flexion to tolerance
- Straight leg raises (three ways: flexion, abduction, adduction)
- Quad sets
- Closed kinetic chain exercises: minisquats, lunges, step-ups

Muscle Stimulation—Electrical muscle stimulation of the quadriceps during voluntary quadriceps exercises (4–6 hr/day)
Neuromuscular/Proprioception Training:

- Eliminate quadriceps avoidance gait
- Retro stepping drills
- Balance training drills

Cryotherapy/Elevation—Apply ice for 20 min/hr; elevate the leg with the knee in full extension (the knee must be above the heart)
Patient Education—Review the postoperative rehabilitation program

- Review instructional video (optional)
- Select an appropriate surgical date

I. IMMEDIATE POSTOPERATIVE PHASE (DAYS 1–7)

Goals:

- Restore full passive knee extension
- Diminish joint swelling and pain
- Restore patellar mobility
- Gradually improve knee flexion
- Reestablish quadriceps control
- Restore independent ambulation

Postoperative Day 1

Brace—Brace/immobilizer applied to the knee locked in full extension during ambulation and sleeping; unlock the brace while sitting, etc.
Weight Bearing—Two crutches, weight bearing as tolerated

Exercises:

- Ankle pumps
- Overpressure into full, passive knee extension
- Active and passive knee flexion (90° by day 5)
- Straight leg raises (flexion, abduction, adduction)
- Quad sets
- Hamstring stretches
- Closed kinetic chain exercises: minisquats, weight shifts

Muscle Stimulation—Use muscle stimulation during active muscle exercises (4–6 hr/day)

Continuous Passive Motion—As needed, 0°–45°/50° (as tolerated and as directed by the physician)
Ice and Evaluation—Apply ice 20 min/hr and elevate the leg with the knee in full extension

Postoperative Days 2–3

Brace—Brace/immobilizer locked at 0° degrees extension for ambulation and unlocked for sitting, etc.
Weight Bearing—Two crutches, weight bearing as tolerated
Range of Motion—Remove the brace and perform ROM exercises 4–6 times per day

Exercises:

- Multiangle isometrics at 90° and 60° (knee extension)
- Knee extension 90°–40°
- Overpressure into extension (knee extension should be at least 0° to slight hyperextension)
- Patellar mobilization
- Ankle pumps
- Straight leg raises (three directions)
- Minisquats and weight shifts
- Quad sets

Muscle Stimulation—Electrical muscle stimulation of quadriceps (6 hr/day)
Continuous Passive Motion—0°–90°, as needed
Ice and Evaluation—Apply ice 20 min/hr and elevate the leg with the knee in full extension

Postoperative Days 4–7

Brace—Brace/immobilizer locked at 0° extension for ambulation and unlocked for sitting, etc.
Weight Bearing—Two-crutch weight bearing as tolerated
Range of Motion—Remove the brace to perform ROM exercises 4–6 times per day, knee flexion to 90° by day 5 and approximately 100° by day 7

Exercises:

- Multiangle isometrics at 90° and 60° (knee extension)
- Knee extension 90°–40°
- Overpressure into extension (full extension 0°–5°/7° hyperextension)
- Patellar mobilization (5–8 times daily)
- Ankle pumps
- Straight leg raises (three directions)
- Minisquats and weight shifts
- Standing hamstring curls
- Quad sets
- Proprioception and balance activities

Neuromuscular Training/Proprioception—OKC passive/active joint repositioning at 90°, 60°; CKC squats/weight shifts with repositioning
Muscle Stimulation—Electrical muscle stimulation (continue 6 hours daily)
Continue Passive Motion—0°–90°, as needed
Ice and Elevation—Apply ice 20 min/hr and elevate the leg with the knee in full extension

(Continued)

Box 19-10

Accelerated Rehabilitation After Reconstruction of the Anterior Cruciate Ligament With a Patellar Tendon Graft—cont'd

II. EARLY REHABILITATION PHASE (WEEKS 2–3)

Criteria to Progress to Phase II:

- Quadriceps control (ability to perform good quad set and SLR)
- Full passive knee extension
- PROM 0°–90°
- Good patellar mobility
- Minimal joint effusion
- Independent ambulation

Goals:

- Maintain full passive knee extension (at least 0°–5°/7° hyperextension)
- Gradually increase knee flexion
- Diminish swelling and pain
- Demonstrate muscle control and activation
- Restore proprioception/neuromuscular control
- Normalize patellar mobility

Week 2

Brace—Continue locked brace for ambulation and sleeping
Weight Bearing—As tolerated (goal is to discontinue crutches 10–14 days postoperatively)
Passive Range of Motion—Self-ROM stretching (4–5 times daily) with emphasis on maintaining full PROM

- Restore patient's symmetric extension

KT2000 Test—15-lb anterior-posterior test only

Exercises:

- Muscle stimulation superimposed on quadriceps exercises
- Isometric quadriceps sets
- SLR (4 planes)
- Leg press (0°–60°)
- Knee extension 90°–40°
- Half squats (0°–40°)
- Weight shifts
- Front and side lunges
- Hamstring curls standing (AROM)
- Bicycle (if ROM allows)
- Proprioception training
- Overpressure into extension
- PROM 0°–100°
- Patellar mobilization
- Well-leg exercises
- Progressive resistance extension program—start with 1 lb and advance 1 lb/wk

Proprioception/Neuromuscular Training:

- OKC passive/active joint repositioning 90°, 60°, 30°
- CKC joint repositioning during squats/lunges
- Initiate squats on tilt board

Swelling Control—Ice, compression, elevation

Week 3

Brace:

- Discontinue locked brace (some patients use AROM brace for ambulation)
- If the patient continues to use a brace, unlock for ambulation

Passive Range of Motion—Continue ROM stretching and overpressure into extension (ROM should be 0°–100°/105°)

- Restore patient's symmetric extension

Exercises:

- Continue all exercises as in week 2
- PROM 0°–105°
- Bicycle for ROM stimulus and endurance
- Pool walking program (if incision is closed)
- Eccentric quadriceps program 40°–100° (isotonic only)
- Lateral lunges (straight plane)
- Front step-downs
- Lateral step-overs (cones)
- Stair Stepper machine
- Advance proprioception drills, neuromuscular control drills
- Continue passive/active reposition drills (CKC, OKC)

III. PROGRESSIVE STRENGTHENING/NEUROMUSCULAR CONTROL PHASE (WEEKS 4–10)

Criteria to Enter Phase III:

- AROM 0°–115°
- Quadriceps strength >60% of contralateral side (isometric test at 60° of knee flexion)
- Unchanged KT test bilateral values (+1 or less)
- Minimal to no full joint effusion
- No joint line or patellofemoral pain

Goals:

- Restore full knee ROM (0°–125°) symmetric motion
- Improve lower extremity strength
- Enhance proprioception, balance, and neuromuscular control
- Improve muscular endurance
- Restore limb confidence and function

Brace—No immobilizer or brace, may use knee sleeve to control swelling/support
Range of Motion:

- Self-ROM (4–5 times daily using the other leg to provide ROM) with emphasis on maintaining 0° of passive extension
- PROM 0°–125° at 4 weeks

KT2000 Test—Week 4, 20-lb anterior and posterior test

Week 4

Exercises:

- Advance isometric strengthening program
- Leg press 0°–100°
- Knee extension 90°–40°
- Hamstring curls (isotonics)
- Hip abduction and adduction
- Hip flexion and extension
- Lateral step-overs
- Lateral lunges (straight plane and multiplane drills)
- Lateral step-ups
- Front step-downs
- Wall squats
- Vertical squats
- Standing toe/calf raises
- Seated toe/calf raises
- Biodex stability system (balance, squats, etc.)

Box 19-10

Accelerated Rehabilitation After Reconstruction of the Anterior Cruciate Ligament With a Patellar Tendon Graft—cont'd

Week 4—cont'd
- Proprioception drills
- Bicycle
- Stair Stepper machine
- Pool program (backward running, hip and leg exercises)

Proprioception/Neuromuscular Drills:
- Tilt board squats (perturbation)
- Passive/active OKC repositioning
- CKC repositioning on tilt board

Week 6
KT2000 Test—20- and 30-lb anterior and posterior test

Exercises:
- Continue all exercises
- Pool running (forward) and agility drills
- Balance on tilt boards
- Progress to balance and ball throws
- Wall slides/squats

Week 8
KT2000 Test—20- and 30-lb anterior and posterior test

Exercises:
- Continue all exercises listed in weeks 4–6
- Leg press sets (single leg) 0°–100° and 40°–100°
- Plyometric leg press
- Perturbation training
- Isokinetic exercises (90°–40°, 120°–240°/sec)
- Walking program
- Bicycle for endurance
- Stair Stepper machine for endurance
- Biodex stability system
- Training on tilt board

Week 10
KT2000 Test—20- and 30-lb and manual maximum test
Isokinetic Test—Concentric knee extension/flexion at 180°
  and 300°/sec

Exercises:
- Continue all exercises listed in weeks 6, 8, and 10
- Plyometric training drills
- Continue stretching drills
- Progress strengthening exercises and neuromuscular training

IV. ADVANCED ACTIVITY PHASE (WEEKS 11–16)
Criteria to Enter Phase IV:
- AROM 0°–125° or greater
- Quadriceps strength 75% of contralateral side, knee extension flexor-to-extensor ratio 70%–75%
- No change in KT values (comparable to contralateral side, within 2 mm)
- No pain or effusion
- Satisfactory findings on clinical examination
- Satisfactory results on isokinetic test (values at 180°)
  - Quadriceps bilateral comparison 75%
  - Hamstrings equal bilaterally

- Quadriceps peak torque/body weight 65% at 180°/sec in males and 55% at 180°/sec in females
- Hamstrings/quadriceps ratio 66%–75%
- Hop test (80% of contralateral leg)
- Subjective knee scoring (modified Noyes system) of 80 points or better

Goals:
- Normalize lower extremity strength
- Enhance muscular power and endurance
- Improve neuromuscular control
- Perform selected sport-specific drills

Exercises:
- May initiate running program (weeks 10–12) (physician's decision)
- May initiate light sport program (golf) (physician's decision)
- Continue all strengthening drills
  - Leg press
  - Wall squats
  - Hip abduction/adduction
  - Hip flexion/extension
  - Knee extension 90°–40°
  - Hamstring curls
  - Standing toe/calf raises
  - Seated toe/calf raises
  - Step down
  - Lateral step-ups
  - Lateral lunges
- Neuromuscular training
  - Lateral step-overs (cones)
  - Lateral lunges
  - Tilt board drills
  - Sports RAC repositioning on tilt board

Weeks 14–16
- Advance program
- Continue all drills above
- May initiate lateral agility drills
- Backward running

V. RETURN-TO-SPORT PHASE (WEEKS 17–22)
Criteria to Enter Phase V:
- Full ROM
- Unchanged KT2000 test (within 2.5 mm of opposite side)
- Isokinetic test that fulfills criteria
- Quadriceps bilateral comparison (80% or greater)
- Hamstring bilateral comparison (110% or greater)
- Quadriceps torque–body weight ratio (55% or greater)
- Hamstrings-quadriceps ratio (70% or greater)
- Proprioceptive test (100% of contralateral leg)
- Functional test (85% or greater of contralateral side)
- Satisfactory findings on clinical examination
- Subjective knee scoring (modified Noyes system) (90 points or better)

Goals:
- Gradually return to full unrestricted sports
- Achieve maximal strength and endurance

(Continued)

Box 19-10

Accelerated Rehabilitation After Reconstruction of the Anterior Cruciate Ligament With a Patellar Tendon Graft—cont'd

Goals—cont'd
- Normalize neuromuscular control
- Advance skill training

Tests—KT2000, isokinetic, and functional tests before return

Exercises:
- Continue strengthening exercises
- Continue neuromuscular control drills
- Continue plyometric drills
- Advance running and agility program
- Advance sport-specific training
  - Running/cutting/agility drills
  - Gradual return to sport drills

6-MONTH FOLLOW-UP
- Isokinetic test
- KT2000 test
- Functional test

12-MONTH FOLLOW-UP
- Isokinetic test
- KT2000 test
- Functional test

AROM, Active range of motion; *CKC,* closed kinetic chain; *OKC,* open kinetic chain; *PROM,* passive range of motion; *ROM,* range of motion; *SLR,* straight leg raise.

Box 19-11

Rehabilitation Protocol Following Reconstruction of the Anterior Cruciate Ligament With the Semitendinosus

I. IMMEDIATE POSTOPERATIVE PHASE

Goals:
- Protect the ACL reconstruction
- Reduce swelling and inflammation
- Restore and maintain full extension
- Gradually restore knee flexion
- Activate the quadriceps muscle
- Independent ambulation
- Patient education and protection of the graft harvest site

Day 1

Brace—Locked at 0° extension for ambulation
Weight Bearing—Two crutches as tolerated (at least 50% WB)
Range of Motion:
- Full passive extension (0°–90°)
- Obtain hyperextension if present on opposite side—goal is symmetric motion

Exercises:
- Ankle pumps
- Passive knee extension to 0° or equal to opposite side (hyperextension)
- Straight leg raise (flexion)
- Hip abduction/adduction
- Knee extension 90°–40°
- Quad sets
- No hamstring stretching

Muscle Stimulation—Stimulation of quadriceps (4–6 hr/day) during active exercises
Continuous Passive Motion—0°–90°
Ice and Evaluation—Apply ice 20 min/hr and elevate the leg with the knee in extension

Days 2–7

Brace—Locked at 0° extension for ambulation

Weight Bearing—Two crutches as tolerated
Range of Motion—Patient out of brace 4–5 times daily to perform self-ROM 0°–90°/100°

Exercises:
- Intermittent ROM exercises (0°–90°)
- Patellar mobilization
- Ankle pumps
- Straight leg raises (four directions)
- Standing weight shifts and minisquats (0°–30° ROM)
- Knee extension 90°–40°
- Continue quad sets

Muscle Stimulation—Electrical stimulation of quadriceps (6 hr/day)
Continuous Passive Motion—0°–90°
Ice and Elevation—Apply ice 20 min/hr and elevate the leg with the knee in extension

II. MAXIMUM-PROTECTION PHASE (WEEKS 2–8)

Goals:
- Absolute control of external forces and protect graft
- Nourish articular cartilage
- Decrease swelling
- Prevent quadriceps atrophy

Week 2

Brace—Locked at 0° for ambulation only, unlocked for self-ROM (4–5 times daily)
Weight Bearing—As tolerated (goal to discontinue crutches 7–10 days postoperatively)
Range of Motion—Self-ROM (4–5 times daily) with emphasis on maintaining 0° passive extension
KT2000 Test—(15-lb anterior-posterior test only)

Exercises:
- Multiangle isometrics at 90°, 60°, 30°
- Leg raises (four planes)

Box 19-11

Rehabilitation Protocol Following Reconstruction of the Anterior Cruciate Ligament With the Semitendinosus—cont'd

Exercises—cont'd
- No hamstring curls
- Knee extension 90°–40°
- Mini squats (0°–40°) and weight shifts
- Lunges
- Leg press (0°–60°)
- PROM/AAROM 0°–105°
- Patellar mobilization
- No hamstring and calf stretching
- Proprioception training
- Well-leg exercises
- PRE program—start with 1 lb, advance 1 lb/wk

Swelling Control—Ice, compression, elevation

Week 4
Brace—Locked at 0° for ambulation only, unlocked for self-ROM (4–5 times daily)
Range of Motion—Self-ROM (4–5 times daily) with emphasis on maintaining 0° passive extension

Exercises:
- Same as week 2
- PROM 0°–125°
- Bicycle for ROM stimulus and endurance
- Pool walking program, swimming
- Initiate eccentric quadriceps exercise 40°–100° (isotonic only)
- Leg press (0°–60°)
- Emphasize CKC exercise
- StairMaster
- Elliptical

KT2000 Test—(week 4, 20-lb anterior and posterior test)

Week 6
Brace—Discontinue use of drop locked brace

Exercises:
- Same as week 4
- Hamstring curls (light resistance)
- Pool program
- AROM 0°–115°
- PROM 0°–125°
- Emphasize CKC exercises
- Bicycle

KT2000 Test—(week 6, 20- and 30-lb anterior and posterior test)

Week 8
Brace—Consider use of functional brace

Exercises:
- Continue PRE program
- Initiate light hamstring PREs

KT2000 Test—(Week 8, 20- and 30-lb anterior and posterior test)

III. MODERATE-PROTECTION PHASE (WEEKS 10–16)
Goals:
- Maximal strengthening for quadriceps/lower extremity
- Protect patellofemoral joint

Week 10
Exercises:
- Knee extension (90°–40°)
- Leg press (0°–60°)
- Mini squats (0°–45°)
- Lateral step-ups
- Hamstring curls
- Hip abduction/adduction
- Toe/calf raises
- Bicycle
- StairMaster
- Wall squats
- Lunges
- Pool running
- Proprioceptive training
- Continue PRE progression (no weight restriction)

Weeks 12–14
Exercise—Continue all above exercises
Testing—Isokinetic test (180° and 300°/sec, full ROM, 10/15 reps)
KT2000 Test—Total displacement at 15, 20, and 30 lb, manual maximal test
Maintain/Begin Running—If patient fulfills criteria

IV. LIGHT-ACTIVITY PHASE (MONTHS 4–5)
Criteria to Enter Phase IV:
- AROM 0°–125°
- Quadriceps strength 70% of contralateral side, knee flexor/extensor rated 70%–79%
- No change in KT scores (+2 or less)
- Minimal/no effusion
- Satisfactory findings on clinical examination

Goals:
- Development of strength, power, endurance
- Begin gradual return to functional activities

Exercises—Initiate light straight line running (physician's decision)

Exercises:
- Emphasize eccentric quadriceps work
- Continue CKC exercises, step-ups, minisquats, leg press
- Continue knee extension 90°–40°
- Hip abduction/adduction
- Initiate plyometric program
- Initiate running program
- Initiate agility program
- Sport-specific training and drills
- Hamstring curls and stretches
- Calf raises
- Bicycle for endurance
- Pool running (forward/backward)
- Walking program
- StairMaster
- High-speed isokinetics

(Continued)

Box 19-11

Rehabilitation Protocol Following Reconstruction of the Anterior Cruciate Ligament With the Semitendinosus—cont'd

Testing:
- Isokinetic test (180° and 300°/sec, Full ROM, 10/15 reps)
- KT2000 test—Total displacement at 15, 20, and 30 lb, manual maximal test

Criteria for Running:
- Isokinetic test—>85% of opposite leg (quadriceps), >90% of opposite leg (hamstring)
- Isokinetic test—Quadriceps torque/body weight (180°/sec) (60%–65% for males) (50%–55% for females)
- KT2000 test—Unchanged
- No pain/swelling
- Satisfactory findings on clinical examination

Functional Drills:
- Straight line running
- Jog to run
- Walk to run

V. RETURN-TO-SPORT PHASE (MONTHS 6–7)

Goals:
- Achieve maximal strength and endurance
- Return to sport activities

- Continue strengthening program for 1 year from surgery*:
  - *For Quadriceps:*
    - Knee extensions
    - Wall squats
    - Leg press
    - Step-ups
  - *For Strength:*
    - Hamstring curls
    - Calf raises
    - Hip abduction
    - Hip Adduction
  - *For Endurance:*
    - Bicycle
    - StairMaster
    - Elliptical
    - Swimming
  - *For Stability:*
    - High-speed hamstrings
    - High-speed hip flexion/extension
    - Balance drills
    - Backward running

AAROM, Active assisted range of motion; *ACL,* anterior cruciate ligament; *AROM,* active range of motion; *CKC,* closed kinetic chain; *PRE,* progressive resistance exercise; *PROM,* passive range of motion.
*Pick one.

Table 19-10 Differences in Anterior Cruciate Ligament Rehabilitation Programs Between Patellar Tendon Autograft and Allograft or Hamstring Autograft

Patellar Bone-Tendon-Bone Autograft	Allograft or Hamstring Autograft
WBAT (with crutches) immediately	NWB for 4 weeks 25% WB from 4–5 weeks 50% WB from 5–6 weeks 100% WB at 6 weeks *or* PWB (with crutches) in brace locked in full extension for 1 week WBAT (with crutches) in brace locked in full extension from 1–2 weeks
Full ROM unloaded knee extension can begin as early as 2 weeks postoperatively	Full ROM unloaded knee extension can begin about 6 weeks postoperatively
Bilateral hopping can begin around 10 weeks	Bilateral hopping can begin around 12 weeks
Single-leg hopping can begin around 12 weeks	Single-leg hopping can begin around 14 weeks

NWB, Non–weight bearing; *PWB,* partial weight bearing; *ROM,* range of motion; *WBAT,* weight bearing as tolerated; *WB,* weight bearing.

delay in hamstring activation,[153] reduced cocontraction of the quadriceps and hamstring,[81] muscle fatigue,[153,154] reduced gastrocnemius recruitment,[153] and insufficient ankle and hip balance and control.[153,154]

Several types of programs have been proposed to address these factors, including plyometric programs,[151,152] wobble board training,[81,154] and perturbation training.[110] The results of studies using plyometric[151] or wobble board[154] training programs indicate that athletes participating in these training regimens have a reduced incidence of ACL injuries. A perturbation training study[110] demonstrated that ACL-deficient athletes were more successful in returning to sports if their rehabilitation included perturbation training. Wobble board and perturbation training programs progressively challenge the athlete's balance and thereby train the athlete to develop strategies that maintain control of the ankle, knee, and hip. Plyometric training improves the athlete's ability to control abduction/adduction forces, especially when landing from a jump.[152] Plyometric training also improves hamstring strength[152] and hamstring activation time.[81] It is important to note that all three types of training are performed functionally with weight bearing through the lower extremity and are controlled "high"-speed activities rather than traditional strength-training exercises. Because of the benefits, these activities should not only be used for ACL prevention programs but also be incorporated into the functional progression, as appropriate, after ACL injuries or reconstruction.

Posterior Cruciate Ligament Injuries

Injury to the PCL is still relatively uncommon in the athletic population. An athlete is much more likely to injure the ACL or MCL. The literature on rehabilitation after PCL injury or surgery is therefore limited.[24]

Tibiofemoral and patellofemoral articular cartilage damage can develop in a PCL-deficient knee and lead to very debilitating pain and dysfunction.[24] Although these degenerative changes do not occur in all PCL-deficient knees, it is a complication that must be considered when one is trying to decide whether surgery is the best option for the athlete.[155] Retropatellar pain can develop and become quite disabling in this patient population. This pain may be a result of the excessive quadriceps activity that occurs in an attempt to control the posterior tibial translation that takes place after the PCL is damaged. There is still much discussion on the topic of whether to reconstruct the PCL in patients with an isolated tear. However, if quadriceps strengthening programs do not control the laxity in athletes with a PCL-deficient knee, surgery becomes the best option.

When surgical reconstruction of the PCL is performed, a variety of tissues can be used. Autografts of bone–patellar tendon–bone, semitendinosus, or the medial head of the gastrocnemius can be used. Patellar tendon or Achilles tendon allografts can also be used. However, the surgical techniques for reconstruction are quite varied, and no particular technique is presently viewed as the gold standard. In fact, Anderson and Noyes[24] stated that data demonstrating the ability of any operative procedure to restore posterior stability at all angles of knee flexion are still incomplete.

The greatest concern after PCL reconstructive surgery is protection of the graft in the early stages of rehabilitation, which can be more difficult than after ACL reconstruction. In general, all the time frames for progression of the rehabilitation program are slightly slower after PCL reconstruction than after ACL reconstruction. The initial goals in the first 3 to 4 weeks of the postoperative rehabilitation program are to control inflammation/effusion, develop quadriceps control, maintain patellar mobility, and minimize stress on the graft. Most protocols call for bracing of the knee and limit weight bearing for 4 to 6 weeks. Isolated open chain hamstring exercise is strictly controlled for 8 to 12 weeks to limit the amount of posterior tibial translation stress that is applied to the reconstructed PCL. Athletes are usually progressed to full weight bearing in the 6- to 10-week range as long as they have good quadriceps control and adequate ROM (especially extension) and the knee joint is not acutely inflamed.

Clinical Pearl #3

Following reconstruction of an ACL- or PCL-deficient knee, patellofemoral dysfunction is one of the most common complications. Therefore, in planning and monitoring the rehabilitation program for athletes with these surgeries, care should be taken to avoid potentiating this complication. A simple rule of thumb is that all athletes who have undergone ligament reconstruction are patellofemoral problems waiting to happen.

As the rehabilitation program is advanced, closed chain activities are emphasized so that cocontractions of the lower extremity musculature aid in preventing posterior tibial translation. Because of the increasing posterior shear stress that occurs as the depth of closed chain activities increases, it has been recommended that the extent of knee flexion be limited to less than 45° during the initial introduction of such activities to the rehabilitation program.[156] Biomechanical analysis of wall squats and lunges by Escamilla et al[157,158] provides further considerations for reducing PCL load when using these activities. Normally, the recommended technique for wall squats and lunges is to not allow the knee to move anterior to the foot. "Shortening" up both the wall squat and the lunge (allowing the knee to move anterior to the foot) produced less calculated load on the PCL than when performing the exercise with the normally recommended technique. Care must be exercised, though, when using "shortened" lunges to not irritate the patellofemoral joint since shortened lunges significantly increase stress on the patellofemoral joint.[159]

Like ACL reconstruction, progression of athletes through the late stages of rehabilitation (sports activity stage) should be based on lack of effusion, improving subjective scores, improving strength, and improving control and symmetry in acceleration, deceleration, and landing activities. The time of return to full activity and sports is extremely variable and individualized to each athlete. Variables that affect the timing of return to sport include the type of surgery, other structures involved in the surgery, age and condition of the athlete, type of activities that the athlete wishes to return to, and other complications that might have occurred during rehabilitation. If the athlete is going to be able to return to full function, it generally takes more than 6 months and is usually closer to 12 months.

An example of a rehabilitation protocol after a two-tunnel autograft reconstruction is shown in Table 19-11. Rehabilitation for single-tunnel reconstructions is similar, but progression of weight bearing and ROM is often more conservative.

Medial Collateral Ligament Injuries

MCL injuries receive less attention today because of nonoperative management of them and their frequent involvement with ACL injuries, which receive more attention. Isolated grade I and II MCL injuries are always managed nonoperatively, and general symptom-driven guidelines for knee rehabilitation are followed. Bracing is often used initially to control valgus stress on the knee. Depending on the severity of the injury, the brace might be set to limit knee ROM. Brace settings vary from allowing full extension to blocking 15° of extension. Usually up to 90° of flexion is allowed. The patient is allowed to bear partial weight immediately if it is pain free. Weight bearing is progressed as tolerated, and full weight bearing is allowed by 3 to 6 weeks for most grade II injuries. For grade I injuries, full activity is usually permitted in 3 to 4 weeks, and for grade II injuries, full activity is allowed in 6 to 8 weeks. To return to sport, the athlete should have (1) full, painless knee ROM, (2) no joint pain or functional instability, (3) normal muscle strength, and (4) normal levels of functional ability.

Grade III MCL injuries can be managed either operatively or nonoperatively. Traditionally, grade III MCL injuries have been managed with 2 to 4 weeks of non–weight bearing and bracing with ROM limitations. Immediately

Table 19-11 **Rehabilitation Protocol After Posterior Cruciate Ligament Two-Tunnel Autograft Reconstruction**

	Week 1	Weeks 2–6	Weeks 6–12	Months 3–5	Months 6–7
Functional progression	PWB with 2 crutches and braced locked at 0°	PWB (single crutch to FWB with brace locked at 0°	FWB with no brace	Begin jogging, progressing to running	Return to sport
Criteria	As postoperative pain allows	No increase in effusion Pain controlled Good quadriceps recruitment	PROM 0°–120° Normal patellar mobility SLR without extensor lag Isometric quadriceps strength 70% of contralateral side	No increase in effusion No pain Full AROM Eccentric control with one-leg minisquat Leg press strength >70% Before initiating running, functional tests >70%, and no KT1000 change	No increase in effusion Functional tests >85% Isokinetic tests >85% Pain free KT1000 unchanged Self-report functional measures
Evaluation	Pain Effusion Patellar mobility PROM Passive extension Quadriceps recruitment Incision/portals	Pain Gait AROM extension PROM flexion Effusion Patellar mobility Quadriceps recruitment Incision/portals	Pain Gait AROM extension Quadriceps isometric strength PROM flexion Effusion Flexibility Balance KT1000	Pain AROM Effusion KT1000 Leg press strength test One-leg minisquat Self-report functional measures	Pain Effusion Functional tests Isokinetic tests KT1000 Self-report functional measures Proprioception tests
Treatment	Pain management Inflammation management Patellar mobilization Passive extension to 0° Passive flexion to 60° Quadriceps sets with NMES or biofeedback Active knee extension 60°–0° SLR Hamstring and calf stretching	Continue previous treatment PROM 0°–90° progressing to 120° Knee extension PRE 50°–0° Leg press 0°–60° Total Gym squats to 0°–60° Gait training (weight shifts) Progress to minisquats 0°–45° Scar mobility	Continue previous activities Proprioception exercises Stationary bike for endurance Single-leg balance activities Lateral step-ups 0°–60° Wall squats 0°–60° Initiate lunge progression 0°–45° Begin active knee flexion against gravity ≈9 weeks	Continue previous activities with emphasis on quadriceps strengthening Jogging progression Initiate hamstring curls Begin light agility drills Double-leg hop drills Begin running ≈4 months	Emphasize quadriceps strengthening Aerobic conditioning Running progression Single-leg hop drills Plyometric training Cutting drills Sport-specific activities
Goals	PROM 0°–60° 50% WB Control effusion/inflammation Good quadriceps recruitment Maintain patellar mobility	AROM 0°–120° FWB SLR without extensor lag Isometric quadriceps strength 70% of contralateral side	Full AROM Normal gait No increase in effusion with 20–30 minutes of biking or ambulating	No pain or increase in effusion with increased exercise load 85% with function and strength tests	Return to sport

Adapted from Wilk, K.E., Andrews, J.R., Clancy, W.G., et al. (1999): Rehabilitation programs for the PCL-injured and reconstructed knee. J. Sport Rehabil., 8:333–361.

AROM, Active range of motion; *FWB*, full weight bearing; *NMES*, neuromuscular electrical stimulation; *PRE*, progressive resistance exercise; *PWB*, partial weight bearing; *PROM*, passive range of motion; *ROM*, range of motion; *SLR*, straight leg raise; *WB*, weight bearing.

after the injury the brace might even be locked at approximately 45°. The brace is then opened to allow 0° to 90° of motion for the rest of the bracing period (4 to 6 weeks). Gentle ROM and strengthening exercises can be performed while the athlete is wearing the brace. Several studies report excellent results of isolated grade III MCL injuries that are managed nonoperatively and in which early motion activities are emphasized. After the initial 4 to 6 weeks of rehabilitation, an athlete with a grade III MCL injury can begin to progress through a more complete program of rehabilitation. Care should be taken to minimize valgus stress on the knee. It is not unusual for athletes with grade III MCL injuries to continue to exhibit some residual valgus laxity; however, this laxity does not appear to cause any functional limitations. These athletes can return to sport in 3 to 6 months, depending on their response to rehabilitation. An example of a rehabilitation protocol after an MCL injury is shown in Table 19-12.

Table 19-12 Rehabilitation Protocol for Isolated Medial Collateral Ligament Sprains Grades I, II, and III

	Week 1	Weeks 2–3	Weeks 4–8
Functional progression	Begin WB without crutches, grades I and II	Advance strengthening exercises	Return to sport, grades I and II
Criteria	Full knee extension present during gait No limp No pain at the MCL No increased effusion Full active extension ROM	No pain with exercises No increased effusion/edema Patellar mobility normal Full AROM	No tenderness Functional testing >85% Quadriceps strength >85%
Evaluation	Pain Effusion/edema Quadriceps recruitment ROM Patellar mobility	Pain Effusion/edema Patellar mobility Quadriceps recruitment AROM Standing balance, grades I and II	Functional testing Isokinetic testing Self-report functional measure
Treatment	Pain management Control of effusion/edema Quadriceps recruitment/biofeedback ROM exercises Flexibility exercises NWB, grade III only Rehabilitation brace, grades II and III	Pain management Control of effusion/edema Mobilization of the patella Quadriceps strengthening AROM exercises Proprioception exercises Endurance exercises	Strengthening exercises Endurance exercises Sport-specific drills
Goals	Maximize ROM Good quadriceps recruitment Control valgus stress 75%–100% WB, grades I and II	Full ROM Absence of pain FWB, grades I and II Normal patellar mobility	Discontinue brace, grade II Begin WB, grade III, and progress through criteria beginning week 1 Return to sport, grades I and II

AROM, Active range of motion; *FWB,* full weight bearing; *MCL,* medial collateral ligament; *NWB,* non–weight bearing; *ROM,* range of motion; *WB,* weight bearing.

Meniscal Injuries

Meniscal lesions have been treated by total meniscectomy, partial meniscectomy, and most recently, meniscal repair. Long-term outcomes of total meniscectomy have been disappointing because of the degenerative articular changes that occur in knees following this procedure.[160,161] For this reason, whenever possible meniscal lesions are treated by partial meniscectomy or repair. Meniscal transplantation with either an allograft or synthetic material is also a possible option. However, athletes who are candidates for this procedure are rarely allowed to return to high-impact, strenuous sports.[1624]

Partial meniscectomy is performed by removing only the damaged portion of the meniscus. Maintaining as much of the meniscus as possible is thought to aid in minimizing long-term degenerative changes at the knee. Rehabilitation after partial meniscectomy is driven by symptoms. The guidelines discussed in the section on the overview of knee rehabilitation principles show the rehabilitation process for an athlete who has undergone partial meniscectomy. Usually, athletes are able to return to sports rapidly, often within 3 weeks, after uncomplicated partial meniscectomy. An example of a rehabilitation protocol after partial meniscectomy is shown in Table 19-13.

Repair of the meniscus is a viable surgical option when the tear is located in a region of the meniscus with a blood supply. Greater understanding of the overall function of the meniscus has led surgeons to prefer to repair rather than remove parts of the meniscus whenever possible. Repairs are most often performed on the peripheral third of the meniscus because this area has a blood supply to allow healing of the repair site. Repairs can be performed arthroscopically or through a small incision at the knee.

The technique on the meniscus itself can be performed in a variety of ways.

Rehabilitation after meniscal repair is much more guarded than that after simple partial meniscectomy with regard to protection of the repair site. Table 19-14 shows an example of a rehabilitation program after a meniscal repair, and Box 19-12 outlines the program used by Andrews and Wilk following repair of complex meniscal tears. In the first 4 weeks after surgery the athlete progresses from non–weight bearing to full weight bearing. In determining the athlete's weight-bearing progression, the type of tear should be considered. With peripheral tears, weight bearing in extension can actually approximate the tear margins, so it can begin as the surgical pain dissipates. With radial tears and other complex tear repairs, weight-bearing progression is slower since even in full extension the axial load can disrupt the repair.[162] If a knee brace is used, it is often locked in full extension during weight-bearing activities. Knee flexion increases pressure on the posterior horn of the menisci, especially in weight bearing, so locking the brace in extension in this early phase of rehabilitation reduces the risk of exposing the repair to damaging forces.[163] The brace can be removed and full ROM attempted while the athlete is still non–weight bearing; however, aggressive flexion is still not performed. As the effusion decreases, active flexion should continue to progress, but if flexion measurements plateau, more aggressive passive flexion can be initiated at 4 weeks. If a brace is used, it is usually removed in the 4- to 6-week range, and the athlete is permitted full weight bearing if minimal joint effusion, full active extension ROM, at least 90° of flexion, and good quadriceps control are demonstrated.

Table 19-13 **Rehabilitation Protocol for Partial Meniscectomy**

	Week 1	Weeks 2–3	Weeks 4–8
Functional progression	Begin FWB without crutches	Advance strengthening exercises	Return to sport
Criteria	Full extension present during gait No limp No increased effusion/edema No increased pain Quadriceps control Full active extension ROM	Absence of pain No increased effusion/edema	Full AROM No effusion Functional testing >85% Quadriceps strength >85%
Evaluation	Pain Gait Quadriceps recruitment AROM Patellar mobility Surgical incisions/portals Effusion/edema	Pain Gait Effusion/edema Surgical incisions/portals Quadriceps recruitment AROM Patellar mobility Standing balance	Functional testing Isokinetic testing Self-report functional measure
Treatment	Pain management Control of effusion/edema Quadriceps recruitment ROM exercises Flexibility exercises	Effusion/edema reduction Strengthening exercises Endurance exercises Proprioception exercises Flexibility exercises	Strengthening exercises Endurance exercises Sport-specific drills
Goals	Maximum ROM Normal patellar mobility SLR without extensor lag Full passive extension	FWB Full ROM No pain with strengthening exercises	Return to sport

AROM, Active range of motion; *FWB,* full weight bearing; *ROM,* range of motion; *SLR,* straight leg raise.

Table 19-14 **Rehabilitation Protocol for Meniscus Repair**

	Weeks 1–3	Weeks 4–11	Weeks 12–15	Weeks 16–24
Functional progression	Begin partial to full WB with a brace locked in full extension	Begin full WB without a brace	Begin jogging	Begin cutting and jumping activities
Criteria	As postoperative pain allows No increased effusion	SLR with no extensor lag Effusion continues to decrease Full extension during gait	Absence of effusion Absence of patellofemoral pain No gait deviations	No increased effusion with running No pain Isokinetic testing >85% Functional testing >85%
Evaluation	Pain Effusion Patellar mobility Quadriceps recruitment AROM/PROM Passive extension Incision/portals	Pain Effusion Patellar mobility Quadriceps recruitment AROM/PROM Standing balance	Gait Isokinetic testing Functional testing Effusion Self-report functional status	Gait Isokinetic testing Functional testing Effusion Self-report functional status
Treatment	Control of pain Control of effusion/edema Patellar mobility AROM Quadriceps recruitment with biofeedback/electrical stimulation Passive extension FWB in a brace locked at 0°	AROM/PROM Quadriceps recruitment/strengthening General strengthening Advance closed chain exercises (no flexion greater than 60°) Endurance exercise Proprioception exercises	Strengthening exercises Endurance exercises Proprioception exercises	Strengthening exercises Endurance exercises Sport-specific drills
Goals	AROM 0°–90° Full passive extension Full WB in brace SLR with no extensor lag	Full AROM No gait deviations	Absence of effusion No pain	Return to sport

Adapted from McLaughlin, J., DeMaio, M., Noyes, F.R., et al. (1994): Rehabilitation after meniscus repair. Orthopedics, 17:463–471.
AROM, Active range of motion; *PROM,* passive range of motion; *SLR,* straight leg raise; *WB,* weight bearing.

Box 19-12

Rehabilitation Program Following Repair of Complex Meniscal Tears

I. MAXIMUM-PROTECTION PHASE (WEEKS 1–6)

Goals:

- Control inflammation/effusion
- Allow early healing
- Full passive knee extension
- Gradual increase in knee flexion
- Independent quadriceps control

Stage 1: Immediate Postsurgical Days 1–10

Swelling Control—Ice, compression, elevation

Brace:

- Locked at 0° for ambulation and sleeping only
- May be unlocked while sitting, etc.

Range of Motion:

- Passive 0°–90°
- Able to restore extension and hyperextension
- Patellar mobilizations
- Stretching of hamstrings and calf

Strengthening Exercises:

- Quad sets
- SLR flexion
- Hip abduction/adduction
- Knee extension 60°–0°

Weight Bearing:

- Toe touch with two crutches
- Avoid active knee flexion beyond 90° of flexion

Stage 2: Weeks 2–4

Swelling Control—Continue use of ice and compression

Brace—Locked for ambulation and sleeping

Range of Motion Guidelines—Gradually increase PROM as tolerated

- Week 2—0°–100°
- Week 3—0°–110°
- Week 4—0°–120°

Weight-Bearing Guidelines—Continue to lock brace

- Week 2—25%–50% WB
- Week 3—50%–75% WB
- Week 4—FWB as toleration

Continue PROM exercises and stretching

Strengthening Exercises:

- Multiangle quadriceps isometrics
- SLR (all four planes)
- Knee extension 90°–0°
- CKC weight shifts

Avoid twisting, deep squatting, and stooping for 12 weeks

Avoid hamstring strengthening for 8 weeks

Stage 3: Weeks 5–6

Weight bearing—As tolerated

Exercises:

- Initiate CKC exercise, such as:
  - ½ squat 0°–45°
  - Leg press 0°–60°
  - Wall squat 0°–60°

- Initiate proprioception training:
  - Tilt board squats
  - Biodex stability
- Continue CKC exercise
- Initiate hip abduction/adduction and hip flexion/extension on multi-hip machine

II. MODERATE-PROTECTION PHASE (WEEKS 7–12)

Goals:

- Establish full PROM
- Diminish swelling/inflammation
- Reestablish muscle control
- Promote proper gait pattern

Weeks 7–10

Swelling Control—Continue use of ice and compression as needed

Range of Motion:

- Continue ROM and stretching
- Week 7: PROM 0°–125°/130°

Brace—Continue use of brace for 8 weeks

Advance Strengthening Exercises:

- Leg press 70°–0°
- Knee extension 90°–40°
- Hip abduction/adduction
- Wall squats 0°–70°
- Vertical squats 0°–60°
- Lateral step-ups
- Front step-downs

Balance/Proprioception Training:

- Biodex stability
- Squats on rocker board
- Cup walking

Bicycle (if ROM permits)

Pool program

Avoid twisting, pivoting, running, and deep squatting

Weeks 10–12

Continue all exercises listed above

Initiate "light" hamstring curls

Initiate toe/calf raises

III. CONTROLLED-ACTIVITY PHASE (WEEKS 13–18)

Goals:

- Improve strength and endurance
- Maintain full ROM
- Gradually increase applied stress

Week 13

Continue all strengthening exercises listed above

Initiate Stair Stepper

Toe/calf raises

Advance balance training

Progress to isotonic strengthening program

Initiate front lunges

Initiate pool running (forward and backward)

Initiate walking program

(Continued)

Box 19-12

Rehabilitation Program Following Repair of Complex Meniscal Tears—cont'd

Week 16

Continue strengthening and stretching program
Advance walking program
Initiate running and cutting in pool

IV. RETURN-TO-SPORT PHASE (MONTHS 6–8)

Goals:
- Improve strength and endurance
- Prepare for unrestricted activities
- Progress to agility and cutting drills

Criteria to Progress to Phase IV:
- Full nonpainful ROM
- No pain or tenderness
- Satisfactory findings on clinical examination
- Satisfactory results on isokinetic test

Exercises:
- Continue and advance all strengthening exercises and stretching drills
  - Advance isotonic program
  - Wall squats
  - Leg press
  - Lateral step-ups
  - Knee extensions 90°–40°
  - Hamstring curls
  - Hip abduction/adduction
  - Bicycle, Stair Stepper, Elliptical machine
- Deep squatting: 5½ months
- Initiate straight line running: 6 months
- Initiate pivoting and cutting: 7 months
- Initiate agility training: 7 months
- Gradually return to sport: 7–8 months

CKC, Closed kinetic chain; *FWB*, full weight bearing; *PROM*, passive range of motion; *ROM*, range of motion; *SLR*, straight leg raise; *WB*, weight bearing.

If the athlete's repair is progressing with no complications 4 to 6 weeks postoperatively, the rehabilitation program can be increased to include more aggressive strengthening and ROM exercises. Although closed chain strengthening exercises, including squats and leg presses, can begin at this time, no such loaded exercise should be performed any deeper than 60° of knee flexion before 12 weeks after surgery.[163] All strengthening exercises (open or closed chain) must be performed in ranges that do not cause joint line or posterior corner symptoms. In athletes who have undergone peripheral repair, straight line jogging can be considered between 12 and 16 weeks after surgery if the athlete has no effusion, gait is normal, ROM is full, flexibility is normal, and strength deficits are less than 20%. When the athlete has successfully adapted to the jogging program, progressive hopping and cutting activities can be added (usually around 16 to 20 weeks after surgery). This begins the final rehabilitation phase of sport-specific progression activities. This final phase will last 4 to 6 weeks and allow the athlete to return to full competition by 6 months postoperatively. If the athlete has undergone repair of a complex tear, the entire rehabilitation program progression is usually slower to allow more healing time.

Rehabilitation After Combined Injuries of the Knee

When more than one structure is involved in a knee injury, rehabilitation of this type of combined injury is controlled by first analyzing which structures are involved. With combined injuries at the knee, the rehabilitation program guidelines are controlled by the more serious of the injuries (Table 19-15). One of the most important initial steps that the rehabilitation specialist can take is to determine which injury/surgical procedure is the one that will control the speed of the rehabilitation process. Fortunately, combined injuries at the knee that cause serious damage to multiple structures are not common. However, when this type of situation does occur, the rehabilitation specialist must determine

Table 19-15 Rehabilitation of Combined Injuries

Surgery	Dominant Rehabilitation Protocol
ACL and partial meniscectomy	ACL
ACL and meniscal repair	ACL in first 3 months, the meniscus in later rehabilitation stages
ACL and MCL	ACL with bracing
ACL and PCL	PCL
ACL and articular cartilage	Articular cartilage
ACL and posterolateral corner	ACL modified to protect the posterior corner
PCL and articular cartilage	Articular cartilage with motion restrictions for the PCL
PCL and posterolateral corner	PCL modified to protect the posterior corner

ACL, Anterior cruciate ligament; *MCL*, medial collateral ligament; *PCL*, posterior cruciate ligament.

which exercises are safe for an individual patient. The specialist must always remember that some exercises might be indicated for one part of the multiple-structure injury and contraindicated for another part of such injury.

The general guidelines for the inflammatory process and tissue healing times should be kept in mind with any rehabilitation program. With injuries to multiple structures, the inflammatory process and its common complications, such as loss of ROM and excessive scar formation, can be more significant because of greater trauma at the joint. The initial goals of rehabilitation in patients with injuries to multiple structures are still decreasing inflammation, regaining patellar mobility, and reestablishing quadriceps control (not necessarily strength). ROM exercises in these patients should be limited depending on the structures involved, but often at least limited ROM exercises are instituted.

One of the more common multiple-structure injuries is damage to the ACL and MCL. When the ACL is damaged in combination with an MCL injury, the MCL is frequently left to heal on its own. The exception to this practice is when significant joint laxity is still present after the ACL graft is put in place. Such laxity is seen if injury to the posterior oblique ligament has also occurred at the knee. In this type of situation the surgeon may choose to reconstruct or repair the MCL as well. When injuries to both structures have occurred, rehabilitation follows the ACL rehabilitation protocol, with no significant valgus load being placed on the knee. Frequently with this type of combined injury a rehabilitation brace is used for a longer time to aid in controlling valgus stress at the knee. Because of the longer time in a brace and the increased trauma to the knee from the combination injury, ROM work must be emphasized to limit the complication of loss of ROM.

If both the ACL and PCL are injured, rehabilitation generally follows the PCL rehabilitation protocol. Often, very significant trauma to the knee is required to rupture both the ACL and the PCL, so postoperative complications, such as loss of ROM, can be a problem. Open chain exercises involving the knee are frequently limited to low-weight reeducation-type exercises to minimize anterior and posterior tibial translation at the knee. Strengthening is accomplished through closed chain exercises. These closed chain exercises are emphasized as the patient's weight-bearing status allows. Correctly performing exercises in a closed chain fashion minimizes anterior and posterior tibial translation because of the compression of weight bearing and cocontractions of the hip, thigh, and leg musculature. In doing a closed chain activity such as a minisquat, the athlete needs to keep the knee between 0° and 60° of flexion while maintaining the trunk upright. This minimizes increasing hip flexion angles, which if not controlled can increase the muscular activity of the hamstrings. If a closed chain exercise is performed incorrectly, excessive hamstring activity might increase posterior translation of the tibia.

The posterolateral corner of the knee joint can be injured in conjunction with other ligament injuries at the knee. If the posterolateral corner is surgically reconstructed, care must be taken to avoid stress on the reconstruction. This includes avoiding hyperextension at the knee, guarding against excessive varus stress on the knee, and controlling posterior tibial translation stress early in the rehabilitation period.[164] When one works on regaining a patient's extension, support should be given to the tibia so that stress on the posterolateral corner is minimized. Some of the more traditional methods of increasing extension might have to be altered or avoided if the posterolateral corner is involved. If the posterolateral corner and the ACL are both reconstructed, the ACL rehabilitation protocol times guide the rehabilitation, but resistive hamstring exercises might be delayed by several weeks. Additionally, deep flexion closed chain exercises and strong open chain quadriceps contractions between 60° and 130° should be delayed for several weeks longer than with a traditional ACL rehabilitation protocol. Some surgeons might also delay full weight bearing by 2 to 3 weeks.

If the posterolateral corner and the PCL are both reconstructed, flexion ROM might be limited early in the rehabilitation program. In an athlete with any combined ligament injury that involves the posterolateral corner, return to full athletic activities might be delayed from several weeks to several months. This delay varies according to the particular surgeon and the surgical procedure used, but it is common for a posterolateral reconstruction to slightly prolong the rehabilitation period (Box 19-13).

Box 19-13

Accelerated Rehabilitation Following Combined Posterior Cruciate Ligament Reconstruction With a Patellar Tendon Graft and Posterolateral Corner Reconstruction

PREOPERATIVE PHASE

Goals:
- Diminish inflammation, swelling, and pain
- Restore normal ROM (gradual knee extension)
- Restore voluntary muscle activation
- Provide patient education to prepare the patient for surgery

Brace—Elastic wrap or knee sleeve to reduce swelling
Weight Bearing—As tolerated with or without crutches

Exercises:
- Ankle pumps
- Passive knee extension (gradual progression)
- Passive knee flexion to tolerance
- SLR, pillow squeezes
- Quad sets
- Closed kinetic chain exercises: mini squats, lunges, step-ups

Muscle Stimulation—Electrical muscle stimulation of the quadriceps during voluntary quadriceps exercises (4–6 hr/day)

Neuromuscular/Proprioception Training:
- Eliminate a quadriceps avoidance gait
- Retro stepping drills
- Joint repositioning (passive/active repositioning)

Cryotherapy/Elevation—Apply ice 20 min/hr, elevate the leg with the knee in full extension (the knee must be above the heart)

Patient Education:
- Review the postoperative rehabilitation program
- Review the instructional video (optional)
- Select an appropriate surgical date

I. IMMEDIATE POSTOPERATIVE PHASE (DAYS 1–7)

Goals:
- Gradual passive knee extension
- Diminish joint swelling and pain
- Restore patellar mobility
- Gradually improve knee flexion
- Reestablish quadriceps control
- Restore independent ambulation

(Continued)

Box 19-13

Accelerated Rehabilitation Following Combined Posterior Cruciate Ligament Reconstruction With a Patellar Tendon Graft and Posterolateral Corner Reconstruction—cont'd

Day 1

Brace—EZ Wrap brace/immobilizer applied to knee and locked in full extension during ambulation

Weight Bearing—Two crutches, weight bearing as tolerated

Exercises:

- Ankle pumps
- Overpressure into passive knee extension
- No active knee flexion—passive knee flexion only
- SLR (flexion, abduction), pillow squeezes
- Quad sets
- Hamstring stretches
- Closed kinetic chain exercises: minisquats, weight shifts

Muscle Stimulation—Use muscle stimulation during active muscle exercises (4–6 hr/day)

Continuous Passive Motion—As needed, 0°–45°/50° (as tolerated and as directed by the physician)

Ice and Evaluation—Apply ice 20 min/hr and elevate the leg with the knee in full extension

Days 2–3

Brace—EZ Wrap brace/immobilizer locked at 0° extension for ambulation and unlocked for sitting, etc.

Weight Bearing—Two crutches, weight bearing as tolerated

Range of Motion:

- Remove the brace and perform ROM exercises 6–8 times per day
- Perform frequent bouts of ROM to regain knee flexibility

Exercises:

- Multiangle isometrics at 90° and 60° (knee extension)
- Knee extension 90°–40°
- Overpressure into extension (knee extension should be at least 0°)
- Emphasize restoring knee extension
- Patellar mobilization
- Ankle pumps
- SLR, pillow squeezes
- Minisquats and weight shifts
- Quad sets

Muscle Stimulation—Electrical muscle stimulation of the quadriceps (6 hr/day)

Continuous Passive Motion—0°–90°, as needed

Ice and Evaluation—Apply ice 20 min/hr and elevate the leg with the knee in full extension

Days 4–7

Brace—EZ Wrap brace/immobilizer locked at 0° extension for ambulation and unlocked for sitting, etc.

Weight Bearing—Two-crutch weight bearing as tolerated

Range of Motion—Remove the brace to perform ROM exercises 6–8 times per day, knee flexion 90° by day 5, approximately 100° by day 7

Exercises:

- Multiangle isometrics at 90° and 60° (knee extension)
- Knee extension 90°–40°
- Overpressure into extension

- Patellar mobilization (5–8 times daily)
- Ankle pumps
- SLR, pillow squeezes
- Minisquats and weight shifts
- Quad sets
- Proprioception and balance activities

Neuromuscular training/proprioception:

- OKC passive/active joint repositioning at 90°, 60°
- CKC squats/weight shifts with repositioning on sports RAC

Muscle Stimulation—Electrical muscle stimulation (continue 6 hours daily)

Continue Passive Motion—0°–90°, as needed

Ice and Elevation—Apply ice 20 min/hr and elevate the leg with the knee in full extension

II. EARLY REHABILITATION PHASE (WEEKS 2–3)

Criteria to Progress to Phase II:

- Quadriceps control (ability to perform good a quad set and SLR)
- Full passive knee extension
- PROM 0°–90°
- Good patellar mobility
- Minimal joint effusion
- Independent ambulation

Goals:

- Gradual increase to full passive knee extension
- Gradually increase knee flexion
- Diminish swelling and pain
- Muscle control and activation
- Restore proprioception/neuromuscular control
- Normalize patellar mobility

Week 2

Brace—Continue with a locked brace for ambulation

Weight Bearing—As tolerated (goal is to discontinue crutches 10–14 days postoperatively)

Passive Range of Motion—Self-ROM stretching (6–8 times daily) with emphasis on maintaining full PROM

Exercises:

- Muscle stimulation superimposed on quadriceps exercises
- Quad sets
- SLR (four planes)
- Leg press (0°–60°)
- Knee extension 90°–40°
- Half squats (0°–40°)
- Weight shifts
- Front and side lunges
- Unicam bicycle (low-intensity cycling)
- Proprioception training
- Overpressure into extension
- PROM from 0°–105°
- Patellar mobilization
- Well-leg exercises
- Progressive resistance extension program—start with 1 lb, advance 1 lb/wk

Box 19-13

Accelerated Rehabilitation Following Combined Posterior Cruciate Ligament Reconstruction With a Patellar Tendon Graft and Posterolateral Corner Reconstruction—cont'd

Proprioception/Neuromuscular Training:
- OKC passive/active joint repositioning 90°, 60°, 30°
- CKC joint repositioning during squats/lunges
- Initiate squats

Swelling Control—Ice, compression, elevation

Week 3

Brace—Discontinue locked brace (some patients use a ROM brace for ambulation)

Passive Range of Motion—Continue ROM stretching and overpressure into extension (ROM should be 0°–100°/105°)

Exercises:
- Continue all exercises as in week 2
- PROM 0°–105°
- Bicycle for ROM stimulus and endurance (emphasize ROM on bike)
- Pool walking program (if incision is closed)
- Eccentric quadriceps program 40°–100° (isotonic only)
- Lateral lunges (straight plane)
- Front step-downs
- Lateral step-overs (cones)
- Progress proprioception drills, neuromuscular control drills
- Frequent bouts of ROM exercises

III. PROGRESSIVE STRENGTHENING/NEUROMUSCULAR CONTROL PHASE (WEEKS 4–10)

Criteria to Enter Phase III:
- AROM 0°–115°
- Quadriceps strength >60% of contralateral side (isometric test at 60° knee flexion)
- Unchanged KT test bilateral values (+1 or less)
- Minimal to no full joint effusion
- No joint line or patellofemoral pain

Goals:
- Restore full knee ROM (0°–125°)
- Improve lower extremity strength
- Enhance proprioception, balance, and neuromuscular control
- Improve muscular endurance
- Restore limb confidence and function

Brace—No immobilizer or brace; may use knee sleeve to control swelling/support

Range of Motion:
- Self-ROM (4–5 times daily using the other leg to provide ROM) with emphasis on maintaining 0° passive extension
- PROM 0°–125° at 4 weeks

KT2000 Test—Week 4, 20-lb anterior and posterior test

Week 4

Exercises:
- Progress isometric strengthening program
- Leg press (0°–100°)
- Knee extension 90°–40°

- Hip abduction and adduction
- Hip flexion and extension
- Lateral step-overs
- Lateral lunges (straight plane and multiplane drills)
- Lateral step-ups
- Front step-downs
- Wall squats
- Vertical squats
- Standing toe/calf raises
- Seated toe/calf raises
- Biodex stability system (balance, squats, etc.)
- Proprioception drills
- Bicycle
- Stair Stepper machine
- Pool program (backward running, hip and leg exercises)

Proprioception/Neuromuscular Drills:
- Tilt board squats (perturbation)
- Passive/active repositioning OKC
- CKC repositioning on a tilt board
- CKC lunges

Week 6

KT2000 Test—20- and 30-lb anterior and posterior test

Exercises:
- Continue all exercises
- Pool running (forward) and agility drills
- Balance on tilt boards
- Progress to balance and ball throws
- Wall slides/squats

Week 8

KT2000 Test—20- and 30-lb anterior and posterior test

Exercises:
- Continue all exercises listed in weeks 4–6
- Leg press sets (single leg) 0°–100° and 40°–100°
- Plyometric leg press
- Perturbation training
- Isokinetic exercises (90°–40°) (120°–240°/sec)
- Walking program
- Bicycle for endurance
- Stair Stepper machine for endurance
- Biodex stability system

Week 10

KT2000 Test—20- and 30-lb and manual maximum test
Isokinetic Test—Concentric knee extension/flexion at 180° and 300°/sec

Exercises:
- Continue all exercises listed in weeks 6, 8 and 10
- Plyometric training drills
- Continue stretching drills
- Progress strengthening exercises and neuromuscular training

(Continued)

Box 19-13

Accelerated Rehabilitation Following Combined Posterior Cruciate Ligament Reconstruction With a Patellar Tendon Graft and Posterolateral Corner Reconstruction—cont'd

IV. ADVANCED-ACTIVITY PHASE (WEEKS 11–16)

Criteria to Enter Phase IV:

- AROM 0°–125° or greater
- Quadriceps strength 75% of contralateral side, knee extension flexor-extensor ratio 70%–75%
- No change in KT values (comparable to contralateral side, within 2 mm)
- No pain or effusion
- Satisfactory findings on clinical examination
- Satisfactory results on isokinetic test (values at 180°)
  - Quadriceps bilateral comparison 75%
  - Hamstrings equal bilaterally
  - Quadriceps peak torque–body weight ratio of 65% at 180°/sec (males) and 55% at 180°/sec (females)
  - Hamstrings-quadriceps ratio 66%–75%
- Hop test (80% of contralateral leg)
- Subjective knee scoring (modified Noyes system) 80 points or better

Goals:

- Normalize lower extremity strength
- Enhance muscular power and endurance
- Improve neuromuscular control
- Perform selected sport-specific drills

Exercises:

- May initiate running program (weeks 10–12) if good quadriceps control and ROM
- May initiate light sport program (golf)
- Continue all strengthening drills
  - Leg press
  - Wall squats
  - Hip abduction/adduction
  - Hip flexion/extension
  - Knee extension 90°–40°
  - Initiate hamstring curls
  - Standing toe/calf raises
  - Seated toe/calf raises
  - Step-downs
  - Lateral step-ups
  - Lateral lunges
- Neuromuscular training
  - Lateral step-overs (cones)
  - Lateral lunges
  - Tilt board drills

Weeks 14–16

Advance program

Continue all drills above

May initiate lateral agility drills

Backward running

V. RETURN-TO-SPORT PHASE (WEEKS 17–22)

Criteria to Enter Phase V:

- Full ROM
- Unchanged KT2000 test (within 2.5 mm of opposite side)
- Isokinetic test that fulfills criteria
- Quadriceps bilateral comparison (80% or greater)
- Hamstring bilateral comparison (110% or greater)
- Quadriceps torque–body weight ratio (55% or greater)
- Hamstrings-quadriceps ratio (70% or greater)
- Proprioceptive test (100% of contralateral leg)
- Functional test (85% or greater of contralateral side)
- Satisfactory findings on clinical examination
- Subjective knee scoring (modified Noyes system) 90 points or better

Goals:

- Gradual return to full unrestricted sports
- Achieve maximal strength and endurance
- Normalize neuromuscular control
- Advance skill training

Tests—KT2000, isokinetic, and functional tests before return

Exercises:

- Continue strengthening exercises
- Continue neuromuscular control drills
- Continue plyometrics drills
- Advance running and agility program
- Advance sport-specific training
  - Running/cutting/agility drills
  - Gradual return-to-sport drills

6-MONTH FOLLOW-UP

Isokinetic test

KT2000 test

Functional test

12-MONTH FOLLOW-UP

Isokinetic test

KT2000 test

Functional test

AROM, Active range of motion; *CKC*, closed kinetic chain; *OKC*, open kinetic chain; *PROM*, passive range of motion; *ROM*, range of motion; *SLR*, straight leg raise.

With ACL reconstruction and associated meniscal repairs, the ACL rehabilitation protocol is followed in an attempt to limit morbidity. However, care must be taken when closed chain activities are performed early in rehabilitation. This type of loaded knee flexion can put the meniscal repair in danger of being damaged.

For this reason, as closed chain exercises are introduced and the loads and depth are progressed, the activity should be adjusted to avoid any joint line symptoms. Some surgeons also require that weight-bearing guidelines be slightly altered from the typical ACL rehabilitation protocol to protect the repair.

Articular Cartilage Injuries

Symptomatic articular cartilage lesions and osteochondral injuries of the knee pose a significant challenge to physicians and rehabilitation specialists. The true incidence of these injuries is unknown.[165] Mechanisms of injury for trauma-related lesions include impaction, shearing, and avulsion. Although the clinical significance of bone bruises (occult subchondral trabecular microfractures) is not fully understood, these lesions have been reported in 80% of patients with acute ACL tears.[166] Treatment options for symptomatic osteochondral lesions include nonsurgical treatment, arthroscopic lavage and débridement, abrasion arthroplasty, microfracture, mosaicplasty or osteoarticular autograft transfer, articular cartilage autographs, autologous chondrocyte implantation, and allografts.[167]

Conservative management of symptomatic individuals has limited indications, and the relief obtained from arthroscopic lavage and débridement appears to be short-lived.[168] Abrasion arthroplasty and microfracture, though differing in technique, are both methods used to introduce bleeding from subchondral bone into the lesion. The clot that forms over the region reorganizes into predominantly fibrocartilaginous tissue.[167] In mosaicplasty the lesion is filled with osteochondral plugs taken from low-load/contact areas of the joint. Autologous chondrocyte implantation is a two-step surgical procedure. During initial arthroscopic inspection of the lesion, a chondral biopsy specimen is obtained. This sample is sent to a laboratory* where the chondrocytes are placed in a culture that allows them to multiply until approximately 12 million cells are present.[168] During the second surgical procedure, a periosteal flap is placed over the defect, and the cell culture is injected into the defect to fill the space between the flap and subchondral bone. Because of a lack of long-term studies with sufficient numbers of patients, there is no clear consensus on which procedure—microfracture, mosaicplasty, or autologous chondrocyte transplantation—is superior.[167] Regardless of the surgical procedure used, the rehabilitation program must be designed so that the healing lesion receives enough stress during the initial postoperative period to enhance healing while excessive stress, especially shear force, is avoided (Box 19-14). This is accomplished primarily by unloaded joint ROM. Joint motion enhances articular cartilage healing, and use of a continuous passive motion machine for 6 to 8 hr/day during the first 4 to 8 weeks after surgery has been advocated.[169]

Rehabilitation guidelines continue to evolve as our understanding of articular cartilage healing and surgical techniques improve. However, specific rehabilitation parameters depend not only on the type of surgical procedure used but also on the location of the lesion. Decisions regarding safe rehabilitation activities and progression depend on an understanding of what surfaces are involved, as well as during what portion of ROM the lesion is in contact with the opposite articular surface. In general, during the first 2 weeks after surgery the athlete will be non–weight bearing.[168-170] Depending on the location and size of the lesion, as well as the procedure performed, toe-touch weight bearing may begin between the second and fourth weeks. Weight bearing may be progressed to partial weight bearing between the sixth and eighth weeks and to full weight bearing with crutches around 8 weeks after surgery. Some protocols require the use of a brace locked at 0° during this weight-bearing progression.[168] Large or multiple lesions in weight-bearing regions of the femur

---

*Available from Genzyme Tissue Repair, Cambridge, MA.

Box 19-14
Early Rehabilitation of Articular Cartilage Lesions

Unloaded range of motion is critical to enhance healing of the cartilage repair

Emphasize active and active assisted range of motion when not in continuous passive motion

---

or tibia may require non–weight-bearing status for 8 weeks.[169] When full weight bearing is allowed, athletes may discontinue the use of crutches if they have at least 0° to 100° of motion; if effusion, when present, is minimal and stable; if they are able to perform a straight leg raise without an extensor lag; and if they do not experience an increase in symptoms.[170]

During the protective rehabilitation phase (1 to 8 weeks), controlled ROM activities are critical.[168-170] Such activities can include passive, active assisted, and unloaded active ROM. As stated earlier, the use of a continuous passive motion machine is highly recommended for at least 4 weeks. If the athlete does not have access to a continuous passive motion machine, it is recommended that 500 repetitions of appropriate motion activities be performed three times a day.[169] Isometric exercises for the quadriceps and hamstrings can be performed at joint angles that do not load the region of the lesion. Biofeedback and electrical stimulation may be useful in activating the quadriceps during these multiangle isometrics. If the chondral defect was located on the patella or femoral sulcus (or both), isometrics may need to be limited to 0°.[169] Ice, compression, and elevation should be used to reduce joint effusion. In many cases a stationary bike with minimal or no resistance can be used for ROM exercise when the athlete has gained enough knee motion to allow normal pedaling.[168,169] Pool ROM activities can be initiated when the incisions have healed[169]; however, the athlete must be careful to maintain the appropriate weight-bearing status, especially when entering and exiting the pool.

During the transition rehabilitation phase, the athlete is allowed to progress from partial to full weight-bearing status. Low-load leg presses, Total Gym activities at lower angles of inclination, and treadmills with unloading devices may be useful in assisting the athlete in the transition from partial to full weight acceptance on the involved lower extremity.[169,170] Progression of weight-bearing activities in the pool is also useful. When the athlete can discontinue the use of crutches (see earlier guidelines), the focus of the rehabilitation program can shift toward controlled strength training, proprioceptive, and balance activities. The athlete can begin a minisquat program, leg presses (0° to 60°), and Total Gym strengthening exercises.[168,169] Open chain knee extension exercises should be avoided in most athletes with patellar lesions during this phase of rehabilitation (and quite possibly throughout the entire rehabilitation process).[169] Athletes with tibial or femoral lesions may be allowed to begin open chain knee extension exercises in this phase.[168] If allowed, these exercises should be progressed very slowly in terms of load, and ROM may need to be limited. Because of relatively high tibiofemoral compression forces, lunges[28] and hopping drills should be avoided during this stage,[169] but it may be possible to begin lateral step-ups.[168] Stationary bicycling and treadmill walking can be used to begin aerobic conditioning.[168] The transition phase will commonly last until about 12 to 16 weeks after surgery.

Box 19-15

Rehabilitation Program After a Femoral Condyle Microfracture Procedure (Medium to Large Lesion)

I. PROTECTION PHASE (WEEKS 1–4)

Goals:

- Reduce swelling and inflammation
- Protect and promote the healing articular cartilage
- Restore full passive knee extension
- Gradually restore knee flexion
- Reestablish voluntary quadriceps control

Weeks 1–2

Brace—Use elastic wrap to control swelling and inflammation

Weight Bearing:

- Non–weight bearing weeks 1–2
- Use of crutches to control weight-bearing forces

Inflammation Control—Use of ice and compression for 15–20 minutes 6–8 times daily

Range of Motion:

- Immediate motion
- Full passive knee extension
- Passive and active assisted knee flexion (3–5 times daily) to promote articular cartilage healing
- Week 1: 0°–90° or beyond (to tolerance)
- Week 2: 0°–105° or beyond (to tolerance)
- Flexibility exercises: stretch hamstrings, calf, and quadriceps

Strengthening Exercises:

- Quad sets
- Straight leg raises (four directions)
- Multiangle quadriceps exercises
- Electrical muscle stimulation of quadriceps
- Bicycle when ROM permits
- Proprioception and balance training

Functional Activities:

- Gradual return to daily activities
- Monitor for swelling, pain, and loss of motion

B. Weeks 3–4

Weight Bearing:

- Toe-touch WB week 3
- 25% WB week 4
- Weight bearing on crutches

Range of Motion:

- Gradually advance knee flexion
- Week 3: 0°–115°/125°
- Week 4: 0°–125°/130°+

- Maintain full passive knee extension
- Continue stretches for quadriceps, hamstrings, gastrocnemius
- Perform active assisted and active ROM (4–5 times daily)

Strengthening Exercises:

- Bicycle (1–2 times daily)
- Low-intensity bicycle—longer duration
- Quad sets
- Straight leg flexion
- Hip abduction/adduction
- Hip flexion/extension
- Light hamstring curls
- Pool program (when incisions are closed)
- Proprioception and balance training
- No OKC resisted knee extension

Inflammation Control—Continue use of ice, elevation, and compression (4–5 times daily)

Functional Activities:

- Gradually return to functional activities
- No sports or impact loading

II. INTERMEDIATE PHASE (WEEKS 5–8)

Goals:

- Protect and promote articular cartilage healing
- Gradually increase joint stress and loading
- Improve lower extremity strength and endurance
- Gradually increase functional activities

Weight Bearing:

- 50% WB week 6
- 5% WB week 7
- FWB as tolerated week 8

Flexibility Exercises—Continue stretching hamstrings, quadriceps, and calf

Strengthening Exercises:

- Initiate functional rehabilitation exercises
- Minisquats and leg press week 6
- Closed kinetic chain exercises (step-ups, lunges) week 8
- Vertical squats, wall squats, leg press
- Bicycle, Elliptical (low intensity, long duration)
- Initiate PREs (physician will determine)
- Hip abduction/adduction, extension/flexion
- Hamstring strengthening (light)
- Pool program

Any increase in effusion or symptoms will necessitate a reduction in rehabilitation intensity.

From 4 to about 6 months postoperatively the rehabilitation program should focus on continued progressive strengthening and endurance exercises. The intensity of the activities begun in the transitional rehabilitation phase can be increased, and a lunge program can be initiated. A jogging progression may be initiated between the fifth and sixth months.[168] After the sixth month, athletes may be allowed to begin sport-specific drills as long as they have full ROM, quadriceps and hamstring strength within 10%

of the uninvolved leg, and no pain or effusion. At this time a hop program tailored to the requirements of the sport can be initiated; as indicated earlier, any evidence of pain or effusion suggests the need to reduce the impact and load intensity of the program. After surgery, return-to-sport rates are lower for articular cartilage injuries than for other knee pathologies,[171] but for low-impact sports, athletes can generally return after 6 months, whereas return to high-impact sports will usually require at least 1 year.[168] The rehabilitation program followed by Andrews and Wilk after a postoperative microfracture procedure is outlined in Box 19-15.

Box 19-15

Rehabilitation Program After a Femoral Condyle Microfracture Procedure (Medium to Large Lesion)—cont'd

- Initiate walking program (light walking) (physician will determine)
- Proprioception and balance training

Functional Activities:
- Gradually increase walking program
- Progression based on monitoring of swelling, pain, and motion

III. LIGHT-ACTIVITY PHASE (WEEKS 8–16)
Goals:
- Improve muscular strength/endurance
- Increase functional activities
- Gradually increase loads applied to joint
- Control compression and shear forces

Criteria to Enter Phase III:
- Full non-painful ROM
- Strength within 20% of contralateral limb
- Able to walk 1.5 miles or bike for 20–25 minutes without symptoms

Exercises:
- Continue PREs
- Continue functional rehabilitation exercises
- Balance and proprioception drills
- Bicycle and elliptical
- Neuromuscular control drills
- Initiate light running program (physician will determine)
- Continue all stretches of lower extremity

Functional Activities:
- Gradually increase walking distance/endurance
- Pool running week 10
- Light running weeks 12–16
- Advance running program weeks 16–18
- Progression based on monitoring patient's swelling, pain, and motion (physician will determine)

IV. RETURN-TO-SPORT PHASE (WEEKS 16–26)
Goals:
- Gradual return to full unrestricted functional activities
- Actual time frames may vary based on extent of injury and surgery
- Physician will advise rate of progression

Exercises:
- Continue functional rehabilitation exercises
- Continue flexibility exercises
- Restrict deep squatting with resistance and heavy knee extensions
- Monitor jumping activities closely

Functional Activities:
- Low-impact sports (cycling, golf) weeks 6–8
- Moderate-impact sports (jogging, tennis, aerobics) weeks 12–16
- High-impact sports (basketball, soccer, volleyball) weeks 16–26
- Actual return to sports or strenuous activities will be determined by physician and rehabilitation team

FWB, Full weight bearing; *OKC*, open kinetic chain; *PRE*, progressive resistive exercise; *ROM*, range of motion; *WB*, weight bearing.

RETURN TO SPORT

Success in sports depends on a multitude of factors; likewise, the decision of when the athlete is ready to return to sport should be determined by a number of measures. Most of the work related to this decision-making process has been developed for determining the readiness of athletes following ACL reconstruction; however, all athletes should be assessed for their readiness to return to sport regardless of their injury. Although the intensity and formality of this process vary with the injury and length of time that has been missed, athletes should not be allowed to return to sport if they cannot participate safely. In postsurgical cases, tissue healing time certainly plays a role in the decision-making process, but time alone should not determine return to sport activities. Measures that shape these decisions include self-report measures, arthrometry, strength tests, functional tests, observational analysis of sport-specific tasks, and when possible, preinjury measures of strength and function. Another basic, but important criterion is normal ROM. Depending on the sport, an athlete may be able to get by with a small restriction in flexion, but the ability to fully extend the knee is critical for all athletes because lack of extension interferes with normal locomotion.

Numerous self-report outcome measures are available for assessing athletes' perception of their function. Although differences exist, these instruments generally contain measures of pain and other symptoms, as well as measures of the impact that the injury has on activities of daily living and sports participation. The Lysholm scale, the Knee Outcome Survey–Activities of Daily Living Scale, the Knee Injury and Osteoarthritis Outcome Score, the International Knee Documentation Committee 2000 Subjective Knee Evaluation Form, and the Cincinnati Knee Rating Scale are examples of instruments used for ligamentous, meniscal, and articular cartilage injuries.[172,174] The Lower Extremity Functional Scale and the Anterior Knee Pain Scale are examples of instruments designed for those with anterior knee pain.[174] The reliability, validity, and responsiveness of all these instruments have been established.

Arthrometry

Arthrometry has long been used as a measure of success or failure for ACL and PCL reconstructions. Arthrometers provide the clinician with a quantifiable method of testing ligamentous laxity of the ACL and PCL. Introduced in 1983 by Daniel et al,[175] the KT1000 was one of the first commercially produced arthrometers used clinically for measuring anterior-posterior

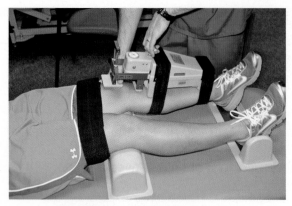

FIGURE 19-30 KT1000 arthrometer.

laxity (Fig. 19-30).[176] A number of other devices have been developed, but the KT1000 (and KT2000, a KT1000 with an X-Y plotter) remains one of the most commonly cited and clinically used arthrometers.

A number of investigations have been undertaken to evaluate the validity and reliability of arthrometry.[176-180] When one interprets, compares, and applies these results, several factors that must be considered are the displacement force used, the displacement difference considered diagnostic, and study design issues (single testers, multiple testers, etc.).

The reliability of arthrometry can be estimated by a statistical technique called intraclass correlation coefficients (ICCs). Depending on the formula used, this test provides either a measure of reproducibility of individual evaluators or the reproducibility of a measure between evaluators. ICCs can range from 0 (totally unreliable) to 1 (perfect reliability). Reported ICCs for ACL testing with a KT1000 or a KT2000 range from 0.65 to 0.99.[62,181-184] In general, results from testers experienced in arthrometry are more reliable than those from novices, and serial measures between testers are less reliable than serial measures from the same tester. The active quadriceps tests are generally less reliable than any of the passive displacement force tests. The reliability results of the common passive displacement forces (67 N, 89 N, 134 N, maximum manual) are mixed, with no particular displacement force being consistently more reliable than the others.

PCL arthrometry appears to be somewhat less reliable than ACL arthrometry. Huber et al[185] reported ICCs ranging from 0.59 to 0.84 for PCL testing with a KT1000. Similar to ACL testing, results from novice testers were generally less reliable than those from experienced testers, and the reliability of results between different testers was less than that for serial measures from the same tester.

Regardless of the accuracy and reliability reported in the literature, clinicians performing arthrometry must be meticulous in their measurement technique. Daniel[186] suggests that the two greatest sources of error in KT1000 measurements are inappropriate patellar pad stabilization and lack of muscle relaxation. Other key points suggested by Daniel to reduce measurement error include proper lower extremity alignment, accurate placement of the arthrometer, and consistent speed and direction of the application of force.[186]

Even though arthrometry provides a measure of an important facet in reconstruction outcome, studies have failed to demonstrate consistent associations between arthrometry and other measures, including functional hop tests and self-report outcome measures.[187-190] The results from these studies suggest that one should not rely solely on arthrometric scores to define reconstruction success or failure.

Strength Testing

Assessment of strength is another key component for determining when an athlete is ready to progress to more demanding activities. Strength can be measured isokinetically, isometrically, or isotonically. Isometric testing is generally more valuable during the earlier phases of rehabilitation when the need to protect the joint is greater. The knee has been studied isokinetically more than any other joint.[191] Isokinetic testing can provide the clinician with valuable information about the isolated strength of muscles groups, either those damaged by injury or those that provide support to injured joints. Isokinetic testing of the knee has been shown to be extremely reliable, with ICCs as high as 0.99[192] for concentric contraction in asymptomatic subjects. Most of the studies reviewed by Perrin[193] had ICCs between 0.80 and 0.99. For eccentric contraction measures, isokinetic testing is still reliable, but not to the same extent that concentric testing is, especially in subjects with knee injuries.[194] With eccentric testing, Steiner et al[194] reported ICCs ranging from 0.58 to 0.96 for average peak torque, with symptomatic subjects scoring lower. To ensure high retest reliability the clinician should make sure that the dynamometer axis is closely matched to the knee joint axis and that the athlete is positioned identically each time that the test is performed.[193] This includes accurate placement of the resistance pad of the dynamometer on the leg. The joint should be tested only through pain-free motion. Allowing the athlete to warm up and perform practice repetitions at the testing speed also improves the reliability of the test.[193]

Isokinetic testing provides information on torque (peak or average), total work, and power. When test results of the quadriceps are compared with those of the hamstrings (agonist-to-antagonist comparisons), it is important to apply a gravity correction factor.[193] The often-quoted normal concentric peak torque hamstring-to-quadriceps ratio is 60%. This ratio for gravity-corrected measures is fairly accurate for slower testing velocities (60°/sec), but as testing velocities increase, the ratio is usually greater than 60% because the decrease in hamstring torque with increasing velocities is usually less than that of the quadriceps.[191,193] Dvir[191] has suggested that the hamstring-to-quadriceps ratio is not generally as important as the ratio developed by dividing the involved side measure by the uninvolved side measure. To illustrate this point, if an athlete produces 100 Nm of torque with the right quadriceps and 60 Nm of torque with the right hamstrings, the hamstring-to-quadriceps ratio is 60%. If an athlete produces a left quadriceps torque of 200 Nm and left hamstring torque of 120 Nm, the left side hamstring-to-quadriceps ratio is also 60%. A side-to-side comparison of the hamstring-to-quadriceps ratios would suggest that the legs were equal, but there is certainly a large deficit in torque production by the right thigh musculature. Therefore, in most instances it is recommended that injured-side muscle group test results be compared with results from the same muscle group on the uninjured side. Another form of the hamstring-to-quadriceps ratio called the functional hamstring-quadriceps ratio has been proposed.[195] The ratio for knee extension is determined by dividing the eccentric hamstring torque by the concentric quadriceps torque. The ratio for knee flexion is determined by dividing the

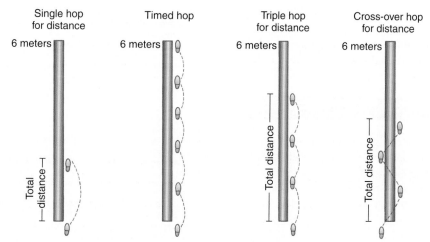

FIGURE 19-31 Four tests for appraising functional stability. *(From Noyes, F.R., Barber, S.D., and Mangine, R.E. [1991]: Abnormal lower limb symmetry determined by function hop tests after anterior cruciate ligament rupture. Am. J. Sports Med., 19:513–518.)*

concentric hamstring torque by the eccentric quadriceps torque. Proponents of these ratios suggest that they are more in line with how the thigh muscles function during activities; however, these ratios are not immune to the same problems illustrated earlier for the conventional hamstring-to-quadriceps ratio.

In making side-to-side comparisons it is important to consider the following testing principles. Placement of the dynamometer resistance pad must be the same on both legs, and both knees should be tested through the same ROM. The isokinetic total work measure is determined by the area under the torque curve. The y-axis for this measure is torque, and the x-axis is ROM. Thus, if the uninjured side is tested through a greater ROM, the total work for that side could be higher merely because it was performed through a greater ROM and not because it produced a higher torque curve.[193]

Isotonic strength testing is usually performed with a 1 repetition maximum (1 RM). Because of the variety of equipment available on the market, it is difficult to provide general measures of reliability for isotonic testing. Isotonic strength tests of seated knee extension, hamstring curls, and single-leg press can provide side-to-side comparisons of strength. In addition to this comparison, the 1 RM can indexed to the athlete's body weight. This is a particularly important consideration when assessing the single-leg press result because athletes should be able to lift at least their body weight when considering progression to more demanding activities.

As a general rule of thumb, if the athlete has strength deficits of greater than 15% to 20%, regardless of whether it was measured isokinetically or isotonically, the athlete will probably have difficulty performing more demanding sport activities such as sprinting, cutting, and jumping. Advancing activities despite such deficits in strength places the knee at risk for the development of pain (especially patellofemoral pain), effusion, and reinjury.

Functional Tests

Functional testing of the lower extremity aids in determining the functional capabilities of the knee joint during sports activities. Functional tests assist in determining limitations that are not evident with strength testing or arthrometry. Common functional tests include a variety of hop tests such as the single-leg hop

for distance, single-leg triple hop for distance, single-leg cross-over hop for distance, and the single-leg 6-m hop for time testing (Fig. 19-31).[196] Intraclass correlation coefficients for these examples range from 0.82 to 0.92 for patients with ACL reconstructions.[173] Single-limb functional tests are commonly analyzed with a limb symmetry index (LSI), which is derived by dividing the involved extremity score by the uninvolved extremity score.

Most of the research efforts related to functional tests of the knee have been concerned primarily with the use of these tests for examining the function of the knee after a ligamentous injury. However, a few functional tests have been described for examination of athletes with patellofemoral dysfunction. Loudon et al[197] reported the intrarater reliability of the following tests: crossover lunge (ICC = 0.82), 8 inch-step-down (ICC = 0.94), single-leg press (ICC = 0.82), bilateral squat (ICC = 0.79), and balance and reach (ICC = 0.83). The number of correctly performed repetitions that the subject completed in 30 seconds served as the measure for all these tests. In the unilateral tests, subjects with patellofemoral dysfunction performed significantly fewer repetitions with the involved lower extremity than with the uninvolved side. LSIs for subjects with patellofemoral problems ranged from 80% to 90%, whereas LSIs for those without patellofemoral problems ranged from 95% to 100%.

Standard agility tests such as the T-test (see Figs. A22-8 and 22-9 [in Chapter 22 Appendix] on Expert Consult @ www.expertconsult.com) can also be used as functional tests; however, even though the results of these tests can be compared with published norms of similar athletes or with preinjury times if available, these tests do not lend themselves to making side-to-side comparisons. Myer et al[139] described a modification of the T-test that they suggest does allow side-to-side comparison. Their modification turns the shuffle component of the test into a unidirectional test that allows comparison of the athlete's times based on the starting point of the test.

Similar to the rule of thumb for the strength test, LSI deficits in these different functional tests of greater than 15% to 20% indicate that the athlete is not ready to return to sport. Observation of the athlete's performance on any functional test is also important in evaluation of the test result. Even if the athlete's LSI deficit is less than 15%, if one observes substitutions, a lack of symmetry in performance, or a lack of confidence in cutting or landing on the involved lower extremity, the athlete is probably going to have difficulty in attempting to return to sport. Lower extremity functional tests are described in further detail in Chapter 22.

Clinical Pearl #4

When can an athlete return to play? The answer should be based at least in part on muscle strength, self-report functional measures, functional tests, observational analysis, and arthrometry. If strength and functional side-to-side comparison tests show deficits of greater than 15% to 20%, the athlete will probably have difficulty returning to sport. However, even scores higher than 85% on any one or all tests do not necessarily mean that an athlete will not experience any difficulty returning to sport. It is always easier to determine who is not ready to return to sport than it is to determine who is ready.

CONCLUSION

- Rehabilitation of the lower extremity should incorporate the appropriate balance of closed and open chain exercises along an increasing continuum of difficulty.
- In choosing exercises, one must understand the effect that the exercises will have on both the tibiofemoral and patellofemoral joints.
- Controlled motion, muscle recruitment, restoration of joint arthrokinematics, and control of inflammation should be the focus of any early-phase rehabilitation program regardless of the injury.
- The transition and advanced phases of rehabilitation should focus on developing muscle strength, power, endurance, and balance.
- Progression through all phases of rehabilitation should be guided by the athlete's ability to meet specific criteria and not simply by time alone.
- Functional testing and other measurements, such as arthrometry, self-reported functional status, and strength testing, should be used to assist in determining when an athlete can return to sport.

REFERENCES

1. Grood, E.S., Noyes, F.R., Butler, D.L., et al. (1981): Ligamentous and capsular restraints preventing straight medial and lateral laxity in intact human cadaver knees. J. Bone Joint Surg. Am., 63:1257–1269.
2. Fuss, F.K. (1992): Principles and mechanisms of automatic rotation during terminal extension in the human knee joint. J. Anat., 180:297–304.
3. Takeda, Y., Xerogeanes, J.W., Livesay, G.A., et al. (1994): Biomechanical function of the human anterior cruciate ligament. Arthroscopy, 10:140–147.
4. Fiebert, I., Gresly, J., Hoffman, S., et al. (1994): Comparative measurements of anterior tibial translation using a KT-1000 knee arthrometer with the leg in neutral, internal rotation, and external rotation. J. Orthop. Sports Phys. Ther., 19:331–334.
5. King, S., Butterwick, D.J., and Cuerrier, J.P. (1986): The anterior cruciate ligament: A review of recent concepts. J. Orthop. Sports Phys. Ther., 8:110–122.
6. Norkin, C.C., and Levange, P.K. (1992): The knee complex. In: Joint Structure and Function: A Comprehensive Analysis, 2nd ed. Philadelphia, Davis. pp. 337–377.
7. Lutz, G.E., Stuart, M.J., and Sim, F.H. (1990): Rehabilitative techniques for athletes after reconstruction of the anterior cruciate ligament. Mayo Clin. Proc., 65:1322–1329.
8. Fu, F.H., Harner, C.D., Johnson, D.L., et al. (1993): Biomechanics of knee ligaments: Basic concepts and clinical application. J. Bone Joint Surg. Am., 75:1716–1727.
9. Henning, C.E., Lynch, M.A., and Glick, K.R. (1985): An in vivo strain gauge study of elongation of the anterior cruciate ligament. Am. J. Sports Med., 13:22–26.
10. Beynnon, B.D., Fleming, B.C., Johnson, R.J., et al. (1995): Anterior cruciate ligament strain behavior during rehabilitation exercises in vivo. Am. J. Sports Med., 23:24–34.
11. Beynnon, B.D., Johnson, R.J., Fleming, B.C., et al. (1997): The strain behavior of the anterior cruciate ligament during squatting and active flexion-extension: A comparison of an open and closed kinetic chain exercise. Am. J. Sports Med., 25:823–829.
12. Beynnon, B.D., and Fleming, B.C. (1998): Anterior cruciate ligament strain in-vivo: A review of previous work. J. Biomech., 31:519–525.
13. Escamilla, R.F., Fleisig, G.S., Zheng, N., et al. (1998): Biomechanics of the knee during closed kinetic chain and open kinetic chain exercises. Med. Sci. Sports Exerc., 30:556–569.
14. Kvist, J., and Gillquist, J. (2001): Sagittal plane knee translation and electromyographic activity during closed and open kinetic chain exercises in anterior cruciate ligament–deficient patients and control subjects. Am. J. Sports Med., 29:72–82.
15. Yack, H.J., Collins, C.E., and Whieldon, T.J. (1993): Comparison of closed and open kinetic chain exercise in the anterior cruciate ligament–deficient knee. Am. J. Sports Med., 21:49–54.
16. Yack, H.J., Riley, L.M., and Whieldon, T.R. (1994): Anterior tibial translation during progressive loading of the ACL-deficient knee during weight-bearing and nonweight-bearing isometric exercise. J. Orthop. Sports Phys. Ther., 20:247–253.
17. Ericson, M.O., and Nisell, R. (1986): Tibiofemoral joint forces during ergometer cycling. Am. J. Sports Med., 14:285–290.
18. Kaufman, K.R., An, K., Litchy, W.J., et al. (1991): Dynamic joint forces during knee isokinetic exercise. Am. J. Sports Med., 19:305–316.
19. Nisell, R., Ericson, M.O., Nemeth, G., et al. (1989): Tibiofemoral joint forces during isokinetic knee extension. Am. J. Sports Med., 17:49–54.
20. Gollehon, D.L., Torzilli, P.A., and Warren, R.F. (1987): The role of the posterolateral and cruciate ligaments in the stability of the human knee. J. Bone Joint Surg. Am., 69:233–242.
21. Grood, E.S., Stowers, S.F., and Noyes, F.R. (1988): Limits of movement in the human knee. J. Bone Joint Surg. Am., 70:88–97.
22. Fowler, P.J., and Lubliner, J. (1995): Functional anatomy and biomechanics of the knee joint. In Griffin L.Y. (ed.): Rehabilitation of the Injured Knee. St. Louis, Mosby.
23. Skyhar, M.J., Warren, R.F., Ortiz, G.J., et al. (1993): The effects of sectioning the posterior cruciate ligament and posterolateral complex on the articular pressures within the knee. J. Bone Joint Surg. Am., 75:694–699.
24. Anderson, J.K., and Noyes, F.R. (1995): Principles of posterior cruciate ligament rehabilitation. Orthopedics, 18:493–500.
25. Wilk, K.E. (1994): Rehabilitation of isolated and combined posterior cruciate ligament injuries. Clin. Sports Med., 13:649–677.
26. Castle, T.H., Noyes, F.R., and Grood, E.S. (1992): Posterior tibial subluxation of the posterior cruciate–deficient knee. Clin. Orthop. Relat. Res., 284:193–202.
27. Ohkoshi, Y., Yasuda, K., Kaneda, K., et al. (1991): Biomechanical analysis of rehabilitation in the standing position. Am. J. Sports Med., 19:605–611.
28. Stuart, M.J., Meglan, D.A., Lutz, E.S., et al. (1996): Comparison of intersegmental tibiofemoral joint forces and muscle activity during various closed chain exercises. Am. J. Sports Med., 14:792–799.
29. Durselen, L., Claes, L., and Kiefer, H. (1995): The influence of muscle forces and external loads on cruciate ligament strain. Am. J. Sports Med., 23:129–136.
30. Markolf, K.L., Mensch, J.S., and Amstutz, H.C. (1976): Stiffness and laxity of the knee: The contributions of the supporting structures. J. Bone Joint Surg. Am., 58:583.
31. Soderberg, G.L. (1986): Kinesiology: Application to Pathological Motion. Baltimore, Williams & Wilkins.
32. Soames, R.W. (1995): Skeletal system. In Gray's Anatomy, 38th ed. New York, Churchill Livingstone.
33. Lane, J.G., Irby, S.E., Kaufman, K., et al. (1994): The anterior cruciate ligament in controlling axial rotation. Am. J. Sports Med., 22:289–293.
34. Arnoczky, S.P. (1994): Meniscus. In Fu, F.H., Harner, C.D., and Vince, K.G. (eds.): Knee Surgery, Vol. 1. Baltimore, Williams & Wilkins, pp. 131–140.
35. Barber, F.A. (1994): Accelerated rehabilitation for meniscus repairs. Arthroscopy, 10:206–210.
36. Fukubayashi, T., and Kurosawa, H. (1980): The contact area and pressure distribution pattern of the knee. Acta Orthop. Scand., 51:871–879.
37. McLaughlin, J., DeMaio, M., Noyes, F.R., et al. (1994): Rehabilitation after meniscus repair. Orthopedics, 17:463–471.
38. Fairbank, T.J. (1948): Knee joint changes after meniscectomy. J. Bone Joint Surg. Br., 30:664–670.
39. Kawai, Y., Fukubayashi, T., and Nishino, J. (1989): Meniscal suture: An experimental study in the dog. Clin. Orthop. Relat. Res., 243:286–293.
40. Markolf, K.L., Bargar, W.L., Shoemaker, S.C., et al. (1981): The role of joint load in knee stability. J. Bone Joint Surg. Am., 63:570–585.
41. Arnheim, D.D. (1989): The knee and related structures. In: Modern Principles of Athletic Training, 7th ed. St. Louis, Times Mirror/Mosby College Publishing.
42. Hungerford, D.S., and Barry, M. (1979): Biomechanics of the patellofemoral joint. Clin. Orthop. Relat. Res., 144:9–15.
43. Reilly, D.T., and Martens, M. (1972): Experimental analysis of the quadriceps muscle force and patellofemoral joint reaction force for various activities. Acta Orthop. Scand., 43:126–137.
44. Steinkamp, L.A., Dillingham, M.F., Markel, M.D., et al. (1993): Biomechanical considerations in patellofemoral joint rehabilitation. Am. J. Sports Med., 21:438–444.
45. Fulkerson, J.P., and Hungerford, D.S. (1990): Biomechanics of the patellofemoral joint. In Disorders of the Patellofemoral Joint, 2nd ed. Baltimore, Williams & Wilkins. pp. 25–39.

46. Goodfellow, J., Hungerford, D.S., and Zindel, M. (1976): Patellofemoral joint mechanics and pathology: 1. Functional anatomy of the patellofemoral joint. J. Bone Joint Surg. Br., 58:287–290.

47. Huberti, H.H., and Hayes, W.C. (1984): Patellofemoral contact pressure. J. Bone Joint Surg. Am., 55:715–724.

48. Dahlkvist, N.J., Mayo, P., and Seedhom, B.B. (1982): Forces during squatting and rising from a deep squat. Eng. Med., 11:69–76.

49. Ericson, M.O., and Nisell, R. (1987): Patellofemoral joint forces during ergometer cycling. Phys. Ther., 67:1365–1369.

50. Flynn, T.W., and Soutas-Little, R.W. (1995): Patellofemoral joint compressive forces in forward and backward running. J. Orthop. Sports Phys. Ther., 21:277–282.

51. Scott, S.H., and Winter, D.A. (1990): Internal forces at chronic running injury sites. Med. Sci. Sports Exerc., 22:357–369.

52. Goh, J.C., Lee, P.Y.C., and Bose, K. (1995): A cadaver study of the function of the oblique part of vastus medialis. J. Bone Joint Surg. Br., 77:225–231.

53. Lieb, F.J., and Perry, J. (1968): Quadriceps function: An anatomical and mechanical study using amputated limbs. J. Bone Joint Surg. Am., 50:1535–1548.

54. Reynolds, L., Levin, T.A., Medeiros, J.M., et al. (1983): EMG activity of the vastus medialis oblique and the vastus lateralis in their role in patellar alignment. Am. J. Phys. Med., 62:61–70.

55. Beckman, M., Craig, R., and Lehman, R.C. (1989): Rehabilitation of patellofemoral dysfunction in the athlete. Clin. Sports Med., 8:841–861.

56. Host, J.V., Craig, R., and Lehman, R.C. (1995): Patellofemoral dysfunction in tennis players. Clin. Sports Med., 14:177–203.

57. Hughston, J.C., Walsh, W.M., and Puddu, G. (1984): Patellar Subluxation and Dislocation. Philadelphia: Saunders pp. 1–20.

58. Eng, J.J., and Pierrynowski, M.R. (1993): Evaluation of soft foot orthotics in the treatment of patellofemoral pain syndrome. Phys. Ther., 73:62–68.

59. Doucette, S.A., and Child, D.D. (1996): The effect of open and closed chain exercise and knee joint position on patellar tracking in lateral patellar compression syndrome. J. Orthop. Sports Phys. Ther., 23:104–110.

60. Doucette, S.A., and Goble, E.M. (1992): The effect of exercise on patellar tracking in lateral patellar compression syndrome. Am. J. Sports Med., 20:434–440.

61. Ingersoll, C.D., and Knight, K.L. (1991): Patellar location changes following EMG biofeedback or progressive resistive exercises. Med. Sci. Sports Exerc., 23:1122–1127.

62. Brosky, J.A., Nitz, A.J., Malone, T.R., et al. (1999): Intrarater reliability of selected clinical outcome measures following anterior cruciate ligament reconstruction. J. Orthop. Sports Phys. Ther., 19:39–48.

63. Gough, J.V., and Ladley, G. (1971): An investigation into the effectiveness of various forms of quadriceps exercises. Physiotherapy, 57:356–361.

64. Pocock, G.S. (1963): Electromyographic study of the quadriceps during resistive exercise. J. Am. Phys. Ther. Assoc., 43:427–434.

65. Soderberg, G.L., and Cook, T.M. (1983): An electromyographic analysis of quadriceps femoris muscle setting and straight leg raising. Phys. Ther., 63:1434–1438.

66. Karst, G.M., and Jewett, P.D. (1993): Electromyographic analysis of exercises proposed for differential activation of medial and lateral quadriceps femoris muscle components. Phys. Ther., 73:286–295.

67. Cerny, K. (1995): Vastus medialis oblique/vastus lateralis muscle activity ratios for selected exercises in person with and without patellofemoral pain syndrome. Phys. Ther., 75:672–683.

68. Gryzlo, S.M., Patek, R.M., Pink, M., et al. (1994): Electromyographic analysis of knee rehabilitation exercises. J. Orthop. Sports Phys. Ther., 20:36–43.

69. Hanten, W.P., and Schulthies, S.S. (1990): Exercise effect on electromyographic activity of the vastus medialis oblique and vastus lateralis muscles. Phys. Ther., 70:561–565.

70. Karst, G.M., and Willett, G.M. (1995): Onset timing of electromyographic activity in the vastus medialis oblique and vastus lateralis muscle in subjects with and without patellofemoral pain syndrome. Phys. Ther., 75:813–823.

71. Schaub, P.A., and Worrell, T.W. (1995): EMG activity of six muscles and VMO:VL ratio determination during a maximal squat exercise. J. Sport Rehabil., 4:195–202.

72. Voight, M.L., and Wieder, D.L. (1991): Comparative reflex response times of vastus medialis obliquus and vastus lateralis in normal subjects and subjects with extensor mechanism dysfunction. Am. J. Sports Med., 19:131–137.

73. Worrell, T.W., Connelly, S., and Hilvert, J. (1995): VMO:VL ratios and torque comparisons at four angles of knee flexion. J. Sport Rehabil., 4:264–272.

74. Boling, M., Pauda, D., Blackburn, J.T., et al. (2006): Hip adduction does not affect VMO EMG amplitude or VMO:VL ratios during dynamic squat exercise. J. Sport Rehabil., 15:195–205.

75. Song, C.Y., Lin, Y.F., Wei, T.C., et al. (2009): Surplus value of hip adduction in leg-press exercise in patients with patellofemoral pain syndrome: A randomized controlled trial. J. Orthop. Sports Phys. Ther., 89:409–418.

76. Powers, C.M. (1998): Rehabilitation of patellofemoral joint disorders: A critical review. J. Orthop. Sports Phys. Ther., 28:345–354.

77. Speakman, H.G.B., and Weisberg, J. (1977): The vastus medialis controversy. Physiotherapy, 63:249–254.

78. Lieb, F.J., and Perry, J. (1971): Quadriceps function: An electromyographic study under isometric conditions. J. Bone Joint Surg. Am., 53:749–758.

79. Grood, E.S., Suntay, W.J., Noyes, F.R., et al. (1984): Biomechanics of the knee-extension exercise. J. Bone Joint Surg. Am., 66:725–733.

80. Sprague, R.B. (1982): Factors related to extension lag at the knee joint. J. Orthop. Sports Phys. Ther., 3:178–181.

81. Lloyd, D.G. (2001): Rationale for training programs to reduce anterior cruciate ligament injuries in Australian football. J. Orthop. Sports Phys. Ther., 31:645–654.

82. Buchanan, T.S., Kim, A.W., and Lloyd, D.G. (1996): Selective muscle activation following rapid varus/valgus perturbations at the knee. Med. Sci. Sports Exerc., 28:870–876.

83. Kennedy, J.C., Alexander, I.J., and Hayes, K.C. (1982): Nerve supply of the human knee and its functional importance. Am. J. Sports Med., 10:329–335.

84. Spencer, J.D., Hayes, K.C., and Alexander, I.J. (1984): Knee joint effusion and quadriceps reflex inhibition in man. Arch. Phys. Med. Rehabil., 65:171–177.

85. Hardy, M.A. (1989): The biology of scar formation. Phys. Ther., 69:1014–1024.

86. Quillen, W.S., and Gieck, J.H. (1988): Manual therapy: Mobilization of the motion restricted knee. Athl. Train., 23:123–130.

87. McConnell, J. (1986): The management of chondromalacia patellae: A long-term solution. Aust. J. Physiother., 32:215–223.

88. Rowinski, M.J. (1985): Afferent neurobiology of the joint. In Gould J.A., and Davies, G.J. (eds.): Orthopedic and Sports Physical Therapy. St. Louis, Mosby.

89. Threlkeld, A.J., Horn, T.S., Wojtowicz, G.M., et al. (1989): Kinematics, ground reaction force, and muscle balance produced by backward running. Orthop. Sports Phys. Ther., 11:56–63.

90. Kramer, P.G. (1986): Patella malalignment syndrome: Rationale to reduce excessive lateral pressure. J. Orthop. Sports Phys. Ther., 8:301–309.

91. Aminaka, N., and Gribble, P.A. (2005): A systematic review of the effects of therapeutic taping on patellofemoral pain syndrome. J. Athl. Train., 40:341–351.

92. Derasari, A., Brindle, T.J., Alter, K.E., and Sheehan, F.T. (2010): McConnell taping shifts the patella inferiorly in patients with patellofemoral pain: A dynamic magnetic resonance imaging study. Phys. Ther., 90:411–419.

93. Bizzini, M., Childs, J.D., Piva, S.R., and Delitto, A. (2003): Systematic review of the quality of randomized controlled trials for patellofemoral pain syndrome. J. Orthop. Sports Phys. Ther., 33:4–20.

94. Watson, C.J., Propps, M., Galt, W., et al. (1999): Reliability of McConnell's classification of patellar orientation in symptomatic and asymptomatic subjects. J. Orthop. Sports Phys. Ther., 19:378–385.

95. Souza, R.B., Draper, C.E., Fredericson, M., and Powers, C.M. (2010): Femur rotation and patellofemoral joint kinematics: A weight-bearing magnetic resonance imaging analysis. J. Orthop. Sports Phys. Ther., 40:277–285.

96. Bahr, R., Fossan, B., Loken, S., et al. (2006): Surgical treatment compared with eccentric training for patellar tendinopathy (jumper's knee) a randomized, controlled trial. J. Bone Joint Surg. Am., 88:1689–1698.

97. Frohm, A., Saartok, T., Halvorsen, K., et al. (2007): Eccentric treatment for patellar tendinopathy: A prospective randomised short-term pilot study of two rehabilitation protocols. Br. J. Sports Med., 41:e7.

98. Purdam, C.R., Jonsson, P., Alfredson, H., et al. (2004): A pilot study of the eccentric decline squat in the management of painful chronic patellar tendinopathy. Br. J. Sports Med., 38:395–397.

99. Visnes, H., and Bahr, R. (2007): The evolution of eccentric training as treatment for patellar tendinopathy (jumper's knee): A critical review of exercise programmes. Br. J. Sports Med., 41:217–223.

100. Woodley, B.L., Newsham-West, R.J., and Baxter, G.D. (2007): Chronic tendinopathy: Effectiveness of eccentric exercise. Br. J. Sports Med., 41:188–198.

101. Young, M.A., Cook, J.L., Purdam, C.R., et al. (2005): Eccentric decline squat protocol offers superior results at 12 months compared with traditional eccentric protocol for patellar tendinopathy in volleyball players. Br. J. Sports Med., 39:102–105.

102. Zwerver, J., Bredeweg, S.W., and Hof, A.L. (2007): Biomechanical analysis of single-leg decline squat. Br. J. Sports Med., 41:264–268.

103. Friden, T., Zatterstrom, R., Anders, L., et al. (1991): Anterior cruciate–insufficient knees treated with physiotherapy. Clin. Orthop. Relat. Res., 263:190–199.

104. Snyder-Mackler, L., DeLuca, P.F., Williams, P.R., et al. (1994): Reflex inhibition of the quadriceps femoris muscle after injury or reconstruction of the anterior cruciate ligament. J. Bone Joint Surg. Am., 76:555–560.

105. Gross, M.T., Tyson, A.D., and Burns, C.B.B. (1993): Effect of knee angle and ligament insufficiency on anterior tibial translation during quadriceps muscle contraction: A preliminary report. J. Orthop. Sports Phys. Ther., 17:133–143.

106. Beard, D.J., Anderson, J.L., Davies, S., et al. (2001): Hamstrings vs. patella tendon for anterior cruciate ligament reconstruction. A randomised controlled trial. Knee, 8:45–50.

107. Engle, R.P. (1988): Hamstring facilitation in anterior instability of the knee. Athl. Train., 23:226–228,285.

108. Engle, R.P., and Canner, G.G. (1989): Proprioceptive neuromuscular facilitation (PNF) and modified procedures for anterior cruciate ligament (ACL) instability. J. Orthop. Sports Phys. Ther., 11:230–236.

109. Engle, R.P., and Canner, G.C. (1989): Rehabilitation of symptomatic anterolateral knee instability. J. Orthop. Sports Phys. Ther., 11:237–244.

110. Fitzgerald, G.K., Axe, M.J., Snyder-Mackler, L., et al. (2000): The efficacy of perturbation training in nonoperative anterior cruciate ligament rehabilitation programs for physically active individuals. Phys. Ther., 80:128–140.

111. Hsieh, Y.F., Draganich, L.F., Ho, S.H., et al. (2002): The effects of removal and reconstruction of the anterior cruciate ligament on the contact characteristics of the patellofemoral joint. Am. J. Sports Med., 30:121–127.

112. Steiner, M.E., Koskinen, S.K., Winalski, C.S., et al. (2001): Dynamic lateral patellar tilt in the anterior cruciate ligament–deficient knee. Am. J. Sports Med., 29:593–599.

113. Noyes, F.R. (1989): Rules for surgical indications in ACL surgery. In: 1989 Advances on the Knee and Shoulder. Cincinnati: Cincinnati Sports Medicine and Deaconess Hospital.

114. Eastlack, M.E., Axe, M.J., and Snyder-Mackler, L. (1999): Laxity, instability, and functional outcome after ACL injury: Copers versus noncopers. Med. Sci. Sports Exerc., 31:210–215.

115. Noyes, F.R., Matthews, D.S., Mooar, P.A., et al. (1983): The symptomatic anterior cruciate–deficient knee. Part II: The results of rehabilitation, activity modification, and counseling on functional disability. J. Bone Joint Surg. Am., 65:154–162.

116. Noyes, F.R., Matthews, D.S., Mooar, P.A., et al. (1983): The symptomatic anterior cruciate–deficient knee. Part I: The long-term functional disability in athletically active individuals. J. Bone Joint Surg. Am., 65:163–174.

117. Limbird, T.J., Shiavi, R., Frazer, M., et al. (1988): EMG profiles of knee joint musculature during walking: Changes induced by anterior cruciate ligament deficiency. J. Orthop. Res., 6:630–638.

118. Noyes, F.R., Barber-Westin, S., and Roberts, C. (1994): Use of allografts after failed treatment of rupture of the anterior cruciate ligament. J. Bone Joint Surg. Am., 76:1019–1031.

119. Fowler, P.S. (1994): The ACL injury. In: 1994 Advances on the Knee and Shoulder. Cincinnati, Cincinnati Sports Medicine and Deaconess Hospital.

120. Millett, P.J., Wickiewicz, T.L., and Warren, R.F. (2001): Motion loss after ligament injuries to the knee. Am. J. Sports Med., 29:664–675.

121. Kocher, M.S., Saxon, H.S., Hovis, W.D., et al. (2002): Management and complications of anterior cruciate ligament injuries in skeletally immature patients: Survey of the Herodicus Society and the ACL Study Group. J. Pediatr. Orthop., 22:452–457.

122. Micheli, L.J., Rask, B., and Gerberg, L. (1999): Anterior cruciate ligament reconstruction in patients who are prepubescent. Clin. Orthop. Relat. Res., 364:40–47.

123. Carey, J.L., Dunn, W.R., Dahm, D.L., et al. (2009): A systematic review of anterior cruciate ligament reconstruction with autograft compared with allograft. J. Bone Joint Surg. Am., 91:2242–2250.

124. Foster, T.E., Wolfe, B.L., Ryan, S., et al. (2010): Does the graft source really matter in the outcome of patients undergoing anterior cruciate ligament reconstruction? An evaluation of autograft versus allograft reconstruction results: A systematic review. Am. J. Sports Med., 38:189–199.

125. Goldblatt, J.P., Fitsimmons, S.E., Balk, E., et al. (2005): Reconstruction of anterior cruciate ligament: Meta-analysis of patellar tendon versus hamstring tendon autograft. Arthroscopy, 21:791–803.

126. Krych, A.J., Jackson, J.D., Hoskins, T.L., et al. (2008): A meta-analysis of patellar tendon autograft versus patellar tendon allograft in anterior cruciate ligament reconstruction. Arthroscopy, 24:292–298.

127. Noyes, F.R., Butler, D.L., Grood, E.S., et al. (1984): Biomechanical analysis of human ligament grafts used in knee-ligament repairs and reconstructions. J. Bone Joint Surg. Am., 66:344–352.

128. Cooper, D.E., Deng, X.H., Burstein, A.L., and Warren, R.F. (1993): The strength of the central third patellar tendon graft: A biomechanical study. Am. J. Sports Med., 21:818–824.

129. Amiel, D., Kleiner, J.B., and Akeson, W.H. (1986): The natural history of the anterior cruciate ligament autograft of patellar tendon origin. Am. J. Sports Med., 14:449–462.

130. Arnoczky, S.P., Tarvin, G.B., and Marshall, J.L. (1982): Anterior cruciate ligament replacement using patellar tendon. J. Bone Joint Surg. Am., 64:217–224.

131. Clancy, W.G., Narechania, R.G., Rosenberg, T.D., et al. (1981): Anterior and posterior cruciate ligament reconstruction in rhesus monkeys. J. Bone Joint Surg. Am., 63:1270–1284.

132. Arnoczky, S.P., Warren, R.F., and Ashlock, M.A. (1986): Replacement of the anterior cruciate ligament using a patellar tendon allograft. J. Bone Joint Surg. Am., 68:376–385.

133. van Grinsven, S., van Cingel, R.E.H., Holla, C.J.M., et al. (2010): Evidence-based rehabilitation following anterior cruciate ligament reconstruction. Knee Surg. Sports Traumatol. Arthrosc., 18:1128–1144.

134. Cascio, B.M., Culp, L., and Cosgarea, A.L. (2004): Return to play after anterior cruciate ligament reconstruction. Clin. Sports Med., 23:395–408.

135. Eitzen, I., Moksnes, H., Snyder-Mackler, L., et al. (2010): A progressive 5-week exercise therapy program leads to significant improvement in knee function early after anterior cruciate ligament injury. J. Orthop. Sports Phys. Ther., 40:705–721.

136. Mangine, R.E., Noyes, F.R., and DeMaio, M. (1992): Minimal protection program: Advanced weight bearing and range of motion after ACL reconstruction—Weeks 1 to 5. Orthopedics, 15:504–515.

137. Snyder-Mackler, L., DeLitto, A., Bailey, S.I., et al. (1995): Strength of the quadriceps femoris muscle and functional recovery after reconstruction of the anterior cruciate ligament. J. Bone Joint Surg. Am., 77:1166–1173.

138. Andersson, D., Samuelsson, K., and Karlsson, J. (2009): Treatment of anterior cruciate ligament injuries with special reference to surgical technique and rehabilitation: An assessment of randomized controlled trials. Arthroscopy, 25:653–685.

139. Myer, G.D., Paterno, M.V., Ford, K.R., et al. (2006): Rehabilitation after anterior cruciate ligament reconstruction: Criteria-based progression through the return-to-sport phase. J. Orthop. Sports Phys. Ther., 36:385–402.

140. Beynnon, B.D., Pope, M.H., Wertheimer, C.M., et al. (1992): The effect of functional knee-braces on strain on anterior cruciate ligament in vivo. J. Bone Joint Surg. Am., 74:1298–1312.

141. Vailas, J.C., and Pink, M. (1993): Biomechanical effects of functional knee bracing. Sports Med., 15:210–218.

142. Branch, T., Hunter, R., and Reynolds, P. (1988): Controlling anterior tibial displacement under static load: A comparison of two braces. Orthopedics, 11:1249–1252.

143. Cook, F.F., Tibone, J.E., and Redfern, F.C. (1989): A dynamic analysis of a functional brace for anterior cruciate ligament insufficiency. Am. J. Sports Med., 17:519–524.

144. Mishra, D.V., Daniel, D.M., and Stone, M.L. (1989): The use of functional knee braces in the control of pathologic anterior knee laxity. Clin. Orthop. Relat. Res., 241:213–220.

145. Nemeth, G., Lamontagne, M., Tho, K.S., et al. (1997): Electromyographic activity in expert downhill skiers using functional knee braces after anterior cruciate ligament injuries. Am. J. Sports Med., 25:635–641.

146. Wojtys, E.M., Kothari, S.U., and Huston, L.J. (1996): Anterior cruciate ligament functional brace use in sports. Am. J. Sports Med., 24:539–546.

147. DeVita, P., Lassiter, T., Hortobagyi, T., et al. (1998): Functional knee brace effects during walking in patients with anterior cruciate ligament reconstruction. Am. J. Sports Med., 26:778–784.

148. Risberg, M.A., Holm, I., Steen, H., et al. (1999): The effect of knee bracing after anterior cruciate ligament reconstruction: A prospective, randomized study with two years' follow-up. Am. J. Sports Med., 27:76–83.

149. Wright, R.W., and Fetzer, G.B. (2007): Bracing after ACL reconstruction. Clin. Orthop. Relat. Res., 455:162–168.

150. Styf, J. (1999): The effects of functional bracing on muscle function and performance. Sports Med., 28:77–81.

151. Hewett, T.E., Lindenfeld, T.N., Riccobene, J.V., et al. (1999): The effect of neuromuscular training on the incidence of knee injury in female athletes: A prospective study. Am. J. Sports Med., 27:699–706.

152. Hewett, T.E., Stroupe, A.L., Nance, T.A., et al. (1996): Plyometric training in female athletes: Decreased impact forces and increased hamstring torques. Am. J. Sports Med., 24:765–773.

153. Wilk, K.E., Arrigo, C., Andrews, A.R., et al. (1999): Rehabilitation after anterior cruciate ligament reconstruction in the female athlete. J. Athl. Train., 34:177–193.

154. Cerulli, G., Benoit, D.L., Caraffa, A., et al. (2001): Proprioceptive training and prevention of anterior cruciate ligament injuries in soccer. J. Orthop. Sports Phys. Ther., 31:655–660.

155. Rubenstein, R.A., and Shelbourne, K.D. (1993): Diagnosis of posterior cruciate ligament injuries and indications for nonoperative and operative treatment. Oper. Tech. Sports Med., 1:118–127.

156. Noyes, F.R., and Barber-Westin, S. (2006): Two-strand posterior cruciate ligament reconstruction with quadriceps tendon–patellar bone autograft: Technical considerations and clinical results. Instr. Course Lect., 55:509–528.

157. Escamilla, R.F., Zheng, N., Imamura, R., et al. (2009): Cruciate ligament force during the wall squat and one-leg squat. Med. Sci. Sports Exerc., 41:408–417.

158. Escamilla, R.F., Zheng, N., Imamura, R., et al. (2010): Cruciate ligament forces between short-step and long-step forward lunge. Med. Sci. Sports Exerc., 42:1932–1942.

159. Escamilla, R.F., Zheng, N., Macleod, T.D., et al. (2008): Patellofemoral joint force and stress between a short- and long-step forward lunge. J. Orthop. Sports Phys. Ther., 38:681–690.

160. Krause, W.R., Pope, M.H., Johnson, R.J., et al. (1976): Mechanical changes in the knee after meniscectomy. J. Bone Joint Surg. Am., 58:599–604.

161. McGinty, J.B., Guess, L.F., and Marvin, R.A. (1977): Partial or total meniscectomy: A comparative analysis. J. Bone Joint Surg. Am., 59:763–766.

162. Heckmann, T.P., Barber-Westin, S.D., and Noyes, F.R. (2006): Meniscal repair and transplantation: Indications, techniques, rehabilitation, and clinical outcome. J. Orthop. Sports Phys. Ther., 36:795–814.

163. Starke, C., Kopf, S., Petersen, W., et al. (2009): Meniscal repair. Arthroscopy, 25:1033–1044.

164. Irrgang, J.J., and Fitzgerald, G.K. (2000): Rehabilitation of the multiple-ligament–injured knee. Clin. Sports Med., 19:545–569.

165. Buckwalter, J.A. (1998): Articular cartilage: Injuries and potential for healing. J. Orthop. Sports Phys. Ther., 18:192–202.

166. Johnson, D.L., Urban, W.P., Caborn, D.N.M., et al. (1998): Articular cartilage changes seen with magnetic resonance imaging–detected bone bruises associated with acute anterior cruciate ligament rupture. Am. J. Sports Med., 16:409–414.

167. Alleyne, K.R., and Galloway, M.T. (2001): Management of osteochondral injuries of the knee. Clin. Sports Med., 10:343–364.

168. Gillogly, S.D., Voight, M., and Blackburn, T. (1998): Treatment of articular cartilage defects of the knee with autologous chondrocyte implantation. J. Orthop. Sports Phys. Ther., 18:241–251.

169. Sledge, S.L. (2001): Microfracture techniques in the treatment of osteochondral injuries. Clin. Sports Med., 20:365–377.

170. Irrgang, J.J., and Pezzullo, D. (1998): Rehabilitation following surgical procedures to address articular cartilage lesions in the knee. J. Orthop. Sports Phys. Ther., 28:232–240.

171. Hambly, K., Bobic, V., Wondrasch, B., et al. (2006): Autologous chondrocyte implantation postoperative care and rehabilitation: Science and practice. Am. J. Sports Med., 34:1020–1038.

172. Logerstedt, D.S., Snyder-Mackler, L., Ritter, R.C., et al. (2010): Knee pain and mobility impairments: Meniscal and articular cartilage lesions. J. Orthop. Sports Phys. Ther., 40:A1–A35.

173. Logerstedt, D.S., Snyder-Mackler, L., Ritter, R.C., et al. (2010): Knee stability and movement coordination impairments: Knee ligament sprain. J. Orthop. Sports Phys. Ther., 40:(4):A1–A37.

174. Watson, C.J., Propps, M., Ratner, J., et al. (2005): Reliability and responsiveness of the Lower Extremity Functional Scale and the Anterior Knee Pain Scale in patients with anterior knee pain. J. Orthop. Sports Phys. Ther., 35:136–146.

175. Daniel, D.M., Stone, M.L., Malcom, L., et al. (1983): Instrumented measurement of ACL disruption. Orthop. Res. Soc., 8:12–17.

176. Hanten, W.P., and Pace, M.B. (1987): Reliability of measuring anterior laxity of the knee joint using a knee ligament arthrometer. Phys. Ther., 67:357–359.

177. Bach, B.R., Warren, R.F., Flynn, W.M., et al. (1990): Arthrometric evaluation of knees that have a torn anterior cruciate ligament. J. Bone Joint Surg. Am., 12:1299–1306.

178. Daniel, D.M., Malcom, L.L., Losse, G., et al. (1985): Instrumented measurement of anterior laxity of the knee. J. Bone Joint Surg. Am., 67:720–726.

179. Daniel, D.M., Stone, M.L., Sachs, R., et al. (1985): Instrumented measurement of anterior knee laxity in patients with acute anterior cruciate ligament disruption. Am. J. Sports Med., 13:401–407.

180. Liu, S.H., Ost, L., Henry, M., et al. (1995): The diagnosis of acute complete tears of the anterior cruciate ligament: Comparison of MRI, arthrometry, and clinical examination. J Bone Joint Surg. Br., 77:586–588.

181. Ballantyne, B.T., French, A.K., Heimsoth, S.L., et al. (1995): Influence of examiner experience and gender on interrater reliability of KT-1000 arthrometer measurements. Phys. Ther., 75:898–906.

182. Berry, J., Kramer, K., Binkley, J., et al. (1999): Error estimates in novice and expert raters for the KT-1000 arthrometer. J. Orthop. Sports Phys. Ther., 29:49–55.

183. Myrer, J.W., Schulthies, S.S., and Fellingham, G.W. (1996): Relative and absolute reliability of the KT-2000 arthrometer for uninjured knees. Am. J. Sports Med., 24:104–108.

184. Queale, W.S., Snyder-Mackler, L., Handling, K.A., et al. (1994): Instrumented examination of knee laxity in patients with anterior cruciate deficiency: A comparison of the KT-2000, Knee Signature System, and Genucom. J. Orthop. Sports Phys. Ther., 19:345–351.

185. Huber, F.E., Irrgang, J.J., Harner, C., et al. (1997): Intratester and intertester reliability of the KT-1000 arthrometer in the assessment of posterior laxity of the knee. Am. J. Sports Med., 25:479–485.

186. Daniel, D.M. (1990). The accuracy and reproducibility of the KT-1000 knee ligament arthrometer. Available at http://medmetric.com/acc.htm. Accessed 10/6/2011.

187. Bach, B.R., Jones, G.T., Hager, C.A., et al. (1995): Arthrometric results of arthroscopically assisted anterior cruciate ligament reconstruction using autograft patellar tendon substitution. Am. J. Sports Med., 23:179–185.

188. Neeb, T.B., Aufdemkampe, G., Wagener, J.H.D., et al. (1997): Assessing anterior cruciate ligament injuries: The association and differential value of questionnaires, clinical tests, and functional tests. J. Orthop. Sports Phys. Ther., 26:324–331.

189. Sgaglione, N.A., Warren, R.F., Wickiewicz, T.L., et al. (1990): Primary repair with semitendinosus tendon augmentation of acute anterior cruciate ligament injuries. Am. J. Sports Med., 18:64–73.

190. Tyler, T.F., McHugh, M.P., Gleim, G.W., et al. (1999): Association of KT-1000 measurements with clinical tests of knee stability 1 year following anterior cruciate ligament reconstruction. J. Orthop. Sports Phys. Ther., 29:540–545.

191. Dvir, Z. (1995): Isokinetics: Muscle Testing Interpretation and Clinical Applications. Edinburgh, Churchill Livingstone.

192. Levene, J.A., Hart, B.A., Seeds, R.H., et al. (1991): Reliability of reciprocal isokinetic testing of the knee extensors and flexors. J. Orthop. Sports Phys. Ther., 14:1221–1227.

193. Perrin, D.H. (1993): Isokinetic Exercise and Assessment. Champaign, IL, Human Kinetics.

194. Steiner, L.A., Harris, B.A., and Krebs, D.E. (1993): Reliability of eccentric isokinetic knee flexion and extension measurements. Arch. Phys. Med. Rehabil., 74:1327–1335.

195. Aagaard, P., Simonsen, E.B., Magnusson, S.P., et al. (1998): A new concept for isokinetic hamstring:quadriceps muscle strength ratio. Am. J. Sports Med., 26:231–237.

196. Noyes, F.R., Barber, S.D., and Mangine, R.E. (1991): Abnormal lower limb symmetry determined by function hop test after anterior cruciate ligament rupture. Am. J. Sports Med., 19:513–518.

197. Loudon, J.K., Wiesner, D., Goist-Foley, H.L., et al. (2002): Intrarater reliability of functional performance tests for subjects with patellofemoral pain syndrome. J. Athl. Train., 37:256–261.

20

Lower Leg, Ankle, and Foot Rehabilitation

Edward P. Mulligan, PT, DPT, OCS, SCS, ATC

CHAPTER OBJECTIVES

- Explain the arthrokinematic considerations that influence motion in the joints of the foot and ankle.
- Explain the concentric and eccentric action of muscles in the lower leg, ankle, and foot.
- Recognize structural abnormalities in alignment of the lower leg, rearfoot, and forefoot.

- Describe key components in evaluation of injuries involving the lower leg, ankle, and foot
- Describe common athletic pathologies and rehabilitative management of lower leg, ankle, and foot injuries.
- Explain the biomechanical principles and clinical practice of orthotic therapy.

The lower leg, ankle, and foot contain 26 bones, all working as one unit to propel the body. The foot has three components: rearfoot, midfoot, and forefoot. The structure of the rearfoot and midfoot is provided by the tarsal bones. The rearfoot contains the subtalar joint, with the talus resting on top of the calcaneus. In the midfoot, the navicular and cuboid articulate with the talus and calcaneus to form the transverse tarsal joint. The three cuneiform bones are located within the midfoot. Five metatarsal and 14 phalangeal bones make up the structure of the forefoot. The shape of the joint, orientation of its axis, supporting ligaments, and subtle accessory motions at the joint surface are important determinants of normal biomechanical behavior. Treatment of pathologic hypomobility or hypermobility is predicated on a thorough understanding of these principles and their functional intimacy.

ARTHROKINEMATIC CONSIDERATIONS

Tibiofibular Joint

The tibiofibular joint provides accessory motion to allow greater freedom of movement in the ankle. Fusion or hypomobility of this joint can restrict or impair ankle function. During ankle plantar flexion, the fibula slides caudad at the superior and inferior tibiofibular joint and the lateral malleolus rotates mediad to cause an approximation of the two malleoli. With dorsiflexion, the opposite accessory motions provide a slight spread of

the malleoli and accommodate the wider portion of the anterior talus. Accessory motion of the tibiofibular joint also occurs with supination (calcaneal inversion) and pronation (calcaneal eversion). The head of the fibula slides distally and posteriorly with supination and proximally and anteriorly during pronation.

Talocrural Joint

The talocrural articulation is a synovial joint with a structurally strong mortice and supporting collateral ligaments. The concave surface of the mortice is made up of the distal tibial plafond and the tibial (medial) and fibular (lateral) malleoli. Within the mortice sits the convex surface of the talar dome. The joint derives ligamentous support from the deltoid ligament medially and the anterior talofibular, calcaneofibular, and posterior talofibular ligaments laterally.

The lateral malleolus is positioned distally and posteriorly relative to the medial malleolus, which causes the axis of motion for the ankle joint to run in a posterolateral inferior to anteromedial superior direction (Fig. 20-1). This oblique orientation allows triplanar motion. Sagittal plane plantar flexion and dorsiflexion make up the primary movements of the joint and are coupled with adduction and abduction, respectively. Because the axis is nearly parallel to the transverse plane, inversion and eversion are negligible components of motion. The available range of motion is typically defined as approximately 20° of dorsiflexion (with the knee flexed) and 50° of plantar flexion.

A small amount of talocrural physiologic accessory motion also accompanies plantar flexion and dorsiflexion. As the foot plantar-flexes, the body of the talus glides anteriorly. Conversely, as the foot dorsiflexes, the direction of talar glide is posterior. Maximal stability with angular and torsional stress occurs in the close-packed position of maximal dorsiflexion, in which the talus slides posteriorly and wedges within the mortice. The resting position of the ankle joint is 10° of plantar flexion (Table 20-1).

Subtalar Joint

The talocalcaneal articulation provides the triplanar motions of pronation and supination. The medial and lateral collateral, interosseous talocalcaneal, and posterior and lateral talocalcaneal ligaments support the joint.

The joint axis runs from dorsal, medial, and distal to plantar, lateral, and proximal. It is oriented approximately 16° from the sagittal plane and 42° from the transverse plane (Fig. 20-2). Because of this axis of orientation, the joint provides the triplanar motions of pronation and supination. The pronation components of motion in an open kinetic chain are calcaneal dorsiflexion, abduction, and eversion. Conversely, open kinetic chain supination consists of calcaneal plantar flexion, adduction, and inversion. Functionally, however, the subtalar joint operates as a closed kinetic chain. Closed kinetic chain motion occurs when the distal segment is fixed and the proximal segment becomes mobile, as when the foot is in contact with the ground. The distal or terminal joints meet with considerable resistance, which prohibits or restrains free motion. During the weight-bearing portion of the stance phase of gait, friction and ground reaction forces prevent the abduction-adduction and

plantar flexion–dorsiflexion elements of open kinetic chain subtalar motion. To counteract these forces, the talus functions to maintain the transverse and sagittal plane motions of supination and pronation. Thus, in closed kinetic chain motion, subtalar joint pronation consists of talar plantar flexion–adduction and calcaneal eversion, whereas subtalar joint supination consists of talar dorsiflexion-abduction and calcaneal inversion (Fig. 20-3). Note that the calcaneal direction of movement is unaffected by the open chain versus the closed chain type of motion (Table 20-2).

The subtalar joint couples the function of the foot with the rest of the proximal kinetic chain. The prime function of the subtalar joint is to permit rotation of the leg in the transverse plane during gait. Rotation of the talus on the calcaneus allows the foot to become a directional transmitter and torque converter to the kinetic chain.[1] These characteristics allow the foot to be a loose adaptor to the terrain in midstance and a rigid lever for propulsion.

Because the subtalar joint is angulated approximately 45° from the transverse plane, 1° of inversion or eversion occurs for every 1° of tibial internal or external rotation. This relationship can be observed in gait. As the subtalar joint

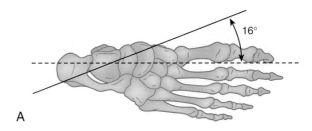

A

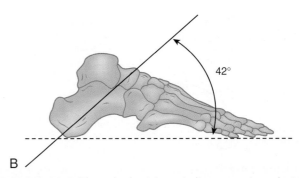

B

FIGURE 20-2 The subtalar joint axis lies approximately 16° from the sagittal plane (**A**) and 42° from the transverse plane (**B**). *(Reproduced by permission from Mann, R.A. [1982]: Biomechanics of running. In: American Academy of Orthopaedic Surgeons: Symposium on the Foot and Leg in Running Sports. St. Louis, Mosby.)*

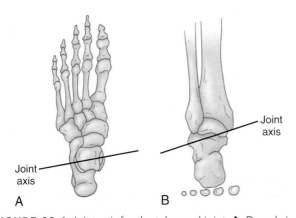

FIGURE 20-1 Joint axis for the talocrural joint. **A,** Dorsal view. **B,** Posterior view. The axis of orientation runs in a posterolateral inferior to anteromedial superior direction.

Table 20-1 Treatment Considerations With Respect to Joint Position

Joint	Close-Packed Position	Resting Position	Capsular Pattern
Talocrural	Maximal dorsiflexion	10° plantar flexion	Plantar flexion restricted more than dorsiflexion
Subtalar	Maximal supination	Neutral	Increasing loss of varus until fixed in valgus
Midtarsal	Maximal supination	STJ neutral	Limitations in adduction and inversion
First MTP	Maximal dorsiflexion	Slight plantar flexion	Gross limitation in extension; slight limitation in flexion

MTP, Metatarsophalangeal; *STJ,* subtalar joint.

pronates, the tibial tuberosity is seen to be rotating internally (Fig. 20-4). High angles of inclination (>45°) of the subtalar joint axis cause a relative decrease in calcaneal inversion-eversion motion and increased tibial rotation motion that leads to posture-related pathologies secondary to poor absorption of ground reaction forces. Conversely, an athlete with a low angle of inclination (<45°) of the subtalar joint demonstrates a relative increase in calcaneal mobility that results in more foot-related overuse and fatigue problems secondary to the calcaneal hypermobility.

The physiologic accessory motions of the subtalar joint occur in the frontal plane. The convex portion of the posterior calcaneus glides laterally during inversion (supination) and medially during eversion (pronation). The close-packed position of the subtalar joint is maximal supination, whereas the resting position is the subtalar neutral position. From its neutral position the subtalar joint can supinate approximately two times as much as it can pronate. This motion is measured in the frontal plane of calcaneal inversion and eversion. Normal subtalar range of motion is approximately 30°, with two thirds of that motion being represented as calcaneal inversion and one third as calcaneal eversion. Normal gait requires at least 8° to 12° of supination and 4° to 6° of pronation.

Midtarsal Joint

The midtarsal joint consists of the talonavicular and calcaneocuboid articulations. They derive their ligamentous support from the calcaneonavicular (spring), deltoid, dorsal talonavicular, and calcaneocuboid (long and short plantar) ligaments.

The midtarsal joint has two separate axes, longitudinal and oblique. Functionally, these two axes work together to result in triplanar motion. The longitudinal axis is essentially parallel to the sagittal and transverse planes, which allows only the frontal plane motions of inversion and eversion, whereas the oblique axis is parallel to the frontal plane, which allows motion in the sagittal (plantar flexion–dorsiflexion) and transverse (adduction-abduction) planes (Fig. 20-5). Because the oblique axis is angulated about equally from the sagittal and transverse planes, plantar flexion–adduction and dorsiflexion-abduction are coupled equally.

From a clinical standpoint, motion in the midtarsal joint cannot be reliably quantified. Midtarsal joint motion is dictated by the position of the subtalar joint. When the subtalar joint is pronated, the axes of the talocalcaneal and calcaneocuboid joints are parallel, which allows the midtarsal joint to unlock and become an adaptor with increased mobility. As the subtalar joint supinates, motion of the midtarsal joint decreases as the two axes diverge and "lock" the forefoot on the rearfoot in preparation for its rigid lever function during the propulsive phase of gait (Fig. 20-6).

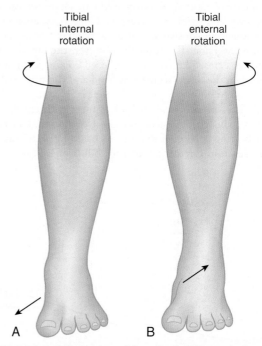

FIGURE 20-4 Relationship of the subtalar joint to the lower leg during gait. **A,** Subtalar pronation. **B,** Subtalar supination.

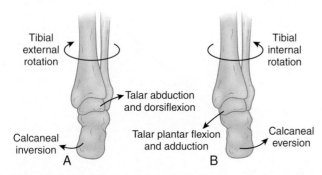

FIGURE 20-3 Closed chain subtalar motion. **A,** Supination. **B,** Pronation.

Table 20-2 Calcaneal and Talar Motion in Open (Non–Weight-Bearing) and Closed (Weight-Bearing) Kinetic Chain

Motion of Foot	Open Chain Component (Non–Weight-Bearing Motion)	Closed Chain Component (Weight-Bearing Motion)
Pronation	Calcaneal eversion	Calcaneal eversion
	Calcaneal abduction	Talar adduction
	Calcaneal dorsiflexion	Talar plantar flexion
Supination	Calcaneal inversion	Calcaneal inversion
	Calcaneal adduction	Talar abduction
	Calcaneal plantar flexion	Talar dorsiflexion

The position of the midtarsal joint is dictated by ground reaction forces during the initial contact and midstance phases of gait and by muscular activity on the joint during the propulsive phase of gait.[2] The standard clinical index for determining midtarsal joint position is to compare the plantar plane position of the central three metatarsal heads with the plantar plane position of the neutral rearfoot when the midtarsal joint is maximally pronated about both its axes.

Physiologic accessory motions of the midtarsal joint that can be evaluated manually include dorsal and plantar glides of the navicular on the talus and the cuboid on the calcaneus. Dorsal glide of the navicular on the talus accompanies supination, and a plantar glide accompanies pronation.

Tarsometatarsal, Metatarsophalangeal, and Interphalangeal Joints

The first ray represents a functional articulation consisting of the bones of the medial column. The joint axis runs in a distolateral to proximomedial direction, almost parallel to the transverse plane. Motion occurs primarily in the sagittal (plantar flexion–dorsiflexion) and frontal (inversion-eversion) planes. The axis is angulated 45° from both these planes, so for every 1° of plantar flexion, 1° of eversion occurs (Fig. 20-7).

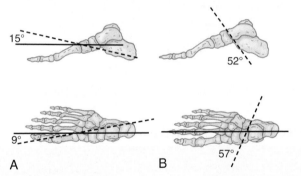

FIGURE 20-5 Axes of motion for the midtarsal joints. **A,** Longitudinal axis. **B,** Oblique axis.

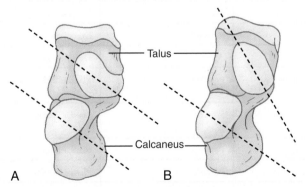

FIGURE 20-6 Axis of the transverse tarsal joint. **A,** When calcaneus is in eversion, the conjoint axes between the talonavicular and calcaneocuboid joints are parallel to one another, so increased motion occurs in the transverse tarsal joint. **B,** When the calcaneus is in inversion, the axes are no longer parallel, and there is decreased motion with increased stability of the transverse tarsal joint. *(Reproduced by permission from Mann, R.A. [1982]: Biomechanics of running. In American Academy of Orthopaedic Surgeons: Symposium on the Foot and Leg in Running Sports. St. Louis, Mosby.)*

First ray motion begins in the late stance phase of gait and continues late into propulsion. As with the midtarsal joint, first ray motion is influenced by the position of the subtalar joint. With the subtalar joint in pronation, the amount of motion of the first ray is increased. As the subtalar joint supinates, motion of the first ray decreases. The normal extent of movement is 0.5 to 1 cm (a thumb width) in the plantar and dorsal directions and is dynamically controlled by the peroneus longus.[2]

The clinical standard for determining the neutral position of the first ray is to evaluate the position of the first metatarsal relative to the three central metatarsal heads. It should lie in the same transverse plane, neither plantar-flexed nor dorsiflexed.

The fifth ray operates about an independent axis with the same directional orientation as the subtalar joint. The central three metatarsophalangeal (MTP) joints have their axis oriented parallel to the frontal and transverse planes. Consequently, only plantar flexion–dorsiflexion motion takes place in the sagittal plane.

The first MTP joint represents the articulation between the first metatarsal and the proximal phalanx of the big toe. Minimal normal first MTP range of motion with the first ray stabilized is about 20° to 30° of hyperextension. Without stabilization, the first MTP joint should hyperextend to at least 60° to 70°. The MTP joints also have an additional vertical axis, parallel to the frontal and sagittal planes, to allow abduction and adduction of the joints.

Physiologic accessory motions of the MTP joints include plantar and dorsal glide. Plantar glide of the convex first metatarsal accompanies extension, whereas dorsal glide accompanies toe flexion.

Clinical Pearl #1

The ideal foot is cosmetically acceptable, structurally neutral, and free of impairments. It fits comfortably into all shoes, promotes normal lower quarter biomechanics, and allows pain-free function.

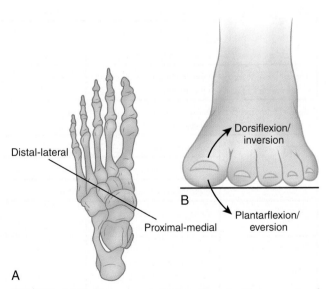

FIGURE 20-7 First ray axis and motion. **A,** First ray axis of motion, dorsal view. **B,** First ray motion.

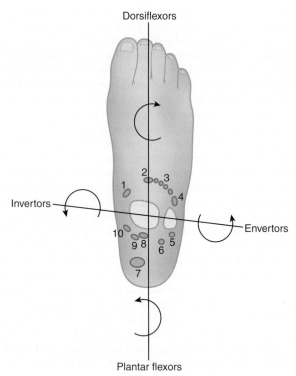

FIGURE 20-8 Motion diagram of the ankle showing the tibialis anterior (*1*), extensor hallucis longus (*2*), extensor digitorum longus (*3*), peroneus tertius (*4*), peroneus brevis (*5*), peroneus longus (*6*), Achilles tendon (*7*), flexor hallucis longus (*8*), flexor digitorum longus (*9*), and tibialis posterior (*10*). *(From Magee, D.J.* [1987]: Orthopedic Physical Assessment. Philadelphia, Saunders.)

MUSCULAR FUNCTION OF THE LOWER LEG, ANKLE, AND FOOT

The phasic action of the muscles of the lower leg and foot can be determined by examining the musculotendinous unit's excursion from its origin to its insertion relative to the axis on which it acts (Fig. 20-8). Each muscle group has specific functions that control or provide the necessary forces to create movement. The muscles of the leg and foot can be divided into subgroups or compartments. Where the tendon lies relative to the talocrural and subtalar axes dictates the motions that they create in the open chain and control in the closed chain (Table 20-3; Fig. 20-9).

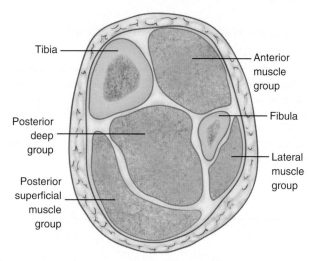

FIGURE 20-9 Cross section of the lower leg muscle groups.

Table 20-3 Lower Leg Muscle Groups and Their Relationship to the Joint Axes and Subsequent Action

Group	Muscle(s)	Tendon Location Relative to the STJ	STJ Motion	Location of the Tendon Location Relative to the TCJ	TCJ Motion
Anterior pretibial	Anterior tibialis	Medial	Supination	Anterior	Dorsiflexion
	Extensor hallucis longus	On axis	—	Anterior	Dorsiflexion
	Extensor digitorum longus	Lateral	Pronation	Anterior	Dorsiflexion
Lateral	Fibularis longus Fibularis brevis	Lateral	Pronation	Posterior	Plantar flexion
Superficial posterior	Gastrocnemius Soleus	Medial	Supination	Posterior	Plantar flexion
Deep posterior	Posterior tibialis	Medial	Supination	Posterior	Plantar flexion
	Flexor digitorum longus	Medial	Supination	Posterior	Plantar flexion
	Flexor hallucis longus	Medial	Supination	Posterior	Plantar flexion
Dorsal intrinsics	Extensor hallucis brevis Extensor digitorum brevis	—	—	—	—
Plantar intrinsics	Flexor digitorum brevis Flexor hallucis brevis Adductor hallucis Abductor hallucis Lumbricales	—	—	—	—

STJ, Subtalar joint; TCJ, talocrural joint.

Posterior Superficial Muscle Group

The posterior superficial muscle group is composed of the gastrocnemius, soleus, and plantaris muscles. These muscles originate from above and below the knee joint and have a common insertion by way of the Achilles tendon on the posterior aspect of the calcaneus. In the open kinetic chain, the triceps surae provides flexion of the knee, plantar flexion of the ankle, and supination of the subtalar joint. With closed kinetic chain function, the gastrocnemius and soleus are active throughout the stance phase of gait. Initially, at heel strike, the gastrocnemius and soleus contract eccentrically to decelerate tibial internal rotation and forward progression of the tibia over the foot. Later, during midstance and heel-off, they provide subtalar joint supination (externally rotating the tibia) and ankle plantar flexion.

Posterior Deep Muscle Group

The posterior deep muscles of the lower part of the leg include the posterior tibialis, flexor digitorum longus, and flexor hallucis longus. The posterior tibialis is a strong invertor (as a component of triplanar supination) of the subtalar joint and functions to control and reverse pronation during gait. It decelerates subtalar joint pronation and tibial internal rotation at heel strike and then reverses its function to accelerate subtalar joint supination and tibial external rotation during stance. The posterior tibialis also maintains the stability of the midtarsal joint in the direction of supination around its oblique axis during the stance phase of gait.

The flexor digitorum longus functions as a supinator of the subtalar joint and flexor of the second through fifth MTP joints in the open kinetic chain. When the foot is in contact with the ground and the digits are stable, the flexor digitorum longus actively stabilizes the foot as a weight-bearing platform for propulsion. If the flexor digitorum longus works unopposed by the action of the intrinsic muscles, clawing of the toes results.

The flexor hallucis longus has a function similar to that of the flexor digitorum longus in that it flexes the first MTP joint in the open kinetic chain. Both these long flexors help support the medial longitudinal arch.

Lateral Muscle Group

The lateral muscle group includes the peroneus longus and brevis. The peroneus longus, because of its attachment to the first metatarsal and medial cuneiform on the plantar surface, functions to pronate the subtalar joint and to plantar-flex and evert the first ray in the open kinetic chain. In the closed kinetic chain, the peroneus longus has many important functions. It provides support to the transverse and lateral longitudinal arches. During the latter portion of midstance and early heel-off, it actively stabilizes the first ray and everts the foot to transfer body weight from the lateral to the medial side of the foot.

The peroneus brevis is primarily an evertor in open kinetic chain motion. During gait it functions in concert with the peroneus longus. Its primary role is to stabilize the calcaneocuboid joint and thereby allow the peroneus longus to work efficiently over the cuboid pulley.

Anterior Muscle Group

The pretibial muscles include the anterior tibialis, extensor digitorum longus, extensor hallucis longus, and peroneus tertius. As a group they are active during the swing phase and the heel-strike to foot-flat phases of gait.

The anterior tibialis is primarily a dorsiflexor of the talocrural joint in open kinetic chain function. During gait, the anterior tibialis basically operates concentrically in the swing phase and eccentrically in the stance phase. At the end of toe-off, the anterior tibialis begins to contract concentrically to initiate dorsiflexion of the ankle and first ray, to assist in ground clearance at midswing, and then to supinate the foot slightly during late swing in preparation for heel strike. When the foot hits the ground, the anterior tibialis reverses its role to decelerate or control plantar flexion to foot flat, prevent excessive pronation, and supinate the midtarsal joint's longitudinal axis. A weak anterior tibialis can lead to "foot slap," or uncontrolled pronation in gait.

In non–weight-bearing function, the long extensors (extensor digitorum and hallucis longus) provide dorsiflexion of the ankle and extension of the toes. Because these tendons pass lateral to the subtalar joint axis, unlike the anterior tibialis, they provide a pronatory force at the joint. In fact, a prime responsibility of the long extensors is to hold the oblique axis of the midtarsal joint in a pronated position at heel strike and then to assist in controlled deceleration of plantar flexion to foot flat.

Clinical Pearl #2

The action of a muscle can be determined by examining the musculotendinous unit's excursion from origin to insertion relative to the axis on which it acts.

Intrinsic Muscle Group

Generally, the intrinsic muscles of the foot act together during most of the stance phase of gait. Their function is to stabilize the midtarsal joint and digits while keeping the toes flat on the ground until liftoff. An unstable, pronated midtarsal joint during midstance makes the intrinsic muscles work harder and longer. This phenomenon explains the common complaint of foot fatigue in athletes with a hypermobile foot.

CLINICAL EXAMINATION

The section on clinical examination of the lower leg, ankle, and foot is presented in the online appendix of this chapter on Expert Consult @ www.expertconsult.com.

LOWER LEG, ANKLE, AND FOOT INJURIES AND THEIR MANAGEMENT

Lower Leg Injuries

Tennis Leg

Originally thought to be a tear of the plantaris muscle, *tennis leg* has now been proved through surgical exploration to be a musculotendinous lesion of the medial gastrocnemius head (Fig. 20-10). Because this injury is more common in the fourth to sixth decades of life, the examiner will need to rule out the presence of thrombophlebitis, compartment syndrome, or intermittent claudication masking as musculoskeletal calf pain. Entrapment of the popliteal artery may need to

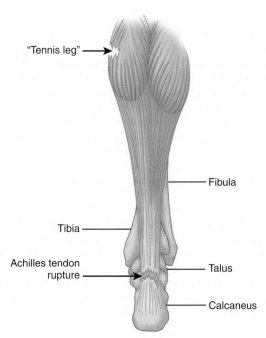

"Tennis leg"

Fibula

Tibia

Achilles tendon rupture

Talus

Calcaneus

FIGURE 20-10 Tennis leg and Achilles tendon injury.

be differentiated by diminished distal pulses and exertional calf pain during ambulation in a younger athlete. The usual mechanism of injury is sudden extension of the knee with the foot in a dorsiflexed position. This places tremendous tensile stress on the two-joint expansion of the gastrocnemius. Middle-aged athletes or those with previous degenerative changes in this anatomic area may be predisposed to this type of trauma.

The athlete feels a sudden, sharp twinge in the upper medial aspect of the calf and immediately has difficulty with full weight bearing. Typically, rapid swelling and ecchymosis occur, with point tenderness or a palpable defect found at the site of the lesion.

Acute care consists of immediate first aid measures, including analgesic medication, ice, compression, and elevation of the injured area. The ankle is placed in mild plantar flexion to alleviate stress on the area of injury. A non–weight-bearing crutch gait may initially be necessary, depending on the severity of the injury.

Gradual, gentle static stretching is initiated early in the subacute phase to align the healing scar tissue. Friction massage of the area also prevents random alignment of the collagen fibers. As the athlete progresses to full weight bearing, heel lifts can be placed in the shoe to protect against weight-bearing stress. As flexibility of the Achilles tendon improves, the height of the lifts can gradually be reduced. Instructions for maintaining calf flexibility and education regarding appropriate warm-up techniques should be provided to reduce the risk for recurrence. Table 20-4 presents further details about progression of rehabilitation for Achilles tendon–related pathology.

Achilles Tendon Rupture

The Achilles tendon complex is prone to injury with a sudden and powerful eccentric contraction of the gastrocnemius-soleus muscles (considered together as the triceps surae). This mechanism is best demonstrated during jumping and landing activities

in which the knee is extending while the ankle is dorsiflexing eccentrically. The tendon usually ruptures at a point just proximal to the calcaneus (see Fig. 20-10). Vascular impairment, nonspecific degeneration leading to tissue necrosis, and the use of injectable corticosteroids may weaken this area and predispose it to injury.

The athlete reports an audible snap and the sensation of being kicked in the leg. Plantar flexion weakness and pain, swelling, and a palpable defect are usually noted immediately. The diagnosis is confirmed by a positive Thompson test (see Fig. 7-4); with the athlete prone and the knee flexed and the foot relaxed, a firm squeeze of the calf should produce calcaneal plantar flexion. The test is positive if no movement of the foot occurs. This test has very high sensitivity and specificity.[3]

Acute care consists of the application of ice with the ankle immobilized in slight plantar flexion. A non–weight-bearing crutch gait should be used until the severity of the injury has been determined. Table 20-4 provides a treatment rationale for lesions of the triceps surae mechanism.

Optimal treatment of acute Achilles tendon rupture has not been definitively established. Surgical (open or percutaneous) versus conservative (nonoperative casting or functional bracing) management decisions are based on the site and thickness of the tear in conjunction with the goals and ambitions of the patient. Both methods of management have produced acceptable results.

It is generally accepted that surgical intervention will lower the likelihood of rerupture whereas nonoperative management decreases the risk for other complications (infection, adhesions, deep vein thrombosis, and skin lesions). A metaanalysis of randomized controlled trials found that the complication rate can be reduced with percutaneous approaches.[4] In percutaneous surgery, the surgeon makes several small incisions rather than one large one as for an open approach. Regardless of whether the issue is resolved with surgery, recent research has been quite harmonious in the endorsement of functional bracing (allowing protected mobilization) as opposed to strict cast immobilization during the first 4 to 8 weeks.[5]

Another concept of postoperative management is the introduction of early mobilization. Protected-arc, active plantar flexion range-of-motion activities may be started as early as 2 to 4 weeks after injury. This allows collagen fibers to be laid down along the lines of stress. A 1-inch heel lift is used when weight bearing is allowed, and the height of the lift is gradually decreased as dorsiflexion range of motion improves. Multiple studies have shown that this early-motion protocol minimizes tendon elongation and improves patient satisfaction without having a negative impact on rerupture rates.[5,6] Early weight bearing and functional bracing may also provide an earlier return of strength but probably do not make any significant difference in calf atrophy or long-term outcome.

Nonoperative management is still indicated for older, nonathletic patients with minimally displaced ruptures who are concerned about the potential surgical complications. However, the principles of early weight bearing and functional bracing should still be applied. For these individuals, the typical protocol is a short period of immobilization in an equinus position with slow, but progressive lowering of heel position as protected weight bearing is allowed.

Table 20-4 Gastrocnemius–Soleus Rehabilitation and Treatment

Parameter	Immediate (Acute) Phase	Intermediate (Subacute) Phase	Terminal (Chronic) Phase	Return-to-Sport (Functional) Phase
Goal	Rest Control inflammation and pain Promote healing Create "flexible" scar	Increase pain-free ROM Restore contractile capability	Increase musculotendinous tensile strength Modify, correct, or control abnormal biomechanics	Preparation and training for specific sport or activity
Modalities	Ice massage NSAIDs Gentle transverse friction massage to prevent adhesion formation HVGS in the shortened position	Heat before rehabilitation Ice after rehabilitation Ultrasound (pulsed vs. continuous) Myofascial soft tissue mobilization techniques	Heat before rehabilitation Ice after rehabilitation Iontophoresis Deep transverse friction massage to improve gliding between tissue planes	Intervention sequence: Passive and active local tissue and systemic warm-up Rehabilitation activity or exercise Static stretching Cool down Cryotherapy
ROM/flexibility	Immobilization or pain-free ROM, depending on type and severity of pathology	Temperature-assisted, prolonged-duration, low-intensity, static stretching NWB gastroc/soleus towel stretches	Low-intensity static stretching of the involved musculotendinous unit Weight-bearing knee bent/straight wall leans Slant board stretching	Assess capability, tolerance, and response to ballistic motion and dynamic stretching of the involved tissue
Exercise rationale	These exercises may have to be delayed 2-6 weeks with surgically repaired ruptures Isometrics progressing from submaximal to maximal intensity in protected ROM (knee flexed and/or ankle in plantar flexion)	NWB submaximal to maximal effort isokinetics in progressively larger arcs of motion; concentric contractions at highest attainable speeds in a velocity spectrum to minimize tensile stress in this early phase	Weight-bearing concentric and eccentric isotonic exercise at increasing speeds of contraction as tolerated by the tissue's symptomatic response	Functional rehabilitation activities—toe walking Plyometric progressions—hopping, bounding, depth jumps, and box drills Sport-specific training
Proprioceptive rehabilitation	BAPS board training in NWB positions if not immobilized	BAPS board training in partial weight bearing to FWB with increasing levels of ROM difficulty	BAPS board training in FWB with resistance via posterior peg overload	Balance board training
Alternative conditioning	Upper body ergometer	Gravity-reduced running with assistance of unloading device or floatation device in water	Gravity-reduced running Stationary cycling	Stair climber Stationary cross-country skier
Complementary exercise	Hip-knee-trunk strengthening and conditioning activities	Dorsiflexion, inversion, and eversion strengthening Exercise of foot intrinsic musculature	Lower extremity stretching and continuance of previous phase activities	Ensure normal plantar flexion–to-dorsiflexion strength ratios and muscle balance—3-4:1—at slow speeds of concentric contraction
Activity education-modification	Controlled immobilization and rest as needed Examine athletic shoes, training surface, and training regimens	Trial of low-amplitude rebounder running	Flat training surfaces only; avoid hilly and cambered terrains or muddy surfaces	Careful increases in training regimens, with program not increasing by more than 5%/wk in intensity, duration, or frequency
Orthotic care	Crutches as necessary; weight-bearing status dictated by severity of pathology	Viscoelastic heel lift inserts to reduce stress on the Achilles tendon and decrease ground reaction forces	Orthotic insert to control excessive or abnormal compensatory subtalar joint motion, if necessary	Orthotic and/or taping techniques

BAPS, Biomechanical Ankle Platform System; FWB, full-weight bearing; HVGS, high-voltage galvanic stimulation; NSAIDs, nonsteroidal antiinflammatory drugs; NWB, non–weight bearing; ROM, range of motion.

Tendinopathies

Tendinous lesions of the muscles of the lower part of the leg occur frequently in athletes involved in activities of a repetitious nature. Microtraumatic damage caused by overuse, fatigue, or biomechanical abnormalities may occasionally be manifested by an inflammatory but, more commonly, a degenerative reaction of these tendons. For more on tendiopathies, see Chapter 7.

ACHILLES TENDINOPATHY

The Achilles tendon is the common tendon of the gastrocnemius and soleus muscles. It inserts into the posterosuperior aspect of the calcaneus and is a frequent site of pathology in competitive and recreational athletes. It is surrounded by the paratenon, which functions as an elastic sleeve that envelops the tendon and allows free movement against surrounding tissues. In areas in which the tendon passes over zones of potential pressure and friction, the paratenon is replaced by a synovial sheath or bursa.

The major blood supply to the Achilles tendon is provided through the paratenon. An area of reduced vascularity is found 2 to 6 cm proximal to the insertion. This region of relative avascularity may play an etiologic role in the frequent onset of symptoms at this level.

Macroscopic and microscopic histologic evaluation of Achilles disease typically shows a degenerative as opposed to an inflammatory condition. The essence of the tendinopathy is a failed healing response with haphazard collagen fibrils and an increase in noncollagenous matrix that results in a larger tendon diameter consisting of smaller, irregular, and crimped or wavy collagen fibers.[7]

The onset of Achilles tendinopathy is usually gradual and insidious, although many precipitating factors have been implicated. These factors may include poor flexibility, prolonged subtalar joint pronation, inappropriate footwear, or the use of fluoroquinolone antibiotics, and they are usually magnified by excessive overload from an alteration or increase in the frequency, duration, or intensity of the activities. The athlete complains of a dull, aching pain during or after activity. On physical examination, slight edema or tendon thickening may be present. Point tenderness is usually elicited 2 to 3 cm proximal to the calcaneal attachment. Because this is a contractile lesion, pain usually increases with passive dorsiflexion and resisted plantar flexion. Crepitation may be noted in plantar flexion movements in the subacute and chronic stages.

Clinical Pearl #3

Degenerative tendinopathies in middle-aged athletes are difficult to manage and often take months to fully resolve. "Weekend warriors" are the most susceptible because they often have "18-year-old ambitions in a 38-year-old body."

Table 20-5 presents a suggested rationale for the conservative management and treatment of tendinopathies and peritendinitis. The four stages of injury define potential entry points into the treatment system. An athlete could initially be seen at any one of these stages. Progression from one stage to the next is variable and dictated by time, symptoms, and individual response.

As is usually true, the best treatment of microtraumatic injuries such as Achilles tendinitis is prevention of onset. The frequency or severity of degenerative Achilles injuries may be reduced if some suggested guidelines are followed:

- Select appropriate footwear. The athletic shoe should have a firm, notched heel counter to decrease tendon irritation and control rearfoot motion. The midsole should have a moderate heel flare, provide adequate wedging, and allow flexibility in the forefoot. It is also important to maintain a relatively consistent heel height in all shoes worn during the day.

- Avoid training errors. Achilles tendon microtrauma can be magnified by errors in training. Steady, gradual increases of no more than 5% to 10% per week in training mileage and speed on appropriate terrain should be emphasized. Running on hills or inclines should be approached in a cautious manner after the symptoms have completely subsided. Use of cross-training principles may also reduce cumulative stress on the Achilles tendon.

- Ensure gastrocnemius-soleus flexibility. The talocrural joint should have 10° of dorsiflexion with the knee joint extended and 20° with the knee flexed. Normal gait requires 10° of dorsiflexion just before heel-off, during which the subtalar joint is in neutral position and the knee is extending in stance phase.

- Control pronation forces. Abnormal compensatory pronation forces can cause a whipping or bowstring effect on the medial edge of the Achilles tendon. Orthotic correction may be indicated if this abnormal pronation has a structural origin. Taping techniques to correct a convex medial tendon orientation in a compensatory pronated stance may also be beneficial.[8]

- Restore the eccentric tensile capabilities of the triceps surae complex. Numerous studies have found that a program of progressive heel drops (Fig. 20-11) accelerates recovery and improves clinical outcomes in athletes with midsubstance Achilles tendinopathy.[9] It is important to note that a mild, temporary level of discomfort should occur during exercise. Table 20-6 provides a rationale for manipulable variables that can be used to properly prescribe and advance the heel drop program. These factors include the influence of gravity, speed of contraction, range of motion, and bilateral versus unilateral contribution to the exercise.

- Perform postural screening for any biomechanical malalignment to detect any abnormalities that could adversely affect the kinetic chain and increase stress on the Achilles tendon. Such conditions include leg length discrepancies, cavus foot resulting from metatarsal forefoot equinus, ankle equinus, tibial varum, and rotational influences of the femur or tibia (Box 20-1).

ANTERIOR TIBIALIS TENDINOPATHY

An inflammatory response of the anterior tibialis tendon occurs when it cannot absorb deceleration forces during the heel-strike phase to the foot-flat phase of gait. Uncontrolled or excessive pronation following heel strike stretches the anterior tibialis as it attempts to control the speed of forefoot loading.

Conditions that predispose the anterior tibialis to overuse usually include training errors and physical abnormalities. Frequently, the combination of excessive extrinsic force placed on intrinsic abnormalities produces stress that cannot be dissipated or tolerated by the athlete. Extrinsic factors include dramatic

Table 20-5 Rehabilitation and Treatment of Lower Leg Tendinopathy

Parameter	Immediate (Acute) Phase	Intermediate (Subacute) Phase	Terminal (Chronic) Phase	Return-to-Sport (Functional) Phase
Goal	Relative rest Control inflammation and pain Promote healing	Rehabilitation of musculotendinous unit Increase ROM Maintain muscle contractile capability	Increase musculotendinous tensile, eccentric strength Modify, correct, or control abnormal biomechanics	Preparation and training for specific sport or activity
Modalities	Ice massage cryotherapy NSAID and acetaminophen for short-term pain relief Glyceryl trinitrate patch Gentle transverse friction massage Cold laser	Active warm-up or heat before rehabilitation activities Cool-down activities or ice after rehabilitation activities Ultrasound (pulsed vs. continuous) Myofascial soft tissue mobilization techniques	Heat before rehabilitation Ice after rehabilitation Iontophoresis/phonophoresis Deep transverse friction massage to improve gliding between tissue planes Platelet-rich plasma injections	Modality sequence: Passive-active tissue and systemic warm-up Static stretching activity or exercise Dynamic stretching Cool down Cryotherapy
ROM—flexibility	Pain-free ROM exercises	Temperature-assisted, prolonged-duration, low-intensity, static stretching	Low-intensity, static stretching progressing to dynamic stretching of involved musculotendinous unit	Assess capability, tolerance, and response to ballistic motion of involved tissue
Exercise rationale	Subsymptom threshold isometrics	Submaximal to maximal effort isotonic or isokinetic exercise in progressively larger arcs of motion	Eccentric exercise at increasing speeds of contraction as governed by symptomatic response of tissue	Functional rehabilitation activities and plyometric progressions Sport-specific training
Proprioceptive rehabilitation	BAPS board training in non–weight-bearing positions	BAPS board training in partial to full weight bearing with increasing levels of ROM difficulty	BAPS board training in full weight bearing with resistance overload on appropriate muscle groups	Balance board training
Alternative conditioning	Upper body ergometer	Stationary cycling Gravity-reduced walking/running with assistance of unloading device or floatation device in water	Progression of gravity-reduced walking/running	Ensure cross-training with alternative aerobic conditioning devices such as elliptical trainers, stair climbers, or stationary cross-country skiers
Complementary exercise	Hip-knee-trunk strengthening and conditioning activities	Exercise for foot intrinsic musculature such as toe curls, towel sweeps	Short-foot exercises	Ensure normal agonist-antagonist strength ratios and muscle balance
Activity education-modification	Controlled immobilization and rest as needed Educate regarding athletic shoes, training surface, and training regimens	Trial of low-amplitude rebounder running	Flat training surfaces only; avoid hilly and cambered terrains or muddy surfaces	Careful increases in training regimens; program not increased by more than 5%-10%/wk in intensity, duration, or frequency
Orthotic care	Heel lift if appropriate	Shock-attenuating inserts to decrease ground reaction forces (especially with rigid cavus feet)	Orthotic insert to control excessive or abnormal compensatory subtalar joint motion	Orthotic and/or taping techniques

BAPS, Biomechanical Ankle Platform System; *NSAID*, nonsteroidal antiinflammatory drug; *ROM*, range of motion.

increases in mileage, overstriding, and excessive hill running, all of which can cause fatigue and injury. An athlete with a tight Achilles complex requires increased muscular output of the anterior tibialis to overcome the inherent posterior tautness. This condition is then magnified by uphill running, which necessitates full dorsiflexion range of motion. In downhill running, increased eccentric forces are necessary to control forefoot loading over an increased range of motion. If the anterior tibialis has undergone adaptive shortening in response to chronic

hyperpronation, the musculotendinous unit cannot provide the necessary range of motion and absorption of tensile forces needed during the early stance phase.

This injury is characterized by pain and swelling over the dorsum of the foot. Crepitation along the tendon or at its point of insertion onto the navicular may be present. Examination reveals pain with stretching into the extremes of plantar flexion and pronation and pain-inhibited weakness during manual muscle testing of anterior tibialis function.

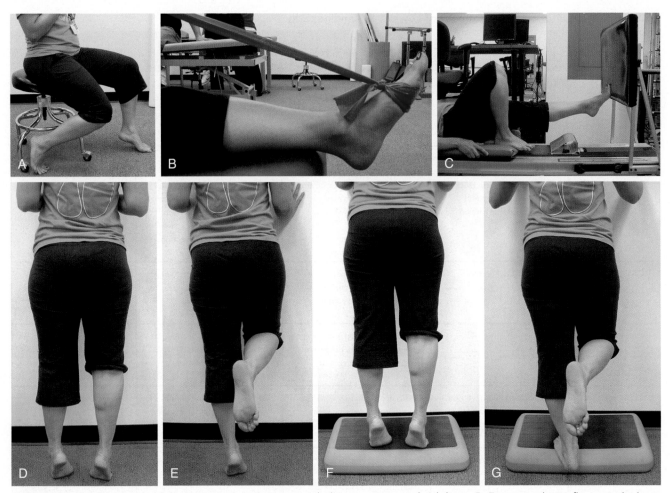

FIGURE 20-11 Eccentric heel drop progression. **A,** Non–weight-bearing eccentric heel drops. **B,** Eccentric plantar flexion with elastic tubing resistance. **C,** Eccentric heel drops in a gravity-eliminated position. **D,** Bilateral weight-bearing heel drops. **E,** Unilateral weight-bearing heel drops. **F,** Bilateral weight-bearing heel drops with the toes on an elevated surface. **G,** Unilateral weight-bearing heel drops with the toes on an elevated surface.

Table 20-6 Progression Variables in Eccentric Training

Position	Involvement	Arc of Motion	Speed	Resistance
Sitting	Bilateral → unilateral	Partial → full ROM	Slow → fast	Manual resistance or cuff weights
Long sitting	Unilateral	Partial → full ROM	Slow → fast	Thera-Band
Incline	Bilateral → unilateral	Partial → full ROM	Slow → fast	% of BW
Standing	Bilateral → unilateral	Partial → full ROM	Slow → fast	BW +10% BW +5-10 lb/wk

BW, Body weight; *ROM,* range of motion.

Table 20-5 summarized the treatment rationale for lower leg tendinopathies. Prime consideration should be given to correcting soft tissue imbalances, improving eccentric muscular capabilities, and selecting appropriate footwear. Shoe selection should focus on midsole materials that attenuate shock and accommodate orthotic additions. A heel lift may be used for athletes with structural equinus, or varus posting may be indicated if forefoot varus or supinatus is prolonging the pronation process.

Clinical Pearl #4

In chronic tendinopathy conditions, the exercise rehabilitation program must gradually reintroduce tensile strain through eccentric stress and plyometric progression to restore function, reduce tendon volume, and normalize histologic neovascularization.

Box 20-1

**Management of Achilles Tendinopathy:
Key Considerations in Rehabilitation**

Typically a degenerative (not inflammatory) condition

Iontophoresis and/or low-level laser therapy

Heel lift and/or tape support to unload stress on the tendon

Control abnormal subtalar joint motion with tape and/or orthotics

Stretching and/or soft tissue mobilization to ensure adequate dorsiflexion range of motion

Restoration of tensile capability through a graded eccentric loading program

Gradual introduction of plyometric progression

Careful increases in training regimens, with the program not increased by more than 5% to 10% per week in intensity, duration, or frequency

---

PERONEAL TENDINOPATHY

Degenerative lesions of the peroneal tendons or inflammation of their protective sheaths is common in athletes who for compensatory reasons overuse this musculature. The pathology is secondary to chronic lateral ankle sprains or occurs in athletes with hypermobile first rays. In both situations, the peroneal muscle tendons are worked excessively in an attempt to provide stability. Any mechanical stress caused by abnormal forefoot structures that force the foot into a valgus position can also amplify this inflammatory response.

Pain and swelling typically occur in the area just posterior to the lateral malleolus. Occasionally, symptoms are manifested at the musculotendinous junction. Tendon crepitus may be present in more chronic conditions. Pain and weakness are evident with passive overstretching of these contractile structures and when resistance is provided to plantar flexion and eversion of the first ray. When compared with peroneal longus tendinopathy, peroneal brevis tendinopathy is more affected by resistance to calcaneal eversion and ankle plantar flexion. The differential diagnosis includes peroneal subluxation, inversion ankle sprain, sural nerve entrapment, and subacute lateral compartmental syndrome, with subsequent management differing for each of these conditions.

Rehabilitation is aimed at providing relief of symptoms and identifying the causative factors. Muscular imbalances between the anterior or posterior tibialis and peroneals should be explored. A metatarsal pad with a first ray cutout or a lateral heel wedge (or both) can provide biomechanical compensation for structural abnormalities. Transverse friction massage can be used to reduce symptoms and promote healing. Table 20-5 presents further treatment considerations.

POSTERIOR TIBIALIS TENDINOPATHY

Posteromedial shin pain secondary to athletic overuse can be caused by inflammatory microtrauma to the tendon of the posterior tibialis. Periosteal irritation and tibial stress reactions may also be suspected.

Medial tibial stress, whether tendinitis or periostitis, is generally the result of abnormal hyperpronation biomechanics (Fig. 20-12). The muscles in the superficial posterior compartment contract in a stretched position and are overworked in an attempt to stabilize the foot during propulsion. Common predisposing factors include improper training on crowned or

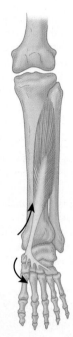

FIGURE 20-12 Etiology of posterior tibialis tendinitis: excessive traction stress placed on the posterior tibialis tendon with hyperpronation.

banked surfaces, inappropriate footwear, and any structural condition that increases the varus attitude of the lower extremity.

Pain and swelling are present over the posteromedial crest of the tibia along the origin of the posterior tibialis. Tenderness and crepitation may be found anywhere along the course of the tendon as it passes behind the medial malleolus and inserts distally on the navicular and first cuneiform. Manual resistance to plantar flexion and inversion localizes the complaint. In subacute phases, repeated unilateral heel raises, which require plantar flexion and supination of the calcaneus, can be a source of symptom aggravation.

It is important to rule out a tibial stress reaction, in which pain is present at the junction of the lower and middle thirds of the posteromedial aspect of the tibia, in the differential diagnosis. Tibial stress fractures can occur in this area if the osteoblastic activity in bone cannot keep pace with the osteoclastic stress placed on it. At approximately 2 weeks after awareness of symptoms, a fracture through the tibial cortex may become evident on radiographs. Before this finding, a bone scan reveals increased calcium uptake in the area of injury. Clinical differentiation is accomplished by detection of tenderness in areas devoid of muscle on the tibial shaft or by percussion and tuning fork vibration techniques.

Treatment is aimed at alleviating abnormal pronation by using a semirigid orthosis with a medial heel wedge. Attention should also be given to the training regimen and to finding shoes with a stable, firm, and snug heel counter.

In an older athlete, dysfunction of the tibialis posterior tendon is the most common cause of acquired adult flatfoot deformity. This pathology can arise from an acute traumatic injury, systemic disease, or chronic tendon degeneration. Like the more proximal dysfunction, it may be treated with symptom-alleviating modalities, exercise-based interventions, and control of destructive hyperpronatory forces with the use of appropriate footwear and orthotic therapy. Ice, nonsteroidal antiinflammatory medication, and rest will offer analgesic benefit, and eccentric training of the posterior tibialis may enhance the value of medially posted orthoses.[10] Elastic tubing–resisted subtalar inversion plus foot adduction with a controlled deceleration back to the starting position is demonstrated in Figure 20-13 with a medial sweep exercise (Box 20-2).

FLEXOR HALLUCIS LONGUS TENDINOPATHY

An athlete (e.g., en pointe dancers) who must perform repetitive push-off maneuvers is especially prone to the development of tendinopathy in the long flexor of the great toe. Hyperpronation during propulsion also places excessive stress on the tendon as it contracts from a lengthened position. This condition is similar to posterior tibial tendinopathy and can be differentiated with selected manual muscle testing. Pain with passive extension of the first MTP joint while the ankle

is dorsiflexed or with resistance to flexion of the great toe while the ankle is plantar-flexed confirms the diagnosis. The condition is managed with appropriate varus posting and tape restriction for excessive dorsiflexion of the first MTP joint. Stretching of the flexor hallucis longus (simultaneous ankle dorsiflexion and great toe extension) may prevent the development of hallux rigidus.[11]

FLEXOR DIGITORUM LONGUS TENDINOPATHY

The flexor digitorum longus is another musculotendinous unit in the superficial posterior compartment that is susceptible to overuse microtrauma. Pain is usually present in the posteromedial third of the leg as a result of overuse from forced, resistive dorsiflexion of the toes during propulsion. The resultant cramping sensation in the forefoot and toes can be relieved with a viscoelastic metatarsal pad, which dorsally displaces the metatarsal heads and reduces the extension angle of the lesser four MTP joints. A more rigid sole in the athletic shoe may also help prevent excessive forced hyperextension of the digits during propulsion. Exercise rehabilitation focuses on correcting any intrinsic muscular imbalances that allow toe-clawing deformities and that require the flexor digitorum longus to work harder. The intrinsic muscles of the foot can be isolated for emphasis with repetitive toe-curling exercises. Functionally, the intrinsic muscles of the foot can be trained to maintain arch integrity without toe clawing with short-foot exercise in both weigh-bearing and non–weight-bearing positions (Fig. 20-14).

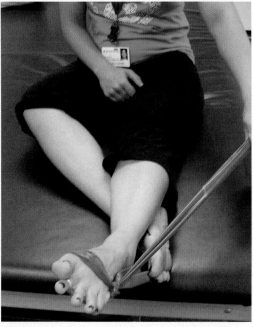

FIGURE 20-13 Elastic tubing–resisted medial sweep subtalar inversion and foot adduction with a controlled deceleration back to a starting position of subtalar eversion and foot abduction.

Box 20-2
Exercises to Improve Control of Pronation
BAPS board training with anteromedial and/or posteromedial overload
Marble pick-ups with the toes and medial towel sweeps with the foot
Supro dance—arch lift and drop
Unilateral balancing activities progressing from stable to unstable surfaces
Unilateral stance with frontal plane motion in the opposite lower extremity
Bilateral progressing to unilateral stance trunk rotation with appropriate resistance and speed of motion

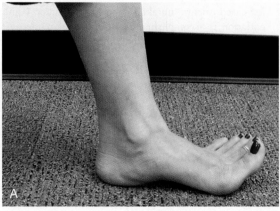
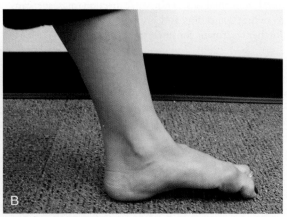

FIGURE 20-14 Short-foot exercise. **A,** Correct. **B,** Incorrect.

Clinical Pearl #5

Strong evidence supports the off-label use of glyceryl trinitrate patches at 1.25 mg/day in individuals with chronic tendinopathy conditions to relieve pain during activities of daily living and increase tendon strength.

Compartmental Compression Syndromes

The lower part of the leg has four osseofascial compartments: the anterior, lateral, superficial posterior, and deep posterior compartments. The anterior compartment is the most common site of compression ischemia. It is bordered by the interosseous membrane posteriorly; the tibia and fibula medially and laterally; and a tough, nonexpansive fascial covering anteriorly. If pressure increases within the compartment, no space is left for expansion or accommodation. With increasing pressure, circulation and tissue function can be quickly compromised. Two types of anterior compartmental compression syndrome are recognized: acute and chronic.

ACUTE COMPARTMENTAL COMPRESSION SYNDROME

This condition is usually traumatic in onset. Contusions, crush injuries, fractures, or severe overexertion can cause a rapid increase in compartmental volume from bleeding or muscular swelling. Increased intercompartmental pressure leads to venous collapse and increased resistance to arterial circulation. These physiologic changes produce ischemic pain and, ultimately, tissue necrosis if the process is left uninterrupted.

The athlete's chief complaint is intense pain that is disproportionate to the injury and not relieved by rest. Palpation reveals a "woody tension" over the muscles of the anterior compartment, and passive plantar flexion evokes pain. In advanced stages, neurologic changes may be evident, and the dorsalis pedis and anterior tibial pulses may be diminished. Table 20-7 presents the neurologic changes manifested in the later stages of lower leg compartment syndrome.

This condition is considered an orthopedic emergency because early muscle damage occurs in the first 4 to 6 hours and irreversible tissue damage occurs within 18 hours after injury. Acute care consists of the application of ice without compression and monitoring of neurovascular status. If pain and swelling do not respond to conservative treatment, emergency surgical fasciotomy must be performed.

CHRONIC EXERTIONAL COMPARTMENTAL SYNDROME

Recurrent, exertional compartmental syndrome has the same pathophysiology as acute compartmental syndrome, but its manifestation and care are different (Table 20-8). The athlete

complains of lower leg pain and tightness that occur at a constant interval after the initiation of physical activity. The symptoms subside with rest but return on resumption of the activity. Most athletes have bilateral involvement with mild edema, tenderness, and occasional paresthesia. The diagnosis is confirmed with a measurement of intercompartmental fluid pressure at rest and during activity. Pedowitz et al[12] defined the compartmental pressure criteria for diagnosis of chronic exertional compartment syndrome as shown in Box 20-3.

The only consistently successful conservative intervention is cessation of activity; however, for many athletes this option is unrealistic. Conservative intervention strategies may include lower leg stretching, manual therapy, soft tissue manipulation, and balancing of plantar flexion–dorsiflexion strength. Any alterations in the training program that decrease muscular workloads, including a reduction in body weight, may also be helpful. Bevel-heeled shoes, softer training surfaces, and energy-absorbing orthoses may accomplish this goal. Lesser weight-bearing aerobic activities such as cycling may be better tolerated because of decreased elevations in compartment pressure. If conservative measures fail, surgical fasciotomy is indicated. To prevent scarring and adhesions, postoperative rehabilitation begins a few days after surgery and consists of active range of motion, gentle stretching, and stationary cycling, with return to sport expected within 2 to 3 months.

Ankle Injuries

Pathologic trauma to the ligamentous structures of the ankle is a common athletic injury. The majority of these injuries occur on the lateral side of the joint with an inversion mechanism of injury. In the neutral position of 0° dorsiflexion, the calcaneofibular ligament is taut, but as the foot plantar-flexes, the anterior talofibular ligament tightens as its fibers become parallel to the axis. Eighty percent to 90% of ankle sprains occur as a result of this plantar flexion–inversion mechanism. Initial damage is to the anterior talofibular ligament because of the direction of force, and further stress affects the calcaneofibular and posterior talofibular ligaments. The posterior talofibular ligament is

Table 20-7 Late Neurologic Changes in Compression Syndromes

Compartment	Area of Paresthesia	Area of Weakness
Anterior	First dorsal web space	Dorsiflexion (footdrop)
Lateral	Anterior lateral aspect of leg	Eversion (peroneals)
Deep posterior	Medial arch	Inversion
Superficial posterior	Sural nerve distribution	Plantar flexion

Table 20-8 Symptoms in Acute Versus Recurrent Compartmental Syndromes

	Recurrent	Acute
Pathology	Reversible changes	Irreversible tissue damage possible
Effect of rest	Decrease in symptoms	No change in symptoms
Nature of complaint	Cramping, aching	Intense pain
Involvement	Often bilateral	Usually unilateral

Box 20-3

Diagnostic Criteria for the Presence of Exertional Compartment Syndrome (One of the Following Three Criteria Must Be Present)

1. Preexercise pressure >15 mm Hg
2. Postexercise pressure >30 mm Hg at 1 minute following cessation of activity
3. Postexercise pressure >20 mm Hg at 5 minutes following cessation of activity

Table 20-9 Mechanism of Ankle Injuries

Mechanism of Injury	Comments	Ligamentous Injury (Progression of Increasing Severity of Pathology)	Potential Bony Lesions
Plantar flexion–inversion	Typical ankle sprain	ATF → ATF and CF→ ATF, CF, and PTF	Transverse fracture of the lateral malleolus Avulsion fracture of the base of the fifth metatarsal Medial malleolus fracture
Supinated position–adduction force Plantar flexion–inversion and rotation Supinated position–eversion force	Crossover cut on a plantar-flexed and inverted foot	ATF and tibfib → ATF, tibfib, and CF	Spiral fracture of the lateral malleolus or fracture of the neck of the fibula
Pure inversion	Rare; landing on another's foot	CF → CF and ATF → CF, ATF, and PTF	
Pronation: abduction-eversion-dorsiflexion Pronated position–eversion force	Open cut	Deltoid → deltoid, tibfib, and interosseus membrane	Avulsion fracture of medial malleolus Fibular fracture above the mortise line

ATF, Anterior talofibular ligament; *CF,* calcaneofibular ligament; *PTF,* posterior talofibular ligament; *tibfib,* anterior and posterior tibiofibular ligaments.

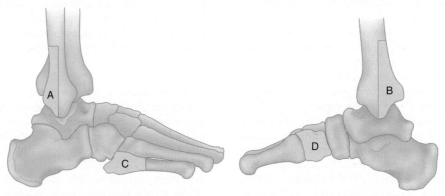

FIGURE 20-15 Ottawa Ankle Rule. Radiographs should be obtained if pain is present in the zone around the malleoli with point tenderness in area *A* or *B*, if pain is present in the zone around the midfoot with point tenderness in the area of *C* or *D*, or if the individual is unable to immediately bear weight. *A,* Distal 6 cm of the posterior edge of the fibula or tip of the lateral malleolus; *B,* distal 6 cm of the posterior edge of the tibia or tip of the medial malleolus; *C,* base of the fifth metatarsal; *D,* navicular.

not involved or injured until the other two ligaments have ruptured and some degree of lower extremity rotation has occurred. Injuries to the medial side of the joint and the deltoid ligament are less frequent and typically involve a hyperpronation force, such as when an athlete plants the foot and then cuts in the opposite direction. Table 20-9 outlines the common mechanisms of injury to bony and ligamentous structures of the ankle.

Clinical Pearl #6

Lateral ankle sprains are notorious for their high likelihood of recurrence. Residual instability rates have been estimated to be 10% to 60% but can be reduced by addressing neuromuscular and proprioceptive impairments that allow a persistent sense of instability and "giving way."

Inversion Sprains

The sign and symptoms of ligamentous ankle injuries vary according to the severity of injury, the tissues involved, and the extent of their involvement. Varying degrees of pain, swelling,

point tenderness, and functional disability are usually evident. Following inversion trauma, radiographic studies of the joint and bone structure are of paramount importance. Bony lesions must be ruled out before decisions about appropriate management of the injury can be made. The Ottawa Ankle Rules are a sensitive means of detecting bony lesions (Fig. 20-15). Unstable bimalleolar fractures, proximal fibular fractures, and avulsion-type fractures all are possible and may require surgical fixation or longer periods of immobilization.

Table 20-10 outlines some criteria for assessing the severity of injury in athletes with lateral ankle sprains. This grading process provides a basis for logically estimating the rate and intensity at which the athlete can progress through the phases of treatment and rehabilitation, as well as for estimating the length of time before the athlete can return to full participation.

TREATMENT AND REHABILITATION

The mechanical or functional disability associated with ankle sprains can be the result of various abnormalities. Mechanical disability can be caused by anterior, posterior, or varus instability of the talus in the ankle mortise; instability or adhesion formation in the subtalar joint; or an inferior tibiofibular diastasis. Even

Table 20-10 Signs and Symptoms of Lateral Ankle Sprains

Grade	Severity	Involvement	Functional Status	Swelling	Pain/Tenderness	Ligament Laxity
I	Mild	Usually only the ATF	Maintenance of joint integrity produces minimal functional disability	Variable, but usually slight	Mild, localized pain over the ATF	Negative anterior drawer and talar tilt
II	Moderate	ATF and CF	Moderate disability, with difficulty in heel and toe walking	Variable, but more than in grade I and resultant ecchymosis	Moderate pain and tenderness over involved ligaments	Laxity evident but distinct end points to stress
III	Severe	ATF and CF; possibly PTF	Functional disability, with loss of ROM and complete inability to bear weight	Anterolateral and spreading diffusely around the joint	Marked tenderness on palpation	Positive anterior drawer or talar tilt

ATF, Anterior talofibular ligament; *CF,* calcaneofibular ligament; *PTF,* posterior talofibular ligament; *ROM,* range of motion.

in the absence of mechanical disability, functional instability (a general sense of "giving way") may persist because of peroneal neuromuscular deficits or motor incoordination secondary to articular deafferentation.[13]

Each potential problem must be addressed in the treatment and rehabilitation program. The damaged ligaments must be allowed to heal as a "flexible" restraint, the contractile elements must regain their dynamic stabilization capability, and the proprioceptive system must be completely restored. Table 20-11 suggests a treatment plan for the conservative management of inversion ankle sprains. Numerous resources have proved the value of a comprehensive, supervised rehabilitation program that emphasizes restoration of proprioception to reduce the risk for recurrent injury.[14] Each athlete's injury is unique, and progression through the various stages of rehabilitation may have to be altered, depending on the severity of the tissue trauma, history, and goals of rehabilitation. Figures 20-16 to 20-29 illustrate some of the rehabilitation procedures used in the restoration of normal ankle joint function after ligamentous injury.

The goal of management is to provide dynamic stability to a potentially unstable joint. During the acute immobilization phase, emphasis is placed on controlling symptoms and maintaining general conditioning and neuromuscular continuity. Various modalities are used to minimize effusion and decrease pain. Edema within the ankle joint distorts the capsule's normal configuration and adversely affects articular mechanoreceptor function. Ice, focal compression around the periphery of the fibular malleolus, electrotherapy, and gentle effleurage with the ankle elevated all facilitate anesthesia and reduction of edema and reverse the neural inhibition of the dynamic stabilizers surrounding the joint. Support of the injured ligaments is provided by a neutral orthosis, Gibney strapping (open basket-weave taping with a horseshoe pad to compress extracellular fluid back into the circulation), and a posterior splint to maintain Achilles tendon flexibility. The posterior splint also positions the talocrural joint in the closed-pack position, which limits the intracapsular space available for swelling. Because strict immobilization is no longer recommended, cautious and gentle motion in protected arcs can be initiated with Biomechanical Ankle Platform System* (BAPS) board activity (Fig. 20-16).

*Available from Camp International, Jackson, Michigan.

Clinical Pearl #7

Following acute ankle trauma, maintenance of the closed-pack position of maximal dorsiflexion minimizes the intracapsular space available to accommodate swelling and maintains posterior talar accessory glide mobility.

Clinical Pearl #8

A critical element in reducing acute ankle swelling is the use of elevation. However, the reduction in edema as a result of elevation or intermittent compression lasts less than 5 minutes after return to a gravity-dependent position. This underscores the importance of constant compression as the athlete becomes ambulatory and the limb more frequently assumes a gravity-dependent position.

Early mobilization allows earlier return to function without an increase in pain, residual symptoms, or rate of reinjury.[15,16] Pain with active inversion may be modulated by mobilization with a movement technique in which the distal end of the fibula is translated in a posterosuperior direction (Fig. 20-17). This may correct the positional fault of an anteriorly displaced fibula during active inversion and allow improved, pain-free motion. Taping can be used to maintain this fibular position (Fig. 20-18) and reduce the risk for reinjury.[17,18] Evidence also suggests that a manipulative distractive thrust at the talocrural joint during the acute phase may decrease pain, increase dorsiflexion range of motion, and ultimately improve function (Fig. 20-19).[19-22] A preliminary clinical prediction rule has been derived to forecast which individuals are most likely to benefit from this intervention. The presence of symptoms that are worse when standing and later in the day, navicular drop greater than 5 mm, and hypomobility at the distal tibiofibular joint seem to have the highest probability of achieving an improvement in status following a grade V mobilization technique.[23] Isometric exercises are also started during this phase to minimize or retard atrophy.

Table 20-11 Conservative Management of Ankle Sprains

Parameter	Immediate (Acute) Phase	Intermediate (Subacute) Phase—After Immobilization	Terminal Phase	Return-to-Sport (Functional) Phase
Goals	Protect joint integrity; Control the inflammatory response; Control pain, edema, and spasm	Optimal stimulation for tissue regeneration	Functional progression of weight-bearing activities; Proprioceptive retraining; Correct/control biomechanics	Preparation for return to sport or activity
Weight-bearing status	Weight bearing to tolerance	Progression toward full weight bearing	Full weight bearing	Full weight bearing
Modalities	Ice; Intermittent/constant compression; Elevation; TENS or HVGS; Effleurage in an elevated position; Grade III/IV mobilization; Cold laser	Cryotherapy (ice, ROM, ice); Contrast baths	Cryokinetics (ice–weight-bearing activities–ice) as needed	Ice after participation
External support	Neutral orthotic; Gibney open basket-weave taping; Posterior splint	Stirrup splint with heel-lock support; Friction massage at the site of the lesion	Stirrup splint with heel-lock support	Taping; Stirrup or Lace-up brace; Active ankle orthosis; Orthotic
Manual therapy	High-velocity, low-amplitude distractive thrust at the talocrural joint; Fibular mobilization with movement	Posterior talar glides; Friction massage at the site of the lesion	Midtarsal mobilizations as necessary	—
ROM/flexibility	—	Achilles stretching in the sitting and standing positions	Achilles stretching in supinated positions	—
Non–weight-bearing exercise	Isometrics	Alphabet ROM; Toe curls and marble pick-ups; Four-direction surgical tubing exercises; Submaximal isokinetics in short arcs	Full-arc isokinetics	—
Weight-bearing exercise	—	Weight-bearing ROM—trunk twists/squats; Shuttle squats/heel raises/toe raises; Soleus pumps; Lunge steps; Tubing side steps	Heel raise progression; Hops in gravity-eliminated positions (shuttle, Total Gym, leg press machines); Contralateral kicks; Short-foot exercises	Marching, running, sidestepping, backpedaling, carioca, etc.; Plyometric drills
Proprioception, agility, balance drills	—	BAPS board in progressive weight-bearing positions with and without overload; Stork stands; Single-plane tilt boards	BAPS in full weight bearing with and without overload; ProFitter or slide board; Multiaxial tilt or balance boards; Tubing-resisted walkaways/runaways	Jump rope/jump platform; Four-square hopping drills; Functional running patterns; Running in place tubing drills
Complementary alternative exercises	Gluteus medius and maximus strengthening	Pool therapy; Stationary cycling	Elliptical trainer; Treadmill; Stair climber	Stationary cross-country skier; Lateral step-ups

BAPS, Biomechanical Ankle Platform System; HVGS, high-voltage galvanic stimulation; ROM, range of motion; TENS, transcutaneous electrical nerve stimulation.

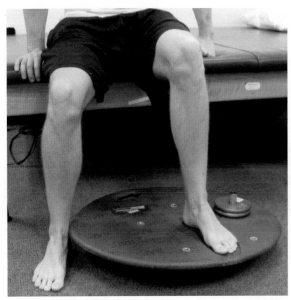

FIGURE 20-16 Biomechanical Ankle Platform System board with posterolateral overload.

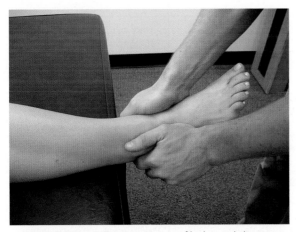

FIGURE 20-17 Posterosuperior fibular mobilization.

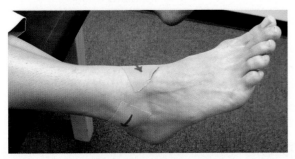

FIGURE 20-18 Fibular taping.

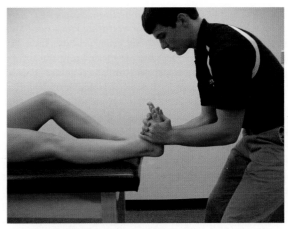

FIGURE 20-19 Talocrural distractive manipulation.

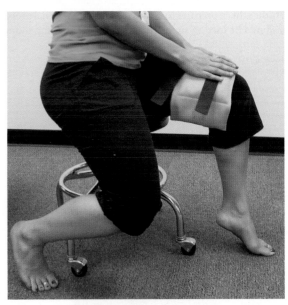

FIGURE 20-20 Soleus pumps.

The weight-bearing status of the athlete is allowed to progress as symptoms and healing allow. Emphasis should be placed on maintaining a normal heel-to-toe gait and on keeping weight-bearing forces below the level at which pain and symptoms occur. Early, pain-free weight bearing will maintain proprioceptive input, prevent stiffness, and provide a means for an active muscle pump to mobilize effusion.

In the intermediate or postimmobilization phase, attention is focused on the healing ligaments. Subpathologic stress through joint mobilization is placed on the injured ligaments to stimulate organized collagen formation along the direction of normal fibers. Care must be taken to not place traction forces on the joint with ankle weight resistance on the foot. Closed chain rehabilitation in a weight-bearing position is preferred because it can provide compressive force that facilitates cocontraction and augment stability.

Weight bearing should progress in this stage to full weight bearing without assisted ambulation. The use of stirrup-type splints with heel-lock protection to limit excessive calcaneal inversion is indicated. Exercise rehabilitation may include Achilles tendon stretching; open chain, cryotherapy-assisted active range of motion progressing toward submaximal effort isokinetics in limited arcs; and weight-bearing functional activities such as soleus pumps, stork stands, stationary cycling, and elastic tubing–resisted exercises (Figs. 20-20 to 20-22).

In the terminal phase of rehabilitation, progressive weight-bearing activities with emphasis on restoring kinesthetic awareness and proximal hip strength are given priority. Table 20-12 outlines many exercise variables for modulating the difficulty and challenge of proprioceptive, unilateral-stance balancing activities. Bullock-Saxton[24] showed that hip muscle function is compromised with severe ankle sprains. Gluteus maximus muscle recruitment may be delayed during hip extension in gait, and gluteus medius weakness may increase frontal plane inversion stress on the ankle secondary to a Trendelenburg gait. Tubing-resisted sidestepping is an excellent exercise to redevelop this strength deficit (Fig. 20-23). Physical agents are used at this point only as needed, but after rehabilitation, ice is generally necessary. Exercise rehabilitation becomes aggressive and includes slant board Achilles tendon stretching without allowing subtalar joint substitution, short-foot balancing activities, full-arc isokinetics, and heel raises (Fig. 20-24). Balance and motor coordination are enhanced with the use of a ProFitter,* balance board, and DynaDisc† (Figs. 20-25 and 20-26).

As the athlete prepares to return to sport, a functional progression should be used to simulate the stresses, forces, and motions

inherent in the activity that caused the original injury. Elastic tubing resistance to weight-bearing activities improves ankle strength and coordination and stimulates proprioception for the entire lower extremity (Fig. 20-27). Progression from resistance in marching to running to motion on inclines can be used (Fig. 20-28). Tubing resistance can be applied from all directions,

---

*Available from ProFitter, Calgary, Alberta, Canada.
†Available from Exertools, Novato, California.

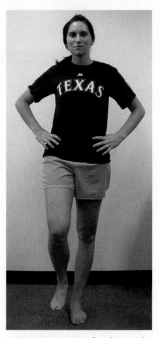

FIGURE 20-21 Stork stands.

Table 20-12 Activity Variables for Proprioceptive Balance Training

Balance/Perturbation Training Variable	Options
Gravitational influence	Full (antigravity) vs. partial (gravity minimized)
External support	Presence vs. absence of bracing, taping, orthotic insoles
Shoe status	Shoe vs. barefoot vs. short foot
Stance position	Bilateral vs. unilateral, wide vs. narrow base of support, staggered vs. symmetric foot placement
Knee position	Locked in hyperextension vs. unlocked in slight flexion
Visual input	Eyes open vs. eyes closed Stability, consistency, and/or distortions in visual background
Vestibular input	Position of head and presence or absence of cervical movement
Arm position	Hands on hips vs. hands folded across chest vs. hands overhead
Surface stability	Stable vs. labile surface, moving vs. stationary surface, uniaxial vs. multiaxial movement
Surface inclination	Uphill (dorsiflexed) vs. downhill (plantar flexed) vs. cambered (inverted vs. everted)
Dynamic movements	Addition of lower or upper extremity movements in the sagittal, frontal, transverse, or diagonal planes
Overload	Manual or mechanical perturbation and overloads in the anterior/posterior or medial/lateral directions

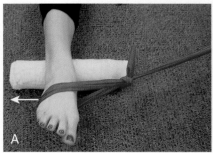
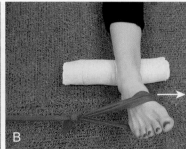
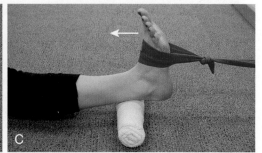

FIGURE 20-22 Surgical tubing–resisted exercises. **A**, Eversion. **B**, Inversion. **C**, Dorsiflexion.

and progression is based on pain-free exercise without effusion or a tendency of the ankle to roll over. Tape or external support should not be used during these controlled activities to allow full rehabilitative benefit. Clinical plyometrics on the Shuttle 2000-1 or with four-square hopping also represents an excellent means of recreating athletic activity (Fig. 20-29). Finally, a functional movement progression that includes backpedaling, sidestepping, cariocas, pivoting, and cutting should be used to assess readiness for return to sport.

Orthotic and external support should be provided to prevent recurrence of trauma. Athletes with an uncompensated rearfoot varus, compensated forefoot valgus, or a rigidly plan-tar-flexed first ray alter their gait pattern with prolonged or excessive supination in midstance and are extremely suscepti-ble to reinjury. Because it takes at least 20 weeks for a ligament to regain its normal histologic characteristics, ankle taping or ankle support should be provided for at least 5 to 6 months after injury during participation in athletics (Box 20-4).

POSTSURGICAL MANAGEMENT OF LATERAL ANKLE RECONSTRUCTIONS

Sometimes surgical repair or reconstruction after lateral ligamentous injury is necessary to provide joint stability. Table 20-13 outlines common reconstructive or reparative

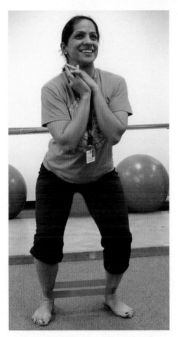

FIGURE 20-23 Tubing-resisted sidestepping.

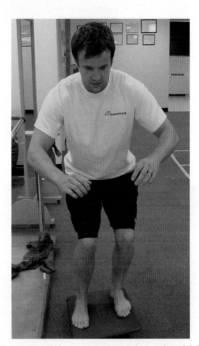

FIGURE 20-25 Balancing on a multiaxial wobble board.

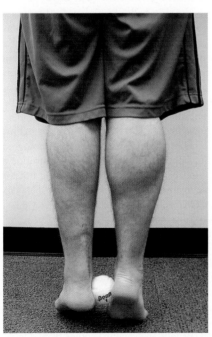

FIGURE 20-24 Heel raise.

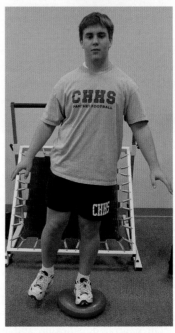

FIGURE 20-26 Balance training on DynaDisc.

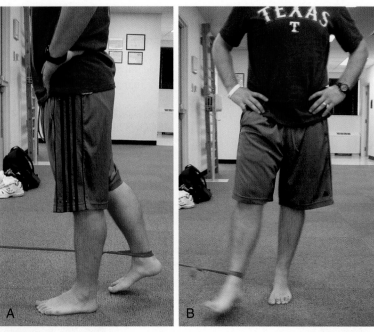

FIGURE 20-27 Contralateral kicks. **A,** Frontal plane motion. **B,** Sagittal plane motion.

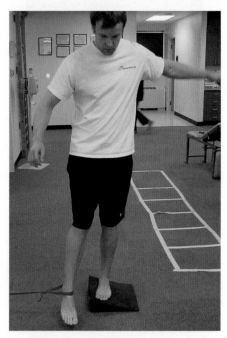

FIGURE 20-28 Proprioceptive training on an inclined surface.

surgical procedures used for the management of chronic lateral ankle instability. It is generally agreed that direct anatomic repair procedures that reproduce the anterior talofibular and calcaneofibular orientation are superior mechanical restraints to anterior talar displacement and tilt without compromising subtalar joint range of motion, sacrificing peroneal function, or altering rearfoot mechanics. Postoperative therapeutic management of these procedures involves principles similar to those used for the conservative care of grade III ankle injuries. Typically, a short leg cast or brace is applied for 6 weeks with the ankle in neutral dorsiflexion and mild eversion.

During the first 2 weeks the athlete uses a non–weight-bearing crutch gait. In the final 4 weeks of immobilization, partial weight bearing on crutches is allowed. Strict immobilization is discontinued at 6 weeks, and active assisted range-of-motion exercises in the sagittal plane are begun. At 8 weeks, active range-of-motion exercises for calcaneal inversion and eversion are begun, along with resistive exercises for the plantar flexors and dorsiflexors. When the athlete can walk without a detectable limp, functional rehabilitation progression may commence. Return to sport is expected after 4 to 6 months.

Syndesmotic (High Ankle) Sprains

Even though the distal tibiofibular and talocrural joints share geographic proximity, injuries to these articulations are quite distinct. Injury to the syndesmotic tibiofibular joint accounts for 1% to 11% of all ankle instability cases.[25] High-intensity athletic activities that demand frequent cutting and twisting (football, rugby, lacrosse) or are characterized by limited mobility in a boot (hockey and skiing) have been reported to be associated with the highest incidence of this injury.[26]

The primary role of the syndesmosis is to maintain congruency of the tibiotalar interface under physiologic axial loads. Ligamentous support comes from the anterior tibiofibular ligament, posterior tibiofibular ligament, and interosseus membrane. These ligaments collectively prevent diastasis and check excessive external rotation of the fibula.

The two most commonly cited mechanisms of injury are forced external rotation of the foot on the tibia and hyperdorsiflexion. The external rotation force comes in two varieties. First, the foot is fixed in a toe-out position during an open cut and the lateral aspect of the knee sustains a direct blow while the body is turning away from the foot. The other mechanism of injury occurs when a player is prone on the ground with the foot fixed in an externally rotated position and a force on the knee or heel (usually in a pileup) comes from a lateral direction

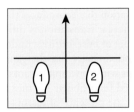

Side to side: Hop laterally between two quadrants.

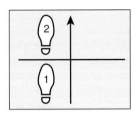

Front to back: Hop forward and backward between two quadrants.

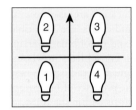

Four square: Hop from square to square in a circular pattern. Sets are performed clockwise and counterclockwise.

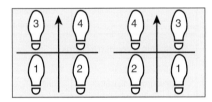

Triangles: Hop within three different quadrants. There are four triangles, each requiring a different diagonal hop.

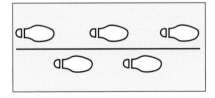

Crisscross: Hop in an X pattern.

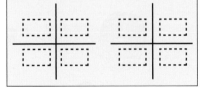

Straight-line hop: Hop forward and then backward along a 15- to 20-ft. line.

Line zigzag: Hop from side to side across a 15- to 20-ft. line while moving forward and then backward.

Disconnected squares: While performing the first five patterns, hop into squares marked in the quadrants.

FIGURE 20-29 Four-square hopping ankle rehabilitation. The eight basic hopping patterns in the four-square ankle rehabilitation program are arranged in order of increasing difficulty. The *arrows* denote the direction that the athlete is facing. Number 1 is the starting point. *(From Toomey, S.J. [1986]: Four-square ankle rehabilitation exercises. Physician Sportsmed., 14:281.)*

(Fig. 20-30).[27] A hyperdorsiflexion injury is most common in running or jumping sports when the foot is planted and the athlete falls, is pushed forward, or comes to an abrupt stop.

The classic feature of this sprain is tenderness on palpation over the anterior and posterior tibiofibular ligaments. Given the mechanism, it is not unusual to find concurrent medial ankle pain in the area of the deltoid ligament. As the severity of the injury increases, tenderness extends proximally over the antero-medial portion of the fibula at the insertion of the interosseous membrane (IOM). A mild amount of swelling is usually seen just proximal to the ankle joint axis within the first 24 hours.

Range of motion is typically limited in both directions of sagittal plane motion, with an empty or painful end-feel at terminal dorsiflexion. A soft or boggy end-feel with valgus stress suggests concomitant deltoid ligament laxity.

The combination of swelling, tenderness, laxity, weight-bearing reluctance, and radiographic findings allows the injury to be classified on a grade I to III continuum. In the absence of a fracture, the West Point Ankle Grading System is an ordinal categorization system that classifies the injury in a range from minimal (grade I), to moderate (grade II), to definite (grade III) instability.[28]

Three radiographic indicators are used to evaluate for syndesmotic injury. These indicators are the tibiofibular clear space, medial clear space, and tibiofibular overlap. Table 20-14 provides normative values. For athletes in whom the response of symptoms becomes stagnant, a radiograph may be used at a later date to evaluate for the presence of heterotopic ossification or development of a synostosis within the IOM.

Numerous special tests have been described for syndesmotic injuries, yet relatively little is known regarding their diagnostic utility. Compression of the proximal end of the tibia and fibula may cause a symptomatic diastasis distally. Simultaneous ankle dorsiflexion with foot external rotation reproduces the mechanism of injury and is somewhat reliable in reproducing the

mortise separation that reproduces the pain. Manual assessment of excessive fibular translation is difficult to interpret and may have a high rate of false-positive findings.[29]

Syndesmotic injuries run the gamut from simple sprains to frank diastasis with concomitant ankle fractures. Surgery is generally indicated for a fibular fracture at least 2 inches above the ankle joint in the presence of disruption of the deltoid ligament

---

Box 20-4

Management of Inversion Ankle Sprains

Aggressively manage acute swelling.
Normalize the gait pattern as soon as possible.
Maintain a closed-pack position of neutral dorsiflexion during the acute and subacute healing phases.
Use manual therapy to restore normal tibiofibular and talocrural joint arthrokinematics.
Address structural abnormalities that would cause compensatory supination in gait:
- Compensated forefoot valgus
- Uncompensated rearfoot varus
- Greater than 10° tibial varum without adequate compensatory calcaneal eversion range of motion

Reestablish proprioceptive and kinesthetic skills and awareness
Enhance gluteus medius and peroneal frontal plane muscle control and stabilization ability.

Table 20-13 Surgical Procedures for Lateral Ankle Instability

Nonanatomic Tenodesis Reconstructions	
Watson-Jones procedure	Peroneus brevis tendon used to reconstruct the anterior talofibular ligament
Evans procedure	Peroneus brevis tendon rerouted to limit inversion at the ankle and subtalar joints
Chrisman-Snook procedure	Anterior talofibular and calcaneofibular ligaments reconstructed with half of the peroneus tendon
Anatomic Repairs	
Modified Brostrom procedure	Direct repair of the anterior talofibular and calcaneofibular ligaments with reinforcement of the extensor retinaculum and lateral talocalcaneal ligament
Anatomic Reconstructions	
Developed to allow restoration of anatomy when ligamentous attenuation makes direct repair difficult	Use of periosteal flaps, gracilis or plantaris autograft, or allograft

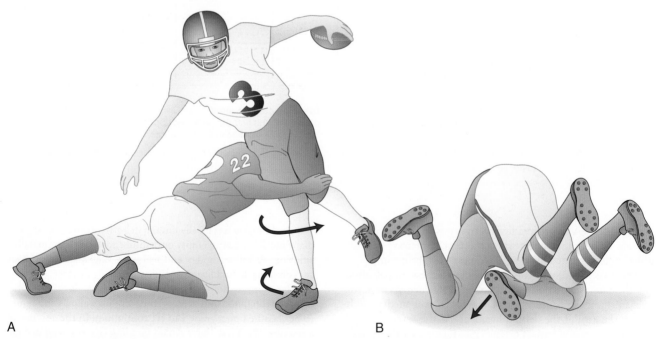

A   B

FIGURE 20-30 Typical mechanisms of injury for distal tibiofibular sprains/fractures. **A,** The foot is fixed in a position of external rotation with the ankle dorsiflexing while a lateral force at the trunk or hip causes internal rotation of the lower limb. **B,** The athlete is in a prone position and sustains a direct blow to the lateral aspect of the leg that forces the dorsiflexed ankle into excessive external rotation.

or with a complete diastasis. Conversely, acute stable sprains (absence of significant radiographic mortise widening with external rotation stress) can be managed with a nonoperative rehabilitation program. Progression of conservative management is determined by individual symptomatic response, whereas postsurgical rehabilitation programs are governed by tissue-healing rates. To ensure adequate protection following surgical intervention it is customary to immobilize the ankle in a boot for the first 6 weeks. Progressive weight bearing can begin over the next 2 to 6 weeks in a stirrup splint, with hardware removal at 8 to 12 weeks if metal cortical screws were used for fixation. Ironically, surgical fixation of unstable grade II and III syndesmosis injuries may allow earlier return to sport because of the early anatomic reduction, secure healing environment for the damaged ligaments, and potential to avoid chronic, latent diastasis.

Table 20-14 Syndesmotic Injury Imaging Criteria

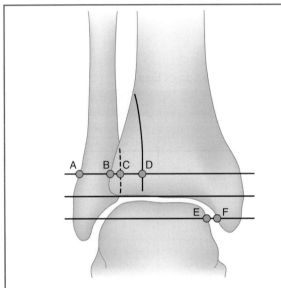

A: Lateral fibular border
B: Lateral tibial border
C: Medial fibular border
D: Lateral border of the posterior tibial malleolus (incisura fibularis)
E: Medial talar border
F: Lateral medial malleolus border
CD: Tibiofibular clear space
BC: Tibiofibular overlap
EF: Medial clear space

Radiographic Finding	View	Measured at:	Normal Parameters
Tibiofibular clear space	AP	1 cm above the tibial plafond	<6 mm or <44% of the width of the fibula
Tibiofibular overlap	AP	1 cm above the tibial plafond	>6 mm or >24% of the width of the fibula
	Mortise	—	>1 mm
Medial clear space	Mortise	At the level of the talar dome	>4 mm or >2 mm than on the uninvolved side

AP, Anteroposterior.

Clinical Pearl #9

Restoration of normal tibiofibular arthrokinematics is essential for normal ankle function. Positional faults and limited translation of accessory motion of the fibula onto the tibia will cause pain or limited motion, or both.

Although it is generally agreed that syndesmotic injuries are associated with a longer recovery time than lateral ankle sprains are, there is no consensus in the literature regarding their optimal management. Many questions still need to be considered in designing the rehabilitation program. The need for immobilization, the necessity of weight-bearing restriction, time frames for healing, return-to-sport parameters, and the inherent lower extremity alignment are all factors that should be considered carefully. A rationale for determining the severity of distal tibiofibular injuries is provided in Table 20-15. Both conservative and postsurgical rehabilitation should use a similar philosophic approach. Table 20-16 provides a general management perspective to guide the rehabilitation process. As with any protocol, each athlete has unique needs, and the individual circumstance will dictate the recovery process. Immobilization and weight-bearing status are governed by the severity of symptoms, degree of instability, and ability to normalize gait. A period of non–weight bearing may be required, with secure, compressive fixation in a walking boot as partial weight-bearing ambulation is allowed. In individuals with latent instability, this period may be prolonged by an additional 2 to 3 weeks.

End-range dorsiflexion and eversion range-of-motion exercises should be introduced with caution. Weight-bearing rotational exercises are also reserved for the lateral stages of rehabilitation. Dynamic stability can be enhanced with an emphasis on restoring eccentric control of pronatory forces by the posterior tibialis and dorsiflexion forces by the triceps surae. Proprioceptive balancing activities are an important aspect of the rehabilitative process. Table 20-12 outlines many of the variables that can be used to provide appropriate challenge without overloading the stress that can be tolerated by the injured tissues. Distal ankle compression can be provided by any combination of circumferential straps at the distal tibiofibular joint, medial subtalar sling straps, or stirrup bracing.

The prognosis for return to sport generally correlates with the grade of injury. Numerous authors have reported that athletes with grade I or II distal tibiofibular injuries take an average of 4 to 6 weeks to resume unrestricted competition. Nussbaum et al[30] developed a return-to-sport prediction formula with a 95% confidence interval via linear regression analysis in athletic subjects without fracture or frank diastasis. The equation is based on the distance from the tip of the lateral malleolus to the most proximal point of tenderness on the anterior portion of the IOM. The formula forecasts that the time to return to sport equals 5 + (0.93 × [length of tenderness in centimeters]) + 3.72 days. Possible complications that should be monitored for a minimum of 6 months include heterotopic ossification, syndesmotic calcification, or the development of anterior impingement syndrome secondary to fibrous scar formation.[30]

Table 20-15 Grading of Injury Severity Based on Clinical Findings for Tibular Injuries

Finding	Grade I—Sprain Without Diastasis	Grade II—Sprain With Latent Diastasis	Grade III—Sprain With Frank Diastasis
Symptoms	Mild point tenderness over the tibiofibular ligaments	Point tenderness extends proximally over the IOM	Significant tenderness and inability to bear weight
Stability (manual fibular translation)	Mild laxity with a stable end point to stress	Moderate laxity with a soft end point to stress	Notable laxity with absence of an end point
X-ray imaging	Stable with stress radiographs	Mild laxity present with stress but absent with plain radiographs	Instability and/or fracture evident on plain radiographs
Management Strategy			
Weight bearing	Weight bearing to tolerance	Progress to full weight bearing after 1-2 weeks	Minimum of 2-3 weeks of non–weight bearing
Immobilization	0-3 days	3-7 days	7+ days

IOM, Interosseous membrane.

Table 20-16 General Rehabilitation Management Strategies for Syndesmotic Ankle Sprain Injuries

	Acute Phase	Subacute Phase	Return-to-Sport Phase
Emphasis	Joint protection and control of the initial inflammatory response	Restoration of strength, mobility, and neuromuscular control	Restoration of activity-specific skills
Management of symptoms	Protection: boot, posterior splint, and/or stirrup brace Rest Ice Compression wrap Elevation with retrograde massage	Contrast thermal therapy Intermittent compression	Ice after rehabilitation or activity
Criteria for progression*	Pain-free ambulation Pain and swelling under control	Normal gait pattern Pain-free activities of daily living, including low-level plyometrics (gentle hop for 10 repetitions)	Use outcome measurement tools and/or functional tests to determine readiness for sport
Fitness maintenance	Upper body ergometer Aquatic therapy	Cycling on a "tall" seat or NuStep with limited knee flexion to minimize dorsiflexion stress	—
ROM	—	Pain-free active range of motion BAPS board initially limiting posteromedial contact and adding weight-bearing stress as tolerated	—
Manual therapy	Grade I-II joint mobilization	Grade III-IV joint mobilization	—
Therapeutic exercise	Proximal hip/knee strengthening Foot intrinsic muscle strengthening	EARLY: Four-way elastic tubing exercises within pain-free range of eversion and dorsiflexion LATER: Short-foot exercises Progression from bilateral flatfoot to unilateral full-arc heel raises Non–weight-bearing squats (shuttle, Total Gym, leg press) progressing to decline retro squats to front squats Lunges Lateral step-ups	Functional running progression and agility drills with careful progression from sagittal to frontal to rotational activities in the transverse plane
Proprioceptive activities	—	Bilateral progressing to unilateral balancing activities	Dynamic balancing activities and increasing plyometric overloads

*No temporal criteria for progression after nonoperative interventions; however, the phase of healing and tissue tolerance constraints should be recognized and honored.
BAPS, Biomechanical Ankle Platform System; *ROM*, range of motion.

REHABILITATION OF POSTIMMOBILIZATION FRACTURES

Rehabilitation following cast removal after ankle fractures is focused on restoring joint mobility. The immobilization time necessary for ensuring union of fractures causes capsular restriction, muscular atrophy, and proprioceptive deficits. Emphasis is then placed on joint mobilization and appropriate exercises to strengthen and mobilize the soft tissues. The mechanics of the fracture and its surgical fixation must be understood and appreciated to avoid excessive force or stress on the initial injury. For joint mobilization techniques that may be used to restore accessory joint motion and normal joint arthrokinematics, see Figures A20-22 to A20-38 (in Appendix 5) on Expert Consult @ www.expertconsult.com.

Clinical Pearl #10

Joint mobilization is indicated for capsular restrictions in motion and is applied in a pain-free manner with short lever arms. Stretching is indicated for soft tissue extensibility and is applied as both a warm-up and cool-down activity to produce gentle tension in the muscles. High-velocity, low-amplitude thrusts within the physiologic range are indicated to reset afferent input to the joint and make minor adjustments in joint alignment.

Subluxation of the Peroneal Tendons

The peroneal tendons lie in a deep groove posterior to the lateral malleolus. They are subject to subluxation out of this groove if a forceful and sudden contraction of the peroneals from a position of dorsiflexion and inversion occurs and causes rupture of the peroneal retinaculum. This is commonly seen in sporting activities that require cutting maneuvers such as skiing, soccer, basketball, tennis, gymnastics, and football.[31]

This injury is commonly confused with inversion ankle sprains because of its location and similar symptoms. The athlete relates a feeling of tenderness, instability, and swelling in an area around the lateral malleolus. Subluxation of the peroneal tendons can be differentiated from inversion sprains if the athlete has intense retromalleolar pain with resistive dorsiflexion and eversion or, in those with a chronic condition, exhibits marked instability and audible snapping of the tendon in and out of its groove.

Conservative management is generally an option only for an acute, nonathletic injury.[31] For chronic conditions or for failure of restricted weight bearing and immobilization for 2 to 6 weeks to stabilize the complaint, a surgical intervention should be elected. Surgical procedures attempt to reconstruct or reinforce the damaged peroneal retinaculum (retinaculoplasty), use bony procedures to deepen the groove behind the lateral malleolus, or reroute the tendons under the calcaneofibular ligament (or any combination of the three).

Postoperatively, the patient is immobilized in a short leg cast with a non–weight-bearing gait for 3 to 4 weeks. During the next 3 to 4 weeks, a short leg walking boot is used with progression toward full weight bearing. Bony block procedures may be managed with a slightly longer period of immobilization before progressive weight bearing. Active range-of-motion exercises can usually begin at 3 to 4 weeks with gradual return to sport by 3 to 4 months.

Calcaneal Injuries

Heel Bruises

Contusion injuries of the heel and calcaneal fat pad are among the most disabling in sports. Athletes who require frequent landings from jumps (volleyball, basketball, and track athletes) seem especially prone to this type of injury. Runners with a leg length discrepancy who overstride on the side of the short leg and as a result experience increased impact force at the heel-strike area are also especially vulnerable to this type of trauma. Contusion injuries that cause subperiosteal bleeding and tender scar formation are sensitive to tissue compression and pressure on nerve endings in the area. Bone scans can be used to rule out a stress fracture in more chronic conditions that did not have a precipitating traumatic event.

The athlete will complain of severe pain on the plantar aspect of the calcaneus that is greatly aggravated by weight bearing. Treatment must include some element of rest to minimize continued, repetitive trauma. As the athlete returns to sport, the heel should be taped and placed in a heel cup. The tape and heel cup strengthen and support the columnar septa and lobules, which provide the calcaneal fat pad with its impact-absorbing qualities. It is also helpful if a shoe with good shock-attenuating midsole qualities in the rearfoot is selected for participation.

Posterior Ankle Impingement Syndrome

Posterior ankle impingement syndrome is a clinical disorder characterized by posterior ankle pain during forced plantar flexion.[32] The symptoms may be the result of acute trauma or chronic repetitive stress. Although fracture of the talar trigonal process and synchondrosis of the os trigonum (Fig. 20-31) are the most common causes of this impingement syndrome, the clinician should also consider other causes such as flexor hallucis

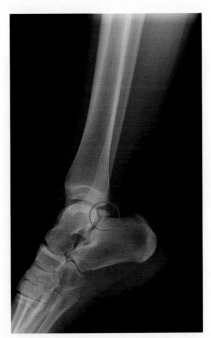

FIGURE 20-31 Os trigonum causing posterior ankle impingement syndrome. *(Copyright © 1994-2011 by WebMD LLC. Marc A Molis, MD "Ankle Impingement Syndrome." From: http://emedicine.medscape.com/.)*

tenosynovitis and osteochondrosis at the tibiotalar or subtalar articulations. This injury is most likely to occur in athletes who function on their toes (e.g., ballet dancers, gymnasts, divers) or who need end-range plantar flexion (downhill running, kicking, or sliding into a base) to perform an activity. Clinical diagnosis is based on the location of the symptoms and reproduction of the symptoms with quick, passive hyper–plantar flexion maneuvers, supported by imaging studies. A nonoperative course of care involves rest from offending activities, avoidance of high-heeled shoes, antiinflammatory medication, and taping techniques to limit end-range plantar flexion. Failure to improve in refractory cases may require surgical excision.

Calcaneal Apophysitis

Traction epiphyseal injuries (also known as Sever disease) during active growth spurts are common in active adolescents (boys more often than girls). The strong pull from the triceps surae causes painful inflammation from repetitive microtrauma on the unossified apophysis.[33] Continued stress results in disruption of the circulation and possible microfractures of the fragile calcified cartilage. The young athlete complains of pain on the posterior aspect of the heel at the insertion point of the Achilles tendon that is aggravated by activity and relieved by rest. Manual compression (medial to lateral squeezing) may best reproduce the complaint during clinical examination (Fig. 20-32). This condition is a self-limited entity that ends at skeletal maturity when the epiphysis closes. Until then, judicious rest, gentle stretching, appropriate footwear, and the insertion of bilateral heel lifts can help alleviate injurious stress.

Retrocalcaneal Bursitis

Long-distance running and repetitive jumping can result in bursal inflammation between the Achilles tendon and calcaneus. This condition is aggravated by excessive compensatory pronation, which can lead to cumulative trauma and pressure in the

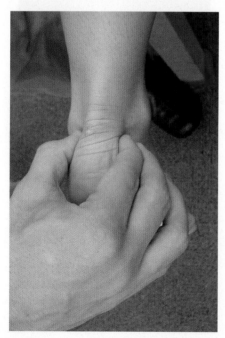

FIGURE 20-32 Manual compression of the calcaneus reproducing pain from calcaneal apophysitis.

posterolateral aspect of the heel. A bony enthesophyte on the superior calcaneal tuberosity may irritate the retrocalcaneal bursa and distal Achilles tendon, particularly during dorsiflexion, whereas bony prominences on the posterolateral calcaneal tuberosity (Haglund deformity, Fig. 20-33) may irritate the superficial calcaneal bursa, particularly with firm or ill-fitting heel counters.[34]

This condition is most common in older or less active populations and is characterized by pain and swelling in the posterolateral and posterosuperior aspects of the heel. Retrocalcaneal tenderness is elicited anterior to the Achilles tendon but posterior to the talus.

Ice, antiinflammatory medication, and orthotic control of the hypermobile calcaneus are used in treatment. If the subcutaneous bursa is involved, modification of the heel counter collar should also be done. Shoe selection should place a high priority on a stable heel counter. Structural predisposition may be alleviated by a heel lift. In chronic conditions that have not responded to conservative management, resection of the exostosis or excision of the inflamed bursa (or both) may be necessary.

Plantar Fasciosis

Plantar fasciosis is one of the most common foot conditions treated by health care providers. It has been estimated that the incidence of plantar fasciosis is about 10% over the course of a lifetime. The pathology is typically caused by repetitive microtrauma with subsequent collagen degeneration at the origin of the plantar fascia on the medial calcaneal tubercle. Histologic evaluation of 50 surgical cases has supported the contention that plantar fasciosis is a degenerative and not an inflammatory condition.[35] Chronic overuse and irritation can lead to bone formation in response to the traction forces of the plantar fascia and the muscles attaching to the calcaneal tuberosity.

The plantar fascia is a dense, multilayered fibrous connective tissue on the sole of the foot. It is made up of three bands (medial, central, and lateral) that are approximately 2 to 4 mm thick. The medial band is the thickest of the three and the one most commonly involved in the pathology. The fascia originates from the medial calcaneal tubercle and courses distally to insert onto the plantar plates of the MTP joints and the base of the proximal phalanges. The fascia is deep to the subcalcaneal fat pad but superficial to the first plantar layer containing the abductor hallucis, flexor digitorum brevis, and adductor digiti

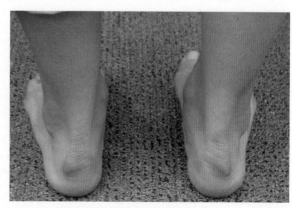

FIGURE 20-33 Haglund deformity.

quinti. In addition, a number of proximate neurologic structures can also cause plantar heel pain. The medial calcaneal nerve arises from the posterior tibial nerve at the level of the medial malleolus and supplies sensation to the medial plantar aspect of the foot. Just below the malleolus it bifurcates into plantar and calcaneal branches. The plantar branches on the sole of the foot run between the flexor digitorum brevis and the quadratus plantae in the plantar layers. The plantar branch splits into medial and lateral divisions, and compression in this area can also be a cause of heel pain.

The plantar fascia has three important functional roles. First, it helps attenuate ground reaction forces early in the stance phase of gait and then provides a truss support to the medial longitudinal arch in midstance. During propulsion, the plantar fascia stabilizes the foot and arch via the windlass mechanism. The windlass mechanism is activated by toe extension during propulsion to put tension on the fascia and passively maintain the height of the arch.

Many etiologic factors have been associated with predisposition of an individual to the onset of plantar fasciosis. The risk factor with the strongest evidence of correlation is obesity or a high body mass index (BMI), particularly in non-athletic populations. When the BMI is higher than 25kg/m^2, the risk for plantar fasciosis is increased fivefold to sixfold.[36] The biomechanical explanation for this phenomenon involves the fascia's truss support role. The plantar fascia is essentially a tie-rod that connects at each end of the medial longitudinal arch. As body weight increases, a greater superior vector load is applied to the arch. This load is then resisted by the plantar fascia's increased tension to prevent migration of the proximal and distal attachments.

Many other musculoskeletal risk factors have also been associated with plantar fasciosis. Moderate evidence supports the fact that both pes cavus and pes planus feet seem to be more susceptible to the problem.[37] A planus foot has perpetually increased tension on the fascia because of its pronated position, whereas a cavus foot has an inherently tight, shortened fascia causing a bowstring-like load. Many sources have noted the association between gastrocnemius-soleus tightness and the presence of plantar fasciosis.[36] A significant percentage of individuals with plantar fasciosis have at least a 5° limitation in ankle dorsiflexion range of motion, and the risk for plantar fasciosis is 23 times higher if dorsiflexion range of motion is less than 0°.[36,38] The theory behind this increased risk with Achilles tightness is that it holds the subtalar in varus and limits pronation or, conversely, causes a compensatory substitution at the midtarsal joint that increases the availability of sagittal plane motion not afforded at the ankle.

Other musculoskeletal risk factors linked to plantar fasciosis include restrictions in first MTP dorsiflexion mobility[39] and intrinsic toe flexor weakness.[40] The last etiologic factor to consider is the patient's age. Plantar fasciosis is much more prevalent in middle-aged adults, perhaps supporting the theory that its pathology is degenerative in nature. It may be that collagen is more tolerant in youth and needs to be more significantly abused in training or activities to manifest the symptoms. The condition is further stressed if a majority of the day is spent in a standing position. For younger patients with overtraining at the root of their onset, it is wise to counsel against sprinting and uphill running and to recommend that harder training surfaces be avoided.

Patients with plantar fasciosis are rather homogeneous in their clinical findings. They often report a gradual, insidious onset and complain of sharp heel pain at the origin of the fascia. This symptom is most noticeable after prolonged non–weight bearing. Fasciosis patients often relate that the worst steps of the day are their first ones. This painful event usually subsides quickly with gentle activity but gradually returns and worsens as the day progresses. Activities that are particularly aggravating include stair climbing, walking barefoot, and plyometric activities such as running and jumping. Common objective findings noted during examination include varus malalignment, point tenderness at the fascial origin, decreased ankle and first MTP range of motion, and an altered gait pattern. Many individuals will assume a hypersupinated gait to avoid weight-bearing pressure on the painful area and may have difficulty performing a unilateral heel raise. The most predictive provocation test is forceful great toe extension in a standing position that reproduces the discomfort at the origin of the fascia. This maneuver has been shown to be very specific but lacks sensitivity (Fig. 20-34).[36]

Clinical Pearl #11

Chronic plantar fasciitis often results in stalagmite calcification at the insertion of the medial calcaneal tubercle; however, the heel spur isn't the problem—it's the reaction to the problem.

Many conditions cause plantar heel pain but can be differentiated with a thorough history and examination. Plantar fasciosis is certainly the most common cause of heel pain, but other conditions must be ruled out. Less common causes can be divided into neurogenic, soft tissue, skeletal, and systemic illness groups. Neurogenic causes may include the aforementioned calcaneal or plantar nerve entrapment and S1 radiculopathy. Soft tissue disorders that mimic fasciosis include calcaneal fat pad atrophy, Achilles tendinopathies, and subcalcaneal bursitis. Common skeletal conditions that are manifested in a similar manner include calcaneal stress fractures, Sever disease (calcaneal apophysitis), Haglund deformity, and bone bruises. Finally, additional laboratory or medical work-up may be needed to rule out systemic causes of plantar heel pain such as Reiter syndrome, ankylosing spondylitis, rheumatoid arthritis, and psoriasis.

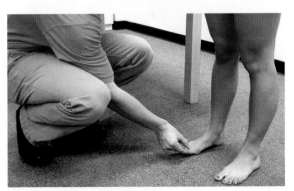

FIGURE 20-34 Windlass test.

The most common condition that mimics plantar fasciosis is tarsal tunnel syndrome, which is caused by entrapment of the posterior tibial nerve as it passes behind the medial malleolus. The chief complaint is usually a burning or throbbing pain with paresthesias in the medial ankle and arch area. Tenderness may be present posterior to the medial malleolus, and symptoms can sometimes be reproduced with a Tinel tapping test. The examiner may notice weakness of the interphalangeal flexors and a sensory deficit in the medial arch and medial side of the plantar surface of the foot. The best differentiation, however, is the location of the symptoms. Plantar fasciosis is most notable on the bottom of the foot, whereas tarsal tunnel symptoms are more evident on the medial side of the foot and ankle.

In general, 80% to 90% of individuals with plantar fasciosis respond well to conservative treatment over a period of 6 to 12 months.[41,42] Initial intervention goals should focus on decreasing pain, minimizing strain on the plantar fascia, and identifying and addressing predisposing risk factors. The most important early intervention may be rest or simply avoiding or reducing activities that aggravate the symptoms. The patient's activities that best reproduce the asterisk sign should be reduced in intensity, duration, frequency, or any combination of the three.

Ice massage has anesthetic value, but most therapeutic modalities and physical agents have not proved effective in the management of fasciosis. The exception is iontophoresis. Numerous studies have demonstrated that iontophoresis with dexamethasone or a 5% dilution of acetic acid has short-term value in reducing pain.[36] Other therapeutic modalities such as ultrasound, low-intensity laser, and electron-generating insoles (magnet therapy) have not been shown in randomized controlled trials to be more effective than sham or placebo treatments in alleviating pain.[36] There is clinical consensus (though limited research support) that one of the more effective early interventions is soft tissue massage and stretching against a firm, cylindrical structure (rolling pin, aerosol can, Coke bottle, etc.) before standing or walking after a period of prolonged non–weight bearing. This intervention consistently reduces the "first step" pain complaint typical in this population.

A critical element in the management of plantar fasciosis, particularly in those with a cavus foot, is stretching of the triceps surae and the plantar fascia itself. Even greater benefits with respect to pain and function are achieved by intrinsic plantar

fascial stretching the first thing in the morning before weight bearing or after prolonged sitting (Fig. 20-35).[36] In addition, increasing first MTP range of motion can be accomplished by stretching and joint mobilization (Fig 20-36). For a planus foot, intuitive reasoning would suggest that training the muscles that control and reverse pronation (posterior tibialis, anterior tibialis, and peroneals) at the subtalar joint would reduce tension on the plantar fascia. Others have emphasized the importance of strengthening the intrinsic muscles of the foot,[36] which may include foot sweeps, toes curls, marble pick-ups, and short-foot exercises.

The final element in management that should be considered by the care provider is external support. This could include the appropriate use of shoes, orthotics, taping, and night splints. Most practitioners recommend a shoe with a firm heel counter and straight last. The midsole should be flared and beveled to enhance stability and have adequate shock attenuation. If the gastrocnemius/soleus is tight, an elevated heel is a desirable temporary measure as long as it does not affect flexibility of the midfoot and forefoot.

A number of taping techniques are effective in providing short-term relief of symptoms.[36] Low-Dye taping techniques (Fig. 20-37) are particularly beneficial for individuals with compensatory forefoot varus deformities, and calcaneal taping

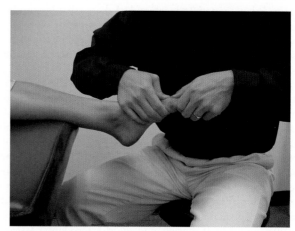

FIGURE 20-36 Traction-translation mobilization of the first metatarsophalangeal joint to increase mobility.

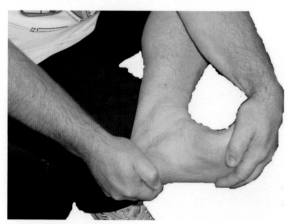

FIGURE 20-35 Intrinsic plantar fascia stretch.

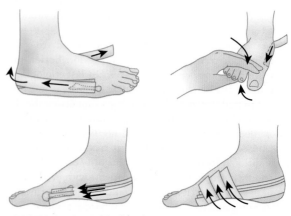

FIGURE 20-37 Modified Low-Dye taping technique.

(Fig. 20-38) is helpful in controlling compensatory rearfoot motion. Relief with plantar taping support is a good indicator of the potential efficacy of an orthotic device.[43] Many studies have also supported the use of orthotics for patients with plantar fasciosis. Both accommodative and customized semi-rigid devices have been shown to decrease pain and improve function.[36]

Clinical Pearl #12

Arch (Low-Dye) taping is effective because it both exerts a biomechanical antipronation effect and appropriately alters neuromuscular activity.

In individuals with more chronic symptoms (longer than 6 months), there is good evidence for the use of night splints.[36] The splint is used to maintain the ankle and toes in a dorsiflexed position during the night to prevent physiologic creep of the fascia while non–weight bearing.

A number of medical interventions either augment the care provided by allied health care providers or are used when conservative measures fail to alleviate pain and restore function. Such interventions include nonsteroidal antiinflammatory drugs, topical medications, extracorporeal shock wave therapy, and partial surgical releases in recalcitrant cases (Boxes 20-5 and 20-6).

Box 20-5

Management of Plantar Fasciitis in a Rigid Cavus Foot—Emphasis on Stretching

Avoidance or minimization of the intensity, duration, and frequency of irritating activities

Improvement in rearfoot and forefoot mobility

Restoration of first metatarsophalangeal joint mobility through stretching and mobilization

Gastrocnemius-soleus stretching with control of hyperpronation tendencies

Intrinsic plantar fascia stretching

Massage and mobilization of tight plantar fascia soft tissue

An accommodative orthosis to redirect plantar contact pressure to more tolerant areas of the foot

---

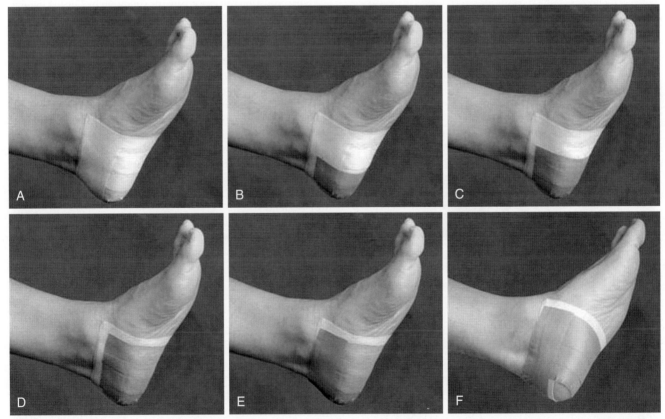

FIGURE 20-38 Calcaneal taping technique. When the cover roll is applied (**A**), taping with Leukotape follows. Piece 1 is applied just distal to the lateral malleolus while pulling the calcaneus medially and is attached to the medial aspect of the foot distal to the medial malleolus (**B**). Pieces 2 and 3 follow the same pattern with overlap of approximately one third of the tape width while moving in the distal direction (**C** and **D**). Piece 4 goes around the back of the heel, starting distal to the lateral malleolus, wraps around the posterior aspect of the calcaneus, and is anchored distal to the medial malleolus (**E**). Piece 4 also serves as an anchor for the first three pieces (**F**).

(From Hyland, M.R., Webber-Gaffney, A., Cohen, L., and Lichtman, P.T. [2006]: Randomized controlled trial of calcaneal taping, sham taping, and plantar fascia stretching for the short-term management of plantar heel pain. J. Orthop. Sports Phys. Ther., 36:364–371.)

Foot Injuries

Tarsometatarsal Injuries

The tarsometatarsal joint is an articulation (Lisfranc joint) that consists of the three cuneiforms and the cuboid as they join with the five metatarsals. Transverse ligamentous supports span the base of the metatarsals with the exception of the first and second metatarsals. Midfoot sprains, dislocations, and fracture-dislocations, though not common, can occur in athletic competition. The joint can be injured through direct and indirect mechanisms. The direct crushing type of injury is less common and predictable in its pathology. Indirect injuries usually occur as a result of an axial load placed on the heel with the foot in plantar flexion, which causes hyperextension stress on the weaker dorsal ligaments of the joint (Fig. 20-39).

Box 20-6

Management of Plantar Fasciitis in a Flexible Planus Foot—Emphasis on Strengthening

Avoidance or minimization of the intensity, duration, and frequency of irritating activities

Strengthening of the muscles that control and reverse pronation

Strengthening of the intrinsic muscles of the foot

Appropriate shoe wear that provides rearfoot stability and forefoot mobility

Taping to reduce strain on the plantar fascia

Semirigid to rigid biomechanical orthotic device to control compensatory pronation tendencies

---

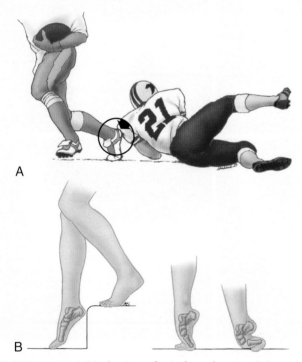

FIGURE 20-39 Mechanism of a Lisfranc fracture-dislocation. **A,** Axial load applied to heel with the foot fixed in equinus. **B,** Axial load applied by body weight with the ankle in extreme equinus. *(From Heckman, J.D. [1991]: Fractures and dislocations of the foot. In Rockwood, C.A. Jr., Green, D.P., and Bucholz, R.W. [eds.]: Rockwood and Green's Fractures in Adults, 3rd ed. Philadelphia, Lippincott, p. 2143.)*

Midfoot sprains have subtle findings on examination that make diagnosis difficult. Swelling is usually mild. Pain with passive forefoot abduction and pronation and tenderness on palpation are reliable indicators of this injury. The athlete will have pain during or be unable to perform unilateral heel raises, jumps, or cutting maneuvers. After an acute injury, initial evaluation should also include a circulatory assessment of the dorsalis pedis pulse because the artery courses over the proximal head of the second metatarsal and may be susceptible to injury in a severe dislocation.

Following open or closed reduction, the foot is immobilized for a period, the length of which depends on the severity of the injury. Rehabilitation and weight-bearing progression can commence after immobilization with gradual progression of functional activities on the toes. Medial midfoot sprains tend to progress at a slower rate and take longer to return to sport.

Tarsal Tunnel Syndrome

Tarsal tunnel syndrome is an entrapment neuropathy of the posterior tibial nerve as it passes through the osseofibrous tunnel between the flexor retinaculum (laciniate ligament) and medial wall of the talus, calcaneus, and medial malleolus (Fig. 20-40). Osseous prominences, edema, or compensatory reactions to rearfoot deformities can narrow the confines of the tarsal tunnel and compress the medial plantar branch of the posterior tibial nerve. Hyperpronation can exacerbate the condition by causing tightening of the overlying flexor retinaculum or the calcaneonavicular ligaments. Direct trauma, ganglia, lipomas, chronic inflammation, or postsurgical or posttraumatic fibrosis in this area can also give rise to a space-occupying lesion that can alter neurologic function.

The athlete reports intermittent neuritic symptoms (burning, tingling, numbness, or pain) in the medial aspect of the foot that are aggravated by prolonged weight-bearing activity or holding the ankle in maximal dorsiflexion and eversion with the toes extended for 5 to 10 seconds. A positive Tinel sign may be elicited with tapping or compression over the affected nerve to reproduce the symptoms. In advanced stages, weakness in toe flexion and atrophy of the abductor hallucis may be evident.

The athlete should be placed in an orthosis to control abnormal subtalar motion and be instructed in modification of activity. Therapeutic modalities such as ultrasound, phonophoresis,

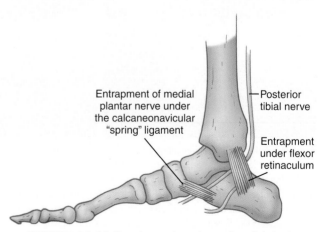

Entrapment of medial plantar nerve under the calcaneonavicular "spring" ligament

Posterior tibial nerve

Entrapment under flexor retinaculum

FIGURE 20-40 Tarsal tunnel syndrome (medial view).

and ice massage may be tried in an attempt to reduce edema and fibrosis in the area of entrapment. Resistant cases may require surgical release of the tissue that is causing compression.

Cuboid Syndrome

Cuboid syndrome describes partial displacement of the cuboid bone by the pull of the peroneus longus. Its onset can be gradual or traumatic. Acute pain and hypomobility can be induced with trauma or a powerful contraction with the foot in a plantar-flexed and inverted position. Gradual onset is more typical in a hyperpronated foot. In these circumstances the peroneus longus is at a mechanical disadvantage, and it pulls the lateral portion of the cuboid dorsally and the medial portion in a plantar direction.

The signs and symptoms of this injury include lateral foot pain that is particularly noticeable in the propulsive phase of gait. Assessment of joint accessory motion will reveal hypomobility at the calcaneocuboid joint. Application of adduction or supination distraction stress at the calcaneocuboid joint may confirm the diagnosis (Fig. 20-41).[44] Treatment is directed at restoring normal arthrokinematics and protecting against further trauma or aggravation. Following ice massage or a cold whirlpool bath, the athlete is positioned for bony manipulation. With the athlete prone and the knee mildly flexed to protect against excessive traction of the superficial peroneal nerve, a dorsal thrust with the thumbs placed on the medial portion of the cuboid is used to relocate the cuboid back into more appropriate alignment (Fig. 20-42). Following restoration of bony congruency, a segmental balance (cuboid) pad may be used to unload stress on the fourth metatarsal and its cuboid articulation. In athletes with chronic hyperpronation, Low-Dye taping or medial heel wedges can be used to counteract the damaging pull of the peroneus longus.

Metatarsal Stress Fractures

Metatarsal stress fractures occur when osteoclastic activity is greater than osteoblastic activity. Stress overload caused by prolonged pronation and excessive hypermobility of the first ray can begin a cycle of injury (Fig. 20-43). Hughes[45] has noted that predisposition for stress fractures is greatest in those with forefoot varus and decreased ankle dorsiflexion range of motion. Both conditions result in pronation during the propulsive phase of gait, which places considerable stress on the central three metatarsals, especially the second. Metatarsal stress fractures are most likely to occur in a deconditioned athlete or in runners and dancers with sudden changes in training surfaces or athletic footwear.

Pain and swelling are localized over the metatarsal and increase with activity and decrease with rest. Percussion and active flexion-extension of the toes also exacerbate the complaint. In the early or prodromal period a radiograph may be negative but a bone scan may reveal the injury because of its heightened sensitivity in revealing the injury. Computed tomography may further define whether the fracture is complete.

Treatment is straightforward. The athlete must rest from weight-bearing or aggravating activities and find alternative (low-impact) methods of conditioning. In those in whom pain is present during ambulation or who are suspected of noncompliance in reducing activity levels, a short leg walking cast may be appropriate. During this convalescence period the clinician may want to further investigate factors that might affect bone health such as diet, drug use, and menstrual irregularities. On return to sport, orthoses, tape, or a felt cutout to float the affected metatarsal should be used to relieve osteoclastic stress.

During the subacute phase it is important for the athlete to correct the muscular, flexibility, and conditioning deficits that may have led to the initial injury.

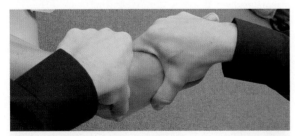

FIGURE 20-41 Calcaneocuboid stress. Provocative adduction stress at the midtarsal joint.

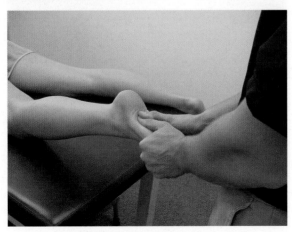

FIGURE 20-42 Cuboid manipulation.

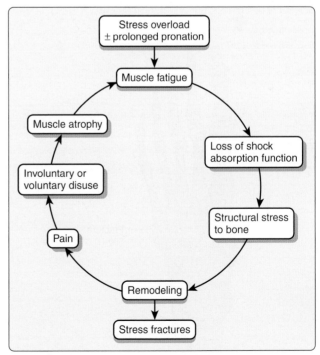

FIGURE 20-43 Injury cycle of stress fractures. *(From Taunton, J.E., Clement, D.B., and Webber, D. [1981]: Lower extremity stress fractures in athletes. Physician Sportsmed., 9:85.)*

Proximal Diaphyseal Fracture of the Fifth Metatarsal

Weight-bearing forces are great on the fifth metatarsal because of its many soft tissue attachments. Tension on the bone from the peroneus brevis, cubometatarsal ligament, lateral band of the plantar fascia, and fibularis tertius can lead to stress reactions in the area of the proximal diaphysis. This area is also susceptible to a complete (Jones) fracture with acute inversion trauma. Both injuries are notoriously unpredictable in healing, and nonunion and reinjury occur frequently (Fig. 20-44).[46] Early intramedullary screw fixation results in lower failure rates and shorter times until both clinical union and return to participation than does non–weight-bearing short leg cast immobilization in recreationally active patients.[47] The first 4 weeks are spent in a removable walking boot to allow active range of motion and progressive weight bearing. Stair Stepper training progressing to running activities can begin at 4 to 5 weeks if pain and swelling allow, with return to sport in an average of 8 weeks.[48] Conservative management requires 6 to 8 weeks of non–weight-bearing cast immobilization before rehabilitation measures can commence. Full athletic participation is contraindicated until the fracture site has fully consolidated. When healing is complete, a semi-rigid orthosis with an extended carbon fiber plate or steel shank should be considered as a prophylactic measure.[48]

Compression Neuropathy of the Interdigital Nerve

Compression and shearing forces at the bifurcation of the neurovascular bundle between the metatarsal heads can result in the formation of a benign tumor of fibrous tissue called a Morton intermetatarsal neuroma (Fig. 20-45). Pinching and squeezing of the neurovascular bundle between the metatarsal heads and transverse metatarsal ligament occur in a hypermobile foot during midstance and propulsion.

The chief complaint is numbness, tingling, or a burning sensation in the forefoot that radiates to the toes. The lesion is usually located between the third and fourth metatarsals and is often described as a lump on the bottom of the foot or a feeling of walking on a rolled-up or wrinkled sock. Pain can be relieved by removal of shoes and is aggravated by manual compression of the metatarsal head (Gauthier test). A clicking or reproduction of symptoms can be elicited with simultaneous compression of the metatarsal heads in the transverse plane and plantar pressure in the interdigital space of the affected MTP joints (Mulder sign) (Fig. 20-46).

Some success has been achieved with a metatarsal pad placed just proximal to the metatarsal heads, which increases their spatial spread and alleviates pressure. Shoe selection should ensure a wide toe box, and orthotic inserts may be used to control hypermobility. Anesthetic injections can provide diagnostic confirmation of the problem, and corticosteroid, dilute alcohol, and sclerosing injections may provide relief of symptoms. Surgical decompression of the nerve or dorsal excision of the neuroma is indicated when conservative measures fail.[49]

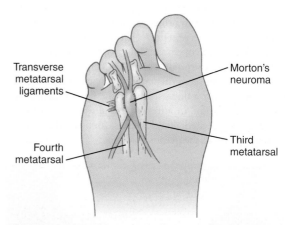

FIGURE 20-45 Plantar view of an interdigital neuroma.

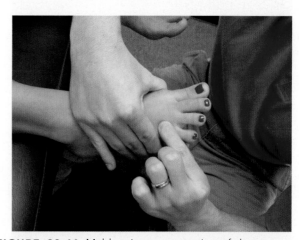

FIGURE 20-46 Mulder sign: compression of the metatarsal head along with plantar pressure over the interdigital nerve to elicit pain or clicking with dorsal glide. A positive test will create a localized complaint on the plantar surface of the foot with paresthesias possibly radiating into the affected toes.

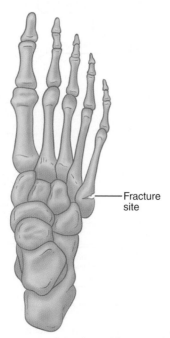

FIGURE 20-44 Proximal diaphyseal fracture of the fifth metatarsal (dorsal view).

Turf Toe

Acute hyperdorsiflexion injuries to the first MTP joint occur as the toes are pressed down into an unyielding surface just before toe-off. This force causes hyperextension of the MTP joint as the phalanx is jammed into the metatarsal. Repetitive trauma of this nature results in plantar capsule tears, articular cartilage damage, and possible fracture of the medial sesamoid bone. Chronic trauma can lead to metatarsalgia with ligamentous calcification and hallux rigidus.

Sudden acceleration under high loads against unyielding surfaces and axial loads delivered through the heel with the ankle plantar-flexed and the big toe maximally dorsiflexed are common mechanisms of injury. Athletes who wear shoes that are extremely flexible and offer minimal support are especially prone to this injury. In addition, athletes who wear a longer shoe to achieve greater width effectively lengthen the lever arm forces acting on the joint and subject the feet to repetitive trauma.

The athlete has a tender, red, and swollen first MTP joint that exhibits increased pain with passive toe extension. Chronic stress may result in MTP instability with evidence of sesamoid injury or proximal migration of the sesamoids secondary to capsular disruption.[50] Initial management calls for rest, ice, compression, elevation, and support of the injured joint. Tape immobilization can be used to limit the excessive extension and valgus stress that irritate the joint (Fig. 20-47). Rehabilitation procedures may include ultrasound to mobilize scar tissue and active range-of-motion exercises with the first ray stabilized. Figure 20-48 demonstrates exercise to increase active range of motion for a hypomobile first MTP joint.

In the subacute stage, gentle plantar-dorsal glides of the first phalanx may be indicated to improve arthrokinematic mobility. On return to sport, the athlete should possess at least 90° of painless passive toe extension and have been screened for appropriate shoe selection. A steel spring plate in the toe box or rigid taping into plantar flexion should be used initially when resuming full participation. Grade III injuries with complete disruption of the plantar structures may require direct primary repair of the plantar capsuloligamentous complex, and it is expected that 4 months will be needed before return to sport and 6 to 12 months until the athlete is capable of performance at preinjury levels.[51]

Sesamoiditis

The two small sesamoid bones of the foot on the plantar surface of the first metatarsal head are embedded within the tendon of the flexor hallucis brevis. The sesamoids function to absorb and redistribute weight-bearing forces, decrease friction, and protect and enhance the power production of the short toe flexor. The medial or tibial sesamoid is often bipartite, and its appearance can be confused with a fracture. *Sesamoiditis* is a generic term for numerous conditions involving the sesamoids, including osteonecrosis, chondromalacia, and mechanical overload resulting in inflammation and possible avascular changes.[52]

Athletes most prone to medial sesamoid pathology are those with a rigid pes cavus, forefoot equinus, tight Achilles tendon, and plantar-flexed first ray.[52] Sesamoid pain also occurs in athletes with normal foot structure but whose activities require repetitive maximal dorsiflexion of the first MTP joint, which results in excessive impact loading stress on the sesamoids.

The athlete usually complains of tenderness and swelling of the first metatarsal head and pain with weight bearing and passive dorsiflexion or active plantar flexion of the first MTP joint. Pressure from improperly placed cleats on an athletic shoe may be a source of further aggravation.

Initial treatment in the acute stage involves ice massage, antiinflammatory medications or cortisone injections, and rest. Pulsed phonophoresis and iontophoresis are alternative methods of combating the inflammatory response and may be of value in reducing symptoms. Definitive treatment must include relief of weight-bearing stress on the affected area. A custom-molded orthotic device with proximal elevation and a first ray cutout combined with a Morton extension or carbon fiber forefoot plate to reduce forefoot motion and eliminate loading in the dorsiflexed position can provide this relief.[52]

ORTHOTIC THERAPY

The section on orthotic therapy can be found in the online appendix to this chapter on Expert Consult @ www.expertconsult.com.

Step 1: Prepare the plantar surface of the foot and toe with tape adherent. Encircle the first phalanx and midfoot with anchor strips. Do not extend the anchor strip to the IP joint; this would cause the MTP joint to extend during the taping technique.

Step 2: Using precut moleskin or 1″ inelastic tape, run a checkrein on the plantar-medial surface of the foot to limit dorsiflexion and adduction of the first MTP joint. Enclose the checkrein with elastic tape.

Step 3: Modify the athletic shoe. Ensure proper length to decrease the lever arm effect on the joint. Place a spring steel, polyethylene, or orthoplast insert in the shoe to increase the rigidity of the distal forefoot.

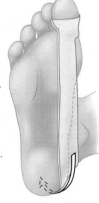

FIGURE 20-47 Turf toe taping technique to prevent excessive hyperextension of the first metatarsophalangeal (*MTP*) joint. *IP*, Interphalangeal.

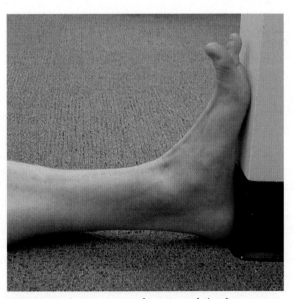

FIGURE 20-48 Active range of motion of the first metatarsophalangeal joint with the first metatarsal head stabilized.

RETURN TO SPORT

The final component of lower leg rehabilitation is the functional progression and testing program, which must precede return to sport. The concept of functional progression mandates a logical and ordered sequence of rehabilitative activities leading back to previous performance. Athletes must be educated to appreciate that they cannot simply resume the activities that led to the initial injury when the pain and swelling have subsided. Even return of normal strength, flexibility, and endurance does not automatically ensure safe resumption of activity. Rehabilitative exercise programs cannot duplicate the speed, force, and stress that normal high-speed athletic activities demand.

Clinical Pearl #13

Tissues remodel according to stimulus imposed on them. Consequently, selection of rehabilitation activities should be based on the unique functional requirement of the athlete and the desired outcome.

For these reasons, the athlete must be gradually guided back to activity by breaking down the component movements of the sport and addressing them in inverse order of difficulty. An example of such progression for an athlete with a lower extremity injury might be the following:

Non–weight-bearing exercise
Partial weight-bearing exercise
Full weight-bearing exercise
Balance training on a table surface
Walking
Balance training on a labile surface
Alternating walking-jogging
Jogging
Running
Jumping and hopping
Backpedaling
Figure-of-eight running
Cutting and twisting
Zigzag running
Plyometrics

The program is structured according to the specific demands of the athlete's sport and the pathologic stress of the injury. Modifications are appropriate, depending on the goals and aspirations of the athlete. Specific criteria that dictate progression from one functional level to the next must be defined precisely. It is the responsibility of the rehabilitation professional to provide the framework and specifics by which the athlete will function and progress.

When the athlete has completed the functional progression program and is psychologically prepared to return to sport, an objective evaluation of physical readiness should be performed. Because physical characteristics alone are inadequate to predict functional capacity, objective functional testing is used to assist the clinician in determining the capabilities of the foot and ankle joints during sporting activities. These tests attempt to recreate in a controlled environment the forces that an athlete will encounter when unrestricted activity is allowed.

Criteria for return to sport should include absence or control of pain, swelling, and spasm; normal range of motion; 85% to 90% of strength; and functional normality with appropriate control, carriage, and confidence. Table 20-17 is a sample functional evaluation form used for lower leg injuries. It contains testing maneuvers and activities that can be used to judge an athlete's readiness to perform with symmetric functional normality.

Finally, a number of self-report outcome measurement tools are available to gauge an athlete's status and progress. The established reliability, validity, and responsiveness of these assessment tools lend confidence to the decision-making process in determining the effectiveness of treatment interventions and the readiness for safe resumption of athletic activities. Outcome instruments that have met these criteria include the Foot and Ankle Ability Measure, Foot Function Index, Foot Health Status Questionnaire, Foot and Ankle Disability Index, and Lower Extremity Functional Scale.[53,54]

Clinical Pearl #14

The athlete's own sense of function is probably the single best predictor of the ability to return to sport. When self-confidence and carriage are restored, functional testing can be used to determine the athlete's physical capability.

CONCLUSION

Arthrokinematic Considerations

- Motion about a joint occurs in a direction that is perfectly perpendicular to the orientation of its axis.
- The resting position of a joint is the position at which to initiate treatment because the intracapsular space is large, ligamentous support is lax, and arthrokinematic spin, glide, and roll are maximized.
- The closed-pack position of a joint is a position that is dynamically stable because the joint surfaces are maximally congruent and ligamentous support is taut.
- Physiologic accessory motions are necessary for full, pain-free range of motion.
- Accessory motion at the tibiofibular joints is necessary for full and pain-free talocrural and subtalar joint motion.
- The talocrural joint is a structurally congruent mortise joint that facilitates primarily sagittal plane motion.
- The talus moves passively on the calcaneus at the subtalar joint to couple the function of the foot with the rest of the proximal kinetic chain.
- The position of the subtalar joint influences the mobility of the midtarsal joint and first ray while coupling the transverse plane rotation of the proximal kinetic chain.
- Interaction at the axes of the midtarsal joint allow the foot to be both a mobile adaptor and rigid lever during the gait cycle.

Muscular Function

- The muscles of the foot and leg work in a triplanar fashion, with their impact being determined by their location relative to the each joint axis that they cross.

Table 20-17 Foot and Ankle Functional Testing Form

Name _____   Involved Extremity_____

HOP/JUMP TESTS

Test	Parameter	Uninvolved	Involved	% Deficit
Unilateral standing long jump Unilateral standing triple jump	Distance in inches	_____ inches _____ inches	_____ inches _____ inches	
Single-leg 20-foot hop	Time in seconds	_____ sec	_____ sec	
Single-leg 20-foot crossover hop	Time in seconds	_____ sec	_____ sec	
Four-square hop	# of hops in _____ sec	_____ hops	_____ hops	
Single-leg vertical jump	Height in inches	_____ inches	_____ inches	

EXCURSION TESTS

Test	Parameter	Uninvolved	Involved	% Deficit
Single-leg knee flexion	Knee flexion depth Ankle dorsiflexion position	_____ degrees _____ degrees	_____ degrees _____ degrees	
Hip rotation in unilateral stance	Degree of CW rotation Degree of CCW rotation	_____ degrees _____ degrees	_____ degrees _____ degrees	
Hip adduction in unilateral stance	Linear distance lateral foot is from wall	_____ cm	_____ cm	
Knee abduction in unilateral stance	Linear distance from medial foot to plumb line dropping from medial knee	_____ cm	_____ cm	

STRENGTH TESTS

Test	Parameter	Uninvolved	Involved	% Deficit
Single leg squats @ _____% BW	Amount and type of resistance	_____ reps	_____ reps	
Unilateral heel raises	Amount and type of resistance	_____ reps	_____ reps	
Unilateral toe raises	Amount and type of resistance	_____ reps	_____ reps	

FUNCTIONAL TESTS

Test	Parameter	Uninvolved	Involved	% Deficit
Stork stand	Time	_____ sec	_____ sec	
Stance reach	Direction and distance	_____ inches	_____ inches	
Functional movement screen: bilateral deep squat	0-3 ordinal scale score			
Functional movement screen: hurdle step	0-3 ordinal scale score			
Functional movement screen: in-line lunge	0-3 ordinal scale score			
Shuttle run	Time	_____ sec	_____ sec	
_____ yd dash	Time	_____ sec	_____ sec	

SUMMARY:

RECOMMENDATIONS:

FUNCTIONAL SCORE = _____% ____ Full participation ____ Participation with restrictions _____ No participation

BW, Body weight; *CW,* clockwise; *CCW,* counterclockwise.

- The functional articulation of the first ray is controlled by the peroneus longus and provides a means of stabilizing the medial aspect of the foot during midstance
- The muscles of the foot and leg work eccentrically early in the early stance phase of gait to control pronation and then reverse their function in late stance to concentrically accelerate propulsion.

Clinical Examination

- A thorough subjective history provides information regarding the stage, intensity, nature, and severity of the injury while allowing the clinician to hone in on provocative maneuvers or special tests that may best reproduce the complaint.
- Identification of structural abnormalities or deviations may predict impairments or functional limitations.
- Normal gastrocnemius flexibility allows 10° of dorsiflexion with the knee extended and the subtalar joint in a neutral position. Normal soleus flexibility would allow an additional 10° of dorsiflexion motion when the knee is unlocked to slacken gastrocnemius.
- Normal subtalar motion allows approximately 10° of calcaneal eversion and 20° of calcaneal inversion from a position in which the bisection of the calcaneus is parallel to the bisection of the distal third of the leg.
- Ideal biomechanical structure requires that the posterior calcaneal bisection be parallel to the bisection of the distal third of the leg, the plantar plane of the rearfoot be parallel to the plantar plane of the central three metatarsal heads, and the first and fifth metatarsal heads be parallel to the central three metatarsal heads when the subtalar joint is in a neutral position.
- Observational gait analysis is a powerful examination tool that can be used in conjunction with static examination techniques to detect the source of pathology, impairments, or functional limitations.
- Prolonged or excessive subtalar hyperpronation during the stance phase of gait can be caused by a variety of skeletal or soft tissue abnormalities, asymmetries, and deviations.
- Special ligamentous tests can be used to detect excessive laxity at the inferior tibiofibular, talocrural, and midtarsal joints.

Lower Leg, Ankle, and Foot Injuries/Management

- Tendinopathies are typically the result of abnormal anatomic structure, altered biomechanics, and improper training techniques or progression. Treatment should be aimed at restoring the tensile, eccentric capability of the involved musculotendinous unit.
- Rehabilitation of inversion sprains should focus on dynamic frontal plane muscular control, protection and support of the lateral ligaments, and restoration of proprioceptive abilities.
- Rehabilitation of high ankle sprains at the tibiofibular joint is a slow process and should focus on protection against rotational forces of the tibia on a fixed foot.
- Restoration of motion following prolonged immobilization may require manual intervention, including specific graded soft tissue and joint mobilization techniques.

- A cavus foot with plantar fasciosis typically responds more slowly to conservative intervention, and emphasis should be placed on restoring joint mobility and soft tissue flexibility at the talocrural and first metatarsophalangeal joints.
- A planus foot with plantar fasciitis responds best to dynamic strengthening of the muscles that control subtalar pronation and orthotic correction or tape support along the medial longitudinal arch.

Orthotic Therapy

- Orthotic therapy is an important adjunct to the physical rehabilitation of injuries to the foot and ankle.

Return to Sport

- A process that includes the patient's self-report of function and objective measurement of physical capabilities should be used in determining progression of treatment and safe return to occupational or athletic activities.

REFERENCES

1. Root, W.L., Orient, W.P., and Weed, J.N. (1977): Clinical Biomechanics, Vol. II: Normal and Abnormal Function of the Foot. Los Angeles, Clinical Biomechanics.
2. Seibel, M.O. (1988): Foot Function. Baltimore, Lippincott Williams & Wilkins.
3. Maffulli, N. (1998): The clinical diagnosis of subcutaneous tear of the Achilles tendon. A prospective study in 174 patients. Am. J. Sports Med., 26:266–270.
4. Khan, R.J., Fick, D., Keough, A., et al. (2005): Treatment of Achilles tendon ruptures. A meta-analysis of randomized controlled trials. J. Bone Joint Surg. Br., 87:2202–2210.
5. Suchak, A.A., Spooner, C., Reid, D.C., and Jomha, N.D. (2006): Postoperative rehabilitation protocols for Achilles tendon ruptures: A meta-analysis. Clin. Orthop. Relat. Res., 445:216–221.
6. Metz, R., Verleisdonk, E.J., van der Heijden, G.J., et al. (2008): Acute Achilles tendon rupture: Minimally invasive surgery versus nonoperative treatment with immediate full weightbearing—a randomized controlled trial. Am. J. Sports Med., 36:1688–1694.
7. Longo, U.G., Ronga, M., and Maffulli, N. (2009): Achilles tendinopathy. Sports Med. Arthrosc. Rev., 17:112–116.
8. Smith, M., Brooker, S., Vicenzino, B., and McPoil, T. (2004): The use of anti-pronation taping to assess suitability of an orthotic prescription: Case report. Aust. J. Physiother., 50:111–113.
9. Carcia, C.R., Martin, R.L., Houck, J., Wukich, D.K.Orthopaedic Section of the American Physical Therapy Association. (2010): Achilles pain, stiffness, and muscle power deficits: Achilles tendinitis. J. Orthop. Sports Phys. Ther., 40:(9):A1–A26.
10. Bowring, B., and Chockalingam, N. (2010): Conservative treatment of tibialis tendon dysfunction. A review. Foot, 20:18–26.
11. Michelson, J., and Dunn, L. (2005): Tenosynovitis of the flexor hallucis longus. A clinical study of the spectrum of presentation and treatment. Foot Ankle Int., 26:291–303.
12. Pedowitz, R.A., Hargens, A., Mubarak, S.J., and Gershuni, D.H. (1990): Modified criteria for the objective diagnosis of chronic syndrome of the leg. Am. J. Sports Med., 18:35–40.
13. Freeman, M.A.R., Dean, M.R.E., and Hanham, I.W.F. (1965): The etiology and prevention of functional instability of the foot. J. Bone Joint Surg. Br., 47:678–685.
14. Zech, A., Hübscher, M., Vogt, L., et al. (2010): Balance training for neuromuscular control and performance enhancement: A systematic review. J. Athl. Train., 45:392–403.
15. Bleakley, C.M., O'Connor, S.R., Tully, M.A., et al. (2010): Effect of accelerated rehabilitation on function after ankle sprain: Randomised controlled trial. BMJ, May 10;340:c1964.
16. Eiff, M.P., Smith, A.T., and Smith, G.E. (1994): Early mobilization versus immobilization in the treatment of lateral ankle sprains. Am. J. Sports Med., 22:83–87.
17. Moiler, K., Hall, T., and Robinson, K. (2006): The role of fibular tape in the prevention of ankle injury in basketball: A pilot study. J. Orthop. Sports Phys. Ther., 36:661–668.
18. Vicenzino, B., Paungmali, A., and Teys, P. (2007): Mulligan's mobilization-with-movement, positional faults and pain relief: Current concepts for a critical review of the literature. Man. Ther., 12:98–108.
19. Eisenhart, A.W., Gaeta, T.J., and Yens, D.P. (2003): Osteopathic manipulative treatment in the emergency department for patients with acute ankle injuries. J. Am. Osteopath. Assoc., 103:417–421.
20. López-Rodríguez, S., Fernández de-Las-Peñas, C., Alburquerque-Sendín, F., et al. (2007): Immediate effect of manipulation of the talocrural joint on stabilometry and bardodometry in patients with ankle sprain. J. Manipulative Physiol. Ther., 30:186–192.
21. Pellow, J.E., and Brantingham, J.W. (2001): The efficacy of adjusting the ankle in the treatment of subacute and chronic grade I and grade II ankle inversion sprains. J. Manipulative Physiol. Ther., 24:17–24.

22. Whitman, J.M., Childs, J.D., and Walker, V. (2005): The use of manipulation in a patient with an ankle sprain injury not responding to conventional management: A case report. Man. Ther., 10:224–231.

23. Whitman, J.M., Cleland, J.A., Mintken, P.E., et al. (2009): Predicting short-term response to thrust and nonthrust manipulation and exercise in patients post inversion ankle sprain. J. Orthop. Sports Phys. Ther., 39:188–200.

24. Bullock-Saxton, J.E. (1994): Local sensation and altered hip muscle function following severe ankle sprain. Phys. Ther., 74:17–31.

25. Lin, C.F., Gross, M.L., and Weinhold, P. (2006): Ankle syndesmosis injuries: Anatomy, biomechanics, mechanism of injury, and clinical guidelines for diagnosis and intervention. J. Orthop. Sports Phys. Ther., 36:372–384.

26. Williams, G.N., Jones, M.H., and Amendola, A. (2007): Syndesmotic ankle sprains in athletes. Am. J. Sports Med., 35:1197–1207.

27. Norkus, S.A., and Floyd, R.T. (2001): The anatomy and mechanism of syndesmotic sprains. J. Athl. Train., 36:68–73.

28. Gerber, J.P., Williams, G.N., Scoville, C.R., et al. (1998): Persistent disability associated with ankle sprains: A prospective examination of an athletic population. Foot Ankle Int., 19:653–660.

29. Alonso, A., Khoury, L., and Adams, R. (1998): Clinical tests for ankle syndesmosis injury: Reliability and prediction of return to function. J. Orthop. Sports Phys. Ther., 27:276–284.

30. Nussbaum, E.D., Hosea, T.M., Sieler, S.D., et al. (2001): Prospective evaluation of syndesmotic ankle sprains without diastasis. Am. J. Sports Med., 29:31–35.

31. Roth, J.A., Taylor, W.C., and Whalden, J. (2010): Peroneal tendon subluxation: The other lateral ankle injury. Br. J. Sports Med., 44:1047–1053.

32. Maquirriain, J. (2005): Posterior ankle impingement syndrome. J. Am. Acad. Orthop. Surg., 13:365–371.

33. Hendrix, C.L. (2005): Calcaneal apophysitis (Sever disease). Clin. Podiatr. Med. Surg., 22:55–62.

34. Aronow, M.S. (2005): Posterior heel pain (retrocalcaneal bursitis, insertional and non-insertional Achilles tendinopathy). Clin. Podiatr. Med. Surg., 22:19–43.

35. Lemont, H., Ammirati, K.M., and Usen, N. (2003): Plantar fasciitis: A degenerative process (fasciosis) without inflammation. J. Am. Podiatr. Med. Assoc., 93:234–237.

36. McPoil, T.G., Martin, R.L., Cornwall, M.W., et al. (2008): Heel pain—plantar fasciitis: Clinical practice guidelines linked to the international classification of function, disability, and health from the orthopaedic section of the American Physical Therapy Association. J. Orthop. Sports Phys. Ther., 38(4):A1–A18.

37. Irving, D.B., Cook, J.L., and Menz, H.B. (2006): Factors associated with chronic plantar heel pain: A systematic review. J. Sci. Med. Sport, 9:11–12.

38. Riddle, D.L., Pulisic, M., and Sparrow, K. (2004): Impact of demographic and impairment-related variables on disability associated with plantar fasciitis. Foot Ankle Int., 25:311–317.

39. Creighton, D.S., and Olson, V.L. (1987): Evaluation of range of motion of the first metatarsophalangeal joint in runners with plantar fasciitis. J. Orthop. Sports Phys. Ther., 8:357–361.

40. Allen, R.H., and Gross, M.T. (2003): Toe flexors strength and passive extension range of motion of the first metatarsophalangeal joint in individuals with plantar fasciitis. J. Orthop. Sports Phys. Ther., 33:468–478.

41. Baxter, D.E., and Thigpen, C.M. (1984): Heel pain—operative results. Foot Ankle, 5:16–25.

42. Wolgin, M., Cook, C., Graham, C., and Mauldin, D. (1994): Conservative treatment of plantar pain: Long-term follow-up. Foot Ankle Int., 15:97–102.

43. Healy, K., and Chen, K. (2010): Plantar fasciitis: Current diagnostic modalities and treatment. Clin. Podiatr. Med. Surg., 27:369–380.

44. Jennings, J., and Davies, G.J. (2005): Treatment of cuboid syndrome secondary to lateral ankle sprains: A case series. J. Orthop. Sports Phys. Ther., 35:409–415.

45. Hughes, L.Y. (1985): Biomechanical analysis of the foot and ankle to developing stress fractures. J. Orthop. Sports Phys. Ther., 7:96–101.

46. Chuckpaiwong, B., Queen, R., Easley, M.E., and Nunley, J.A. (2008): Distinguishing Jones and proximal diaphyseal fractures of the fifth metatarsal. Clin. Orthop. Relat. Res., 466:1966–1970.

47. Vu, D., McDiarmid, T., Aukerman, D., and Brown, M. (2006): Clinical inquiries. What is the most effective management of acute fractures of the base of the fifth metatarsal. J. Fam. Pract., 55:713–717.

48. Porter, D.A., Duncan, M., and Meyer, S.F. (2005): Fifth metatarsal Jones fracture fixation with a 4.5-mm cannulated stainless steel screw in the competitive and recreational athlete. Am. J. Sports Med, 33:726–733.

49. Clinical Practice Guideline Forefoot Disorders Panel Thomas, J.L., Blitch, E.L., Chaney, D.M., et al. (2009): Diagnosis and treatment of forefoot disorders. Section 3. Morton's intermetatarsal neuroma. J. Foot Ankle Surg, 48:251–256.

50. Anderson, R.B., Hunt, K.J., and McCormick, J.J. (2010): Management of common sports-related injuries about the foot and ankle. J. Am. Acad. Orthop. Surg., 18:546–556.

51. McCormick, J.J., and Anderson, R.B. (2010): Rehabilitation following turf toe injury and plantar plate repair. Clin. Sports Med., 29:313–323.

52. Cohen, B.E. (2009): Hallux sesamoid disorders. Foot Ankle Clin. N. Am., 14:91–104.

53. Hale, S., and Hertel, J. (2005): Reliability and sensitivity of the foot and ankle disability index in subjects with chronic ankle instability. J. Athl. Train., 40:35–40.

54. Martin, R.L., and Irrgang, J.L. (2007): A survey of self-report outcome instruments for the foot and ankle. J. Orthop. Sports Phys. Ther., 37:72–84.

21

Clinical Gait Assessment

R. Barry Dale, PT, PhD, DPT, ATC, SCS, OCS, CSCS

CHAPTER OBJECTIVES

- Define gait and describe its various phases.
- Discuss the various joint angular kinematics and muscle activation requirements in the various phases of gait.
- Explain the procedure for static assessment of standing posture.

- Discuss various methods for clinical gait assessment.
- Describe common gait abnormalities.

Walking becomes almost automatic at an early age and occurs with very little thought or effort. Because walking is a routine part of everyday life, it is often taken for granted until it becomes challenged because of injury or disease. Coincidently and unfortunately, morbidity and mortality rates increase dramatically when one's mobility becomes compromised.[1,2]

Abnormal gait patterns arise from traumatic injuries, diseases, or conditions of neurologic or musculoskeletal origin. Deviations in gait may also be associated with aberrant yet subclinical biomechanical abnormalities of the lower extremities. Clinicians should have a working knowledge of normal gait and possess the basic skills necessary to detect abnormal walking patterns. For example, information attained from gait assessment allows the clinician to determine functional abnormalities within joints of the lower extremities. Altogether, information from gait assessment should complement detailed examination of the individual joints of the lower extremities and spine. Therapeutic interventions are implemented according to the findings from such examinations.

This chapter provides an overview of the gait cycle. The purposes of this chapter are to present terminology describing human gait and the basic techniques of gait analysis, discuss normal characteristics of standing static posture, and discuss various pathologies in joints of the lower extremities and how they influence gait. A detailed presentation of gait is beyond the scope of this chapter, and the reader is referred to other sources for more specific information.[3]

TERMINOLOGY

Walking, or gait, could be described as "a series of catastrophes narrowly averted," the act of falling forward and catching oneself,[4] and the process of getting from point A to point B.[5] Gait is a continuous activity that is cyclic and repetitive. As is the case with other continuous activities, individuals are normally able to start or stop their gait with volition. Gait begins from a static standing position (see the section on static standing posture) as the person moves the center of mass forward. This forward excursion of the center of mass must be countered by forward movement of the base of support, or the person would not be able to maintain an upright position and would subsequently fall. The gait cycle occurs from one heel strike to the next heel strike on the same lower extremity (Fig. 21-1).[4-10]

The feet serve as the base of support and, unlike static postures, must move with the body during gait. During walking, at least one foot is always in contact with the ground (unlike running, which has a flight phase characterized by neither foot being in contact with the ground) (Fig. 21-2). Each forward movement of a foot is a step.[4-12] A stride consists of two steps, right and left, and represents the gait cycle.[4-12] The heel is the most commonly used point of reference because the heel is—or should be—the first point of contact with the supporting surface.

A stride can be further dissected into a stance phase, in which a foot is in contact with the ground, and a swing phase, characterized by the foot moving forward. Once the swing foot makes contact with the ground, it enters the stance phase again (Figs. 21-3 and 21-4). Thus, a complete gait cycle for each foot contains stance and swing phases. The phases of gait and the overall gait process contain various observable or measurable gait parameters.

Gait parameters may be recorded from kinematic or kinetic measurements. Kinematic gait evaluation assesses joint range of motion (ROM) and time and distance parameters without consideration of the forces involved.[7] Kinematic assessments

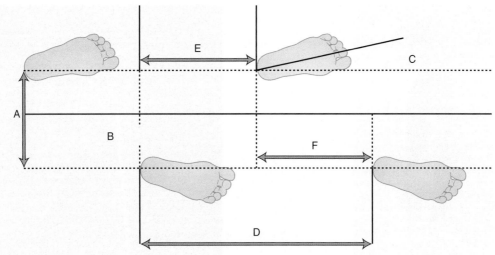

FIGURE 21-1 Temporal gait measurements taken with footprint impression techniques. *A*, Width of the base of support (step width); *B*, line of progression; *C*, foot (toe) angle; *D*, gait cycle, also stride length; *E*, left step length; *F*, right step length.

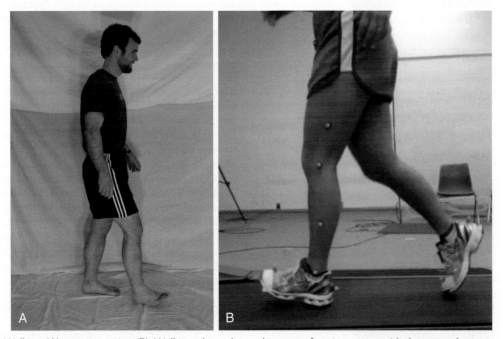

FIGURE 21-2 Walking (**A**) versus running (**B**). Walking always has at least one foot in contact with the ground, as opposed to running, which has a flight phase (no foot is in contact with the ground).

may be qualitative or quantitative and require relatively minimal equipment to perform. Kinetic assessments, in contrast, quantify the forces and muscle activity that occur during gait. Although kinetic assessments may be performed in the clinic, most take place in special research laboratories equipped with motion analysis systems, electromyography, force plates, and sophisticated walkways (Fig. 21-5). Even though laboratory gait analysis of kinetic gait parameters offers additional information about an athlete's gait, the focus of this chapter is on the techniques and terminology associated with clinical kinematic gait assessment. It is recommended that athletes be referred for more sophisticated analysis if the gait abnormalities are too complicated for clinical assessment.

A CLOSER LOOK AT THE GAIT PHASES

The overall gait cycle for the right lower extremity begins with right foot contact, which initiates double support, followed by right single support, double support again, and the right swing phase (a swing phase consists of an initial or acceleration swing phase, midswing phase, and terminal or deceleration phase) (Fig. 21-6). It is important to refer to the side (i.e., right or left) of the lower extremity when referring to the phases of gait. In addition, it is easier to consider only one lower extremity at a time as it undergoes the gait cycle until a level of comfort is achieved with the terminology associated with gait. See Table 21-1 for a comparison of gait terminologies. Caution should be used when

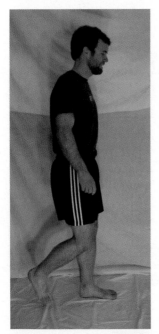

FIGURE 21-3 Swing phase.

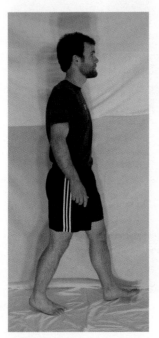

FIGURE 21-4 Stance phase.

interpreting the kinematic data presented because they vary considerably with altered walking speeds.[5,7,15]

Stance Phase

Recall that stance phase implies that a foot is in contact with the ground, which normally accounts for approximately 60% of the gait cycle.[10,11] A closer look at the stance phase reveals a portion of stance in which both feet are in contact with the ground, called the double-support phase, and a portion in which only one foot is in contact with the ground, called the single-support phase (Fig. 21-7). The double-support phase may be further divided

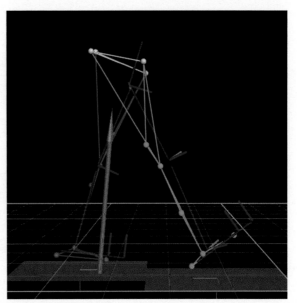

FIGURE 21-5 This graphic depicts three-dimensional kinematic and kinetic data from a gait laboratory. Note the ground reaction force (*red arrow*) during the stance phase of the left lower extremity (*red lines* connecting the *red spheres*). *(Photo courtesy Dr. R. Barry Dale and the University of Tennessee at Chattanooga Department of Physical Therapy.)*

into initial double-support and terminal double-support phases (Figs. 21-8 and 21-9).[5-7,12] This terminology qualifies portions of double support by describing the functional activity in the lower extremities: (1) on heel contact with the ground in which the lower extremity comes to a stop (initial double support) and (2) when the heel leaves the surface as the foot thrusts against the ground to prepare the lower extremity for the forward propulsion of swing phase (terminal double support).[5-7,12] Each lower extremity counters the opposite lower extremity during these phases of double support. Consider the following example: when the right heel makes contact with the ground, the foot is stopping, or braking, whereas the left foot is accelerating, or thrusting, to prepare for the swing phase. Thus, during these periods of double support, each lower extremity acts the opposite of its counterpart.

Angular Kinematics and Muscle Activity: Initial Double Support

Recall that double support inherently implies that both feet are in contact with the ground. One limb is decelerating (initial double support) while the other is preparing to accelerate (terminal double support). In the following descriptions, the reference limb is in the initial double-support phase. Initial double support technically occurs between ipsilateral heel contact and contralateral toe-off and accounts for approximately the first 10% of the gait cycle (see Fig. 21-8).[16]

The ankle, immediately before contact with the ground, is in a neutral position (not particularly in dorsiflexion or plantar flexion). When the heel makes contact with the ground, the ankle dorsiflexors act eccentrically to control the foot as it comes to rest on the ground at approximately 7° of plantar flexion.[12] The knee is in extension on contact and moves to about 20° of flexion under eccentric control of the knee extensors.[12] The hip is flexed to approximately 30° on heel contact and is controlled by the hip extensors, which serve to control forward momentum of the trunk.[14] The pelvis is in

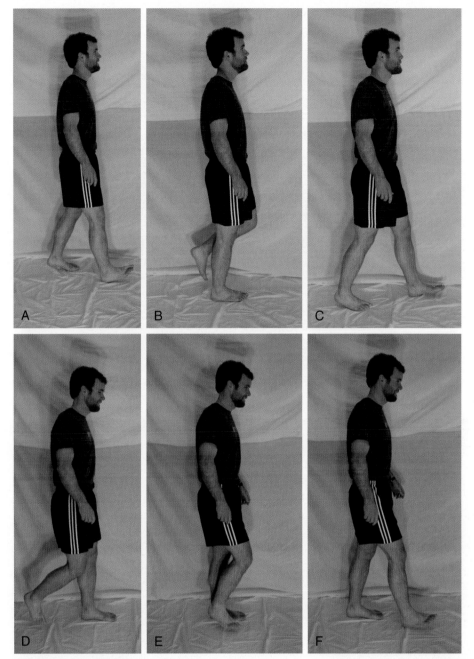

FIGURE 21-6 Composite of the entire gait cycle. **A,** Right initial double support. **B,** Right single support. **C,** Right terminal double support. **D,** Right initial swing phase. **E,** Right midswing phase. **F,** Right terminal swing phase.

Table 21-1 **Comparison of Gait Terminologies**

	Perry/Ranchos Los Amigos[11]	Wall[12]	Hoppenfeld[13]	Whittle[14]

Stance	Initial double stance:
	   Initial heel contact
	   Loading response
		Braking double support	Heel strike	Loading response

	Single limb support:
	   Midstance
	   Terminal stance
		Single support	Foot flat
			Midstance
				Midstance

	Terminal double stance
	   Preswing
		Thrusting double support	Push-off	Terminal stance
				   Preswing

Swing	Initial swing Midswing Terminal swing	Swing	Acceleration swing Midswing Deceleration swing	Initial swing Midswing Terminal swing

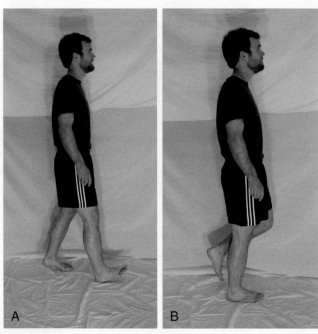

FIGURE 21-7 Double (**A**) versus single (**B**) support.

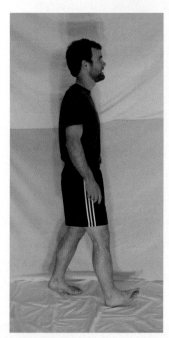

FIGURE 21-8 Initial double-support phase (right foot).

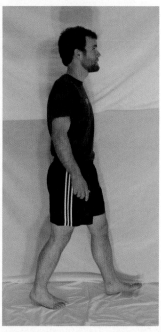

FIGURE 21-9 Terminal double-support phase (right foot).

neutral during initial double support. Eccentric actions of the ankle dorsiflexors and knee and hip extensors provide the braking characteristics, or controlled antagonistic motions, of this phase.

Angular Kinematics and Muscle Activity: Single Support

From initial double support, the foot that recently made contact with the ground begins to bear the entire weight of the body as the contralateral foot leaves the ground during the early swing phase. The foot remaining in contact with the ground is in the single-support phase (see Fig. 21-7).

The ankle moves from the plantar flexion associated with initial double support to approximately 10° of dorsiflexion during the single-support phase. The plantar flexors serve to control momentum of the tibia as it rotates forward on the fixed ankle.

The knee moves from 20° of flexion during the initial double-support phase to full extension in single support. This movement is initiated by concentric activity of the knee extensors, which is facilitated by plantar flexor stabilization of the tibia. The body's forward momentum produces the final degrees of knee extension during the single-support phase.[11]

In the single-support phase, the hip moves to a neutral position by extending from its flexed position during the initial double-support phase. The hip extensors activate to concentrically produce this movement.

The pelvis moves from neutral during initial double support to a laterally tilted position that is away from the leg that is in late single support. The gluteus medius of the leg in single support eccentrically controls this excursion.

Angular Kinematics and Muscle Activity: Terminal Double Support

The stance leg moves from single support into terminal double support as the contralateral swing leg makes contact with the ground (thus, the contralateral leg is entering the initial double-support phase). Terminal double support prepares the leg for the swing phase and occurs between contralateral heel contact and ipsilateral toe-off (see Fig. 21-9).[16]

Ankle motion moves from dorsiflexion to plantar flexion in the transition from the single-support to the terminal double-support phase. Plantar flexion reaches approximately 20° at the end of double support as the leg accelerates into the initial swing phase. Concentric activity of the plantar flexors produces this movement.

The knee moves from extension during single support to approximately 35° of flexion at the end of double support. Concentric plantar flexor activity, change in body position, and gravity contribute to this motion.[11]

Hip motion progresses from neutral to approximately 20° of extension at the onset of the terminal double-support phase, which is produced by the continued activity of the hip extensors. At the end of terminal double support, the hip flexes under the influence of concentric hip flexor activity.

The pelvis is level during single support but tilts downward toward the lower extremity that is in terminal double support. Posterior pelvic rotation approaches approximately 4° during terminal double support.

Swing Phase

The advancing lower extremity is not in contact with the ground during the swing phase, which accounts for 40% of the gait cycle.[10] The swing phase consists of three subphases: initial, midswing, and terminal (see Table 21-1 for comparative terminology).[3] The initial swing phase (Fig. 21-10) immediately follows terminal double support as the toe leaves the supporting surface (toe-off). The midswing phase follows the initial phase (Fig. 21-11). During midswing, the lower extremity reaches terminal velocity. However, the lower extremity continues forward until it approaches the end of its excursion of motion and begins to decelerate. The terminal swing phase occurs when the lower extremity slows in preparation for contact with the ground (Fig. 21-12). A discussion of the initial, midswing, and terminal swing subphases follows.

Angular Kinematics and Muscle Activity: Acceleration Swing Phase

During the initial swing phase, also known as the acceleration swing phase, the foot leaves contact with the ground (see Fig. 21-10). The toe should be the last portion of the foot that has contact with the ground, which is known as toe-off. Dorsiflexion of the ankle occurs during initial swing as it moves to 10° of plantar flexion from the approximately 20° of plantar flexion obtained in terminal double support. The dorsiflexors work concentrically to produce this motion.

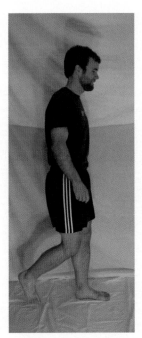

FIGURE 21-10 Initial swing phase (right foot).

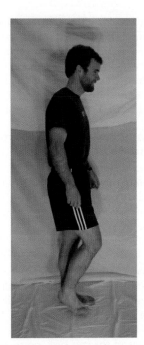

FIGURE 21-11 Midswing phase (right foot).

The knee is flexed to about 35° during initial swing, which is caused by tibial inertia from rapid hip flexion and concentric knee flexor activity.[11] Hip flexion reaches approximately 20° as a result of concentric hip flexor activity. The pelvis is in posterior rotation but begins to rotate anteriorly as it follows the swing leg in its forward motion.

Angular Kinematics and Muscle Activity: Midswing Phase

During the midswing phase, the lower extremity continues its forward flight (see Fig. 21-11). In midswing, limb velocity plateaus with respect to the initial swing phase. The ankle continues to dorsiflex

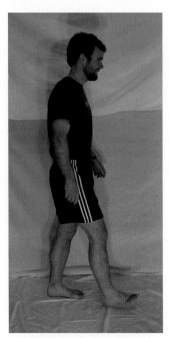

FIGURE 21-12 Terminal swing phase (right foot).

and attains a neutral position from concentric activity of the dorsiflexors. At the beginning of midswing, the knee has reached approximately 60° of flexion, and the knee then begins to extend under the influence of gravity and its forward momentum. Eccentric knee flexor activity serves to control this movement. Hip flexion continues to increase to approximately 30° from concentric activity of the hip flexors. The pelvis is level and in neutral rotation.

Angular Kinematics and Muscle Activity: Terminal Swing Phase

The terminal, or deceleration, swing phase is the final subphase of the lower extremity's forward flight path (see Fig. 21-12). The limb must slow in preparation for contact with the ground. The terminal swing phase ends with heel contact, which begins the double-support stance phase again.

The ankle continues in a neutral position that remains until heel contact. The knee continues to extend and reaches 0° at the end of swing phase, controlled by eccentric knee flexor activity. Hip flexion reaches 30°, but muscle activity shifts from concentric hip flexion to eccentric hip extension, which decelerates the limb in preparation for contact with the ground. The pelvis rotates forward approximately 4° during the terminal swing phase.

The descriptions of the gait cycle portrayed in this section are concise and intended to provide a basic overview. For more information on the gait cycle, the reader is referred to additional sources.[11,12,17,18]

ASSESSMENT

Static Assessment of Standing Posture

Upright standing posture is discussed before gait analysis techniques because upright standing is the posture in which walking occurs. In addition to its potential effect on gait, abnormal posture appears to play a role in predisposition to injury.[19-21] Deviations from normal posture are considered abnormalities or

malalignments. Sometimes postural abnormalities cause deviations in gait, but it is important to note that not all gait deviations are caused by postural abnormalities. Furthermore, not all gait deviations are evident in a static postural assessment. The clinician should perform both static standing posture and dynamic gait assessments for a comprehensive clinical picture of the athlete.

Clinical postural assessment is subjective. Whenever feasible, the athlete should remove as much clothing as possible to allow visualization of anatomic landmarks. It may be helpful to mark various landmarks with a grease pen, a water-based marker, or colored stickers to aid visual assessment (see Box 21-1 for list of common landmarks to assess during evaluation of posture). A plumb line should be used to provide the examiner with a true reference to vertical. Photography and videography increase the reliability of postural assessment.[22,23] Image-processing applications such as Image J* have been validated for photographic assessment.[24,25] In addition, a posture grid† placed in the background of the respective view allows quantification of deviations in posture (Fig. 21-13). Static postures should be assessed from the anterior, lateral, oblique, and posterior views. These respective views provide a comprehensive postural assessment.

Anterior View

The plumb line in the anterior view is in the sagittal plane. The plumb line should pass from the middle of the cranium and bisect the body into right and left portions as it passes down the midline of the trunk (Fig. 21-14). Plumb line assessment allows the clinician to detect subtle deviations in posture associated with asymmetry.

---

*Image J is an open-source image processing and analysis tool written in Java. It runs as 32- or 64-bit modes on Linux, Mac OS X, and Windows (http://rsbweb.nih.gov/ij/). One can import video files and then analyze individual frames with various analysis tools within the application. The angle-drawing tool is particularly helpful to estimate joint angle kinematics.
†Some photographic editing applications allow the superimposition of gridlines on photographs. This would serve as a substitute for a physical posture grid and plumb line.

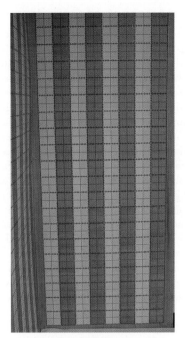

FIGURE 21-13 Posture grid.

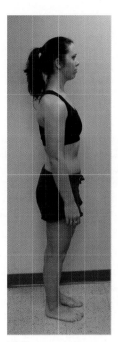

FIGURE 21-15 Posture assessment: lateral view.

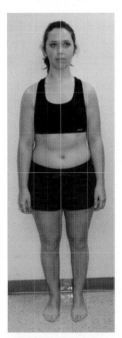

FIGURE 21-14 Posture assessment: anterior view.

Beginning proximally, the position of the head, jaw, and nose is assessed. The head and neck should be in a neutral position and straight on the shoulders. Abnormal findings commonly include cervical rotation or lateral flexion to one side. A normal jaw posture implies that the lips are approximated with the teeth slightly apart while the tongue rests on the roof of the mouth posterior to the upper row of teeth. The nose is aligned with the manubrium and xiphoid process of the sternum.

The shoulders should be even in height, although the dominant shoulder may appear somewhat lower in well-developed individuals. Trapezius muscle bulk is equal on both sides but may be somewhat increased on the dominant shoulder.

The lower extremities should also have symmetry in the anterior view. Two particular judgments are ankle position and leg interspace.[22] Ankle position is assessed by observing the medial longitudinal arch and the positions of the talus and navicular. If the person is flat-footed, the talus and navicular may appear relatively low in position, which is known as pes planus. A high arch, or pes cavus, is another abnormality observable from the anterior view. The position of the calcaneus also contributes to ankle posture but is obscured in the anterior view and must be assessed posteriorly (see the posterior view section). The leg interspace is the space between the lower extremities during normal standing. If an athlete has genu valgum (knock-kneed), the interspace is quite small in comparison to someone with genu varum (bowlegged).[22]

Lateral View

The lateral view of static standing posture should be made from both sides of the body. A straight line (plumb line) is placed at the center of the cranium and should run posterior to the ear, pass through the acromion process at the shoulder, split the lateral epicondyle of the humerus at the elbow, bisect the high point of the iliac crest, pass through the lateral femoral condyle at the knee, and complete its course anterior to the lateral malleolus at the ankle (Fig. 21-15).

As the athlete stands, specifically assess posture at different regions from the lateral view. Begin at the athlete's head and observe the chin, which should be in a neutral position and not excessively forward. Altogether, the chin and head should be balanced above the shoulders with an erect cervical spine. The spine has four normal curves: two kyphoses and two lordoses. Kyphosis is a natural rounding at the thoracic and sacral regions of the spine. Conversely, lordosis is a "backward" bending of the spine at the cervical and lumbar regions. All areas of the spine should be observed for excessive curvature. A normal lateral view consists of a slightly rounded thoracic region, an erect trunk with a flat abdomen, and a curved lumbar region.

The knees should be in alignment with the greater trochanter of the hip and the lateral malleolus of the distal end of the tibia. If the knee is posterior to a line drawn from the greater trochanter to the lateral malleolus, hyperextension or recurvatum is present.[22] Conversely, if the knee is forward of this imaginary line, the knee is excessively flexed.

Oblique View

An oblique view occurs at a 45° angle between the anterior and lateral views (Fig. 21-16). Watson and Mac Donncha recommended using the oblique view to supplement lateral assessment of the position of the scapula and spinal kyphoses and lordoses[22] because an abducted scapula may hamper the ability to detect abnormalities in spinal kyphosis and lordosis in the lateral view.

Posterior View

Postural assessment from the posterior view is similar to that in the anterior view. Shoulder position, knee interspace, and ankle position are all assessed, in addition to the overall symmetry of the body (Fig. 21-17). The major advantages of the posterior view are additional information regarding heel position and scoliosis screening of the spine.

Ankle position in the posterior view allows assessment of the heel. If the heel is tilted inward, such as occurs with pes planus, the term *hindfoot valgus* is used to describe the abnormality. Conversely, a heel tilted outward is termed *hindfoot varus*. These foot positions may also be present during gait, as discussed later.

Posterior postural views allow screening for scoliosis. Scoliosis is a lateral and sometimes rotatory curvature of the spine resulting in a "C"- or "S"-shaped curve as assessed from the posterior view.[22] Beginning proximally, shoulder and scapular symmetry are observed. Scoliosis may cause one shoulder to be elevated on one side. In addition, skin creases around spinous processes may be also be present on the convex sides of the curvatures.[22]

Clinical Assessment of Gait Parameters

Clinical gait analysis and assessment are the processes related to information gathering and clinical interpretation of the data collected, respectively.[26] Most often, limited time, space, and equipment are available to gather information, and consequently the clinician is forced to use visual inspection as the primary judgment tool.[10] Visual inspection alone, however, is limited because the information is temporarily stored in the clinician's memory. The clinician must decide whether the gait pattern observed is normal by comparing the observed gait with a mental image of what is considered to be "normal." Thus, previous gait assessment experience is invaluable because the quality of information gathered is highly dependent on the clinician's experience and skill.[27] Although observational gait analysis tends to be subjective, various measurements may be taken to increase objectivity.

Combining subjective gait observation with quantitative methods of measuring gait parameters increases objectivity during gait assessment. Methods of observation are presented and techniques that enhance objectivity are discussed in the sections that follow. Clinical gait analysis may be qualitative or quantitative.[10]

Regardless of whether the assessments are qualitative or quantitative, recording the performance with videotape allows the clinician to analyze gait outside the initial evaluation and document the current status of the athlete's condition.[6,16] Videotaped gait analysis also improves the reliability of observational gait assessments.[9,15,28-30] Reliability particularly increases when clinicians have considerable experience analyzing gait from videotape.[28] Recording gait with videotape also allows the clinician to derive general gait parameters and estimate joint ROM.[31] Use of slow-motion videotape analysis allows determination of the percentage of time spent in right and left single-limb support, swing phase, and double support.[6,16] Furthermore, videotape analysis is comparable, if not superior, to other methods of analysis when the athlete is wearing footwear.[28]

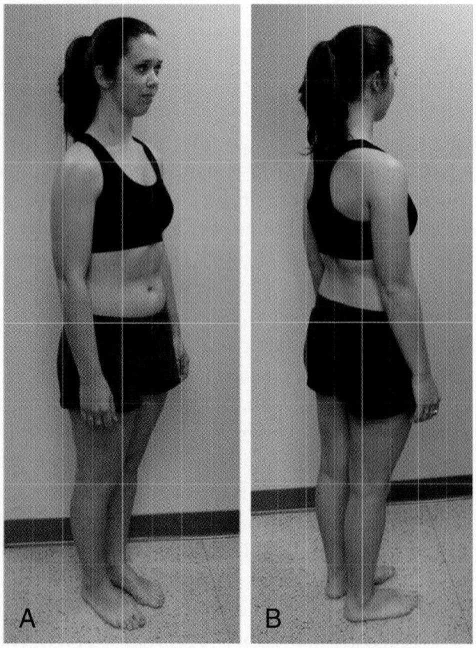

FIGURE 21-16 A and **B,** Posture assessment: oblique views.

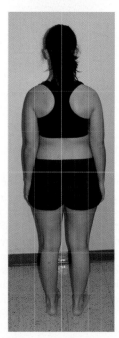

FIGURE 21-17 Posture assessment: posterior view.

Quantitative gait assessment requires proper recording methods to ensure reliability of the assessment. A stopwatch can be combined with methods that physically record the steps taken during the gait cycle, such as footprint impressions, which is an inexpensive and clinically useful technique (see Fig. 21-22).

A stopwatch can directly or indirectly determine the time taken to walk a given distance, cycle time, cadence, walking speed, step time, stride time, and stride length (stride length may be calculated from walking speed and stride time). For example, the clinician quantifies stride time by pressing the lap button for each heel strike of one extremity as the patient walks a given distance.[6,16] This gives an indication of respective stride times during the distance walked.

Adequate joint mobility, motor control, muscle strength, and metabolic capacity allow a person to walk "normally." Impairments in one or more of these factors can adversely affect walking ability. However, it may be difficult to relate abnormal findings to clinical rehabilitation when using even the most sophisticated means of gait analysis.[32] This is perhaps due to a difference in how gait has traditionally been analyzed, which is on the impairment level, versus how it affects the overall ability of an individual (disability level). Mulder et al argue that most gait assessment and analysis techniques, from the most complex to the most simplistic, focus on the impairment level, which often does not provide a functional view of gait.[32] Routine clinical gait analysis is commonly performed on an obstacle-free course, and the surface is usually level, which perhaps provides a limited view of gait and motor performance. However, this is not to say that gait assessment is altogether obsolete or useless. Rather, newer approaches to qualify gait in the context of function are under study.[32]

Examples of newer technologies include portable force platforms used by Footmaxx (Roanoke, VA) and the GAITrite system (Havertown, PA).[33] These technologies provide relatively quick feedback on the gait cycle and are considerably less expensive than laboratory methods (Fig. 21-18, *A* and *B*).

Observation and Visual Inspection of Gait

Gait observation follows assessment of static standing posture and also includes the same views used for static posture assessment: anterior, lateral, and posterior. The ordering of views is not important as long as a systematic approach is used. Clinical experience will help the practitioner develop a preferred system for performing gait observation. In addition, the clinician should get an overall or gross assessment of how the athlete moves as a unit. From there, a comprehensive review of the bilateral joints involved in the gait process should take place over repeated bouts of the athlete walking. The clinician may wish to observe one extremity at a time followed by the contralateral extremity or perhaps comparatively observe anatomic regions between the extremities. Paper or electronic evaluation forms assist the examiner in systematic gait observation. Such forms have been proprietarily developed by the Ranchos Los Amigos Pathokinesiology Laboratory[34] and the Rivermead Rehabilitation Centre.[35]

The athlete may be observed while walking back and forth on a stretch of floor space (walkway) or on a treadmill. Recommended distances for observing gait on a walkway range from 8 m (26 feet) up to 12 m (39 feet), depending on the walking speed of the athlete.[27] The width of the walkway should be 3 m (10 feet) for observation and a little wider, 4 m (13 feet), if videotaped.[27]

ANTERIOR VIEW

The anterior view allows assessment of movement in the frontal plane (Fig. 21-19) and permits the clinician to appreciate the stance leg and its acceptance of body weight. Although actual forces cannot be appreciated with observation, injured lower extremity joints often cannot fully accept the compressive loads associated with weight bearing. Injury may shorten the amount of time spent in stance phase on the affected lower extremity. Additionally, the base of support should be observed as well for width.

As the athlete walks toward the clinician, each joint is systematically observed from the feet up to pelvis. Whether the clinician begins at the feet or pelvis is a personal choice, although it is best to adopt a particular routine to ensure that nothing is omitted from the assessment. The feet are observed for their foot or "toe angle," which should be outward by approximately 5° to 7°.[36] Foot contact goes through several stages during stance phase. The heel makes first contact with the surface as the ankle is in a neutral position. This is followed by contact of the lateral aspect of the

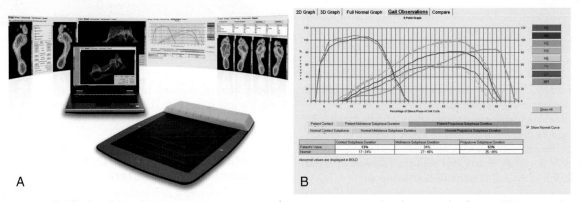

FIGURE 21-18 A, The FootMaxx Metascan system consists of a sensor, computer hardware, and software. This system is primarily used for orthotic prescription but offers basic gait analysis of the stance phase. **B,** Information obtained from the FootMaxx Metascan for the stance phase of gait. *(Courtesy FootMaxx, Roanoke, VA).*

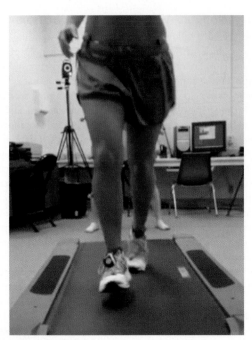

FIGURE 21-19 An anterior view of gait allows assessment of movement in the frontal plane.

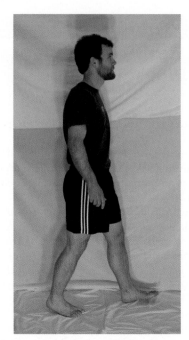

FIGURE 21-20 A lateral view of gait allows assessment of movement in the sagittal plane.

foot from a supinated position as the ankle plantar-flexes; thus, the fifth metatarsal normally makes contact with the ground before the first metatarsal. As the foot comes to rest on the floor, dorsiflexion and pronation occur and bring the body weight medially through the forefoot and away from the lateral side. Finally, during terminal double support in which the ankle is plantar-flexing, the heel leaves the ground and the forefoot and great hallux push against the surface to accelerate the lower extremity into the swing phase.[11] Genu varus and valgus may be observed, as well as hip rotation. Lateral tilt of the pelvis should be symmetric. The trunk should not lurch toward one side during the gait cycle, a condition often associated with an antalgic gait pattern. Weak hip abductors are associated with the aforementioned "lurch," as well as "pelvic drop" during the stance phase, which can be more subtle than the trunk sway associated with lurching. In addition, circumduction of the leg during the swing phase may be observed from the anterior view, which is associated with a functionally longer leg length (e.g., the knee braced in extension).

LATERAL VIEW

Gait observed from the lateral view allows assessment of ROM excursions in the sagittal plane (Fig. 21-20). These motions include dorsiflexion and plantar flexion at the ankle and flexion and extension at the knee, hip, and trunk. The clinician should note coordination of movement between all of the joints of the lower extremity during the gait cycle. Step lengths should be observed for symmetry and adequacy.

The ankle should move into plantar flexion on heel strike. As the body moves over the fixed foot in single support, dorsiflexion occurs. Pronation occurs with dorsiflexion, which reaches its maximum at the onset of terminal support, followed by rapid plantar flexion at the end of terminal double support.

POSTERIOR VIEW

The posterior view is similar to the anterior view. All structures and symmetries observed in the anterior view should be qualified in the posterior view as well. The posterior view allows

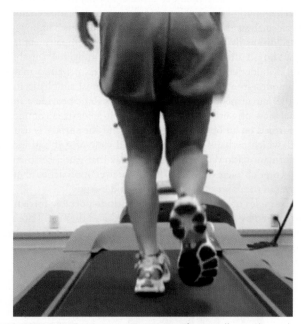

FIGURE 21-21 A posterior view of gait allows direct heel observation.

observation of the heel, particularly its rise and position during the gait cycle (Fig. 21-21). Posterior assessment also allows observation of the transition from the stance to the swing phase.

Quantitative Methods for Determining Temporal Gait Parameters

Besides observing gait for obvious deviations, temporospatial gait parameters are perhaps the most cost-effective and simplest to assess in a clinical setting. Temporal gait parameters, which pertain to time, may be used to describe normal walking ability and include cadence, step and stride times, walking speed,

Table 21-2 Gait Parameter Values for Women Walking at Normal Speed

Parameter	Age (yr)	n	Mean ± SD
Walking speed (cm/sec)	15-19	15	123.9 ± 17.5
	20-29	15	124.1 ± 7.1
	30-39	15	128.5 ± 19.1
Cadence (steps/sec)	15-19	15	2.09 ± 0.18
	20-29	15	2.08 ± 0.15
	30-39	15	2.13 ± 0.17
Step length (cm)	15-19	15	59.3 ± 4.3
	20-29	15	59.1 ± 6.3
	30-39	15	59.7 ± 5.3
Stride length (cm)*	15-19	15	≈119.0
	20-29	15	≈118.0
	30-39	15	≈120.0
Stride time (sec)†	15-19	15	≈1.05
	20-29	15	≈1.04
	30-39	15	≈1.07

Data from Oberg, T., Karsznia, A., and Oberg, K. (1993): Basic gait parameters: Reference data for normal subjects, 10-79 years of age. J. Rehabil. Res. Dev., 30:210–223.
*Derived from step length values (step length multiplied by 2).
†Derived from cadence values [cadence (steps/sec) divided by 2].

Table 21-3 Gait Parameter Values for Men Walking at Normal Speed

Parameter	Age (yr)	n	Mean ± SD
Walking speed (cm/sec)	15-19	15	135.1 ± 13.3
	20-29	15	122.7 ± 11.1
	30-39	15	131.6 ± 15
Cadence (steps/sec)	15-19	15	2.02 ± 0.2
	20-29	15	1.98 ± 0.13
	30-39	15	2.00 ± 0.14
Step length (cm)	15-19	15	66.0 ± 4.8
	20-29	15	61.6 ± 3.5
	30-39	15	64.9 ± 4.6
Stride length (cm)*	15-19	15	≈132.0
	20-29	15	≈123.0
	30-39	15	≈130.0
Stride time (sec)†	15-19	15	≈1.01
	20-29	15	≈0.99
	30-39	15	≈1.00

Data from Oberg, T., Karsznia, A., and Oberg, K. (1993): Basic gait parameters: Reference data for normal subjects, 10-79 years of age. J. Rehabil. Res. Dev., 30:210–223.
*Derived from step length values (step length multiplied by 2).
†Derived from cadence values [cadence (steps/sec) divided by 2].

Table 21-4 Normal Values for Base of Support and Foot (Toe) Angle While Walking

Parameter	Mean Value
Base of support (step width)	≈5.0-10.0 cm[13,37]
Foot (toe) angle	≈5.0°-7.0°[36]

and affected and unaffected static stance times. Spatial parameters include various angles and distances, including step and stride length, width of the base of support, and foot (toe) angle. All parameter measurements may be compared between the extremities or compared within the same extremity at different time points (initial evaluation, time of discharge, and various points in time between the two). In addition, cadence, stride length, and walking speed are gait parameters that have been normalized for gender, age, and walking speed (Tables 21-2 and 21-3). Other parameters have values considered normal as well (Table 21-4). Because walking speed has an impact on all kinematic and kinetic gait parameters, it should always be calculated and reported during clinical assessment of any gait parameter so that the information obtained from interpretation of clinical gait analysis is meaningful.[18]

Injury, as discussed in the next section, often diminishes the ability to bear compressive loads during the support phases of gait, especially single support. This may be roughly assessed statically by having the athlete stand on one foot for as long as possible (Box 21-2).[10,38] The amount of time spent in unilateral support should be approximately symmetric between the lower extremities.

Footprint impressions may be made with a variety of methods (see the following section and Box 21-3). Shoes may be left on the patient, although it is best to perform the analysis with the patient walking barefoot. The athlete walks on a paper (butcher paper) runway, and the ink marks give impressions of heel and forefoot contact (Fig. 21-22).

TEMPORAL PARAMETERS

Cadence and cycle time can easily be measured in the clinic. The clinician instructs the athlete to walk and, once up to full speed, counts the number of steps taken during a given period (could range from 10 seconds up to a minute). The distance should allow for acceleration and deceleration during the initial and final portions of the walk, respectively. Cadence, or the number of steps per minute, is calculated by multiplying the number of steps taken by 60 and dividing by the amount of time observed [cadence = (number of steps × 60)/time (seconds)].[27] For example, an athlete taking 14 steps in 10 seconds would have a cadence of 84 steps per minute [cadence = (14 steps × 60)/10 seconds) = 84 steps per minute]. Cycle time is the amount of time spent in the gait cycle and is expressed in seconds. Since the gait cycle is composed of two steps, cycle time is calculated by multiplying the amount of time (seconds) by 2 (steps) and then dividing by the number of steps counted [cycle time (seconds) = time (seconds) × 2 steps/number of counted steps]. Our same athlete would have a gait cycle time of 1.43 seconds [cycle time (seconds) = (10 seconds × 2 steps)/14 steps = 1.43 seconds].

Walking speed is the distance walked during a certain period divided by the time taken to walk that particular distance. Thus, speed (meters/second) is calculated by timing the subject while moving from a starting point to a finishing point. The distance from the starting to the finishing point is divided by the amount of time needed to cover the distance (distance/time). For example, if our athlete covers 6 m in 4 seconds, walking speed would be 1.5 m/sec (6 m/4 sec = 1.5 m/sec).

Because the major factors affecting walking speed are stride length and step rate, walking speed may be calculated by multiplying stride length by one half of the cadence value (velocity = stride length $\times$ 0.5 cadence).[17] For example, an athlete with stride length of 1.4 m and a cadence of 100 steps per minute would have a walking speed of 70 m/min.

Step time may be recorded with a multimemory stopwatch while the athlete walks a predetermined distance.[6,16] The lap button is pressed at every heel contact as the athlete walks (Box 21-4). Each extremity's step times are summed and then divided by the number of laps to give an average step time. It is important to note which step was recorded first. Unlike stride length, which may be calculated by using cadence and walking speed or walking speed and stride time, step length cannot be determined from step time and walking speed (see the section on deriving temporal data).[39]

Box 21-2

Affected and Unaffected Static Stance Times

SUPPLIES NEEDED
Multimemory stopwatch
Parallel bars, sturdy plinth, or wall

INSTRUCTIONS
Affected static stance time
- Have the athlete stand on the injured lower extremity. Begin the stop watch when the unaffected extremity leaves the floor. Keep time up to 30 seconds.

Unaffected static stance time
- Have the athlete stand on the uninjured lower extremity. Begin the stop watch when the affected extremity leaves the floor. Keep time up to 30 seconds.

From Nelson, A.J. (1974): Functional ambulation profile. Phys. Ther., 54:1059–1065.

Box 21-3

Moleskin Method of Footprint Impressions

SUPPLIES NEEDED
Moleskin
Liquid ink or water-based paint
Sheet of paper (0.9 m wide by 6 m long)
Stopwatch

INSTRUCTIONS
Place moleskin on the heel and toe of the patient's shoe or foot. Wet the moleskin with ink. Have the stopwatch ready and begin timing the patient walking down the paper runway. Press the lap button at every heel contact for the given distance.

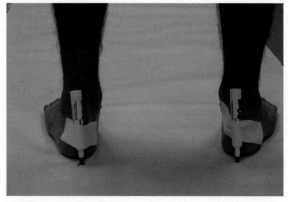

FIGURE 21-22 Felt-tip markers attached to the lower extremities will record heel strike or other aspects of foot contact during gait.

Box 21-4

Recording Temporal Gait Parameters With a Multimemory Stopwatch

SUPPLIES NEEDED
Multimemory stopwatch
Walkway of 10 m

INSTRUCTIONS
Observe the athlete from a lateral view. Mark a line 2 m beyond the beginning and 2 m shy of the end of the runway to allow for acceleration and deceleration, respectively. Have the athlete begin walking on the 10-m runway, press the start button as the athlete passes the first 2-m mark and then the lap button on the first right heel contact after the athlete passes the first 2-m mark. Press the lap button at every heel contact until the final 2 m is reached, and press the stop button as the final 2-m mark is reached.

Average left step time: Time between lap 1 and lap 2, lap 3 and lap 4, lap 5 and lap 6, etc. Sum these times and divide by the number of laps to get an average step time.

Average right step time: Time between lap 2 and lap 3, lap 4 and lap 5, lap 6 and lap 7, etc. Sum these times and divide by the number of laps to get an average step time.

Walking speed: Divide 6 m by the time necessary to walk 6 m. This time is the total time expired on the stopwatch.

Stride time (seconds per stride): Sum the average right and left step times.

Average stride length: Calculate by multiplying walking speed and stride time.

Data from Youdas, J.W., Atwood, A.L., Harris-Love, M.O., et al. (2000): Measurements of temporal aspects of gait obtained with a multimemory stopwatch in persons with gait impairments. J. Orthop. Sports Phys. Ther., 30:279–286; and Wall, J.C., and Scarbrough, J. (1997): Use of a multimemory stopwatch to measure the temporal gait parameters. J. Orthop. Sports Phys. Ther., 25:277–281.

Footprint Impression Techniques

Impression techniques capture the athlete's footprints during a bout of walking. Footprint analysis allows the clinician to directly measure step and stride lengths, width of the base of support or step width, and foot or toe angle.

Create a walkway with at least 6 m of paper (plain or butcher paper 0.9 m wide) or other media on which the athlete will walk. Altogether, the athlete will walk at least 10 m (see Box 21-4), with the first and final 2 m allowing for acceleration and deceleration, respectively.[8,17] Time should be recorded with a stopwatch during the analysis. Footprints may be made with ink-soaked moleskin or ink pads attached to the patient's heel and forefoot or great toe or with felt-tip markers attached to the athlete's shoes or feet (see Fig. 21-22 and Box 21-3); alternatively, the athlete can step barefoot into water, baby powder, chalk, or water-based paint before walking on an absorbent paper runway.[40-42]

The base of support and foot (toe) angle are relatively easy to measure once the athlete's footprints have been recorded (see Fig. 21-1). The base of support is a width measurement made from the distance between one heel and the other perpendicular to the line of progression. The foot (toe) angle is the angle of the foot with respect to the line of progression of gait. The line of progression is drawn as a line extending forward through measured midpoints of the base of support (see Fig. 21-1).

Stride and step lengths are then measured. The distance measured between consecutive heel contacts of the same foot is the stride length. Step length, however, is measured from consecutive heel contacts. In other words, left step length is the distance measured from right heel contact to left heel contact along the line of progression (see distance E in Fig. 21-1).

It is important to consider standardizing step and stride lengths to the athlete's height or lower extremity length.[43] This is important because height and lower extremity length linearly increase step and stride lengths, which makes it difficult to compare different individuals with the same pathology. In young adults without pathology, step length corresponds to about 75% of leg length.[43]

Deriving Temporal Data

Stride length can be calculated from cadence and walking speed.[17] Stride length is equivalent to velocity divided by 0.5 cadence (speed/0.5 cadence). Our athlete with a gait velocity of 70 m/min and a cadence of 100 steps per minute would have a calculated stride length of 1.4 m: (70 m/min)/(0.5) × 100 steps per minute = stride length of 1.4 m.

Stride length can also be derived from walking speed and stride time. Stride time is the amount of time from consecutive heel contacts of the same foot. Stride time may be calculated from the time to produce a number of strides divided by the number of strides taken or by summing the average right and left step times.[5,6,16] Thus, an athlete who produces five strides in 6 seconds has a stride time of 1.2 seconds (a stride is completed every 1.2 seconds). Stride length is equal to the product of stride time and walking speed.[5] However, the walking speed used here must be converted to meters per second as opposed to meters per minute. This simple conversion may be done by dividing by 60 (60 seconds equals 1 minute). Now that walking speed is converted to meters per second, it may be multiplied by stride time to give an appropriate stride length. For example, our athlete walking 70 m/min would walk 1.17 m/sec. This walking speed of 1.17 m/sec multiplied by 1.2 seconds yields a stride length of 1.4 m.

Injury to the lower extremities often causes gait parameters that are outside normal ranges. Additionally, injury may also cause asymmetries when comparing one extremity with the other. Common gait deviations are now reviewed.

Common Gait Deviations

It is important to understand that gait analysis does not determine the cause of gait abnormalities; rather, gait deviations are compensational strategies for various pathologies.[27] For example, deviations in gait associated with joint pathology often occur as a result of diminished joint ROM during the swing phase or as a result of pain from weight bearing during the stance phase. Compensation for these gait deviations include decreased stride length and diminished time spent in weight-bearing stance phases. Decreased time spent in stance phase affects step time (and perhaps length). These deviations are manifested as the familiar "antalgic" gait pattern, or "hopping," noticed during gait.[13] In the following sections, only common deviations in gait that are observable during routine clinical assessment are presented. It is important to note that joint trauma resulting in decreased weight acceptance during the stance phase may be present in each of the joints examined. Motion analysis and other sophisticated means of gait assessment may be indicated in some athletes for detailed analysis of gait deviation.

Hip

The hip joint largely affects the ability to walk normally. Joint pathologies that diminish hip ROM may cause multiple deviations. The more common gait deviations associated with hip joint hypomobility are insufficient extension and excessive abduction. Weakness of the hip abductors and extensors affect normal gait as well.

Insufficient hip extension may occur from pain associated with joint trauma, hip flexor muscle strain or contracture, or a tight iliotibial band. Weight-bearing capacity decreases because the stance phase is altered to accommodate for the lack of hip extension. Postural compensations such as increased lordosis or increased knee flexion serve to allow the trunk to maintain an upright position.[17]

Excessive hip abduction may be caused by ipsilateral and contralateral pathologies.[17] Two common pathologies resulting in excessive ipsilateral hip abduction include shortened hip abductor musculature and a shortened lower extremity in an individual with severe leg length discrepancy. Contralateral pathology of the hip adductors following strain or contracture can also result in excessive hip abduction.[17]

Individuals with weakness of the hip abductor or extensor muscles may walk with a lurch, or asymmetric compensatory trunk movements.[13] Abductor weakness results in an asymmetric shift toward the affected side during the stance phase. Similarly, an extension lurch causes excessive trunk extension during the stance phase of the affected lower extremity.

Knee

The most common gait deviations at the knee occur from either decreased ROM or quadriceps weakness. Insufficient flexion and extension are the more frequent ROM problems encountered. Most commonly, the knee is maintained in a "loose-packed" position of slight flexion throughout the gait cycle. Quadriceps weakness, a common result of reflex inhibition, often occurs with joint trauma (see Chapter 2).

Insufficient knee extension affects the gait cycle in a number of ways.[11] The athlete avoids the normal excursions of knee motion during the gait cycle, which is typically manifested as diminished knee extension during heel contact and terminal double support just before toe-off. A compensation for decreased knee extension is to shorten stride length, which results in an overall increase in the number of steps needed to cover the same relative distance (if stride length decreases, the number of steps needed to cover a distance must increase if velocity remains the same). This may or may not increase cadence because walking speed will most likely adjust downward. This type of deviation is commonly associated with a knee flexion contracture.

Insufficient knee flexion results in a "stiff leg" gait pattern. Here, the knee extensors are not able to eccentrically absorb force, and it is transmitted from the tibia to the femur. Microtrauma and macrotrauma to the femur and hip joint may result from long-term insufficient knee flexion. Disruption of the anterior cruciate ligament is associated with anterior translation of the tibia on the femur. Individuals may cope with the instability by "stiffening the knee," which decreases knee flexion during gait.[44]

Quadriceps weakness often prevents eccentric control of the lower extremity on impact with the ground. The compensation for this weakness is to maintain the knee locked in extension by using the inherent anatomic stability of the of the knee's "screw-home" mechanism. Another compensatory action is for the athlete to manually push the knee into extension during the stance phase.[13]

Ankle and Foot

Several deviations can occur at the ankle and foot. Excessive plantar flexion, excessive dorsiflexion, biomechanical foot abnormalities, and weakness of the dorsiflexor muscles are the more common deviations seen at the ankle and foot.

Excessive plantar flexion can occur as a result of muscle weakness or tissue hypomobility. Weakness of the dorsiflexors mostly affects ankle position during midswing and initial contact. Foot clearance becomes compromised because the ankle remains plantar-flexed during midswing. The knee and hip compensate by increased flexion, which results in a "steppage" gait pattern. The tissue hypomobility associated with plantar flexion contractures affects gait during the stance and swing phases. Excessive plantar flexion is commonly associated with a shortened stride length.[17]

Increased dorsiflexion may occur as a result of tissue hypomobility or weakness of the plantar flexor muscles or as a compensation for excessive knee flexion. From a functional standpoint, excessive dorsiflexion has a negative impact on stance phase more than on swing phase. Tissue hypomobility of the ankle joint or the dorsiflexors pulls the tibia relatively forward, which increases knee flexion.[17] Knee flexion and ankle dorsiflexion are related in the stance phase of gait in that an increase in one concomitantly increases the other.

Anatomic foot dysfunction adversely affects the stance phase of gait more than the swing phase. Common foot dysfunctions are excessive eversion and inversion. Excessive eversion or valgus occurs with pes planus, with the first metatarsal contacting the ground before the fifth metatarsal. The medial aspect of the foot bears most of the weight during the stance phase as pronation increases and supination decreases. Excessive inversion or varus commonly occurs with pes cavus. In the case of excessive inversion, the lateral aspect of the heel and the fifth metatarsal

dominate and contact the ground as supination increases and pronation decreases. This gives the clinical impression of one walking on the outside of the foot.

Common traumatic injuries such as ankle sprains result in loss of motion while hampering the ability of the joints to bear weight. Plantar flexion and dorsiflexion decrease, which shortens the stance phase on the affected side. Step time, but not necessarily length, may also shorten on the unaffected side as a result of the inability to maintain a normal stance phase on the affected side.

Finally, weak dorsiflexors are not able to control the forefoot in its descent to the ground. This causes the foot to come in contact with the ground too quickly, which gives the clinical impression of a "foot slap" shortly after heel contact.

CONCLUSION

- Clinical gait assessment can be challenging, a basic understanding of the gait cycle is prerequisite to attempting clinical gait assessment.
- The overall gait cycle for the right lower extremity begins with initial right foot contact, which initiates double support, followed by right single support, double support again, and right swing phase (the swing phase consists of the initial or acceleration swing phase, midswing phase, and terminal or deceleration phases).
- The clinician should perform both static standing posture and dynamic gait assessments to obtain a comprehensive clinical picture of the athlete.
- Familiarity with normal upright static standing posture allows better appreciation of the dynamic process of gait. Static standing posture should be viewed from the anterior, posterior, lateral, and oblique views. A posture grid, plumb line, and photography aid in the objectivity and reliability of postural assessments.
- Gait assessment requires the collection of kinematic data, kinetic data, or both. Kinematic data are the easiest to produce in the clinical setting. In addition to gait observation, various temporospatial measurements increase objectivity and may be performed relatively easily in the clinic.
- Common gait abnormalities should be appreciated. Most gait deviations arise from pathology at the hip, knee, and ankle. Athletes with severe disturbances in gait may need referral to a facility capable of kinetic and kinematic assessments.

ACKNOWLEDGEMENT

The author wishes to thank Dr. James Wall for his contribution to the field of clinical gait analysis and for his influence on the development of this chapter.

REFERENCES

1. Abellan van Kan, G., Rolland, Y., Andrieu, S., et al. (2009): Gait speed at usual pace as a predictor of adverse outcomes in community-dwelling older people. An International Academy on Nutrition and Aging (IANA) Task Force. J. Nutr. Health Aging, 13:881–889.
2. Dumurgier, J., Elbaz, A., Ducimetiere, P., et al. (2009): Slow walking speed and cardiovascular death in well functioning older adults: Prospective cohort study. BMJ, 339:b4460.
3. Perry, J., and Burnfield, J.M. (2010): Gait Analysis: Normal and Pathological Function 2nd ed. Thorofare, NJ, Slack.
4. Magee, D.J. (1992): Gait assessment. In Orthopedic Physical Assessment. 2nd ed. Philadelphia, Saunders, pp. 563–578.

5. Wall, J.C., and Kirtley, C. (2001): Strategies for clinical gait assessment. Orthop. Phys. Ther. Clin. North Am., 10:35–54.

6. Youdas, J.W., Atwood, A.L., Harris-Love, M.O., et al. (2000): Measurements of temporal aspects of gait obtained with a multimemory stopwatch in persons with gait impairments. J. Orthop. Sports Phys. Ther., 30:279–286.

7. Wall, J.C., and Brunt, D. (1997): Clinical gait analysis: Temporal and distance parameters. In Van Deussen, J.V. (ed.): Assessment in Occupational Therapy and Physical Therapy. Havertown, PA, CIR Systems.

8. Oberg, T., Karsznia, A., and Oberg, K. (1993): Basic gait parameters: Reference data for normal subjects, 10-79 years of age. J. Rehabil. Res. Dev., 30:210–223.

9. Eastlack, M.E., Arvidson, J., Snyder-Mackler, L., et al. (1991): Interrater reliability of videotaped observational gait-analysis assessments. Phys. Ther., 71:465–472.

10. Norkin, C. (2000): Gait analysis. In Sullivan, S., and Shcmitz, T. (eds.): Physical Rehabilitation: Assessment and Treatment. Philadelphia, Davis, pp. 257–307.

11. Perry, J., and Burnfield, J.M. (2010): Gait cycle. In Gait Analysis: Normal and Pathological Function, 2nd ed. Thorofare, NJ, Slack, pp. 3–6.

12. Wall, J.C. (1999): Walking. In Durward B.R., Baer, G.D., and Rowe, P.J. (eds.): Functional Human Movement: Measurement and Analysis. Oxford, Butterworth Heinemann, pp. 93–105.

13. Hoppenfeld, S. (1976): Examination of gait. In Physical Examination of the Spine and Extremities. East Norwalk, CT, Appleton-Century-Crofts, pp. 133–141.

14. Whittle, M.W. (2002): Normal gait. In Whittle, M.W. (ed.): Gait Analysis: An Introduction. Oxford, Butterworth Heinemann, pp. 42–88.

15. Krebs, D.E., Edelstein, J.E., and Fishman, S. (1985): Reliability of observational kinematic gait analysis. Phys. Ther., 65:1027–1033.

16. Wall, J.C., and Scarbrough, J. (1997): Use of a multimemory stopwatch to measure the temporal gait parameters. J. Orthop. Sports Phys. Ther., 25:277–281.

17. Perry, J., and Burnfield, J.M. (2010): Gait analysis systems. In Gait Analysis: Normal and Pathological Function, 2nd ed. Thorofare, NJ, Slack, pp. 403–405. .

18. Simoneau, G.G. (2002): Kinesiology of walking. In Neumann D. A. (ed.): Kinesiology of the Musculoskeletal System. St. Louis, Mosby, pp. 523–569.

19. Watson, A.W. (2001): Sports injuries related to flexibility, posture, acceleration, clinical defects, and previous injury, in high-level players of body contact sports. Int. J. Sports Med., 22:222–225.

20. Shambaugh, J.P., Klein, A., and Herbert, J.H. (1991): Structural measures as predictors of injury to basketball players. Med. Sci. Sports Exerc., 23:522–527.

21. Cowan, D.N., Jones, B.H., Frykman, P.N., et al. (1996): Lower limb morphology and risk of overuse injury among male infantry trainees. Med. Sci. Sports Exerc., 28:945–952.

22. Watson, A.W., and Mac Donncha, C. (2000): A reliable technique for the assessment of posture: assessment criteria for aspects of posture. J. Sports Med. Phys. Fitness, 40:260–270.

23. Fortin, C., Ehrmann Feldman, D., Cheriet, F., and Labelle, H. (2011): Clinical methods for quantifying body segment posture: A literature review. Disabil. Rehabil., 33:367–383.

24. Abramoff, M.D., Magelhaes, P.J., and Ram, S.J. (2004): Image Processing with Image J. Biophotonics Int., 11(7):36–42.

25. Rasband, W. and Image, J. http://rsb.info.nih.gov/ij/. Accessed August 23, 2010.

26. Rose, G.K. (1983): Clinical gait assessment: A personal view. J. Med. Eng. Technol., 7:273–279.

27. Whittle, M.W. (2002): Methods of gait analysis. In Whittle, M.W. (ed.): Gait Analysis: An Introduction, 3rd ed. Oxford, Butterworth Heinemann, pp. 127–161.

28. Hughes, K.A., and Bell, F. (1994): Visual assessment of hemiplegic gait following stroke: Pilot study. Arch. Phys. Med. Rehabil., 75:1100–1107.

29. Wall, J.C., and Crosbie, J. (1996): Accuracy and reliability of temporal gait measurement. Gait Posture, 4:293–296.

30. Brunnekreef, J.J., van Uden, C.J., van Moorsel, S., and Kooloos, J.G. (2005): Reliability of videotaped observational gait analysis in patients with orthopedic impairments. BMC Musculoskelet. Disord., 6:17.

31. Stuberg, W.A., Colerick, V.L., Blanke, D.J., and Bruce, W. (1988): Comparison of a clinical gait analysis method using videography and temporal-distance measures with 16-mm cinematography. Phys. Ther., 68:1221–1225.

32. Mulder, T., Nienhuis, B., and Pauwels, J. (1998): Clinical gait analysis in a rehabilitation context: Some controversial issues. Clin. Rehabil., 12:99–106.

33. Webster, K.E., Wittwer, J.E., and Feller, J.A. (2005): Validity of the GAITRite walkway system for the measurement of averaged and individual step parameters of gait. Gait Posture, 22:317–321.

34. Rancho Los Amigos National Rehabilitation Center Pathokinesiology Service and Physical Therapy Department (2001): Observational Gait Analysis Handbook. Downey, CA, Los Amigos Research and Education Institute.

35. Lord, S.E., Halligan, P.W., and Wade, D.T. (1998): Visual gait analysis: The development of a clinical assessment and scale. Clin. Rehabil., 12:107–119.

36. Lemke, M.R., Wendorff, T., Mieth, B., et al. (2000): Spatiotemporal gait patterns during over ground locomotion in major depression compared with healthy controls. J. Psychiatr. Res., 34:277–283.

37. Lehmann, J.F. (1982): Gait analysis: Diagnosis and management. In Kottke, F.J., Stillwell, G.K., Lehmann, J.F. (eds.): Krusen's Handbook of Physical Medicine and Rehabilitation. Philadelphia, Saunders.

38. Nelson, A.J. (1974): Functional ambulation profile. Phys. Ther., 54:1059–1065.

39. Singleton, S., Keating, S., McDowell, S., et al. (1992): Predicting step time from step length and velocity. Aust. J. Physiother., 31:43–46.

40. Cerny, K. (1983): A clinical method of quantitative gait analysis. Suggestion from the field. Phys. Ther., 63:1125–1126.

41. Clarkson, B.H. (1983): Absorbent paper method for recording foot placement during gait. Suggestion from the field. Phys. Ther., 63:345–346.

42. Shores, M. (1980): Footprint analysis in gait documentation. An instructional sheet format. Phys. Ther., 60:1163–1167.

43. Judge, J.O., Davis, R.B., 3rd, and Ounpuu, S. (1996): Step length reductions in advanced age: The role of ankle and hip kinetics. J. Gerontol. A. Biol. Sci. Med. Sci., 51:M303–M312.

44. Rudolph, K.S., Eastlack, M.E., Axe, M.J., and Snyder-Mackler, L. (1998): Basmajian Student Award Paper: Movement patterns after anterior cruciate ligament injury: A comparison of patients who compensate well for the injury and those who require operative stabilization. J. Electromyogr. Kinesiol., 8:349–362.

Section V

Restoration of Athletic Performance

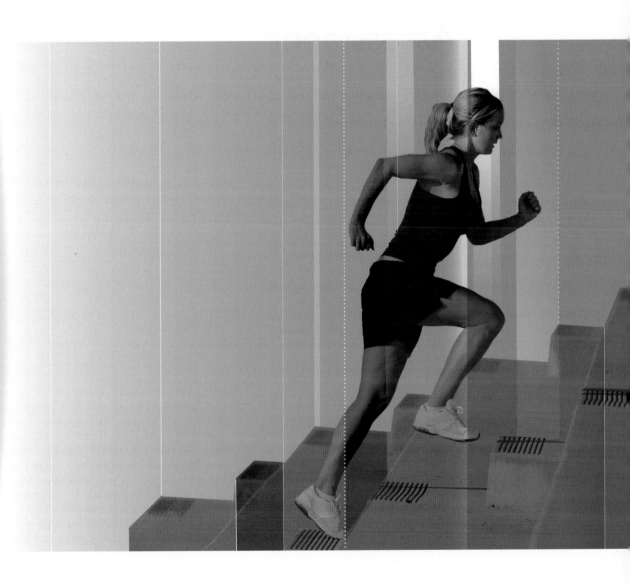

481

22

Functional Movement Assessment

Barb Hoogenboom, PT, EdD, SCS, ATC, Michael L. Voight, PT, DHSc, OCS, SCS, ATC, CSCS, FAPTA, and Gray Cook, PT, MS, OCS, CSCS

CHAPTER OBJECTIVES

- Explain the benefits of a functional, comprehensive movement screening process versus the traditional impairment-based evaluation approach.

- Differentiate between movement, testing, and assessment.

- Explain how poor movement patterns and dysfunctional movement strategies can result in injury or reinjury.

- Explain the use and components of the Functional Movement Screen and the Selective Functional Movement Assessment.

- Describe and score the movement patterns of the Functional Movement Screen and the Selective Functional Movement Assessment and interpret how the results from each can have an impact on clinical interventions.

- Articulate the difference between movement screening and specific functional performance tests.

- Apply specific functional performance test to clinical practice.

INTRODUCTION

Movement is at the core of the human journey. It is foundational to the human experience and allows us to interact with our environment in ways different from other mammals. Movement, which begins in the womb, is the basis of early growth and development. It proceeds in a highly predictable manner in infants and young children and is known as the developmental sequence or traditional motor development. When an individual reaches a certain age, full integration of reflexive behavior allows the development of purposive, highly developed, and unique mature motor programs. We continue to move functionally throughout a lifetime until the effects of aging alter the normalcy of movement.

Motion Versus Movement

Because movement is complex, it must be differentiated from the simpler construct of motion. The authors believe that many professionals lack a true understanding of movement; they err on the side of quantitative assessment of motion and fail to understand the hierarchic progression from general, fundamental move-

ment patterns to specific, highly specialized movements. These highly specialized movements have complex, fine-tuned motor programs that support their consistency and intricacy. Most rehabilitation and medical professionals have been trained to measure isolated joint motion with goniometers, inclinometers, linear measurements, or ligament laxity tests. These types of motion assessment are not wrong, but rather represent only a piece of a much bigger puzzle of "movement" and the inherent stability and mobility demands that are part of the synchronous, elegant, coordinated activities that make up activities of daily living, work tasks, and sport maneuvers. Mere motion measurements cannot capture the whole spectrum of human movement, nor the complexity of human function.

Systems Approach to Movement

The premise of this chapter and the chapter that follows is that impairment-based, highly specialized motion assessment is far too limiting and in fact predisposes practitioners to errors in professional judgment. It is too narrow of an approach that focuses on small, discrete pieces of an integrated functional task or movement. The alternative of a more functional, comprehensive movement screen is vitally important for understanding human function and identifying impairments and dysfunctional movement patterns that diminish the quality of function. In many cases, weakness or tightness of a muscle or group is often identified and then treated with isolated stretching or strengthening activities instead of using a standard movement pattern that could address several impairments at once. Likewise, many professionals often focus on a specific region of complaint instead of beginning by identifying a comprehensive movement profile and relating the profile to dysfunction.

Fundamentals First

Where does one start with the examination and assessment of something as complex as human function? Standard, frequently used, fundamental or general movements would seem the logical place to start. To prepare an athlete for the wide variety of activities needed to participate in the demands of sport, analysis of fundamental movements should be incorporated into preparticipation screening. Assessment of fundamental movements can help the rehabilitation professional determine who possesses or lacks the ability to perform a wide variety of essential movements. The authors believe that assessment of fundamental or composite movements is necessary before the assessment of highly specific or specialized motions or movements. Consider the following statements in the context of assessment of an athlete:

- What appears to be muscular weakness may in fact be muscular inhibition.
- Identifiable weakness in a prime mover may be the result of a dysfunctional stabilizer or group of muscular stabilizers.
- Diminished function in an agonist may actually be dysfunction of the antagonist.
- What is described as muscular tightness may in fact be protective muscle tone leading to guarding and inadequate muscle coordination during movement.
- "Bad" technique might be the only option for an individual performing poorly selected, "off-target" exercises.
- Diminished general fitness may be related to the increased metabolic demand required by patients who use inferior neuromuscular coordination and compensations.

It is vital that fundamental, essential movements be examined to develop a working hypothesis regarding the source of the dysfunction. This approach allows the rehabilitation professional to see the big picture and attempt to discern the cause of the dysfunction rather than just identifying and treating specific, isolated impairments. This fundamental first approach, typically used when teaching a motor skill, holds true for assessment and correction of movement.

The Mobility-Stability Continuum

Movement becomes less than optimal (dysfunctional) as a result of breakdowns in parts of the movement system. Typically, such breakdowns are described as mobility or stability dysfunction. Unfortunately, the terms *mobility* and *stability* are not universally defined and can imply different things to clinicians with different backgrounds. For this reason it is important to describe the approach of the authors regarding descriptions of mobility and stability.

Mobility dysfunction can be broken down into two unique subcategories:

- *Tissue extensibility dysfunction* involves tissues that are extraarticular. Examples include active or passive muscle insufficiency, neural tension, fascial tension, muscle shortening, scarring, and fibrosis.
- *Joint mobility dysfunction* involves structures that are articular or intraarticular. Examples include osteoarthritis, fusion, subluxation, adhesive capsulitis, and intraarticular loose bodies.

Stability dysfunction may include an isolated muscular weakness or joint laxity, but it is frequently more complex and refers to multiple systems that are involved in the complex construct known as motor control. To account for the complexity of a stability problem, the term *stability motor control dysfunction* (SMCD) is used. SMCD is an encompassing, broad description of problems in movement pattern stability. Traditionally, stability dysfunction is often addressed by attempting to concentrically strengthen the muscle groups identified as stabilizers of a region or joint. This approach neglects the concept that true stabilization is reflex driven and relies on proprioception and timing rather than isolated, gross muscular strength. By using the term SMCD to distinguish stability problems, the clinician is forced to consider the central nervous system (CNS), peripheral nervous system, motor programs, movement organization, timing, coordination, proprioception, joint and postural alignment, structural instability, and muscular inhibition, as well as the absolute strength of the stabilizers. The concepts of mobility and stability are discussed further in the context of the Selective Functional Movement Assessment (SFMA) later in this chapter.

The purpose of this chapter as part of a sports medicine rehabilitation text is to provide the context for and convince the reader of the importance of a timely, accurate, and reproducible functional movement assessment. Though a part of examination, isolated measurements and quantitative assessments are not enough to capture the essence of functional movement in activities of life.

MOVEMENT SCREENING, TESTING, AND ASSESSMENT

Athletic trainers screen during the preseason. Physical therapists are involved in screening, prevention, and wellness initiatives. Physicians serve patients by medically or surgically fixing problems but also attempt to prevent repeat injury. The number one risk for injury is previous injury.[1-6] What contributes to this paradigm? Poor screening that does not identify athletes at risk for injury? Poor rehabilitation that does not finish the job? Poor or untested surgical or medical interventions that do not get to the root of the problem? Each is a possibility, and all disciplines may be responsible for unsuccessfully preparing or providing the building blocks for full return to movement normalcy. It is the job of all health professionals to adequately screen, test, assess, and identify movement dysfunction and offer solutions to restore movement efficiency and normalcy.

At this point it is important to distinguish between screening, testing, and assessment (Table 22-1). This chapter is written to enhance the reader's ability to comprehensively assess the movement (recall the previous discussion of movement versus motion) of patients, athletes, and clients. Many would argue

Table 22-1 Differences Between Screening, Testing, and Assessment

Term	Definition	Meaning
Screening	A system for selecting suitable people; to protect somebody from something unpleasant or dangerous	To create grouping and classification; to check risk
Testing	A series of questions, problems, or practical tasks to gauge knowledge, experience, or ability; measurement with no interpretation needed	To gauge ability
Assessment	To examine something; to judge or evaluate it; to calculate a value based on various factors	To estimate inability

Table 22-2 Outcomes of Movement Assessment

Outcome	Description
Acceptable	Movement is good enough to allow the individual to be cleared for activity without an increase in risk for injury.
Unacceptable	Movements are dysfunctional and the individual may be at risk for injury unless movement patterns are improved.
Painful	Screening movements produce pain. Currently injured regions require additional, more advanced movement and physical assessment, including imaging, by a qualified health care provider.

that assessment of movement is important before embarking on a physical performance endeavor because the ability to move provides the foundation for the ability to perform physical fitness activities, work and athletic tasks, and basic activities of daily living. It is important to be able to distinguish dysfunctional movement from normal movement during preparticipation or preseason screening, as well as during postinjury or postoperative rehabilitation. It is also important to acknowledge that training through or despite poor movement patterns reinforces poor quality of movement and is likely to increase the risk for injury and predispose to greater levels of dysfunction.[4-6] Even highly skilled athletes may have fundamental imperfections in movement.

The authors of this chapter propose that the astute sports medicine professional combine the tasks of screening, testing, and assessment to systematically ascertain the risk, ability, or inability of each athlete, patient, or client. The outcome of such a logical and refined procedure would provide the caregiver the best possible information to formulate opinions regarding readiness for participation or return to sport.

Therefore, screening might come first in the assessment process, and the outcome of a useful, practical movement screening tool or approach would allow the provider to do the following:

- Demonstrate movement patterns that produce pain within expected ranges of movement
- Identify individuals with nonpainful but limited movement patterns who are likely to demonstrate higher potential risk for injury with exercise and activity
- Identify specific exercises and activities to avoid until competency in the required movement is achieved
- Identify and logically link screening movements to the most effective and efficient corrective exercise path to restore movement competency
- Build a description of standardized, fundamental movement patterns against which broader movement can be compared

Sahrmann, Kendall, and Janda have each offered valuable perspectives regarding human movement, posture, and function.[7-9] They have been instrumental in describing examination of structural as well as functional symmetry or lack thereof. Rehabilitation professionals have progressed from examination of isolated muscles and posture[7] to appreciation of the necessity of examining complex movement patterns.[9]

There are numerous ways in which slight subtleties in movement patterns contribute to specific muscle weaknesses. The relationship between altered movement patterns and specific muscle weaknesses requires that remediation address the changes to the movement pattern; the performance of strengthening exercises alone will not likely affect the timing and manner of recruitment during functional performance.

—Dr. Shirley Sahrmann

The transition from analysis of motion to analysis of functional movement and movement patterns helps rehabilitation providers discern the underlying cause of the dysfunction or imbalance. This paradigm shift propels rehabilitation providers toward the big picture, cause-and-effect, and regional interdependence thinking necessary for success in the twenty-first century.

Most would agree that it is difficult to qualitatively discern the quality of movement unless provided with a framework for making a judgment. Systematic screening, testing, and assessment of movement require not only a framework but also benchmarks or criteria that define the proper method of performing a movement. The authors of this chapter propose three possible general outcomes of movement assessment (Table 22-2) as determined by comparison between the movement performed by the athlete and predetermined descriptors of success.

Training through or despite identified "poor" movement patterns reinforces poor quality and increases the risk for injury even during low-stress activities and the possibility of progression to greater movement dysfunction. Training and functional exercise techniques and strategies are covered in the next chapter (Chapter 23); however, it is important to note here that that poor movement patterns must be identified and addressed before embarking on high-level functional training.

MOVEMENT RELATED TO INJURY POTENTIAL AND RETURN FROM INJURY

The greatest risk for injury is a history of previous injury,[1-6] and this fact has been demonstrated in a wide variety of populations and athletes. Yet how might this relate to an uninjured athlete or worker? Are there certain "markers" or performance measures that could separate high-quality, proper or correct movement from low-quality, improper or incorrect movements? Conceptually, if movement is dysfunctional, all activities, including activities of daily living, work tasks, and athletic performance built on that dysfunction, may be flawed and predispose the individual to increased risk for the development of even greater dysfunction. This statement is true even when dysfunctional base movements are masked by apparently acceptable, age-appropriate, and even highly skilled performance. It is possible to move poorly and not experience pain and, conversely, to move well and yet experience pain. Over time, poor movement patterns and dysfunctional movement strategies are likely to produce pain. An example might be a gymnast with an exaggerated lordosis that is functional for her sport but is likely, over time, to result in facet joint compression in the lumbar spine and decreased flexibility of the hip flexors. It is important to note that although poor movement patterns may increase risk for injury with activity, good movement patterns do not guarantee decreased risk for injury. It is the job of the astute health care professional to target and address identifiable risk factors, such as tight muscles, weak muscles, or poor balance or coordination during movement, and their biomechanical influences on movement. When poor movement patterns are addressed, proper movement must be enhanced with appropriate strength, endurance, coordination, and skill development, but proper movement comes *first*!

THE FUNCTIONAL MOVEMENT SCREEN AND THE SELECTIVE FUNCTIONAL MOVEMENT ASSESSMENT

The two movement assessment systems described in this chapter work together and use some common patterns of movement, but each possesses unique aspects. They serve to provide common language and "thinking" between a wide variety of health and fitness professions. Both are about the assessment of *quality* and not so much about the assessment of *quantity* of movement. Both stress the clinician's ability to rate performance quality, rank and describe the greatest dysfunction, and measure, if necessary, within the context of foundational, general movements.

The Functional Movement Screen

The Functional Movement Screen (FMS) is a predictive, but not diagnostic functional screening system. The FMS is an evaluation or screening tool created for use by professionals who work with patients and clients for whom movement is a key part of exercise, recreation, fitness, and athletics. It may also be used for screening within the military, fire service, public safety, industrial laborers, and other highly active workers. This screening tool fills the void between preparticipation/preplacement screening and specific performance tests by examining individuals in a more general dynamic and functional capacity. Research has suggested that tests that assess multiple facets of function such as balance, strength, range of motion (ROM), and motor control simultaneously may assist professionals in identifying athletes at risk for injury.[10-12]

The FMS, described by Cook et al,[13,14] is composed of seven fundamental movement patterns that require a balance of mobility and stability for successful completion. These functional movement patterns were designed to provide observable performance tasks that relate to basic locomotive, manipulative, and stabilizing movements. The tests use a variety of common positions and movements appropriate for providing sufficient challenge to illuminate weakness, imbalance, or poor motor control. It has been observed that even individuals who perform at high functional levels during normal activities may be unable to perform these simple movements if appropriate mobility or stability is not present.[10,11] An important aspect of this assessment system is its foundation on principles of proprioception

Box 22-1

Seven Movement Patterns of the Functional Movement Screen

1. Deep squat
2. Hurdle step
3. In-line lunge
4. Shoulder mobility test
5. Active straight leg raise
6. Trunk stability push-up
7. Rotatory stability test

Table 22-3 Scoring System for the Functional Movement Screen

A Score of...	Is Given If...
0	At any time during testing the athlete has pain anywhere in the body. *Note:* The clearing tests consider only pain, which would indicate a "positive" clearing test and requires a score of 0 for the test with which it is associated.
1	The person is unable to complete the movement pattern or is unable to assume the position to perform the movement.
2	The person is able to complete the movement but must compensate in some way to complete the task.
3	The person performs the movement correctly, without any compensation.

and kinesthesia. Proprioceptors must function in each segment of the kinetic chain and associated neuromuscular control must be present for efficient movement patterns to occur.

The FMS is not intended for use in individuals displaying pain during basic movement patterns or in those with documented musculoskeletal injuries. Painful movement is covered subsequently in the section on the SFMA. The FMS is for healthy, active people and for healthy, inactive people who want to increase their physical activity. Interrater reliability of the FMS has been reported by Minick et al[15] to be high, which means that the assessment protocol can be applied and reliable scores obtained by trained individuals when standard procedures are adhered to.

The FMS consists of seven movement patterns that serve as a comprehensive sample of functional movement (Box 22-1). Additionally, three clearing tests, each associated with one of the FMS movement patterns, assess for pain with shoulder rotation motions, trunk extension, or trunk flexion.

A kit for FMS testing is available commercially (www.performbetter.com); however, simple tools such as a dowel, 2 × 0.6 inches board, tape, tape measure, a piece of string or rope, and a measuring stick are enough to complete the testing procedures. When conducting the screening tests, athletes should not be bombarded with multiple instructions about how to perform the tests; rather, they should be positioned in the start position and offered simple commands to allow achievement of the test movement while observing their performance. The FMS is scored on an ordinal scale, with four possible scores ranging from 0 to 3 (Table 22-3). The clearing tests mentioned earlier consider only pain, which would indicate a positive clearing test and requires a score of 0 for the test with which it is associated. Three is the highest or best score that can be achieved on any single test, and 21 is the best total score that can be achieved.

The majority of the movements test both the right and left sides, and it is important that the sides be scored independently. The lower score of the two sides is recorded and used for the total FMS score, with note made of any imbalances or asymmetry occurring during performance of the task (Fig. 22-1). The creators of the FMS suggest that when in doubt, the athlete should be scored low.

Seven Movement Patterns of the Functional Movement Assessment

THE DEEP SQUAT (Fig. 22-2, A to C)

The squat is a movement needed in most athletic events; it is the "ready position" that is required for many power movements

FMS™ Test	Right	Left	Score	(for bilateral tests, choose lowest score to record)
Overhead deep squat	X	X		
Trunk stability push-up	X	X		
Hurdle step: described by the LE stepping over the hurdle				
In-line lunge: described using the LE in front				
Shoulder mobility: described using the upper UE				
Active straight leg raise				
Rotary stability: described by the UE performing the movement				

Total Score _____ /21

FIGURE 22-1 Functional Movement Screen (FMS) scoring sheet. *LE,* Lower extremity; *UE,* upper extremity.

such as jumping and landing. The deep squat assesses bilateral, symmetric mobility and stability of the hips, knees, ankles, and core. The overhead position of the arms (holding the dowel) also assesses the mobility and symmetry of the shoulders and thoracic spine. To perform a deep squat, the athlete starts with the feet at approximately shoulder width apart in the sagittal plane. The dowel is grasped with both hands, and the arms are pressed overhead while keeping the dowel in line with the trunk and the elbows extended. The athlete is instructed to descend slowly and fully into a squat position while keeping the heels on the ground and the hands above the head.

THE HURDLE STEP (Fig. 22-3, A and B)

The hurdle step is designed to challenge the ability to stride, balance, and perform a single-limb stance during coordinated movement of the lower extremity (LE). The athlete assumes the start position by placing the feet together and aligning the toes just in contact with the base of the hurdle or 2- × 6-inch board. The height of the hurdle or string should be equal to the height of the tibial tubercle of the athlete. The dowel is placed across the shoulders below the neck, and the athlete is asked to step up and over the hurdle, touch the heel to the floor (without accepting weight) while maintaining the stance leg in an extended position, and return to the start position. The leg that is stepping over the hurdle is scored.

IN-LINE LUNGE (Fig. 22-4, A and B)

The in-line lunge attempts to challenge the athlete with a movement that simulates dynamic deceleration with balance and lateral challenge. Lunge length is determined by the tester by measuring the distance to the tibial tubercle. A piece of tape or a tape measure is placed on the floor at the determined lunge distance. The arms are used to grasp the dowel behind the back with the top arm externally rotated, the bottom arm internally rotated, and the fists in contact with the neck and low back region. The hand opposite the front or lunging foot should be on top.

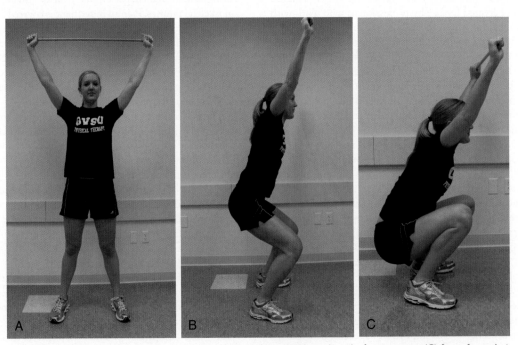

FIGURE 22-2 Overhead deep squat maneuver: beginning (**A**), midrange (**B**), and end of movement (**C**) from frontal view (**A**) and side view (**B** and **C**).

The dowel must begin in contact with the thoracic spine, back of the head, and sacrum. The athlete is instructed to lunge out and place the heel of the front/lunge foot on the tape mark. The athlete is then instructed to slowly lower the back knee enough to touch the floor while keeping the trunk erect and return to the start position. The front leg identifies the side being scored.

SHOULDER MOBILITY (Fig. 22-5, A to C)

This mobility screen assesses bilateral shoulder ROM by combining rotation and abduction/adduction motions. It also requires normal scapular and thoracic mobility. Begin by determining the length of the hand of the athlete by measuring from the distal wrist crease to the tip of the third digit. This distance is used during scoring of the test. The athlete is instructed to make a fist with each hand with the thumb placed inside the fist. The athlete is then asked to place both hands behind the back in a smooth motion (without walking or creeping them upward)— the upper arm in an externally rotated, abducted position (with a flexed elbow) and the bottom arm in an internally rotated, extended, adducted position (also with a flexed elbow). The tester measures the distance between the two fists. The flexed (uppermost) arm identifies the side being scored.

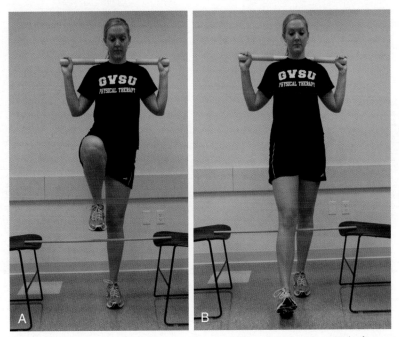

FIGURE 22-3 Hurdle step maneuver: midmotion (**A**) and end motion (**B**) before return.

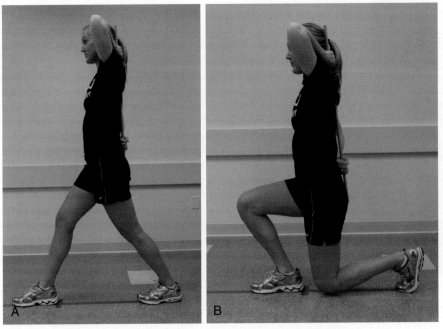

FIGURE 22-4 In-line lunge: beginning (**A**) and end (**B**) of maneuver.

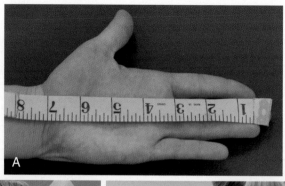

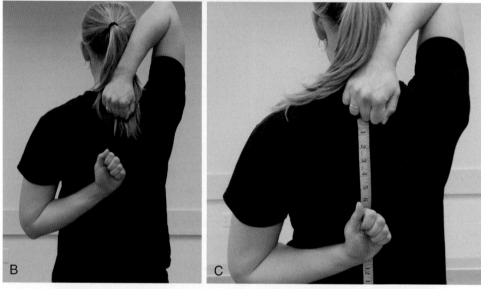

FIGURE 22-5 Shoulder mobility test: hand measurement (**A**), at end of motion (**B**), and how motion is related to hand measurement (**C**).

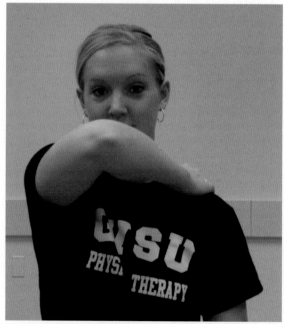

FIGURE 22-6 Screening test for shoulder, also known as the Yocum test. If positive for pain, the athlete scores "0" on the shoulder mobility test.

Shoulder Clearing Test (Fig. 22-6). After the previous test is performed, the athlete places a hand on the opposite shoulder and attempts to point the elbow upward and touch the forehead (Yocum test). If painful, this clearing test is considered positive and the previous test must be scored as 0.

ACTIVE STRAIGHT LEG RAISE (Fig. 22-7)
This test assesses the ability to move the LE separately from the trunk, as well as tests for flexibility of the hamstring and gastrocnemius. The athlete begins in a supine position, arms at the side. The tester identifies the midpoint between the anterior superior iliac spine (ASIS) and the middle of the patella and places a dowel on the ground, held perpendicular to the ground. The athlete is instructed to slowly lift the test leg with a dorsiflexed ankle and a straight knee as far as possible while keeping the opposite leg extended and in contact with the ground. Make note to see where the LE ends at its maximal excursion. If the heel clears the dowel, a score of 3 is given; if the lower part of the leg (between the foot and the knee) lines up with the dowel, a score of 2 is given; and if the patient is only able to have the thigh (between the knee and the hip) line up with the dowel, a score of 1 is given.

TRUNK STABILITY PUSH-UP (Fig. 22-8, *A* and *B*)
This test assesses the ability to stabilize the spine in anterior/posterior and sagittal planes during a closed chain upper body movement. The athlete assumes a prone position with the

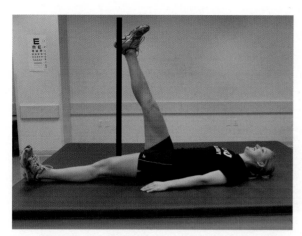

FIGURE 22-7 Active straight leg raise test, end of motion.

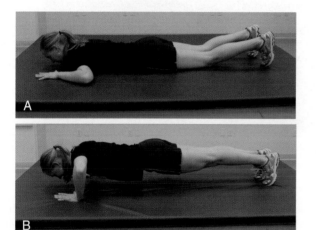

FIGURE 22-8 Trunk stability push-up test: beginning of motion (**A**) and midmotion (**B**). Note that the hand position is for a score of 3 for females (thumbs at chin); to score a 2, females start with the thumbs at clavicular height. In males a score of 3 is achieved with the thumbs at forehead level and a 2 with the thumbs at chin level.

Table 22-4 Alignment Criteria for a Trunk Stability Push–Up by Gender

Position Level	Male	Female
III	Thumbs aligned with the forehead	Thumbs aligned with the chin
II	Thumbs aligned with the chin	Thumbs aligned with the clavicle

The athlete receives a score of 1 if unable to perform a push-up at level II.

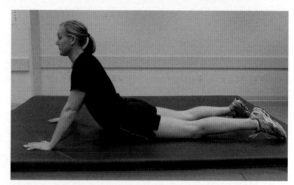

FIGURE 22-9 Screening (clearing) test for spinal extension. If positive for pain, the athlete scores 0 on the trunk stability push-up.

feet together, toes in contact with the floor, and hands placed shoulder width apart (level determined by gender per criteria described later) (Table 22-4), as though ready to perform a push-up from the ground. The athlete is instructed to perform a single push-up in this position with the body lifted as a unit. If unable, the hands should be moved to a less challenging position per criteria and a push-up attempted again. The chest and stomach should come off the floor at the same instance, and no lag should occur in the lumbar spine.

A clearing examination is performed at the end of the trunk stability push-up test and graded as pass or fail, failure occurring when pain is experienced during the test. Spinal extension is cleared by using a full-range prone press-up maneuver from the beginning push-up position (Fig. 22-9); if pain is associated with this motion, a score of 0 is given.

ROTARY STABILITY (Fig. 22-10, A to D)
The rotary stability test is a complex movement that requires neuromuscular control of the trunk and extremities and the ability to transfer energy between segments of the body.

It assesses multiplane stability during a combined upper extremity (UE) and LE motion. The athlete assumes the staring position of quadruped with the shoulders and hips at 90° of flexion. The athlete is instructed to lift a hand off the ground and extend the same-side shoulder (allowing the elbow to flex) while concurrently lifting the knee off the ground and flexing the hip and knee. The athlete needs to raise the extremities only approximately 6 inches from the floor while bringing the elbow and knee together (Fig. 22-10, A and B) until they touch and then return them to the ground. The test is repeated on the opposite side. The UE that moves during testing is scored. Completion of this task allows a score of 3. If unable to perform, the athlete is cued to perform the same maneuver with the opposite LE and UE (Fig. 22-10, C and D), which allows a score of 2 to be awarded. Inability to perform a diagonal (level II) stability test results in a score of 1.

A clearing examination is performed at the end of this test and again is scored as positive if pain is reproduced. From the beginning position for this test, the athletes rock back into spinal flexion and touches the buttocks to the heels and the chest to the thighs (Fig. 22-11). The hands should remain in contact with the ground. Pain on this clearing test overrides any score for the rotary stability test and causes the athlete to receive a score of 0.

A total score of 21 is the highest possible score on the FMS, which implies excellent and symmetric (in tests that are performed bilaterally) performance of the variety of screening maneuvers. Total FMS scores have been investigated in relation to injury in NFL football players[11] and female collegiate soccer, basketball, and volleyball players.[10] Kiesel et al[11] reported a 51% probability of football players sustaining a serious injury over the course of one season with scores less than a 14, and Chorba et al[10]

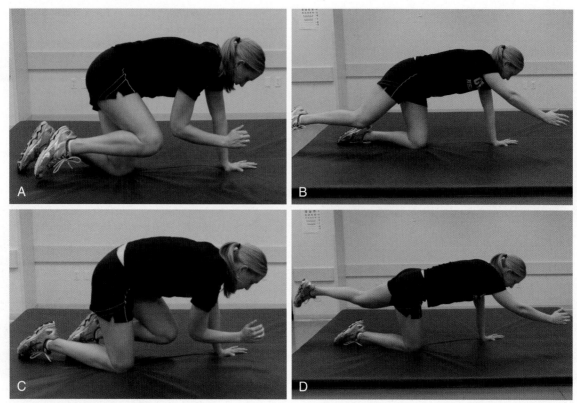

FIGURE 22-10 Rotary stability test: flexed position for a score of 3 (**A**), extended position for a score of 3 (**B**), flexed position for a score of 2 (**C**), and extended position for a score of 2 (**D**).

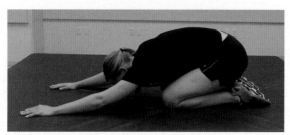

FIGURE 22-11 Screening test for spinal flexion. If positive for pain, the athlete scores 0 on the rotary stability test.

found a significant correlation between low FMS scores (<14) in female athletes and injury. Furthermore, a score of 14 or less on the FMS resulted in an elevenfold increase in the chance of sustaining injury in professional football players and a fourfold increase in the risk for lower extremity injury in female collegiate athletes.[10,11] Okada et al[16] investigated the relationship between the FMS and tests of core stability and functional performance. Significant correlations between some of the FMS screening tests and performance tests of the upper and lower quarter were reported, but these correlations were not consistent among all screening maneuvers. No significant correlations were found between measures of core stability and FMS variables.

The Selective Functional Movement Assessment

Musculoskeletal pain is the reason that most patients seek medical attention. The contemporary understanding of pain has moved beyond the traditional tissue damage model to include the cognitive and behavioral facets. Most scientists accept that pain alters motor function, although the mechanism of these changes has not been clearly identified. The CNS response to painful stimuli is complex, but motor changes have consistently been demonstrated and seem to be influenced by higher centers, consistent with a change in transmission of the motor command. The human body migrates to predictable patterns of movement in response to injury and in the presence of weakness, tightness, or structural abnormality. Richardson et al[17] summarized the evidence that pain alters motor control at higher levels of the CNS than previously thought by stating,

> *Consistent with the identification of changes in motor planning, there is compelling evidence that pain has strong effects at the supraspinal level. Both short- and long-term changes are thought to occur with pain in the activity of the supraspinal structures including the cortex. One area that has been consistently found to be affected is the anterior cingulated cortex which has long thought to be important in motor responses with its direct projections to motor and supplementary motor areas.*[17]

The SFMA is a movement-based diagnostic system for clinical use. This system is used by professionals working with patients experiencing pain on movement. The goal of the SFMA is to observe and capture the patterns of posture and function for comparison against a baseline. It uses movement to provoke symptoms, demonstrate limitations, and offer information regarding movement pattern deficiency related to the patient's primary complaint. The SFMA uses a series of movements with a specific organizational method to rank the quality of functional movements and, when suboptimal, identify the source of provocation of symptoms during movement. The SFMA has been refined and expanded to help the health care professional in musculoskeletal examination, diagnosis, and treatment geared toward choosing the optimal rehabilitative and therapeutic interventions. It helps the clinician identify the most dysfunctional movement patterns, which are then assessed in detail. By identifying all facets of dysfunction within multiple patterns, specific targeted therapeutic interventions designed to capture or illuminate tightness, weakness, poor mobility, or poor stability can be chosen. Thus, the facets of movement identified to most represent or define the dysfunction and thereby affected movement can be addressed. Manual therapy and corrective exercises are focused on movement dysfunction, not pain.

The SFMA is one way of quantifying the qualitative assessment of functional movement and is not a substitute for the traditional examination process. Rather, the SFMA is the first step in a functional orthopedic examination process that serves to focus and direct choices made during the remaining portions of the examination that are pertinent to the functional needs of the patient. The approach taken with the SFMA places less emphasis on identifying the source of the symptoms and more on identifying the cause. An example of this assessment scheme is illustrated by a runner with low back pain. Frequently, the symptoms associated with low back pain are not examined in light of other secondary causes such as hip mobility. Lack of mobility at the hip may be compensated for by increased mobility or instability of the spine. The global approach taken by the SFMA would identify the cause of the low back dysfunction.

The authors believe that it is important to start with a whole-body functional approach such as the SFMA before specific impairment assessments to direct the evaluation in a systematic and constructive manner. Unfortunately, a functional orthopedic examination often involves provocation of symptoms. Provocation of symptoms may occur during the interplay of posture tests, movement in transition, and specific movement tests. Production of these symptoms creates the road map that the clinician will follow to a more specific diagnosis:

- When symptoms have been provoked, the clinician should work backward to a more specific breakdown of the component parts of the movement.
- Inconsistencies observed between provocation of symptoms that are not the result of symptom magnification may suggest a stability problem.
- Consistent limitations and provocation of symptoms can be indicative of a mobility problem.

The functional assessment process emphasizes analysis of function to restore proper movement for specific physical tasks. Use of movement patterns and the application of specific stress and overpressure assist in determining whether dysfunction or pain (or both) are present. The movement patterns will reaffirm hypotheses or redirect the clinician to the cause of the musculoskeletal problem. As an example, the SFMA standing rotation test (Fig. 22-12) is performed with the patient's feet planted side by side and stationary. The subject makes a complete rotation with segments of the entire body first in one direction and then in the other. When consistent production of pain in the left thoracic spine is noted during standing left rotation, the same maneuver can be repeated in the seated posture (Fig. 22-13). The two motions, though similar in demands for spinal rotation, have several differences; with the hips and lower

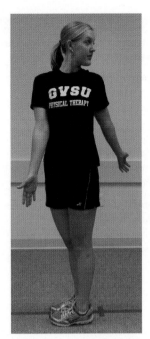

FIGURE 22-12 Total-body rotation test while standing.

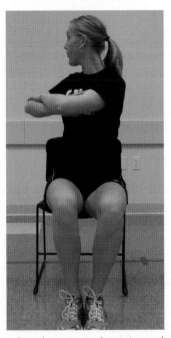

FIGURE 22-13 Spinal rotation in the sitting, unloaded position.

extremities removed from the movement, an entirely different level of postural control may result.

When nearly the same provocation of symptoms and limitations at the same degree of left rotation are noted during both standing and seated, the cause may be an underlying mobility problem somewhere in the spine. Alternatively, if the seated rotation does not produce a consistent limitation and provocation of symptoms in the same direction and to the same degree, a stability problem might be present. This change in position results in a different degree of postural alignment, muscle tone, proprioception, muscle activation or inhibition, and reflex stabilization. The clinician must investigate the lower body component of this

Movement Patterns of the Selective Functional Movement Assessment

SEVEN BASIC MOVEMENTS
1. Cervical spine assessment
2. Upper extremity movement pattern assessment
3. Multisegmental flexion assessment
4. Multisegmental extension assessment
5. Multisegmental rotation assessment
6. Single-leg stance (standing knee lift) assessment
7. Overhead deep squat assessment

FOUR OPTIONAL MOVEMENTS
1. Plank with a twist
2. Single-leg squat
3. In-line lunge with lean, press, and lift
4. Single-leg hop for distance

Table 22-5 Scoring System for the Selective Functional Movement Assessment Based on Function and Pain Reproduction

Label of Outcome of Pattern Performance	Description of Outcome
Functional nonpainful	Unlimited, unrestricted movement that is performed without pain or increased symptoms
Functional painful	Unlimited, unrestricted movement that reproduces or increases symptoms or brings on secondary symptoms
Dysfunctional painful	Movement that is limited or restricted in some way because of lack of mobility, stability, or symmetry; reproduces or increases symptoms; or brings on secondary symptoms
Dysfunctional nonpainful	Movement that is limited or restricted in some way because of lack of mobility, stability, or symmetry and is performed without pain or increased symptoms

problem. When consistency or inconsistency is observed with respect to limitation of movement or provocation of symptoms, the clinician should continue to look for other instances that support the suspicion.

Maintaining or restoring proper movement of specific segments is key to preventing or correcting musculoskeletal pain. The SFMA also identifies where functional exercise may be beneficial and provides feedback regarding the effectiveness of such exercise. A functional approach to exercise uses key specific movements that are common to the patient regardless of the specific activity or sport. Exercise that uses repeated movement patterns required for desired function is not only realistic but also practical and time efficient. Such functional exercises are discussed in Chapter 23.

Scoring System for the Selective Functional Movement Assessment

The hallmark of the SFMA is the use of simple, basic movements to reveal natural reactions and responses by the patient. These movements should be viewed in both loaded and unloaded conditions whenever possible and bilaterally to examine functional symmetry. The SFMA uses seven basic movement patterns (Box 22-2) to rate and rank the two variables of pain and function. In addition, four optional tests can be used to further refine movement dysfunction.

The term *functional* describes any unlimited or unrestricted movement. The term *dysfunctional* describes movements that are limited or restricted in some way because of lack of mobility, stability, or symmetry within a given movement pattern. *Painful* denotes a situation in which the selective functional movement reproduces symptoms, increases symptoms, or brings about secondary symptoms that need to be noted. Therefore, by combining the words *functional, dysfunctional, painful,* and *nonpainful,* each pattern of the SFMA must be scored with one of four possible outcomes (Table 22-5).

Basic Movements in the Selective Functional Movement Assessment

The seven basic movements or motions included in the SFMA screen look simple but require good flexibility and control. They are referred to as *top-tier* tests or patterns.

A patient who is (1) unable to perform a movement correctly, (2) shows a major limitation in one or more of the movement patterns, or (3) demonstrates an obvious difference between the left and right side of the body has exposed a significant finding that may be the key to correcting the problem. The seven basic movements of the SFMA are described in the following sections.

CERVICAL SPINE ASSESSMENT (Fig. 22-14, *A* to *C*)
● The cervical spine is cleared for pain and dysfunction by the patient actively demonstrating three patterns of motion: flexion (both upper and lower cervical), extension, and cervical rotation with side bending.

UPPER EXTREMITY MOVEMENT PATTERN ASSESSMENTS (Fig. 22-15, *A* and *B*)
● The UE movement pattern assessments check for total ROM in the shoulder:
  ● Pattern 1 assesses internal rotation, extension, and adduction of the shoulder (Fig. 22-15, *A*).
  ● Pattern 2 assesses external rotation, flexion, and abduction of the shoulder (Fig. 22-15, *B*).
● UE pain provocation patterns:
  ● Pattern 1 is the Yocum impingement test to help identify rotator cuff impingement (see Fig. 22-6).
  ● Pattern 2 is the shoulder adduction crossover maneuver for identifying acromioclavicular joint dysfunction and posterior shoulder tightness (Fig. 22-16).

MULTISEGMENTAL FLEXION ASSESSMENT (Fig. 22-17)
● The multisegmental flexion assessment tests for normal flexion in the hips and spine. The patient assumes the starting position by standing erect with the feet together and the toes pointing forward. The patient then bends forward at the hips and spine and attempts to touch the ends of the fingers to the tips of the toes without bending the knees.

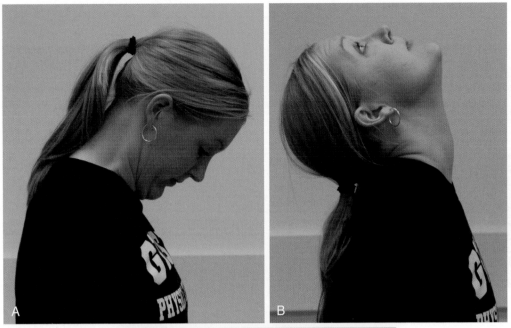

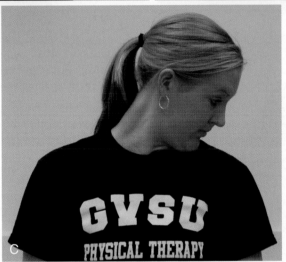

FIGURE 22-14 Cervical spine assessment: flexion (**A**), extension (**B**), and combined side bending/rotation (**C**).

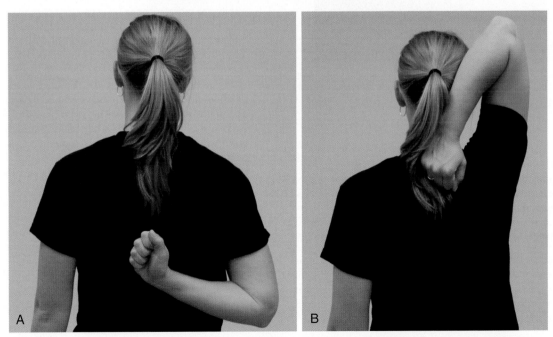

FIGURE 22-15 Shoulder mobility tests. **A,** Internal rotation, adduction, and extension. **B,** External rotation, abduction, and flexion.

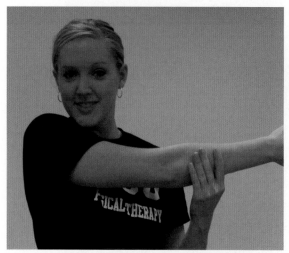

FIGURE 22-16 Shoulder clearing test 2: horizontal adduction/crossover maneuver.

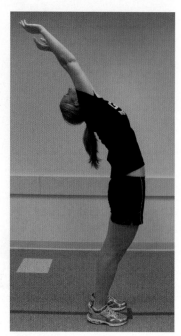

FIGURE 22-18 Multisegmental extension test: end of maneuver. Note the anterior shift of the pelvis, extension of the upper extremities, and distribution of spinal curves.

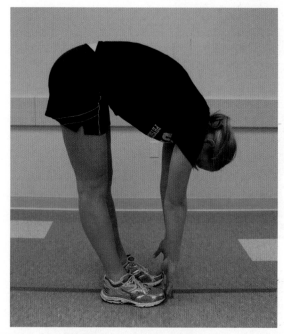

FIGURE 22-17 Multisegmental flexion test: end of maneuver. Note the straight legs, posterior weight shift, and distributed spinal curves.

- Observe for the following criteria to be met:
  - Posterior weight shift
  - Touching the toes
  - Uniform curve of the lumbar spine
  - No lateral spinal bending

MULTISEGMENTAL EXTENSION ASSESSMENT (Fig. 22-18)

- The multisegmental extension assessment tests for normal extension in the shoulders, hips, and spine. The patient assumes the starting position by standing erect with the feet together and the toes pointing forward. The patient should raise the arms directly overhead and observe the response.

- The arms are then lowered back to the starting position while the examiner looks for synchrony and symmetry of scapular motion.
- The ability to move one body part independently of another is called *dissociation*. Dissociation problems can be caused by poor stabilizing patterns that do not allow full mobility and stability at the same time. If the patient can maintain stability only by limiting limb or trunk movement, the patient is functionally rigid rather than dynamically stable. The patient may appear to have a restriction in mobility when in fact the true dysfunction is inadequate postural or motor control. As the patient raises the arms overhead, the clinician observes for the ability to move only one body part and that bilateral symmetry is present. The ideal response is for the patient to raise the arms 180° with the pelvis maintaining a neutral position.
- The patient raises the arms back up to over the head with the elbows in line with the ear. The midhand line should clear the posterior aspect of the shoulder at the end range of shoulder flexion. The elbows should remain extended and in line with the ears. At this point have the patient bend backward as far as possible while making sure that the hips go forward and the arms go back simultaneously. The spine of the scapula should move posteriorly enough to clear the heels. Both ASISs should move anteriorly, past the toes.
- Observe for the following criteria to be met:
  - The ASIS must clear the toes. Forward rotation of the pelvis will pull the lumbar spine out of a neutral position into extension. The pelvis slides forward by shifting body weight toward the front of the feet and again pulls the lumbar spine out of neutral.
  - Symmetric spinal curves should be present and the spine of the scapula must clear a vertical line drawn from the patient's heels.
  - Arms/elbows in line with the ears represent 180° of shoulder flexion.

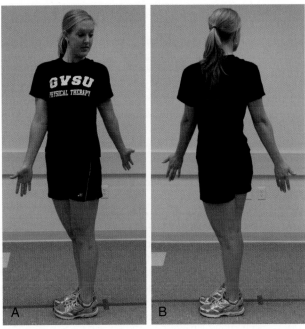

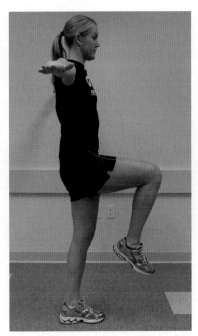

FIGURE 22-19 Multisegmental rotation test: start of maneuver (**A**) and end of maneuver (**B**). Note the rotation at the pelvis and trunk and the upright posture.

FIGURE 22-20 Single-limb stance, eyes open.

MULTISEGMENTAL ROTATION ASSESSMENT (Fig. 22-19, A and B)

- The multisegmental rotation assessment examines the total rotational motion available from the foot to the top of the spine. Usually, rotation occurs as a result of many parts contributing to the total motion. This assessment tests rotational mobility in the trunk, pelvis, hips, knees, and feet. The patient assumes a starting position by standing erect with the feet together, toes pointing forward, and arms relaxed to the sides at about waist height. The patient then rotates the entire body as far as possible to the right while the foot position remains unchanged. The patient returns to the starting position and then rotates toward the left.
  - There should be at least 50° of rotation from the starting position of the pelvis and lower quarter bilaterally.
  - In addition to the 50° of pelvic rotation, there should also be at least 50° of rotation from the thorax bilaterally, for a combined total of 100° of total-body rotation from the starting position.
- Observe for the following criteria to be met:
  - Pelvis rotating greater than 50°
  - Trunk rotating greater than 50°
  - No loss of body height with the rotation testing
  - *Note:* Because both sides are tested simultaneously with the feet together, the externally rotating hip is also extending and can thus limit motion. Close attention should be paid to each segment of the body. One area may be hypermobile because of restriction in an adjacent segment. Rotation should be symmetric on each side (within 10°)

SINGLE-LEG STANCE (STANDING KNEE LIFT) ASSESSMENT (Fig. 22-20)

- The single-leg stance assessment evaluates the ability to independently stabilize on each leg in a static and dynamic posture. The static portion of the test looks at the fundamental

foundation for control of movement. The patient assumes the starting position by standing erect with the feet together, toes pointing forward, and arms raised out to the side at shoulder height. The patient should be instructed to stand tall before testing. The patient should lift the right leg up so that the hip and knee are both flexed to 90°. The patient should maintain this posture for 10 seconds. The test is repeated on the left leg. The examiner should look to see whether the patient maintains a level pelvis (no Trendelenburg position present).

- The test is repeated again with the eyes closed. The body has three main systems that contribute to balance: visual, vestibular, and somatosensory. When the eyes are closed and vision is eliminated, the patient must rely on the other two systems to maintain an upright posture.
- To further test the patient's single-leg stance in a dynamic task, proceed to dynamic leg swings (Fig. 22-21, A and B). For dynamic leg swings, the patient is instructed to stand with the feet together, toes pointing forward, and hands resting on the hips. The patient flexes the right hip and begins to swing the right leg back and forth into flexion and extension of the hip while maintaining good posture and balance for 10 seconds. The test is repeated on the other leg.
  - Foot position should remain unchanged throughout the movement, and the hands should remain resting on the hips.
  - Look for loss of posture or height when moving from two to one leg. Any of the three portions of the test are scored as dysfunctional if the patient loses posture.

OVERHEAD DEEP SQUAT ASSESSMENT (same as used in the Functional Movement Screen) (see Fig. 22-2, A to C)

- The overhead deep squat assessment tests for bilateral mobility of the hips, knees, and ankles. When combined with the overhead upper extremity position, this test also assesses bilateral mobility of the shoulders, as well as extension of the thoracic spine.

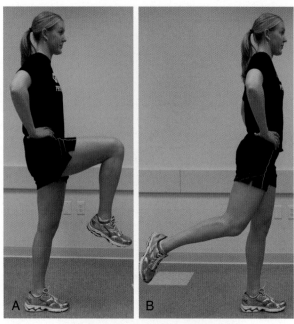

FIGURE 22-21 Dynamic leg swings: flexion position (**A**) and extension position (**B**).

- The patient assumes the starting position by placing the instep of the feet in vertical alignment with the outside of the shoulders. The feet should be in the sagittal plane, with no external rotation of the feet. The patient then raises the arms overhead, arms abducted slightly wider than shoulder width and the elbows fully extended. The patient slowly descends as deeply as possible into a full squat position. The squat position should be attempted while maintaining the heels on the floor, the head and chest facing forward, and the hands overhead. The knees should be aligned over the feet with no valgus collapse.
- Hand width should not increase as the patient descends into the squat position.
- The UEs and hands should not deviate from the plane of the tibias as the squat is performed.
- The ability to perform this test requires closed chain dorsiflexion of the ankles, flexion of the hips and knees, extension of the thoracic spine, and flexion abduction of the shoulders.

Each movement is graded with a notation of functional nonpainful, functional painful, dysfunctional painful, or dysfunctional nonpainful (see Table 22-5). All responses other than functional nonpainful are then assessed in greater detail to help refine the movement information and direct the clinical testing. Detailed algorithmic SFMA breakouts are available for each of the movement patterns, but they are beyond the scope of this chapter to describe in detail.

Optional Movements of the Selective Functional Movement Assessment

In addition to the SFMA top-tier or base assessments, four optional assessments have recently been added to further refine the movement dysfunction. They serve to illuminate movement dysfunction in higher-functioning patients. For more information on these optional movements, see Figures A22-1 through A22-4 (in Appendix 22) on Expert Consult @ www.expertconsult.com.

When dysfunction or symptoms, or both, have been provoked in a functional manner, it is necessary to work backward to more specific assessments of the component parts of the functional movement by using special tests or ROM comparisons. As the gross functional movement is broken down into its component parts, the clinician should examine for consistencies and inconsistencies, as well as the level of dysfunction, in each test with respect to the optimal movement pattern. Provocation of symptoms, as well as limitations in movement or an inability to maintain stability during movements, should be noted.

Further Refinement of Movement Dysfunction: Using the Breakouts

When dysfunction is noted, the clinician can use the SFMA to systematically dissect each of the major pattern dysfunctions with breakout algorithms. The breakouts provide an algorithmic approach to testing all areas potentially involved in the dysfunction to isolate limitations or determine dysfunction by the process of elimination. The breakouts include active and passive movements, weight-bearing and non–weight-bearing positions, multiple-joint and single-joint functional movement assessments, and unilateral and bilateral challenges. By performing parts of the test movements in both loaded and unloaded conditions, the clinician can draw conclusions about the interplay between the patient's available mobility and stability. If any of the top-tier movements are restricted when performed in the loaded position (e.g., limited or in some way painful before the end of ROM), a clue is provided regarding functional movement. For example, if a movement is performed easily (does not provoke symptoms or have any limitation) in an unloaded situation, it would seem logical that the appropriate joint ROM and muscle flexibility exist and therefore a stability problem may be the reason why the patient cannot perform the movement in a loaded position. In this case, a patient has the requisite available biomechanical ability to go through the necessary ROM to perform the task, but the neurophysiologic response needed for stabilization that creates dynamic alignment and postural support is not available when the functional movement is performed.

If the patient is observed to have limitation, restriction, or pain when unloaded, the patient displays consistent abnormal biomechanical behavior of one or more joints and would therefore require specific clinical assessment of each relevant joint and muscle complex to identify the barriers that are restricting movement and may be responsible for the provocation of pain. Consistent limitation and provocation of symptoms in both the loaded and unloaded conditions may be indicative of a mobility problem. True restrictions in mobility often require appropriate manual therapy in conjunction with corrective exercise.

The SFMA breakout testing applies the same categorizations as its top-tier assessment, with isolated focus on each pattern demonstrating pain or dysfunction. This focus helps identify gross limitations in mobility and stability. Recall that the SFMA uses specific descriptors to identify dysfunction in both mobility and stability, as described earlier in this chapter.

- Tissue extensibility dysfunction involves tissues that are extraarticular. Examples can include active or passive muscle insufficiency, neural tension, fascial tension, muscle shortening, scarring, and fibrosis.
- Joint mobility dysfunction involves structures that are articular or intraarticular. Examples can include osteoarthritis, fusion, subluxation, adhesive capsulitis, and intraarticular loose bodies.

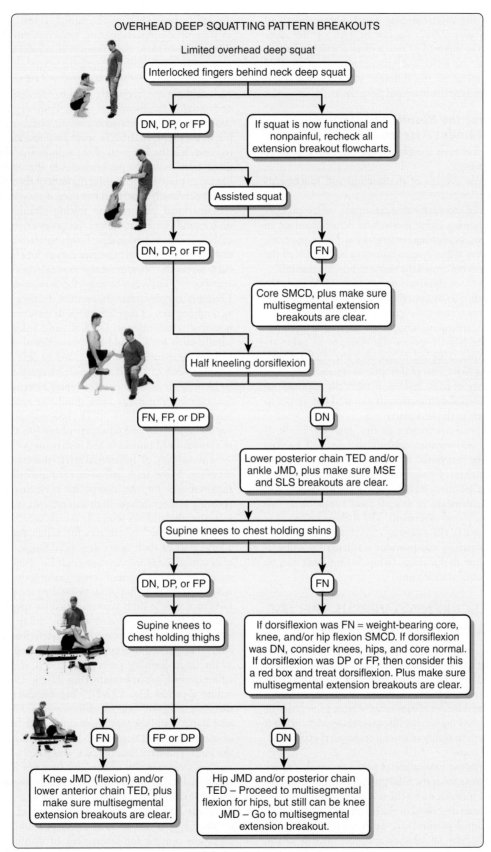

FIGURE 22-22 Overhead deep squat pattern breakout. *DN*, Dysfunctional nonpainful; *DP*, dysfunctional painful; *FN*, functional nonpainful; *FP*, functional painful; *JMD*, joint mobility dysfunction; *MSE*, multisegmental extension; *SLS*, single limb stance; *SMCD*, stability motor control dysfunction; *TED*, tissue extensibility dysfunction.

An example of the overhead deep squat pattern breakout can be found in Figure 22-22. As can be seen on the algorithm, the clinician is directed to move from a weighted to an unweighted posture, and active and passive movements are used to systematically isolate all the different variables that could cause dysfunction during the overhead deep squat.

How to Interpret the Results of Selective Functional Movement Assessment

When the SFMA has been completed, the clinician should be able to do the following:

1. Identify the major sources of dysfunction and movements that are affected.
2. Identify patterns of movement that cause pain, with reproduction of pain indicating either mechanical deformation or an inflammatory process affecting nociceptors in the symptomatic structures. The key followup question must be "Which of the functional movements caused the tissue to become painful?"
3. When the pattern of dysfunction has been identified, the problem is classified as dysfunction of either mobility or stability to determine where intervention should commence.

With the SFMA, treatment is not about alleviating mechanical pain; rather, the SFMA guides the clinician to begin by choosing interventions designed to improve the dysfunctional nonpainful patterns first. This philosophy of intervention does not ignore the source of pain; instead, it takes the approach of removing the mechanical dysfunction that caused the tissues to become symptomatic in the first place.

Pain-free functional movement is the goal for all. It is requisite for work performance, athletic success, and healthy aging. The pain-free functional movement necessary to allow participation in activities of daily living, work, and athletics has many components: posture, ROM, muscle performance, and motor control. Impairments in any of these components can potentially alter functional movement. The authors believe that the SFMA incorporates the essential elements of many daily, work, and sports activities and provides a schema for addressing movement-related dysfunction. (More information can be found at www.Rehabeducation.com.)

MOVEMENT SCREENING VERSUS SPECIFIC FUNCTIONAL PERFORMANCE TESTS

The fundamental movement screening tests described in this chapter do not assess the whole of function. They do not include power tasks, running, jumping, acceleration, or deceleration, which are important facets of almost all sports and must therefore be examined before return of an athlete to practice or competition. The following section discusses the evidence that is available and the current utility of several common specific functional performance tests.

Professionals involved with athletes perform a wide variety of functional performance tests. Objective, quantitative assessment of functional limitations by the use of functional performance testing has been described in the literature for more than 20 years.[18-24] Functional performance assessment may be used in an attempt to describe an athlete's aptitude, identify talent, monitor performance, describe asymmetry or dysfunction, and determine readiness to participate in sports. Before sports participation athletes are frequently timed in a 40-yard dash, measured for vertical jump abilities, or assessed for performance

on agility tests such as the timed T-test. This often occurs as part of a preparticipation examination. After progressing through postinjury or postsurgical rehabilitation, patients are assessed for their ability to perform functional tasks such as step-downs, hopping, jumping, landing, and cutting. Functional tests such as these are frequently used to simulate sporting activities or actions in the context of whole-body dynamic movement to contribute to the decision regarding whether an athlete is fit or physically prepared to begin sport participation or ready to return to sport. It is the assertion of the authors that these specific functional tests should be performed only after movement screening has taken place and successful mastery of the fundamental movements previously described has been demonstrated.

Functional performance testing should examine athletes under conditions that imitate the necessary functional demands of their sports. Functional performance tests use dynamic skills or tasks to assess multiple components of function, including muscular strength, neuromuscular control/coordination, and joint stability.[25,26] They can be used for assessment of patients after LE injury, surgery, muscular contusions, overuse conditions such as tendinopathy or patellofemoral dysfunction, anterior cruciate ligament reconstruction (ACLR), and ankle instability.[19-21,26,27] Ideally, such tests should be time efficient and simple, require little or inexpensive equipment, and be able to be performed in a clinical setting.[11,21,28] If at all possible, such tests should be able to identify subjects at risk for injury or reinjury.[28-31] Above all, functional performance tests should be objective, reliable, and sensitive to change.[19,24,27,29,32] The root requirement for establishing the objectivity and reliability of any functional test is the use of standardized protocols and instructions.[27]

The validity of functional performance tests is difficult to establish. Many tests assess or examine only a portion of the requirements for the composite performance of a complex sporting activity. Single-limb assessments may have advantages in evaluating athletes who rely on unilateral limb performance, such as runners,[33] or athletes for whom running accounts for a large part of their sport demands. Single-limb tasks or hops offer considerable information regarding functional readiness in a wide variety of athletes because many sports entail single-limb weight acceptance, hopping, or landing as a part of their performance. Single-limb assessments offer specific benefits in the realm of objectivity because of their ability to provide within-subject, between-limb comparisons, described as a *biologic baseline*, versus having to use population-derived norms. Tests such as the single-limb leg press (Fig. 22-23), step-down performed either to the front or laterally (Fig. 22-24, A to C),[27,34] squat (see online appendix Fig. A22-2),[35] hop for distance, triple hop for distance, crossover hop for distance (Fig. 22-25, A to C),[18,20,21] stair hop,[29,30] and the 6-m timed single-limb hop[20,21] are examples of commonly used single-limb tests that allow establishment of the limb symmetry index (LSI), which helps identify existing or residual postoperative asymmetry between limbs.[20,21,25,29,30] The functional status of the knee has been categorized as "compromised" if the LSI is less than 85%.[18,20,21]

Single-limb tasks offer a wide variety of imposed demands on the LE that can be used at various times during the rehabilitation process for assessment of symmetry, recovery, and readiness to resume sports participation.[27,29,30] The triple hop for distance has been demonstrated to be a strong predictor of both power (as measured by vertical jump) and isokinetic strength.[22,25,36] Sekir et al[26] describe a lateral single-limb hop test that may be an important facet of functional assessment for athletes who rely on repetitive lateral movements for sport proficiency. Several researchers also advocate assessment of lateral movement during single-limb hop testing or the side-cutting maneuver because it may be more valid for athletes who move and cut laterally.[37,38] Several authors[18,20,21,29,30] have related the LSI to functional status; for example, a lower LSI after ACLR is related to poorer function, and improvements in raw scores on the single-limb hop test, as well as the LSI, represent functional recovery over 52 weeks after ACLR. Noyes et al[20,21] suggested that the LSI should be higher than 85% before return to sport. Loudon et al[27] suggested that in the case of patellofemoral pain syndrome, the LSI should be closer to 90% to prevent reinjury. Bilateral assessments, including squats, leg presses, and two-legged jumps such as the drop jump (Fig. 22-26, *A* to *C*) or tuck jump (Fig. 22-27, *A* to *C*), may be more valid for assessing athletes in whom two-legged jumping and landing tasks are important.[31,33] Most athletic skills require a combination

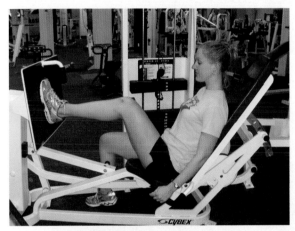

FIGURE 22-23 Single-leg press.

of vertical, horizontal, and lateral movement by one or both LEs. Probably the most important requirement for successful sport performance is a series of highly developed motor control strategies to allow speed and agility during performance.[33] If an LE reach, jump, hop, or agility test could be used to objectively screen athletes' neuromuscular performance and suggest intervention before either sport participation or return to sport, that functional performance test would be valuable for preventing injury or decreasing the likelihood of reinjury.[12,21,28,31,37]

The authors know of no single optimal, valid, and reliable test that can determine an athlete's readiness for participation or return to sport. Given the wide variation and complexity of the demands of sport, this is not surprising! Many professionals suggest the use of functional test batteries or a series of functional tests that are related to the specific demands of a specific sport or that can be related to the probable mechanisms of injury for a specific pathology. A combination of two or more tests is recommended for relevant, sensitive, responsive functional assessment.[18,20,21,39,40] Bjorklund et al[39] proposed a functional test instrument (battery) named the Test for Athletes with Knee Injuries (TAK) that they describe as valid, reliable, and sensitive for use after ACLR. The TAK is composed of eight evaluations, including jogging, running, single-limb squat, rising from sitting (single leg), bilateral squat, single-limb hop for distance, single-limb vertical jump (performed plyometrically), and the single-limb crossover hop (8 m). The authors present suggested scoring criteria for each test that take into account qualitative assessment of performance of the eight tests. This is just one such example of combining several functional performance tests into a series for examination of a group of patients. Clearly, all functional performance tests are not relevant for all athletes, and it is the role of the rehabilitation professional to select valid, reliable, sensitive, and relevant functional performance tests. For additional examples of functional performance tests, see Figures A22-5 through A22-9 (in Appendix 22) on Expert Consult @ www.expertconsult.com.

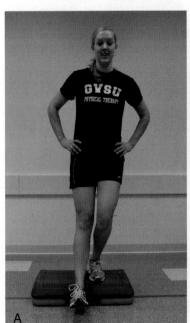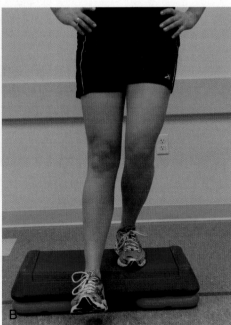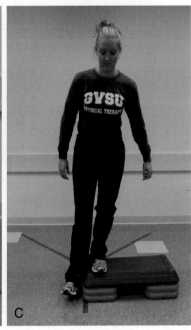

FIGURE 22-24 Step-down test. Monitor for lower extremity biomechanics and control. **A,** Front step down; note the trunk and hands. **B,** Front step-down close-up; note the alignment of the stance knee. **C,** Lateral step-down with same qualitative criteria.

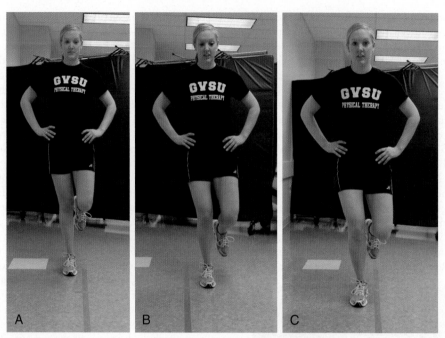

FIGURE 22-25 Crossover hop for distance: start (**A**), lateral movement (**B**), and final lateral movement (**C**). *Note:* the athlete must "stick" or control the landing. The athlete attempts to go as far as possible in the combined three hops.

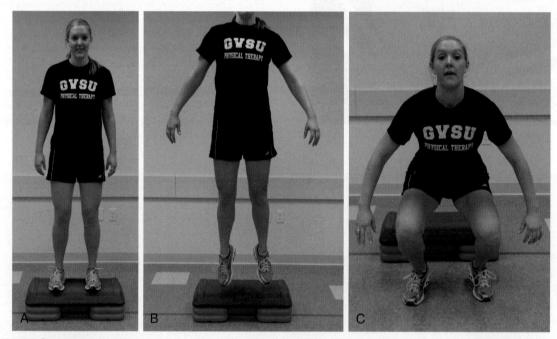

FIGURE 22-26 Drop jump assessment: start position (**A**), midposition (**B**), and landing (**C**). Note the deep flexion angle in landing and alignment of the hips and knees.

CONCLUSION

Movement Scoring Systems

- One of the most difficult decisions that must be made by rehabilitation providers is whether an athlete is ready to participate in sports or safely return to sport participation.
- Acceptance plus use of fundamental movement screening systems such as the FMS and the SFMA is sweeping across the country. These screens offer valuable information

to professionals regarding the fundamental functional abilities of an athlete in the realm of *movement* by identifying compensatory movements or deficits in mobility or stability.

Functional Performance Tests

- Functional performance tests or test batteries can be used to assess athletes of all ages and skill levels who participate in a wide variety of sports.

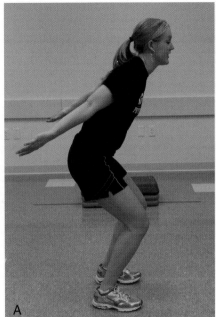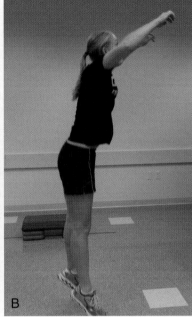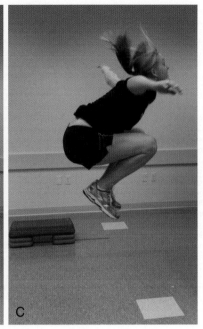

FIGURE 22-27 Tuck jump assessment: beginning of movement (**A**), midmovement (**B**), and in air in a tucked position (**C**). Note that this test must be observed from the side and the front to analyze performance.

- Frequently, functional performance tests assess a facet or single part the vast demands of any given sport, and therefore the validity of such tests is hard to determine. Though not providing a complete picture of athletic function, these tests are essential tools for the rehabilitation professional. It is critical that the rehabilitation professional be familiar with the use of such screens and tests to discern readiness for participation.

- Skillful combinations of movement screening, functional performance testing, and sport-specific movement testing offer the best assessment of an athlete's readiness for return to sport.

Future Research

- Although evidence regarding tests and systems that are objective, valid, and reliable is beginning to mount (Minick, DiMattia, Loudon, and others), many questions regarding the big picture of return to function exist. Does the FMS relate to core stability? Does it predict performance in athletics or merely identify potential for injury? Which functional performance measures are best used for athletes who participate in certain sports? Normative scores for the FMS and other functional performance tests by age and gender would be very helpful for comparison between athletes.

- As the published evidence on functional testing continues to accumulate, rehabilitation professionals will have to keep abreast of changes and adapt their use of screens and tests accordingly.

REFERENCES

1. Fuller, C., and Drawer, S. (2004): The application of risk management in sports. Sports Med., 19:2108–2114.
2. Paterno, M.V., Schmitt, L.C., Ford, K.R., et al. (2010): Biomechanical measures during landing and postural stability predict second anterior cruciate ligament injury after anterior cruciate ligament reconstruction and return to sport. Am. J. Sports Med., 38:1968–1978.
3. Reed, F.E. (2004): The preparticipation athletic exam process. South. Med. J., 97:871–872.
4. Van Mechelen, W., Hlobil, H., Kemper, H.C., et al. (1992): Incidence, severity, etiology, and prevention of sports injuries. Sports Med., 14:82–89.
5. Van Mechelen, W., Twisk, J., Molendjk, A., et al. (1996): Subject related risk factors for sports injuries: A 1-year prospective study in young adults. Med. Sci. Sports Exerc., 28:1171–1179.
6. Watson, A.W. (2001): Sports injuries related to flexibility, posture, acceleration, clinical deficits, and previous injury in high-level players of body contact sports. Int. J. Sports Med., 22:220–225.
7. Kendall, F.P. (2005): Muscle Testing and Function, 5th ed. Philadelphia, Lippincott Williams & Wilkins.
8. Page, P., Frank, C.C., and Lordner, R. (2011): Assessment and Treatment of Muscle Imbalance: The Janda Approach. Champaign, IL, Human Kinetics.
9. Sahrmann, S.A. (2002): Diagnosis and Treatment of Movement Impairment Syndromes. St. Louis, Mosby.
10. Chorba, R.S., Chorba, D.J., Bouillon, L.E., et al. (2010): Use of a functional movement screening tool to determine injury risk in female collegiate athletes. N. Am. J. Sports Phys. Ther., 5:47–54.
11. Kiesel, K., Plisky, P.J., and Voight, M.L. (2007): Can serious injury in professional football be predicted by a preseason functional movement screen? N. Am. J. Sports Phys. Ther., 2:147–152.
12. Plisky, P.J., Rauh, M.J., Kaminski, T.W., and Underwood, F.B. (2006): Star excursion balance test as a predictor of lower extremity injury in high school basketball players. J. Orthop. Sports Phys. Ther., 36:911–919.
13. Cook, G., Burton, L., and Hoogenboom, B. (2006): Pre-participation screening: The use of fundamental movements as an assessment of function—Part 1. N. Am. J. Sports Phys. Ther., 1:62–72.
14. Cook, G., Burton, L., and Hoogenboom, B. (2004): Pre-participation screening: The use of fundamental movements as an assessment of function—Part 2. N. Am. J. Sports Phys. Ther., 1:132–139.
15. Minick, K.I., Kiesel, K.M., Burton, L., et al. (2010): Interrater reliability of the functional movement screen. J. Strength Cond. Res., 24:479–486.
16. Okada, T., Huxel, K.C., and Nesser, T.W. (2011): Relationship between core stability, functional movement, and performance. J. Strength Cond. Res., 25:252–261.
17. Richardson, C., Hodges, P., and Hides, J. (2004): Therapeutic Exercise for Lumbopelvic Stabilization: A Motor Control Approach for the Treatment and Prevention of Low Back Pain, 2nd ed. Philadelphia, Churchill Livingstone.
18. Barber, S.D., Noyes, F.R., Mangine, R.E., et al. (1990): Quantitative assessment of functional limitation in normal and anterior cruciate ligament–deficient knees. Clin. Orthop. Relat. Res., 255:204–214.
19. Bolgla, L.A., and Keskula, D.R. (1997): Reliability of lower extremity functional performance tests. J. Orthop. Sports Phys. Ther., 26:138–142.
20. Noyes, F.R., Barber, S.D., and Mangine, R.E. (1991): Abnormal lower limb symmetry determined by functional hop tests after anterior cruciate ligament rupture. Am. J. Sports Med., 19:513–518.
21. Noyes, F.R., Barber-Westin, S.D., Fleckenstein, C., et al. (2005): The drop-jump screening test: Difference in lower limb control by gender and effect of neuromuscular training in female athletes. Am. J. Sports Med., 33:197–207.

22. Petschnig, R., Baron, R., and Albrecht, M. (1998): The relationship between isokinetic quadriceps strength test and hop tests for distance and one-legged vertical jump test following anterior cruciate ligament reconstruction. J. Orthop. Sports Phys. Ther., 28:23–31.

23. Risberg, M.A., and Ekeland, A. (1994): Assessment of functional tests after anterior cruciate ligament surgery. J. Orthop. Sports Phys. Ther., 19:212–217.

24. Ross, M.D., Langford, B., and Whelan, P.J. (2002): Test-retest reliability of 4 single-leg hop tests. J. Strength Cond. Res., 16:617–622.

25. Hamilton, R.T., Shultz, S.J., Schmitz, R.J., and Perrin, D.H. (2008): Triple-hop distance as a valid predictor of lower limb strength and power. J. Athl. Train., 43:144–151.

26. Sekir, U., Yildiz, Y., Hazneci, B., et al. (2008): Reliability of a functional test battery evaluating functionality, proprioception, and strength in recreational athletes with functional ankle instability. Eur. J. Phys. Rehabil. Med., 44:407–415.

27. Loudon, J.K., Waiesner, D., Goist-Foley, L.H., et al. (2002): Intrarater reliability of functional performance tests for subjects with patellofemoral pain syndrome. J. Athl. Train., 37:256–261.

28. Myer, G.D., Ford, K.R., and Hewett, T.E. (2008): Tuck jump assessment for reducing anterior cruciate ligament injury risk. Athl. Ther. Today, 13:(5):39–44.

29. Hopper, D.M., Goh, S.C., Wentworth, L.A., et al. (2002): Test-retest reliability of knee rating scales and functional hop tests one year following anterior cruciate ligament reconstruction. Phys. Ther. Sport, 3:10–18.

30. Hopper, D.M., Strauss, G.R., Boyle, J.J., and Bell, J. (2008): Functional recovery after anterior cruciate ligament reconstruction: A longitudinal perspective. Arch. Phys. Med. Rehabil., 89:1535–1541.

31. Padua, D.A., Marshall, S.W., Boling, M.C., et al. (2009): The landing error scoring system (LESS) is a valid and reliable clinical assessment tool of jump-landing biomechanics: The JUMP-ACL study. Am. J. Sports Med., 37:1996–2002.

32. Brosky, J., Nitz, A., Malone, T., et al. (1999): Intrarater reliability of selected clinical outcome measures following anterior cruciate ligament reconstruction. J. Orthop. Sports Phys. Ther., 29:39–48.

33. Meylan, C., McMaster, T., Cronin, J., et al. (2009): Single-leg lateral, horizontal, and vertical jump assessment: Reliability, interrelationships, and ability to predict sprint and change-of-direction performance. J. Strength Cond. Res., 23:1140–1147.

34. Piva, S.R., Fitzgerald, K., Irrgang, J.J., et al. (2006): Reliability of measures of impairments associated with patellofemoral pain. BMC Musculoskelet. Disord., 7:33–46.

35. DiMattia, M.A., Livengood, A.L., Uhl, T.L., et al. (2005): What are the validity of the single-leg-squat test and its relationship to hip abduction strength? J. Sport Rehabil., 14:108–123.

36. Wilk, K.E., Romaniello, W.T., Soscia, S.M., et al. (1994): The relationship between subjective knee scores, isokinetic testing and functional testing in the ACL-reconstructed knee. J. Orthop. Sports Phys. Ther., 20:60–73.

37. Hewett, T.E., Myer, G.D., Ford, K.R., and Slauterbeck, J.R. (2006): Preparticipation physical examination using a box drop vertical jump test in young athletes: The effects of puberty and sex. Clin. J. Sport Med., 16:298–304.

38. Zebis, M.K., Andersen, L.L., Bencke, J., et al. (2009): Identification of athletes at future risk of anterior cruciate ligament ruptures by neuromuscular screening. Am. J. Sports Med., 37:1967–1973.

39. Bjorklund, K., Andersson, L., and Dalen, N. (2009): Validity and responsiveness of the test of athletes with knee injuries: The new criterion based functional performance test instrument. Knee Surg. Sports Traumatol. Arthrosc., 17:435–445.

40. Gustavsson, A., Neeter, C., Thomee, P., et al. A test battery for evaluation of hop performance in patients with ACL injury and patients who have undergone ACL reconstruction. Knee Surg. Sports Traumatol. Arthrosc., 14:778-788.

23

Functional Training and Advanced Rehabilitation

Michael L. Voight, PT, DHSc, OCS, SCS, ATC, CSCS, FAPTA,
Barb Hoogenboom, PT, EdD, SCS, ATC, and Gray Cook, PT, MS, OCS, CSCS

CHAPTER OBJECTIVES

- Define and discuss the importance of proprioception in the neuromuscular control process.
- Define and discuss the different levels of motor control by the central nervous system and the neural pathways responsible for transmission of afferent and efferent information at each level.
- Apply a systematic functional evaluation designed to provoke symptoms.
- Demonstrate consistency between functional and clinical testing information (combinatorial power).

- Apply a three-step model designed to promote the practical systematic thinking required for effective therapeutic exercise prescription and progression.
- Define and discuss objectives of a functional neuromuscular rehabilitation program.
- Develop a rehabilitation program that uses various exercise techniques for development of neuromuscular control.

FUNCTION AND FUNCTIONAL REHABILITATION

The basic goal in rehabilitation is to restore and enhance function within the environment and to perform specific activities of daily living (ADLs). The entire rehabilitation process should be focused on improving the functional status of the patient. The concept of functional training is not new, nor is it limited to function related to sports. By definition, *function* means having a purpose or duty. Therefore, *functional* can be defined as performing a practical or intended function or duty. Function should be considered in terms of a spectrum because ADLs encompass many different tasks for many different people. What is functional to one person may not be functional to another. It is widely accepted that to perform a specific activity better, one must practice that activity. Therefore, the functional exercise progression for return to ADLs can best be defined as breaking the specific activities down into a hierarchy and then performing them in a sequence that allows acquisition or reacquisition of that skill. It is important to note that although people develop different levels of skill, function, and motor control, certain fundamental tasks are common to nearly all individuals (barring pathologic conditions and disability). Lifestyle, habits, injury, and other factors can erode the fundamental components of movement without obvious alterations in higher-level function and skill. Ongoing higher-level function is a testament to the compensatory power of the neurologic system. Imperfect function and skill create stress in other body systems. Fundamental elements can first be observed during the developmental progression of posture and motor control. The sequence of developmental progression can also give insight into the original acquisition of skill. The ability to assess retention or loss of fundamental movement patterns is therefore a way to enhance rehabilitation. The rehabilitation process starts with a two-part appraisal that creates perspective by viewing both ends of the functional spectrum:

- The current level of function (ADLs, work, and sports/recreation) relative to the patient's needs and goals
- The ability to demonstrate the fundamental movement patterns that represent the foundation of function and basic motor control

Objectives of Functional Rehabilitation

The overall objective of a functional exercise program is to return patients to their preinjury level as quickly and as safely as possible by resolving or reducing the measurable dysfunction within fundamental and functional movement patterns. Specific training activities are designed to restore both dynamic joint stability and ADL skills.[1] To accomplish this objective, a basic tenet of exercise physiology is used. The SAID (specific adaptations to imposed demands) principle states that the body will adapt to the stress and strain placed on it.[2] Athletes cannot succeed if they have not been prepared to meet all the demands of their specific activity.[2] Reactive neuromuscular training (RNT) helps bridge the gap from traditional rehabilitation via proprioceptive and balance training to promote a more functional return to activity.[2] The SAID principle provides constructive stress, and RNT creates opportunities for input and integration. The main objective of the RNT program is to facilitate the unconscious process of interpreting and integrating the peripheral sensations received by the central nervous system (CNS) into appropriate motor responses. This approach is enhanced by the unique clinical focus on pathologic orthopedic and neurologic states and their functional representation. This special focus forces the clinician to consider evaluation of human movement as a complex multisystem interaction and the logical starting point for exercise prescription. Sometimes this will require a breakdown of the supporting mobility and stability within a pattern. Regardless of the specific nature of the corrective needs, all the functional exercises follow a simple but very specific path. First, the functional exercise program is driven by a functional screening or assessment that produces a baseline of movement (see Chapter 22). The process of screening and assessment will rate and rank patterns. It will provide valuable information about dysfunction in movement patterns such as asymmetry, difficulty with movement, and pain. Screening and assessment will therefore identify faulty movement patterns that should not be exercised or trained until corrected. Second, the functional framework will assist in making the best possible choices for corrective categories and exercises. No single exercise is best for a movement problem, but there is an appropriate category of corrective exercises to choose from. Third, following the initial session of corrective exercises, the movement pattern should be rechecked for changes against the original baseline. Fourth, when an obvious change is noted in the key pattern, the screening or assessment is repeated to survey other changes in movement and identify the next priority. By working on the most fundamental pattern, it is possible to see other positive changes. Therefore, these four steps provide the framework that makes corrective exercise successful:

- The screening and assessment direct the clinician to the most fundamental movement dysfunction.
- One or two of the most practical corrective exercises from the appropriate category should be chosen and applied.
- When the exercise has been taught and is being performed correctly, check for improvement in the dysfunctional basic movement pattern as revealed by specific tests in the screening or assessment.

This concept is called the *functional continuum*. Most patients seek care because of an obvious source of pain or dysfunction. What is not obvious is the true cause of the pain or dysfunction,

Table 23-1 Four Phases of the Functional Continuum

Phase	Description
Subconscious dysfunction	This is the initial phase when most patients are first seen by the clinician. Patients are totally unaware of their true dysfunction (it is in their subconscious) or are convinced that the problem lies elsewhere.
Conscious dysfunction	This is what happens after a movement assessment is performed. Patients are now aware of their true dysfunction (it is in their conscious), and they can start to address the real cause.
Conscious function	This phase is entered once patients can perform the correct functional pattern, but it is not automatic (it is functional only with conscious control). They still need conscious effort to perform a good pattern of movement.
Subconscious function	The final stage occurs when patients can perform a functional pattern automatically (it is in their subconscious control) without having to think about the correction.

ascertainment of which is the purpose of functional movement assessment (see Chapter 22). By looking at movement as a whole, all the compensations and conscious sources of pain and dysfunction can be highlighted and addressed. Patients fall into one of four phases on a functional continuum (Table 23-1).

Exercise prescription choices must continually represent the specialized training of the clinician through a consistent and centralized focus on human function and consideration of the fundamentals that make function possible. Exercise applied at any given therapeutic level must refine movement, not simply create general exertion in the hope of increased tolerance of movement.[3] Moore and Durstine state, "Unfortunately, exercise training to optimize functional capacity has not been well studied in the context of most chronic diseases or disabilities. As a result, many exercise professionals have used clinical experience to develop their own methods for prescribing exercise."[4] Experience, self-critique, and specialization produce seasoned clinicians with intuitive evaluation abilities and innovations in exercise that are sometimes difficult to follow and even harder to ascertain; however, common characteristics do exist. Clinical experts use parallel (simultaneous) consideration of all factors influencing functional movement. RNT as a treatment philosophy is inclusive and adaptable and has the ability to address a variety of clinical situations. It should also be understood that a clinical philosophy is designed to serve, not to be served. The treatment design demonstrates specific attention to the parts (clinical measurements and isolated details) with continual consideration of the whole (restoration of function).[3] Moore and Durstine follow their previous statement by acknowledging that "experience is an acceptable way to guide exercise management, but a systematic approach would be better."[4] We use the three Rs as a way to understand the type of treatment phases that a patient will undergo (Table 23-2).

Table 23-2 Three Rs of Treatment Phases

R	Description
Reset	Most problems require resetting of the complete system to break them out of their dysfunctional phase. By just jumping to exercises, the results can be less than optimal. Types of treatments that would be considered a reset include joint mobilization, soft tissue mobilization, and various soft tissue techniques.
Reinforce	After the system has been reset, many dysfunctions will need support or reinforcement while proper patterns are being introduced. Types of reinforcement devices include taping, bracing, orthotics, postural devices, and static and dynamic stretching.
Reload	The last phase of treatment is the exercise implementation or reload phase, in which the new software is loaded into the central nervous system and a true functional pattern of motion can be reprogrammed.

Box 23-1

Three-Phase Rehabilitation Model

1. Proprioception and kinesthesia
2. Dynamic stability
3. Reactive neuromuscular control

Box 23-2

Four Principles for Prescription of Exercise

Functional evaluation and assessment in relation to dysfunction (disability) and impairment
Identification and management of motor control
Identification and management of osteokinematic and arthrokinematic limitations
Identification of current movement patterns followed by facilitation and integration of synergistic movement patterns

---

The Three-Phase Model for Prescription of Exercise

The purpose of this chapter is to demonstrate a practical model designed to promote the systematic thinking required for effective prescription of therapeutic exercise and progression at each phase of rehabilitation.[3] The approach is a serial (consecutive) step-by-step method that will, with practice and experience, lead to parallel thinking and multilevel problem solving. The (redundant) purpose of this method is to reduce arbitrary trial-and-error attempts at prescribing effective exercise and lessen protocol-based thinking. It will give the novice clinician a framework that will guide but not confine clinical exercise prescription. It will provide experienced clinicians with a system to observe their particular strengths and weaknesses in dosage and design of exercise. Inexperienced and experienced clinicians alike will develop practical insight by applying the model and observing the interaction of the systems that produce human movement. The focus is specifically geared to orthopedic rehabilitation and the clinical problem-solving strategies used to develop an exercise prescription through an outcome-based goal-setting process. All considerations for therapeutic exercise prescription will give equal importance to conventional orthopedic exercise standards (biomechanical and physiologic parameters) and neurophysiologic strategies (motor learning, proprioceptive feedback, and synergistic recruitment principles). This three-phase model (Box 23-1) will create a mechanism that necessitates interaction between orthopedic exercise approaches and optimal neurophysiologic techniques. It includes a four-principle foundation that demonstrates the hierarchy and interaction of the founding concepts used in rehabilitation (both orthopedic and neurologic). For all practical purposes, these four categories help demonstrate the efficient and effective continuity necessary for formulation of a treatment plan and prompt the clinician to maintain an inclusive, open-minded clinical approach.

This chapter is written with the clinic-based practitioner in mind. It will help the clinician formulate an exercise philosophy. Some clinicians will discover reasons for success that were intuitive and therefore hard to communicate to other professionals. Others will discover a missing step in the therapeutic exercise design process. Much of the confusion and frustration encountered by rehabilitation specialists is due to the vast variety of treatment options afforded by ever improving technology and accessibility to emerging research evidence. To effectively use the wealth of current information and what the future has yet to bestow, clinicians must adopt an operational framework or personal philosophy about therapeutic exercise. If a clinical exercise philosophy is based on technology, equipment, or protocols, the scope of problem solving is strictly confined. It would continually change because no universal standard or gauge exists. However, a philosophy based solely on the structure and function of the human body will keep the focus (Box 23-2) uncorrupted and centralized. Technologic developments can enhance the effectiveness of exercise only as long as the technology, system, or protocol remains true to a holistic functional standard. Known functional standards should serve as governing factors that improve the clinical consistency of the clinician and rehabilitation team for prescription and progression of training methods. The four principles for exercise prescription (see Table 23-3) are based on human movement and the systems on which it is constructed (see Box 23-2). The intent of these four distinct categories is to break down and reconstruct the factors that influence functional movement and to stimulate inductive reasoning, deductive reasoning, and the critical thinking needed to develop a therapeutic exercise progression. It is hoped that these factors will serve the intended purpose of organization and clarity, thereby giving due respect to the many insightful clinicians who have provided the foundation and substance for construction of this practical framework.[3]

PROPRIOCEPTION, RECEPTORS, AND NEUROMUSCULAR CONTROL

Success in skilled performance depends on how effectively an individual detects, perceives, and uses relevant sensory information. Knowing exactly where our limbs are in space and how much muscular effort is required to perform a particular action is critical for successful performance of all activities requiring intricate coordination of the various body parts. Fortunately, information about the position and movement of various body parts is available from peripheral receptors located in and around articular structures and the surrounding musculature. A detailed discussion of proprioception and neuromuscular control is also presented in Chapter 24.

Joints: Support and Sensory Function

In a normal healthy joint, both static and dynamic stabilizers provide support. The role of capsuloligamentous tissues in the dynamic restraint of joints has been well established in the literature.[5-15] Although the primary role of these structures is mechanical in nature by providing structural support and stabilization to the joint, the capsuloligamentous tissues also play an important sensory role by detecting joint position and motion.[8,16-18] Sensory afferent feedback from receptors in the capsuloligamentous structures projects directly to the reflex and cortical pathways, thereby mediating reactive muscle activity for dynamic restraint.[5,6,8,17,19] The efferent motor response that ensues from the sensory information is called *neuromuscular control*. Sensory information is sent to the CNS to be processed, and appropriate motor strategies are executed.

Physiology of Proprioception

Sherrington[18] first described the term *proprioception* in the early 1900s when he noted the presence of receptors in the joint capsular structures that were primarily reflexive in nature. Since that time, mechanoreceptors have been morphohistologically identified around articular structures in both animal and human models. In addition, the well-described muscle spindle and Golgi tendon organs are powerful mechanoreceptors. Mechanoreceptors are specialized end-organs that function as biologic transducers for conversion of the mechanical energy of physical deformation (elongation, compression, and pressure) into action nerve potentials yielding proprioceptive information.[10] Although receptor discharge varies according to the intensity of the distortion, mechanoreceptors can also be described in terms of their discharge rates. Quickly adapting receptors cease discharging shortly after the onset of a stimulus, whereas slowly adapting receptors continue to discharge while the stimulus is present.[8,10,20] Around a healthy joint, quickly adapting receptors are responsible for providing conscious and unconscious kinesthetic sensations in response to joint movement or acceleration, whereas slowly adapting mechanoreceptors provide continuous feedback and thus proprioceptive information related to joint position[10,20,21] (see Chapter 24 for examples of quickly and slowly adapting receptors).

When stimulated, mechanoreceptors are able to adapt. With constant stimulation, the frequency of the neural impulses decreases. The functional implication is that mechanoreceptors detect change and rates of change, as opposed to steady-state conditions.[22] This input is then analyzed in the CNS to determine joint position and movement.[23] The status of the musculoskeletal structures is sent to the CNS so that information about static versus dynamic conditions, equilibrium versus disequilibrium, or biomechanical stress and strain relationships can be evaluated.[24,25] When processed and evaluated, this proprioceptive information becomes capable of influencing muscle tone, motor execution programs, and cognitive somatic perceptions or kinesthetic awareness.[26] Proprioceptive information also protects the joint from damage caused by movement exceeding the normal physiologic range of motion (ROM) and helps determine the appropriate

balance of synergistic and antagonistic forces. This information generates a somatosensory image within the CNS. Therefore, the soft tissues surrounding a joint serve a double purpose: they provide biomechanical support to the bony partners making up the joint by keeping them in relative anatomic alignment, and through an extensive afferent neurologic network, they provide valuable proprioceptive information.

CENTRAL NERVOUS SYSTEM: INTEGRATION OF MOTOR CONTROL

The response of the CNS falls into three categories or levels of motor control: spinal reflexes, brainstem processing, and cognitive cerebral cortex program planning. The goal of the rehabilitation process is to retrain the altered afferent pathways and thereby enhance the neuromuscular control system. To accomplish this goal, the objective of the rehabilitation program should be to hyperstimulate the joint and muscle receptors to encourage maximal afferent discharge to the respective CNS levels.[21,27-30]

First-Level Response: Muscle

When faced with an unexpected load, the first reflexive muscle response is a burst of electromyographic (EMG) activity that occurs between 30 and 50 msec. The afferent fibers of both the muscle spindle and the Golgi tendon organ mechanoreceptors synapse with the spinal interneurons and produce a reflexive facilitation or inhibition of the motor neurons.[28,30,31] The monosynaptic stretch reflex is one of the most rapid reflexes underlying limb control. The stretch reflex occurs at an unconscious level and is not affected by extrinsic factors. These responses can occur simultaneously to control limb position and posture. Because they can occur at the same time, are in parallel, are subconscious, and are not subject to cortical interference, they do not require attention and are thus automatic.

At this level of motor control, activities to encourage short-loop reflex joint stabilization should dominate.[15,21,27,30] These activities are characterized by sudden alterations in joint position that require reflex muscle stabilization. With sudden alterations or perturbations, both the articular and muscular mechanoreceptors will be stimulated to produce reflex stabilization. Rhythmic stabilization exercises encourage monosynaptic cocontraction of the musculature, thereby producing dynamic neuromuscular stabilization.[32] These exercises serve to build a foundation for dynamic stability.

Second-Level Response: Brainstem

The second level of motor control interaction is at the level of the brainstem.[25,28,33] At this level, afferent mechanoreceptors interact with the vestibular system and visual input from the eyes to control or facilitate postural stability and equilibrium of the body.[21,25,27-29] Afferent mechanoreceptor input also works in concert with the muscle spindle complex by inhibiting antagonistic muscle activity under conditions of rapid lengthening and periarticular distortion, both of which accompany postural disruption.[26,30] In conditions of disequilibrium in which simultaneous neural input exists, a neural pattern is generated that affects the muscular stabilizers and thereby returns equilibrium to the body's center of gravity.[28] Therefore, balance is influenced by the same peripheral afferent mechanism that mediates joint proprioception and is at least partially dependent on an individual's inherent ability to integrate joint position sense with neuromuscular control.[34]

It is important that these activities remain specific to the types of activities or skills that will be required of the athlete on return to sport.[35] Static balance activities should be used as a precursor to more dynamic skill activity.[35] Static balance skills can be initiated when the individual is able to bear weight on the lower extremity. The general progression of static balance activities is to move from bilateral to unilateral and from eyes open to eyes closed.[21,28,35-37] With balance training, it is important to remember that the sensory systems respond to environmental manipulation. To stimulate or facilitate the proprioceptive system, vision must be disadvantaged, which can be accomplished in several ways (Box 23-3).

Third-Level Response: Central Nervous System/Cognitive

Appreciation of joint position at the highest or cognitive level needs to be included in an RNT program. These types of activities are initiated on the cognitive level and include programming motor commands for voluntary movement. Repetitions of these movements will maximally stimulate the conversion of conscious programming to unconscious programming.[21,25,27-29,38] The term for this type of training is the *forced-use paradigm*. By making a task significantly more difficult or asking for multiple tasks, the CNS is bombarded with input. The CNS attempts to sort and process this overload information by opening additional neural pathways. When the individual goes back to a basic ADL task, the task becomes easier. This information can then be stored as a central command and ultimately be performed without continuous reference to conscious thought as a triggered response.[21,27-29,39] As with all training, the single greatest obstacle to motor learning is the conscious mind. We must get the conscious mind out of the act!

Closed-Loop, Open-Loop, and Feedforward Integration

Why is a coordinated motor response important? When an unexpected load is placed on a joint, ligamentous damage occurs in 70 to 90 msec unless an appropriate response ensues.[40-42]

Therefore, reactive muscle activity that provides sufficient magnitude in the 40- to 80-msec time frame must occur after loading begins to protect the capsuloligamentous structures. The closed-loop system of CNS integration may not be fast enough to produce a response to increase muscle stiffness. There is simply no time for the system to process the information and provide feedback about the condition. Failure of the dynamic restraint system to control abnormal force will expose the static structures to excessive force. In this case, the open-loop system of anticipation becomes more important in producing the desired response. Preparatory muscle activity in anticipation of joint loading can influence the reactive muscle activation patterns. Anticipatory activation increases the sensitivity of the muscle spindles, thereby allowing the unexpected perturbations to be detected more quickly.[43]

Very quick movements are completed before feedback can be used to produce an action to alter the course of movement. Therefore, if the movement is fast enough, a mechanism such as a motor program would have to be used to control the entire action, with the movement being carried out without any feedback. Fortunately, the open-loop control system allows the motor control system to organize an entire action ahead of time. For this to occur, previous knowledge needs to be preprogrammed into the primary sensory cortex (Box 23-4).

In the open-loop system, a program that sets up some kind of neural mechanism or network that is preprogrammed organizes movement in advance. A classic example of this occurs in the body as postural adjustments are made before the intended movement. When an arm is raised into forward flexion, the first muscle groups to fire are not even in the shoulder girdle region. The first muscles to contract are those in the lower part of the back and legs (approximately 80 msec passes before noticeable activity occurs in the shoulder) to provide a stable base for movement.[44] Because the shoulder muscles are linked to the rest of the body, their contraction affects posture. If no preparatory compensations in posture were made, raising the arm would shift the center of gravity forward and cause a slight loss of balance. The feedforward motor control system takes care of this potential problem by preprogramming the appropriate postural modification first rather than requiring the body to make adjustments after the arm begins to move.

Lee[45] demonstrated that these preparatory postural adjustments are not independent of the arm movement but rather are part of the total motor pattern. When the arm movements are organized, the motor instructions are preprogrammed to adjust posture first and then move the arm. Therefore, arm movement and postural control are not separate events but instead are different parts of an integrated action that raises the arm while maintaining balance. Lee showed that these EMG preparatory postural adjustments disappear when the individual leans against some type of support before raising the arm. The motor control system recognizes that advance preparation for postural control is not needed when the body is supported against the wall.

It is important to remember that most motor tasks are a complex blend of both open- and closed-loop operations. Therefore, both types of control are often at work simultaneously. Both feedforward and feedback neuromuscular control can enhance dynamic stability if the sensory and motor pathways are frequently stimulated.[21] Each time that a signal passes through a sequence of synapses, the synapses become more capable of transmitting the same signal.[14,46] When these pathways are "facilitated" regularly, memory of that signal is created and can be recalled to program future movements.[14,47]

Conclusion: Relationship to Rehabilitation

A rehabilitation program that addresses the need for restoring normal joint stability and proprioception cannot be constructed until one has total appreciation of both the mechanical and sensory functions of the articular structures.[27] Knowledge of the basic physiology of how these muscular and joint mechanoreceptors work together in the production of smooth, controlled coordinated motion is critical in developing a rehabilitation training program. This is because the role of the joint musculature extends well beyond absolute strength and the capacity to resist fatigue. With simple restoration of mechanical restraints or strengthening of the associated muscles, the smooth coordinated neuromuscular controlling mechanisms required for joint stability are neglected.[27] The complexity of joint motion necessitates synergy and synchrony of muscle firing patterns, thereby permitting proper joint stabilization, especially during sudden changes in joint position, which is common in functional activities. Understanding of these relationships and functional implications will allow the clinician greater variability and success in returning patients safely back to their playing environment.

FOUR PRINCIPLES FOR THERAPEUTIC EXERCISE PRESCRIPTION

The functional exercise program follows a linear path from basic mobility to basic stability to movement patterns. Corrective exercise falls into one of the three basic categories: mobility, stability, and retraining of movement patterns. Mobility exercises focus on joint ROM, tissue length, and muscle flexibility. Stability exercises focus on the basic sequencing of movement. These exercises target postural control of the starting and ending positions within each movement pattern. Movement pattern retraining incorporates the use of fundamental mobility and stability into specific movement patterns to reinforce coordination and timing.

The corrective exercise progression always starts with mobility exercises. Because many poor movement patterns are associated with abnormalities in mobility, restoration of movement needs to be addressed first. Mobility exercises should be performed bilaterally to confirm limitation and asymmetry of mobility. Clinicians should never assume that they know the location or side in which mobility is restricted. Rather, both sides should always be checked and mobility cleared before advancing the exercise program. If the assessment reveals a limitation or asymmetry, it should be the primary focus of the corrective exercise program. Treatments that promote mobility can involve manual therapy, such as soft tissue and joint mobilization and manipulation. Treatments of mobility might also include any modality that improves tissue pliability or freedom of movement. If no change in mobility is appreciated, the clinician should not proceed to stability work. Rather, all mobility problems should continue to be worked on until a measurable change is noted. Mobility does not need to become full or normal, but improvement must be noted before advancing. The clinician can proceed to a stability exercise only if the increased mobility allows the patient to get into the appropriate exercise posture and position. The stability work should reinforce the new mobility, and the new mobility makes improved stabilization possible because the new mobility provides new sensory information. If there is any question about compromised mobility, each exercise session should always return to mobility exercises before moving to stability exercises. This will ensure that proper tissue length and joint alignment are available for the stabilization exercises.

When no limitation or asymmetry is present during the mobility corrective exercises, one can move directly to stability corrective exercises. When mobility has been restored, it needs to be controlled. Stability exercises demand posture, alignment, balance, and control of forces within the newly available range and without the support of compensatory stiffness or muscle tone. Stability exercises should be considered as challenges to posture and position rather than being conventional strength exercises.

We propose four principles for therapeutic exercise prescription, which will be described as the *four Ps* in this section. These principles serve to guide decisions for selecting, advancing, and terminating therapeutic exercise interventions. Application of these four principles in the appropriate sequence will allow the clinician to understand the starting point, a consistent progression, and the end point for each exercise prescription. This sequence is achieved by using functional activities and fundamental movement patterns as goals. By proceeding in this fashion, the clinician will have the ability to evaluate the whole before the parts and then discuss the parts as they apply. Table 23-3 lists and describes the principles for therapeutic exercise prescription.

Clinical Pearl #2

The true art of rehabilitation is to understand the whole of synergistic functional movement and the therapeutic techniques that will have the greatest positive effect on that movement in the least amount of time.

The Four Ps

The four Ps represent the four principles for therapeutic exercise: purpose, posture, position, and pattern (Table 23-4). They serve as quick reminders of the hierarchy, interaction, and application of each principle. The questions of what, when, where, and how for functional movement assessment and exercise prescription are addressed in the appropriate order (see Table 23-4).

Table 23-3 Four Principles for Therapeutic Exercise Prescription

Principle	Description
Functional evaluation and assessment in relation to dysfunction (disability) and impairment	The evaluation must identify a functional problem or limitation resulting in diagnosis of a functional problem. Observation of whole movement patterns tempered by practical knowledge of key stress points and common compensatory patterns will improve the efficiency of evaluation.
Identification and management of motor control	Rehabilitation can be greatly advanced by understanding functional milestones and fundamental movements such as those demonstrated during the positions and postures paramount to growth and development. These milestones serve as key representations of functional mobility and control, as well as play a role in the initial setup and design of the exercise program.
Identification and management of osteokinematic and arthrokinematic limitations	The skills and techniques of orthopedic manual therapy are beneficial in identifying specific arthrokinematic restrictions that would limit movement or impede the motor-learning process. Management of myofascial and capsular structures will improve osteokinematic movement, as well as allow balanced muscle tone between the agonist and antagonist. It will also help the clinician understand the dynamics of the impairment.
Identification of current movement patterns followed by facilitation and integration of synergistic movement patterns	When restrictions and limitations are managed and gross motion is restored, application of proprioceptive neuromuscular facilitation–type patterning will further improve neuromuscular function and control. Consideration of synergistic movement is the final step in restoration of function by focusing on coordination, timing, and motor learning.

Table 23-4 Memory Cues and Primary Questions Associated with the Four Principles for Prescription of Therapeutic Exercise

Principle	Memory Cue	Memory Cue Definition	Primary Questions
Functional evaluation and assessment	Purpose	Used during both the evaluation process and the exercise prescription process to keep the clinician intently focused on the greatest single factor limiting function	"*What* functional activity is limited?" "*What* does the limitation appear to be—a mobility problem or a stability problem?" "*What* is the dysfunction or disability?" "*What* fundamental movement is limited?" "*What* is the impairment?"
Identification of motor control	Posture	Helps the clinician remember to consider a more holistic approach to exercise prescription	"*When* in the development sequence is the impairment obvious?" "*When* do the substitutions and compensations occur?" "*When* in the developmental sequence does the patient demonstrate success?" "*When* in the developmental sequence does the patient experience difficulty?" "*When* is the best possible starting point for exercise with respect to posture?"
Identification of osteokinematic and arthrokinematic limitations	Position	Describes not only the location of the anatomic structure (joint, muscle group, ligament, etc.) where impairment has been identified but also the positions (with respect to movement and load) in which the greatest and least limitations occur	"*Where* is the impairment located?" "*Where* among the structures (myofascial or articular) does the impairment have its greatest effect?" "*Where* in the range of motion does the impairment affect position the greatest?" "*Where* is the most beneficial position for the exercise?"
Integration of synergistic movement patterns	Pattern	Cues the clinician to continually consider the functional movements of the human body that occur in unified patterns that occupy three-dimensional space and cross three planes (frontal, sagittal, and transverse)	"*How* is the movement pattern different on bilateral comparison?" "*How* can synergistic movement, coordination, recruitment and timing be facilitated?" "*How* will this affect the limitation in movement?" "*How* will this affect function?"

Purpose

The word *purpose* is simply a cue to be used during both the evaluation process and the exercise prescription process to keep the clinician intently focused on the greatest single factor limiting function. The primary questions to ask for this principle appear in Table 23-4. It is not uncommon for clinicians to attempt to resolve multiple problems with the initial exercise prescription. However, the practice of identifying the single greatest limiting factor will reduce frustration and also not overwhelm the patient. Other factors may have been identified in the evaluation, but a major limiting factor or a single weak link should stand out and be the focus of the initial therapeutic exercise intervention.

Table 23-5 Three Levels of Functional Evaluation

Level	Name	Description
I	Functional activity assessment	Combined movements common to the patient's lifestyle and occupation are reproduced. They usually fit the definition of a general or specific skill.
II	Functional or fundamental movement assessment	The clinician takes what is learned through the observation of functional movements and breaks the movements down to the static and transitional postures seen in the normal developmental sequence.
III	Specific clinical measurement	Clinical measurements are used to identify and quantify specific problems that contribute to limitations in motion or control.

Alterations in the limiting factor may produce positive changes elsewhere, which can be identified and considered before the next exercise progression.

The functional evaluation process should take on three distinct layers or levels (Table 23-5). Each of the three levels should involve qualitative observations followed by quantitative documentation when possible. Normative data are helpful, but bilateral comparison is also effective and demonstrates the functional problem to the patient at each level. Many patients think that the problem is simply symptomatic and structural in nature and have no example of dysfunction outside of pain with movement. Moffroid and Zimny suggest that "Muscle strength of the right and left sides is more similar in the proximal muscles whereas we accept a 10% to 15% difference in strength of the distal muscles.... With joint flexibility, we accept a 5% difference between goniometric measurements of the right and left sides."[48]

The functional activity assessment involves a reproduction of combined movements common to the patient's lifestyle and occupation. These movements usually fit the definition of a general or specific skill. The clinician must have the patient demonstrate a variety of positions and not just positions that correspond to the reproduction of symptoms.[49] Static postural assessment is included, as well as assessment of dynamic activity. The quality of control and movement is assessed. Specific measurement of bilateral differences is difficult, but demonstration and observation are helpful for the patient. The clinician should note the positions and activities that provoke symptoms, as well as the activities that illustrate poor body mechanics, poor alignment, right-left asymmetries, and inappropriate weight shifting. When the clinician has observed gross movement quality, it may be necessary to also quantify movement performance. Repetition of the activity for evaluation of endurance, reproduction of symptoms, or demonstration of rapidly declining quality will create a functional baseline for bilateral comparison and documentation.

Next is the functional or fundamental movement assessment. The clinician must take what is learned through the observation of functional movements and break the movements down into the static and transitional postures seen in the normal developmental sequence. This breakdown will reduce activities to the many underlying mobilizing and stabilizing actions and reactions that constitute the functional activity. More simply stated, the activity is broken down into a sequence of primary movements that can be observed independently. It must be noted that these movements still involve multiple joints and muscles.[49] Assessment of individual joints and muscle groups will be performed during clinical measurements. Martin notes, "The developmental sequence has provided the most consistent base for almost all approaches used by physical therapists."[48] This is a powerful statement, and because true qualitative measurements of normal movement in adult populations are limited, the clinician must look for universal similarities in movement. Changes in fundamental movements can effect significant and prompt changes in function and must therefore be considered functional as well. Because the movement patterns of most adults are habitual and specific and thus are not representative of a full or optimal movement spectrum, the clinician must first consider the nonspecific basic movement patterns common to all individuals during growth and development. The developmental sequence is predictable and universal in the first 2 years of life,[50] with individual differences seen in the rate and quality of the progression. The differences are minimal in comparison to the variations seen in the adult population with their many habits, occupations, and lifestyles. In addition to diverse movement patterns, the adult population has the consequential complicating factor of a previous medical and injury history. Each medical problem or injury has had some degree of influence on activity and movement. Thus, evaluation of functional activities alone may hide many uneconomical movement patterns, compensations, and asymmetries that when integrated into functional activities, are not readily obvious to the clinician. By using the fundamental movements of the developmental progression, the clinician can view mobility and static and dynamic stability problems in a more isolated setting. Although enormous variations in functional movement quality and quantity are seen in specific adult patient populations, most individuals have the developmental sequence in common.[50] The movements used in normal motor development are the building blocks of skill and function.[50] Many of these building blocks can be lost while the skill is maintained or retained at some level (though rarely optimal). We will refer to these movement building blocks as *fundamental movements* and consider them precursors to higher function. Bilateral comparison is helpful when the clinician identifies qualitative differences between the right and left sides. These movements (like functional activities) can be compared quantitatively as well.

Finally, clinical measurements will be used to identify and quantify specific problems that are contributing to limitation of motion or limitation of control. Clinical measurements will first classify a patient through qualitative assessment. The parameters that define that classification must then be quantified to reveal impairment. These classifications are called hypermobility and hypomobility and help create guides for treatment that consider the functional status, anatomic structures, and the severity of symptoms. The clinician should not proceed into exercise prescription without proper identification of one of these general categories. The success or failure of a particular exercise treatment regimen probably depends more on this classification than on the choice of exercise technique or protocol.

When the appropriate clinical classification is determined, specific quantitative measurements will define the level of involvement within the classification and set a baseline for exercise treatment. Periodic reassessment may identify a different major limiting factor or a weak link that may require reclassification,

---

Specific Skill

Because both functional movement and functional performance have been appropriately addressed, the restoration of skill becomes a process of sensory motor learning techniques and positive feedback experiences.

Functional Performance and General Skill Performance

Only consider this if all functional movement quality and quantity is within normal or functional limits. If structural or physiologic barriers (that cannot be addressed) limit movement, then proceed into performance and consider current fundamental movement as an acceptable plateau.

Functional or Fundamental Movement

This is always the first consideration for all functional evaluation and exercise intervention and this involves restoring movement by addressing the clinical classification and level of involvement. The isolated improvement is then integrated into the fundamental movement and reassessed.

FIGURE 23-1 Different levels of function.

followed by specific measurement. The new problem or limitation would then be inserted as the purpose for a new exercise intervention. A simple diagram (Fig. 23-1) will help the clinician separate the different levels of function so that intervention and purpose will always be at the appropriate level and assist in the clinical decision making related to exercise prescription.[51]

Posture

Posture is a word to help the clinician consider a more holistic approach to exercise prescription. The primary questions to ask for this principle appear in Table 23-4. Janda[52] stated an interesting point when discussing posture and the muscles responsible for its maintenance. Most discussions on posture and the musculature responsible for posture generally refer to erect standing. However, "...erect standing position is so well balanced that little or no activity is necessary to maintain it."[52] Therefore, "basic human posture should be derived from the principal movement pattern, namely gait. Since we stand on one leg for most of the time during walking, the stance on one leg should be considered to be the typical posture in man; the postural muscles are those which maintain this posture." Janda reported that 85% of the gait cycle is spent in the single-leg stance and 15% in the double-leg stance. "The muscles that maintain erect posture in standing on one leg are exactly those that show a striking tendency to get tight."[53] Infants and toddlers use tonic holding before normal motor development and maturation produce the ability to use cocontraction as a means of effective support. "Tonic holding is the ability of tonic postural muscles to maintain a contraction in their shortened range against gravitational or manual resistance."[54] An adult orthopedic patient may revert to some level of tonic holding after injury or in the presence of pain and altered proprioception. Likewise, adults who have habitual postures and limited activity may adopt tonic holding for some postures. Just as Janda uses single-leg stance to observe postural function with greater specificity than the more conventional double-leg erect standing, the developmental progression can offer greater understanding by examination of the precursors to single-leg stance.[55] As stated earlier, fundamental movements are basic representations of mobility, stability, and dynamic stability and include the transitional postures used in

Box 23-5
Most Common Postures Used in Corrective Exercise
Supine and prone
Prone on elbows
Quadruped
Sitting and unstable sitting
Kneeling and half kneeling
Symmetric and asymmetric stance
Single-leg stance

growth and development. From supine to standing, each progressive posture imposes greater demands on motor control and balance. The most common postures used in corrective exercise are listed in Box 23-5.

This approach will help the clinician consider how the mobility or stability problem that was isolated in the evaluation has been (temporarily) integrated by substitution and compensation by other body parts. The clinician must remember that motor learning is a survival mechanism. The principles that the clinician will use in rehabilitation to produce motor learning have already been activated by the functional response to the impairment. Necessity or affinity, repetition, and reinforcement have been used to avoid pain or produce alternative movements since onset of the symptoms. Therefore, a new motor program has been activated to manage the impairment and produce some level of function that is usually viewed as dysfunction. It should be considered a natural and appropriate response of the body reacting to limitation or symptoms. The body will sacrifice quality of movement to maintain a degree of quantity of movement. Taking this into consideration, two distinct needs are presented.

POSTURE FOR PROTECTION AND INHIBITION

The clinician must restrict or inhibit the inappropriate motor program. In the case of a control or stability problem, the patient must have some form of support, protection, or facilitation. Otherwise, the inappropriate program will take over in an attempt to protect and respond to the postural demand. Although most adult patients function at the necessary skill level, on evaluation many qualitative problems are noted. Inappropriate joint loading and locking, poor tonic responses, or even tonic holding can be observed with simple activities. Some joint movements are used excessively, whereas others are unconsciously avoided. Many primary stability problems exist when underlying secondary mobility problems are present. Moreover, in some patients the mobility problem precedes the stability problem. This is a common explanation for microtraumatic and overuse injuries. It is also why bilateral comparison and assessment of proximal and distal structures are mandatory in the evaluative process. With a mobility problem, a joint is not used appropriately because of weakness or restriction. The primary mobility problem may be the result of compromised stability elsewhere. Motor programs have been created to allow a patient to push on despite the mobility or stability problem. The problems can be managed by mechanical consideration of the mobility and stability status of the patient in the fundamental postures.

For primary stability problems, mechanical support or other assistance must be provided. This can be done simply by partial or complete reduction of stress, which may include non–weight bearing or partial weight bearing of the spine and extremities or temporary bracing. If the stability problem is only in a particular range of movement, that movement must be managed. If an underlying mobility problem is present, it must be managed and temporarily taken out of the initial exercise movement. The alteration in posture can effectively limit complete or partial motion with little need for active control by the patient. The patient must be trained to deal with the stability problem independently of the mobility problem or be at a great mechanical advantage to avoid compensation. The secondary mobility problem, when managed, should be reintroduced in a nonstressful manner so that the previous compensatory pattern is not activated.

Manual articular and soft tissue techniques, when appropriate, can be used for the primary mobility problem, followed by movement to integrate any improved range and benefit from more appropriate tone. If the limitation in mobility seems to be the result of weakness, one should make sure that the proximal structures have the requisite amount of stability before strengthening and then proceed with strengthening or endurance activities with a focus on recruitment, relaxation, timing, coordination, and reproducibility. Note that the word *resistance* was not used initially. Resistance is not synonymous with strengthening and is only one of many techniques used to improve functional movement in early movement reeducation. However, the later sections on position and pattern will address resistance in greater detail. Posture should be used to mechanically block or restrict substitution of stronger segments and improve quality at the segment being exercised.

POSTURE FOR RECRUITMENT AND FACILITATION

The clinician must facilitate or stimulate the correct motor program, coordination, and sequence of movement. Although verbal and visual feedback is helpful through demonstration and cueing, kinesthetic feedback is paramount to motor learning.[56] Correct body position or posture will improve feedback. The posture and movement that occur early in the developmental sequence require a less complex motor task and activate a more basic motor program. This will create positive feedback and reinforcement and mark the point (posture) at which appropriate and inappropriate actions and reactions meet. From this point,

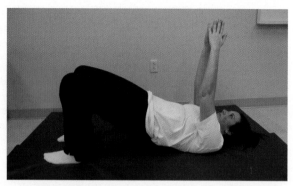

FIGURE 23-2 Supine bridging movement.

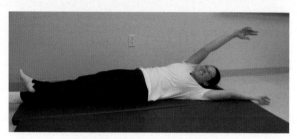

FIGURE 23-3 Rolling to prone.

the clinician can manipulate frequency, intensity, and duration or advance to a more difficult posture in the appropriate sequence.

The clinician must also consider developmental biomechanics by dividing movement ability into two categories—internal forces and external forces. Internal forces include the center of gravity, base of support, and line of gravity. External forces include gravity, inertia of the body segment, and ground reaction forces. Accordingly, the clinician should evaluate the patient's abilities in the same manner by first observing management of the mass of the body over the particular base provided by the posture. The clinician then advances the patient toward more external stresses such as inertia, gravity, and ground reaction forces. This interaction will require various degrees of acceleration production, deceleration control, anticipatory weight shifting, and increased proprioception. Resistance and movement can stress static and dynamic postures, but the clinician should also understand that resistance and movement could be used to refine movement and stimulate appropriate reactions.[56] Postures must be chosen that reduce compensation and allow the patient to exercise below the level at which the impairment hinders movement or control. This is easily accomplished by creating self-limited exercises.[3] Such exercises require passive or active "locking" by limiting movement of the area that the patient will most likely use to substitute or "cheat" with during exercise.

To review, posture identifies the fundamental movements used in growth and development. These movements serve as steps toward the acquisition of skill and are also helpful in the presence of skill when quality is questionable. Figures 23-2 through 23-5 illustrate a few examples of these types of movements.

By following this natural sequence of movement, the clinician can observe the point at which a mobility or stability problem will first limit the quality of a whole movement pattern. The specific posture of the body is as important as the movement that is introduced onto that posture. Clinicians may already know the movement pattern that they want to train, but they also need to consider the posture of the body as the fundamental neuromuscular platform when making a corrective exercise choice. The posture is the soil and the movement

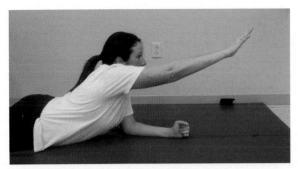

FIGURE 23-4 Prone on elbows with reaching.

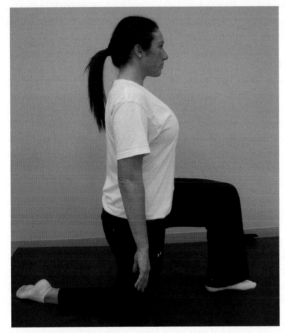

FIGURE 23-5 Half-kneeling position.

is the seed. A chop pattern with the arms can be performed while supine, seated, half kneeling, tall kneeling, and standing. Each posture will require different levels of stability and motor control.

When stability and motor control is the primary problem, a posture must be selected to start the corrective exercise process. A patient with a mild knee sprain or even a total knee replacement may demonstrate segmental rolling to one side but "logroll" to the other simply to avoid using a flexion-adduction–medial rotation movement pattern with the involved lower extremity. The clinician has now identified where success and failure meet in the developmental sequence. The knee problem creates a dynamic stability problem in the developmental sequence long before partial or full weight bearing is an issue. It must therefore be addressed at that level. The patient is provided with an example of how limited knee mobility can greatly affect movement patterns (such as rolling) that seem to require little of the knee. However, by restoring the bilateral segmental rolling function, measurable qualitative and quantitative improvements in many gait problems can be achieved. With use of postural progression, the earliest level of functional limitation can easily be identified and incorporated into the exercise program. Limitations can also be placed on the posture and movement (the self-limited concept) to control postural compensation and focus. If rolling from prone to supine does not present a problem, a more complex posture can be assumed. The obvious next choice would be

to move to quadruped. From the all-fours position, alternate arms and legs can be lifted to an extended and flexed position. They can also be tucked into a flexed and extended position by bringing the alternate knee to the alternate elbow. This causes a significant motor control load by moving from four points of stability to two. The load becomes even greater as movement of the extremities causes weight shifting, which must be managed continuously. If the movements are not compromised, the next progressive posture would be half kneeling with a narrow base. If this narrow-base half-kneeling posture demonstrates asymmetry and dysfunction, this is the posture for which the corrective exercise will be developed. Slightly widening the base improves control, and as control is developed, the base can be narrowed to challenge motor control.

Clinical Pearl #3

The clinician must define postural levels of success and failure to identify the postural level at which therapeutic exercise intervention should start. Otherwise, the clinician could potentially prescribe exercise at a postural level at which the patient makes significant amounts of inappropriate compensation and substitution during exercise.

Position

The word *position* describes not only the location of the anatomic structure (e.g., joint, muscle group, or ligament) at which impairment has been identified but also the location (with respect to movement and load) at which the greatest and least limitations occur. The limitations can be either reduced strength and control or restricted movement. The primary questions to ask for this principle appear in Table 23-4. Orthopedic manual assessment of joints and muscles in various functional positions will demonstrate the influence of the impairment and symptoms throughout the range of movement. The clinician will identify various deficits. Each will be qualified or quantified through assessment and objective testing and then addressed through the appropriate dosage and positioning for exercise.

Purpose is the obvious reason for exercise intervention, whereas posture describes the orientation of the body in space. Position refers to the specific mobilizing or stabilizing segment. Attention should be paid to positions of body segments not directly involved in the posture or movement pattern. For the single-leg bridge (Fig. 23-6), the hip is moving toward extension. If ROM were broken down into thirds, this exercise would involve only the extension third of movement. The flexion third and middle third of movement are not needed because no impairment was identified in those respective ranges. Not only was the hip in extension, but the knee was also in flexion. This is important because the hamstring muscle will try to assist hip extension in the end range of movement when gluteal strength is not optimal. However, the hamstrings cannot assist hip extension to any significant degree because of active insufficiency. Likewise, the lumbar extensors cannot assist the extension pattern because of the passive stretch placed on them via maximal passive hip flexion. Hip extension proprioception is now void of any inappropriate patterning or compensation from the hamstrings or spinal erectors through the positional use of active and passive insufficiency.[57]

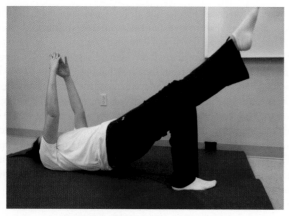

FIGURE 23-6 Single-leg bridge.

Qualitative measures will provide specific information about exercise start and finish position, movement speed and direction, open and closed chain considerations, and the need for cueing and feedback. Close observation of the osteokinematic and arthrokinematic relationships for movement and bilateral comparison is the obvious starting point. Specific identification of the structure and position represents mobility observed by selective tension (active, passive, and resisted movements), and the end-feel of the joint structures would provide specific information about the mechanical nature of the limitations and symptoms.[58] Assessment of positional static and dynamic control will reveal limitations in stability and provide a more specific starting point for exercise.

Quantitative measures will reveal a degree of deficit, which can be recorded in the form of a percentage through bilateral comparison and compared with normative data when possible. ROM, strength, endurance, and recovery time should be considered along with many other (quantitative) clinical parameters to describe isolated or positional function. This will provide clear communication and specific documentation for goals, as well as be a tracking device for the effectiveness of treatment, information that will help define the baseline for initial exercise considerations. As stated earlier, any limitation in mobility or stability will require bilateral comparison, in addition to clearing of the joints above and below. The proximal and distal structures must also be compared with their contralateral counterparts. This central point of physical examination is often overlooked. Cyriax[58] noted, "Positive signs must always be balanced by corroborative negative signs. If a lesion appears to lie at or near one joint, this region must be examined for signs identifying its site. It is equally essential for the adjacent joints and the structures around them to be examined so that, by contrast, their normality can be established. These negative findings then reinforce the positive findings emanating elsewhere; then only can the diagnosis be regarded and established."

After position and movement options have been established, a trial exercise session should be used to observe and quantify performance before prescription of exercise. Variables, including intensity and duration, can be used to establish strength or endurance baselines. Bilateral comparison should be used to document a deficit in performance, which is also recorded as a percentage. A maximum repetition test (with

or without resistance) to fatigue, onset of symptoms, or loss of exercise quality is a common example. This will allow close tracking of home exercise compliance and help establish a rate of improvement. If all other factors are addressed, the rate of improvement should be quite large. This is the benefit of correct dosage in prescription of exercise position and appropriate workload. Most of the significant improvement is not due to training volume, tissue metabolism, or muscle hypertrophy but to the efficient adaptive response of neural factors.[59] These factors can include motor recruitment efficiency, improved timing, increased proprioceptive awareness, improved agonist/antagonist coordination, appropriate phasic and tonic response to activity, task familiarity, and motor learning, as well as psychologic factors. Usually, greater deficits are associated with more drastic improvement. Treatments should be geared to stimulate these changes whenever possible.

Pattern

The primary questions to ask for the pattern principle appear in Table 23-4. The word *pattern* will serve as a cue to the clinician to continually consider the functional movements of the human body occurring in unified patterns that occupy three-dimensional space and cross three planes (frontal, sagittal, and transverse).[3] Sometimes this is not easily ascertained by observing the design and use of fixed-axis exercise equipment and the movement patterns suggested in some rehabilitation protocols. The basic patterns of proprioceptive neuromuscular facilitation (PNF), for both the extremities and the spine, are excellent examples of how the brain groups movement. Muscles of the trunk and extremities are recruited in the most advantageous sequence (proprioception) to create movement (mobility) or control (stability) movement. Not only does this provide efficient and economical function, but it also effectively protects the respective joints and muscles from undue stress and strain. Voss et al[60] clearly and eloquently stated, "The mass movement patterns of facilitation are spiral and diagonal in character and closely resemble the movements used in sports and work activities. The spiral and diagonal character is in keeping with the spiral rotatory characteristics of the skeletal system of bones and joints and the ligamentous structures. This type of motion is also in harmony with the topographical alignment of the muscles from origin to insertion and with the structural characteristics of the individual muscles." When a structure within the sequence is limited by impairment, the entire pattern is limited in some way. The clinician should document the limited pattern, as well as the isolated segment causing the pattern to be limited. The isolated segment is usually identified in the evaluation process and outlined in the "position" considerations. The resultant effect on one or more movement patterns must also be investigated. A review of the basic PNF patterns can be beneficial to the rehabilitation specialist. When a structure is evaluated, one should look at the basic PNF patterns involving that structure. Multiple patterns can be limited in some way, but usually one pattern in particular will demonstrate significantly reduced function. Obviously, poor function in a muscle group or joint can limit the strength, endurance, and ROM of an entire PNF pattern to some degree. However, the clinician must not simply view reduced function of a PNF pattern as an output problem. It should be equally viewed as an input problem. When muscle and joint functions are not optimal, mechanoreceptor and muscle spindle functions are not optimal. This can create an input or proprioceptive problem and greatly distort joint position and muscle tension information, which distorts the initial information (before movement is initiated), as well as feedback (once movement is in progress). Therefore, the clinician cannot consider only functional output. Altered proprioception, if not properly identified and outlined, can unintentionally become part of the recommended exercises and therefore be reinforced. The clinician must focus on synergistic and integrated function at all levels of rehabilitation. An orthopedic outpatient cannot afford to have a problem simply isolated three times a week for 30 minutes only to reintegrate the same problem at a subconscious level during necessary daily activities throughout the remaining week. PNF-style movement pattern exercise can often be taught as easily as an isolated movement and will produce a significantly greater benefit. Therapeutic exercise is no longer limited by sets as repetitions of the same activity. Successive intervals of increasing difficulty (though not physically stressful) that build on the accomplishment of an earlier task will reinforce one level of function and continually be a challenge for the next. A simple movement set focused on isolation of a problem can quickly be followed by a pattern that will improve integration. The integration can be followed by a familiar fundamental movement or functional activity that may reduce the amount of conscious and deliberate movement and give the clinician a chance to observe subcortical control of mobility and stability, as well as appropriate use of phasic and tonic responses.

Clinical Pearl #4

By continuously considering the pattern options, as well as pattern limitations, the clinician will be able to refine the exercise prescription and reduce unnecessary supplemental movements that could easily be incorporated into pattern-based exercise.

Direction, speed, and amount of resistance (or assistance) will be used to produce more refined patterns. Manual resistance, weighted cable or elastic resistance, weight-shifting activities, and even proprioceptive taping can improve recruitment and facilitate coordination. The clinician should refrain from initially discussing specific structural control such as pelvic tilting or scapular retraction. Instead, the clinician should use posture and position to set the initial movement and design proprioceptive feedback to produce a more normal pattern whenever possible.

REESTABLISHING PROPRIOCEPTIOIN AND NEUROMUSCULAR CONTROL

Although the concept and value of proprioceptive mechanoreceptors have been documented in the literature, treatment techniques focused on improving their function have not generally been incorporated into the overall rehabilitation program. The neurosensory function of the capsuloligamentous structures has taken a back seat to the mechanical structural role. This is mainly due to lack of information about how mechanoreceptors contribute to the specific functional activities and how they can be specifically activated.[61,62]

Effects of Injury on the Proprioceptive System

After injury to the capsuloligamentous structures, it is thought that partial deafferentation of the joint occurs as the mechanoreceptors become disrupted. This partial deafferentation may be due to either direct or indirect injury. Direct effects of trauma would include disruption of the joint capsule or ligaments, whereas posttraumatic joint effusion or hemarthrosis[19] illustrate indirect effects.

Whether from a direct or indirect cause, the resultant partial deafferentation alters the afferent information received by the CNS and therefore the resulting reflex pathways to the dynamic stabilizing structures. These pathways are required by both the feedforward and feedback motor control systems to dynamically stabilize the joint. A disruption in the proprioceptive pathway will result in an alteration in position and kinesthesia.[63,64] Barrett[65] showed an increase in the threshold for detection of passive motion in a majority of patients with anterior cruciate ligament (ACL) rupture and functional instability. Corrigan et al,[66] who also found diminished proprioception after ACL rupture, confirmed this finding. Diminished proprioceptive sensitivity has likewise been shown to cause giving way or episodes of instability in the ACL-deficient knee.[67] Therefore, injury to the capsuloligamentous structures not only reduces the mechanical stability of the joint but also diminishes the capability of the dynamic neuromuscular restraint system. Consequently, any aberration in joint motion and position sense will affect both the feedforward and feedback neuromuscular control systems. Without adequate anticipatory muscle activity, the static structures may be exposed to insult unless the reactive muscle activity can be initiated to contribute to dynamic restraint.

Restoration of Proprioception and Prevention of Reinjury

Although it has been demonstrated that a proprioceptive deficit occurs after knee injury, both kinesthetic awareness and reposition sense can be at least partially restored with surgery and rehabilitation. A number of studies have examined proprioception after ACL reconstruction. Barrett[65] measured proprioception after autogenous graft repair and found that proprioception was better after repair than in an average patient with an ACL deficiency but still significantly worse than in a normal knee. He further noted that patient satisfaction was more closely correlated with proprioception than with clinical score.[65] Harter et al[68] could not demonstrate a significant difference in the reproduction of passive positioning between the operative and nonoperative knee at an average of 3 years after ACL reconstruction. Kinesthesia has been reported to be restored after surgery, as detected by a threshold for detection of passive motion in the midrange of motion.[63] A longer threshold for detection of passive motion was observed in a knee with a reconstructed ACL than in the contralateral uninvolved knee when tested at the end ROM.[63] Lephart et al[69] found similar results in patients after arthroscopically assisted ACL reconstruction with a patellar-tendon autograft or allograft. The importance of incorporating a proprioceptive element in any comprehensive rehabilitation program is justified from the results of these studies.

Methods to enhance proprioception after injury or surgery could improve function and decrease the risk for reinjury. Ihara and Nakayama[70] demonstrated a reduction in neuromuscular lag time with dynamic joint control after a 3-week training period on an unstable board. Maintenance of equilibrium and an improvement in reaction to sudden perturbations on the unstable board improved neuromuscular coordination. This phenomenon was first reported by Freeman and Wyke in 1967 when they stated that proprioceptive deficits could be reduced with training on an unstable surface.[51] They found that proprioceptive training through stabilometry, or training on an unstable surface, significantly reduced episodes of giving way after ankle sprains. Tropp et al[53] confirmed the work of Freeman and Wyke by demonstrating that the results of stabilometry could be improved with coordination training on an unstable board.

Relationship of Proprioception to Function

Barrett[65] demonstrated the relationship between proprioception and function. Their study suggested that limb function relied more on proprioceptive input than on strength during activity. Blackburn and Voight[33] also found high correlation between diminished kinesthesia and the single-leg hop test. The single-leg hop test was chosen for its integrative measure of neuromuscular control because a high degree of proprioceptive sensibility and functional ability is required to successfully propel the body forward and land safely on the limb. Giove et al[71] reported a higher success rate in returning athletes to competitive sports with adequate hamstring rehabilitation. Tibone et al[72] and Ihara and Nakayama[70] found that simple hamstring strengthening alone was not adequate; it was necessary to obtain voluntary or reflex-level control of knee instability for return to functional activities. Walla et al[73] found that 95% of patients were able to successfully avoid surgery after ACL injury when they could achieve "reflex-level" hamstring control. Ihara and Nakayama[70] found that the reflex arc between stressing the ACL and hamstring contraction could be shortened with training. With the use of unstable boards, the researchers were able to successfully decrease the reaction time. Because afferent input is altered after joint injury, proprioceptive sensitivity to retrain these altered afferent pathways is critical for shortening the time lag in muscular reaction to counteract the excessive strain on the passive structures and guard against injury.

Restoration of Efficient Motor Control

How do we modify afferent/efferent characteristics? The mechanoreceptors in and around the respective joints offer information about change in position, motion, and loading of the joint to the CNS, which in turn stimulates the muscles around the joint to function.[70] If a time lag exists in the neuromuscular reaction, injury may occur. The shorter the time lag, the less stress on the ligaments and other soft tissue structures around the joint. Therefore, the foundation of neuromuscular control is to facilitate the integration of peripheral sensations related to joint position and then process this information into an effective efferent motor response. The main objective of the rehabilitation program for neuromuscular control is to develop or reestablish the afferent and efferent characteristics around the joint that are essential for dynamic restraint.[21]

Several different afferent and efferent characteristics contribute to efficient regulation of motor control. As discussed earlier, these characteristics include the sensitivity of the mechanoreceptors and facilitation of the afferent neural pathways, enhancement of muscle stiffness, and production of reflex muscle activation. The specific rehabilitation techniques must also take into consideration the levels of CNS integration. For the rehabilitation program to be complete, each of the three levels must be addressed to produce dynamic stability. The plasticity of the neuromuscular system permits rapid adaptations during the rehabilitation program that enhance preparatory and reactive activity.[21,40,46,69,70,74]

> ### Clinical Pearl #5
>
> Specific rehabilitation techniques that produce adaptations to enhance the efficiency of neuromuscular techniques include balance training, biofeedback training, reflex facilitation through reactive training, and eccentric and high-repetition/low-load exercises.[21]

THE THREE-PHASE REHABILITATION MODEL

The following is a three-phase model designed to progressively retrain the neuromuscular system for complex functions of sports and ADLs (Table 23-6). The model phases are successively more demanding and provide sequential training toward the objective of reestablishment of neuromuscular control. This three-phase model has also been described as RNT. Ideally, the phases should be followed in order and should use the four rehabilitation considerations mentioned earlier (the four Ps) at each phase. Application of the four Ps at each phase is crucial to place successive demands on the athlete during rehabilitation. In addition, progression of exercise is guided by the four-by-four design. The four-by-four method of therapeutic exercise design refers to the four possible exercise positions combined with the four types of resistance used (Table 23-7).

The difficulty of any exercise can be increased by either changing the position (non–weight bearing being the easiest and standing being the toughest) or changing the resistance (unloaded with core activation being the easiest and loaded without core activation being the hardest). It is important to remember that exercises that present too much difficulty will

Table 23-6 Three-Phase Rehabilitation Model

Phase	Description	Objective
1	Restore static stability through proprioception and kinesthesia	Restoration of proprioception
2	Restore dynamic stability	Encourage preparatory agonist-antagonist cocontraction
3	Restore reactive neuromuscular control	Initiate reflex muscular stabilization

force the patient to revert back to a compensation pattern. Therefore, the first set of exercises following a change in mobility will give all the information that one needs to know by producing one of three responses:

- **It is too easy.** The patient can perform the movement for more than 30 repetitions with good quality.
- **It is challenging, but possible.** The patient can perform the movement 8 to 15 times with good quality of movement and no signs of stress. Between 15 and 30 repetitions, however, there is a sharp decline in quality as demonstrated by a limited ability to maintain full ROM, balance, stabilization, and coordination, or the patient just becomes physically fatigued.
- **It is too difficult.** The patient has sloppy, stressful, poorly coordinated movement from the beginning, and it only gets worse.

Using this as a corrective exercise base, the clinician can observe the response and act accordingly. If the initial choice of exercise is too difficult, decrease the difficulty, observe the response to the next set, and repeat the process. If the initial exercise is too easy, increase the difficulty, observe the response to the next set, and repeat the process. Increasing difficulty rarely means increased resistance. A more advanced posture, a smaller base of support, or a more complex or involved movement pattern is usually indicated to increase the difficulty. A typical example would be some form of activity with a rolling movement pattern moving to a quadruped exercise, then going to a half-kneeling activity, and finally progressing to movement with a single-leg stance.

Phase I: Restore Static Stability Through Proprioception and Kinesthesia

Functional neuromuscular rehabilitation activities are designed to both restore functional stability about the joint and enhance motor control skills. The RNT program is centered on stimulation of both the peripheral and central reflex pathways to the skeletal muscles. The first objective that should be addressed in the RNT program is restoration of proprioception. Reliable kinesthetic and proprioceptive information provides the foundation on which dynamic stability and motor control is based. It has already been established that altered afferent information received by the CNS can alter the feedforward and feedback motor control systems. Therefore, the first objective of the RNT program is to restore the neurosensory properties of

Table 23-7 Four-by-Four Method for Design of Therapeutic Exercise

The Four Positions	The Four Types of Resistance
Non–weight bearing (supine or prone)	Unloaded with core activation
Quadruped	Unloaded without core activation
Kneeling (half kneeling or tall kneeling)	Loaded with core activation
Standing (lunge, split, squat, single leg)	Loaded without core activation

the damaged structures while at the same time enhancing the sensitivity of the secondary peripheral afferents.[69]

To facilitate appropriate kinesthetic and proprioceptive input into the CNS, joint reposition exercises should be used to provide maximal stimulation of the peripheral mechanoreceptors. The use of closed kinetic chain activities creates axial loads that maximally stimulate the articular mechanoreceptors via the increase in compressive force.[10,55] The use of closed chain exercises not only enhances joint congruency and neurosensory feedback but also minimizes shearing stress about the joint.[75] At the same time, the muscle receptors are facilitated by the change in both length and tension.[10,55] The objective is to induce unanticipated perturbations and thereby stimulate reflex stabilization. Persistent use of these pathways will decrease the response time when an unanticipated joint load occurs.[76] In addition to weight-bearing exercises, active and passive joint-repositioning exercises can be used to enhance the conscious appreciation of proprioception. Rhythmic stabilization exercises can be included early in the RNT program to enhance neuromuscular coordination in response to unexpected joint translation. The intensity of the exercises can be manipulated by increasing either the weight loaded across the joint or the size of the perturbation (Tables 23-8 and 23-9). The addition of a compressive sleeve, wrap, or taping about the joint can also provide additional proprioceptive information by stimulating the cutaneous mechanoreceptors.[21,65,77,78] Figures 23-7 through 23-10 provide examples of exercises that can be begun in this phase.

Phase II: Restore Dynamic Stability

The second objective of the RNT program is to encourage preparatory agonist-antagonist cocontraction. Efficient coactivation of the musculature restores the normal force couples that are necessary to balance joint forces, increase joint congruency, and thereby reduce the loads imparted onto the static structures.[21] The cornerstone of rehabilitation during this phase is postural stability training. Environmental conditions are manipulated to produce a sensory response (Box 23-6). The use of unstable surfaces allows the clinician to use positions of compromise to produce maximal afferent input into the spinal cord and thus produce a reflex response. Dynamic coactivation of the muscles about the joint to produce a stabilizing force requires both the feedforward and feedback motor control systems. To facilitate these pathways, the joint must be placed in positions of compromise for the patient to develop reactive stabilizing strategies. Although it was once believed that the speed of the stretch reflexes could not be directly enhanced, efforts to do so have been successful in human and animal studies. This has significant implications for reestablishing the reactive capability of the dynamic restraint system. Reducing electromechanical delay between joint loading and protective muscle activation can increase dynamic stability. In the controlled clinical environment, positions of vulnerability can be used safely (see Tables 23-8 and 23-9). Figures 23-11 and 23-12 provide examples of exercises that can be implemented in this phase.

Proprioceptive training for functionally unstable joints after injury has been documented in the literature.[38,53,70,79] Tropp et al[53] and Wester et al[80] reported that ankle disk training significantly reduced the incidence of ankle sprains. Concerning the mechanism of the effects, Tropp et al[53] suggested that unstable surface training reduced the proprioceptive deficit. Sheth et al[79]

Table 23-8 Upper Extremity Neuromuscular Exercises

Phase I: Proprioception and Kinesthesia	Phase II: Dynamic Stabilization	Phase III: Reactive Neuromuscular Control
Goals		
Normalize motion	Enhance dynamic functional stability	Improve reactive neuromuscular abilities
Restore proprioception and kinesthesia	Reestablish neuromuscular control	Enhance dynamic stability
Establish muscular balance	Restore muscular balance	Improve power and endurance
Diminish pain and inflammation	Maintain normalized motion	Gradual return to sport/throwing
Stability Exercises		
Joint repositioning	PNF D$_2$ Flex/Ext	PNF D2 Flex/Ext
Movement awareness	Supine	RS with T-band
RS	Side lying	Perturbation RS
RI	Seated	Perturbation RS—eyes closed
SRH	Standing	90°/90°
PNF D$_2$ Flex/Ext	PNF D$_2$ Flex/Ext at end range	ER at end-range RS
PNF D$_2$ Flex/Ext RS, SRH, RI	90°/90 ER at end range	ER Conc/Ecc
Side-lying RS, SRH, RI	Scapular strengthening	ER Conc/Ecc RS
Weight bearing (axial compression)	Scapular PNF—RS, SRH	ER/IR Conc/Ecc
Weight-bearing RS, RI	ER/IR at 90° abduction—eyes closed	ER/IR Conc/Ecc RS
Standing while leaning on hands	PNF D$_2$ Flex/Ext—eyes closed	Eyes closed
Quadruped position	Balance beam	Standing on one leg
Tripod position	PNF D$_2$ Flex/Ext—balance beam	Reactive plyoballs
Biped position	Slide board—side to side	Push-ups on unstable surface
Axial compression with ball on wall	Slide board push-ups	UE plyometrics
OTIS	Axial compression—side to side	Two-handed overhead throw
	Axial compression—unstable surfaces	Side-to-side overhead throw
	Plyometrics—two handed (light and easy)	One-handed baseball throw
	Two-handed chest throw	Endurance
	Two-handed underhand throw	Wall dribble
		Wall baseball throw
		Axial compression circles
		Axial compression—side/side
		Sports-specific
		Underweighted throwing
		Overweighted throwing
		Oscillating devices
		Boing
		Body Blade

Conc, Concentric; *Ecc,* eccentric; *ER,* external rotation; *Ext,* extension; *Flex,* flexion; *IR,* internal rotation; *OTIS,* oscillating techniques for isometric stabilization; *PNF,* proprioceptive neuromuscular facilitation; *RI,* reciprocal isometrics; *RS,* rhythmic stabilization; *SRH,* slow reversal hold; *UE,* upper extremity.

demonstrated changes in healthy adults in patterns of contraction of the inversion and eversion musculature before and after training on an unstable surface. They concluded that the changes would be supported by the concept of reciprocal Ia inhibition via the mechanoreceptors in the muscles. Konradsen and Ravin[81] also suggested from their work that afferent input from the calf musculature was responsible for dynamic protection against sudden ankle inversion stress. Pinstaar et al[82] reported that postural sway was restored after 8 weeks of ankle disk training when performed three to five times a week. Tropp and Odenrick[39] also showed that postural control improved after 6 weeks of training when performed 15 minutes per day. Bernier and Perrin,[54] whose program consisted of balance exercises progressing from simple to complex sessions (3 times a week for 10 minutes), also found that postural sway was improved after 6 weeks of training. Although each of these training programs do have some differences, postural control improved after 6 to 8 weeks of proprioceptive training in subjects with functional instability of the ankle.

Phase III: Restore Reactive Neuromuscular Control

Dynamic reactive neuromuscular control activities should be initiated into the overall rehabilitation program after adequate healing and dynamic stability have been achieved. The key objective is to initiate reflex muscular stabilization.

Progression of these activities is predicated on the athlete satisfactorily completing the activities that are considered prerequisites for the activity being considered. With this in mind, progression of activities must be goal oriented and specific to the tasks that will be expected of the athlete.

The general progression of activities to develop dynamic reactive neuromuscular control is from slow-speed to fast-speed activities, from low-force to high-force activities, and from controlled to uncontrolled activities. Initially, these exercises should evoke a balance reaction or weight shift in the lower extremities and ultimately progress to a movement pattern.

Table 23-9 Lower Extremity Neuromuscular Exercises

Phase I: Proprioception and Kinesthesia	Phase II: Dynamic Stabilization	Phase III: Reactive Neuromuscular Control
Goals		
Normalize motion	Enhance dynamic functional stability	Improve reactive neuromuscular abilities
Restore proprioception and kinesthesia	Reestablish neuromuscular control	Enhance dynamic stability
Establish muscular balance	Restore muscular balance	Improve power and endurance
Diminish pain and inflammation	Maintain normalized motion	Gradual return to activities, running, jumping, cutting
Develop static control and posture		
Stability Exercises		
Bilateral to unilateral	Oscillating techniques for isometric stabilization (OTIS)	Squats
Eyes open to eyes closed	AWS	Assisted
Stable to unstable surfaces	PWS	AWS
Level surfaces	MWS	PWS
Foam pad	LWS	MWS
Controlled to uncontrolled	Chops/lifts	LWS
PNF	ITIS	Chops/lifts
Rhythmic stabilization	PACE	Lunges (front and lateral)
Rhythmic isometrics	PNF	AWS
Slow reversal hold	Rhythmic stabilization	PWS
	Rhythmic isometrics	MWS
	Slow reversal hold	LWS
	Stable to unstable surface	Stationary walking with unidirectional WS
	Rocker board	Stationary running
	Wobble board	PWS
	BAPS	MWS
	Balance beam	LWS
	Foam rollers	AWS
	Dyna-disc	Mountain climber
		CKC side to side
		Fitter
		Slide board
		Plyometrics
		Jumps in place
		Standing jumps
		Bounding
		Multiple hops and bounds
		Hops with rotation
		Bounds with rotation
		Resisted lateral bounds
		Box jumps
		Depth jumps
		Multidirectional training
		Lunges
		Rock wall
		Clock drill
		Step-tos
		Four-square
		Agility training

AWS, Anterior weight shift; *BAPS,* biomechanical ankle platform system; *CKC,* closed chain kinetic; *ITIS,* impulse techniques for isometric stabilization; *LWS,* lateral weight shift; *MWS,* medial weight shift; *PACE,* partial-arc controlled exercise; *PNF,* proprioceptive neuromuscular facilitation; *PWS,* posterior weight shift; *WS,* weight shift.

A sudden alteration in joint position induced by either the clinician or the athlete may decrease the response time and serve to develop reactive strategies to unexpected events. These reactions can be as simple as static control with little or no visible movement or as complex as a dynamic plyometric response requiring explosive acceleration, deceleration, or change in direction. The exercises will allow the clinician to challenge the patient by using visual or proprioceptive input, or both, via tubing (oscillating techniques for isometric stabilization) and other devices (e.g., medicine balls, foam rolls, or visual obstacles). Although these exercises will improve physiologic parameters, they are specifically designed to facilitate neuromuscular reactions. Therefore, the clinician must be concerned with the kinesthetic input and quality of the movement patterns rather than the particular number of sets and repetitions. When fatigue occurs, motor control becomes poor and all training effects are lost.

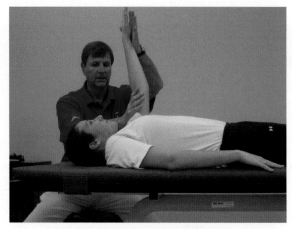

FIGURE 23-7 Rhythmic stabilization.

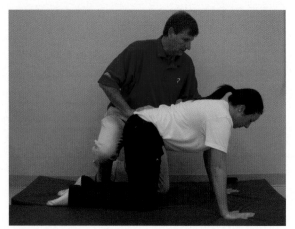

FIGURE 23-8 Quadruped position with manual perturbations.

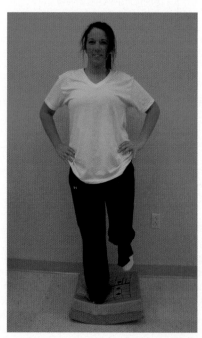

FIGURE 23-9 Single-leg balance on an unstable (foam) base.

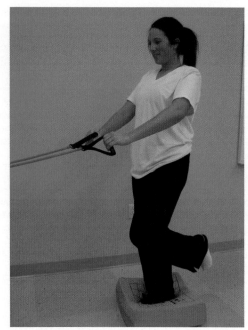

FIGURE 23-10 Single-leg balance with oscillating techniques for isometric stabilization.

Box 23-6
Balance Variables That Can Be Manipulated in the Dynamic Stability Phase to Produce a Sensory Response
Bilateral to unilateral stance
Eyes open to eyes closed
Stable to unstable surfaces

Therefore, during the exercise progression, all aspects of normal function should be observed, including isometric, concentric, and eccentric muscle control; articular loading and unloading; balance control during weight shifting and changes in direction; controlled acceleration and deceleration; and demonstration of both conscious and unconscious control (see Tables 23-8 and 23-9). Figures 23-13 through 23-15 are examples of exercises that can be implemented in this phase.

When dynamic stability and reflex stabilization have been achieved, the focus of the neuromuscular rehabilitation program is to restore ADL and sport-specific skills. It is essential that the exercise program be specific to the patient's needs. The most important factor to consider during rehabilitation of patients is that they should be performing functional activities that simulate their ADL requirements. This rule applies not only to the specific joints involved but also to the speed and amplitude of movement required in ADLs. Exercise and training drills that will refine the physiologic parameters required for return to preinjury levels of function should be incorporated into the program. The progression should be from straight plane to multiplane movement patterns. ADL movement does not occur along a single joint or plane of movement. Therefore, exercise for the kinetic chain must involve all three planes simultaneously. Emphasis in the RNT program must be placed on progression from simple to complex neuromotor

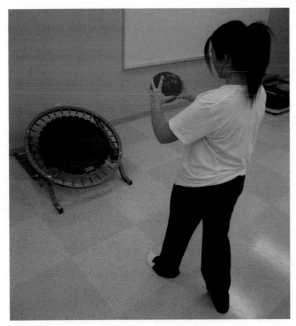

FIGURE 23-11 Plyoback, two-handed upper extremity chest pass.

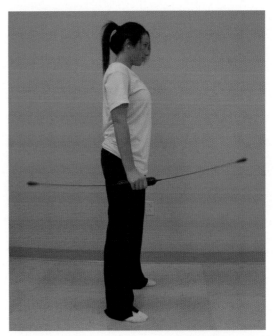

FIGURE 23-13 Dynamic training; Body Blade–low position.

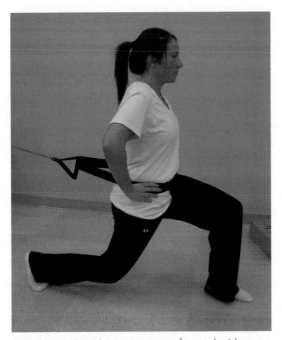

FIGURE 23-12 Lunging movement, forward with sport cord resistance.

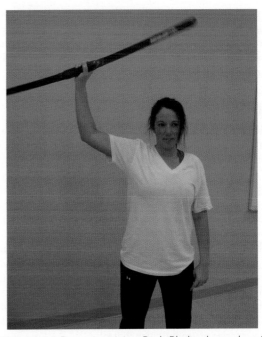

FIGURE 23-14 Dynamic training; Body Blade–elevated position.

patterns that are specific to the demands placed on the patient during function. The functional progression breaks an activity down into its component parts so that they can be performed in a sequence that allows acquisition or reacquisition of the activity. Basic conditioning and skill acquisition must be achieved before advanced conditioning and skill acquisition. The training program should begin with simple activities, such as walking/running, and then progress to highly complex motor skills requiring refined neuromuscular mechanisms, including proprioceptive and kinesthetic awareness, which provides reflex joint

stabilization. A significant amount of controlled chaos should be included in the program. Unexpected activities during ADLs are by nature unstable. The more patients rehearse in this type of environment, the better they will react under unrehearsed conditions. The clinician needs to learn how to categorize, prioritize, and plan effectively because corrective exercises will evolve and equipment will change. The clinician's professional skill must be based in a systematic approach. Just being great at a technique is not good enough. Technical aspects of exercise will change. The clinician should not worry. This system is not based on exercise.

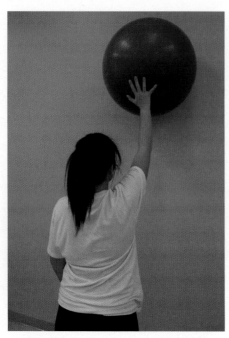

FIGURE 23-15 Elevated wall dribble.

It is based on human movement, not equipment, techniques, or trends. The final and most important consideration of this phase is to make the rehabilitation program fun. The first three letters of functional are FUN. If the program is not fun, compliance will suffer and so will the results.

CONCLUSION

- Increased attention has been devoted to the development of balance, proprioception, and neuromuscular control in the rehabilitation and reconditioning of athletes after injury.
- It is believed that injury results in altered somatosensory input, which influences neuromuscular control.
- If static and dynamic balance and neuromuscular control are not reestablished after injury, the patient will be susceptible to recurrent injury and performance may decline.
- The three-phase model for reactive neuromuscular training may be an excellent method to assist athletes in regaining optimal neuromuscular performance and high-level function after injury or surgery.
- The three-phase model consists of restoring static stability through proprioception and kinesthesia, dynamic stability, and reactive neuromuscular control.
- Current information has been synthesized to produce a new perspective for therapeutic exercise decisions. This new perspective was specifically designed to improve treatment efficiency and effectiveness and have a focus on function.
- The four principles of purpose, posture, position, and pattern assist problem solving by providing a framework that categorizes clinical information in a hierarchy.
- The four principles serve as quick reminders of the hierarchy, interaction, and application for each therapeutic exercise prescription principle. The questions of what, when, where, and how for functional movement assessment and exercise prescription are answered in the appropriate order.

- Functional evaluation and assessment = purpose.
- Identification of motor control = posture.
- Identification of osteokinematic and arthrokinematic limitations = position.
- Integration of synergistic movement patterns = pattern.
- The clinician should always ask whether the program makes sense. If it does not make sense, it is probably not functional and therefore not optimally effective.
- Clinical wisdom is the result of experience and applied knowledge. Intense familiarity and practical observation improve application. To be of benefit, the knowledge available must be organized and tempered by an objective and inclusive framework. It is hoped that this framework will provide a starting point to better organize and apply each clinician's knowledge and experience of functional exercise prescription.

REFERENCES

1. Barnett, M., Ross, D., Schmidt, R., and Todd, B. (1973): Motor skills learning and the specificity of training principle. Res. Q., 44:440–447.
2. McNair, P.J., and Marshall, R.N. (1994): Landing characteristics in subjects with normal and anterior cruciate ligament deficient knee joints. Arch. Phys. Med., 75:584–589.
3. Cook, G. (1997): The Four P's (Exercise Prescription): Functional Exercise Training Course Manual. Greeley, CO, North American Sports Medicine Institute Advances in Clinical Education, Nashville, TN.
4. American College of Sports Medicine. (1997): Exercise Management for Persons with Chronic Diseases and Disabilities. Champaign, IL, Human Kinetics.
5. Barrack, R.L., Lund, P.J., and Skinner, H.B. (1994): Knee joint proprioception revisited. J. Sport. Rehabil., 3:18–42.
6. Barrack, R.L., and Skinner, H.B. (1990): The sensory function of knee ligaments. In Daniel, D., Akeson, W., O'Conner J. (eds.): Knee Ligaments: Structure, Function, Injury, and Repair. New York, Raven Press.
7. Ciccotti, M.R., Kerlan, R., Perry, J., and Pink, M. (1994): An electromyographic analysis of the knee during functional activities: I. The normal profile. Am. J. Sports Med., 22:645–650.
8. Functional Movement Service Manual. (1998): Danville, VA, Athletic Testing Services.
9. Grigg, P. (1976): Response of joint afferent neurons in cat medial articular nerve to active and passive movements of the knee. Brain Res., 118:482–485.
10. Grigg, P. (1994): Peripheral neural mechanisms in proprioception. J. Sport Rehabil., 3:1–17.
11. Grigg, P., Finerman, G.A., and Riley, L.H. (1973): Joint position sense after total hip replacement. J. Bone Joint Surg. Am., 55:1016–1025.
12. Grigg, P., and Hoffman, A.H. (1984): Ruffini mechanoreceptors in isolated joint capsule. Reflexes correlated with strain energy density. Somatosens. Res., 2:149–162.
13. Grigg, P., and Hoffman, A.H. (1982): Properties of Ruffini afferents revealed by stress analysis of isolated sections of cat knee capsule. J. Neurophysiol., 47:41–54.
14. Guyton, A.C. (1991): Textbook of Medical Physiology, 6th ed. Philadelphia, Saunders.
15. Skinner, H.B., Barrack, R.L., Cook, S.D., and Haddad, R.J. (1984): Joint position sense in total knee arthroplasty. J. Orthop. Res., 1:276–283.
16. Cross, M.J., and McCloskey, D.I. (1973): Position sense following surgical removal of joints in man. Brain Res., 55:443–445.
17. Freeman, M.A.R., and Wyke, B. (1967): Articular reflexes of the ankle joint. An electromyographic study of normal and abnormal influences of ankle-joint mechanoreceptors upon reflex activity in leg muscles. Br. J. Surg., 54:990–1001.
18. Sherrington, C.S. (1911): The Interactive Action of the Nervous System. New Haven, CT, Yale University Press.
19. Kennedy, J.C., Alexander, I.J., and Hayes, K.C. (1982): Nerve supply to the human knee and its functional importance. Am. J. Sports Med., 10:329–335.
20. Clark, F.J., and Burgess, P.R. (1975): Slowly adapting receptors in cat knee joint: Can they signal joint angle? J. Neurophysiol., 38:1448–1463.
21. Lephart, S. (1994): Reestablishing proprioception, kinesthesia, joint position sense and neuromuscular control in rehab. In Prentice W.E. (ed.): Rehabilitation Techniques in Sports Medicine, 2nd ed. St. Louis, Mosby.
22. Schulte, M.J., and Happel, L.T. (1990): Joint innervation in injury. Clin. Sports Med., 9:511–517.
23. Willis, W.D., and Grossman, R.G. (1981): Medical Neurobiology, 3rd ed. St. Louis, Mosby.
24. Voight, M.L., Blackburn, T.A., and Hardin, J.A., et al. (1996): The effects of muscle fatigue on the relationship of arm dominance to shoulder proprioception. J. Orthop. Sports Phys. Ther., 23:348–352.
25. Voight, M.L., Cook, G., and Blackburn, T.A. (1997): Functional lower quarter exercise through reactive neuromuscular training. In Bandy, W.E. (ed.): Current Trends for the Rehabilitation of the Athlete. Lacrosse, WI, SPTS Home Study Course.

26. Phillips, C.G., Powell, T.S., and Wiesendanger, M. (1971): Protection from low threshold muscle afferents of hand and forearm area 3A of Babson's cortex. J. Physiol., 217:419–446.

27. Borsa, P.A., Lephart, S.M., Kocher, M.S., and Lephart, S.P. (1994): Functional assessment and rehabilitation of shoulder proprioception for glenohumeral instability. J. Sport Rehabil., 3:84–104.

28. Tippett, S., and Voight, M.L. (1995): Functional Progressions for Sports Rehabilitation. Champaign, IL, Human Kinetics.

29. Voight, M.L. (1990): Functional exercise training. Presented at the 1990 National Athletic Training Association Annual Conference, Indianapolis.

30. Voight, M.L. (1994): Proprioceptive concerns in rehabilitation. In Proceedings of the XXVth FIMS World Congress of Sports Medicine. Athens, Greece, The International Federation of Sports Medicine.

31. Voight, M.L., and Draovitch, P. (1991): Plyometric training. In: Muscle Training in Sports and Orthopaedics. New York, Churchill Livingstone.

32. Small, C., Waters, C.L., and Voight, M.L. (1994): Comparison of two methods for measuring hamstring reaction time using the Kin-Com isokinetic dynamometer. J. Orthop. Sports Phys. Ther., 19:335–340.

33. Blackburn, T.A., and Voight, M.L. (1995): Single leg stance: Development of a reliable testing procedure. In: Proceedings of the 12th International Congress of the World Confederation for Physical Therapy, Washington, DC.

34. Swanik, C.B., Lephart, S.M., Giannantonio, F.P., and Fu, F. (1997): Reestablishing proprioception and neuromuscular control in the ACL-injured athlete. J Sport Rehabil., 6:183–206.

35. Rine, R.M., Voight, M.L., Laporta, L., and Mancini, R. (1994): A paradigm to evaluate ankle instability using postural sway measures (Abstract). Phys. Ther., 74:S72.

36. Voight, M.L., Rine, R.M., Apfel, P., et al. (1993): The effects of leg dominance and AFO on static and dynamic balance abilities (Abstract). Phys. Ther., 73:S51.

37. Voight, M.L., Rine, R.M., Briese, K., and Powell, C. (1993): Comparison of sway in double versus single leg stance in unimpaired adults (Abstract). Phys. Ther., 73:S51.

38. Tropp, H., Askling, C., and Gillquist, J. (1985): Prevention of ankle sprains. Am. J. Sports Med., 13:259–262.

39. Tropp, H., and Odenrick, P. (1988): Postural control in single limb stance. J. Orthop. Res., 6:833–839.

40. Beard, D.J., Dodd, C.F., Trundle, H.R., et al. (1993): Proprioception after rupture of the ACL: An objective indication of the need for surgery? J. Bone Joint Surg. Br., 75:311.

41. Pope, M.H., Johnson, D.W., Brown, D.W., and Tighe, C. (1972): The role of the musculature in injuries to the medial collateral ligament. J. Bone Joint Surg. Am., 61:398–402.

42. Wojtys, E., and Huston, L. (1994): Neuromuscular performance in normal and anterior cruciate ligament–deficient lower extremities. Am. J. Sports Med., 22:89–104.

43. Dunn, T.G., Gillig, S.E., Ponser, E.S., and Weil, N. (1986): The learning process in biofeedback: Is it feed-forward or feedback? Biofeedback Self Regul., 11:143–155.

44. Belen'kii, V.Y., Gurfinkle, V.S., and Pal'tsev, Y.I. (1967): Elements of control of voluntary movements. Biofizika, 12:135–141.

45. Lee, W.A. (1980): Anticipatory control of postural and task muscles during rapid arm flexion. J. Mot. Behav., 12:185–196.

46. Hodgson, J.A., Roy, R.R., DeLeon, R., et al. (1994): Can the mammalian lumbar spinal cord learn a motor task? Med. Sci. Sports Exerc., 26:1491–1497.

47. Schmidt, R.A. (1988): Motor Control and Learning. Champaign, IL, Human Kinetics.

48. Scully, R., and Barnes, M. (1989): Physical Therapy. Philadelphia, Lippincott.

49. Cook, G., and Fields, K. (1997): Functional Training for the Torso. Colorado Springs, CO, National Strength and Conditioning Association, pp. 14–19.

50. Sullivan, P.E., Markos, P.D., and Minor, M.D. (1982): An Integrated Approach to Therapeutic Exercise: Theory and Clinical Application. Reston, VA, Reston Publishing.

51. Freeman, M.A.R., and Wyke, B., (1966): Articular contributions to limb reflexes. Br. J. Surg., 53:61–69.

52. Janda, V. (1987): Muscles and motor control in low back pain: Assessment and management. In Twomey, L. (ed.): Physical Therapy of the Low Back. New York, Churchill Livingstone, pp. 253–278.

53. Tropp, H., Ekstrand, J., and Gillquist, J. (1984): Factors affecting stabilometry recordings of single leg stance. Am. J. Sports Med., 12:185–188.

54. Bernier, J.N., and Perrin, D.H. (1998): Effect of coordination training on proprioception of the functionally unstable ankle. J. Orthop. Sports Phys. Ther., 27:264–275.

55. Clark, F.J., Burgess, R.C., Chapin, J.W., and Lipscomb, W.T. (1985): Role of intramuscular receptors in the awareness of limb position. J. Neurophysiol., 54:1529–1540.

56. Voight, M.L., and Cook, G. (1996): Clinical application of closed kinetic chain exercise. J. Sport Rehabil., 5:25–44.

57. Kendall, F.P., McCreary, K.E., and Provance, P.G. (1993): Muscle Testing and Function, 4th ed. Baltimore, Williams & Wilkins.

58. Cyriax, J. (1982): Textbook of Orthopedic Medicine, Vol. I, Diagnosis of Soft Tissue Lesions, 8th ed. London, Bailliere Tindall.

59. Baechle, T.R. (1994): Essentials of Strength Training and Conditioning. Champaign, IL, Human Kinetics.

60. Voss, D.E., Ionta, M.K., and Myers, B.J. (1985): Proprioceptive Neuromuscular Facilitation: Patterns and Techniques, 3rd ed. Philadelphia, Harper & Row.

61. Gandevia, S.C., and McCloskey, D.I. (1976): Joint sense, muscle sense and their contribution as position sense, measured at the distal interphalangeal joint of the middle finger. J. Physiol., 260:387–407.

62. Glenncross, D., and Thornton, E. (1981): Position sense following joint injury. Am. J. Sports Med., 21:23–27.

63. Barrack, R.L., Skinner, H.B., and Buckley, S.L. (1989): Proprioception in the anterior cruciate deficient knee. Am. J. Sports Med., 17:1–6.

64. Skinner, H.B., Wyatt, M.P., Hodgdon, J.A., et al. (1986): Effect of fatigue on joint position sense of the knee. J. Orthop. Res., 4:112–118.

65. Barrett, D.S. (1991): Proprioception and function after anterior cruciate reconstruction. J. Bone Joint Surg. Br., 3:833–837.

66. Corrigan, J.P., Cashman, W.F., and Brady, M.P. (1992): Proprioception in the cruciate deficient knee. J. Bone Joint Surg. Br., 74:247–250.

67. Borsa, P.A., Lephart, S.M., Irrgang, J.J., et al. (1997): The effects of joint position and direction of joint motion on proprioceptive sensibility in anterior cruciate ligament deficient athletes. Am. J. Sports Med., 25:336–340.

68. Harter, R.A., Osternig, L.R., Singer, S.L., et al. (1988): Long-term evaluation of knee stability and function following surgical reconstruction for anterior cruciate ligament insufficiency. Am. J. Sports Med., 16:434–442.

69. Lephart, S.M., Pincivero, D.M., Giraldo, J.L., and Fu, F. (1997): The role of proprioception in the management and rehabilitation of athletic injuries. Am. J. Sports Med., 25:130–137.

70. Ihara, H., and Nakayama, A. (1986): Dynamic joint control training for knee ligament injuries. Am. J. Sports Med., 14:309–315.

71. Giove, T.P., Miller, S.J., Kent, B. E., et al. (1983): Non-operative treatment of the torn anterior cruciate ligament. J. Bone Joint Surg. Am., 65:184–192.

72. Tibone, J.E., Antich, T.J., Funton, G.S., et al. (1986): Functional analysis of anterior cruciate ligament instability. Am. J. Sports Med., 14:276–284.

73. Walla, D.J., Albright, J.P., McAuley, E., et al. (1985): Hamstring control and the unstable anterior cruciate ligament–deficient knee. Am. J. Sports Med., 13:34–39.

74. Wojtys, E., Huston, L.J., Taylor, P.D., and Bastian, S.D. (1996): Neuromuscular adaptations in isokinetic, isotonic, and agility training programs. Am. J. Sports Med., 24:187–192.

75. Voight, M.L., Bell, S., and Rhodes, D. (1992): Instrumented testing of tibial translation during a positive Lachman's test and selected closed-chain activities in anterior cruciate deficient knees. J. Orthop. Sports Phys. Ther., 15:49.

76. Ognibene, J., McMahon, K., Harris, M., et al. (2000): Effects of unilateral proprioceptive perturbation training on postural sway and joint reaction times of healthy subjects. In: Proceedings of the National Athletic Training Association Annual Meeting. Champaign, IL, Human Kinetics.

77. Matsusaka, N., Yokoyama, S., Tsurusaki, T., et al. (2001): Effect of ankle disk training combined with tactile stimulation to the leg and foot in functional instability of the ankle. Am. J. Sport Med., 29:25–30.

78. Perlau, R.C., Frank, C., and Fick, G. (1995): The effects of elastic bandages on human knee proprioception in the uninjured population. Am. J. Sports Med., 23:251–255.

79. Sheth, P., Yu, B., Laskowski, E.R., et al. (1997): Ankle disk training influences reaction times of selected muscles in a simulated ankle sprain. Am. J. Sports Med., 25:538–543.

80. Wester, J.U., Jespersen, S.M., Nielsen, K.D., et al. (1996): Wobble board training after partial sprains of the lateral ligaments of the ankle: A prospective randomized study. J. Orthop. Sports Phys. Ther., 23:332–336.

81. Konradsen, L., and Ravin, J. B. (1991): Prolonged peroneal reaction time in ankle instability. Int. J Sports Med., 12:290–292.

82. Pinstaar, A., Brynhildsen, J., and Tropp, H. (1996): Postural corrections after standardized perturbations of single limb stance: Effect of training and orthotic devices in patients with ankle instability. Br. J. Sports Med., 30:151–155.

24

Proprioception and Neuromuscular Control

Todd S. Ellenbecker, DPT, MS, OCS, SCS, CSCS, George J. Davies, DPT, MEd, SCS, ATC, CSCS, and Jake Bleacher, PT, MS, CSCS

CHAPTER OBJECTIVES

- Define proprioception, kinesthesia, and other related aspects by using terminology consistent with the expanded classic definitions contained in this chapter.

- Identify the different types and functions of mechanoreceptors in the upper and lower extremities.

- List and describe clinical measurements of proprioception and kinesthesia in the upper and lower extremities.

- Identify factors associated with diminished proprioception and the effects of injury, disuse, and aging on neuromuscular control and joint stability in the upper and lower extremities.

- Design and implement progressive proprioception training programs that meet the functional demands of the patient and are appropriate for the patient's level of skill and recovery when returning from an upper or lower extremity injury.

Human beings are unique in their capacity to propel themselves through their environment in an upright posture. This ability is achieved through a complex interaction of lower limb muscle activity coordinated by the central nervous system (CNS). To maintain balance and postural control we rely on sensory information from the periphery from our visual, vestibular, and somatosensory systems. The nervous system integrates this peripheral afferent information to maintain postural control during stance.

Control of locomotion, including walking or running, occurs through complex neural pathways in the spinal cord called central pattern generators or limb controllers. These motor programs for locomotion are automatic but are modulated by the CNS through feedback and feedforward mechanisms. The feedforward mechanism operates on the premise of initiating a motor response in anticipation of a load or activity that will disrupt the integrity of a joint and gauges the response from previous experiences. In contrast, the feedback system operates directly in response to a potentially destabilizing event by using a normal reference point to monitor the muscle activity necessary to restore homeostasis.[1]

Both feedback and feedforward systems rely on processing of afferent information from the periphery at different levels of the CNS (spinal cord, brainstem and cerebellum, and cerebral cortex), with the end result being coordinated muscle activity during movement to maintain joint stability.[1] The motor response varies depending on joint position, type of force, direction of force, and which higher center predominates in processing the information.

Segmental spinal reflexes involve the processing of afferent input between peripheral receptors in the muscle spindle and Golgi tendon organs at the musculotendinous junction with the efferent output of motor neurons in the ventral horn of the spinal cord. On the most basic level, monosynaptic reflexes produce an excitatory or inhibitory efferent motor response to the stimulus received from the periphery. Along with the physiologic properties of the muscle itself (length-tension curve), these peripheral receptors potentially assist in modulating muscle stiffness, with muscle tension varying according to the amount of afferent input.[1]

The afferent information received in the cortical area of the brain from peripheral mechanoreceptors produces a voluntary motor response to potential disturbances in functional joint stability. The latency of the response is usually greater than 120 msec and sometimes longer, depending on the amount of information in the environment being processed. In addition to the response to an environmental stimulus, the potential exists for a theorized motor program operating under the assumption that the individual components of performing skilled movements, such as swinging a bat, that require sequential steps would be difficult to enact successfully without having a preprogrammed set of instructions to optimize efficiency, speed, and coordinated muscle activity.[2]

The function of the cerebellum and brainstem is to integrate peripheral feedback from the environment with the motor commands from the cerebral cortex to enable humans to perform skilled and coordinated movement. The action of these neural centers allows the adjustments needed to carry out an intended motor skill with precision and efficiency.[2]

A PubMed search of the terms *proprioception* and *neuromuscular control* was performed in October 2010. The results identified 305 references, the majority (260) of which have been published during the last decade. However, when the search is limited to higher levels of evidence, including randomized controlled trials (RCTs), systematic reviews, and metaanalysis studies, the actual number is 37 high-quality studies. In one such study, Riemann et al[3] performed a literature review to identify sensorimotor assessment techniques, many of which are described throughout this chapter. Their conclusions indicate that the complex interactions and relationships among the individual components of the sensorimotor system make measuring and analyzing specific characteristics and functions difficult. Additionally, the specific assessment techniques used to measure a variable can influence the results obtained. Optimizing the application of sensorimotor research to clinical settings can best be accomplished through the use of common nomenclature to describe the underlying physiologic mechanisms and specific measurement techniques.

DEFINITIONS

Review of the orthopedic and musculoskeletal rehabilitation literature identifies many different versions of definitions for the terms associated with joint proprioception and neuromuscular control. In Goetz's *Textbook of Clinical Neurology*, proprioception is defined as any postural, positional, or kinetic information provided to the CNS by sensory receptors in muscles, tendons, joints, or skin.[4] Other texts define proprioception as "awareness of the position and movements of our limbs, fingers, and toes derived from receptors in the muscles, tendons and joints."[5] Sherrington's classic definition of proprioception is "afferent information arising from the proprioceptive field," and mechanoreceptors or proprioceptors were identified as being the source of the origination of this afferent information.[6]

These original definitions of the term *proprioception* continue to be used today; however, a more advanced definition of the sensory functions that encompass human proprioceptive function is clearly needed. In a classic monograph titled *Physiologie des Muskelsinnes*, Goldsheider[7] proposed that muscle sense be divided into four distinct and separate sensory functions. These functions were described as sensation of passive movements, sensation of active movements, sensation of position, and appreciation or sensation of heaviness and resistance. These original classifications or definitions have been expanded to decrease confusion. The sensation of passive movements is considered to

be a product of sensations induced by external forces that result in a change in limb position with noncontracting muscles. The sensation of active movement (or *kinesthesia* as it is now better known) encompasses the appreciation of change in position of a limb with contracting muscles. Appreciation of the position of a limb in space has been termed *stagnosia*, and finally, in the presence of tension, appreciation of force applied during a voluntary contraction has been termed *dynamaesthesia*.[8] Although these expanded definitions found in the classic literature provide additional information about human proprioception, adaptations of these classic definitions have been suggested and are used for the purposes of this chapter (Box 24-1).

AFFERENT NEUROBIOLOGY OF THE JOINT

Early work on afferent proprioceptive function of the human joint included investigations into the role of joint- and muscle-based afferent receptors in human active and passive movement and detection of joint position.[8] In 1898 Goldsheider proposed that the sensation of passive movements was solely the product of joint-based receptors. This view is still widely accepted today for passive movements.[7,8]

The view up until the 1970s about the sensory feedback of active human movements was that when voluntary movement was initiated by the cerebral cortex, only low-level control was presented by the receptors in muscles and tendons. This sensory information from the muscles and tendons yielded information to the spinal cord and some subcortical extrapyramidal parts of the brain such as the cerebellum but played no contributing role in conscious sensation, which remained in the province of the joint receptors.[8] In the early 1970s, however, important research by Goodwin et al[9] and Eklund[10] independently demonstrated the important role that muscular receptors play in contributing to sensations of active movement qualitatively. This section of the chapter focuses on both joint- and muscle-based afferent receptors to allow the clinician a more complete understanding of the sources of afferent information in the human body. This will later lead to a greater understanding of how specific treatment strategies can be used clinically to improve proprioceptive and neuromuscular function in both upper and lower extremity rehabilitation (Box 24-2).

Box 24-1

Definitions of Proprioception and Associated Functions in Humans

Proprioception: Afferent information, including joint position sense, kinesthesia, and sensation of resistance

Joint position sense: The ability to recognize joint position in space

Kinesthesia: The ability to appreciate and recognize joint movement or motion

Sensation of resistance: The ability to appreciate and recognize force generated within a joint

Neuromuscular control: Appropriate efferent responses to afferent proprioceptive input

Classification of Afferent Mechanoreceptor

Mechanoreceptors are sensory neurons or peripheral afferents located within joint capsular tissues, ligaments, tendons, muscle, and skin.[11,12] Deformation or stimulation of the tissues in which the mechanoreceptors lie produces gated release of sodium, which elicits an action potential.[13] Four primary types of afferent mechanoreceptors have been classified and are commonly present in noncontractile capsular and ligamentous structures in human joints (Table 24-1).

Type I articular receptors are traditionally globular or ovoid corpuscles with a very thin capsule. They are numerous in the capsular tissues of all the limb joints, as well as the apophyseal joints of the vertebral column. Wyke[12] reported that the population of type I receptors appears to be more dense in proximal joints than in distal joints. Type I receptors are typically located in the superficial layers of the joint capsule.

Physiologically, type I receptors are low-threshold, slowly adapting mechanoreceptors. A proportion of type I receptors are always active in every joint position.[12] The resting discharge of type I receptors allows the body to know where the limb is placed and receive constant input on limb position in virtually any joint position. The type I receptor is categorized as both a static and dynamic mechanoreceptor[12] whose discharge pattern signals static joint position, changes in intraarticular pressure, and the direction, amplitude, and velocity of joint movements.

Type II mechanoreceptors are elongated, conical corpuscles with thick multilaminated connective tissue capsules. These type II corpuscles are present in the fibrous capsules of all joints but are reported to be present in greater number in distal joints than in proximal joints.[1] Type II corpuscles are located in the deeper layers of the fibrous joint capsule, particularly at the border between the fibrous capsule and the subsynovial fibroadipose tissue and often alongside articular blood vessels. Type II mechanoreceptors are low-threshold, rapidly adapting receptors and are reported to be entirely inactive in immobile joints.[12] These receptors become activated for very brief moments (1 second or less) at the onset of joint movement. The type II receptor is considered to be a dynamic mechanoreceptor whose brief, high-velocity discharges signal joint acceleration and deceleration during both active and passive joint movements.

The type I and type II mechanoreceptors described in the preceding paragraphs are the primary receptors located in the joint capsule. Type III receptors are primarily confined to the joint ligamentous structures. These type III receptors are found in both intrinsic and extrinsic ligamentous structures[12] and are similar in nature to the Golgi tendon organs found in tendons, as discussed in later sections of this chapter. Type III receptors are found predominantly in the superficial surfaces of the joint ligaments, near their bony attachments. Research delineating the type III mechanoreceptor classifies this receptor as a high-threshold, slowly adapting structure, again similar in nature to the Golgi tendon organ. These type III receptors are completely inactive in immobile joints and become active or stimulated only toward the extreme ranges of joint motion where the ligamentous structures become taut. When considerable stress is generated in the joint ligaments, the type III receptor will become actively stimulated. Wyke[14] also reported that type III receptors become activated with longitudinal traction on the limbs; the receptors remain activated centripetally at a high velocity only if extreme joint displacement or joint traction is maintained.

The final joint receptor to be discussed in this section is the type IV receptor. These receptors are noncorpuscular, unlike type I, II, and III receptors, and are represented by plexuses of small unmyelinated nerve fibers or free nerve endings. Type IV receptors are typically distributed throughout the fibrous joint capsule, adjacent periosteum, and articular fat pads. The type IV receptor represents the pain receptor system of articular tissues and is entirely inactive in normal circumstances. Marked mechanical deformation or chemical irritation such as exposure of the nerve endings to agents such as histamine, bradykinin, and other inflammatory exudates produced by damaged or necrosing tissues can stimulate activation of the type IV receptor.[12,14,15]

Box 24-2

Factors Affecting Joint Proprioception

Fatigue
Immobility
Injury
Surgery
Disuse
Ligamentous laxity
Aging
Arthritis

Table 24-1 Classification of Mechanoreceptors in the Human Body

Type	Location	Threshold	Response	Active
I	Superficial joint capsule Limbs and vertebrae Greater density proximal joints	Low	Slow adapting	Always Static/dynamic
II	Deeper layers of the joint capsule Greater density distal joints	Low	Rapidly adapting	Dynamic only
III	Superficial surface of the joint Ligament	High	Slowly adapting	Dynamic end-range movements Joint traction
IV	Joint capsule, adjacent periosteum Articular fat pads	—	—	Not active in normal circumstances

AFFERENT MECHANORECEPTORS IN THE LOWER EXTREMITY

The distribution of afferent articular nerves in synovial joints consists of medium and large myelinated fibers innervating the small end-organs or mechanoreceptors throughout joint tissue. These nerves represent approximately 55% of the total quantity of articular nerves, with the remaining 45% consisting of small unmyelinated fibers that transmit nociception or pain sensation.[12]

Type I or Ruffini receptors located in the superficial layers of the joint capsule are low-threshold, slowly adapting mechanoreceptors. These receptors respond to changing mechanical stress and are always active because of the gradient pressure difference in the joint capsule. They undergo deformation with natural movement because of their location in the superficial portion of the joint capsule. In the limbs, type I receptors are found to be more densely distributed in the proximal joints of the hip and are not as prevalent in the distal joints of the ankle.[12] Ruffini receptors have also been found in the meniscofemoral, cruciate, and collateral ligaments of the knee.[2]

Type II or pacinian receptors are located in the deep layers of the joint capsule, the meniscofemoral, cruciate, and collateral ligaments of the knee. In addition, type II receptors are located in the intraarticular and extraarticular fat pads of all synovial joints. These pacinian receptors are more prevalent in distal joints such as the ankle and are less densely distributed in proximal joints such as the hip. They function as rapidly adapting, low-threshold receptors and respond to acceleration, deceleration, and passive joint movement but are silent during inactivity and joint movement at constant velocity.[2]

Type III or Golgi tendon organ–like endings are found predominantly in intraarticular and extraarticular joint ligaments, including the collateral ligaments and cruciate ligaments in the knee.[12] These receptors have also been identified in the menisci of the knee.[2] Type III Golgi tendon organ–like endings are structurally identical to the Golgi tendon organ receptors and function as slowly adapting, high-threshold receptors with a function similar to that of the Golgi tendon organs found in tendons.

Type IV free nerve endings function as the pain receptor or nociception system in synovial joints. These type IV receptor nerve endings are found throughout the joints of the extremities in the fibrous capsule and adjacent periosteum and in the articular fat pads and are the most prevalent receptor type in the knee menisci. They are completely inactive in normal situations and are activated by marked mechanical deformation or chemical stimuli resulting from an inflammatory response.[2]

AFFERENT JOINT RECEPTORS IN THE UPPER EXTREMITY

The classification system mentioned earlier for the four primary types of mechanoreceptors found in human noncontractile capsular and ligamentous tissues described by Wyke[12,14] provides generalized information about the location of these receptors in the human body. Vangsness et al[16] studied the neural histology of the human shoulder joint, including the glenohumeral ligaments, labrum, and subacromial bursa. They found two types of mechanoreceptors and free nerve endings in the glenohumeral joint capsular ligaments. Two types of slowly adapting Ruffini end-organs and rapidly adapting pacinian corpuscles were identified in the superior, middle, and inferior portions of the glenohumeral ligaments. The most common mechanoreceptor was the classic Ruffini end-organ in the capsular ligaments of the glenohumeral joint. Pacinian corpuscles were less abundant overall; however, Kikuchi[17] and Shimoda[18] reported that type II pacinian corpuscles were more commonly found in the capsular ligaments of the human glenohumeral joint than in the human knee. Analysis of the coracoclavicular and acromioclavicular ligaments showed equal distribution of type I and II mechanoreceptors. Morisawa et al[13] identified type I, II, III, and IV mechanoreceptors in human coracoacromial ligaments. These reviews show how the capsular ligaments of the glenohumeral joint aid in the provision of afferent proprioceptive input by their inherent distribution of both type I Ruffini mechanoreceptors and the more rapidly adapting pacinian receptors. A rapidly adapting receptor such as the pacinian receptor can identify changes in tension in the joint capsular ligaments but quickly decreases its input once the tension becomes constant.[16] In this way the type II receptor has the ability to monitor acceleration and deceleration of the tension on a ligament.

Several authors have also studied the labrum and subacromial bursa. Vangsness et al[16] reported that no evidence of mechanoreceptors was found in the glenoid labrum; however, free nerve endings were noted in the fibrocartilage tissue in the peripheral half. The subacromial bursa was found to have diffuse, yet copious free nerve endings, with no evidence of larger, more complex mechanoreceptors. Ide et al[19] also studied the subacromial bursa, taken from three cadavers, and found a copious supply of free nerve endings, most of which were present on the roof side of the subacromial arch, which is exposed to impingement-type stress. Unlike the study by Vangsness et al,[16] Ide et al[19] did find evidence of both Ruffini and pacinian mechanoreceptors in the subacromial bursa. Their findings suggest that the subacromial bursa receives both nociceptive and proprioceptive stimuli and may play a role in regulation of shoulder movement. Further research into the exact distribution of these important structures in the human shoulder is indicated to give clinicians further information and enhance the understanding of proprioceptive function of the shoulder.

AFFERENT RECEPTORS OF CONTRACTILE STRUCTURES IN THE UPPER EXTREMITY

In addition to the afferent structures found in noncontractile tissues of the human shoulder (joint capsule, subacromial bursa, and intrinsic and extrinsic ligaments), significant contributions to the regulation of human movement and proprioceptive feedback are obtained from receptors located in contractile structures.

Two of the primary mechanisms for afferent feedback from the muscle-tendon unit are the muscle spindle and the Golgi tendon organ.[15,20] Research classifying muscle spindles has traditionally grouped intrafusal muscle fibers into two groups based on the type of afferent projections.[20,21] These two groups consist of nuclear bag and nuclear chain fibers. Nuclear chain fibers project from large afferent axons.[20,21] Nuclear bag fibers are innervated by γ_1 (dynamic) motor neurons and are more sensitive to the rate of change in muscle length, such as that occurring during rapid stretch of a muscle during an eccentric contraction or passive stretch.[20] Intrafusal nuclear chain fibers are innervated by

Table 24-2 Characteristics of the Muscle Spindle

Type	Fiber Length	Motor Axon Type	Function
Nuclear bag	7-8 mm long	Medium size	Stimulation of larger motor fibers increases tension in the bag.
Nuclear chain	4-5 mm long	Small	Stimulation of smaller motor fibers reduces tension on the bag.

γ_2 (static) motor neurons and are more sensitive to static muscle length. The combination of nuclear chain and nuclear bag fibers allows afferent communication from the muscle-tendon unit to remain sensitive over a wide range of joint motion during both reflex and voluntary activation (Table 24-2).

Muscle spindles provide much of the primary information for motor learning, including muscle length and joint position. Upper levels of the CNS can bias the sensitivity of muscle spindle input and sampling.[20] Muscle spindles do not occur in similar density in all muscles in the human body. Spindle density is probably related to muscle function, with greater densities of muscle spindles being reported in muscles that initiate and control fine movements or maintain posture. Muscles that cross the front of the shoulder, such as the pectoralis major and biceps, have a very high number of muscle spindles per unit of muscle weight.[22] Muscles with attachment to the coracoid, such as the biceps, pectoralis minor, and coracobrachialis, also have high spindle densities. Lower spindle densities have been reported for the rotator cuff muscle-tendon units, with the subscapularis and infraspinatus having greater densities than the supraspinatus and teres minor.[22] This lower rotator cuff spindle density probably suggests synergistic mechanoreceptor activation with the scapulothoracic musculature during movement of the glenohumeral joint.[20,23] This coupled or shared mechanoreceptor activation is an example of the kinetic link or proximal-to-distal sequencing that occurs with predictable or programmed movement patterns in the human body.[24] This kinetic link activation concept is further demonstrated by the deltoid/rotator cuff force couple[23] and other important biomechanical features of the human glenohumeral joint and is discussed later in this chapter.

The second major aspect of musculotendinous afferent activity is the Golgi tendon organ. These tendinous mechanoreceptors are present in the human shoulder and respond to the tension generated by muscular contraction.[15,20] Activation of the Golgi tendon organs relays afferent feedback about muscle tension and joint position. Additionally, as a protective mechanism, activation of the tension-sensitive Golgi tendon organ produces a protective mechanism that causes relaxation of the agonist muscle that is undergoing tension, with simultaneous stimulation of antagonistic musculature.

CLINCAL ASSESSMENT OF PROPRIOCEPTION IN THE LOWER EXTREMITY

The two primary tests measuring proprioception and kinesthetic awareness in the knee joint are the threshold to detection of passive motion (TTDPM) for movement sense and reproduction

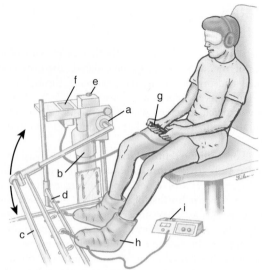

FIGURE 24-1 Proprioceptive testing device. *a*, Rotational transducer; *b*, motor; *c*, moving arm; *d*, stationary arm; *e*, control panel; *f*, digital microprocessor; *g*, handheld disengage switch; *h*, pneumatic compression boot; and *i*, pneumatic compression device. The threshold for detecting passive movement is assessed by measuring angular displacement until the subject senses motion in the knee. *(From Lephart, S.M., Kocher, M.S., Fu, F.H., et al. [1992]: Proprioception following anterior cruciate ligament reconstruction. J. Sport Rehabil., 1:188–196.)*

of angular position for joint position sense. The TTDPM test has been more standardized in the literature.[2,25,26] The method described by Barrack et al[27] and Skinner et al[28] involves placing the subject in a seated position with the leg hanging freely over the seat and suspended by a motorized pulley system in 90° of flexion (Fig. 24-1). Tactile, visual, and auditory cues are eliminated with the use of custom-fitted Jobst air splints and wearing of a blindfold. Initiation of movement into either flexion or extension proceeds at a rate of angular deflection of 0.5°/sec. When subjects initially detect movement to occur, they engage a control switch to indicate that the test leg has been moved.[28]

Testing for joint position sense involves passive movement of the extremity to a specified angle by the clinician, holding of the position for several seconds, and passive return of the extremity to the starting reference position. The patient is then asked to actively move the extremity to the specified angle without visual input. The difference between the actual and replicated angle can be calculated as either an absolute or a real angular error. With absolute error, only the magnitude of the error is determined, and whether the subject overestimates or underestimates knee position is not considered. Real error calculations, however, consider both the magnitude and direction of the error and can be used to determine whether a subject overestimates or underestimates the reference angle.[29] Barrack et al[30] demonstrated through studies on proprioception that extremities with no evidence of pathologic conditions have a high degree of symmetry in joint position sense.

Because essentially no standard protocols have been established for measuring joint position sense or for performing joint replication tests, many variations exist, including apparatuses used for angular measurement, starting reference angle, active or passive reproduction, and open chain (seated) versus closed chain (standing).[31] Lattanzio et al[25] and Marks and Quinney[32] used closed chain weight-bearing joint replications and reported a high degree of accuracy. Their results may be due to the fact that proprioceptive input is greater in the standing weight-bearing position, in which multiple joints are being loaded.

Single-limb postural stability tests have also been used for measuring the amount of sway in individuals with complaints of ankle instability. Tropp et al[33] developed such a test for measuring ankle instability that has been used with variations throughout the years. Individuals stand for 60 seconds on a force platform, and the instantaneous center of pressure is recorded along a graph; the magnitude of sway is compared with that on the uninvolved side.

Single-leg hop tests are often used for assessing stability in patients with pathologic knee or ankle conditions. Variations of the test include single-leg or triple-leg hop tests for distance, the crossover hop test, and the timed hop test. The relationship of hop tests to functional parameters such as instability, proprioception, and leg strength has been inconclusive in studies to date.

ASSESSMENT OF PROPRIOCEPTION AND NEUROMUSCULAR CONTROL IN THE UPPER EXTREMITY WITH SPECIFIC REFERENCE TO THE HUMAN SHOULDER

Determination of which patients require particular emphasis in rehabilitation on restoring proprioception and neuromuscular control requires the use of clinical assessment techniques. In this section, techniques used in research investigations, as well as in clinical applications, to allow the clinician to perform a detailed evaluation are reviewed.

Primary Measures of Proprioception and Neuromuscular Control for the Shoulder

Evaluation of proprioception and neuromuscular control in the human shoulder encompasses both afferent and efferent neural function, as well as the resulting muscular activation patterns.[15] Proprioception for the purposes of this and many other articles, texts, and chapters[2,15,34] consists of three major submodalities: kinesthesia, joint position sense, and sensation of resistance. Separate techniques can be used to assess each of these aspects of proprioception.

Measurement of Kinesthesia

Assessment of glenohumeral joint kinesthesia has been performed with a test called the TTDPM. This test assesses the subject's or patient's ability to detect a passive movement occurring typically at very slow angular velocities.[2,15,35] Elaborate testing devices have been used in several studies that have reported on the TTDPM, such as an instrumented (motorized) shoulder wheel[35] and other devices such as the one used by the University of Pittsburgh, whose characteristics are described next (Fig. 24-2).[2] Extensive research[2,15,36] using the TTDPM test has resulted in the selection and recommendation of slow angular velocities (0.5° to 2°/sec) to enhance the reliability of

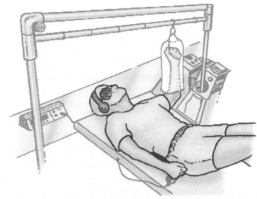

FIGURE 24-2 Upper extremity proprioceptive testing device. *(From Pollack, R. [2000]: Role of shoulder stabilization relative to restoration of neuromuscular control and joint kinematics. In Lephart, S.M., and Fu, F.H. [eds.]: Proprioception and Neuromuscular Control. Champaign, IL: Human Kinetics.)*

data acquisition. In addition to the device used, blindfolds, earphones, and a pneumatic cuff are recommended to eliminate cues from the visual, auditory, and tactile realm. This ensures that only joint kinesthesia is being assessed and not simply visual or auditory responses to perceived movement.

Physiologically, the TTDPM test is designed to selectively stimulate the Ruffini or Golgi-type mechanoreceptors in the articular structures being tested. Testing is typically performed for internal and external rotation of the glenohumeral joint in varying positions of elevation in the scapular and coronal planes. Testing in the literature has been done at the midrange and end-range positions of glenohumeral rotation.[2,15,36] As stated earlier, TTDPM in the human shoulder was measured by Blaiser et al,[34] and passive motion was found to be enhanced (smaller amount of movement before detection) at or near the end range of external rotation versus the midrange of external rotation or internal rotation.

Normative data on 40 healthy college-aged individuals undergoing the TTDPM test were reported by Warner et al[37] from both neutral rotational starting positions and 30° of humeral rotation with 90° of glenohumeral joint abduction. They found an average of 1.5° to 2.2° for all testing conditions, with no significant difference measured between the dominant or preferred hand relative to the nondominant extremity.[38] Allegrucci et al[39] measured shoulder kinesthesia in healthy athletes who performed unilateral upper extremity sports, such as baseball, tennis, or volleyball. The TTDPM test was performed with the shoulder in 90° of abduction and both 0° and 75° of external rotation and compared bilaterally. The results showed that the athletes had greater difficulty detecting passive motion in the dominant extremity than in the nondominant extremity. Consistent with earlier research,[34] Allegrucci et al[39] measured greater sensitivity to passive movement with the shoulder in 75° of external rotation bilaterally than with the shoulder in a more neutral condition. The findings in this study suggest that athletes in unilaterally dominant upper extremity sports may have a proprioceptive deficit in the dominant arm that may interfere with optimal afferent feedback regarding joint position.[39] This finding provides a rationale for proprioceptive upper extremity training in athletes from this population.

Measurement of Joint Position Sense

Joint position sense is the ability of the subject to appreciate where the extremity is oriented in space. Testing procedures to assess joint position sense are called *joint angular replication tests*. These tests typically place the extremity in a particular position to allow the subject to appreciate the spatial orientation of the extremity. After this period of joint positioning, the subject's extremity is returned to a starting position. The subject then reapproximates the position initially selected as closely as possible, without any visual, auditory, or tactile cues. Researchers have used both active[2,15,36,40,41] and passive[41] angular replication tests for assessment of the glenohumeral joint, and various apparatuses have been used to facilitate the accuracy of joint angular replication testing. Voight et al[41] used an isokinetic dynamometer with 90° of abduction and elbow flexion and standard isokinetic stabilization to perform active angular joint replication testing via a fatigue paradigm. They also used the passive mode of the isokinetic dynamometer set at 2°/sec to perform passive joint angular replication testing. Various authors[2,42,43] have used complex three-dimensional spatial tracking devices and multiple positions of active joint angular replication testing to quantify arm position.

In the most clinically applicable research study on active joint angular reproduction, Davies and Hoffman[40] tested subjects in a seated position with an electronic digital inclinometer (EDI).* Reference angles were chosen in several ranges and verified with the EDI; the patient then attempted to replicate the angular position, with the EDI being used to verify the position of the extremity. Angles chosen were greater than 90° and less than 90° of flexion and abduction, external rotation greater than 45° and less than 45°, and internal rotation greater than 45° and less than 45°. Normative data developed by Davies and Hoffman for 100 male subjects without pathologic shoulder conditions showed the average of the seven measurements to be 2.7°.[40] This represents the average difference between the seven reference angles and the actual matched angles by the subjects over the seven measurements.

Regardless of the testing methodology, active joint angular position replication tests primarily involve stimulation of both joint and muscle receptors and provide a thorough assessment of the afferent pathways of the human shoulder.[2,15]

Assessment of Neuromuscular Control of the Shoulder

Several methods have been used by clinicians and researchers to assess neuromuscular control of the shoulder. Widespread use of electromyographic (EMG) studies to measure muscular activity during shoulder rehabilitative exercise,[44-47] functional movement patterns such as the throwing motion[48] and tennis serve and groundstrokes,[49] and abnormal muscular activity patterns during planar motions[50-52] and functional activities[53] is reported in the scientific and clinical literature. Most of these studies comparing muscular activity expressed the contribution or activity of the muscle in terms of the amount of muscle activity relative to the maximal activity assessed via a maximal isolated manual muscle test (MMT). This is commonly referred to as %MMT or %MVC (maximum voluntary contraction) and allows comparison and expression of the relative activity of human muscle activity during activities of daily living (ADLs) and sport-specific movement patterns.[48,49]

---

*Available from Cybex, Inc., Medway, MA.

Muscular Strength Testing

Another important aspect of assessing neuromuscular control is measurement of muscular strength. Methods such as the MMT and the use of handheld dynamometers and isokinetic apparatuses have been used extensively for the documentation of both upper and lower extremity strength. Further discussion is beyond the scope of this chapter; however, the reader is referred to Chapter 25.

Closed Kinetic Chain Upper Extremity Testing

Closed kinetic chain (CKC) upper extremity tests are also used to assess neuromuscular control of the shoulder. Although widespread use of CKC training techniques has been reported in the physical medicine and rehabilitation literature,[54-58] currently existing evaluation methods to properly assess CKC function of the upper extremity are limited.

One of the "gold standards" in physical education for gross assessment of upper extremity strength has been the push-up. This test has been used to generate sport-specific normative data in normal populations,[56,59] but it is not typically considered appropriate for use in patients with shoulder dysfunction. The positional demands placed on the anterior capsule and the increased joint loading limit the effectiveness of this test in musculoskeletal rehabilitation. Modification of the push-up has been reported, and the modified push-up has been used clinically as an acceptable alternative to assess CKC function in the upper extremities.

Davies developed the CKC upper extremity stability test in an attempt to provide a means of assessing the functional ability of the upper extremity more accurately.[56,60,61] The test is initiated in the starting position of a standard push-up for males and modified (off the knees) push-up for females. Two strips of tape are placed parallel to each other, 3 feet apart on the floor. The subject or patient then moves both hands back and forth and touches each line alternatively as many times as possible in 15 seconds. Each touch of the line is counted and tallied to generate the CKC upper extremity stability test score. Normative results have been established, with males averaging 18.5 touches and females averaging 20.5 touches in 15 seconds. The CKC upper extremity stability test has been subjected to a test-retest reliability measure, with an intraclass correlation coefficient of 0.927 being generated, which is indicative of high clinical reliability between sessions with this examination method.[61]

EFFECTS OF AGING, INSTABILITY, AND INJURY ON LOWER EXTREMITY PROPRIOCEPTION

The effects of age and injury have been correlated with diminished proprioceptive sense.[62] Studies[63,64] have shown decreased proprioceptive acuity in older adults with testing, and it has been suggested that this decreased capacity for movement sense results in a higher incidence of falling and joint degeneration in this population. However, it has also been found that with regular physical activity, the age-related decline in proprioception can be lessened through dampening of the effect of disuse atrophy on the neuromuscular system.[2] In addition to age-related deficits, injuries to the lower extremity joints sustained as a result of repetitive microtrauma or a single traumatic event can create an environment in which degenerative changes occur in the joint along with disruption of the neuromuscular response. The presence of pain and inflammation in a joint produces an inhibitory effect on neuromuscular activation with decreased afferent mechanoreceptor signals.[65] Hurley and Newham[66] and Sharma and Pai[67] demonstrated arthrogenous muscle inhibition in patients with degenerative arthritis. The inability to achieve full voluntary muscle contraction may lead to continued overload on the joints through the loss of dynamic control and attenuation of force.

Loss of capsuloligamentous stability has been shown to cause proprioceptive deficits as a result of inadequate activation of mechanoreceptors leading to delayed muscle reaction latencies. Barrack et al[68] found decreased proprioception in a group of ballet dancers and attributed this clinical loss of proprioception to the hyperlaxity found in the ligamentous restraints in this population. It is theorized that without adequate tension in the capsuloligamentous restraints, insufficient stimulation of the mechanoreceptors used for proprioception occurs and results in decreased motor control. A study by Garn and Newton[69] also showed that individuals suffering from chronic ankle instability have diminished proprioception with a low threshold for passive plantar flexion. A similar study by Lentell et al[70] tested subjects with chronic lateral ankle instability who demonstrated decreased passive movement sense, with the uninvolved ankle being used as the control. Subjects in this study demonstrated no evidence of everter strength contributing to the functional instability. Therefore, the chronic instability was due to loss of mechanoreceptor function from ligamentous laxity and the resultant delayed muscular reflex. Lephart and Fu[2] and Nawoczenski et al[71] confirmed this decreased muscular stabilization in a study involving subjects with ankle instability. The results of their studies supported this loss of motor control, with a delay in onset latency in the peroneal muscles when subjected to sudden inversion stress.

Effects of Knee Injury on Proprioception

Degenerative arthritis in the knee causes pain, inflammation, and muscular inhibition, which results in decreased functional performance during gait and weight-bearing activities.[2] When combined with pain and altered muscle activity, the inadequate ligamentous tension resulting from narrowing of the joint space contributes to the interruption in afferent signals for proprioception and neuromuscular control. The goal of joint replacement surgery is to restore function through resurfacing joints, retensioning soft tissue structures, and ultimately restoring dynamic stability. Research performed by Warren et al[72] and Barrett et al[73] suggested that joint replacement surgery may actually improve joint position sense, with subjects showing significant improvement in position sense 6 months postoperatively. Furthermore, correlations have been made between improved functional outcomes and gait parameters and proprioceptive scores, thus suggesting a relationship between restoration of proprioception and improved functional outcomes.

The results of studies to date on the selection of joint prostheses and the effects of retaining versus sacrificing the posterior cruciate ligament (PCL) on proprioception have been inconclusive. However, it has been theorized that by restoring joint integrity and retensioning soft tissue structures, retention of the PCL will enhance dynamic joint stability through preservation of the neural reflexive pathway.[73–75]

Studies in the literature have consistently demonstrated decreases in proprioceptive sense and altered muscle patterns after rupture of the anterior cruciate ligament (ACL).[1,2,29] Loss of stability of the ACL causes alterations in muscle activity and reflex patterns, primarily the ACL-hamstring reflex. Measuring the ACL-hamstring reflex in patients with ACL rupture, Beard et al[76] showed significant reflex latency delays that were directly correlated with functional instability. Using EMG studies, Limbird et al[77] showed variations in muscle activation patterns with increased hamstring activation and concomitant decreased quadriceps activity with joint loading during gait. Andriacchi and Birac[78] had similar findings in patients performing normal activities of ambulation, stair climbing, and jogging. With the loss of stability and neural sensory input, many individuals experience functional disability in performance of normal ADLs.

EFFECTS OF PATHOLOGIC SHOULDER CONDITIONS ON PROPRIOCEPTION AND NEUROMUSCULAR CONTROL

In this section the normal afferent neurobiology of the joint and periarticular structures is reviewed, and examples of how proprioception and neuromuscular control are affected in pathologic conditions of the shoulder are provided. Examples of both glenohumeral joint instability and pathologic rotator cuff conditions are presented, as well as dysfunction of the scapulothoracic joint.

Effects of Glenohumeral Joint Instability on Proprioception

Several studies have addressed the influence of glenohumeral joint instability on proprioception. One of the most common clinical maladies seen by clinicians is anterior glenohumeral joint instability. Speer et al[79] studied the effects of a simulated Bankart lesion in cadavers. Coupled anterior/posterior translations were assessed in the presence of sequentially applied loads of 50 N in the anterior, posterior, superior, and inferior directions. The effects of a simulated Bankart lesion were small increases (maximum of 3.4 mm) in anterior and inferior translation of the humeral head relative to the glenoid in all positions of elevation and in posterior translation at 90° of elevation only.[79] The relevance of this article to the current discussion on proprioception is that Speer et al[79] concluded that detachment of the anterior inferior labrum from the glenoid (Bankart lesion) alone does not create large enough increases in humeral head translation to allow anterior glenohumeral joint dislocation. They indicated that permanent stretching or elongation of the inferior glenohumeral ligament may also occur and is necessary to produce full dislocation of the glenohumeral joint. This elongation or permanent stretching of the ligamentous structures may lead to alterations in the intrinsic tensile relationships of the glenohumeral joint capsule and capsular ligaments. The authors concluded that capsular elongation may be responsible for the high incidence of anterior reconstructions that fail to address anterior glenohumeral joint instability and do not fully restore normal capsular tension in the anterior structures.

Blaiser et al[34] examined the proprioceptive ability of subjects without known pathologic shoulder conditions and compared them with individuals with clinically determined generalized joint laxity. Individuals with greater glenohumeral joint laxity were found to have less sensitive proprioception than were those with less glenohumeral joint laxity. The authors found enhanced proprioception at or near the end range of external rotation, a position at which the anterior capsular structures have greater internal tension. They concluded that decreased joint angular reposition sense is one characteristic in individuals with increased glenohumeral joint laxity.

Smith and Brunolli[35] examined kinesthesia after glenohumeral joint dislocation in 8 subjects and compared their inherent joint position sense with that in 10 normal subjects by using an instrumented modification of a shoulder wheel. Their results indicated a significant decrease in joint awareness in the involved shoulders after shoulder dislocation in comparison to all uninvolved shoulders tested in the study.

Barden et al[80] tested subjects with multidirectional instability (MDI) for joint angular replication in multiple positions, including overhead reaching and abduction with external rotation. Subjects with MDI exhibited significantly greater hand position error than did control subjects without instability. This study showed significant proprioceptive deficits in patient with MDI.

Lephart et al[36] studied glenohumeral joint proprioception in 90 subjects in three experimental groups. One group consisted of 40 normal college-aged subjects, another group consisted of 30 patients with anterior instability, and the third group included 20 subjects who underwent surgical reconstruction for shoulder instability. No significant difference was found between extremities (dominant versus nondominant) in the normal subjects' proprioceptive ability; however, subjects with anterior instability had significant differences between the normal and unstable shoulders. Finally, Lephart et al[36] found no significant difference in the operated extremity versus the uninjured extremity after reconstructive surgery. This study was performed at least 6 months after subjects underwent open or arthroscopic repair for chronic, recurrent shoulder anterior instability. The authors concluded that these results provide evidence, consistent with the studies mentioned earlier, for partial deafferentation leading to proprioceptive deficits when the capsuloligamentous structures are damaged. Reconstructive surgery in this experiment appeared to restore normal joint proprioception 6 months or more after the surgical procedure.

Safran et al[81] used a testing device to study 21 collegiate baseball pitchers to determine whether bilateral differences in joint angular replication (JAR) and kinesthesia were present between extremities. They found that JAR was more accurate in the nondominant extremity when moving from a position of 75° of external rotation into internal rotation. Measurements were taken in 90° of abduction. No difference in proprioceptive ability was observed when moving from 75° of external rotation to end range of motion (ROM) between the extremities. Six collegiate pitchers with reports of shoulder pain were tested by Safran et al[81] and found to have a kinesthetic deficit in the injured dominant shoulder versus the nondominant shoulder when moving from neutral rotation into internal rotation. These results show JAR to be bilaterally symmetric from 75° of external rotation to end ROM between extremities in healthy skilled baseball pitchers despite increases in laxity and training effects. Additionally, despite a small sample size, Safran et al[81]

did show very importantly that pitchers with a recent report of injury involving the shoulder do have kinesthetic deficits in the injured arm that may affect further performance.

The finding of reduced proprioception in unstable shoulders has prompted researchers to examine the effect of surgical stabilization procedures on restoring proprioception following surgery. Rokito et al[82] studied the effects of two open surgical procedures for recurrent unidirectional anterior instability. Thirty subjects underwent an open inferior capsular shift procedure involving an approach that detached the subscapularis from the lesser tuberosity to gain exposure. Twenty-five underwent anterior capsulolabral reconstruction with a transverse splitting approach to the subscapularis for exposure. At 6 months postoperatively patients underwent proprioceptive testing, and the group with transverse splitting of the subscapularis had no deficits in proprioception and mean strength with respect to the contralateral uninvolved extremity. However, the group that underwent open capsular shift with subscapularis detachment had significant deficits in proprioception and mean strength that did not return to full functional values until 1 year postoperatively. This study shows that deficits in proprioception and strength following an open approach with detachment of the subscapularis require up to 1 year for return to the same functional level as the contralateral baseline extremity.

Effects of Glenohumeral Joint Instability on Neuromuscular Control

Lephart and Fu[2] defined neuromuscular control as the unconscious efferent response to an afferent signal concerning dynamic joint stability. Several studies highlighting changes in neuromuscular control in subjects with glenohumeral joint instability have been published. Glousman et al,[53] using an indwelling EMG electrode, studied the muscular activity patterns of normal healthy baseball pitchers and compared them with throwers with anterior glenohumeral joint instability. The results of the study showed marked increases in muscular activation of the supraspinatus and biceps muscle, as well as selective increases in the infraspinatus muscle during the early cocking and follow-through phases.[53] Also of interest was the finding of decreased muscular activation of the pectoralis major, latissimus dorsi, subscapularis, and serratus anterior muscles in the throwing athletes with anterior glenohumeral joint instability. This study showed neuromuscular compensations in the group with glenohumeral joint instability, as evidenced by increased activation of the primary dynamic stabilizers. Inhibition of the serratus anterior in the group with anterior instability may decrease scapular stability and further jeopardize joint congruity through improper scapulothoracic muscle sequencing.

McMahon and et al[83] tested normal shoulders and those with anterior instability and monitored them via indwelling EMG muscular activation patterns. Planar motions of flexion, abduction, and scapular-plane elevation (scaption) were studied in 30° increments. Significant decreases in serratus anterior muscle activity were measured in all three planar motions in the group of subjects with anterior glenohumeral joint instability. None of the other muscles—rotator cuff, deltoid, or scapular—showed a significant difference in testing during standard planar movement patterns. This study clearly shows the importance of the scapulothoracic musculature and dynamic stabilization during both aggressive overhead and common ADL-type movement patterns.

Finally, Kronberg et al[50] used intramuscular electrodes to compare shoulder muscle activity in patients with generalized joint laxity and normal control subjects. Increased subscapularis muscular activity was measured during internal rotation in the subjects with increased glenohumeral joint laxity, as well as increased middle and anterior deltoid activity during abduction and flexion. These studies clearly show the increased demand required by the dynamic stabilizers in subjects with joint laxity and glenohumeral joint instability. Application of the resistive exercise progressions and use of the kinetic chain exercise series listed later in this chapter have these research-based rationales and can directly enhance neuromuscular control of the shoulder complex.

Effects of Rotator Cuff Dysfunction on Neuromuscular Control in the Shoulder

Research similar to that discussed in the preceding section in which muscular activation patterns in patients with rotator cuff impingement were measured has been published. Ludewig and Cook[51] studied 52 male construction workers, 26 of whom had unilateral shoulder impingement and 26 had no symptoms of impingement or other pathologic shoulder condition. Similar to subjects in the previously discussed research studies on glenohumeral joint instability, those with unilateral impingement demonstrated a decrease in serratus anterior muscle activation during active elevation of the arm in comparison to normal, uninjured subjects.[51] Additionally, increases in upper and lower trapezius muscle activity were found in the subjects with unilateral impingement. This altered neuromuscular control mechanism also resulted in abnormal scapular posturing consisting of decreased upward rotation with elevation, increased anterior tipping, and increased medial rotation. These scapular modifications are thought to be contributing factors to rotator cuff impingement and demonstrate the importance of optimal and coordinated muscular control of the scapulothoracic and glenohumeral joints.

EFFECTS OF FATIGUE ON LOWER EXTREMITY PROPRIOCEPTION

Muscle fatigue reduces the force-generating capacity of the neuromuscular system, which essentially leads to increased laxity in the knee joint.[84] Skinner et al[28] found an increase in laxity of the ACL measured with a KT1000* arthrometer after a fatigue protocol. Similarly, Weisman et al[85] found increased laxity in the medial collateral ligament in athletes at a university after participation in various sporting activities. Furthermore, studies in the literature[2,28,86,87] have shown a decrease in the sensitivity of muscle receptors under fatigue conditions. The consequences of decreased proprioceptive sense from fatigue can be deleterious because of the possibility of sustaining injuries under these conditions when higher-level activities are performed. Skinner et al[28] studied the effects of fatigue on joint position sense and knee angle reproduction in a group of healthy, highly trained male recruits in the Special Forces division of the Navy. Subjects underwent an interval running program followed by isokinetic measurement of knee extension and flexion. Fatigue was

determined by the percent decrement in work output measured from pretraining to posttraining conditions on an isokinetic device. The authors concluded that after fatigue ensues, values on angular replication tests are significantly decreased, but no significant changes were noted in the threshold of movement sense. They determined that loss of muscle receptor efficiency as a result of fatigue played a key role in angular replication errors. The authors concluded that the dual role of afferent input by the receptors in the contractile and noncontractile elements of the knee is important for proprioceptive sense.

Lattanzio et al[25] conducted a study involving healthy male and female subjects performing three different cycling protocols (ramp, continuous, and interval training) at a percentage of their Vo_2max. In this study, methods for determining the threshold for detection of movement were similar, but angular replications were performed with subjects in the standing weight-bearing position instead of the seated open kinetic chain (OKC) protocol used in the study of Skinner et al. The results of the study of Lattanzio et al[25] were similar to those of Skinner et al, with statistically significant decrements in joint replication in male subjects after the three different fatigue protocols. Female subjects similarly showed significant differences in joint replication after the continuous and interval programs, but not with the ramp protocol for joint angular replication. The conclusions drawn by the authors of this study were that anatomic gender differences possibly account for the variation in proprioception in response to fatigue.

Finally, Barrack et al[30] and Barrett et al[73] studied the effects of total knee replacement on knee joint proprioception. This research paradigm is of particular interest because insertion of a total knee joint prosthesis results in removal of most joint receptors in the human knee. Both groups of investigators found no significant loss of proprioception in the extremity that underwent total knee replacement in comparison to the contralateral extremity 6 months postoperatively. These groups of authors both concluded that their research again points to the important role that muscle-based mechanoreceptors play in knee joint proprioception.

EFFECTS OF MUSCULAR FATIGUE ON UPPER EXTREMITY PROPRIOCEPTION AND NEUROMUSCULAR CONTROL

The role of specific afferent receptors in the human body has been examined with different methods to better understand the role of joint and muscular afferents. Provins[62] reported a decrease in the ability to detect passive motion of the finger when digital nerves containing both joint and cutaneous afferents were blocked by local anesthesia. He concluded that both types of afferent feedback may be equally important when joint proprioception is analyzed.

Zuckerman et al[88] injected lidocaine into the subacromial space and glenohumeral joint to assess proprioception in young and old male subjects. They found no adverse effects from the injection of lidocaine in either location and proposed that compensatory extracapsular feedback ensured intact proprioception after injection. No differences in joint position sense and TTDPM testing were noted between the dominant and nondominant extremity; however, a decline in proprioception with age was measured in the young (20 to 30 years of age) and older (50 to 70 years of age) subjects.

---

*Available from Medmetric Corporation, San Diego, CA.

Several studies have been performed on the human shoulder to investigate the effect of muscular fatigue on various indices of joint proprioception and neuromuscular control. Carpenter et al[89] tested subjects using a TTDPM test with the shoulder in 90° of abduction and 90° of external rotation. After an isokinetic fatigue protocol, subjects' detection of passive motion was marred or decreased by 171% for internal rotation and 179% for external rotation. In preexercise testing, Carpenter et al found increased sensitivity when moving into external rotation versus internal rotation but no difference between the dominant and nondominant extremities.[89] These authors concluded that the effect of muscular fatigue on joint proprioception may play a role in injury and decrease athletic performance.

Voight et al[41] tested subjects with an active and passive joint angular replication protocol after isokinetically induced muscular fatigue of the glenohumeral joint internal and external rotators. No significant difference in shoulder joint angular replication was found between the dominant and nondominant extremities. Significant decreases in accuracy were noted after muscular fatigue in both the active and passive joint angular replication tests. Pederson et al[90] tested the ability of healthy subjects to discriminate movement velocity of the glenohumeral joint in the transverse plane. The results of their study showed that subjects had a decrement in discrimination of movement velocity after a hard isokinetic horizontal flexion/extension exercise fatigue protocol versus a light exercise condition.

Myers et al[91] used an active angular replication test and neuromuscular control test to examine the effects of muscle fatigue in normal shoulders. A concentric isokinetic internal and external rotation fatigue protocol was used. Fatigue of the internal and external rotators of the shoulder decreased subjects' accuracy in detecting both midrange and end-range absolute angular error but did not have a negative effect on neuromuscular control in a bilaterally assessed unilateral CKC stability-type test measuring postural sway velocity.

Additional research by Myers et al[92] has demonstrated that patients with anterior glenohumeral instability have alterations in muscle activation. Therefore, clinicians can implement therapeutic exercises that address the suppressed muscles as the scientific foundation of a rehabilitation program. Myers et al[93,94] found that capsuloligamentous injury to the shoulder decreases proprioceptive input to the CNS and thereby results in decreased neuromuscular control. Consequently, clinicians need to address the mechanical instability but also implement functional rehabilitation interventions to return an athlete to competition. Tripp et al[95] demonstrated that functional fatigue affects the acuity of the entire upper extremity.

Lin et al[96] investigated the effects of scapular taping on shoulder proprioception and EMG activity in several muscles of the shoulder complex. The magnitude of proprioceptive feedback was significantly lower in the taping conditions. The results suggest that scapular tape affects the activity of the shoulder muscles and ultimately that these effects are related to the proprioceptive feedback provided by the tape. Further research will continue to be needed to better understand and demonstrate the efficacy of shoulder and scapular taping because it is a very popular technique with many anecdotal reports demonstrating effectiveness; however, high-level research support for this technique is limited at this time.

The consistent finding in these studies of a decrement in proprioception after muscular fatigue has led researchers to emphasize the importance of the muscle-based receptors. The use of active joint angular positioning tests has been reported to stimulate both joint and muscle mechanoreceptors and is considered to be a more functional assessment of the afferent pathways.[2,15,91] The exact mechanism by which muscle-based proprioception is affected is not entirely clear or known. Muscle fatigue is thought to desensitize the muscle spindle threshold and thereby lead to decrements in both joint position sense and neuromuscular control. Djupsjobacka et al[97-99] reported alterations in muscle spindle output in the presence of lactic acid, potassium chloride, arachidonic acid, and bradykinin. Intramuscular concentrations of these substances are altered during muscular exertion and fatigue. This consistent relationship has provided further rationale and support for improvement in muscular endurance of the dynamic stabilizers of the glenohumeral joint. This topic is covered in detail in the application section of this chapter.

EFFECTS OF TRAINING ON PROPRIOCEPTION IN THE LOWER EXTREMITY

Some studies in the literature have investigated the notion of injury prevention and improvement in neuromuscular stabilization through proprioceptive training. A review of research in this section will provide the reader with important references that support the use of proprioceptive training of the lower part of the body for both injury prevention and rehabilitation.

In a prospective study by Cerulli et al,[100] 600 semiprofessional and amateur soccer players were monitored for three seasons to determine the frequency of ACL injury in players who underwent a progressive proprioceptive training program and in a control group who performed only traditional strengthening exercises. The results showed significant differences between the experimental and control groups, with the proprioception training group sustaining fewer lesions of the ACL than the control group who performed traditional strengthening exercises.

Osborne et al[101] studied the effects of ankle disk training in eight individuals who sustained an inversion ankle sprain within the preceding years and who had not received any formal rehabilitation. The subjects performed 15 minutes of daily training on a disk with the involved leg in an 8-week training program. After completion of the 8-week training program, the subjects were tested for onset latencies with surface EMG electrodes on the muscles of the ankle influencing stability to measure the motor response to a simulated inversion sprain on a platform. The results showed significant improvements in anterior tibialis latency times in both the trained and untrained control ankles.

A similar study by Eils and Dieter[102] showed significant improvements in muscle reaction times and patterns of muscle coactivation in 30 subjects with chronic ankle sprains. The subjects performed a multistation proprioceptive exercise program that included 12 stations with various devices once weekly for 6 weeks. The frequency of once per week and the types of exercises were chosen for their ability to be implemented easily into a rehabilitation program. The exercises included a Biodex balance system,* inversion boards, minitrampoline, and ankle disk. The subjects performing the exercises showed significant improvement over the control group in position sense and reported subjective improvements in functional stability.

---

*Available from Biodex, Shirley, NY.

Friden et al[31] conducted a study in subjects with ACL deficiencies who performed traditional lower extremity strengthening exercises and in subjects who performed traditional rehabilitation along with perturbation training. The perturbation program consisted of progressive exercises using rocker boards and roller boards, with advancement to the next phase after successful completion of the task without evidence of instability or pain. After the training program, the perturbation group was found to have significantly greater success with subjective reports of stability during completion of higher-level activities than did the traditional training group. Beard et al[76] conducted a similar study but used hamstring reflex latencies and the Lyshom rating scale for measuring functional outcomes. They concluded that the group that underwent perturbation training had improved functional outcomes in knee stability while performing ADLs. Additionally, numerous studies have evaluated the effectiveness of neuromuscular training programs, including perturbation training, in patients with ACL injuries.[52,103-107] Numerous studies have also evaluated the effectiveness of neuromuscular training programs, including perturbation training, in patients with chronic/functional ankle instability.[108-111]

One very important aspect inherent in most lower extremity proprioceptive training programs is inclusion of the entire lower extremity kinetic chain in the exercise. Most proprioceptive exercises in the literature described herein use multiple joint-training positions and CKC positioning environments that allow the entire lower extremity kinetic chain to be included. Research[112-114] has emphasized the importance of examining the entire kinematic chain from the trunk and hip musculature throughout the lower extremity for postural control mechanisms in rehabilitation and prevention of injury. Furthermore, using absolute angular error measurements, Miura et al[115] found that local and general fatigue affects knee proprioception, decreases muscular power, and has effects on different mechanisms in the proprioceptive pathway. Consequently, to prevent injury caused by a fatigue-induced decline in proprioception, local muscle training by itself is not enough, but neuromuscular training, including central programming, is essential for the entire lower extremity kinetic chain.

NEUROMUSCULAR TRAINING FOR REHABILITATION AND PREVENTION OF SPORTS INJURIES

Zech et al[116] performed a systematic review of the use of neuromuscular training for rehabilitation of sports injuries. Fifteen studies met the inclusion criteria and demonstrated the effectiveness of neuromuscular training in increasing functionality and decreasing the incidence of recurrence after ankle and knee injuries. However, no studies demonstrated the effectiveness of neuromuscular training in rehabilitating sports injuries in the shoulder, only for lower body injuries. Though used inherently and recommended for shoulder rehabilitation, this systematic review showed much less scientific support for the use of neuromuscular control exercises in the upper extremity. Hübscher et al[117] performed a systematic review of the use of neuromuscular training for rehabilitation of sports injuries. Thirty-two articles were identified, but only seven methodically well conducted studies were included in the review. Multiintervention training was effective in reducing the risk for lower limb injuries. Balance training alone decreased the incidence of ankle sprains in athletes. Interestingly, exercise interventions were more effective in athletes with a history of sports injuries than in those without. This probably relates to the concept of inadequate rehabilitation following the initial sports injury. Additional research on the use of balance training to improve neuromuscular control was performed by Zech et al.[118] They completed a systematic review of balance training for neuromuscular control and enhancement of performance. Twenty RCTs met the inclusion criteria. Balance training was effective in improving postural sway and functional balance, and larger effect sizes were demonstrated for training programs of longer duration. It is controversial whether balance training was effective in improving jumping performance, agility, and neuromuscular control.

CLINICAL APPLICATION: TECHNIQUES TO IMPROVE LOWER EXTREMITY PROPRIOCEPTION AND NEUROMUSCULAR CONTROL

Lower extremity injuries occur often in competitive and recreational sports. These injuries are sometimes caused by physical contact with another individual, but they usually result from a noncontact injury in which the external forces in the environment exceed the internal forces of the body.[100] Some of the more common injuries involve damage to the ligamentous and cartilaginous components in the knee and ankle. Injuries that do not involve another person occur when the player or individual attempts to suddenly change the rate of speed or course of direction or when an obstacle in the external environment causes overload on the static joint restraints. The questions that have received recent attention in the literature are the degree to which these injuries can be prevented and, once an individual is injured, the ways in which recurrent injuries to an existing compromised system can be prevented through dynamic neuromuscular stabilization.[119]

For a patient with ACL deficiency, neuromuscular training is achieved through coordinated muscle activation in response to controlled perturbation forces imparted on the joint. One strategy for dynamic stabilization is cocontraction of opposing muscle groups to essentially stabilize the knee in a rigid posture. This strategy may be successful for simple tasks, but with higher-level activities such as sports, stabilization is achieved through selective motor recruitment that is dependent on the task. A force feedback mechanism in which stability is achieved through varied patterns of muscle recruitment, depending on the situational needs of the task, has been discussed.[1,2] This theory acknowledges that different patterns of movement require varied muscular stabilization, depending on the direction, speed, and amount of force occurring at the joint.

At the University of Delaware, Snyder-Mackler et al[1,120] designed a rehabilitation program based on the premise of achieving dynamic muscular stabilization during normal and higher-level skills through neuromuscular perturbation training. They use the term *copers* for individuals who successfully perform varied high-level activities without experiencing functional instability. In copers, the muscular strategies used for joint stability allow normal joint movement, whereas deleterious compressive and shear forces at the joint are minimized. The term given to individuals who are unsuccessful in maintaining joint stability during lower extremity weight-bearing tasks is *noncopers*. In the group of noncopers, a cocontraction stiffening strategy is used with all tasks, which results in inefficient movement strategies and functional instability. Furthermore, with this inadequate coping mechanism, progressive deterioration of joint surfaces and capsuloligamentous restraints occurs as a result of excessive shear and compressive forces at the joint.[1,2]

The faculty at the University of Delaware designed a program using the guidelines of Fitzgerald et al to implement a neuromuscular training program for patients with ACL deficiency in an attempt to restore functional stability during higher-level sporting activities. In selection of individuals for the program, certain criteria had to be met to ensure a successful outcome of the training.

The program is designed to identify individuals who would be successful rehabilitation candidates through a screening process. The criteria include isolated injury to the ACL, infrequent episodes of instability (<1), a passing score on functional hop tests, and a passing percentage on two subjective rating scales for functional knee impairment. Before a stabilization program is initiated, the early focus of rehabilitation is on decreasing joint effusion, restoring ROM, and increasing quadriceps and hamstring strength to allow stabilization through muscle recruitment.[1] When these goals have been met, an advanced neuromuscular training program can be initiated. The program is progressive in nature and designed for specificity of sport or activity.

The program consists of 10 treatment sessions at a frequency of two to three times per week and is progressive in nature with three phases of implementation (early phase, sessions 1 to 4; middle phase, sessions 5 to 7; and late phase, sessions 8 to 10). Progression of the program is based on the symptomatic patient response (i.e., increased effusion or pain), which is used as a guideline, and the ability of the patient to perform successful motor strategies to counteract the perturbation force, which includes no episodes of falling or instability. All three phases include the use of rocker boards, roller boards, and platforms with an introduction to sport-specific agility drills in the middle to later stages.

In the early phase of perturbation training, patients are subjected to perturbation forces on all three devices in slow predictable directions with the use of verbal cues as necessary for the onset and direction of the forces. Initially, the direction of the applied forces is in the anterior/posterior and medial/lateral directions with progression to diagonal and rotational planes. The clinical implication of this phase thus involves the application of progressive variable perturbation forces in multiple directions (sagittal, transverse, and frontal planes) in a controlled manner to retrain the nervous system in a number of applications or situational needs while avoiding the use of rigid cocontraction strategies.[2]

The middle phase of training continues with perturbation training and requires successful adaptation of strategies in the early phase. Variations in the parameters of training, including predictability, speed, amplitude, intensity, and direction of force, are advanced, along with the implementation of light sport-specific drills while the individual is wearing a functional knee brace. In the last phase of treatment, sport-specific movements are emphasized with the use of agility drills. Initially, training

begins in straight planes and then moves to variable-direction drills such as cutting and changing direction on command. The drills are initially performed at 50% and progress to 100% in the later stages. Examples of some of the agility drills are side shuffles, shuttle running, and cutting maneuvers at 45° and 90° angles. With no evidence of instability, patients then perform sport-specific activities while undergoing perturbations on roller boards and platforms to simulate the competitive demands of the sporting environment. Before returning to full athletic competition, athletes are required to pass a posttreatment ACL screening involving measures similar to those used during prescreening for acceptance into the program.[2]

GUIDELINES FOR IMPLEMENTING LOWER EXTREMITY PROPRIOCEPTIVE TRAINING

Regardless of whether surgery or conservative care is chosen to restore stability and function to a degenerative or unstable joint, rehabilitation is crucial for reestablishing neuromuscular control or dynamic stability in a compromised joint. The loss of neuromuscular control results from damage to the mechanoreceptors within the capsuloligamentous structures of the joint and from interruption of the afferent sensory pathways that play a crucial role in producing smooth, coordinated movement.[2]

Several considerations are important when a rehabilitation program is designed to restore proprioception and dynamic stability. In selecting exercises for training, a focus on restoring function to the individual should remain at the forefront. Exercises chosen should then focus on an individual's deficits in strength, ROM, and balance and, most importantly, on the individual's ability to meet the demands of stability while performing daily or sporting activities.

Traditionally, a combination of OKC and CKC exercises have been used in rehabilitation. OKC exercises have been defined as movements in which the distal segment is free to move in space, and CKC movements occur when the distal segment is fixed or meets considerable resistance.[121] Emphasis on the use of CKC exercises has predominated because they are thought to more closely resemble the functional demands placed on the lower extremity during a variety of activities. Another advantage of CKC exercises is the simultaneous movement of multiple joints, which requires cocontraction of opposing muscle groups to control joint movement. CKC exercises can also reduce shear forces across joint surfaces as a result of the stability of joint-through-joint compression forces and cocontraction of opposing muscle groups. The advantage of OKC exercises is their ability to isolate targeted muscle groups for strengthening.

In a study by Snyder-Mackler et al,[122] isolated OKC quadriceps strengthening was found to be superior to CKC exercises in improving quadriceps function in patients after ACL surgery because the involvement of other muscle groups in performing the CKC exercises did not isolate the quadriceps as effectively. In fact, most functional activities, such as ambulation, use a combination of both OKC and CKC muscle activation patterns, and therefore both should be incorporated in the design of a successful program.

In the early stages of rehabilitation, the development of an exercise program should identify deficits in ROM, strength, and joint effusion, and progression should not exceed the rate of natural healing or limitations in the involved structures. Any number of exercises will elicit proprioception training based on the fact that deformation of the joint mechanoreceptors occurs with active, active assisted, and passive movements and provides sensory input to improve neural mechanisms.[2] Performing ROM exercises on an immobilized joint and weight shifting early after an ankle sprain or surgery on the ACL are examples of early forms of proprioception training.

When sufficient healing has taken place in the subacute stages of recovery, initiation of resistance exercises for building muscular strength and endurance will enable sufficient muscle recruitment patterns for the dynamic stabilization needed for advanced forms of training. Proprioceptive training in this stage may involve two-legged stance exercises on an unstable surface such as the Biodex stability balance system (Fig. 24-3), which can be advanced to a functional squatting movement pattern. The exercise progression can include single-leg stance (Fig. 24-4) and single-leg stance with partial squatting on the machine with the benefit of a visual cursor to assess weight distribution so that compensatory patterns can be avoided.

Other exercises that are beneficial for proprioception involve the use of rocker boards for directional perturbations to activate selective muscle recruitment patterns in a variety of planes of movement. These training techniques can be advanced to sport-specific activities such as tossing a ball against a trampoline while manual perturbations are applied to the board (Fig. 24-5). Movement patterns such as a straight plane or multidirectional lunge are also useful for selective motor recruitment in functional or sport-related activities (Figs. 24-6 and 24-7). These patterns can be performed on balance pads or exercise mats to enhance motor control through maintenance of balance while performing initially slow and then more rapid movements beyond the base of support (Fig. 24-8).

The goal of proprioceptive training is to reestablish stability or dynamic neuromuscular control and should emphasize

return to functional or sport-specific activity. In the later stages of training, exercise should focus on restoring and ideally optimizing the adaptive neuromuscular response to situational needs. If stabilization training has yielded the appropriate muscular response toward the final stages of

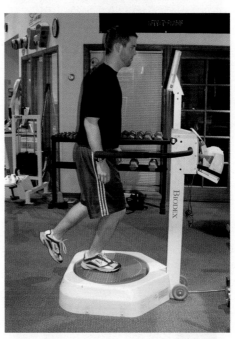

FIGURE 24-4 Single-leg balance on Biodex balance system. The level of difficulty is progressed by decreasing the stability of the platform or removing visual cues by having the patient close his eyes.

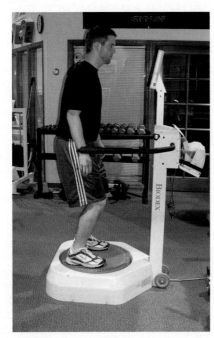

FIGURE 24-3 Incorporating functional movements such as the squat on the Biodex balance system.

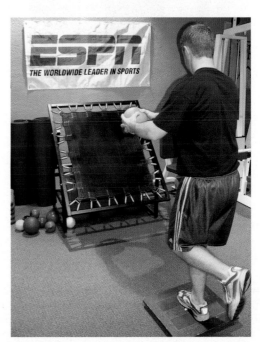

FIGURE 24-5 Chest pass with a weighted ball incorporates plyometric exercises with proprioceptive exercise, with difficulty being increased by manual perturbations of the rocker board while the patient throws and catches the ball.

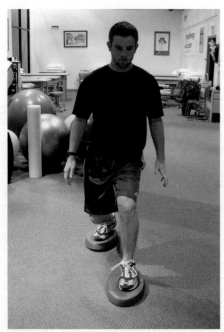

FIGURE 24-6 Combination of proximal pelvic control with lower extremity proprioception while the patient performs lunges on Thera-Band balance pads.

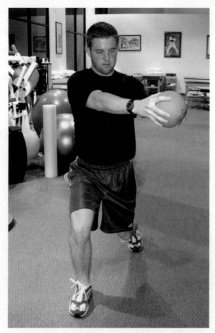

FIGURE 24-7 A lunge being performed with rotation of the torso while a weighted ball is held outside the base of support for the integration of upper and lower extremity movement patterns.

rehabilitation, more advanced exercises incorporating sport-specific drills should be performed. Exercises on a Fitter board* or slide board can be performed to challenge the patient with higher-velocity movements while performing sport-specific drills involving full body movement patterns on a yielding surface (Figs. 24-9 and 24-10). Agility drills, including

*Available from Fitter International, Calgary, Alberta, Canada.

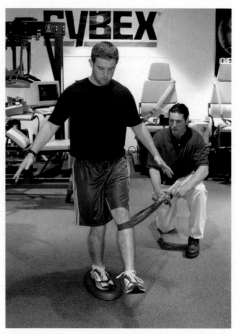

FIGURE 24-8 Single-leg balance on Thera-Band balance pads while opposite extremity movements are resisted beyond the base of support in functional planes.

progressively quicker changes in direction while pivoting on the involved extremity, should be incorporated in the final stages of rehabilitation for athletes who perform such maneuvers in the competitive arena.

CLINICAL APPLICATION: TECHNIQUES TO IMPROVE PROPRIOCEPTION AND NEUROMUSCULAR CONTROL OF THE UPPER EXTREMITY WITH SPECIFIC REFERENCE TO THE SHOULDER

Application of the basic science information on proprioception and neuromuscular control of the shoulder to clinical practice allows clinicians to most appropriately provide stability to the glenohumeral joint and optimize shoulder girdle arthrokinematics. Several areas are covered in this section, including the use of CKC and joint approximation exercises, joint oscillation exercises, postoperative interventions, and techniques to improve muscular endurance of the rotator cuff and scapular musculature.

Closed Kinetic Chain (Joint Approximation) Exercises

Exercises that produce approximation of the glenohumeral joint and are characterized by a fixed distal aspect of the extremity are typically referred to as joint approximation or CKC upper extremity exercises. The approximation of the joint surfaces and the multiple joint loading inherent in CKC exercises are reported to increase mechanoreceptor stimulation[2,123] and produce muscular cocontraction. The presence of muscular cocontraction around the human shoulder is particularly

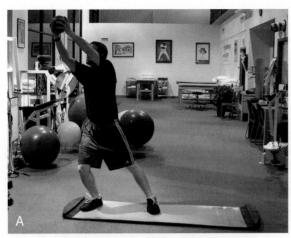
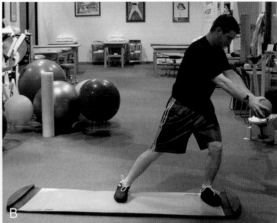

FIGURE 24-9 Dynamic balance on a slide board incorporating upper body movements with resistance in proprioceptive neuromuscular facilitation patterns. **A,** Reaching high. **B,** Reaching low.

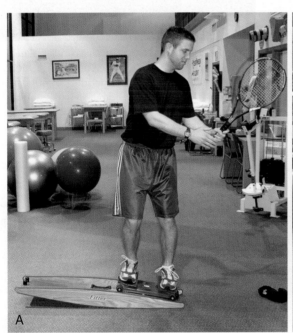
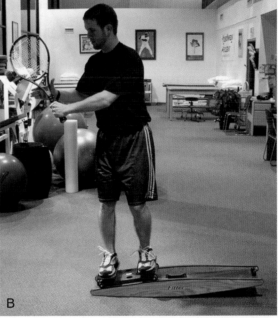

FIGURE 24-10 Dynamic balance on a Fitter board with sport-specific drills such as the ground stroke in tennis. **A,** Forehand. **B,** Backhand.

beneficial because of the important role that the musculature surrounding the scapulothoracic joint plays in stabilizing and controlling movement of the shoulder.[124,125]

Significantly less EMG research has been published on upper extremity CKC exercise than on upper extremity OKC exercise. Moesley et al[46] published a comprehensive analysis of the scapular muscles during traditional rehabilitation exercises. Two CKC upper extremity exercises were included in their analysis. These exercises were the push-up with a plus and the press-up. The push-up with a plus includes maximal protraction of the scapula during the end of the ascent phase of a modified push-up and produces very high levels of serratus anterior muscle activity. The press-up exercise did not elicit high levels of muscular activity in the trapezius or serratus but instead produced high activation levels in the pectoralis

minor. Decker et al[126] confirmed the importance of the plus position for serratus anterior activation and concluded that exercises emphasizing scapular upward rotation and accentuated protraction produce the highest levels of muscular activity in the serratus anterior.

Kibler et al[125] published EMG research on a series of very low level CKC exercises for the upper extremity, including weight-bearing upper extremity weight shifts and exercises on the rocker board or biomechanical ankle platform system with the upper extremity. Muscle activation levels during these exercises were very low in the rotator cuff, deltoid, and scapular muscles; however, low levels of activity were present in virtually all these muscles during these activities. This indicates that high degrees of coactivation and cocontraction are inherent in this type of exercise.

Research has demonstrated the important role that joint compression plays in glenohumeral joint CKC exercise. Warner et al[37] studied the effects of applying a 5-, 25-, and 50-lb compressive force to cadaveric shoulder specimens. These amounts of compression resulted in decreases in anterior humeral head translation in neutral elevation from 11 to 2 mm with 5 and 25 lb of compressive force and from 21.5 to 1.4 mm at 45° of abduction, respectively. This study shows the potential benefit of a compressive load in the provision of glenohumeral joint stability and points out the important application that CKC exercises may have in enhancement of neuromuscular control in patients with glenohumeral joint instability.

Application of CKC exercises clinically is facilitated by a thorough review of glenohumeral joint anatomy. It is imperative that the clinician realize the osseous relationship of the glenohumeral joint. The human glenoid is oriented slightly inferiorly with the arm held at the side and tilted anteriorly 30° from the coronal plane of the body.[127,128] This anterior version of the scapula is aligned with 30° of retrotorsion of the humeral head, and optimal bony congruity occurs with the arm placed in the scapular plane.[128] Understanding these important relationships will guide the clinician in shoulder positioning and ROM selection during joint approximation exercises with the arm placed in the scapular plane.[128]

Research on CKC upper extremity training is limited. Lephart et al[86] used five neuromuscular control exercises that emphasized joint positioning, joint approximation and compression, and muscular cocontraction in one experimental group, in addition to traditional OKC shoulder rehabilitation exercises in patients with glenohumeral joint instability. They found significant improvements in kinesthetic ability, scapular slide testing, and isokinetically documented protraction and retraction strength in the group that performed these neuromuscular control exercises during rehabilitation.

Application of these concepts in patients with rotator cuff dysfunction and glenohumeral joint instability is pictured in Figures 24-11 to 24-15. Guidelines for the time-based sets of exercise depend on the patient, with the ability of the patient to maintain the desired scapulothoracic stabilization being a governing factor. Careful monitoring of the medial and inferior borders of the scapula is important to ensure proper neuromuscular control and avoid the development of undesired motor patterning.[124] Sets of exercises lasting up to 30 or 45 seconds are desired in the later stages of rehabilitation.

Joint Oscillation Exercises

Rehabilitative exercises involving joint oscillation have increased in popularity in recent years. Appliances such as the Bodyblade,* BOING (body oscillation integrates neuromuscular gain),† and resistance bar‡ have facilitated the use of joint oscillation exercises. Rapid oscillation of these devices coupled with external loads such as light weights, manual resistance, and TheraTubing‡ can provide additional emphasis on particular muscle groups during these exercises. Figures 24-16 to 24-19 show exercises using oscillatory devices or manual contact that require the rotator cuff and scapular musculature to respond to external cues

---

*Available from Hymanson, Inc., Playa Del Rey, CA.
†Available from OPTP, Minneapolis, MA.
‡Available from Hygenic Corp., Akron, OH.

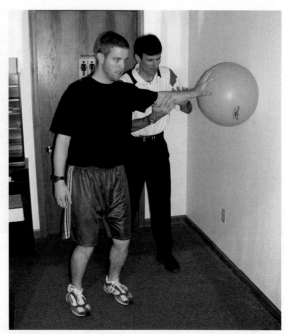

FIGURE 24-11 Closed chain wall scapular-plane rhythmic stabilization. The patient's arm is placed on a medicine ball or small exercise ball in varying degrees of abduction in the scapular plane. The clinician performs rhythmic stabilization with the patient remaining as stable as possible over the ball; varying the position of the hand contacts by progressing further toward the patient's hand increases the intensity of the exercise.

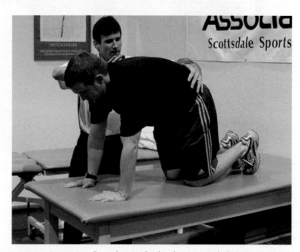

FIGURE 24-12 Quadruped rhythmic stabilization exercise progression with instruction to maintain scapular protraction or the "plus" position during repeated multidirectional challenges.

induced via the oscillation and stretch imparted during the exercise. The ability of these time-based exercises to promote local muscular endurance is increased by manipulation of set duration and rest cycles.[129] Progression to the external rotation oscillation exercise in Figure 24-17 by using the 90° abducted scapular-plane position is followed as rehabilitation progresses to more closely approximate the glenohumeral and scapulothoracic positions inherent in overhead sport-specific movement

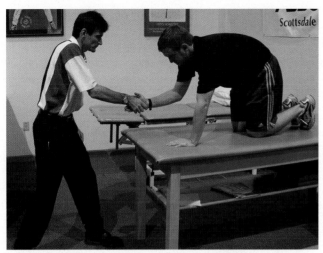

FIGURE 24-13 Tripod rhythmic stabilization technique with the involved extremity in the closed chain position and maintenance of the "plus" position to increase activation of the serratus anterior muscle. The clinician alternately provides multidirectional challenges to the non–weight-bearing limb as the patient attempts to isometrically hold the pictured position.

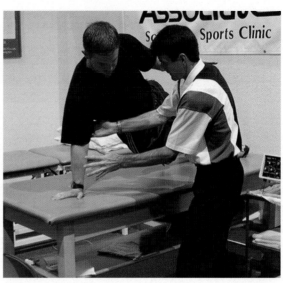

FIGURE 24-15 High-level unilateral scapular stabilization exercise with the patient in a closed chain unilateral scapular-plane stance position with rhythmic stabilization superimposed on the upper extremity to increase the challenge of the exercise.

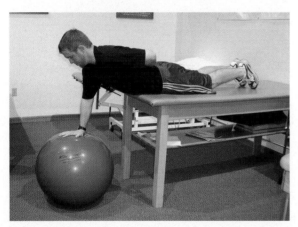

FIGURE 24-14 Unilateral prone exercise ball stabilization exercise. The degree of support is progressively decreased to increase the challenge to the patient by sliding the patient in a cephalad direction.

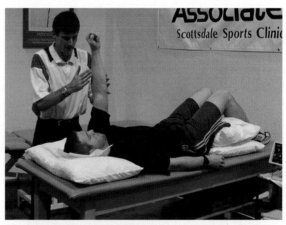

FIGURE 24-16 Supine modified rhythmic stabilization technique performed in 90° of shoulder flexion with scapular protraction.

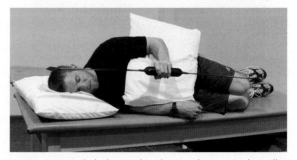

FIGURE 24-17 Side-lying glenohumeral rotational oscillation exercise using the Bodyblade.

patterns.[130] Figure 24-20 shows the push-up with a plus exercise. Care is taken with this exercise to protect the shoulder complex by descending only approximately one half the distance of a standard push-up and then maximally protracting the scapula on the ascent phase to increase activity of the serratus anterior muscle.[46]

Holt et al[131] investigated four different positions of exercise with the Bodyblade and its effect on infraspinatus muscle activity. These four positions included (1) standing with the glenohumeral joint in a neutral abduction/adduction position for internal and external rotation, (2) side-lying position with the glenohumeral joint in neutral abduction/adduction for internal and external rotation (see Fig. 24-17), (3) 90° of glenohumeral joint scapular-plane elevation with stabilization, and (4) 90° of scapular-plane elevation with the unsupported arm.

The results of a repeated-measures analysis of variance showed that the side-lying internal/external rotation oscillatory pattern elicited the highest levels of infraspinatus muscle activation.[131] Further research such as this is needed to guide clinicians in the use of oscillatory-type exercise.

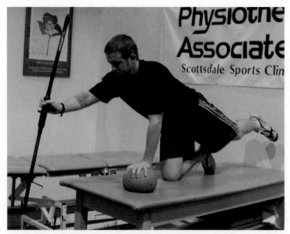

FIGURE 24-18 Biped closed kinetic chain exercise using the Bodyblade to provide joint oscillation in the non–weight-bearing upper extremity and a medicine ball to decrease surface stability of the closed chain upper extremity. Scapular position can be altered in this exercise, depending on the intended goal of muscular activation.

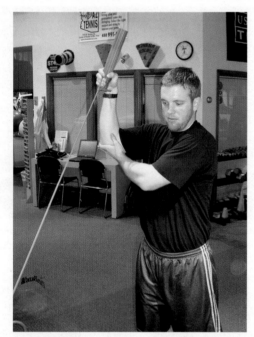

FIGURE 24-19 "Statue of Liberty" external rotation oscillation exercise using Thera-band elastic resistance and a resistance bar for oscillation. A scapular-plane position in 90° of elevation is used while the contralateral extremity provides support to decrease the role of the deltoid in actively holding the exercising extremity in the 90° position.

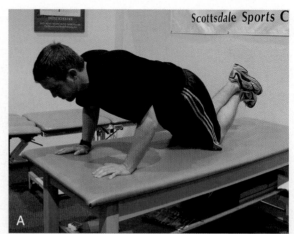

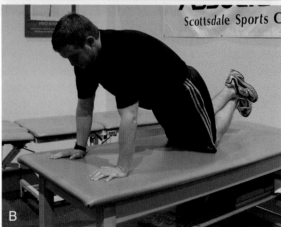

FIGURE 24-20 Push-up with a plus and maximal protraction of the scapula to elicit higher levels of serratus anterior activity. **A,** Starting position. **B,** Ending position of movement.

Thirty-one studies met the inclusion criteria. Many factors influence the training responses and effect sizes demonstrated by the studies. These studies show that gender, training status, exercise protocol, and type of vibration platform all influence the outcomes. It appears that vertical platforms produce chronic adaptations whereas oscillating platforms have a more profound effect on acute responses to the exercises. The results of the vibration exercise can be used by exercise professionals to enhance muscular strength based on the aforementioned criteria. Marin and Rhea[132] also completed a metaanalysis of the effects of vibration training on muscle power. Vertical platforms were more effective than oscillating platforms in producing a larger treatment effect for chronic adaptations. However, age is a moderator of the response to vibration exercise for power. The results of the vibration exercise can be used by exercise professionals to enhance muscular power in selected subjects and specific protocols.

Muscular Endurance Exercise

Exercises to increase endurance and fatigue resistance of the rotator cuff and scapular musculature would have a direct effect on improving performance and enhancing proprioception

Vibration Training on Performance

One of the fastest growing areas focusing on proprioceptive and neuromuscular control deals with the effects of vibration training on performance. Marin and Rhea[132] performed a metaanalysis of the effects of vibration training on muscle strength.

and neuromuscular control. All the exercises described in this chapter can be used to promote local muscular endurance by increasing the work duration and decreasing the rest periods in the exercise format. Exercises using sets of 15 to 20 repetitions and 15 to 20 repetition maximum loading schemes are geared toward improving local muscular endurance.[129] Current practice in orthopedic and sports physical therapy usually includes exercises with this type of prescription or recommendation.[54,57] The use and integration of joint oscillation, joint approximation or closed chain, plyometric, and isotonic and isokinetic training of targeted muscles or muscle groups have clear benefits and research-oriented rationales as outlined in this chapter and other sources.[15,54,57,60,129]

One additional study performed by Ellenbecker and Roetert[121] specifically evaluated the relative muscular fatigue of the rotator cuff with isokinetic testing. Seventy-two elite junior tennis players underwent isokinetic fatigue testing consisting of 20 reciprocal concentric contractions of the internal and external rotators with 90° of glenohumeral joint abduction. The results showed significantly different fatigue responses between the internal and external rotators. Analysis of the relative fatigue ratio, which compares the work performed in the second half of the testing protocol with the work performed in the first half, showed that the internal rotators fatigued to a level of only 83%. The external rotators, however, fatigued to a level of 69% over the 20 testing repetitions.[121] This study demonstrated a greater relative degree of muscular fatigue in the external rotators, even in healthy trained subjects, and provides an important rationale for the inclusion of copious amounts of endurance-oriented training of the external rotators in patients with rotator cuff dysfunction or glenohumeral joint instability.

Chen et al[133] demonstrated the effects of muscular fatigue on glenohumeral joint kinematics. Subjects were studied radiographically as they elevated their shoulders before and after a series of rehabilitation exercises that produced substantial levels of muscular fatigue in the shoulder. They found significantly greater amounts of superiorly directed humeral head translation documented radiographically with arm elevation after fatigue. This study shows the important role that the rotator cuff plays in maintaining glenohumeral joint congruity and stabilizing the humeral head within the glenoid.[34] Repeated attempts to enhance muscular endurance based on these studies, as well as on earlier literature citations linking muscular fatigue of the glenohumeral rotators to decrements in proprioception, are clinically indicated.

Postoperative Applications

The use of treatment techniques to enhance proprioception and neuromuscular control is indicated for the shoulder after surgery. Methods proposed for addressing glenohumeral joint instability include primarily capsular plication and the application of thermal energy to produce capsular shortening, which may acutely alter glenohumeral joint proprioception.[20,134] Myers et al[135] measured joint position sense, kinesthesia, and shoulder function in patients who underwent thermal capsular shrinkage for glenohumeral joint instability. No significant differences were found in active and passive angular reproduction of joint position sense 6 to 24 months postoperatively. The acute effects of thermal capsular shrinkage on glenohumeral joint proprioception are not completely understood; however,

this study shows that full return of proprioceptive function is expected after rehabilitation.

Early postoperative proprioceptive training consists of passive angular joint repositioning in available ROM with the elimination of visual cues. Replication of either the contralateral extremity position or repeated movements can be done passively initially and then be progressed to active angular joint position replication as patient status and tissue healing allow. Early application of the joint approximation exercises and rhythmic stabilization exercises described earlier in this chapter is also beneficial in the early progression after rotator cuff repair and open and arthroscopic stabilization.[136]

Neuromuscular control is a result of the efferent response to the afferent signals generated through the sensory system. Proprioception plays a critical role in this feedback system. When the proprioceptive pathways are injured or disrupted, not only inefficient motor responses but also greater risk for injury are possible, especially in the area of athletics in which overcoming resistance from opposing players is coupled with environmental obstacles in an often fast-paced arena. In preparing athletes for competition, the clinician should consider the effects of fatigue and disuse on proprioception and also their potential impact when designing a comprehensive training or rehabilitation program.

Use of the clinically oriented exercise progressions highlighted in this chapter, including techniques such as joint approximation, joint oscillation, and local muscular endurance applications, provides the framework for objectively based rehabilitation programs using the scientific concepts reviewed in this chapter.

CONCLUSION

Introduction

- More is known about proprioception in the lower extremity than in the upper extremity.
- To maintain balance and postural control, we rely on sensory information from the periphery, as well as from our visual, vestibular, and somatosensory systems.
- Feedforward and feedback mechanisms are responsible for initiating a motor response in anticipation of a stimulus.

Afferent Mechanoreceptor Classification

- Mechanoreceptors are sensory neurons or peripheral afferents located within joint capsular tissues, ligaments, tendons, muscle, and skin.
- Four primary types of afferent mechanoreceptors are commonly present in noncontractile capsular and ligamentous structures in human joints: types I, II, III, and IV.
- Type I and II mechanoreceptors are the primary receptors located in the joint capsule.
- The lower extremity contains types I, II, III, and IV mechanoreceptors, whereas the glenohumeral joint appears to have all four types, which are dependent on the structure. Types I and II predominate in the glenohumeral joint.
- The primary mechanisms for afferent feedback from the muscle-tendon unit are the muscle spindle and the Golgi tendon organ.

Clinical Assessment of Proprioception in the Lower Extremity

- The two primary tests measuring proprioception and kinesthetic awareness in the knee and glenohumeral joint are the threshold to detection of passive motion for movement sense and reproduction of angular position for measuring joint position sense.
- Essentially no standard protocols have been established for measuring joint position sense or for joint replication tests.

Assessment of Proprioception and Neuromuscular Control in the Upper Extremity

- Evidence suggests that athletes performing unilaterally dominant upper extremity movements, such as those involved in baseball, tennis, or volleyball, may have a proprioceptive deficit in the dominant arm that may interfere with optimal afferent feedback regarding joint position.
- Active joint angular position replication tests primarily involve the stimulation of both joint and muscle receptors and provide a thorough assessment of the afferent pathways of the human shoulder.
- Neuromuscular control of the shoulder can be assessed with electromyography, functional movement patterns, abnormal muscular activity patterns during planar motion, functional activities, muscular strength, and closed kinetic chain upper extremity tests.
- Evaluation methods to assess closed chain function of the upper extremity are limited. Those that have been used include the push-up and the closed kinetic chain stability test.

Effects of Aging, Instability, and Injury on Lower Extremity Proprioception

- Age and injury result in diminished proprioception.
- Loss of capsuloligamentous stability causes proprioceptive deficits because of inadequate activation of mechanoreceptors, which results in delayed muscle reaction latencies.
- Some evidence suggests that total knee replacement results in improved proprioception scores, although the effects of sacrificing or retaining the posterior cruciate ligament are inconclusive.
- Proprioceptive sense is decreased and muscle patterns are altered after rupture of the anterior cruciate ligament.

Effects of Pathologic Shoulder Conditions on Proprioception and Neuromuscular Control

- Damage to the capsuloligamentous structures of the shoulder leads to deficits in proprioception.
- Glenohumeral joint instability and rotator cuff dysfunction result in changes in neuromuscular control patterns.

Effects of Fatigue on Lower Extremity Proprioception

- Muscle fatigue reduces the force-generating capacity of the neuromuscular system, which essentially leads to increased laxity in the knee joint.

- Evidence shows a decrease in the sensitivity of muscle receptors with fatigue. The consequences of decreased proprioceptive sense as a result of fatigue can be deleterious because of the possibility of sustaining injuries under these conditions when higher-level activities are performed.

Effects of Muscular Fatigue on Upper Extremity Proprioception and Neuromuscular Control

- Evidence suggests that the effect of muscular fatigue on joint proprioception may play a role in injury and decrease athletic performance.
- The consistent finding of a decrement in proprioception after muscular fatigue has led researchers to emphasize the importance of the muscle-based receptors.

Effects of Training on Proprioception in the Lower Extremity

- It appears that proprioception can be enhanced through a proprioception training program.

Techniques to Improve Lower Extremity Proprioception and Neuromuscular Control

- Different patterns of movement require varied muscular stabilization, depending on the direction, speed, and amount of force occurring at the joint.
- Progression of proprioceptive and neuromuscular control training during the early and middle phases of training consists of moving along a continuum in which predictability, speed, amplitude, intensity, and direction of force are modified.

Guidelines for Implementing Lower Extremity Proprioceptive Training

- When one selects exercises for restoring proprioception and dynamic stability, a focus on restoring function to the individual should remain at the forefront. The exercises chosen should then focus on an individual's deficits in strength, ROM, and balance and, most importantly, on the individual's ability to meet the demands of stability while performing daily or sporting activities.
- Any number of exercises will elicit proprioceptive training based on the fact that deformation of the joint mechanoreceptors occurs with active, active assisted, and passive movements and provides sensory input to improve neural mechanisms.
- The goal of proprioceptive training is to reestablish stability or dynamic neuromuscular control and should emphasize a return to functional or sport-specific activity.

Techniques to Improve Proprioception and Neuromuscular Control of the Upper Extremity

- The approximation of joint surfaces and the multiple joint loading inherent in closed kinetic chain exercises are reported to increase mechanoreceptor stimulation and produce muscular cocontraction.

- Patients with rotator cuff dysfunction or glenohumeral joint instability progress on a continuum of difficulty, with the patient's ability to maintain the desired scapulothoracic stabilization being a governing factor. Careful monitoring of the medial and inferior borders of the scapula is important to ensure proper neuromuscular control and avoid the development of undesired motor patterning.

- Exercises to increase endurance and fatigue resistance of the rotator cuff and scapular musculature have a direct effect on improving performance and enhancing proprioception and neuromuscular control.

- Exercises using sets of 15 to 20 repetitions and 15 to 20 repetition maximum loading schemes are geared toward improving local muscular endurance.

REFERENCES

1. Williams, G.N., Chmielewski, T., Rudolph, K.S., et al. (2001): Dynamic knee stability: Current theory and implications for clinical scientists. J. Orthop. Sports Phys. Ther., 31:546–566.
2. Lephart, S.M., and Fu, F.H. (2000): Proprioception and Neuromuscular Control in Joint Stability. Champaign, IL, Human Kinetics.
3. Riemann, B.L., Myers, J.B., and Lephart, S.M. (2002): Sensorimotor system measurement techniques. J. Athl. Train., 37:85–98.
4. Goetz, C.G. (1999): Textbook of Clinical Neurology, 1st ed. Philadelphia, Saunders.
5. Adams, R.D., Victor, M., and Ropper, A.H. (1997): Principles of Neurology, 6th ed. New York, McGraw-Hill.
6. Sherrington, C. (1906): The Integrative Action of the Nervous System. New York, Scribner's Son.
7. Goldscheider, A. (1898): Gesammelte Abhandlungen. II. Physiologie des Muskelsinnes. Leipzig, Germany, Barth.
8. Roland, P.E., and Ladegaard-Pedersen, H. (1977): A quantitative analysis of sensations of tension and of kinesthesia in man: Evidence for a peripherally originating muscular sense and for a sense of effort. Brain, 100:671–692.
9. Goodwin, G.M., McCloskey, D.I., and Matthews, P.B.C. (1972): The contribution of muscle afferents to kinesthesia shown by vibration induced illusions of movement and by the effects of paralyzing joint afferents. Brain, 95:705–748.
10. Eklund, G. (1972): Position sense and state of contraction: The effects of vibration. J. Neurol. Neurosurg. Psychiatry, 35:606–611.
11. Grigg, P. (1994): Peripheral mechanisms in proprioception. J. Sport Rehabil., 3:2–17.
12. Wyke, B. (1972): Articular neurology—A review. Physiotherapy, 58:94–99.
13. Morisawa, Y., Kawakami, T., Uemura, H., et al. (1994): Mechanoreceptors in the coracoacromial ligament. A study of the aging process. J. Shoulder Elbow Surg., 3:S45.
14. Wyke, B.D. (1967): The neurology of joints. Ann. R. Coll. Surg. Engl., 41:25.
15. Myers, J.B., and Lephart, S.M. (2000): The role of the sensorimotor system in the athletic shoulder. J. Athl. Train., 35:351–363.
16. Vangsness, C.T., Ennis, M., Taylor, J.G., et al. (1995): Neural anatomy of the glenohumeral ligaments, labrum, and subacromial bursa. Arthroscopy, 11:180–184.
17. Kikuchi, T. (1968): Histological studies on the sensory innervation of the shoulder joint. J. Iwate Med. Assoc., 20:554–567.
18. Shimoda, F. (1955): Innervation, especially sensory innervation of the knee joint and motor organs around it in early stage of human embryo. Arch. Histol. (Jpn.), 9:91–108.
19. Ide, K., Shirai, Y., Ito, H., et al. (1996): Sensory nerve supply in the human subacromial bursa. J. Shoulder Elbow Surg., 5:371–382.
20. Nyland, J.A., Caborn, D.N.M., and Johnson, D.L. (1998): The human glenohumeral joint: A proprioceptive and stability alliance. Knee Surg. Sports Traumatol. Arthrosc., 6:50–61.
21. Barker, D., Banks, R.W., Harker, D.W., et al. (1976): Studies of the histochemistry, ultrastructure, motor innervation, and regeneration of mammalian intrafusal muscle fibers. Exp. Brain Res., 44:67–88.
22. Voss, H. (1971): Tabelle der absoluten und relativen Muskel-spindelzahlen der menschlichen Skeletmuskulatur. Anat. Anz., 129:562–572.
23. Inman, V.T., Saunders, J.B., and Abbot, L.C. (1944): Observations on the function of the shoulder joint. J. Bone Joint Surg., 26:1–30.
24. Marshall, R.N., and Elliot, B.C. (2000): Long-axis rotation: The missing link in proximal to distal segmental sequencing. J. Sports Sci., 18:247–254.
25. Lattanzio, P.J., Petrella, R.J., Sproule, J.R., et al. (1997): Effects of fatigue on knee proprioception. Clin. J. Sports Med., 7:22–27.
26. Pincivero, D.M., and Coelho, A.J. (2001): Proprioceptive measures warrant scrutiny. Biomechanics, 3:77–86.
27. Barrack, R.L., Skinner, H.B., and Buckley, S.L. (1989): Proprioception in the anterior cruciate–deficient knee. Am. J. Sports Med., 17:1–6.
28. Skinner, H.B., Wyatt, M.P., Hodgdon, J.A., et al. (1986): Effect of fatigue on joint position sense of the knee. J. Orthop. Res., 4:112–118.
29. Beynnon, B.D., Good, L., and Risberg, M.A. (2002): The effect of bracing on proprioception of knees with anterior cruciate ligament injury. J. Orthop. Sports Phys. Ther., 32:11–23.
30. Barrack, R.L., Skinner, H.B., Cook, S.D., et al. (1983): Effect of articular disease and total knee arthroplasty on knee joint-position sense. J. Neurophysiol., 50:684–687.
31. Friden, T., Roberts, M., Ageberg, E., et al. (2001): Review of knee proprioception and the relation to extremity function after an anterior cruciate ligament rupture. J. Orthop. Sports Phys. Ther., 31:568–576.
32. Marks, R., and Quinney, H.A. (1993): Effect of fatiguing maximal isokinetic quadriceps contractions on ability to estimate knee position. Percept. Mot. Skills, 77:1195–2002.
33. Tropp, H., Ekstrand, J., and Gillquist, J. (1984): Factors affecting stabilometry recordings of single limb stance. Am. J. Sports Med., 12:185–188.
34. Blaiser, R.B., Carpenter, J.E., and Huston, L.J. (1994): Shoulder proprioception: Effect of joint laxity, joint position, and direction of motion. Orthop. Rev., 23:45–50.
35. Smith, R.L., and Brunolli, J. (1989): Shoulder kinesthesia after anterior glenohumeral joint dislocation. Phys. Ther., 69:106–112.
36. Lephart, S.M., Warner, J.J.P., Borsa, P.A., and Fu, F.H. (1994): Proprioception of the shoulder joint in healthy, unstable, and surgically repaired shoulders. J. Shoulder Elbow Surg., 3:371–380.
37. Warner, J.J.P., Bowen, M.K., Deng, X., et al. (1999): Effect of joint compression on inferior stability of the glenohumeral joint. J. Shoulder Elbow Surg., 8:31–36.
38. Warner, J.J.P., Lephart, S., and Fu, F.H. (1996): Role of proprioception in pathoetiology of shoulder instability. Clin. Orthop. Relat. Res., 330:35–39.
39. Allegrucci, M., Whitney, S.L., Lephart, S.M., et al. (1995): Shoulder kinesthesia in healthy unilateral athletes participating in upper extremity sports. J. Orthop. Sports. Phys. Ther., 21:220–226.
40. Davies, G.J., and Hoffman, S.D. (1993): Neuromuscular testing and rehabilitation of the shoulder complex. J. Orthop. Sports Phys. Ther., 18:449–457.
41. Voight, M.L., Hardin, J.A., Blackburn, T.A., et al. (1996): The effects of muscle fatigue on and the relationship of arm dominance to shoulder proprioception. J. Orthop. Sports Phys. Ther., 23:348–352.
42. Jerosch, J.G. (2000): Effects of shoulder instability on joint proprioception. In Lephart, S.M., and Fu, F.H. (eds.): Proprioception and Neuromuscular Control in Joint Stability. Champaign, II, Human Kinetics.
43. Slobounov, S.M., Poole, S.T., Simon, R.F., et al. (1999): The efficacy of modern technology to improve healthy and injured shoulder joint sense. J. Sport Rehabil., 8:10–23.
44. Ballantyne, B.T., O'Hare, S.J., Paschall, J.L., et al. (1993): Electromyographic activity of selected shoulder muscles in commonly used therapeutic exercises. Phys. Ther., 73:668–682.
45. Blackburn, T.A., McLeod, W.D., White, B., et al. (1990): EMG analysis of posterior rotator cuff exercises. Athl. Train., 25:40–45.
46. Moesley, J.B., Jobe, F.W., and Pink, M. (1992): EMG analysis of the scapular muscles during a shoulder rehabilitation program. Am. J. Sports Med., 20:128–134.
47. Townsend, H., Jobe, F.W., Pink, M., et al. (1991): Electromyographic analysis of the glenohumeral muscles during a baseball rehabilitation program. Am. J. Sports Med., 19:264–272.
48. DiGiovine, N.M., Jobe, F.W., Pink, M., et al. (1994): An electromyographic analysis of the upper extremity in pitching. J. Shoulder Elbow Surg., 1:15–25.
49. Rhu, K.N., McCormick, J., Jobe, F.W., et al. (1988): An electromyographic analysis of shoulder function in tennis players. Am. J. Sports Med., 16:481–485.
50. Kronberg, M., Brostrom, L.A., and Nemeth, G. (1991): Differences in shoulder muscle activity between patients with generalized joint laxity and normal controls. Clin. Orthop. Relat. Res., 209:181–192.
51. Ludewig, P.M., and Cook, T.M. (2000): Alterations in shoulder kinematics and associated muscle activity in people with symptoms of shoulder impingement. Phys. Ther., 80:276–291.
52. McLeod, T.C., Armstrong, T., Miller, M., and Sauers, J.L. (2009): Balance improvements in female high school basketball players after a 6-week neuromuscular training program. J. Sport Rehabil., 18:465–481.
53. Glousman, R., Jobe, F., Tibone, J., et al. (1988): Dynamic electromyographic analysis of the throwing shoulder with glenohumeral instability. J. Bone Joint Surg. Am., 70:220–226.
54. Ellenbecker, T.S. (1995): Rehabilitation of shoulder and elbow injuries in tennis players. Clin. Sports Med., 14:87–110.
55. Ellenbecker, T.S., and Cappel, K. (2000): Clinical application of closed kinetic chain exercises in the upper extremities. Orthop. Phys. Ther. Clin. North Am., 9:231–245.
56. Ellenbecker, T.S., Manske, R., and Davies, G.J. (2000): Closed kinetic chain testing techniques of the upper extremities. Orthop. Phys. Ther. Clin. North Am., 9:219–245.
57. Wilk, K.E., and Arrigo, C. (1993): Current concepts in the rehabilitation of the athletic shoulder. J. Orthop. Sports Phys. Ther., 18:365–378.
58. Wilk, K.E., Arrigo, C.A., and Andrews, J.R. (1996): Closed and open kinetic chain exercises for the upper extremity. J. Sport Rehabil., 5:88–102.
59. Roetert, E.P., and Ellenbecker, T.S. (1998): Complete Conditioning for Tennis. Champaign, IL, Human Kinetics.
60. Ellenbecker, T.S., and Davies, G.J. (2000): The application of isokinetics in testing and rehabilitation of the shoulder complex. J. Athl. Train., 35:338–350.
61. Goldbeck, T.G., and Davies, G.J. (2000): Test-retest reliability of the closed kinetic chain upper extremity stability test: A clinical field test. J. Sport Rehabil., 9:35–45.
62. Provins, K.A. (1958): The effect of peripheral nerve block on the appreciation and execution of finger movements. J. Physiol., 143:55–67.

63. Kaplan, F.S., Nixon, J.E., Reitz, M., et al. (1985): Age-related changes in joint proprioception and sensation of joint position. Acta Orthop. Scand., 56:72–74.

64. Skinner, H.B., Barrack, R.L., and Cook, S.D. (1984): Age related decline in proprioception. Clin. Orthop. Relat. Res., 184:208–211.

65. Beard, D.J., Kyberd, P.J., Ferguson, C.M., et al. (1993): Proprioception after rupture of the anterior cruciate ligament. J. Bone Joint Surg. Br., 73:311–315.

66. Hurley, M.V., and Newham, D.J. (1993): The influence of arthrogenous muscle inhibition on quadriceps rehabilitation of patients with early, unilateral osteoarthritic knees. Br. J. Rheumatol., 32:127–131.

67. Sharma, L., and Pai, Y.C. (1997): Impaired proprioception and osteoarthritis. Curr. Opin. Rheumatol., 9:253–258.

68. Barrack, R.L., Skinner, H.B., Brunet, M.E., and Cook, S.D. (1983): Joint laxity and proprioception in the knee. Phys. Sports Med., 11:130–135.

69. Garn, S.N., and Newton, R.A. (1988): Kinesthetic awareness in subjects with multiple ankle sprains. Phys. Ther., 68:1667–1671.

70. Lentell, G.G., Baas, B., Lopez, D., et al. (1995): The contributions of proprioceptive deficit, muscle function, and anatomic laxity to functional instability of the ankle. J. Orthop. Sports Phys. Ther., 21:206–215.

71. Nawoczenski, D.A., Owen, G., Ecker, B., et al. (1985): Objective evaluation of peroneal response to sudden inversion stress. J. Orthop. Sports Phys. Ther., 25:107–109.

72. Warren, P.J., Olankun, T.K., Cobb, A.G., and Bentley, G. (1993): Proprioception after knee arthroplasty: The influence of prosthetic design. Clin. Orthop. Relat. Res., 297:182–187.

73. Barrett, D.S., Cobb, A.G., and Bently, G. (1991): Joint proprioception in normal osteoarthritic and replaced knees. J. Bone Joint Surg. Br., 73:53–56.

74. Andriacchi, T.P., and Galante, J.O. (1988): Retention of the posterior cruciate ligament in total knee arthroplasty. J. Arthroplasty, 3(Suppl.):S13–S19.

75. Dorr, L.D., Ochsner, J.L., Growley, J., and Perry J. (1988): Functional comparisons of posterior cruciate retained versus sacrificed in total knee arthroplasty. Clin. Orthop. Relat. Res., 236:36–43.

76. Beard, D.J., Dodd, C.F., Trundle, H.R., and Simpson, A.W. (1994): Proprioception enhancement for anterior cruciate ligament deficiency. J. Bone Joint Surg. Br., 76:654–659.

77. Limbird, T.J., Shiavir, R., Frazer, M., and Borra, H. (1988): EMG profiles of knee joint musculature during walking: Changes induced by anterior cruciate ligament deficiency. J. Orthop. Res., 6:630–638.

78. Andriacchi, T.P., and Birac, D. (1993): Functional testing in the anterior cruciate ligament–deficient knee. Clin. Orthop. Relat. Res., 288:40–47.

79. Speer, K.P., Deng, X., Borrero, S., et al. (1994): Biomechanical evaluation of a simulated Bankart lesion. J. Bone Joint Surg. Am., 76:1819–1826.

80. Barden, J.M., Balyk, R., Raso, J., et al. (2004): Dynamic upper limb proprioception in multidirectional shoulder instability. Clin. Orthop. Relat. Res., 420:181–189.

81. Safran, M.R., Borsa, P.A., Lepahrt, S.M, et al. (2001): Shoulder proprioception in baseball pitchers. J. Shoulder Elbow Surg., 10:438–444.

82. Rokito, A.S., Birdzell, M.G., Cuomoa, F., et al. (2010): Recovery of shoulder strength and proprioception after open surgery for recurrent anterior instability: A comparison of two surgical techniques. J. Shoulder Elbow Surg., 19:564–569.

83. McMahon, P.J., Jobe, F.W., Pink, M.M., et al. (1996): Comparative electromyographic analysis of shoulder muscles during planar motions: Anterior glenohumeral instability versus normal. J. Shoulder Elbow Surg., 5:118–123.

84. Skinner, H.B., Wyatt, M.P., Stone, M.L., et al. (1986): Exercise related knee joint laxity. Am. J. Sports Med., 14:30–34.

85. Weisman, G., Pope, M.H., and Hohnson, R.J. (1980): Cyclic loading in knee ligament injuries. Am. J. Sports Med., 8:24–30.

86. Lephart, S.M., Henry, T.J., Riemann, B.L., et al. (1998): The effects of neuromuscular control exercises on functional stability in the unstable shoulder. J. Athl. Train., 33:S15.

87. Lattanzio, P.J., and Petrella, R.J. (1998): Knee proprioception: A review of mechanisms, measurements, and implications of muscular fatigue. Orthopedics, 21:463–470.

88. Zuckerman, J.D., Gallagher, M.A., Lehman, C., et al. (1999): Normal shoulder proprioception and the effect of lidocaine injection. J. Shoulder Elbow Surg., 8:11–16.

89. Carpenter, J.E., Blaiser, R.B., and Pellizon, G.G. (1998): The effects of muscle fatigue on shoulder joint position sense. Am. J. Sports Med., 26:262–265.

90. Pederson, J., Jonn, J., Hellstrom, F., et al. (1999): Localized muscle fatigue decreases the acuity of the movement sense in the human shoulder. Med. Sci. Sports Exerc., 31:1047–1052.

91. Myers, J.B., Guskiewicz, K.M., Schneider, R.A., et al. (1999): Proprioception and neuromuscular control of the shoulder after muscle fatigue. J. Athl. Train., 34:362–367.

92. Myers, J.B., Ju, Y.Y., Hwang, J.H., et al. (2004): Reflexive muscle activation alterations in shoulders with anterior glenohumeral instability. Am. J. Sports Med., 32:1013–1021.

93. Myers, J.B., and Lephart, S.M. (2000): The role of the sensorimotor system in the athletic shoulder. J. Athl. Train., 35:351–363.

94. Myers, J.B., Wassinger, C.A., and Lephart, S.M. (2006): Sensorimotor contribution to shoulder stability: Effect of injury and rehabilitation. Man. Ther., 11:197–201.

95. Trip, B.L., Yochem, E.M., and Uhl, T.L. (2007): Functional fatigue and upper extremity sensorimotor system acuity in baseball athletes. J. Athl. Train., 42:90–98.

96. Lin, J.J., Hung, C.J., and Yang, P.L. (2011): The effects of scapular taping on electromyographic muscle activity and proprioception feedback in healthy shoulders. J. Orthop. Res., 29:53–57.

97. Djupsjobacka, M., Johansson, H., and Bergenheim, M. (1994): Influences on the gamma muscle spindle system from muscle afferents stimulated by increased intramuscular concentrations of arachidonic acid. Brain Res., 663:293–302.

98. Djupsjobacka, M., Johansson, H., Bergenheim, M., et al. (1995): Influences on the gamma muscle spindle system from muscle afferents stimulated by increased intramuscular concentrations of bradykinin and 5-HT. Neurosci. Res., 22:325–333.

99. Djupsjobacka, M., Johansson, H., Bergenheim, et al. (1995): Influences on the gamma muscle spindle system from contralateral muscle afferents stimulated by KCl and lactic acid. Neurosci. Res., 21:301–309.

100. Cerulli, G., Benoit, D.L., Caraffa, A., et al. (2001): Proprioceptive training and prevention of anterior cruciate ligament injuries in soccer. J. Orthop. Sports Phys. Ther., 31:655–661.

101. Osborne, M.D., Chou, L.S., Laskowski, E.R., et al. (2001): The effect of ankle disk training on muscle reaction time in subjects with a history of ankle sprain. Am. J. Sports Med., 29:627–632.

102. Eils, E., and Dieter, R. (2001): A multi-station proprioceptive exercise program in patients with ankle instability. Med. Sci. Sports Exerc., 33:1991–1998.

103. Risberg, M.A., Mork, M., Jenssen, H.K., and Holm, I. (2001): Design and implementation of a neuromuscular training program following anterior cruciate ligament reconstruction. J. Orthop. Sports Phys. Ther., 31:620–631.

104. Hewett, T.E., Paterno, M.V., and Myer, G.D. (2002): Strategies for enhancing proprioception and neuromuscular control of the knee. Clin. Orthop. Relat. Res., 402:76–94.

105. Mandelbaum, B.R., Silvers, H.J., Watanabe, D.S., et al. (2005): Effectiveness of a neuromuscular and proprioceptive training program in preventing anterior cruciate ligament injuries in female athletes: 2 year follow-up. Am. J. Sports Med., 33:1003–1010.

106. Hurd, W.J., Chmielewski, T.L., and Snyder-Mackler, L. (2006): Perturbation-enhanced neuromuscular training alters muscle activity in female athletes. Knee Surg. Sports Traumatol. Arthrosc., 14:60–69.

107. Biel, A., and Dudzinski, K. (2005): Rehabilitation outcome in patients recovering from reconstruction of the anterior cruciate ligament; a preliminary report. Ortop. Traumatol. Rehabil., 7:401–405.

108. Hale, S.A., Hertel, J., and Olmsted-Kramer, L.C. (2007): The effect of a 4-week comprehensive rehabilitation program on postural control and lower extremity function in individuals with chronic ankle instability. J. Orthop. Sports Phys. Ther., 37:303–311.

109. Wikstrom, E.A., Bishop, M.D., Inamdar, A.D., and Hass, C.J. (2010): Gait termination control strategies are altered in chronic ankle instability subjects. Med. Sci. Sports Exerc., 42:197–205.

110. Gutierrez, G.M., Kaminski, T.W., and Douex, A.T. (2009): Neuromuscular control and ankle instability. P MR, 1:359–365.

111. Kynsburg, A., Panics, G., and Halasi, T. (2010): Long-term neuromuscular training and ankle joint position sense. Acta Physiol. Hung., 97:183–191.

112. Blackburn, J.T., Riemann, B.L., Myers, J.B., and Lephart, S.M. (2003): Kinematic analysis of the hip and trunk during bilateral stance on firm, foam and multiaxial support surfaces. Clin. Biomech. (Bristol, Avon), 18:655–661.

113. Riemann, B.L., Myers, J.B., and Lephart, S.M. (2003): Comparison of the ankle, knee, hip and trunk corrective action shown during single-leg stance on firm, foam, and multiaxial surfaces. Arch. Phys. Med. Rehabil., 84:90–95.

114. Zazulak, B.T., Hewett, T.E., Reeves, N.P., et al. (2007): Deficits in neuromuscular control of the trunk predict knee injury risk; a prospective biomechanical-epidemiologic study. Am. J. Sports Med., 35:1123–1130.

115. Miura, K., Ishibashi, Y., Tsuda, E., et al. (2004): The effect of local and general fatigue on knee proprioception. Arthroscopy, 20:414–418.

116. Zech, A., Hübscher, M., Vogt, L., et al. (2009): Neuromuscular training for rehabilitation of sports injuries: A systematic review. Med. Sci. Sports Exerc., 41:1831–1841.

117. Hübscher, M., Zech, A., Pfeifer, K., et al. (2010): Neuromuscular training for sports injury prevention; a systematic review. Med. Sci. Sports Exerc., 42:413–421.

118. Zech, A., Hübscher, M., Vogt, L., et al. (2010): Balance training for neuromuscular control and performance enhancement: A systematic review. J. Athl. Train., 45:392–403.

119. Lephart, S.M., Pincivero, D.M., Giraldo, J.L., and Fu, F.H. (1997): The role of proprioception in the management and rehabilitation of athletic injuries. Am. J. Sports Med., 25:130–137.

120. Fitzgerals, G.K., Axe, M.J., and Snyder-Mackler, L. (2000): The efficacy of perturbation training in nonoperative anterior cruciate ligament rehabilitation programs for physically active individuals. Phys. Ther., 80:128–140.

121. Ellenbecker, T.S., and Roetert, E.P. (1999): Testing isokinetic muscular fatigue of shoulder internal and external rotation in elite junior tennis players. J. Orthop. Sports Phys. Ther., 29:275–281.

122. Snyder-Mackler, L.A., Delitto, S.L., and Straka, S.W. (1995): Strength of the quadriceps femoris muscle and functional recovery after reconstruction of the anterior cruciate ligament. J. Bone Joint Surg. Am., 77:1166–1173.

123. Palmitier, R.A., An, K.N., Scott, S.G., et al. (1991): Kinetic chain exercise in knee rehabilitation. Sports Med., 11:402–413.

124. Kibler, W.B. (1998): The role of the scapula in athletic shoulder function. Am. J. Sports Med. 26:325–337.

125. Kibler, W.B., Livingstone, B., and Bruce, R. (1995): Current concepts in shoulder rehabilitation. Adv. Oper. Orthop., 3:249–297.

126. Decker, M.J., Hintermeister, R.A., Faber, K.J., and Hawkins, R.J. (1999): Serratus anterior muscle activity during selected rehabilitation exercises. Am. J. Sports Med., 27:784–791.

127. Poppen, N.K., and Walker, P.S. (1976): Normal and abnormal motion of the shoulder. J. Bone Joint Surg. Am., 58:195–201.

128. Saha, A.K. (1983): Mechanism of shoulder movements and a plea for the recognition of "zero-position" of glenohumeral joint. Clin. Orthop. Relat. Res., 173:3–10.
129. Kraemer, W.J., and Fleck, S.J. (2003): Designing Resistance Training Programs, 3 rd ed. Champaign, IL, Human Kinetics.
130. Elliot, B., Marsh, T., and Blanksby, B. (1986): A three dimensional cinematographic analysis of the tennis serve. Int. J. Sport Biomech., 2:260–271.
131. Holt, S., O'Brien, M., Davies, G.J., et al. (2000): An investigation of shoulder muscle electrical activity during Bodyblade exercises. Presented at Wisconsin State Physical Therapy Association Spring Meeting.
132. Marin, P.J., and Rhea, M.R. (2010): Effects of vibration training on muscle strength; a meta-analysis. J. Strength Cond. Res., 24:548–556.
133. Chen, S.K., Simonion, P.T., Wickiewicz, T.L., and Warren, R.F. (1999): Radiographic evaluation of glenohumeral kinematics: A muscle fatigue model. J. Shoulder Elbow Surg., 8:49–52.
134. Lu, Y., Hayashi, K., Edwards, R.B., et al. (2000): The effect of monopolar radiofrequency treatment pattern on joint capsular healing. In vitro and in vivo studies using an ovine model. Am. J. Sports Med., 28:711–719.
135. Myers, J.B., Lephart, S.M., Riemann, B.L., et al. (2000): Evaluation of shoulder proprioception following thermal capsulorraphy. Med. Sci. Sports Exer., 32:S123.
136. Ellenbecker, T.S., and Mattalino, A.J. (1999): Glenohumeral joint range of motion and rotator cuff strength following arthroscopic anterior stabilization with thermal capsulorraphy. J. Orthop. Sports Phys. Ther., 29:160–167.

25

Application of Isokinetics in Testing and Rehabilitation

George J. Davies, DPT, MEd, SCS, ATC, CSCS, and
Todd S. Ellenbecker, DPT, MS, OCS, SCS, CSCS

CHAPTER OBJECTIVES

- Define the terminology used with isokinetics.
- Apply general guidelines regarding the application of isokinetic testing.
- Explain the specific applications of isokinetic assessment of muscular power in the upper extremities.

- Implement the application of isokinetics as part of rehabilitation programs.
- Explain the scientific and clinical rationale for the use of isokinetics in evaluation and rehabilitation of sports injuries.

Isokinetics plays a significant role in the evaluation and rehabilitation of injured athletes. The use of isokinetics has changed as interest in isokinetics has varied over the past 25 years. Isokinetics was developed in the 1960s and used increasingly during the 1970s. However, research on this subject was minimal, and the potential uses and applications of isokinetics were not clearly understood. In the 1980s the field of isokinetics came into its own, with increasing popularity and, most importantly, an increasing body of knowledge through numerous publications that supported the appropriate use of isokinetics in the testing and rehabilitation of athletes. During this period, isokinetics was used increasingly in many different areas and with many different applications. The first book dedicated solely to isokinetics was published in the early 1980s[1]; it provided an overview of the testing and application of isokinetics through a combination of published research and empirically based clinical experience. However, in the 1990s there was a trend away from the use of isokinetics as part of the total evaluation and rehabilitation process. Despite extensive publications on isokinetics (more than 2000 published articles on the use and efficacy of isokinetics, an entire journal dedicated to the art and science of isokinetics [*Isokinetics and Exercise Science*], and four books dedicated exclusively to isokinetics[1-4]), many practicing clinicians have discontinued using isokinetics on the grounds that it is not functional. A PubMed search (performed on 12/16/2010) of the term *isokinetics* identified 4196 references. However, when the search was limited to higher levels of evidence, including

randomized controlled trials, systematic reviews, and metaanalysis studies, the actual number was 513 high-quality studies. More than 220 of these articles have been published in the last decade. Interestingly, when a Google search was performed for the term *isokinetics*, 79,400 citations appeared. Although admittedly most athletes do not sit and flex and extend their knees as a functional activity, there is high correlation between isokinetic testing of the knee and functional testing. Unfortunately, many clinicians are disregarding the extensive documentation of isokinetics in the evaluation and treatment of athletes and are embracing closed kinetic chain (CKC) exercises as a panacea without significant documentation of efficacy. We do not advocate that only isokinetics should be used or that CKC exercises should not be used; we would, however, like to emphasize the need for an integrated approach that uses many modes of testing and rehabilitation.

OVERVIEW AND TERMINOLOGY

Numerous modes of exercise can be used for the evaluation and rehabilitation of athletes, including isometrics, isotonics, plyometrics, isoacceleration, isodeceleration, and isokinetics.

The concept of isokinetic exercise was introduced by James Perrine in the late 1960s, and it proved to be a revolution in exercise training and rehabilitation. Instead of the traditional exercises that were performed at variable speeds against a constant weight or resistance, Perrine developed the concept of

548

isokinetics, which involves a dynamic preset fixed speed with resistance that is totally accommodating throughout the range of motion (ROM). Since the inception of isokinetics, this form of testing and exercise has become increasingly popular in clinical, athletic, and research settings, with the first article describing isokinetic exercise being published in 1967.[5] Since then, numerous articles and research presentations have documented the use of isokinetics for objective testing or for training.

Isokinetics means that exercise is performed at a fixed velocity (ranging from 1°/sec to approximately 1000°/sec) with an accommodating resistance. Accommodating resistance means that isokinetic exercise is the only way to dynamically load a muscle to its maximum capability at every point throughout ROM. Therefore, the resistance varies to exactly match the force applied by the athlete at every point in ROM. This is important because as the joint goes through ROM, the amount of torque that can be produced varies because of the Blix curve (musculotendinous length-to-tension ratio) and because of the physiologic changes in the length-to-tension ratio that occur in the muscle-tendon unit and in biomechanical skeletal leverage. The advantages and limitations of isokinetics are listed in Box 25-1.

Open Kinetic Chain

An open kinetic chain (OKC) assessment or rehabilitation exercise is considered to be an activity in which the distal component of the extremity is not fixed but is free in space.[6] It is questionable whether many exercises are pure OKC, CKC, or combinations of the two. Nevertheless, an operational definition of an OKC test or exercise, within the limitations of this chapter, is one in which the distal end of the extremity is free and not fixed to an object. One of the best examples of the OKC pattern is performance of a knee flexion-to-extension pattern while sitting. This OKC pattern will serve as the model to describe OKC exercises.

Closed Kinetic Chain

A CKC assessment or rehabilitation exercise is considered to be an activity in which the distal component of the extremity is fixed.[6] The fixed end may be either stationary or movable.[6] An example of a CKC exercise in which the distal end is stationary is a squat exercise in which the foot is fixed to the ground. An example of a CKC exercise in which the distal end is movable is an exercise on a leg press system in which the athlete's body is stationary and there is a movable footplate.

Box 25-1

Advantages and Limitations of Isokinetics

ADVANTAGES

Efficiency: It is the only way to load a dynamically contracting muscle to its maximum capability at all points throughout the range of motion.

Safety: Individuals will never meet more resistance than they can handle because the resistance is equal to the force applied.

Accommodating resistance: Accommodating resistance occurs and is predicated on changes in the musculotendinous length-to-tension ratio, changes in skeletal leverage (biomechanics), fatigue, and pain.

Decreased joint compressive force at higher speeds: This is an empiric clinical observation that one of us (G.J.D.) has made in more than 25 years of using isokinetics in testing and rehabilitation of athletes. It occurs because often an athlete exercises at a slow speed and pain develops; however, if the athlete exercises at a faster velocity, pain does not develop. Furthermore, at faster speeds, there is less time for force to develop, and the torque decreases with concentric isokinetics according to the force-velocity curve.

Physiologic overflow through the velocity spectrum: When an athlete exercises at a particular speed, a specificity response takes place, with the greatest power gains occurring at the speed of training; however, a concomitant increase in power gain occurs at other speeds as well. The majority of studies demonstrate that this phenomenon occurs at slower speeds, although some research demonstrates an overflow in both directions from the training speed.

Velocity spectrum training: As a result of the various velocities at which functional and sporting activities are performed, the ability to train at various functional velocities is important because of the specificity of training. It is important to train the muscles neurophysiologically to develop a normal motor recruitment pattern of neural contraction of the muscle.

Minimal postexercise soreness with concentric isokinetic contractions

Validity of the equipment

Reliability of the equipment

Reproducibility of physiologic testing (reliability)

Development of muscle recruitment quickness (time rate of torque development)

Objective documentation of testing

Computer feedback provided so that an athlete can train at submaximal or maximal levels

LIMITATIONS

Isolated joint/muscle testing

Nonfunctional patterns of movement

Limited velocities to replicate the actual speeds of sports performance

Increased compressive force at slower speeds

Increased tibial translation at slow speeds without proximal pad placement

---

Data from Davies, G.J. (1992): A Compendium of Isokinetics in Clinical Usage and Rehabilitation Techniques, 4th ed. Onalaska, WI, S & S Publishers.

The acronyms *OKC* and *CKC* will be used often throughout this chapter in describing both testing and rehabilitation applications of isokinetic exercise.

ISOKINETIC TESTING

In this section some general guidelines and principles of isokinetic testing are described briefly. For more detailed information the reader is referred to *A Compendium of Isokinetics in Clinical Usage and Rehabilitation Techniques*.[7]

The purposes of isokinetic testing are several: to obtain objective records, screen athletes, establish a database, quantify objective information, obtain objective serial reassessments, develop normative data, correlate isokinetic torque curves with pathologic conditions, and use the shape of the curve to individualize the rehabilitation program to a specific athlete's needs.

Isokinetic assessment allows the clinician to objectively assess muscular performance in a way that is both safe and reliable.[8] It produces objective criteria for the clinician and provides reproducible data for assessing and monitoring an athlete's status. Isokinetic testing has been demonstrated to be reliable and valid.[1,9-25]

Absolute and relative contraindications to testing and using isokinetics in rehabilitation must be established, as with any methodology in medicine. Examples of such contraindications are soft tissue–healing constraints, pain, limited ROM, effusion, joint instability, acute strains and sprains, and occasionally, subacute conditions.

A standard test protocol should be established to enhance reliability of the testing. Numerous considerations should be taken into account when devising such a protocol, including the following: (1) educating the athlete regarding the particular requirements of the test, (2) testing the uninvolved side first to establish a baseline and to demonstrate the requirements so that the athlete's apprehension is decreased, (3) providing appropriate warm-ups at each speed, (4) using consistent verbal commands for instructions to the athlete, (5) having a consistent protocol for testing different joints, (6) having properly calibrated equipment, and (7) providing proper stabilization. A standard orthopedic testing protocol should be followed during isokinetic testing.[7] Box 25-2 provides such an example.

Isokinetic testing allows the use of a variety of testing protocols ranging from power to endurance tests (see Davies[7] for a detailed description of the various isokinetic testing protocols). Our primary recommendation is to perform velocity spectrum testing so that the test will assess the muscle's capabilities at different speeds, thus simulating various activities. Frequently, deficits in a muscle's performance may be revealed at one speed and not at others. For example, athletes with a patellofemoral problem often have more deficits in power at slow speeds, whereas after various surgical procedures on the knee, athletes will have fast-velocity deficits.

ISOKINETIC DATA AND ANALYSIS

One of the advantages of isokinetic testing is that it provides numerous objective parameters that can be used to evaluate and analyze an athlete's performance. Various isokinetic testing data that are frequently used to analyze an athlete's performance are peak torque, time rate of torque development, acceleration, deceleration, ROM, total work, average power, and shape of the

---

Box 25-2

Orthopedic Testing Protocol

Educate the athlete: The athlete must first be informed and educated about the purpose, procedures, and requirements of the testing.

Test the uninvolved side first: The uninvolved side is tested first to establish a baseline and to decrease the athlete's apprehension before the involved extremity is tested.

Perform warm-ups: The athlete should perform several submaximal gradient warm-ups and at least one maximal warm-up before each test. The submaximal warm-ups (25%, 50%, and 75%) prepare the extremity for the test and allow the athlete to get a feel for the machine. The maximal effort is performed to create a positive learning transfer from a maximal warm-up to a maximal testing effort. This procedure improves the reliability of the testing sequence.[7,15]

Give consistent verbal commands: Commands should be standardized and remain the same throughout the testing sequence to improve test-retest reliability.

Use standardized test protocols: The recommended testing protocols for each joint have been described in detail. The specific anatomic position and stabilization guidelines, range of motion, speed, and other considerations have been described.[7]

Test at different speeds: We recommend the use of a velocity spectrum testing protocol. Velocity spectrum testing refers to testing at slow (0-60°/sec), intermediate (60-180°/sec), fast (180 to 300°/sec), and functional (300-1000°/sec) contractile velocities. Performing 3 to 5 repetitions at each speed and 20 to 30 repetitions at a fast speed (240-300°/sec) for an endurance test is recommended.

---

torque curves.[26] After these data are collected from the tests and analyzed to determine specific deficits and limitations of the athlete, the results need to be interpreted with use of the criteria presented in Box 25-3.[7,27-29]

Recent research has demonstrated the possible relationship between the isokinetic torque curve and joint function. Bryant et al[30] indicated that specific characteristics of the isokinetic torque curve of the knee extensor (extensor torque smoothness) may provide valuable clinical information regarding joint function. The morphology of knee extension torque-time curves demonstrated that following reconstruction of the anterior cruciate ligament (ACL), the involved knee had significant deficits. Eitzen et al[31] evaluated isokinetic quadriceps strength profiles in ACL-deficient potential copers and noncopers. The results demonstrated that the peak torque did not identify the largest quadriceps muscle strength deficit; rather, it was established at knee flexion angles of less than 40°. This resulted in significant differences in angle-specific torque values between potential copers and noncopers. Furthermore, moderate to strong associations were disclosed between angle-specific torque values and single-legged hop performance, but only for the noncopers. Eitzen et al[31] concluded that interpretation of isokinetic curve profiles seems to be of clinical importance for the evaluation of quadriceps muscle performance after ACL injury. Interestingly, more than a quarter of a century ago in the first book dedicated

Criteria for Interpreting Isokinetic Tests Results

Bilateral comparison: Comparing the involved with the uninvolved extremity is probably the most common evaluation. Bilateral differences of 10% to 15% are thought to represent significant asymmetry. However, this single parameter by itself has limitations.

Unilateral ratios: Comparing the relationship between agonist and antagonist muscles may identify particular weaknesses in certain muscle groups. This parameter is particularly important to assess with velocity spectrum testing because the percent relationships of the muscles change with changing speeds in many muscle groups. (Percent relationship means that the unilateral ratio of antagonistic muscle torque is a certain percentage of agonist muscle torque. This percentage of torque production of the antagonist to the agonist muscle changes throughout the velocity spectrum.)

Torque-to-body weight relationship: Comparing torques with body weight adds another dimension in interpreting test results. Frequently, even though bilateral symmetry and normal unilateral ratios are present, the torque-to-body weight relationship is altered.

Total leg strength: Nicholas et al,[27] Gleim et al,[28] and Boltz and Davies[29] have published articles on the importance of considering the entire kinetic chain concept of total leg strength.

Comparison to normative data: Although the use of normative data is controversial, if properly used relative to a specific population of athletes, it can provide guidelines for testing or rehabilitation.

to isokinetics, entire chapters were dedicated to isokinetic analysis, including angle-specific torques and shapes of the torque curves.[1]

Although it is beyond the scope of this chapter to completely review all aspects of data interpretation, the reader is referred to several key texts[1,3,4] and Ellenbecker and Davies[32] for a more comprehensive review of the basic tenants of interpretation of data from isokinetic tests of the upper and lower extremity, as well as the trunk.

RATIONALE AND NEED FOR ISOKINETIC TESTING AND REHABILITATION

Even though the purpose of this chapter is to describe the rationale and need for isokinetic rehabilitation, a few comments about why CKC exercises should be used instead of just OKC exercises are necessary. Many articles have described the rationale for using CKC exercises,[33-44] particularly in rehabilitating athletes after ACL reconstruction.[42,45-67] However, Crandall et al[68] performed a metaanalysis of 1167 articles published between 1966 and 1993 on the treatment of athletes with ACL injuries and found only 5 articles (and 3 of these articles included data on the same athletes) that met the criteria for metaanalysis of

prospective, randomized, controlled, experimental clinical trials. Consequently, many of the articles that are commonly thought of as "definitive treatment articles" are simply descriptive studies. Therefore, although the benefits of using CKC exercises in rehabilitation have been described quite extensively, few scientifically based prospective, randomized, controlled, experimental clinical trials[69-71] have documented the efficacy of CKC exercises. The reader is referred to a text that outlines these research studies and the application of CKC exercise as a complement to the material presented here on OKC isokinetic training and testing.[6]

The rationale for the use of CKC exercise only is thus founded not on scientific studies that have documented its efficacy but more on unverified empiric observations and descriptive studies.[72]

RATIONAL FOR OPEN KINETIC CHAIN ISOKINETIC ASSESSMENT IN THE LOWER EXTREMITY

Despite the many disadvantages described for OKC assessment, there are still several reasons why OKC exercises should be incorporated in both assessment and rehabilitation, as listed in Box 25-4.[7,8,27,28,52,70,73-83]

The primary purpose for performing OKC isokinetic assessment is the need to test specific muscle groups of a pathologic joint in isolation. Although the muscles do not work in an isolated fashion, a deficit, or "weak link," in a kinetic chain will never be identified unless specific isolated OKC isokinetic testing is performed. Furthermore, on serial retesting, one will not know how the athlete is progressing and whether and when the athlete meets the parameters for discharge. Examples of the importance of performing isolated testing of the kinetic chain to identify specific dysfunctions have been offered by several authors, including Nicholas et al[27] and Gleim et al.[28]

Nicholas et al[27] performed total leg strength isokinetic testing and developed a composite lower extremity score. They evaluated several groups of athletes with various pathologic conditions and determined that certain characteristic patterns of muscle weakness could be correlated with specific pathologic syndromes. Athletes with ankle and foot problems, knee ligamentous instability, intraarticular defects, and patellofemoral dysfunction had an irrefutable deficit in total leg strength ($P < .01$). For example, athletes with ankle and foot problems have statistically significant weakness of the ipsilateral hip abductors and adductors. Furthermore, there was a trend toward ipsilateral weakness of the quadriceps and hamstring muscles, although this trend was not statistically significant.

Gleim et al[28] also determined that the total percent deficit in the injured leg was the one value that was most informative. Typically, when a single muscle group is compared bilaterally, values that fall within 10% are empirically determined to be normal. Because the total leg strength composite score is more sensitive and minimizes variability, Gleim et al[28] suggested that even a 5% difference in bilateral comparison is significant.

It is important to note that the only way to document weakness in muscle groups distant to the site of injury is through performance of isolated OKC testing. Furthermore, specific muscle weakness at the site of injury can be identified only by isolated OKC testing.

Box 25-4

Rationale for Incorporating Open Kinetic Chain Exercises into Assessment and Rehabilitation

It is necessary to perform isolated testing of specific muscle groups usually affected by certain pathologic changes. If the component parts of the kinetic chain are not measured, the weak link will not be identified or adequately rehabilitated, which will affect the entire chain.[773]

Muscle groups away from the specific site of injury must be assessed to determine other associated weaknesses (e.g., disuse or preexisting problems).[27,28]

CKC or total extremity testing may not demonstrate the true weakness that exists; proximal and distal muscles often compensate for weak areas.[73,74]

Performing OKC testing allows the clinician to have significant clinical control. The clinician can control ROM, speed, translational stress (by shin pad placement), varus and valgus force, and rotational force. When CKC exercises are begun, control of these variables decreases, thereby increasing the potential risk for injury to the athlete.

Although most athletes do not sit flexing and extending their knees in an OKC pattern when they are performing, numerous studies (based on a variety of functional assessment tests) demonstrate a correlation between OKC testing and CKC functional performance.[8,75-80]

When an athlete has an injury or dysfunction related to pain, reflex inhibition, decreased ROM, or weakness, abnormal movement patterns often result and create abnormal motor learning. Isolated OKC training can work within the limitations to normalize the motor pattern.

The efficacy of rehabilitation with OKC exercises has been demonstrated in numerous articles throughout the literature.[8,27,52,70,74,79,81-83] The reader is encouraged to check the references for a more detailed description of the studies.

CKC, Closed kinetic chain; *OKC*, open kinetic chain; *ROM*, range of motion.

Box 25-5

Guidelines for Testing or Rehabilitation of an Athlete After Anterior Cruciate Ligament Reconstruction

Know the type of surgery (e.g., whether an autograft or allograft was used).
Know the fixation technique.
Determine the graft status (with KT1000 testing).
Establish testing guidelines for particular pathologic conditions (exceptions always exist).
Respect soft tissue healing times (based on clinical protocols).
Use a proximally placed pad.[86,87]
Limit range of motion (avoid 30° to 0° of knee flexion to extension).[88]
Use faster velocities.[87]

Similar results were reported by Feiring and Ellenbecker[84] with isokinetic open and closed chain testing of 23 athletes 15 weeks after ACL reconstruction. Bilateral comparisons of OKC isokinetic knee extension muscle function ranged from 74% to 77% of the uninjured extremity, whereas the results of CKC isokinetic testing using a leg press extension-type movement pattern ranged between 91% and 93% of the uninjured extremity.

When testing multiple muscle groups and developing a composite score of their force, one sees that the proximal and distal muscles apparently compensate for the weak muscles and tend to demonstrate less of a deficit than actually exists in the area. We have made this empirically based observation for years, but now CKC isokinetic testing that objectively documents and quantifies performance has supported this observation. Again, if a muscle's performance is not measured, a deficit cannot be identified. These research studies and examples provide justification of the need for OKC isokinetic testing.

Another major reason for performing OKC isokinetic testing is the clinical control that it provides. When testing, the clinician controls ROM, speed, translational stress (by shin pad placement), varus and valgus stress, and rotational force. However, when one begins CKC testing, control of these variables decreases, thereby increasing potential risk to the athlete.

An often-cited example is that performance of OKC isokinetic tests on an athlete who has undergone ACL reconstruction can stretch or injure the graft. This is a situation of good science being applied to an inappropriate clinical setting. If the graft were actually to be stretched during OKC testing, the problem is more one of the clinician performing an inappropriate test or testing at an inappropriate time rather than the OKC test itself.[85] Box 25-5 lists guidelines that should be followed when one is testing or rehabilitating an athlete after ACL reconstruction.[86-88]

Correlation of Open Kinetic Chain With Closed Kinetic Chain Functional Performance

In addition to obtaining clinical control, another reason to perform OKC isokinetic testing is because of its correlation with CKC functional performance. Although athletes do not

Another example of the need for isolated testing was illustrated in work by Davies,[73] who performed CKC computerized isokinetic tests on athletes with various knee injuries and also analyzed bilateral comparison data. Dynamic CKC isokinetic testing, which required a linear motion with force production being measured in pounds at slow (10 in/sec), medium (20 in/sec), and fast (30 in/sec) velocities, was done on a Linea computerized CKC isokinetic dynamometer system.* The same athletes were also tested on a Cybex OKC computerized isokinetic dynamometer,† and bilateral analysis of the data was performed. Isolated joint testing was performed to provide rotational force and torque values, which were recorded at slow (60°/sec), medium (180°/sec), and fast (300°/sec) angular velocities. The results of the testing demonstrated that more significant deficits were shown to exist in athletes after OKC isolated joint and muscle testing than after CKC multiple joint and muscle testing (Table 25-1).

---

*Available from Loredan Biomedical, West Sacramento, CA.
†Available from Cybex, Medway, MA.

Table 25-1 Comparisons Between Open Kinetic Chain and Closed Kinetic Chain Computerized Isokinetic Dynamometer Testing of 300 Patients With Various Pathologic Knee Conditions or After Surgery

Cybex (OKC)			Linea (CKC)		
Parameter	Values	Deficit	Parameter	Values	Deficit
Peak torque force	60°/sec (quadriceps)	29%	Peak torque force	10 in/sec	9%
U	142 ft-lb	–	U	462 lb	–
I	101 ft-lb	–	I	420 lb	–
Peak torque (BW) force	60°/sec (quadriceps)	31%	Peak torque (% BW) force	10 in/sec	11%
U	95%	–	U	298 lb	–
I	66%	–	I	266 lb	–
Peak torque force	180°/sec	21%	Peak torque force	20 in/sec	11%
U	99 ft-lb	–	U	374 lb	–
I	78 ft-lb	–	I	331 lb	–
Peak torque (BW) force	180°/sec	25%	Peak torque (% BW)	20 in/sec	11%
U	64%	–	U	239 lb	–
I	48%	–	I	253 lb	–
Peak torque force	300°/sec	20%	Peak torque force	30 in/sec	16%
U	80 ft-lb	–	U	302 lb	–
I	64 ft-lb	–	I	253 lb	–
Peak torque (BW) force	300°/sec	20%	Peak torque (% BW)	30 in/sec	11%
U	51%	–	U	193 lb	–
I	41%	–	I	171 lb	–

BW, Body weight; CKC, closed kinetic chain; I, involved extremity; OKC, open kinetic chain; U, uninvolved extremity.

regularly function by sitting in a chair and flexing and extending their knees and even though some research indicates that there is no functional correlation,[75,89] numerous studies do demonstrate a positive correlation between OKC testing and functional performance.[49,64,76-80,90,91]

Patel et al[90] tested 44 normal subjects and 44 subjects with unilateral ACL deficiency isokinetically to assess knee extension and flexion strength. The group with ACL deficiency had significantly less isokinetic quadriceps strength than the control group did, and this difference in strength was related to a significant decrease in the peak external quadriceps moment during jogging, jog-stop, and jog-cut activities, as well as during stair ascent.[90] Isokinetic quadriceps strength was significantly correlated with the external quadriceps moment for these functional activities in both the ACL-deficient and control groups. This study supports the use of isokinetic muscle testing because of the correlation with basic lower extremity functional measures.

Petschnig et al[91] demonstrated the relationship between isokinetic strength testing and several lower extremity functional tests. A limb symmetry index of 95% or higher was regularly demonstrated in normal subjects and patients after ACL reconstruction via isokinetic testing, hop tests for distance, and one-legged vertical jump tests. Additionally, Jones et al[92] compared isokinetic dynamometry at 60°/sec with functional field tests (seated unilateral leg press, horizontal hop, single-leg vertical, and drop jumps). No significant relationships were identified between the isokinetic variables and the field tests. However, it has previously been demonstrated by Wilk et al[8] that testing at slower speeds does not correlate with functional tests whereas faster speeds (>180°/sec) do in fact correlate with functional hop tests. Moreover,

because of the specificity of the angular velocities involved in functional activities, it relates empirically to faster isokinetic testing velocities. Admittedly, isolated joint testing is performed at velocities slower than functional velocities, but most functional movements are really a summation of velocities through the kinematic chain. Therefore, if each link in the kinematic chain were evaluated independently, the velocities would be much slower than the summated force of the entire kinematic chain—hence the reason to perform faster isolated joint testing.

Sbriccoli et al[93] investigated the neuromuscular response of the knee extensor and flexor muscles in elite and amateur karateka. Elite karateka had higher lower extremity isokinetic torques than amateurs did. Elite karateka demonstrated a typical neuromuscular activation strategy that seems to be dependent on task and skill level. Furthermore, the results in elite karateka suggested an improved ability to recruit fast motor units as a part of training-induced neuromuscular adaptations.

SPECIFIC APPLICATIONS OF ISOKINETIC TESTING IN LOWER EXTREMITY REHABILITATION

A plethora of research exists that provides both the rationale and objective guidance for the use of isokinetics in the rehabilitation of individuals with specific lower extremity conditions, including ACL reconstruction, patellofemoral pain, hip injury, and knee osteoarthritis (OA). A summary of pertinent research in these areas will provide additional framework for the application of isokinetic testing and training in these patient populations.

Use of Isokinetics to Assist in Prognosis Following Anterior Cruciate Ligament Reconstruction and Injury

Karanikas et al[94] investigated the adaptations in walking, running, and muscle strength after ACL reconstruction and examined the interactions between muscle strength and walking and running kinematics. Isokinetics was used for dynamic muscle assessment, and the results demonstrated that adaptation of the motor tasks and muscle strength follows different time patterns. They showed that patients can function normally at submaximal levels; however, with a decrease in muscle strength after ACL reconstruction, documented isokinetically as significant weakness that exceeds a certain threshold in comparison to the uninvolved side, the kinematics of these patients' locomotion strategies was abnormal.

Oiestad et al[95] identified risk factors for knee OA 10 to 15 years after ACL reconstruction. Individuals with low self-reported knee function 2 years postoperatively and loss of quadriceps strength as measured with isokinetics between the 2-year and the 10- to 15-year follow-up had significantly higher odds for symptomatic, radiographically detected knee OA. However, quadriceps muscle weakness, by itself, after ACL reconstruction was not significantly associated with knee OA.

Keays et al[96] used isokinetic testing to evaluate 10 factors involved in the development of OA after ACL reconstruction. The incidence of OA after ACL reconstruction is disturbingly high, with reports of mild to moderate OA developing in nearly 50% of patients 6 years after surgery. The five factors found to be predictive of tibiofemoral OA were meniscectomy, chondral damage, patellar tendon grafting, weak quadriceps, and low quadriceps-to-hamstring strength ratios. The quadriceps deficits and unilateral quadriceps-to-hamstring ratios were evaluated by isokinetic testing. Use of hamstring/gracilis grafts and restoration of quadriceps/hamstring strength balance were associated with less OA of the knee.

Segal et al[97] used isokinetics to evaluate the effect of quadriceps strength and proprioception on risk for knee OA. The finding that quadriceps strength protected against incident symptomatic but not radiographic knee OA regardless of joint position sense (JPS) suggests that strength may be more important than JPS in mediating risk for knee OA. The clinical implications of these findings are interesting because quadriceps strength is often influenced by rehabilitation interventions. Because of the accommodating resistance afforded by isokinetics, it provides an excellent intervention technique that can be used in patients with OA of the knee.

Hiemstra et al[98] used isokinetic testing to demonstrate specific muscle imbalances in a group after ACL reconstruction versus a control group. Angle- and velocity-matched hamstring-quadriceps ratio maps demonstrated systematic variation based on joint angle, velocity, and contraction type for both the control and ACL-reconstructed groups.

Ageberg et al[99] used isokinetics as an outcome measure to determine muscle strength in patients with ACL injuries treated by training only or by ACL reconstruction. No differences were observed between the surgical and nonsurgical treatment groups in muscle strength or functional performance. The lack of difference in patients treated by training and surgical reconstruction or by training only indicates that reconstructive surgery is not a prerequisite for restoring muscle function.

Sekir et al[100] investigated an early versus late start of isokinetic hamstring-strengthening exercise after ACL reconstruction with a patellar tendon graft. The results of this study demonstrated that hamstring and quadriceps strength can be increased by early hamstring strengthening after ACL reconstruction with no negative impact on knee function.

Stefanska et al[101] demonstrated that 13 weeks following ACL reconstruction, patients had significant deficits in peak torque, maximum work, and average power in the injured limb. The deficit exceeded 30% for all measured values on isokinetic testing.

Eitzen et al[102] used a variety of outcome measures, including isokinetics, to assess whether an early 5-week exercise therapy program following ACL injury improves function. A progressive 5-week exercise therapy program led to significant improvement in knee function from before to after the program in patients classified as both potential copers and noncopers. The authors concluded that short-term progressive exercise therapy programs are well tolerated and should be incorporated in early-stage ACL rehabilitation, either to improve knee function before ACL reconstruction or as a first step in further nonoperative management.

Isokinetic Testing Related to Patients With Osteoarthritis of the Knee

One of the most important reasons for locomotor dysfunction and disability in patients with knee OA is muscle weakness in the lower extremity. Isokinetics can be used in the treatment and assessment of functional outcomes in these patients very effectively. Important references in this section provide guidance and rationale for the application of isokinetic testing and training in patients with knee OA.

Diracoglu et al[103] performed bilateral isokinetic testing for knee flexion/extension. Although manual muscle testing (MMT) produced normal or nearly normal results, significantly lower strength values were found in patients with knee OA with isokinetic testing than in healthy subjects. Muscle strength loss cannot be detected during clinical examination but can be identified during isokinetic measurements. This again demonstrates the accuracy of dynamic isokinetic muscle testing versus static muscle testing as an indicator of muscle performance.

Segal et al[97] used isokinetics to evaluate the effect of quadriceps strength and proprioception on risk for knee OA. The finding that quadriceps strength protected against incident symptomatic but not radiographically detected knee OA, regardless of JPS, suggests that strength may be more important than JPS in mediating risk for knee OA. The clinical implications of these findings are interesting because the strength of the quadriceps is often influenced by rehabilitation interventions. Because of the accommodating resistance afforded by isokinetics, it provides an excellent intervention technique that can be used in patients with OA of the knee.

Segal et al[104] also performed isokinetic testing of the quadriceps and hamstrings to examine the relationship between quadriceps strength and worsening of knee joint space narrowing over a 30-month period. It was demonstrated that women with the lowest quadriceps strength had increased risk for whole knee joint space narrowing. However, no associations were found between strength and joint space narrowing in men. Consequently, quadriceps weakness was associated with increased risk for tibiofemoral and whole knee joint space narrowing.

Kean et al[105] examined test-retest reliability and quantified the minimal detectable change (MDC) in quadriceps strength (using isokinetics and isometrics) and voluntary activation in patients with knee OA. Intraclass correlation coefficients (ICCs) for all measures ranged from 0.93 to 0.98. Based on the standard error of measurement for the isokinetic tests, the MDC was 33.90 Nm for quadriceps strength. Therefore, based on maximal quadriceps isokinetic strength testing, the results demonstrated excellent test-retest reliability in patients with knee OA. The findings suggest that these measures are appropriate for use when evaluating change in neuromuscular function of the quadriceps in individual patients.

Rydevik et al[106] compared functioning and disability in patients with hip OA. The patients with hip OA had mild to moderate pain and significantly lower knee extension strength based on isokinetic testing. Their conclusions recommended including quadriceps strengthening and hip ROM exercises when developing rehabilitation programs for patients with hip OA in the aim of improving function and reducing disability.

Isokinetic Testing of the Hip

Because of the positioning, stabilization required, muscle mass, free limb acceleration, and impact artifact caused by the size of the muscle mass, hip testing performed with isokinetics is limited. Julia et al[107] demonstrated very good ICCs (values between 0.75 and 0.96) for concentric and eccentric peak torque values of the hip flexors and extensors. Additionally, they demonstrated no differences between the dominant and nondominant sides of the body, which enables use of the contralateral limb as a reference.

Boling et al[108] compared the concentric and eccentric torque of the hip musculature in individuals with and without patellofemoral pain syndrome (PFPS). Patients with PFPS displayed weakness in eccentric hip abduction and hip external rotation (ER), which may allow increased hip adduction and internal rotation (IR) during functional movements.

With an increase in the past decade in both early recognition and diagnosis of hip injuries, such as acetabular labral tears and femoroacetabular impingement, it is expected that outcomes research profiling hip strength following important new procedures to treat these injuries in elite athletes and young active patients will result in greater application of both isokinetic testing and training of the hip. Further research and publication of normative data in this region will allow greater application of isokinetics to this important joint.

SPECIFIC APPLICATION OF ISOKINETIC ASSESSMENT IN THE UPPER EXTREMITY

Application of isokinetic exercise and testing for the upper extremity is imperative because of the demanding muscular work required in sport-specific activities. The large unrestricted ROM of the glenohumeral joint and its limited inherent bony stability necessitate dynamic muscular stabilization to ensure normal joint arthrokinematics.[109] Objective information on the intricate balance of agonist and antagonist muscular strength at the glenohumeral joint is a vital resource for rehabilitation

and preventive evaluation of the shoulder. Therapeutic exercise and isolated joint testing for the entire upper extremity kinetic chain, including the scapulothoracic joint, are indicated for overuse injury or postoperative rehabilitation of an isolated injury of the shoulder or elbow.[110]

Rationale for the Use of Isokinetics in Assessing Upper Extremity Strength

Unlike the lower extremities, in which most functional and sport-specific movements occur in a CKC environment, the upper extremities function almost exclusively in an OKC format.[43] The throwing motion, tennis serve, and ground stroke are all examples of OKC activities for the upper extremity. OKC muscular strength assessment methodology allows the isolation of particular muscle groups, as opposed to CKC methods, which use multiple joint axes, planes, and joint and muscle segments. Traditional isokinetic upper extremity test patterns are open chain with respect to the shoulder, elbow, and wrist. The velocity spectrum (1°/sec to approximately 1000°/sec) currently available on commercial isokinetic dynamometers provides specificity for testing the upper extremity by allowing the clinician to assess muscular strength at faster, more functional speeds. Table 25-2 lists the angular velocities of sport-specific upper extremity movements.[111-114]

The dynamic nature of upper extremity movements is a critical factor in directing the clinician to the optimal testing methodology for the upper extremity. MMT provides a static alternative for assessment of muscular strength that uses well-developed patient positions and stabilization.[68,115] Despite detailed descriptions of manual assessment techniques, the reliability of MMT is compromised because of differences in the size and strength of clinicians and patients and the subjective nature of the grading system.[116]

Ellenbecker[117] compared isokinetic testing of the shoulder internal and external rotators with MMT in 54 subjects who exhibited symmetric normal grade (5/5) strength by manual assessment. With isokinetic testing, 13% to 15% bilateral differences in ER and 15% to 28% bilateral differences in IR were found. Of particular significance was the large variability in the size of this mean difference between extremities despite the presence of bilateral symmetry on MMT. The use of MMT is an integral part of a musculoskeletal evaluation. MMT provides a time-efficient, gross screening of the strength of multiple muscles by using a static, isometric muscular contraction, particularly in patients with neuromuscular disease or in athletes with large deficits in muscular strength.[116,118] The limitations of MMT appear to be most evident in instances in which only minor impairment of strength is present, as well as in the identification of subtle isolated deficits in strength. Differentiation of agonist and antagonist muscular strength balance is also complicated when manual techniques are used rather than an isokinetic apparatus.[117]

Glenohumeral Joint Testing

Dynamic assessment of the strength of the rotator cuff musculature is of primary importance in rehabilitation and preventive screening of the glenohumeral joint. The rotator cuff forms an integral component of the force couple in the shoulder, as described by Inman et al.[119] The approximating role of

Table 25-2 Upper Extremity Angular Velocities of Functional Activities

Joint	Movement	Sports Activity	Angular Velocity (°/sec)	Source
Shoulder	Internal rotation	Baseball pitching	7000	Dillman et al[111]
Shoulder	Internal rotation	Tennis serve	1000-1500	Shapiro and Steine[112]
Shoulder	Internal rotation	Tennis serve	2300	Dillman et al[111]
Elbow	Extension	Baseball pitching	2500	Dillman et al[111]
Elbow	Extension	Tennis serve	1700	Dillman[113]
Wrist	Flexion	Tennis serve	315	Vangheluwe and Hebbelinck[114]

the supraspinatus muscle for the glenohumeral joint, as well as the inferior (caudal) glide component action provided by the infraspinatus, teres minor, and subscapularis muscles, must stabilize the humeral head within the glenoid cavity against the superiorly directed force exerted by the deltoid muscle with humeral elevation.[120] Muscular imbalances, primarily in the posterior rotator cuff, have been objectively documented in athletes with glenohumeral joint instability and impingement.[121]

Shoulder Internal Rotation and External Rotation Strength Testing

Initial testing and training using isokinetics for rehabilitation of the shoulder typically involve the modified base position. The modified base position is obtained by tilting the dynamometer approximately 30° from the horizontal base position.[1,7] This causes the shoulder to be placed in approximately 30° of abduction (Fig. 25-1). The modified base position places the shoulder in the scapular plane 30° anterior to the coronal plane.[122] The scapular plane is characterized by enhanced bony congruity and a neutral glenohumeral position that results in a midrange position for the capsular ligaments and scapulohumeral musculature.[122] This position does not place the suprahumeral structures in an impingement situation and is well tolerated by athletes.[1]

Isokinetic testing using the modified base position requires consistent testing of the athlete on the dynamometer. Studies have demonstrated significant differences in IR and ER strength with varying degrees of abduction, flexion, and horizontal abduction and adduction of the glenohumeral joint.[123-125] The modified base position requires the athlete to be standing, which compromises both isolation and test-retest reliability. Despite these limitations, valuable data can be obtained early in the rehabilitative process with this neutral, modified base position.[7,126,127]

Isokinetic assessment of IR and ER strength is also done with 90° of glenohumeral joint abduction. Specific advantages of this test position are greater stabilization in either a seated or supine test position on most dynamometers and placement of the shoulder in an abduction angle corresponding to the overhead throwing position used in sports activities.[111,128] As a precursor to using the 90° abducted position, we require initial tolerance of the athlete to the modified base position; 90° abducted isokinetic testing can be performed in either the coronal or the scapular plane. The benefits of use of the scapular plane are similar to those discussed for the modified position and include protection of the anterior capsular glenohumeral ligaments and theoretic

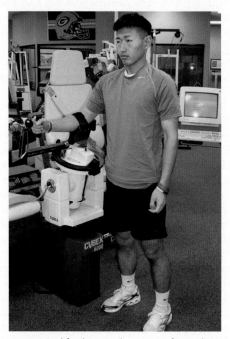

FIGURE 25-1 Modified neutral position for isokinetic testing of shoulder internal or external rotation.

enhancement of the length-tension relationship of the posterior rotator cuff.[123,129,130] Changes in the length-tension relationship and in the line of action of the scapulohumeral and axiohumeral musculature are reported with 90° of glenohumeral joint abduction instead of a more neutral adducted glenohumeral joint position.[1] The 90° abducted position for isokinetic strength assessment is more specific for assessing the muscular functions required for overhead activities.[131]

Heavy emphasis is placed on assessing the IR and ER strength of the shoulder during rehabilitation. The rationale for this apparently narrow focus is provided by an isokinetic training study by Quincy et al.[81] Six weeks of isokinetic training of the internal and external rotators produced statistically significant improvements not only in IR and ER strength but also in flexion-extension and abduction-adduction strength. Isokinetic training for flexion-extension and for abduction-adduction produced improvements only in the position of training. The physiologic overflow of strength caused by training the internal and external rotators provides a rationale for the heavy emphasis on strength development and assessment in rehabilitation.

Table 25-3 Isokinetic Peak Torque–to–Body Weight Ratios in 150 Professional Baseball Pitchers*

	Internal Rotation		External Rotation	
Speed	Dominant Arm	Nondominant Arm	Dominant Arm	Nondominant Arm
180°/sec	27%	17%	18%	19%
300°/sec	25%	24%	15%	15%

Data from Wilk, K.E., Andrews, J.R., Arrigo, C.A., et al. (1993): The strength characteristics of internal and external rotator muscles in professional baseball pitchers. Am. J. Sports Med., 21:61–66.
*Data were obtained on a Biodix isokinetic dynamometer.

Table 25-4 Isokinetic Peak Torque–to–Body Weight and Work–to–Body Weight Ratios in 147 Professional Baseball Pitchers*

	Internal Rotation		External Rotation	
Speed	Dominant Arm	Nondominant Arm	Dominant Arm	Nondominant Arm
210°/sec				
Torque	21%	19%	13%	14%
Work	41%	38%	25%	25%
300°/sec				
Torque	20%	18%	13%	13%
Work	37%	33%	23%	23%

Data from Ellenbecker, T.S., and Mattalino, A.J. (1997): Concentric isokinetic shoulder internal and external rotation strength in professional baseball pitchers. J. Orthop. Sports Phys. Ther., 25:323–328.
*Data were obtained on a Cybex 350 isokinetic dynamometer.

Additional research has identified the IR and ER movement pattern as the preferred testing pattern in athletes with rotator cuff tendinopathy.[132]

Interpretation of Shoulder Internal and External Rotation Testing

BILATERAL DIFFERENCES
As with isokinetic testing of the lower extremities, assessment of the strength of an extremity relative to the contralateral side forms the basis for standard data interpretation. This practice is more complicated in the upper extremities because of limb dominance, particularly in athletes in unilaterally dominant sports. In addition to the complexity caused by limb dominance, isokinetic descriptive studies demonstrate disparities in the degree of limb dominance, as well as in strength dominance, only in specified muscle groups.[26,133-139]

In general, maximum limb dominance of the internal and external rotators of 5% to 10% is assumed in nonathletic persons and athletes engaging in recreational upper extremity sports.[140] Significantly greater IR strength has been identified in the dominant arm in professional,[137,141] collegiate,[26] and high school[139] baseball players, as well as in elite junior[136] and adult[135] tennis players. No difference between extremities has been demonstrated in concentric ER in professional[129,142] and collegiate[26] baseball pitchers or in elite junior[134,136] and adult[135] tennis players. This selective strength development in the internal rotators produces significant changes in agonist-antagonist muscular balance. Identification of such selectivity with isokinetic testing has implications for rehabilitation and prevention of injuries.

USE OF NORMATIVE DATA
Normative or descriptive data can assist clinicians in further analyzing isokinetic test data. Care must be taken to use normative data that are both population and apparatus specific.[11] Tables 25-3 to 25-5 present data using two dynamometer systems from large samples of specific athletic populations. Data are presented with body weight used as the normalizing factor.

UNILATERAL STRENGTH RATIOS (AGONIST TO ANTAGONIST)
Assessment of the balance in muscular strength of the internal and external rotators is of vital importance when one interprets upper extremity strength tests. Alteration of this ER-to-IR ratio has been reported in athletes with glenohumeral joint instability and impingement.[109] The initial description of the ER-to-IR ratio for normal female subjects was published by Ivey et al[143] and confirmed by Davies[1] in both men and women. An ER-to-IR ratio of 66% is the target in normal subjects. Biasing this ratio in favor of the external rotators has been advocated by clinicians,[68,127,144] both for preventing injury in throwing and racquet sport athletes and after injury to or surgery on the glenohumeral joint.

Reports of alteration in the ER-to-IR ratio as a result of selective muscular development of the internal rotators without concomitant ER strength are widespread in the literature.[26,135-139] This alteration has provided clinicians with an objective rationale for the global recommendation of preventive posterior rotator cuff ER-strengthening programs in athletes performing high-level overhead activities.[127,144] Examples of ER-to-IR ratios in specific athletic populations and with specific apparatus are presented in Tables 25-5 and 25-6.

Table 25-5 Isokinetic Peak Torque–to–Body Weight Ratios, Single-Repetition Work-to–Body Weight Ratios, and External Rotation–to–Internal Rotation Ratios in Elite Junior Tennis Players*

	Dominant Arm		Nondominant Arm	
	Peak Torque (%)	Work (%)	Peak Torque (%)	Work (%)
External Rotation (ER)				
Male, 210°/sec	12	20	11	19
Male, 300°/sec	10	18	10	17
Female, 210°/sec	8	14	8	15
Female, 300°/sec	8	11	7	12
Internal Rotation (IR)				
Male, 210°/sec	17	32	14	27
Male, 300°/sec	15	28	13	23
Female, 210°/sec	12	23	11	19
Female, 300°/sec	11	15	10	13
ER/IR Ratio				
Male, 210°/sec	69	64	81	81
Male, 300°/sec	69	65	82	83
Female, 210°/sec	69	63	81	82
Female, 300°/sec	67	61	81	77

Data from Ellenbecker, T.S., and Roetert, E.P. (2003): Age specific isokinetic glenohumeral internal and external rotation strength in elite junior tennis players. J. Sci. Med. Sport, 6:65–72.
*A Cybex 6000 series isokinetic dynamometer and 90° of glenohumeral joint abduction were used. Data are expressed in foot-pounds per unit of body weight for ER and IR measures, with the ER/IR ratio representing the relative muscular balance between the external and internal rotators.

Table 25-6 Unilateral External Rotation–Internal Rotation Ratios in Professional Baseball Pitchers

Speed	Dominant Arm	Nondominant Arm
180°/sec		
Torque	65	64
300°/sec		
Torque	61	70
210°/sec		
Torque	64	74
Work	61	66
300°/sec		
Torque	65	72
Work	62	70

Data from Wilk, K.E., Andrews, J.R., Arrigo, C.A., et al. (1993): The strength characteristics of internal and external rotator muscles in professional baseball pitchers. Am. J. Sports Med., 21:61–66; and Ellenbecker, T.S., and Mattalino, A.J. (1997): Concentric isokinetic shoulder internal and external rotation strength in professional baseball pitchers. J. Orthop. Sports Phys. Ther., 25:323–328.

the limitation of ROM to approximately 120° to avoid glenohumeral joint impingement and the consistent use of gravity correction.[145]

Interpretation of abduction-adduction isokinetic test results involves traditional bilateral comparison, normative data comparison, and unilateral strength ratios. Ivey et al,[143] in testing normal adult women, reported ratios of 50% bilaterally. Similar findings were reported by Alderink and Kluck[133] in high school and collegiate baseball pitchers. Wilk et al[146,147] reported dominant arm abduction-to-adduction ratios of 85% to 95% with a Biodex dynamometer.* They used a windowing technique that removed impact artifacts from the data after free limb acceleration and end-stop impact. Upper extremity testing using long input adapters and fast isokinetic testing velocities can produce a torque artifact that significantly changes the isokinetic test result. Wilk et al[147] recommended windowing the data by excluding all data obtained at velocities outside 95% of the present angular testing velocity. (Because of free limb acceleration and deceleration, only a portion of the entire ROM is truly isokinetic. If the velocities differ from the actual test speed by 5% or more, the data are not valid isokinetic data and should not be used.)

Additional Glenohumeral Joint Testing Positions

Shoulder Abduction and Adduction

Shoulder abduction-adduction strength is an additional pattern frequently evaluated isokinetically because of the key role of the abductors in the Inman force couple[119] and the functional relationship of the adductors to throwing velocity.[29] Specific factors important in this testing pattern are

Shoulder Flexion-Extension and Horizontal Abduction-Adduction

Additional isokinetic patterns used to obtain a more detailed profile of shoulder function are flexion-extension and horizontal abduction-adduction. Both motions are generally tested in a less functional supine position to improve stabilization. Normative data for these testing positions are less prevalent in the literature. Flexion-to-extension ratios reported for normal

---

*Available from Biodex, Shirley, NY.

subjects by Ivey et al[143] are 80% (4:5). Ratios for athletes with shoulder extension–dominant activities are reported to be 50% for baseball pitchers[123] and 75% to 80% for highly skilled adult tennis players.[135] Normative data need to be developed further to define strength more clearly in these upper extremity patterns. Body position and gravity compensation are, again, key factors affecting proper interpretation of the data.

Scapulothoracic Testing (Protraction-Retraction)

In addition to the supraspinatus-deltoid force couple, the serratus anterior–trapezius force couple is of critical importance for thorough evaluation of upper extremity strength. Gross MMT and screening that attempt to identify scapular winging are commonly used in clinical evaluation of the shoulder complex. Davies and Hoffman[74] published normative data on 250 shoulders for isokinetic protraction-retraction testing. An approximately 1:1 relationship of protraction-retraction strength was reported. Testing and training the serratus anterior, trapezius, and rhomboid musculature enhance scapular stabilization and strengthen the primary musculature involved in the scapulohumeral rhythm. Emphasis on promotion of proximal stability to enhance distal mobility is a concept used and recognized by nearly all disciplines of rehabilitative medicine.[83]

Concentric Versus Eccentric Considerations

The availability of eccentric dynamic strength assessment has made a significant impact, primarily in research investigations. Extrapolation of research-oriented isokinetic principles to patient populations has been a gradual process. Eccentric testing of the upper extremity is clearly indicated because of the prevalence of functionally specific eccentric work. Maximal eccentric functional contractions of the posterior rotator cuff during the follow-through phase of the throwing motion and tennis serve provide a rationale for eccentric testing and training in rehabilitation and preventive conditioning.[148] Kennedy et al[149] found mode-specific differences between the concentric and eccentric strength characteristics of the rotator cuff. Saccol et al[150] evaluated shoulder ER and IR strength variables in concentric and eccentric modes in elite junior tennis players. To determine the peak torque–functional ratio, the eccentric strength of ER and the concentric strength of IR were calculated. Elite junior tennis players without shoulder injuries have imbalances in muscle strength during shoulder rotation that alter the normal functional ratio between rotator cuff muscles. This is probably a normal adaptive physiologic response caused by the specificity of training at a high level of performance. Further research on eccentric muscular training is necessary before widespread use of eccentric isokinetics can be applied to patient populations.

The basic characteristics of eccentric isokinetic testing, such as greater force production than with concentric contractions at the same velocity, have been reported for the internal and external rotators.[151-153] This enhanced force generation is generally explained by the contribution of the series elastic (noncontractile) elements of the muscle-tendon unit in eccentric conditions. An increase in postexercise muscle soreness, particularly of latent onset, is a common occurrence after periods of eccentric work. Therefore, eccentric testing would not be the mode of choice during the early inflammatory stages of an overuse injury.[110] Many clinicians recommend the use of dynamic concentric testing before they perform an eccentric test. Both concentric and eccentric isokinetic training of the rotator cuff has produced objective improvements in concentric and eccentric strength in elite tennis players.[152,153]

RELATIONSHIP OF ISOKINETIC TESTING TO FUNCTIONAL PERFORMANCE

Dynamic muscular strength assessment is used to evaluate the underlying strength and balance of strength in specific muscle groups. This information is used to determine the specific anatomic structure that requires strengthening, as well as to demonstrate the efficacy of treatment procedures. Isokinetic testing of the shoulder internal and external rotators has been used as one parameter for demonstrating the functional outcome after rotator cuff repair in select patient populations.[154-157]

Bigoni et al[158] used isokinetics as an outcome measure to determine recovery of strength after rotator cuff tears treated with two different arthroscopic repair techniques. Isokinetic strength testing demonstrated a difference between the two repairs and can therefore be used as a measure to assess the efficacy of surgical procedures. Oh et al[159] evaluated patients with an isokinetic dynamometer following rotator cuff repair. Isokinetic muscle performance testing is a validated and objective method for evaluating muscle function, but it is presently unknown whether it correlates with the severity of rotator cuff tears. Oh et al[159] demonstrated a correlation between isokinetic testing and preoperative isokinetic muscle performance parameters. The isokinetic muscle performance testing deficit was greater in shoulders with larger rotator cuff tears and greater degrees of fatty degeneration/infiltration. Isokinetic muscle performance testing provides objective and quantitative data for estimating the preoperative status of rotator cuff tears and can provide baseline data for postoperative anatomic assessment in patients with rotator cuff disorders.

An additional purpose for isokinetic testing is to determine the relationship of muscular strength to functional performance. Several investigators have tested upper extremity muscle groups and correlated their respective levels of strength with sport-specific functional tests. Pedegana et al[160] found a statistical relationship between elbow extension, wrist flexion, shoulder extension-flexion, and ER strength measured isokinetically and throwing speed in professional pitchers. In a similar study, Bartlett et al[161] found that shoulder adduction correlated with throwing speed. These studies are in contrast to those of Pawlowski and Perrin,[162] who did not find a significant relationship in throwing velocity.

Andrade-Mdos et al[163] established an isokinetic profile of shoulder rotator muscle strength in female handball players. Concentric balance and functional balance ratios did not differ between sides at slower angular velocities, but at faster angular velocities the functional balance ratio in the dominant limb was lower than that on the nondominant side. The results suggest that concentric strength exercises should be used for the internal and external rotators on the nondominant side and that functional exercise should be used to improve eccentric rotation strength for prevention programs.

Edouard et al[164] did not find any significant postoperative correlations between shoulder function (as judged by the Rowe and Walch-Duplay scores) and IR or ER muscle strength. However, it is necessary to objectively measure recovery of rotator cuff strength to adequately strengthen the rotator cuff muscles before resumption of sports activities. Isokinetic strength assessment may thus be a valuable decision support tool for resumption of sports activities and would complement the functional scores studied in this study.

Additionally, Mandalidis et al[56] evaluated the relationship between handgrip isometric strength and isokinetic strength of the shoulder musculature. A positive relationship was found between handgrip isometric strength and isokinetic strength of the shoulder stabilizers. The results of the present findings suggest that handgrip isometric strength can be used to monitor the isokinetic strength of certain muscle groups contributing to the stability of the shoulder joint. However, handgrip strength may account for only approximately 16% to 50% of the variability in isokinetic strength of these muscle groups.

Several studies have examined the relationship between isokinetic strength and the tennis serve in elite players. Ellenbecker et al[152] determined that 6 weeks of concentric isokinetic training of the rotator cuff resulted in a statistically significant improvement in serving velocity in collegiate tennis players. In a similar study, Mont et al[153] found improvements in serving velocity after both concentric and eccentric IR and ER training. A direct statistical relationship between isokinetically measured upper extremity strength and tennis serve velocity was not obtained by Ellenbecker[135] despite earlier studies showing increases in serving velocity after isokinetic training. The complex biomechanical sequence of segmental velocities and the interrelationship of the kinetic chain link with the lower extremities and trunk make delineation and identification of a direct relationship between an isolated structure and a complex functional activity difficult.

Finally, from a distal upper extremity strength perspective, Lin et al[165] used an isokinetic dynamometer to assess dominant arm (elbow) flexor and extensor concentric and eccentric strength. Based on the results of isokinetic tests, regression analysis revealed that a ratio of biceps concentric to triceps concentric strength greater than 0.76 significantly predicted elbow injury. No other ratios or variables were predictive of injury status. Assessment of this ratio may prove useful in a practical setting for training purposes and for both diagnosis and rehabilitation of injury.

Isokinetic testing can provide a reliable, dynamic measurement of isolated joint motions and muscular contributions to assist the clinician in the assessment of underlying muscular strength and strength balance. Integration of isokinetic testing with a thorough, objective clinical evaluation allows the clinician to provide optimal rehabilitation after both overuse injuries and surgery.

APPLICATION OF ISOKINETICS IN DESIGNING REHABILITATION PROGRAMS

Many types of exercise programs are in widespread use for rehabilitating injured athletes. This section focuses on resistive rehabilitation programs, as well as on the specific progression of

Table 25-7 Commonly Used Subjective and Objective Criteria for Patient Progression in a Rehabilitation Program

Subjective Criteria (Symptoms)	Objective Criteria (Signs)
Pain	Anthropometric measurements
Stiffness	Goniometric measurements
Changes in function	Palpable changes in cutaneous temperature Redness Manual muscle testing Isokinetic testing Kinesthetic testing Functional performance testing KT1000 testing

From Davies, G.J. (1992): A Compendium of Isokinetics in Clinical Usage and Rehabilitation Techniques, 4th ed. Onalaska, WI, S & S Publishers.

resistive exercise recommended during rehabilitation. Resistive rehabilitation programs vary from isometric, concentric, and eccentric isotonics to concentric and eccentric isokinetics to isoacceleration and isodeceleration programs. The scientific and clinical rationale for progression through a resistive exercise rehabilitation program is described, including the specific progression and inclusion of isokinetic exercise in the clinical rehabilitation of upper extremity overuse injuries.

Patient Progression Criteria

Progression through the resistive exercise program is predicated on several important concepts, including athlete status, signs and symptoms, time after surgery, and soft tissue–healing constraints. The athlete's progression through the various levels of the resistive exercise program is determined by continual charting and assessment of subjective and objective evaluation criteria (Table 25-7). This resistive exercise progression continuum[7] is based on the concept of a trial treatment. If any adverse changes occur, the rehabilitation program continues at the previous level of intensity of repetitions, sets, or duration without the athlete progressing to the next level of the exercise progression continuum.

If, however, an athlete performs the trial treatment without any negative effects, the athlete progresses gradually to the next higher level in the exercise continuum. An athlete may enter the exercise rehabilitation continuum at any stage, depending on the results of the initial evaluation. Furthermore, an athlete may also progress through several stages from one treatment session to the next, depending primarily on the response to treatment. Before the athlete begins the actual resistive exercise portion of the rehabilitation program, various warm-up exercises and mobilization stretching exercises are appropriate.

Resistive Exercise Progression Continuum

The rehabilitation program is designed along a progression continuum. The program begins with the safest exercises and progresses to more stressful exercises. These are illustrated in Figure 25-2 and Table 25-8.

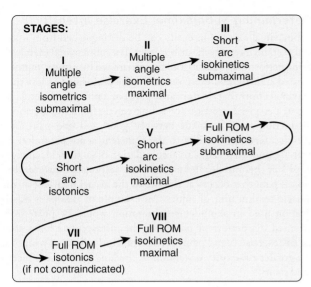

FIGURE 25-2 Stages of Davies' resistive exercise progression continuum. *ROM*, Range of motion. *(From Davies, G.J. [1992]: A Compendium of Isokinetics in Clinical Usage and Rehabilitation Techniques, 4th ed. Onalaska, WI, S & S Publishers.)*

Multiple-Angle Isometrics

The exercise rehabilitation program typically begins with multiple-angle isometrics performed at a submaximal intensity level. The isometrics are performed approximately every 20° through the ROM that is indicated, based on the safe and comfortable ROM demonstrated during examination of the athlete. The rationale for using this particular exercise is the presence of a 20° physiologic overflow with the application of isometrics[7] (Fig. 25-3). Therefore, as an example (Fig. 25-4), if the athlete has a painful arc syndrome, which is common in a shoulder with a pathologic rotator cuff condition, isometrics can be applied every 20° throughout the ROM, and the athlete will still obtain a concomitant strengthening effect throughout the entire ROM without increasing the symptomatic area. The painful arc that is typical in athletes with pathologic rotator cuff conditions occurs between 85° and 135° of elevation, at which point peak forces against the undersurface of the acromion occur.[166] Performing isometric exercise around the painful arc during the rehabilitation process is a prime example of applying isometrics early in rehabilitation of the shoulder after an overuse injury or surgery.

The next consideration with isometric exercise is that the athlete use the rule of 10s: 10-second contractions, 10-second rest, 10 repetitions, and so on. The athlete is usually taught to perform the isometrics in the following sequence: (1) take 2 seconds to gradually build up the desired tension, whether working at a submaximal or maximal intensity level; (2) hold the desired tension of the isometric contraction for 6 seconds, which is the optimal duration for an isometric contraction[167]; and (3) gradually relax and release tension in the muscle over the last 2 seconds (Fig. 25-5). This sequence allows controlled buildup and easing of the contraction with an optimal 6-second isometric contraction.

Gradient Increase and Decrease in Force Production

Gradient increase and decrease in muscle force production are concepts that athletes have taught us over the years. As an example, if an athlete has effusion or pain in a joint and performs a

Table 25-8 Davies' Resistive Exercise Progression Continuum

Exercise Effort (%)	Exercise Program
100	Submaximal multiple-angle isometrics SOAP TT of maximal multiple-angle isometrics
50/50	Submaximal multiple-angle isometrics + maximal multiple-angle isometrics SOAP
100	Maximal multiple-angle isometrics SOAP TT of submaximal short-arc isokinetics
50/50	Maximal multiple-angle isometrics + submaximal short-arc isokinetics SOAP
100	Submaximal short-arc isokinetics SOAP TT of maximal short-arc isokinetics or short-arc isotonics
50/50	Submaximal short-arc isokinetics + maximal short-arc isokinetics SOAP
100	Maximal short-arc isokinetics SOAP TT of submaximal full ROM isokinetics
50/50	Maximal short-arc isokinetics + submaximal full ROM isokinetics SOAP
100	Submaximal full ROM isokinetics SOAP TT of maximal full ROM isokinetics SOAP (full ROM isotonics here if not contraindicated)
50/50	Submaximal full ROM isokinetics + maximal full ROM isokinetics SOAP
100	Maximal full ROM isokinetics SOAP

From Davies, G.J. (1992): A Compendium of Isokinetics in Clinical Usage and Rehabilitation Techniques, 4th ed. Onalaska, WI, S & S Publishers.
ROM, Range of motion; *SOAP*, subjective-objective assessment and plan; *TT*, trial treatment.

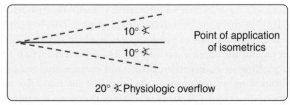

FIGURE 25-3 Isometric exercises and physiologic overflow through the range of motion. *(From Davies, G.J. [1992]: A Compendium of Isokinetics in Clinical Usage and Rehabilitation Techniques, 4th ed. Onalaska, WI, S & S Publishers.)*

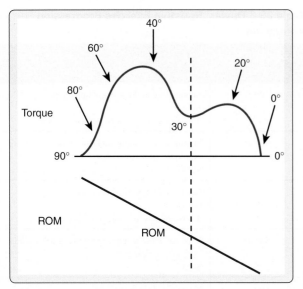

FIGURE 25-4 Application of isometric exercises through the range of motion (ROM) with a "painful" deformation. Isometrics are applied every 20° through the ROM. Note particularly the application of isometrics on each side of the "painful" deformation. *(From Davies, G.J. [1992]: A Compendium of Isokinetics in Clinical Usage and Rehabilitation Techniques, 4th ed. Onalaska, WI, S & S Publishers.)*

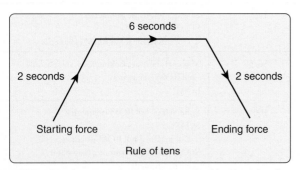

FIGURE 25-5 Isometric contraction applied by the rule of tens. *(From Davies, G.J. [1992]: A Compendium of Isokinetics in Clinical Usage and Rehabilitation Techniques, 4th ed. Onalaska, WI, S & S Publishers.)*

muscle contraction, pain is often induced. It is usually the result of capsular distention from the internal pressure of the effusion. The submaximal muscle contraction places external pressure on the capsule, which is highly innervated,[168] and subsequently increases the pain. However, with a gradient increase in muscle contraction to the desired intensity (submaximal or maximal), an accommodation is often created that either eliminates or minimizes the pain. At completion of the 6-second isometric contraction, a gradient decrease in muscle contraction is performed. Again, when an effusion is present and the athlete suddenly releases the contraction, pain results. This is perhaps due to a rebound type of phenomenon in which effusion in the joint pushes the capsule out and the muscular contraction that was pushing in against the capsule and compressing it causes an "equalizing" of the pressure. At release of the muscular contraction, the external pressure is relieved; therefore, the internal pressure causes a rebound phenomenon in which the capsule is stretched and discomfort results. If the athlete gradually releases the muscle contraction and some type of accommodation occurs, the pain is either eliminated or minimized.

Determining Submaximal Exercise Intensity

Submaximal exercise intensity can be distinguished from maximal exercise intensity in various ways. If a submaximal exercise is being performed, intensity can be determined by using symptom-limited submaximal exercises (exercises performed at less than maximal effort that do not cause pain) or a musculoskeletal rating of perceived exertion for submaximal effort. Furthermore, distinction must be made between good and bad pain after exercise. *Good pain* refers to the transient acute pain after an exercise bout that is due to accumulation of lactic acid, changes in pH in the muscle, and an ischemic response. However, *bad pain* is pain that occurs at the site of the actual injury or at the muscle-tendon unit of injury. An example of this pain classification used in shoulder rehabilitation would be posteriorly oriented discomfort or pain over the infraspinous fossa after an ER exercise (good pain) versus anteriorly directed pain over the greater tuberosity or tendon of the long head of the biceps (bad pain).

Guidelines for Pain During Exercise

The following are guidelines that we use during the rehabilitation program: (1) if no pain is present at the start of an exercise bout but develops after the exercise, that particular exercise is stopped, and modifications are made in the exercise; (2) if pain is present at the start of the exercise and the pain increases, that exercise is terminated; and (3) if pain is present at the start of an exercise and the pain plateaus, the athlete continues the exercise program.

Trial Treatment

When a rehabilitation program includes progression of the athlete through a resistive exercise continuum, a key element is how to determine the progression from one stage to the next in the continuum. One of the keys to this progression is the use of a trial treatment. A trial treatment essentially consists of the athlete performing one set from the next stage in the exercise progression continuum (see Fig. 25-2). After the athlete completes the exercise program at one level of the exercise progression continuum, a trial of the next stage of treatment is performed. The athlete's signs and symptoms are then evaluated at the conclusion of that particular treatment session, as well as at the next scheduled visit, at which time the athlete's condition is reevaluated and a decision made on the basis of the athlete's signs and symptoms. If they have stayed the same or improved, the athlete can progress to the next level of exercise because the trial treatment has demonstrated that the athlete's muscle-tendon unit or joint is ready for the higher exercise intensity. Any negative sequelae such as increased pain or effusion in the joint are an indication that the joint or muscle is not ready for progression, and consequently, the athlete continues to work at the same level of intensity. Further physical therapy is performed to decrease the irritability of the joint or muscle-tendon unit, and during the next visit, a trial treatment is once again attempted to determine whether the athlete's injury can tolerate the progression.

Submaximal Exercise: Fiber Recruitment

Several exercise modes can be performed at a submaximal level to enhance selective fiber recruitment. Preferential muscle fiber recruitment is predicated on the intensity of the muscle contraction to recruit either slow-twitch or fast-twitch A or fast-twitch

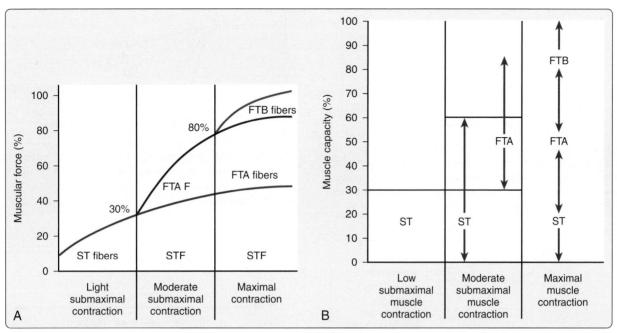

FIGURE 25-6 A and **B,** Preferential muscle fiber recruitment is predicated on the intensity of the muscle contraction. *FTA,* Fast-twitch A; *FTB,* fast-twitch B; *ST,* slow-twitch. *(From Davies, G.J. [1992]: A Compendium of Isokinetics in Clinical Usage and Rehabilitation Techniques, 4th ed. Onalaska, WI, S & S Publishers.)*

B fibers. It is generally accepted that during voluntary contractions of human muscle there is an orderly recruitment of motor units according to the size principle.[169] In mixed muscle containing both slow-twitch and fast-twitch fibers, this implies that involvement of slow-twitch fibers is obligatory, regardless of the power and velocity being generated, with fast-twitch A and fast-twitch B muscle fibers being recruited once higher intensities are generated.[170] Figure 25-6 summarizes this preferential muscular recruitment. Slow-twitch motor units have relatively low contraction velocities and long contraction times that require only low levels of stimulus to contract. In contrast, fast-twitch motor units require a very high intensity stimulus to contract and have very short contraction times. The preferential recruitment of muscle fibers is an important concept for the clinician to understand with regard to the manipulation of submaximal and maximal exercise intensities in rehabilitative exercise. Submaximal exercise can stimulate the slow-twitch muscle fibers and allow athletes to exercise at lower, pain-free intensities early in the rehabilitation process, with progression to higher exercise intensities that preferentially stimulate the fast-twitch fibers occurring later in rehabilitation.

Short-Arc Exercises

The athlete next progresses from static isometric exercises to more dynamic exercises. The dynamic exercises start with short-arc exercises and the ROM within symptom and soft tissue–healing constraints. Short-arc exercises are often started with submaximal isokinetics (Fig. 25-7) because the accommodating resistance inherent in submaximal isokinetic exercise makes it safe for the athlete's healing tissues. With short-arc isokinetics, speeds ranging from 60 to 180°/sec are used (Fig. 25-8). The athlete works with what is called a velocity spectrum rehabilitation protocol (VSRP). When the athlete is performing short-arc isokinetics, slower contractile velocities (60 to 180°/sec)

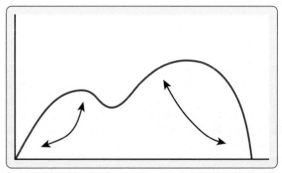

FIGURE 25-7 Short-arc isokinetic exercises being applied at different points in the range of motion. If an isokinetic torque curve has a deformity in the range of motion as illustrated, short-arc isokinetic exercises can be applied to each side of the deformity. *(From Davies, G.J. [1992]: A Compendium of Isokinetics in Clinical Usage and Rehabilitation Techniques, 4th ed. Onalaska, WI, S & S Publishers.)*

are chosen because of the acceleration and deceleration response (Fig. 25-9). Isokinetic exercise contains three major components, as identified in Figure 25-9: acceleration, deceleration, and load range. Acceleration is the portion of the ROM in which the athlete's limb is accelerating to "catch" the preset angular velocity, deceleration is the portion of the ROM in which the athlete's limb is slowing before cessation of that repetition, and the load range is the actual portion of the ROM in which the preset angular velocity is met by the athlete and a true isokinetic load is imparted to the athlete. Load range is inversely related to isokinetic speed. A larger load range is found at slower contractile velocities, and a statistically shorter load range occurs at faster contractile velocities.[171]

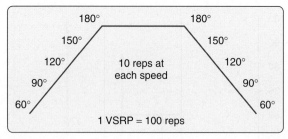

FIGURE 25-8 Short-arc isokinetic velocity spectrum rehabilitation protocol (VSRP) performed at intermediate contractile velocities. *reps,* Repetitions. *(From Davies, G.J. [1992]: A Compendium of Isokinetics in Clinical Usage and Rehabilitation Techniques, 4th ed. Onalaska, WI, S & S Publishers.)*

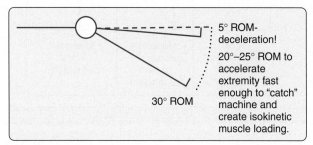

FIGURE 25-9 Acceleration and deceleration range of motion (ROM) with short-arc isokinetic exercise. *(From Davies, G.J. [1992]: A Compendium of Isokinetics in Clinical Usage and Rehabilitation Techniques, 4th ed. Onalaska, WI, S & S Publishers.)*

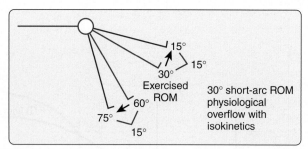

FIGURE 25-10 Thirty-degree short-arc range of motion (ROM) overflow with isokinetics. *(From Davies, G.J. [1992]: A Compendium of Isokinetics in Clinical Usage and Rehabilitation Techniques, 4th ed. Onalaska, WI, S & S Publishers.)*

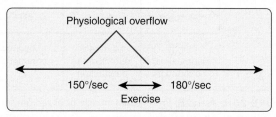

FIGURE 25-11 Physiologic overflow of 30°/sec through the velocity spectrum. *(From Davies, G.J. [1992]: A Compendium of Isokinetics in Clinical Usage and Rehabilitation Techniques, 4th ed. Onalaska, WI, S & S Publishers.)*

Further support for short-arc or limited ROM exercise comes from research by Clark et al.[172] These authors determined the influence of variable range of motion (VROM) training on neuromuscular performance and control of external loads. Subjects trained with either full ROM or partial ROM exercises. The partial ROM exercises demonstrated significant increases in several of the outcome measures, including isokinetic testing in terminal ROM. Analysis of the force-ROM relationship revealed that the VROM intervention enhanced performance at shorter muscle lengths. These findings suggest that VROM training improves gains in terminal and midrange performance, with the result that the athlete has improved ability to control external loading and produce dynamic force.

Consequently, the athlete's available ROM must be evaluated to determine the optimal ROM for exercise. With short-arc isokinetic exercise, there is a physiologic overflow of approximately 30° throughout the ROM (Fig. 25-10). Therefore, when an athlete with a pathologic rotator cuff condition is exercising, an abbreviated ROM in IR-ER can be used in the pain-free range, with overflow into the painful ROM, without actually placing the injured structures into that movement range. Another example of isokinetic exercise for the upper extremities is limitation of external ROM to 90° during isokinetic training, even though the demands on the athletic shoulder in overhead activities exceed the 90° ER. Limiting ER to 90° protects the anterior capsular structures of the shoulder, with physiologic overflow improving strength at ranges of ER exceeded during training.

In addition to ROM, the speed selected with isokinetic exercise is also of vital importance in a VSRP. The speeds in the protocol are designed so that the athlete will exercise at 30°/sec

through the velocity spectrum. The reason for using an interval of 30°/sec in the velocity spectrum is the physiologic overflow with respect to speed that has been identified in isokinetic research (Fig. 25-11).[173-175]

Rest Intervals

When the athlete is performing either submaximal or maximal short-arc isokinetics in a VSRP, the rest interval between each set of 10 training repetitions may be as long as 90 seconds.[89] However, this is not a viable clinical rest time because it takes too much time to complete the exercise session. Consequently, rest intervals are often applied on a symptom-limited basis. If the athlete does complete a total VSRP, a rest period of 3 minutes after completion of the VSRP has been shown to be an effective rest interval[176] (Fig. 25-12). Additional research has provided guidance for selection of rest intervals after isotonic and isokinetic exercise in rehabilitation. According to Fleck,[177] 50% of the adenosine triphosphate and creatine phosphate is restored in 20 seconds after an acute bout of muscular work. Seventy-five percent and 87% of intramuscular stores are replenished in 40 and 60 seconds, respectively. Knowledge of the phosphagen replenishment schedule allows clinicians to make scientifically based decisions on the amount of rest needed or desired after periods of muscular work. Another factor in determining optimal rest intervals with isotonic and isokinetic training is specificity. For example, during rehabilitation of the shoulder of a tennis player, a high-repetition format is used to improve local muscular endurance. Rest cycles are limited to 25 to 30 seconds because that is the time allotted during tennis play for rest between points. Applying activity or sport-specific muscular work rest cycles is an important consideration during rehabilitation.

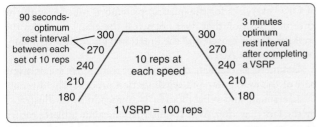

FIGURE 25-12 Optimum rest intervals. *reps*, Repetitions; *VSRP*, velocity spectrum rehabilitation protocol. *(From Davies, G.J. [1992]: A Compendium of Isokinetics in Clinical Usage and Rehabilitation Techniques, 4th ed. Onalaska, WI, S & S Publishers.)*

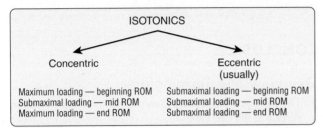

FIGURE 25-13 Concentric and eccentric isotonic muscle loading and submaximal and maximal loading through the range of motion (ROM). *(From Davies, G.J. [1992]: A Compendium of Isokinetics in Clinical Usage and Rehabilitation Techniques, 4th ed. Onalaska, WI, S & S Publishers.)*

When isotonic exercises are performed, they are implemented between isokinetic submaximal and maximal exercises (see Fig. 25-2). The reason is that isotonic muscle loading loads a muscle only at its weakest point in the ROM. Figure 25-13 demonstrates the effects of isotonic muscle loading through the ROM. Consequently, when isotonic muscle exercise is performed through the ROM, a combination of maximal and submaximal loading occurs, whereas with isokinetics, submaximal exercises can be performed throughout the ROM, and loading of the muscle is maximal in intensity throughout the ROM because of the accommodating resistance phenomena inherent in isokinetic exercise.

Full Range-of-Motion Exercises

The athlete next progresses to full ROM isokinetic exercise beginning with submaximal exercise and then progressing to maximal intensity (Fig. 25-14). Straight planar movements are used initially to protect the injured plane of movement. Faster contractile velocities are also used from 180° up to the maximum capabilities of the isokinetic dynamometer. Numerous reasons have been proposed for using faster isokinetic speeds: physiologic overflow to slower speeds, specificity response, motor-learning response, and decreased joint compressive force.[7] Joint compressive force is decreased based on the Bernoulli principle that at faster speeds, there is decreased pressure on the articular surface because of the synovial fluid interface.[178] This is probably due to interfacing of the hydrodynamic pattern of the articular cartilage and movement of the synovial fluid. Another consideration is positioning of the athlete to use the length-tension curve of the muscle. With isokinetic exercise, the athlete's position is often modified to bias the respective muscles, for example, to stretch them to facilitate contraction or to place them in a shortened position if that is the functional position. Obviously, of greatest importance is

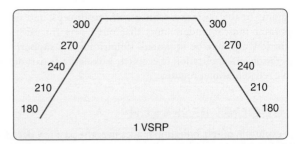

FIGURE 25-14 Full range-of-motion isokinetic velocity spectrum rehabilitation protocol (VSRP) performed at fast contractile velocities. *(From Davies, G.J. [1992]: A Compendium of Isokinetics in Clinical Usage and Rehabilitation Techniques, 4th ed. Onalaska, WI, S & S Publishers.)*

the attempt to replicate the ultimate functional performance position of the individual.

GENERAL ISOKINETIC TRAINING ISSUES

Remaud et al[179] measured neuromuscular adaptations with isotonic versus isokinetic training. Significant increases in strength in both dynamic and static conditions were identified in both groups; however, no significant differences were noted between groups. Remaud et al[179] recommended that either training method can be used. If isokinetic equipment is available and no contraindications are present, these authors recommend using isokinetics because of the accommodating resistance. Accommodating resistance allows maximal muscle loading throughout the entire ROM, thereby improving total work and not just peak torque in the middle of the ROM.

Oliveria et al[180] evaluated the effectiveness of a single training session on power output in different contraction types; however, little is known about the neuromuscular adaptations to reach this enhancement. They demonstrated that a single training session improves neural strategies to contract muscles stronger and faster at the slowest velocity whereas higher velocities present different adaptations and might need more practice to further adaptations.

Isoacceleration and Deceleration

Because functional activities are primarily accelerative and decelerative movement patterns, it is important to try to replicate these patterns when one performs different types of rehabilitation activities. In addition, because of the functional activities involved in various sports, such as the deceleration phase of tennis or baseball that is applied to the posterior rotator cuff or to the forearm or biceps muscles, the potential use of eccentric exercise may also be important. Few studies have demonstrated the efficacy of performing eccentric exercise or eccentric isokinetic rehabilitation programs at this time.[38] Ellenbecker et al[152] reported improvement in IR and ER concentric strength after 6 weeks of eccentric isokinetic training of the internal and external rotators in elite tennis players. Mont et al[153] found improvement in both concentric and eccentric strength with eccentric isokinetic training of the rotator cuff in elite tennis players. Despite the lack of research on eccentric exercise training, particularly in athletes, specific application of eccentric exercise programs to the posterior rotator cuff, quadriceps, and other important muscle-tendon units that must perform extensive eccentric work may be indicated. Empirically, we support the integration and application of eccentric isokinetics as part of the whole rehabilitation program.

OUTCOMES RESEARCH

The evolution of rehabilitation modes over the past few decades can best be described as follows:

1970s: Functional rehabilitation
1980s: OKC assessment and rehabilitation (with emphasis on isokinetics)
1990s: CKC rehabilitation
2000: Integrated assessment and rehabilitation that include both OKC and CKC

Bynum et al[69] published the results of the first prospective, randomized study comparing OKC and CKC exercises. With respect to the parameters listed, their conclusions indicate the following about CKC exercises:

1. Lower mean KT1000 arthrometer side-to-side differences (KT-20, $P = .057$, not significant; KT-max, $P = .018$, significant)
2. Less patellofemoral pain ($P = .48$, not significant)
3. Patients generally more satisfied with the end result ($P = .36$, not significant)
4. Patients returned to activities of daily living sooner than expected ($P = .007$, significant)
5. Patients returned to sports sooner than expected ($P = .118$, not significant)

The authors stated: "As a result of this study, we now use the CKC protocol exclusively after anterior cruciate ligament reconstruction."[69] Surprisingly, Bynum et al[69] came to several conclusions on data that were not statistically significant and probably not clinically significant either. Yet they based their entire protocol exclusively on these findings.

CKC exercises have almost replaced OKC exercises in the rehabilitation of athletes after ACL reconstruction. As indicated earlier, this change is not founded on solid experimental or clinical studies, with limited published prospective, randomized, experimental studies to prove the efficacy of CKC exercises.[10] In contrast, the literature on OKC isokinetics and OKC isotonics is extensive, but most clinicians have ignored past successes with OKC exercises and have chosen to use CKC exercises without documentation.[50]

Snyder-Mackler et al[71] described prospective, randomized clinical trials and the effects of intensive CKC rehabilitation programs and different types of electrical stimulation on athletes after ACL reconstruction. These researchers had previously demonstrated that the strength of the quadriceps femoris muscle correlates well with the function of the knee during the stance phase of gait. In their later study,[71] after an intensive CKC rehabilitation program, they reported residual weakness in the quadriceps that produced alterations in the normal gait function of these athletes. The authors concluded that CKC exercise alone does not provide an adequate stimulus to the quadriceps femoris to permit more normal knee function in the stance phase of gait in most athletes soon after ACL reconstruction. They suggested that the judicious application of OKC exercises for the quadriceps femoris muscle (with the knee in a position that does not stress the graft) improves the strength of this muscle and the functional outcome after reconstruction of the ACL.

Isokinetic assessment and treatment techniques are only one part of the evaluation and rehabilitation process. The diversity in assessment and rehabilitation is tremendous, as illustrated by the fact that after ACL reconstruction, some athletes return to sport after 12 weeks and others return after 12 months. Therefore, we strongly encourage clinicians to use an integrated approach to assessment and rehabilitation, to review the literature critically, and to contribute to the advancement of the art and science of sports medicine by performing research and sharing results through peer-reviewed publications.

CONCLUSION

Overview and Terminology

- The concept of isokinetic exercise was developed by James Perrine in the late 1960s.
- Isokinetics refers to exercise that is performed at a fixed velocity with an accommodating resistance. Accommodating resistance means that the resistance varies to exactly match the force applied by the athlete at every point in the ROM; thus, the muscle is loaded to its maximum capability at every point throughout the ROM.
- Isokinetic exercise contains three major components: acceleration, deceleration, and load range.

Isokinetic Testing

- Isokinetic assessment allows the clinician to objectively assess muscular performance in a way that is both safe and reliable.
- Contraindications to testing and using isokinetics include soft tissue–healing constraints, pain, limited ROM, effusion, joint instability, acute strains and sprains, and occasionally, subacute conditions.
- A standard test protocol should be used to enhance the reliability of testing.
- Isokinetic testing allows a variety of testing protocols ranging from power to endurance tests. Use of velocity spectrum testing is recommended so that the test will assess the muscle's capabilities at different speeds, thus simulating various activities.
- Isokinetic testing provides numerous objective parameters that can be used to evaluate and analyze an athlete's performance.
- Differentiation of the balance in agonist and antagonist muscular strength with manual techniques is not as reliable as using an isokinetic apparatus.
- With isokinetic testing, assessment of the strength of an extremity relative to the contralateral side forms the basis for interpretation of the data.
- It is necessary to perform isolated testing of specific muscle groups usually affected by certain pathologic changes. If the component parts of the kinetic chain are not measured, the weak link will not be identified or adequately rehabilitated, which will affect the entire chain.

Closed Kinetic Chain Versus Open Kinetic Chain Isokinetic Assessment and Rehabilitation

- The benefits of using CKC exercises in rehabilitation have been described quite extensively; however, few scientifically based prospective, randomized, controlled, experimental clinical trials document the efficacy of CKC exercises.
- The primary purpose of performing OKC isokinetic assessment is the need to test specific muscle groups of a pathologic joint in isolation. Although the muscles do not work in an isolated fashion, a deficit, or "weak link," in a kinetic chain will never be identified unless specific isolated OKC isokinetic testing is performed.
- Evidence suggests a correlation between OKC isokinetic testing and CKC functional performance, as well as sport-specific functional tests.

Use of Isokinetics in Upper Extremity Testing and Rehabilitation

- One rationale for using isokinetics in upper extremity testing and rehabilitation is that the upper extremities function almost exclusively in an OKC format.
- Initial testing and rehabilitation of the shoulder should be done in the modified base position before progressing to the 90° abducted position.
- The 90° abducted position for isokinetic strength assessment is more specific for assessing the muscular functions required for overhead activities.
- Research has identified the IR and ER movement patterns as the preferred testing patterns in athletes with rotator cuff tendinopathy.
- Some athletic populations have significantly greater IR than ER strength in the dominant arm, which produces significant changes in agonist-antagonist muscular balance.
- Alteration of the ER-to-IR ratio has been reported in athletes with glenohumeral joint instability and impingement.
- Eccentric testing in the upper extremity is clearly indicated on the basis of the prevalence of functionally specific eccentric work.

Use of Isokinetics in Rehabilitation Programs

- The athlete should progress from static isometric exercises to more dynamic exercises.
- Isometrics are performed at approximately every 20° through the ROM that is indicated. The rationale for 20° is the physiologic overflow that occurs with isometrics.
- Performing isometric exercise around the painful arc during the rehabilitation process is an example of applying isometrics early in the rehabilitation process.
- It is recommended that isometrics be performed by using the rule of tens: 10-second contractions, 10-second rest, 10 repetitions, and so on.
- The 10-second contraction should be performed with a 2-second gradual buildup to the desired tension, which should be held for 6 seconds with gradual relaxation for 2 seconds. This technique can also result in a decrease in the pain that can result from a muscle contraction around an injured area.

- When an athlete progresses through a progressive resistive program trial, treatments can be used to determine whether the athlete is ready to advance to the next stage of an exercise progression continuum.
- Submaximal exercise can stimulate the slow-twitch muscle fibers and allow athletes to exercise at lower, pain-free intensities early in the rehabilitation process, with a progression to higher exercise intensities later in rehabilitation that preferentially stimulate the fast-twitch fibers.
- Dynamic exercises begin with short-arc exercises and the ROM within symptom and soft tissue–healing constraints.
- Short-arc exercises are often started with submaximal isokinetics.
- With short-arc isokinetics, speeds ranging from 60 to 180°/sec are used.
- With short-arc isokinetic exercise, there is a physiologic overflow of approximately 30° through the ROM.
- The speed selected with isokinetic exercise is of vital importance in a VSRP. The speeds in the protocol are designed so that the athlete will exercise 30°/sec through the velocity spectrum. The reason for using an interval of 30°/sec in the velocity spectrum is the physiologic overflow with respect to speed that has been identified with isokinetic research.
- With full ROM exercises, straight planar movements are used initially to protect the injured plane of movement. Faster contractile velocities are also used from 180°/sec up to the maximum capabilities of the isokinetic dynamometer.
- Despite the lack of research on eccentric exercise training, particularly in athletes, specific application of eccentric exercise programs to the posterior rotator cuff, quadriceps, and other important muscle-tendon units that must perform extensive eccentric work may be indicated.

REFERENCES

1. Davies, G.J. (1984): A Compendium of Isokinetics in Clinical Usage and Rehabilitation Techniques. La Crosse. WI, S & S Publishers.
2. Chan, K.M., and Maffulli, N. (1966): Principles and Practice of Isokinetics in Sports Medicine and Rehabilitation. Hong Kong, Williams & Wilkins.
3. Dvir, Z. (1993): Isokinetic Exercise and Assessment. Champaign. IL, Human Kinetics.
4. Perrin, D.H. (1993): Isokinetic Exercise and Assessment. Champaign. IL, Human Kinetics.
5. Hislop, H.J., and Perrine, J.J. (1967): The isokinetic concept of exercise. Phys. Ther., 47:114–117.
6. Ellenbecker, T.S., and Davies, G.J. (2000): Closed Kinetic Chain Exercise. Champaign, IL, Human Kinetics.
7. Davies, G.J. (1992): A Compendium of Isokinetics in Clinical Usage and Rehabilitation Techniques, 4th ed. Onalaska, WI, S & S Publishers.
8. Wilk, K.E., Romaniello, W.T., Soscia, S.M., et al. (1994): The relationship between subjective knee scores, isokinetic (OKC) testing and functional testing in the ACL reconstructed knee. J. Orthop. Sports Phys. Ther., 20:60–73.
9. Barbee, J., and Landis, D. (1984): Reliability of Cybex computer measures. Phys. Ther., 68:737.
10. Farrell, M., and Richards, J.G. (1986): Analysis of the reliability and validity of the kinetic communicator exercise device. Med. Sci. Sports Exerc., 18:44.
11. Francis, K., and Hoobler, T. (1987): Comparison of peak torque values of the knee flexor and extensor muscle groups using the Cybex II and Lido 2.0 isokinetic dynamometers. J. Orthop. Sports Phys. Ther., 8:480–483.
12. Griffin, J.W. (1985): Differences in elbow flexion torque measure concentrically, eccentrically, and isometrically. Phys. Ther., 67:1205.
13. Jackson, A.L., Highgenboten, C., Meske, N., et al. (1987): Univariate and multivariate analysis of the reliability of the kinetic communicator. Med. Sci. Sports Exerc., 19:(Suppl.):23.
14. Johnson, J., and Siegel, D. (1978): Reliability of an isokinetic movement of the knee extensors. Res. Q., 49:88.
15. Mawdsley, R.H., and Knapik, J.J. (1982): Comparison of isokinetic measurements with test repetitions. Phys. Ther., 62:169.
16. Moffroid, M., Whipple, R., Hofkosh, J., et al. (1969): A study of isokinetic exercise. Phys. Ther., 49:735.

17. Molnar, G.E., and Alexander, J. (1973): Objective, quantitative muscle testing in children: A pilot study. Arch. Phys. Med. Rehabil., 54:225–228.

18. Molnar, G.E., Alexander, J., and Gudfeld, N. (1979): Reliability of quantitative strength measurements in children. Arch. Phys. Med. Rehabil., 60:218.

19. Perrin, D.H. (1986): Reliability of isokinetic measures. Athl. Train., 23:319.

20. Reitz, C.L., Rowinski, M.J., and Davies, G.J. (1988): Comparison of Cybex II and Kin-Com reliability of the measures of peak torque, work and power at three speeds. Phys. Ther., 69:782.

21. Snow, D.J., and Johnson, K. (1988): Reliability of two velocity controlled tests for the measurement of peak torque of the knee flexors during resisted muscle shortening and resisted muscle lengthening. Phys. Ther., 68:781.

22. Thorstensson, A., Grimby, G., and Karlsson, J. (1976): Force-velocity relations and fiber composition in human knee extensor muscles. J. Appl. Physiol., 40:12.

23. Timm, K.E. (1988): Reliability of Cybex 340 and MERAC isokinetic measures of peak torque, total work, and average power at five test speeds. Phys. Ther., 69:782.

24. Wessel, J., Mattison, G., Luongo, F., et al. (1988): Reliability of eccentric and concentric measurements. Phys. Ther., 68:782.

25. Wilk, K.E., and Johnson, R.E. (1988): The reliability of the Biodex B-200. Phys. Ther., 68:792.

26. Cook, E.E., Gray, V.L., Savinor-Nogue, E., et al. (1987): Shoulder antagonistic strength ratios: A comparison between college-level baseball pitchers. J. Orthop. Sports Phys. Ther., 8:451–461.

27. Nicholas, J.A., Strizak, A.M., and Veras, G. (1976): A study of thigh muscle weakness in different pathological states of the lower extremity. Am. J. Sports Med., 4:241–248.

28. Gleim, G.W., Nicholas, J.A., and Webb, J.N. (1978): Isokinetic evaluation following leg injuries. Physician Sportsmed., 6:74–82.

29. Boltz, S., and Davies, G.J. (1984): Leg length differences and correlation with total leg strength. J. Orthop. Sports Phys. Ther., 6:23–29.

30. Bryant, A.L., Pua, Y.H., and Clark, R.A. (2009): Morphology of knee extension torque-time curves following anterior cruciate ligament injury and reconstruction. J. Bone Joint Surg. Am., 91:1424–1431.

31. Eitzen, I., Eitzen, T.J., Holm, I., et al. (2010): Anterior cruciate ligament–deficient potential copers and noncopers reveal different isokinetic quadriceps strength profiles in the early stage after injury. Am. J. Sports Med., 38:586–593.

32. Ellenbecker, T.S., and Davies, G.J. (2000): The application of isokinetics in testing and rehabilitation of the shoulder complex. J. Athl. Train., 35:338–350.

33. Arms, S.W., Pope, M.H., Johnson, R.J., et al. (1984): The biomechanics of anterior cruciate ligament rehabilitation and reconstruction. Am. J. Sports Med., 12:8–18.

34. Brask, B., Lueke, R.H., and Soderberg, G.L. (1984): Electromyographical analysis of selected muscles during the lateral step-up exercise. Phys. Ther., 64:324–329.

35. Chandler, T.J., Wilson, G.D., and Store, M.H. (1989): The effects of the squat exercise on knee stability. Med. Sci. Sports Exerc., 21:299–303.

36. Cook, T.M., Zimmerman, C.L., Lux, K.M., et al. (1992): EMG comparison of lateral step-up and stepping machine exercise. J. Orthop. Sports Phys. Ther., 16:108–113.

37. DeCarlo, M., Porter, D.A., Gehlsen, G., et al. (1992): Electromyographic and cinematographic analysis of the lower extremity during closed and open kinetic chain exercise. Isokin. Exerc. Sci., 2:24–29.

38. Draganich, L.F., and Vahey, J.W. (1990): An in vitro study of anterior cruciate ligament strain induced by quadriceps and hamstring forces. J. Orthop. Res., 8:57–63.

39. Graham, V.L., Gehlsen, G.M., and Edwards, J.A. (1993): Electromyographic evaluation of closed and open kinetic chain knee rehabilitation exercises. J. Athl. Train., 28:23–30.

40. Gryzlo, S.M., Pateck, R.M., Pink, M., et al. (1989): Effects of position and speed on eccentric and concentric isokinetic testing of the shoulder rotators. J. Orthop. Sports Phys. Ther., 11:64–69.

41. Hsieh, H., and Walker, P.S. (1976): Stabilizing mechanisms of the loaded and unloaded knee joint. J. Bone Joint Surg. Am., 58:87–93.

42. Ohkoski, Y., and Yasada, K. (1989): Biomechanical analysis of shear force exerted to anterior cruciate ligament during half squat exercise. Orthop. Trans., 13:310.

43. Palmitier, R.A., An, K.N., Scott, S.G., et al. (1991): Kinetic chain exercise in knee rehabilitation. Sports Med., 11:402–413.

44. Reynolds, N.L., Worrell, T.W., and Perrin, D.H. (1992): Effects of a lateral step-up exercise protocol on quadriceps isokinetic peak torque values and thigh girth. J. Orthop. Sports Phys. Ther., 15:151–155.

45. Anderson, A.F., and Lipscomb, A.B. (1989): Analysis of rehabilitation techniques after anterior cruciate reconstruction. Am. J. Sports Med., 17:154–160.

46. DeCarlo, M., Shelbourne, K.D., McCarroll, J.R., et al. (1992): Traditional versus accelerated rehabilitation following ACL reconstruction: A one-year follow-up. J. Orthop. Sports Phys. Ther., 15:309–316.

47. Draganich, L.F., Jaeger, R.J., and Kralj, A.R. (1989): Coactivation of the hamstrings and quadriceps during extension of the knee. J. Bone Joint Surg. Am., 71:1075–1081.

48. Grana, W.A., and Muse, G. (1988): The effect of exercise on laxity in the anterior cruciate ligament deficient knee. Am. J. Sports Med., 16:586–588.

49. Harter, R.A., Osternig, L.R., Singer, K.M., et al. (1988): Long-term evaluation of knee stability and function following surgical reconstruction for anterior cruciate ligament insufficiency. Am. J. Sports Med., 16:434–443.

50. Hefzy, M.S., Grood, E.S., and Noyes, F.R. (1989): Factors affecting the region of most isometric femoral attachments. Part II. The anterior cruciate ligament. Am. J. Sports Med., 17:208–216.

51. Henning, C.E., Lynch, M.A., and Glick, K.R. (1985): An in-vivo strain gauge study of elongation of the anterior cruciate ligament. Am. J. Sports Med., 13:22–26.

52. Kannus, P.M., Jarvinen, M., Johnson, R., et al. (1992): Function of the quadriceps and hamstring muscles in knees with chronic partial deficiency of the ACL. Am. J. Sports Med., 20:162–168.

53. Lutz, G.E., Palmitier, R.A., An, K.N., et al. (1991): Closed kinetic chain exercises for athletes after reconstruction of the anterior cruciate ligament. Med. Sci. Sports Exerc., 23:413.

54. Lutz, G.E., Palmitier, R.A., An, K.N., et al. (1993): Comparison of tibiofemoral joint forces during open kinetic chain and closed kinetic chain exercises. J. Bone Joint Surg. Am., 75:732–739.

55. Maltry, J.A., Noble, P.C., Woods, G.W., et al. (1989): External stabilization of the anterior cruciate ligament deficient knee during rehabilitation. Am. J. Sports Med., 17:550–554.

56. Mandalidis, D., and O'Brien, M. (2010): Relationship between hand-grip isometric strength and isokinetic moment data of the shoulder stabilisers. J. Bodyw. Mov. Ther., 14:19–26.

57. Markolf, K.L., Barger, W.L., Shoemaker, S.C., et al. (1981): Role of joint load in knee stability. J. Bone Joint Surg. Am., 63:579–585.

58. Markolf, K.L., Gorek, J.F., Kabo, J.M., et al. (1990): Direct measurement of resultant forces in the anterior cruciate ligament. J. Bone Joint Surg. Am., 72:557–567.

59. Markolf, K.L., Graff-Radford, A., and Amstutz, H.C. (1978): In-vivo knee stability. J. Bone Joint Surg. Am., 60:664–674.

60. Markolf, K.L., Kochan, A., and Amstutz, H.C. (1984): Measurement of knee stiffness and laxity in patients with documented absence of anterior cruciate ligament. J. Bone Joint Surg. Am., 66:242–253.

61. Markolf, K.L., Mensch, J.S., and Amstutz, H.C. (1976): Stiffness and laxity of the knee. The contributions of the supporting structures. J. Bone Joint Surg. Am., 58:583–594.

62. More, R.C., Karras, B.T., Neiman, R., et al. (1993): Hamstrings: An anterior cruciate ligament protagonist. An in vitro study. Am. J. Sports Med., 21:231–237.

63. Renstrom, P., Arms, S.W., Stanwyck, T.S., et al. (1986): Strain within the anterior cruciate ligament during hamstring and quadriceps activity. Am. J. Sports Med., 14:83–87.

64. Sachs, R.A., Daniel, D.M., Stone, M.L., et al. (1989): Patellofemoral problems after anterior cruciate ligament reconstruction. Am. J. Sports Med., 17:760–764.

65. Shelbourne, K.D., and Nitz, P. (1990): Accelerated rehabilitation after anterior cruciate ligament rehabilitation. Am. J. Sports Med., 18:292–299.

66. Shoemaker, S.C., and Markolf, K.L. (1982): In-vivo rotatory knee stability. J. Bone Joint Surg. Am., 64:208–216.

67. Shoemaker, S.C., and Markolf, K.L. (1985): Effects of joint load on the stiffness and laxity of ligament-deficient knees. J. Bone Joint Surg. Am., 67:136–146.

68. Crandall, D., Richmond, J., Lau, J., et al. (1994): A meta-analysis of the treatment of the anterior cruciate ligament. Presented at the American Orthopedic Society of Sports Medicine, Palm Desert, CA.

69. Bynum, E.B., Barrack, R.L., and Alexander, A.H. (1995): Open versus closed chain kinetic exercises after anterior cruciate ligament reconstruction: A prospective randomized study. Am. J. Sports Med., 23:401–406.

70. Davies, G.J., and Romeyn, R.L. (1992 to present): Prospective, randomized single blind study comparing closed kinetic chain versus open and closed kinetic chain integrated rehabilitation programs of patients with ACL autograft infrapatellar tendon reconstructions. Research in progress.

71. Snyder-Mackler, L., Delitto, A., Bailey, S.L., et al. (1995): Strength of the quadriceps femoris muscle and functional recovery after reconstruction of the anterior cruciate ligament. J. Bone Joint Surg. Am., 77:1166–1173.

72. Crowell, J.R. (1987): College football: To brace or not to brace (Editorial). J. Bone Joint Surg. Am., 69:1.

73. Davies, G.J. (1995): Descriptive study comparing OKC vs. CKC isokinetic testing of the lower extremity in 200 patients with selected knee pathologies. Presented at the World Confederation of Physical Therapy. Washington, DC.

74. Davies, G.J., and Hoffman, S.D. (1993): Neuromuscular testing and rehabilitation of the shoulder complex. J. Orthop. Sports Phys. Ther., 18:449–458.

75. Greenberger, H.B., and Paterno, M.V. (1994): Comparison of an isokinetic strength test and functional performance test in the assessment of lower extremity function. J. Orthop. Sports Phys. Ther., 19:61.

76. Barber, S.D., Noyes, F.R., Mangine, R.E., et al. (1990): Quantitative assessment of functional limitations in normal and anterior cruciate ligament deficient knees. Clin. Orthop. Relat. Res., 225:204–214.

77. Shaffer, S.W., Payne, E.D., Gabbard, L.R., et al. (1994): Relationship between isokinetic and functional tests of the quadriceps. J. Orthop. Sports Phys. Ther., 19:55.

78. Tegner, Y., Lysholm, J., Lysholm, M., et al. (1986): A performance test to monitor rehabilitation and evaluate anterior cruciate ligament injuries. Am. J. Sports Med., 14:156–159.

79. Timm, K.E. (1988): Post-surgical knee rehabilitation: A five year study of four methods and 5,381 patients. Am. J. Sports Med., 16:463–468.

80. Wiklander, J., and Lysholm, J. (1987): Simple tests for surveying muscle strength and muscle stiffness in sportsmen. Int. J. Sports Med., 8:50–54.

81. Quincy, R., Davies, G.J., Kolbeck, K., et al. (2000): Isokinetic exercise: The effects of training specificity on shoulder power. J. Athletic Training, 35:564.

82. Sullivan, E.P., Markos, P.D., and Minor, M.D. (1982): An Integrated Approach to Therapeutic Exercise: Theory and Clinical Application. Reston, VA, Reston Publishing.

83. Davies, G.J. (1995): The need for critical thinking in rehabilitation. J. Sport Rehabil., 4:1–22.

84. Feiring, D.C., and Ellenbecker, T.S. (1995): Open versus closed chain isokinetic testing with ACL reconstructed patients. Med. Sci. Sports Exerc., 17:S106.

85. Maitland, M.E., Lowe, R., and Stewart, S. (1993): Does Cybex testing increase knee laxity after anterior cruciate ligament reconstructions? Am. J. Sports Med., 21:690–695.

86. Jurist, K.A., and Otis, J.C. (1985): Anteroposterior tibiofemoral displacements during isometric extension efforts. Am. J. Sports Med., 13:254–258.

87. Wilk, K.E., and Andrews, J.R. (1993): The effects of pad placement and angular velocity on tibial displacement during isokinetic exercise. J. Orthop. Sports Phys. Ther., 17:23–30.

88. Grood, E.S., Suntay, W.J., Noyes, F.R., et al. (1984): Biomechanics of the knee-extension exercise. J. Bone Joint Surg. Am., 66:725–734.

89. Anderson, M.A., Gieck, J.H., Perrin, D., et al. (1991): The relationship among isometric, isotonic and isokinetic concentric and eccentric quadriceps and hamstring force and three components of athletic performance. J. Orthop. Sports Phys. Ther., 14:114–120.

90. Patel, R.R., Hurwitz, D.E., Bush-Joseph, C.A., et al. (2003): Comparison of clinical and dynamic knee function in patients with anterior cruciate ligament deficiency. Am. J. Sports Med., 31:68–74.

91. Petschnig, R., Baron, R., and Albrecht, M. (1998): The relationship between isokinetic quadriceps strength test and hop tests for distance and one-legged vertical jump test following anterior cruciate ligament reconstruction. J. Orthop. Sports Phys. Ther., 28:23–31.

92. Jones, P.A., and Bampouras, T.M. (2010): A comparison of isokinetic and functional methods of assessing bilateral strength imbalance. J. Strength Cond. Res., 24:1553–1558.

93. Sbriccoli, P., Camomilla, V., DiMario, A., et al. (2010): Neuromuscular control adaptations in elite athletes: The case of top level karateka. Eur. J. Appl. Physiol., 108:1269–1280.

94. Karanikas, K., Arampatzis, A., and Bruggemann, G.P. (2009): Motor task and muscle strength followed different adaptation patterns after anterior cruciate ligament reconstruction. Eur. J. Phys. Rehabil. Med., 45:37–45.

95. Oiestad, B.E., Holm, I., Gunderson, R., et al. (2010): Quadriceps muscle weakness after anterior cruciate ligament reconstruction: A risk factor for knee osteoarthritis? Arthritis Care Res. (Hoboken), 62:1706–1714.

96. Keays, S.L., Newcombe, P.A., Bullock-Saxton, J.E., et al. (2010): Factors involved in the development of osteoarthritis after anterior cruciate ligament surgery. Am. J. Sports Med., 38:455–463.

97. Segal, N.A., Glass, N.A., Felson, D.T., et al. (2010): Effect of quadriceps strength and proprioception on risk for knee osteoarthritis. Med. Sci. Sports Exer., 42:2081–2088.

98. Hiemstra, L.A., Webber, S., MacDonald, P.B., and Kriellaars, D.J. (2004): Hamstring and quadriceps strength balance in normal and hamstring anterior cruciate ligament–reconstructed subjects. Clin. J. Sport Med., 14:274–280.

99. Ageberg, E., Thomee, R., Neeter, C., et al. (2008): Muscle strength and functional performance in patients with anterior cruciate ligament injury treated with training and surgical reconstruction or training only: A two to five-year followup. Arthritis Rheum., 59:1773–1779.

100. Sekir, U., Gur, H., and Akova, B. (2010): Early versus late start of isokinetic hamstring-strengthening exercise after anterior cruciate ligament reconstruction with patellar tendon graft. Am. J. Sports Med., 38:492–500.

101. Stefanska, M., Rafalska, M., and Skrzek, A. (2009): Functional assessment of knee muscles 13 weeks after anterior cruciate ligament reconstruction—pilot study. Orthop. Traumatol. Rehabil., 11:145–155.

102. Eitzen, I., Moksnes, H., Snyder-Mackler, L., and Risberg, M.A. (2010): A progressive 5-week exercise therapy program leads to significant improvement in knee function early after anterior cruciate ligament injury. J. Orthop. Sports Phys Ther., 40:705–721.

103. Diracoglu, D., Baskent, A., Yagci, I., et al. (2009): Isokinetic strength measurements in early knee osteoarthritis. Acta Reumatol. Port., 34:72–77.

104. Segal, N.A., Glass, N.A., Tomer, J., et al. (2010): Quadriceps weakness predicts risk for knee joint space narrowing in women in the MOST cohort. Osteoarthritis Cartilage, 18:769–775.

105. Kean, C.O., Birmingham, T.B., Garland, S.J., et al. (2010): Minimal detectable change in quadriceps strength and voluntary muscle activation in patients with knee osteoarthritis. Arch. Phys. Med. Rehabil., 91:1447–1451.

106. Rydevik, K., Fernandes, L., Nordsletten, L., and Risberg, M.A. (2010): Functioning and disability in patients with hip osteoarthritis with mild to moderate pain. J. Orthop. Sports Phys. Ther., 40:616–624.

107. Julia, M., Dupeyron, A., Laffont, I., et al. (2010): Reproducibility of isokinetic peak torque assessments of the hip flexor and extensor muscles. Ann. Phys. Rehabil. Med., 53:293–305.

108. Boling, M.C., Padua, D.A., and Alexander Creighton, R. (2009): Concentric and eccentric torque of the hip musculature in individuals with and without patellofemoral pain. J. Athl. Train., 44:7–13.

109. Meister, K., and Andrews, J.R. (1993): Classification and treatment of rotator cuff injuries in the overhand athlete. J. Orthop. Sports Phys. Ther., 18:413–421.

110. Davies, G.J., and Ellenbecker, T.S. (1993): Total arm strength rehabilitation for shoulder and elbow overuse injuries. In: Timm, K. E. (ed.), Orthopaedic Physical Therapy Home Study Course. Orthopaedic Section. American Physical Therapy Association, La Crosse, WI.

111. Dillman, C.J., Fleisig, G.S., and Andrews, J.R. (1993): Biomechanics of pitching with emphasis upon shoulder kinematics. J. Orthop. Sports Phys. Ther., 18:402–408.

112. Shapiro, R., and Steine, R.L. (1992): Shoulder rotation velocities. Technical report submitted to the Lexington Clinic, Lexington, KY.

113. Dillman, C.J. (1991): The upper extremity in tennis and throwing athletes. Presented at a United States Tennis Association meeting, Tucson, AZ.

114. Vangheluwe, B., and Hebbelinck, K.M. (1986): Muscle actions and ground reaction forces in tennis. Int. J. Sport Biomech., 2:89–99.

115. Kendall, F.D., and McCreary, E.K. (1983): Muscle Testing and Function, 3rd ed. Baltimore, Lippincott Williams & Wilkins.

116. Wakin, K.G., Clarke, H.H., Elkins, E.C., and Martin, G.M. (1950): Relationship between body position and application of muscle power to movements of joints. Arch. Phys. Med. Rehabil., 31:81–89.

117. Ellenbecker, T.S. (1994): Muscular strength relationship between normal grade manual muscle testing and isokinetic measurement of the shoulder internal and external rotators. J. Orthop. Sports Phys. Ther., 1:72.

118. Nicholas, J.A., Sapega, A., Kraus, H., and Webb, J.N. (1978): Factors influencing manual muscle tests in physical therapy. J. Bone Joint Surg. Am., 60:186.

119. Inman, V.T., Saunders, J.B., de, C.M., and Abbot, L.C. (1944): Observations of the function of the shoulder joint. J. Bone Joint Surg., 26:1–30.

120. Kronberg, M., Nemeth, F., and Brostrom, L.A. (1990): Muscle activity and coordination in the normal shoulder: An electromyographic study. Clin. Orthop. Relat. Res., 257:76–85.

121. Warner, J.P., Micheli, L.J., Arslanian, L.E., et al. (1990): Patterns of flexibility, laxity and strength in normal shoulders and shoulders with instability and impingement. Am. J. Sports Med., 18:366–375.

122. Saha, A.K. (1971): Dynamic stability of the glenohumeral joint. Acta Orthop. Scand., 42:491–505.

123. Hageman, P.A., Mason, D.K., Rydlund, K.W., et al. (1989): Effects of position and speed on eccentric and concentric isokinetic testing of the shoulder rotators. J. Orthop. Phys. Ther., 11:64–69.

124. Soderberg, G.J., and Blaschak, M.J. (1987): Shoulder internal and external rotation peak torque production through a velocity spectrum in differing positions. J. Orthop. Sports Phys. Ther., 8:518–524.

125. Walmsley, R.P., and Szybbo, C. (1987): A comparative study of the torque generated by the shoulder internal and external rotator muscles in different positions and at varying speeds. J. Orthop. Sports Phys. Ther., 9:217–222.

126. Daniels, L., and Worthingham, C. (1986): Muscle Testing: Techniques of Manual Examination, 5th ed. Philadelphia: Saunders.

127. Ellenbecker, T.S., and Derscheid, G.L. (1988): Rehabilitation of overuse injuries in the shoulder. Clin. Sports Med., 8:583–604.

128. Elliot, B., March, T., and Blanksby, B. (1986): A three dimensional cinematographic analysis of the tennis serve. Int. J. Sport Biomech., 2:260–271.

129. Ellenbecker, T.S., Feiring, D.C., Dehart, R.L., and Rich, M. (1992): Isokinetic shoulder strength: Coronal versus scapular plane testing in upper extremity unilateral dominant athletes. Phys. Ther., 72:S80–S81.

130. Greenfield, B.H., Donatelli, R., Wooden, M.J., and Wilkes, J. (1990): Isokinetic evaluation of shoulder rotational strength between the plane of the scapula and the frontal plane. Am. J. Sports Med., 18:124–128.

131. Basset, R.W., Browne, A.O., Morrey, B.F., and An, K.N. (1994): Glenohumeral muscle force and moment mechanics in a position of shoulder instability. J. Biomech., 23:405–415.

132. Holm, I., Brox, J.I., Ludvigsen, P., and Steen, H. (1996): External rotation—best isokinetic movement pattern for evaluation of muscle function in rotator tendinosis. A prospective study with a 2-year follow up. Isokin. Exerc. Sci., 5:121–125.

133. Alderink, G.J., and Kluck, D.J. (1986): Isokinetic shoulder strength in high school and college pitchers. J. Orthop. Sports Phys. Ther., 7:163–172.

134. Chandler, T.J., Kibler, W.B., Stracener, E.C., et al. (1992): Shoulder strength, power, and endurance in college tennis players. Am. J. Sports Med., 20:455–458.

135. Ellenbecker, T.S. (1991): A total arm strength isokinetic profile of highly skilled tennis players. Isokin. Exerc. Sci., 1:9–21.

136. Ellenbecker, T.S. (1992): Shoulder internal and external rotation strength and range of motion of highly skilled junior tennis players. Isokin. Exerc. Sci., 2:1–8.

137. Ellenbecker, T.S., Dehart, R.L., and Boeckmann, R. (1992): Isokinetic shoulder strength of the rotator cuff in professional baseball pitchers. Phys. Ther., 72:S81.

138. Ellenbecker, T.S., and Mattalino, A.J. (1997): Concentric isokinetic shoulder internal and external rotation strength in professional baseball pitchers. J. Orthop. Sports Phys. Ther., 25:323–328.

139. Hinton, R.Y. (1988): Isokinetic evaluation of shoulder rotational strength in high school baseball pitchers. Am. J. Sports Med., 16:274–279.

140. Ohkoski, Y., Yasuda, K., Kaneda, K., et al. (1991): Biomechanical analysis of rehabilitation in the standing position. Am. J. Sports Med., 19:605–610.

141. Brown, L.P., Neihues, S.L., Harrah, A., et al. (1988): Upper extremity range of motion and isokinetic strength of the internal and external shoulder rotators in major league baseball players. Am. J. Sports Med., 16:577–585.

142. Wilk, K.E., Andrews, J.R., Arrigo, C.A., et al. (1993): The strength characteristics of internal and external rotator muscles in professional baseball pitchers. Am. J. Sports Med., 21:61–66.

143. Ivey, F.M., Calhoun, J.H., Rusche, K., et al. (1984): Normal values for isokinetic testing of shoulder strength. Med. Sci. Sports Exerc., 16:127.

144. Wilk, K.E., and Arrigo, C.A. (1993): Current concepts in the rehabilitation of the athletic shoulder. J. Orthop. Sports Phys. Ther., 18:365–378.

145. Hellwig, E.V., Perrin, D.H., Tis, L.L., and Shenk, B.S. (1991): Effect of gravity correction on shoulder external/internal rotator reciprocal muscle group ratios. J. Natl. Athl. Trainers Assoc., 26:154.

146. Wilk, K.E., Arrigo, C.A., and Andrews, J.R. (1991): Standardized isokinetic testing protocol for the throwing shoulder: The throwers series. Isokin. Exerc. Sci., 1:63–71.

147. Wilk, K.E., Arrigo, C.A., and Andrews, J.R. (1992): Isokinetic testing of the shoulder abductors and adductors: Windowed vs. nonwindowed data collection. J. Orthop. Sports Phys. Ther., 15:107–112.

148. Jobe, F.W., Tibone, J.E., Perry, J., et al. (1983): An EMG analysis of the shoulder in throwing and pitching. A preliminary report. Am. J. Sports Med., 11:3–5.

149. Kennedy, K., Altcheck, D.W., and Glick, I.V. (1993): Concentric and eccentric isokinetic rotator cuff ratios in skilled tennis players. Isokin. Exerc. Sci., 3:155–159.

150. Saccol, M.F., Gracitelli, G.C., da Silva, R.T., et al. (2010): Shoulder functional ratio in elite junior tennis players. Phys. Ther. Sport, 11:8–11.

151. Davies, G.J., and Ellenbecker, T.S. (1992): Eccentric isokinetics. Orthop. Phys. Ther. Clin. North Am., 1:297–336.

152. Ellenbecker, T.S., Davies, G.J., and Rowinski, M.J. (1988): Concentric versus eccentric isokinetic strengthening of the rotator cuff: Objective data versus functional test. Am. J. Sports Med., 16:64–69.

153. Mont, M.A., Choen, D.B., Campbell, K.R., et al. (1994): Isokinetic concentric versus eccentric training of the shoulder rotators with functional evaluation of performance enhancement in elite tennis players. Am. J. Sports Med., 22:513–517.

154. Gore, D.R., Murray, M.P., Sepic, S.B., and Gardner, G.M. (1986): Shoulder muscle strength and range of motion following surgical repair of full thickness rotator cuff tears. J. Bone Joint Surg. Am., 68:266–272.

155. Rabin, S.J., and Post, M.P. (1990): A comparative study of clinical muscle testing and Cybex evaluation after shoulder operations. Clin. Orthop. Relat. Res., 258:147–156.

156. Walker, S.W., Couch, W.H., Boester, G.A., and Sprowl, D.W. (1987): Isokinetic strength of the shoulder after repair of a torn rotator cuff. J. Bone Joint Surg. Am., 69:1041–1044.

157. Walmsley, R.P., and Hartsell, H. (1992): Shoulder strength following surgical rotator cuff repair: A comparative analysis using isokinetic testing. J. Orthop. Sports Phys. Ther., 15:215–222.

158. Bigoni, M., Gorla, M., Guerrasio, S., et al. (2009): Shoulder evaluation with isokinetic strength testing after arthroscopic rotator cuff repairs. J. Shoulder Elbow Surg., 18:178–183.

159. Oh, J.H., Yoon, J.P., Kim, J.Y., and Oh, C.H. (2010): Isokinetic muscle performance test can predict the status of rotator cuff muscle. Clin. Orthop. Relat. Res., 468:1506–1513.

160. Pedegana, L.R., Elsner, R.C., Roberts, D., et al. (1982): The relationship of upper extremity strength to throwing speed. Am. J. Sports Med., 10:352–354.

161. Bartlett, L.R., Browne, A.O., Morrey, B.F., and An, K.N. (1994): Glenohumeral muscle force and moment mechanics in a position of shoulder instability. J. Biomech., 23:405–415.

162. Pawlowski, D., and Perrin, D.H. (1989): Relationship between shoulder and elbow isokinetic peak torque, torque acceleration energy, average power, and total work and throwing velocity in intercollegiate pitchers. Athl. Train., 24:129–132.

163. Andrade Mdos, S., Fleury, A.M., de Lira, C.A., et al. (2010): Profile of isokinetic eccentric-to-concentric strength ratios of shoulder rotator muscles in elite female team handball players. J. Sports Sci., 28:743–749.

164. Edouard, P., Beguin, L., Fayolle-Minon, I., et al. (2010): Relationship between strength and functional indexes (Rowe and Walch-Duplay scores) after shoulder surgical stabilization by the Latarjet technique. Ann. Phys. Rehabil. Med., 53:499–510.

165. Lin, Y.C., Thompson, A., Kung, J.T., et al. (2010): Functional isokinetic strength ratios in baseball players with injured elbows. J. Sport Rehabil., 19:21–29.

166. Lucas, D.B. (1973): Biomechanics of the shoulder joint. Arch. Surg., 107:425.

167. Astrand, P., and Rodahl, K. (1977): Textbook of Work Physiology. New York, McGraw-Hill.

168. Rowinski, M.J. (1985): Afferent neurobiology of the joint. In Davies G. J., and Gould J.A. (eds.): Orthopaedic and Sports Physical Therapy. St. Louis, Mosby.

169. Henneman, E., Somjen, G., and Carpenter, D.O. (1965): Functional significance of cell size in spinal motorneurons. J. Neurophysiol., 28:560–580.

170. Green, H.J. (1986): Muscle power: Fibre type, recruitment, metabolism and fatigue. In Jones N.L., McCartney N., and McCoas A.J. (eds.): Human Muscle Power. Champaign, IL, Human Kinetics.

171. Brown, L.E., Whitehurse, M., Findley, B.W., et al. (1995): Isokinetic load range during shoulder rotation exercise in elite male junior tennis players. J. Strength Cond. Res., 9:160–164.

172. Clark, R.A., Humphries, B., Hohmann, E., and Bryant, A.L. (2011): The influence of variable range of motion training on neuromuscular performance and control of external loads. J. Strength Cond. Res., 25:704–711.

173. Caizzo, V.J., Perrine, J.J., Edgerton, V.R., et al. (1980): Alterations in the in-vivo force-velocity. Med. Sci. Sports Exerc., 12:134.

174. Lesmes, G.R., Costill, D.L., Coycle, E.F., and Fine, W.J. (1978): Muscle strengthening and power changes during maximal isokinetic training. Med. Sci. Sports Exerc., 10:266–269.

175. Moffroid, M., and Whipple, R.H. (1970): Specificity of speed of exercise. Phys. Ther., 50:1693–1699.

176. Ariki, P., Davies, G.J., Siweart, M., et al. (1985): Rest interval between isokinetic velocity spectrum rehabilitation sets. Phys. Ther., 65:733–734.

177. Fleck, S. (1983): Interval training: Physiological bases. J. Strength Cond. Res., 5:4–7.

178. Barnam, J.N. (1978): Mechanical Kinesiology. St Louis, Mosby.

179. Remaud, A., Comu, C., and Geuvel, A. (2010): Neuromuscular adaptations to 8-week strength training: Isotonic versus isokinetic mode. Eur. J. Appl. Physiol., 108:59–69.

180. Oliveira, A.S., Corvino, R.B., Goncalves, M., et al. (2010): Effects of a single habituation session on neuromuscular isokinetic profile at different movement velocities. Eur. J. Appl. Physiol., 110:1127–1133.

26

Plyometric Training and Drills

Anthony Cuoco, DPT, MS, CSCS, and Timothy F. Tyler, PT, MS, ATC

CHAPTER OBJECTIVES

- Explain the fundamental basis of plyometric training, its origins, and its applications.
- Describe the mechanical and neuromuscular physiologic processes involved in the stretch-shortening cycle and how it applies to plyometrics.
- Describe the important clinical considerations surrounding the appropriate use of plyometrics in the orthopedic and sports medicine rehabilitation setting.

- Describe and apply important fundamentals for the use of plyometrics as a rehabilitation tool, including pretraining assessment, application of exercise prescription principles, and injury prevention.
- Design a basic plyometric training program at low-, medium-, and high-intensity levels.
- Use a variety of upper and lower extremity plyometric exercises as a part of the rehabilitation process.

Speed and strength are integral components of sports that are found to varying degrees in virtually all athletic movements. Simply stated, the combination of speed and strength is power. For many years, coaches and athletes have sought to improve power to enhance performance. Recently, rehabilitation specialists have implemented techniques to prevent injuries and improve power to optimize postsurgical and postinjury outcomes. Throughout the twentieth century and no doubt long before that, jumping, bounding, and hopping exercises have been used in various ways to enhance athletic performance. In recent years this distinct method of training for power and explosiveness has been termed *plyometrics*. Plyometrics is a form of strength training designed to develop explosive power in athletics.[1] Plyometric exercises stress the rapid generation of (maximal) force, primarily during the eccentric (lengthening) phase of muscle action, and speeding the transition between the eccentric and concentric (shortening) phases. This rapid deceleration-acceleration movement produces an explosive reaction that increases both speed and power.[2] The ultimate aim is to increase muscle performance to absorb and move an applied load throughout its functional range of motion and allow an athlete to translate strength into power more efficiently. The concentric phase of muscle activity during plyometric training has been estimated to result in 18% to 20% more force than a concentric contraction from a resting position.[2,3]

Although the actual term *plyometrics* is relatively new, this particular form of training has been in existence for quite some time. Translated from its Greek origins, it literally means to

increase measurement.[4] Many studies have shown effective, measurable increases in power and jumping ability via plyometric training programs.[5] However, whether improvements in strength and power with plyometric training directly translate into improvements in functional outcome measures in rehabilitation may be questioned in some cases.[6] Plyometric training is often considered the missing link between weight training (strength) and athletic performance (power), with particular emphasis on the speed of activity. Plyometric training was first developed in the Soviet Union for its intense and very effective athletic development program during the 1960s. It came to the attention of the West during the 1970s and, by about 1980, had become a valuable tool in major athletic programs. The term was first applied in 1975 by American track and field coach Fred Wilt to describe the training methods used by Eastern European athletes at the time, which supposedly was the reason for differences between the performance of Eastern and Western athletes. During the 1980s, Donald Chu published the first articles on plyometric training methods in this country, and he has been a leader in this area ever since.[4,7,8] In the early 1990s, George Davies and Kevin Wilk introduced plyometrics into rehabilitation programs.[9,10]

In the early years of plyometric training, most drills focused on developing jumping ability. More recently, some drills have been designed to develop lateral movement qualities and others to improve upper body power, but plyometrics seems to have been focused traditionally on enhancing lower body power. In the past 10 years, plyometrics has been used not only for the lower extremity to increase strength and conditioning but also for the upper extremity as a rehabilitation tool and as part of injury prevention programs.

GENERAL THEORY

The premise behind plyometric training is that the maximum force that a muscle can develop is attained during a rapid eccentric contraction. However, it should be recognized that muscles seldom perform one type of contraction in isolation during athletic movements. When a concentric contraction occurs (muscle shortening) immediately after an eccentric contraction (muscle lengthening), the force generated can be dramatically increased. If a muscle is stretched, much of the energy required to stretch it is lost as heat, but some of this energy can be stored by the elastic components of the muscle. This stored energy is available to the muscle only during a subsequent contraction. It is important to realize that this energy boost is lost if the eccentric contraction is not followed immediately by a concentric effort. To express this greater force the muscle must contract within the shortest time possible. This whole process is usually called the stretch-shortening cycle (SSC) and is the underlying mechanism of plyometric training. Theoretically, the SSC increases power production based on two proposed models: (1) mechanical and (2) neurophysiologic. The mechanical model describes the series elastic component of the musculotendinous unit as the key element of plyometric exercise, whereas the neurophysiologic model involves potentiation of concentric muscle action by use of the stretch reflex. The reflex component of plyometric exercise is based on proprioception provided by the muscle spindles during the stretching (eccentric) action.[4] Even though these two models can be viewed as separate descriptions of plyometric theory, they are in fact tightly interwoven in explaining the mechanisms involved in plyometric training.

CLINICAL RELEVANCY

Overall, the final phase of rehabilitating an injured athlete introduces functional, sport-specific components of athletic performance. Depending on the athlete, this will typically involve increasing metabolic capacity, strength, power, speed, and agility. It is during this final phase that the use of plyometrics is most appropriate. In earlier phases of rehabilitation, the clinician has presumably addressed joint and soft tissue mobility, range of motion, flexibility, biomechanics, balance, proprioception/kinesthesia, endurance, and strength. The challenge of the final, sport-specific phase is designing rehabilitation progression that maximizes neuromuscular and skeletal adaptations without adversely affecting biologic healing. Sport-specific training means that the movement that the patient performs should match, as closely as possible, the movements encountered during competition without jeopardizing the patient's health status. If the patient is a basketball player practicing for rebounding or a volleyball player interested in increasing vertical jump height (VJH), drop jumping or box jumping may be the right exercise. If, however, the patient is a quarterback 6 months after a Bankart repair who is trying to increase throwing velocity, upper body plyometrics may be far more appropriate. In the volleyball and quarterback cases, though, the strength and power generated from both the lower and upper extremities might be considered.

Of course, plyometric training is not appropriate for all patients. For instance, an injured gymnast who is trying to develop the shoulder strength to maintain static, slow-moving positions on the balance beam may not require any plyometric drills. In contrast, one study showed that plyometric training significantly improved VJH in elite volleyball players.[11] Plyometric training is not generally a favored choice of exercise for increasing muscle mass or muscular endurance. Therefore, plyometric training is probably not appropriate for muscles that are predominately type I muscle fibers or that act as stabilizers. In fact, unless the athlete participates in a sport that requires explosive movements (e.g., volleyball, baseball pitching, sprinting, basketball, high jump), there is no compelling reason to introduce plyometrics into the rehabilitation program.

APPLIED ANATOMY/PHYSIOLOGY AND THE BIOMECHANICS OF PLYOMETRICS

Similar to other modes of therapeutic exercise, safe and effective interventions using plyometrics require that clinicians be familiar with applied neuromuscular physiologic principles. The use of plyometrics as a training method is primarily based on two fundamental dynamic qualities of muscle tissue: elasticity and contractility. The capacity of working muscles to generate greater (or maximal) force in a minimal amount of time depends on these tissue qualities, along with neuromuscular control, strength, and flexibility. In fact, most of the early physiologic research relevant to plyometrics was described as a muscle action termed the *stretch-shortening cycle*.[7] Currently, the SSC is the physiologic theory that forms the basis of plyometrics.

Stretch-Shortening Cycle

The SSC can be defined as a phenomenon whereby the natural pattern of lengthening of active muscle produces energy that is stored in the musculotendinous unit for later use in a subsequent shortening, or concentric, contraction of the SSC. It is this eccentric-concentric coupling that forms the basis of the SSC. In an often-referenced study, Cavagna[12] established that concentric muscle performance in an SSC is enhanced greater than that in a pure concentric-only action. In practical terms, plyometrics involves high-velocity eccentric contraction or prestretching of a muscle before an immediate reciprocal concentric contraction of that same muscle (group). The eccentric contraction stores energy that can be used to maximize the amount of power produced during concentric contraction of that muscle or muscle group.[13,14] This storage of elastic energy in musculotendinous tissues contributes to the increased force produced in the subsequent concentric contraction phase and increased efficiency of movement.[15,16] Muscles and tendons have an intrinsic stiffness that resists stretch and then reciprocates with a muscle contraction stimulated by the stretch reflex loop.[13,17] Though an oversimplification, this phenomenon can be visualized as the action of a spring. Biomechanically, one can relate the SSC to the simple action of a person attempting to improve VJH by instinctively performing a partial squat before jumping in place. The simple act of walking or running uses the SSC with each stride, which begins with the loading response through an eccentric contraction of the quadriceps, soleus, and gastrocnemius muscles, followed by a concentric push-off action. Hence, the SSC of plyometric exercise is a natural motion, given the mechanical properties of the musculoskeletal system. The SSC has been studied by many investigators, and it is generally agreed that several important factors of neuromuscular anatomy and physiology should be considered: serial elastic components of muscles and tendons, proprioception, and gross musculotendinous architecture. The eccentric-concentric coupling of the SSC stimulates the proprioceptors of the muscle spindle, Golgi tendon organs (GTOs), and ligament receptors to facilitate recruitment of the motor units required to maximize the concentric power generated during plyometric activity (Box 26-1).[16,18,19]

Histologic Considerations in Skeletal Muscle

Histologically, the level of the fascicles is a fundamental component of the serial elasticity of muscle. Although much research has been conducted on the dynamics of the SSC at the histologic level, the behavior of human skeletal muscle during SSC exercises has not been directly investigated in vivo. It has been well documented in the literature that activated muscle stretched before shortening performs more forcefully.[12] However, the exact mechanisms that mediate the stretch-enhanced performance have been a source of controversy. Kubo et al examined changes in fascicle length and tendon structure in humans during SSC exercises involving the gastrocnemius muscle at both fast and slow speeds with real-time ultrasonography. They found that both fascicle and tendon structures are lengthened at the dorsiflexion phase and shortened at the plantar flexion phase.[20] The stretching ability depends on many factors, but the rate and magnitude of the stretch applied contribute to how much force a muscle can generate.

Though perhaps not as critical in terms of stretching dynamics, the fiber types used for plyometrics are worth reviewing. It is well documented that type II, or fast-twitch, fibers are capable of generating more force than type I, or slow-twitch, fibers can. This is primarily a function of the increased cross-sectional area, larger motor units, and high glycolytic capacity associated with type II fibers.[21-23] The amount of force necessary during the eccentric and subsequent explosive concentric phases of SSC exercise necessitates the recruitment of type II fibers. It should also be noted that type II fibers are also readily fatigable. Although a detailed discussion of the metabolic properties of muscle fiber types is

beyond the scope of this chapter, it is important for the clinician to be aware of the metabolic systems that contribute to optimal performance of muscle tissues during plyometric exercise. Type II fibers are classified further into at least two basic types: type IIa and type IIb. Fast-twitch type IIb fibers are those that rely primarily on the phosphate and glycolytic energy systems and are termed *fast glycolytic fibers*. Type IIa fibers are more like a hybrid between the slow oxidative type I fibers and the type IIb fibers and are termed *fast glycolytic-oxidative fibers*.[21-23] Plyometric exercise should focus on adaptation of these fibers to overload with anaerobic training while still taking into consideration those type IIa fibers that use both the oxidative and glycolytic energy systems. Both the force generation and endurance qualities necessary in functional athletic activity require that the athlete develop both classes of type II fibers. Practically, consider the metabolic demands imposed on a basketball player jumping for consecutive rebounds over a 5-second period, and then consider that same task early and very late in the same game.

Neuromuscular Physiology: Muscle Spindles and Golgi Tendon Organs

Muscle spindles function primarily as stretch receptors, as observed clinically in the performance of standard reflex testing (e.g., the knee jerk). When the patellar tendon is tapped with a reflex hammer, the muscle spindles are stimulated, which causes an immediate concentric contraction of the quadriceps muscle group. This minimal latency time between the quick stretch and subsequent contraction is mediated at the level of the spinal cord as a monosynaptic reflex. Muscle spindles are sensitive to changes in velocity and are innervated by type 1a nerve fibers. These afferent nerve fibers conduct the impulse directly to the spinal cord, where they are immediately conducted via interneurons to alpha motor neurons, which stimulate muscle contraction. The brain is not involved in this spinal reflex loop, contributing to the speed at which the stretch-contraction cycle occurs.[24]

Muscle spindles are located within extrafusal (skeletal) muscle fibers and consist of connective tissue surrounding intrafusal fibers in a capsular structure. Muscle spindles are innervated by myelinated afferent nerve fibers, which enter the capsule of and spiral around the intrafusal fibers. Based on the architecture of the muscle spindle, stretching of the skeletal (extrafusal) fibers also stretches the intrafusal fibers. This stretch increases the firing rate of the afferent fibers innervating the intrafusal fibers, thus "loading" the muscle spindle. When the stretch is released or lessened, the firing rate diminishes. Both primary and secondary afferent fibers are present, and these fibers contribute to the ability of the spindle to detect small changes in length. Thus, the muscle spindle is sensitive to changes in muscle length, as well as to the speed and magnitude of the stretch.[25]

Although the muscle spindle reacts to stretch, it does not simply "turn off" when the muscle is no longer stretched; the fibers continue to send messages when the muscle has begun to concentrically contract and shorten. The central nervous system (CNS) regulates the loading through alpha motor neurons, which modulate spindle activity and thereby make the transition from stretch to contraction smoother.[25] This modulation contributes to muscle tone and thus to the intrinsic stiffness of the muscle. Therefore, the muscle tends to act as a spring that enables the SSC to produce force with precision.

Although the muscle spindle is sensitive to stretch, the GTOs provide complementary information to the CNS about muscle activity. Specifically, length and the degree of tension are monitored by GTOs. GTOs are encapsulated collagen structures typically located at the musculotendinous junction. Each GTO is innervated by nerve fibers that wrap around the collagen bundles. As the collagen bundles are stretched, they straighten and the nerve fibers fire more rapidly. GTOs are sensitive to small changes in muscle tension. Because GTOs surround collagen and not extrafusal muscle fibers, they are not as sensitive to stretch since collagen has a stiffer molecular structure than muscle fiber does. Thus, most of the stretch is absorbed by the muscle fibers and the muscle spindles. This makes GTOs more sensitive to active muscle contraction that stresses the musculotendinous junction to a greater degree.[25]

Gross Musculotendinous Structure

On a gross anatomic and clinical level, muscles and tendons resist stretch as force increases. Muscle stiffness can be defined as change in force over change in muscle length. This inherent stiffness is the resistance to stretch by the fibers of the active muscle and tendons before the changes in activation modulated by the muscle spindles and GTOs described earlier occur. Benn et al[26] described this property of stiffness as the stretch work used in completion of the SSC. Several authors have studied the relationship between SSC performance and muscle stiffness. Goslow et al[27] found that cat tendons with a high degree of stiffness may transfer energy more rapidly to attached muscles, thereby resulting in earlier activation of the stretch reflex and thus more rapid contraction of the muscle. Wilson et al[17] concluded that in humans, a stiffer musculotendinous unit may result in an increased rate of concentric contraction and more rapid transmission of force to the working limbs. In another study these authors concluded that decreased musculotendinous stiffness actually enhances SSC performance in a bench press exercise because more elastic energy can be stored in a less stiff musculotendinous unit. Other studies have concluded that increased musculotendinous stiffness may be more important than the ability to store more elastic energy in terms of enhancing SSC performance in activities such as sprinting.[26] Given these equivocal results, the principle of specificity in terms of exercise mode and the muscles involved may be an important distinction in determining optimal musculotendinous stiffness.

To this point, one can see that the histologic structure of muscle and tendons can both enhance and hinder movement and force-generating capacity. Although the inherent elastic components of the musculotendinous unit can store energy for use in generating force and powerful movement, gross structural aspects may be present that limit the ability of a muscle to maximize the SSC. Neural factors and recruitment of fibers, as well as the metabolic capacities of muscle and the appropriate exercise conditioning, all have an impact on performance.

Finally, Brownstein and Bronner[18] formulated a classification system based on three types of musculotendinous units (Table 26-1). Their theory centers around gross muscle structure (i.e., length of the muscles and tendons).

Fundamentals of Plyometrics

Plyometrics is defined by the SSC and is an inherent part of the functional aspects of athletic movement. The primary basis of plyometrics is to use both the serial elastic (mechanical) and neurophysiologic components described earlier to combine speed and strength in the production of power. Plyometrics has been described as stretch-shortening drills or reactive neuromuscular training. There are basically three phases of a plyometric exercise and the SSC.

The *eccentric phase* (sometimes called the preloading or setting phase) refers to the early moments in the movement in which the muscle spindles are loaded and stretched during an eccentric contraction, such as stepping from a box onto the ground and squatting as one lands to absorb the ground reaction force. This is when storing of elastic energy takes place. The time interval for this phase depends on how much stretch facilitation is desired for the subsequent phases. For rehabilitation, this

Table 26-1 Summary of Three Types of Musculotendinous Units

Type	Example	Characteristics
Muscles with long fascicles and relatively short tendons	Gluteus maximus	This type of muscle is usually located proximally and tends to be large in size. These muscles are typically powerful movers with a large muscle fiber cross-sectional area. They are capable of moving the limb through a wide range of motion and can absorb a significant amount of energy. For the gluteus maximus, stepping off a box and into a squat position smoothly is partially a function of eccentric contracting (lengthening) of the gluteal muscles.
Muscles with long, thick, inelastic tendons	Gastrocnemius (although this muscle type is generally located more proximally)	The tendons have a high degree of stiffness and provide strong control of the distal segment.
Muscles with short fascicles and long, slender tendons	Tibialis anterior	These muscles can store large amounts of elastic energy when stretched rapidly because they are less stiff. Such muscles shorten very little and are more efficient on the length-tension and force-velocity curves. They tend to have more slow-twitch, highly oxidative fibers and are therefore metabolically efficient.

From Brownstein, B., Bronner, S. (1997): Functional Movement. New York, Churchill Livingstone.

phase will most likely be dictated by the range of motion and amount of shock absorption that the athlete's body is capable of withstanding or the amount of eccentric loading that the agonist musculature and passive restraints (e.g., ligaments) can tolerate. From a tissue protection standpoint, this is why so much clinical research has focused on the landing phase of athletic movement. In this area, the primary concern is the potentially poor neuromuscular strategies used during athletic movement. Numerous studies on prevention of injury to the anterior cruciate ligament (ACL) and rehabilitation are concerned with the biomechanics of the landing, or eccentric, phase.[11,28-31]

The *amortization phase* refers to the time between the end of the eccentric contraction and initiation of the concentric, explosive reaction force that accelerates the body or working limb in the desired direction. This phase should be as short as possible because with a long interval there is a risk of losing much of the elastic energy as heat within the muscle.[8] Successful performance of a plyometric drill depends on the ability of the musculotendinous unit to effectively absorb and exploit the stored elastic energy. The rapid stretching (eccentric loading) must be immediately followed by a rapid, explosive concentric contraction to maximize the force generated. The quicker that an athlete can overcome the yielding eccentric force and produce a concentric contraction, the more power that can be produced. The *concentric phase* represents the cumulative effect of the eccentric and amortization phases through a powerful concentric contraction (Box 26-2).[4,32]

It is important to note that many clinicians and strength/conditioning coaches would suggest that most plyometric and athletic injuries occur on landing and not during the jumping (concentric) or takeoff phase. Although this might be true, especially for noncontact ACL injuries, for example, the clinician should nonetheless be cognizant of the potential for muscle, tendon, and soft tissue injury during takeoff when designing plyometric programs for rehabilitation.

CLINICAL CONSIDERATIONS FOR PLYOMETRICS

Although all athletes may not necessarily need to produce explosive strength to excel at a given sport, most athletes undergoing rehabilitation need to regain strength and proprioception after an injury. Even though plyometrics has traditionally been used in the realm of sports that require strength, speed, and power, such as sprinting and other track and field events, all competitive athletes may be able to reduce the risk for future injury by maximizing their dynamic restraint system. Joint stability depends on both passive and dynamic restraint structures. Passive structures, such as the arthrokinematics of articulating surfaces, ligaments, joint capsule, menisci, and labrum, provide support to the musculoskeletal components. The dynamic restraints that provide joint stability include the muscles and neural controls associated with movement. It is often the passive restraints that are damaged in sports and daily activities involving high-velocity movements and perturbations in dynamic balance.[33,34] Unfortunately, even though healing of passive restraints can be addressed through physical therapy, these structures are not easily modified by active conservative treatment on the part of the athlete because the healing process is more passive (modalities, passive range of motion, and manual therapy). Thus, protective and rehabilitative efforts have focused primarily on modifying the dynamic neuromuscular elements, including joint capsule mechanoreceptors. To this end, proprioceptive training, active range of motion, flexibility, and strengthening interventions are typically used to empower the patient to maximize the ability of the dynamic restraints to contribute to stability and prevention of injury. Any displacement that occurs too quickly for reflex reactions to protect a joint requires that the mechanical properties of the musculotendinous unit resist the displacement. Active muscle response to any perturbation that might compromise joint stability is thus an important consideration in rehabilitation for prevention and athletic performance. Plyometric exercises can assist the clinician in addressing these biomechanical demands.

Generally, plyometrics involves ballistic and repetitive movements. Although these exercises and drills are designed to optimize the SSC and improve athletic performance, clinicians need to be cautious in deciding when a patient is ready for safe and effective use of plyometrics. Specifically, a patient must have achieved a certain level of range of motion, neuromuscular control, proprioception, balance, strength, and flexibility before undertaking plyometric exercises. The evaluation process should always consider the treatment goals established for a given patient at the onset of therapy (Box 26-3).

Box 26-2

Summary of the Plyometric Phases

ECCENTRIC PHASE
Preloading or setting period
Muscle spindles "loaded" via stretch/eccentric contraction of agonists

AMORTIZATION PHASE
Interval between the eccentric and concentric phases
Should be short enough to fully use the elastic energy stored in the stretched muscle-tendon complex

CONCENTRIC PHASE
Concentric muscle contraction of agonists
Maximal power generation with explosive movement

Box 26-3

Neuromuscular Assessment Before Initiating Plyometrics

Sufficient resolution of pain to participate in higher-level exercises and activities
No inflammation or joint effusion before or after exercise
Normal range of motion with respect to the uninvolved side
Normal joint alignment and mobility
Soft tissue flexibility, including both contractile and noncontractile structures, within normal limits
Adequate strength for full weight-bearing activity on the involved limb unilaterally if the lower extremity or strength for functional use of the upper extremity, including full weight bearing on the upper extremities if appropriate for function
Normal reflexes
Normal motor control
Balance and proprioception/kinesthetic sense within functional limits of the uninvolved side (e.g., consider the concept of time to stabilization)

Applications in Rehabilitation

Plyometrics is used widely in a less intense manner for the rehabilitation of many athletic injuries. In contrast, some patients progress sufficiently to allow the use of medium- and high-intensity plyometrics before discharge from formal rehabilitation. In addition to increasing conditioning, plyometrics can facilitate improved functional motor patterns, reflexes, and proprioception, all of which are crucial in the attempt to return an athlete to competition (Box 26-4).

In the past 15 years or so, the use of lower extremity plyometrics has received increased attention as an adjunctive modality for the prevention of noncontact ACL injuries. Although research in this area might be considered somewhat limited, it seems that plyometric-oriented exercise programming is an important component in reducing ACL injuries in females.[28,29,35] A growing body of evidence is linking ACL injuries to poor neuromuscular control in injured athletes.[31] It is possible that some athletes may have poor technique during jumping, landing, stopping, or turning that may lead to injury. Neuromuscular control must be developed in all three planes of motion—frontal, sagittal, and transverse—to decrease stress on the ACL and move it to the muscles and tendons. Proper plyometric training can decrease the force and torque placed on the knee.[28,35] Proper technique increases the load placed on the muscles and tendons and removes it from the joint and ligaments. The principles of plyometric training—functional motor patterns, reflexes, and proprioception—are instrumental in the prevention of knee injuries. These same principles can be applied to an upper extremity that is functionally weak and perhaps unstable for competitive athletic loads or has lost position sense.

In fact, Hewett et al examined the effects of a plyometric training program on landing mechanics and leg strength in female athletes involved in jumping sports. The plyometric program was designed to decrease landing force by helping the athletes improve neuromuscular control over the lower extremity during landing. It was also designed to increase VJH. The authors reported that peak landing force during a volleyball block jump decreased by 22%. Horizontal force acting on the knee during landing was reduced by approximately 50%. Hamstring-quadriceps peak torque-strength ratios increased 26% in the nondominant leg and 13% in the dominant leg. Hamstring power increased 44% in the dominant leg and 21% in the nondominant leg. Mean vertical jump increased by 10% overall.[28] This study, as well as others since, has linked the preventive aspect of plyometrics and therapeutic exercise.[29] It suggests that a properly performed plyometric training protocol may help prevent knee injury in female athletes involved in jumping sports, such as volleyball, by increasing knee stabilization during landing and teaching athletes muscular control. Plyometrics may also help correct torque imbalances between the hamstrings and quadriceps and can help increase VJH.

Hewett et al[35] prospectively monitored two groups of female athletes, one trained before sports participation and the other untrained, and a group of untrained male athletes throughout the high school soccer, volleyball, and basketball seasons. Fourteen serious knee injuries occurred in the 1263 athletes tracked through the study. Ten of 463 untrained female athletes sustained serious knee injuries (eight noncontact), 2 of 366 trained female athletes sustained serious knee injuries (zero noncontact), and 2 of 434 male athletes sustained serious knee injuries (one noncontact). The untrained female athletes had a 3.6-fold higher incidence of knee injury than the trained female athletes did and a 4.8-fold higher incidence than the male athletes did. The incidence of knee injury in the trained female athletes was not significantly different from that in the untrained male athletes. A significant difference was seen in the incidence of noncontact injuries between the female groups. In this prospective study a decreased incidence of knee injury was demonstrated in female athletes after a specific plyometric training program.

Although the jumping aspect of plyometric training is important for conditioning, it is the landing of each jump that is vital in the theoretic prevention of knee and lower extremity injuries. Obviously, rehabilitation and conditioning that focus on landing technique only do not involve the entire SSC since there is no concentric phase. Nonetheless, good technique on landing is crucial to avoid a knee going into hyperextension and external rotation, the point of no return. A key concept is that the athlete should land softly and quietly while using the knees and hips as shock absorbers. Another is that the shoulders should be over the knees when the athlete lands. During plyometric training at any intensity, the athlete should be constantly reminded to land softly. Another key concept for prevention of injury and conditioning is that hyperextension should be avoided during all activities such as turning, landing, stopping, cutting, or slowing down. When landing from a depth jump exercise the athlete should "stick" and hold the landing. This is accomplished when balance is maintained for several seconds after landing with no additional steps taken and minimal trunk sway in any direction. Ideally, no foot movement should occur after landing (Box 26-5).

Clearly, proper execution of plyometric exercises requires dynamic stabilization during the amortization phase and landing, as well as during the concentric phase. Some authors have suggested that the components of plyometric landing be measured by time to stabilization (TTS).[36] The intensity of plyometrics, especially jumping modalities, has been studied via electromyographic (EMG), kinematic, and kinetic analysis, but the specific characteristics of many plyometric exercises have not. Ebben et al[36] demonstrated that TTS can be used for progression of

---

Box 26-4

Proposed Beneficial Effects of Plyometrics

Improved proprioception during dynamic movement
Improved speed, strength, and power
Improved reaction time
Increased bone mineral density

Box 26-5

Plyometric Concepts for Prevention of Knee Injuries in Females

"Stick" the landing with minimal trunk or hip-knee sway
Hold the landing for 2 to 5 seconds (as appropriate)
Land softly and quietly
Keep the shoulders over the knees when landing and do not allow the knees to shift anterior to the toes in the sagittal plane
Avoid hyperextension during all activities

plyometric intensity and that it has moderate to high reliability for jumping conditions in both male and female college-aged athletes. Although the average clinician does not have access to the force platform equipment to precisely measure TTS, the concept is important in evaluating a patient's ability to perform and progress through a plyometric program. Briefly, TTS has been used to evaluate ankle stability under varying conditions, including a jump task from bilateral takeoff to single-leg landing, as well as step-down from a box 20 cm high.[36,37] An athlete's or any patient's ability to perform and progress through plyometric exercises should be evaluated with consideration of these concepts.

With the exception of research studying ACL injuries and prevention, there is a relative dearth of controlled studies in the rehabilitation literature on plyometrics. In contrast, many studies in the strengthening and conditioning literature have examined the effectiveness of plyometrics in improving parameters of athletic performance, especially power and VJH.[5,38] Numerous studies have shown improvements in VJH, but a few studies have failed to demonstrate significant improvement in VJH.[5,38] Nonetheless, in terms of rehabilitation in particular, relatively little information is available on the efficacy and evidence-based guidelines for plyometric rehabilitation. Clinicians must therefore combine knowledge of basic science, the available studies on ACL rehabilitation, and outcomes of plyometrics in healthy subjects to optimize results in the athletic population.

As most clinicians would suspect, the literature suggests that the effects of plyometric training in healthy subjects differ depending on training level, gender, age, sport activity, and familiarity with plyometric training.[5] Even in healthy athletes it is generally believed that an individual should have a reasonable amount of flexibility, strength, and agility before starting a plyometric training program. Though perhaps not as important as for other exercise modes used in the athletic training room or clinic, it is critical that specific assessment and testing be conducted before the use of plyometrics. Plyometrics is demanding physically and requires that the individual concentrate on controlling movements both statically and dynamically.

According to some authors, the risk for injury from plyometrics is low,[39] but few studies have actually addressed injury rates associated with plyometric training in healthy individuals. Even though no studies of injury rates have been performed in patients undergoing rehabilitation and using plyometrics, some studies have examined fatigue, inflammation, muscle damage, and recovery times in healthy subjects after SSC exercise. Gollhofer et al[40] found that repeated SSC muscle activity induces fatigue effects associated with a decrease in neural input to the muscle and reduced overall muscle performance. It has been suggested that during fatigue from SSC exercise, the repeated stretch loads might reduce the reflex contribution to the SSC.[41] Avela and Komi studied a group of experienced endurance runners and concluded that fatiguing SSC exercise reduces stretch-reflex sensitivity, which was associated with decreased muscle stiffness.[42] The authors postulated that this would impair the athlete's ability to use the stored elastic energy in the muscle-tendon complex. As discussed previously, plyometric training has a significant eccentric component, and the muscle-damaging effect of eccentric exercise modalities has been well established in the litereature.[43] A recent study demonstrated acute inflammatory responses and reduced jump performance after an intense bout of plyometric training.[44] Other studies have shown evidence of muscle damage by studying serum markers for creatine kinase and collagen breakdown.[45] Overall, some research suggests that plyometric exercise may cause more delayed-onset muscle damage than concentric exercise does, but not as much as eccentric exercise alone does.[45]

Lower extremity plyometric exercises are of particular concern for injury to the feet, ankles, lower part of the legs, knees, hips, and lumbosacral spine. As is the case during most athletic events, injuries are more likely when an individual is fatigued, typically toward the end of an event or exercise session. Sprained ankles and knee injuries are commonly associated with lack of control because of excessive fatigue.[8] Inadequate conditioning, lack of adequate warm-up, poor-quality athletic shoes, inappropriate training surfaces, and low levels of skill may predispose an athlete or patient to injury. Borkowski[39] reported that a preseason plyometric training program in collegiate volleyball players did not cause injuries but actually significantly reduced in-season muscle soreness. Thus, it is clear that proper assessment and testing of athletes before a plyometric program is started and diligent application of the exercise prescription principles of frequency, duration, and intensity are extremely important.

Basic Pretraining Testing

In addition to the physical assessments and strength guidelines mentioned previously, several basic static and dynamic tests can be used to determine a patient's ability to begin a plyometric training program. Voight and Tippett proposed that an individual be able to perform a 30-second one-leg stance with the eyes open and closed before starting a plyometric program.[46] Involved versus uninvolved legs should be compared. Voight and Draovitch recommended that the stork balance test be performed for 30 seconds and that a single-leg half-squat also be evaluated before any jumping plyometric exercises are begun.[47] Although it is important to consider the athlete's ability to perform a single repetition of a dynamic movement, such as a single-leg squat, single-leg heel raise, or standard push-up with proper biomechanics, pretraining testing should closely monitor multiple repetitions and sets of exercise to test for local muscle endurance.

The clinician should be creative in using functional testing to determine whether a patient is prepared to begin a plyometric program. Vertical jumps in place and horizontal long jumps on a shock-absorbing surface are two simple tests that may provide feedback about a patient's status. Particular attention to the involved (injured) side with unilateral testing can prove invaluable in avoiding reinjury or progressing too abruptly by adding a plyometric component to a rehabilitation or training program. Any pain or instability observed during these tests may provide clues to the patient's tolerance of plyometrics. Having the patient perform step-ups and step-downs from progressively increasing heights will also provide some indication of the patient's tolerance. Lateral shuffle and carioca (crossover) drills likewise provide the clinician with ways of testing whether an affected lower limb is prepared to handle plyometrics. Obviously, jogging and running are perhaps the first dynamic movements performed to assess the ability of the affected limb to bear full body weight dynamically. Before incorporating any high-intensity, or shock, plyometric drills such as box jumps or depth jumps, the reader is encouraged to consult sources to determine the height of the box that should be used for an individual's ability.[4,7]

Concerning plyometric training in healthy athletes, five methods are used by various authors to identify the optimal drop height that will increase countermovement jump performance on an individual basis. The two most common methods are the maximum jump height and the reactive strength index.[48] The clinician is reminded that these methods are intended for use in healthy athletes and should be used as a potential guideline; there is no substitute for sound, practical clinical judgment.

Strength and Conditioning Level

In terms of strength, it is generally accepted that a patient should have a sufficient base of strength-training experience. It is important that a sufficient base of strength training may simply be based on movement patterns that are free of dysfunction. For patients with an ankle sprain, perhaps this is simply the ability to perform three sets of 15 repetitions of unilateral heel raises on the involved ankle at full range of motion off the end of a step (with the heels dipping slightly below parallel or to 10° of dorsiflexion). When plyometrics is used for rehabilitation, a great deal of subjective clinical judgment is necessary on the part of the clinician. The reason is that except for perhaps ACL rehabilitation, evidence in the literature supporting the use of various plyometric exercises for rehabilitation is limited. Indeed, it is agreed that plyometric training principles are beneficial for healthy athletes, although there is much room for subjective judgment in terms of how these drills and exercises should progress. Even though plyometrics can be a form of functional training for rehabilitating both the upper and lower extremities, the ballistic nature of most of these exercises makes them inappropriate for the early stages of rehabilitation. One major disadvantage of plyometric training is that joint excursion is difficult to control because of the nature of the activity.

Although it is not necessary or suggested that strength-training programs focus solely on eccentric contractions, it is important that sufficient eccentric strength be established before a plyometric training program is begun, especially for an injured athlete. Studies have shown that force production is increased during eccentric contractions, thus necessitating tolerance of higher loads and preferential recruitment of fast-twitch fibers; in addition, high eccentric loads may reduce neural inhibition and lead to greater generation of concentric force.[49-51] During most athletic pursuits, as well as activities of daily living, movement in the opposite direction, an eccentric motion, precedes movement in the intended direction. In most movements, the eccentric contraction is responsible for decelerating the moving limb. Similarly, the eccentric phase of the plyometric exercise absorbs the energy by decelerating the limb and allows storage of elastic energy. Thus, the clinician should incorporate eccentric work during repetitions of various therapeutic and functional exercises. Emphasis on the eccentric phase of the motion just before the concentric work more closely matches true human movement patterns. Note that the focus on eccentric contraction is not intended to minimize the importance of training with faster concentric contractions as well.

No discussion of strength would be complete without mention of the need for establishing a strength base by using closed kinetic chain exercises before a plyometric exercises program is begun. Indeed, practically all lower extremity plyometric exercises are of the closed chain variety, like the functional movements that they mimic. In the case of jumping and landing, the entire kinetic chain, from the ankles through the knees and hips, as well as the vertebral column, needs to absorb full body weight and maintain stability. As discussed earlier, the serial elastic component is important, but the muscle synergy and neuromuscular coordination required for smooth landing and subsequent explosive movement during athletic activity and plyometrics are probably better served by enhancing closed chain strength.

Strength and power (speed strength) are intrinsically necessary components of plyometric training. Chu and Cordier recommended the power squat test as a good closed chain exercise to determine whether a patient has an adequate speed-strength base for lower extremity plyometrics.[8] The exercise is performed with 6% of the person's body weight. Five squat repetitions are done in 5 seconds, and the depth of each repetition should be close to 90° of knee flexion. If the patient cannot perform the exercise in the allotted time with proper technique, the clinician should continue to emphasize strength training and delay initiation of the plyometric program. For the upper extremities, it has been suggested the athlete be able to perform five repetitions of the bench press at 60% of a one-repetition maximum (1RM) in 5 seconds.[4] For strength training to improve vertical leap performance, Weiss et al concluded that training programs to enhance moderately fast squatting power may improve performance as long as body weight, especially body fat, is not increased.[32] In a related finding, McBride et al concluded that training with light-load jump squats results in increased movement velocity capability and that velocity-specific changes in muscle activity may play a role in this adaptation.[52] Guidelines are not as clear for the upper extremity. Anecdotally, we recommend that the patient have full range of motion, rotator cuff strength at least 75% as strong as that on the uninvolved extremity, and greater than grade 4 of 5 for the prime movers on a manual muscle test.

According Potash and Chu, as well as other authors, for shock- and high-intensity lower extremity plyometrics, it is recommended that a healthy athlete have a 1RM squat of 1.5 times body weight. For high-intensity upper extremity plyometrics, the bench press 1RM is suggested to be at least the athlete's body weight for larger athletes (body weight >100 kg). For smaller athletes (body weight <100 kg), it has been suggested that the bench press 1RM be 1.5 times body weight. Another method suggests that an athlete be able to perform five clap push-ups in a row.[4] Clearly, this requirement is not necessary for plyometrics performed in the early and middle stages of rehabilitation, but it underscores the diligence that is important in evaluating a patient before initiation of plyometrics. By definition, plyometric training involves maximal voluntary contractions. Therefore, plyometrics should be incorporated during the end stages of rehabilitation, when the clinician is preparing an athlete for return to sport or for any patient to achieve maximal functional capacity.

The focus on making sure that a patient has the strength foundation necessary to engage in plyometrics should not overshadow the need for proper endurance and conditioning. Though not an endurance activity per se, a plyometric training session does require a measure of glycolytic endurance because anaerobic or strength/power exercise is more likely to increase lactate levels in the muscle, which decreases the pH of the muscle. The process of removing lactic acid and metabolites from muscle tissue (i.e., recovery) is an oxidative process. Thus, an athlete should have a reasonable measure of endurance to safely avoid fatigue and risk for injury during a plyometric training session.

A plyometric program uses successive sets/repetitions and rest periods, but as the duration of the routine increases (e.g., to 15 to 30 minutes), the athlete will encounter fatigue. Similar to what occurs during an athletic event, there is a need for anaerobic endurance. Specifically, the athlete encounters short bouts of explosive anaerobic activity, with short rest periods, and then must continue to attempt to achieve that performance level for several minutes or even hours. Take as an example a tennis match or a basketball or football game. The same explosive movements are required at the end of the match or game as are necessary in the beginning of the competition. Gollhofer et al found reduced EMG activity during the eccentric phase of SSC exercise with fatigue in healthy subjects.[40] Similarly, Nicol et al concluded that the EMG response of calf muscles to passive stretch was a smaller after submaximal SSC exercise.[41] Strojnik and Komi also found that fatiguing submaximal SSC exercise on a sledge jump apparatus decreases the contractile characteristics of the quadriceps femoris muscle.[53]

Special Clinical Considerations

Anthropometrics

Simply because a patient is an athlete does not mean that the rehabilitation program should progress to high-intensity or even high-volume plyometrics programming. In general, high-intensity drills and high-volume plyometric programs may not be appropriate for larger athletes (>100 kg),[4] particularly if the athlete's body fat level is high. A football lineman, for example, may be at increased risk, especially because his role in competition does not require jumping and leaping movements as much as the role of a running back or wide receiver does. By the same token, an endurance athlete with a low body fat level but low muscle mass might also be at risk for injury with high-impact plyometric exercises. Ugarkovic et al studied anthropometric and strength variables as predictors of jumping performance in elite junior basketball players and concluded that these measures alone are not the best predictors to assess movement performance in homogeneous groups of athletes. They suggest that these factors and especially sport-specific movements and power be used in a comprehensive evaluation.[54] Nonetheless, body structure, body fat measures, and particularly structural abnormalities and previous injuries must be considered. If body fat measurements are not readily available, it is suggested that the body mass index (BMI) be considered as a starting point. The reader is also advised to keep in mind that the BMI is a less appropriate measure in the athletic population because it is not a measure of body fat; that is, it does not take into consideration lean body mass. Vertebral abnormalities, as well as problems with the knees, hips, and ankles, are of special concern for lower extremity drills. Previous shoulder, elbow, wrist, hand, and cervical or thoracic injuries should be considered when contemplating the use of upper extremity plyometrics.

Age and Gender

PEDIATRIC ATHLETES

Prepubescent children (<12 years) and adolescent athletes (12 to 17 years) represent a special population regarding plyometrics. School-age children play games such as leap frog, hopscotch, and jump rope to their own level of comfort without any formal instruction—these activities are plyometric by their very nature and are perfectly normal for healthy children. Although it is generally considered inappropriate for children younger than 12 to engage in formal plyometric training, any activity that includes jumping activities on safe surfaces is probably healthy for growing bones and muscles as long as overuse injuries are avoided. The fact that many young children (<12 years) participate in organized sports such as gymnastics, soccer, hockey, basketball, and football speaks to the safety of low-level, informal plyometric activity. In terms of rehabilitation, we have used low-intensity plyometric drills at low volume for gymnasts, dancers, soccer players, swimmers, and other childhood athletes who intend to return to their sports following physical therapy.

In terms of strength and conditioning, properly designed and supervised plyometric training programs have been used in the adolescent population with safety and effective results. Potdevin et al trained pubescent swimmers for 6 weeks with a plyometric program and observed improved swimming performance as a result of improved dive and turn movements.[55] Rubley et al recently conducted a low-frequency, low-impact plyometric program in female soccer players and observed increased lower body power in terms of kicking distance and VJH.[56] Other studies have also used plyometric training in high school basketball players and soccer players.[57,58]

Weight-bearing exercise with high load intensity is known to have osteogenic effects.[59,60] Children who participate in activities associated with higher loads have been shown to exhibit higher bone mass than have children who participate in activities with lower loads.[61] Witzke and Snow investigated the effects of 9 months of plyometric jump training on bone mineral content, performance, and balance in adolescent girls. They found that moderate- to high-intensity plyometric training improved trochanteric bone mineral content, leg strength, and balance in these adolescent girls.[62]

In summary, pubescent athletes can engage in low- to medium-intensity plyometrics, although it is critical that they have the strength and coordination to tolerate these drills safely without incurring injuries to the epiphyseal (growth) plates and overuse injuries to tendons and other soft tissue. High-intensity (shock) plyometrics such as box jumps are not generally recommended for adolescents. Although sequential age should be considered in terms of maturity, each child should be evaluated for maturity in terms of strength, flexibility, balance, and coordination. Finally, pediatric participants must be psychologically mature enough to follow the instructions of the supervising clinician or strength and conditioning coach.

GENDER

Regarding gender differences, Aura and Komi found that female subjects better use the prestretch phase of SSC at low intensity levels whereas men show greater potentiation of elastic energy at higher prestretch levels. However, males exhibited higher work because of elasticity. They suggested that there may be fundamental differences in neuromuscular function between males and females.[63] In a more recent study, an SSC index derived from upper extremity tests showed significantly higher values in men than in women, although individual differences were more variable in women. The authors concluded that men may have superior ability to use the SSC in the upper extremities.[64] Based on the work of various authors,[28,29,31] it is clear that the neuromuscular patterns exhibited by females during jumping tasks make a strong case for the clinician to use diligence in designing and supervising female athletes during both rehabilitation and training programs involving plyometrics.

MASTERS ATHLETES (MIDDLE AGED AND OLDER)

Generally speaking, middle age begins at 35 years, and most sports organizations offer "masters" athlete categories beginning at approximately 40 years of age. Whether one is working with a weekend warrior or a competitive amateur masters athlete, it is important to evaluate the patient's functional status and goals for rehabilitation. When one considers the anatomic and physiologic changes that are inherent in the aging athlete, the use of plyometric exercises comes with special clinical considerations. First, a through medical history is critical in determining how previous injuries, surgeries, and medical conditions might have an impact on design of the program. Second, it is important to consider the decrease in muscle fiber cross-sectional area, preferential loss of type II muscle fibers, reduction in the number of motor units, changes in neuromuscular recruitment, and the subsequent reductions in strength and especially power that accompany the aging process. Rates of skeletal muscle protein synthesis and therefore rates of recovery decline with age.[65,66] In addition to changes in skeletal muscle and muscle strain injuries, the clinician needs to consider the potential for damage to articular cartilage, knee menisci, intervertebral disks, and tendons, which is more likely in this population. As with plyometric programming for any age group, attention to appropriate levels of exercise intensity, frequency, duration, and volume are especially important in older athletes. Again, understanding each patient's goals in the context of the plyometric program is important. For instance, a 50-year-old man or woman with a history of meniscus injury who would like to improve running performance in a 5-km event might benefit more from hop and bounding-type exercises than from 24-inch box jumps and high-impact plyometrics.

Warm-Up, Stretching, and Flexibility

The importance of warm-up is well documented in the literature, and it is related to many positive effects on athletic performance, including faster relaxation and contraction of both agonist and antagonist muscles, improved rate of force development, and improvement in strength, power, and reaction time.[67] In contrast, stretching has recently come under scrutiny in the literature. Specifically, static stretching has been associated with acute negative effects on muscle power, torque, force, and maximal strength, as well as jump, sprint, and agility performance.[67,68] Dynamic stretching, however, has not been shown to elicit decrements in performance and has, in fact, been shown to improve running peformance.[67] It is important to also note that a metaanalysis of stretching studies concluded that the evidence is not sufficient to recommend eliminating preexercise stretching and that no studies have examined populations who are at increased risk for injury.[69] Overall, the evidence that warm-up and stretching reduce risk for injury is equivocal because studies often combine warm-up, stretching modes, and prestretching and poststretching practices.[69] Ultimately, it is probably important for athletic activities that require increased range of motion (e.g., high hurdles, gymnastics) or high-intensity SSC movements to include appropriate flexibility regimens. Because of the eccentric, or lengthening, nature of the SSC and the subsequent

maximal concentric contraction, it seems important that athletes should possess a level of flexibility conducive to handling the demands of the specific plyometric exercises being performed.

For plyometric warm-up, whole-body movements should be used to raise the heart rate, increase muscle and soft tissue temperature, decrease the viscosity of synovial fluid, and increase overall body temperature enough to generate mild perspiration. The warm-up and stretching should be activity specific and incorporate the dynamic movements associated with that activity. Assuming that no joint structures are limiting range of motion, improved flexibility through appropriate stretching of muscles and soft tissues should aid in the safe performance of demanding plyometric exercises. Prolonged static stretching before and during a plyometric routine may have a negative impact on performance, so this should be considered carefully. Dynamic, ballistic stretching is probably warranted since plyometric activity is ballistic by definition. Additionally, proprioceptive neuromuscular facilitation stretching may be an appropriate adjunct to improvement in flexibility as well. Detailed discussion of stretching and flexibility is beyond the scope of this chapter, and the reader is encouraged to review Chapter 6.

Balance and Proprioception

Proprioception describes the collection of sensory afferent nerves that enhance awareness of posture, movement, joint position, limb velocity, changes in equilibrium and weight, and resistance of objects in relation to the body. Kinesthesia is also important and represents the ability to perceive the extent, direction, and weight of movement.[70] Conscious and unconscious perception of these factors is critical fore safe and effective return of the athlete to competition. Research has shown that during jumping, the leg extensor muscles are activated before the feet contact the ground.[71] Komi described this phenomenon as the preactivation or preinnervation phase.[19] Melvill-Jones and Watt suggested that this preactivation is mediated by higher CNS processes before the person lands and that the correct timing and sequence of the (eccentric) contractions to absorb the force have been learned from previous experience.[71] According to Avela and Komi, many studies have confirmed this theory, and a clear relationship exists between the duration and amount of preactivation and the height of the drop as a result of the person's jumping.[72] Komi et al showed that preactivation rises with increasing running speed.[73] Despite these studies, there is evidence that the vestibular and visual systems also play a role in this process.[42] Finally, it has been shown that the preactivation phase is important in preparing the muscle to resist the high impact force and in preparing for the subsequent push-off after contact.[74] These studies suggest that plyometric training and the motor learning that takes place as a result of repetitive practice can play a critical role in developing proprioception. The speed-strength components of the drills should better prepare a patient to handle these circumstances during functional activity.

As discussed earlier, the concept of TTS is important to consider in plyometric programming, especially with bilateral versus unilateral SSC exercise. For example, plyometric drills, especially in rehabilitation, should progress from bilateral to unilateral modes. There is evidence that the feet touch down at different times, thus suggesting an asymmetry in the landing, with one leg absorbing more energy than the other.[75] In fact, these authors have found bilateral differences in both average and maximum force when drop jumps are performed at less than

0.40 m, which suggests that the feet are placed on the ground at different times; interestingly, symmetry of landing was better with a higher depth jump (0.6 m). Clinicians should, at least grossly, monitor TTS, landing, and takeoff asymmetry when implementing balance and proprioception training as it relates to plyometric exercise even when the intensity is low, as might occur in the rehabilitation setting.

Joint stability depends partially on proper neuromuscular control. Presumably, the clinician has addressed proprioception during the intervention leading up to initiation of a plyometric training program. Nonetheless, the plyometric program should be viewed as a higher-level extension of this component in rehabilitation for a patient to achieve return to maximal functional status. It should be noted that healing and strengthening of the static and dynamic restraints do not necessarily prepare a patient for the demands of athletic endeavors. Indeed, the unanticipated changes in joint positions encountered during athletic events are something that the athlete must be prepared to tolerate. Plyometric training is the next logical step in properly preparing the athlete for return to sport. Although running and changing direction are important aspects of proprioception, these conditions in the athletic training room or clinic do not adequately mimic the functional requirements during competition or even practice drills. Besier et al studied anticipatory effects on knee joint loading during running and cutting maneuvers. They concluded that performance of cutting maneuvers without preplanning may increase the risk for noncontact knee ligament injury. The authors suggested that training should involve drills that familiarize athletes with making unanticipated changes in direction and that plyometrics should be included, as well as helping athletes focus on visual cues to increase the time available for preplanning a movement.[76]

PROGRAMMING AND IMPLEMENTATION

Exercise Surface and Environmental Considerations

Depending on the rehabilitation location, it is likely that only low-level plyometrics will be conducted in the clinical setting. Whenever possible, low-intensity plyometric jumps in place, hops, bounds, and in-depth jumps (>12 inches) should be performed on yielding or shock-absorbing surfaces such as hardwood or spring-loaded flooring. Bounds and hops can be performed outside on level, well-groomed grassy surfaces or artificial turf. Rubberized indoor and outdoor tracks may also be safe surfaces. The typical flooring in an athletic training room or clinic, even if carpeted, is not appropriate for lower extremity plyometrics that involve full body weight. Wrestling or gymnastics mats might also be a good choice, especially for landings involving full body weight. However, these surfaces should not be so thick, soft, or cushioned that they increase the risk for knee or ankle sprain or soft tissue injury. In addition, it is preferable that the athlete perform the plyometric exercises on a surface similar or specific to a given sport.

Although minitrampolines or excessively thick exercise mats might seem appropriate surfaces for lower extremity plyometrics in the early, low-intensity stages of rehabilitation,

they might actually extend the amortization phase and reduce efficient use of the stretch reflex for the SSC. Again, these surfaces are not specific to the surface on which the athlete will be competing.

Obviously, the amount of space needed for the lower extremity is a function of the type of plyometric drills being performed. Some drills may require as much as 100 m, although most bounding and running drills require only about 30 m of straightaway.[4,7,8] If plyometric exercises are performed indoors, ceilings must be high enough to accommodate vertical leaps and in-depth jumps even though a small floor surface area is needed.

Equipment

Footwear

The flooring or playing surface is probably the most important "equipment" needed for plyometric training. Similarly, the footwear worn by the patient/athlete is very important. Footwear should provide good cushioning and sturdy support. A standard cross-training shoe is probably best suited for the performance of lower extremity plyometric exercises, especially if lateral movements will be included. Running shoes are not typically a good choice for plyometric training because the sole is generally narrower and affords minimal lateral support for the ankles. A basketball or tennis shoe might also be a good choice because they typically provide good support for lateral activities, as well as for changes in direction and stop/go activity.

In contrast, our rehabilitation programs for gymnasts, swimmers, and dancers have included a significant amount of barefoot low-intensity plyometric drills. In addition, recent work with a mogul skier was performed with the patient actually wearing her ski boots during the plyometric jumps. For all these athletes, we believed that it was important to establish balance, proprioception, strength, and power in ways specific to the demands of the sport.

Boxes or Platforms, Hurdles, and Other Lower Extremity Items

Boxes have always been a staple of lower extremity plyometric training. The top or landing surfaces of the boxes should be covered with solid rubber, nonslip covers. Typically, these boxes are constructed of ¾-inch plywood or pressboard (pulp) wood. The boxes can vary from 6 to 24 inches or more in height. Plastic cones, hurdles, and physioballs are also useful pieces of equipment. Plyometric or weighted balls are very useful for both upper extremity, core, and lower extremity training. A slide board and strength/jumping/plyometric shoes are likewise useful pieces of equipment. Kraemer et al[44] recently studied the effects of one type of strength shoe and concluded that sprint and plyometric training with the shoe along with weight training significantly increased VJH in young, healthy men who were experienced in both resistance and plyometric training.

Medicine Balls, Pads, and Rebounder for Upper Extremity Tools

Because of greater reliance on open kinetic chain activities, the upper extremities require a different set of equipment for implementing safe and effective plyometric drills. A rebounder or adjustable minitrampoline enables the patient to perform unassisted medicine ball throws and allows the clinician the ability to observe the activity from a variety of angles. The foam pads typically used for balance activity can function as cushioning for the hand/wrist when performing closed chain upper extremity plyometric exercises such as clap push-ups and upper extremity hops. Again, these pads should not be so soft that they interfere with the intended SSC exercise performance.

Warm-Up and Cool-Down

Similar to any other exercise session or higher-level therapy regimen, proper warm-up and stretching are important components for a safer and more effective and efficient plyometric training session. Especially for lower extremity plyometric exercises, a comprehensive warm-up routine might include the following principles:

- Jogging for 5 to 10 minutes raises the heart rate, increases respiration, and raises body temperature (especially with respect to soft tissue and synovial fluid viscosity). Although some stationary biking might be used as an adjunct to warm-up, full weight-bearing activity is absolutely critical to the warm-up for lower extremity plyometric activity.
- All appropriate muscle groups, both primary agonists, antagonists, and stabilizer muscles (e.g., quadriceps, hip flexors, gluteals, hamstrings, and triceps surae, as well as the internal/external hip rotators, peroneals, tibialis anterior, and lumbar spine), should be dynamically engaged in closed chain movements and stretching (if indicated) for 5 to 10 minutes. Dynamic stretch positions that mimic the specific plyometric movements to be performed are clearly indicated here (Box 26-6).
- After the plyometric routine has been completed, a 3- to 5-minute walk/light jog or light stationary bike ride for cool-down is warranted. Stretching for 5 to 15 minutes after a workout is probably an important activity when considering the rehabilitation of specific soft tissue structures.

For upper extremity plyometrics, a brief 5-minute full-body warm-up followed by upper body ergometer exercise for 5 minutes can precede specific dynamic stretches and movements of the upper part of the body in preparation for the program.

Exercise Frequency, Intensity, and Duration

In addition to considering the clinical appropriateness of plyometric exercise in the rehabilitation of an individual athlete, other conditioning activities such as formal sport practice sessions, strength training, and aerobic activity must be taken into account in designing the plyometric training program. As return to sport approaches, the athlete might be engaged in complex training, which describes a combination of resistance exercise followed by biomechanically similar plyometric exercise during the same exercise session. It is believed that power (e.g., VJH) is increased after a heavily loaded resistance exercise because of a postactivation potentiation effect.[77] Although programming of this type is not typically associated with rehabilitation, the clinician might implement a low-intensity version of this technique to enhance preparation for return to sport.

Box 26-6
Dynamic Warm-Up

Jogging or light running for 5 to 10 minutes
Full body weight squats for 15 to 20 repetitions
Lateral and oblique lunges for 15 to 20 repetitions
Carioca for 50 to 100 feet
Lateral shuffles for 50 to 100 feet
High-knee marches with appropriate reciprocal arm swing (elbows in 90° of flexion) three times for 30 feet
Butt-kickers three times for 30 feet
Submaximal high knee (power) skips three times for 30 feet
Upper part of body:
- Upper body ergometer exercise for 5 minutes
- Push-ups, three sets of 5 to 10 repetitions
- Walking on hands in a protracted scapular position/trunk on physioball
- Basketball or volleyball two-handed chest and overhead passes

Frequency

As for principles of traditional exercise prescription, frequency is defined as the number of times per week that plyometric exercises are performed. Typically, one to three sessions are held each week. However, the frequency is primarily a function of the intensity and duration of the workouts and hence the amount of recovery that a patient needs between workouts. For example, the clinician may choose to have a patient perform low-intensity plyometric exercises three times a week while in the athletic training room or clinic. As the patient's condition improves, the sessions would become more intense and last longer (duration) but take place only twice per week.

For comparison, plyometric programming in healthy athletes varies during off-season and in-season periods according to the demands of other conditioning, especially practice sessions and actual competition. For most sports, off-season plyometric routines are performed twice per week, although certain athletes (e.g., track and field) may perform them two to three times per week. During the season, one session per week is appropriate for most sports, whereas track and field athletes may maintain the two- or three-per-week schedule. Regardless of the frequency used, it is recommended that plyometric drills for a given muscle group or groups and joint complex not be performed on 2 consecutive days.[4]

Intensity

Intensity is the amount of stress placed on the individual during a training session. In cardiovascular exercise, intensity is most often measured via the training heart rate, the percentage of maximum oxygen consumption, or a rating of perceived exertion.[78] In strength training and anaerobic sports, intensity is typically measured in terms of the amount of resistance or weight, speed, or the amount of recovery allowed between exercises used for a given routine. The amount of work performed in a given period, or power, may also be used to describe intensity in any type of exercise.

For plyometrics, intensity can mean the amount of stress placed on muscles, joints, and connective tissue or the complexity and amount of work necessary to complete the exercise.[4,8]

The intensity of plyometric drills is typically classified as low, medium, or high. As a general rule in any exercise prescription, volume decreases as intensity increases. However, in an effort to improve conditioning and endurance, the early stages of plyometric exercise (or any exercise) can involve increases in both volume and intensity. When high-intensity levels are reached by the athlete, volume should decrease. The intensity of plyometric drills for the lower extremities has been related to foot contact, direction of jump, speed, jump height, and body weight (Box 26-7).

From an exercise physiology perspective, it has been shown that a plyometric jump-training protocol whereby participants perform 8 sets of 10 repetitions from a 0.8-m ($\approx$31.5 inches) platform elicits oxygen consumption equal to 80% Vo_2max and increased blood lactate to levels that one would expect from an aerobically paced 400-m run. Furthermore, this level of intensity included 3 minutes of passive rest between sets.[79] Although no other studies have directly examined the metabolic or energy systems involved during plyometric training sessions, the clinician should be cognizant of intensity from a metabolic perspective as well. Indeed, many sports-related injuries occur as a result of fatigue.

Generally speaking, bilateral upper extremity and lower extremity exercises are less intense than unilateral or isolateral varieties. Raising box jump and hurdle heights, increasing the resistance of elastic bands, increasing vertical leap height and horizontal distance, using a heavier plyometric (medicine) ball, and increasing the number of hurdles are all examples of manipulating intensity. Chu and Cordier[8] and others classified the types of plyometric exercise into groups according to increasing intensity; however, low- and high-intensity variations exist for each type of drill. For instance, although in-place jumps are generally a lower-intensity activity, a single-leg power vertical jump in place is a high-intensity variation. Similarly, lateral hops over a 6-inch hurdle are of lesser intensity than when the drill is performed with a 12- or 18-inch hurdle.

AQUATIC PLYOMETRICS
Aquatic plyometric exercises represent an interesting option in rehabilitation, strengthening, and conditioning. As opposed to an explosive workout for power that involves high levels of impact force, plyometrics in water allows increasing intensity with low impact and low risk for injury to healing tissues. In addition, there may be the opportunity for plyometric workouts of longer duration and greater frequency. Several studies have observed increased VJH, muscle power, and torque with aquatic plyometrics programming.[80,81] Clearly, this is a specialized area,

and there are safety issues related to slipping on the bottom of the pool's surface and stumbling on any boxes that are placed in the water. Water depth is probably the most important consideration since buoyancy is the key element separating aquatic from land-based plyometrics. For example, studies have shown approximately 50% of a person's body weight is supported by water when submerged to the waist.[80,81]

In addition to the buoyancy factor, plyometrics in water also provides different sensory input for proprioception and kinesthetic awareness because of the hydrostatic pressure. As discussed in the next section, intensity can be manipulated in various ways. The key advantage of aquatic plyometrics is probably that an athlete might be able to perform a typically high-intensity plyometric drill in a low-intensity manner.

CLASSIFICATION OF PLYOMETRIC DRILLS BY INTENSITY
There are basic categories of plyometric movements. It is important for the clinician to recognize opportunities to design and implement low-, medium-, and high-intensity exercises in each of the basic categories. For instance, although depth jumps are considered a high-intensity drill, working on neuromuscular control with a 6-inch box is a low-intensity drill in the rehabilitation setting. The critical difference between plyometrics in rehabilitation and traditional plyometrics in healthy athletes is that exercises are not always performed with maximum effort. However, rehabilitation plyometric drills can be performed with maximum power output in the latter stages. In addition, a patient might concurrently perform maximal-effort ankle plyometric drills while working on low- to medium-intensity submaximal jumps for the entire lower chain.

As a general rule, any unilateral version of a plyometric drill is more intense than its bilateral counterpart. Jumps in place are probably the most basic lower extremity drill and tend to be low intensity (e.g., ankle plyometrics), although squat jumps and tuck jumps should probably be considered medium to high intensity, depending on the athlete's rehabilitation progress. By definition, this exercise is repetitive with no rest between jumps.[4] Although many see obtaining maximum vertical height as the basic objective of jumps in place, the clinician is advised to use such jumps as a diagnostic for how well the patient tolerates repetitive SSC exercise early in rehabilitation. Standing jumps are probably the next level of plyometric activity. These exercises can be for both vertical and horizontal components and are generally viewed as maximal jump attempts.[4] A clinical example is the single-leg hop test for return to sport. Forward and lateral hurdle jumps are also examples.

As the athlete approaches return to athletic activity, it is important to incorporate multiple jumps and hops. A hop is a movement that is initiated and completed with a one-foot or two-foot landing.[82] Hops are not maximal-effort jumps and are repeated for a specific time, fixed height (e.g., a 6- or 12-inch hurdle), or distance. When compared with the maximal-distance or vertical jumps that are used to train for explosive power, hops are typically focused on speed and agility. Clearly, the clinician's objective with plyometric hops (and bounds) is to establish the readiness of the athlete in terms of neuromuscular recruitment, dynamic balance, and proprioception for repetitive loading with speed and agility. Excellent examples of unilateral tests/exercises are the figure-of-eight test, lateral hop test, 6-m crossover hop test, and square hop test.[83]

Bounds usually represent a series of movements whereby the athlete lands on alternating feet, but single-leg and bilateral bounding is also an option.[4,82] The focus on these drills is both horizontal distance and speed for greater repetitions.[4] In strengthening and conditioning, bounding drills are typically measured over distances greater than 30 m (≈100 feet). The clinician is strongly recommended to incorporate low- and medium-intensity bounding drills in the clinic over short distances to monitor the patient's response to this type of loading before return to sport. Many sports require the ability to bound in varying degrees, whether it is a basketball player's drive to the hoop or a soccer or football player leaping over a tackling defender.

High-intensity plyometric exercises such as depth and box jumps are sometimes referred to as shock response. Naturally, the height of the box, weight of the athlete, landing surface, and the clinician's instructions to the patient determine just how intense the exercise ultimately becomes. Box jumps can be performed unilaterally or bilaterally and, like hurdles, incorporate multiple jumping movements. Depth jumps, in contrast, are more intense box jumps in that the landing from a box is followed by an immediate jump vertically, horizontally, or to another box.[4,82] They are typically performed repetitively, in sets and repetitions just as one might design a basic strength-training program. As with any plyometric exercise, the volume of both box and depth jumps is critical to monitor and calibrate, depending on the individual's ability and the established goals of the rehabilitation program.

Generally speaking, low-intensity drills will be performed in the athletic training room or clinic. They might include jumps in place, standing jumps, low-intensity/short-distance hops, and low-height box jumps. Chu and Cordier[8] recommended that low-intensity depth jumps, known as jump or drop-downs, be performed in the athletic training room or clinic to improve eccentric strength. The patient simply steps off (does not jump) and lands on the ground without rebounding with a jump. In other words, this amounts to performing the first two phases of the SSC (i.e., preloading/eccentric and amortization), although the amortization phase is purposely too long and elastic energy is being lost as heat in the musculotendinous unit. As condition improves, the athlete progresses to completing the concentric phase (e.g., depth jumps) while attempting to decrease the amortization phase and increase the height or distance achieved by the concentric phase jump.

The listing in Box 26-8 is a sample of some low-, medium-, and high-intensity plyometric drills. More important than the exercise per se is how the intensity of an exercise is implemented (e.g., jump to a 6-inch versus an 18-inch box). The reader is encouraged to consult the referenced sources and other works for a more complete presentation of the many exercises and drills for both the upper and lower extremities.[4,8,84]

Duration

Duration describes how long an exercise session lasts. Although on the surface this would seem appropriate only for cardiovascular conditioning, it is useful for plyometric sessions as well. It is true that volume and intensity will ultimately determine the duration of a session; however, duration is an excellent indicator of the patient's conditioning level. Specifically, if the patient's plyometric sessions are taking 30 minutes instead of the 20 minutes planned, the clinician should examine the recovery times between exercises. For example, perhaps the patient needs 5 minutes of rest between drills when only 2 to 3 minutes

---

Box 26-8

Categories of Plyometric Drills by Intensity With Examples

LOW INTENSITY

Lower extremity: squat jump, jump to box, ankle bounces, lateral low hurdle/cone jumps, standing bilateral vertical leap and reach, aquatic drills

Upper extremity: medicine ball chest pass, bilateral overhead throw

MEDIUM INTENSITY

Lower extremity: split squat jumps, bilateral hurdle jumps, lateral hops, lateral box jumps, double- and single-leg pike jump, double-leg tuck jump, standing triple jump, zigzag cone hops, double-leg hop, alternate leg bounds, combination bounds, aquatic drills

Upper extremity: medicine ball push-up, standing or kneeling side throw, backward throw

HIGH INTENSITY

Lower extremity: in-depth jumps, box jumps, single-leg vertical power jump, single-leg tuck jump

Upper extremity: drop push-up, medicine ball push-up

---

was planned. This could be an indication that the current program is too intense for the patient, that the patient needs to do more cardiovascular conditioning work, or that the patient is not anaerobically fit enough to tolerate this level of training volume or intensity. If the latter is the case, perhaps this patient needs to participate in more high-volume, moderate-intensity strength training to improve oxidative-glycolytic capacity, or strength-endurance.

Traditionally, plyometric sessions are geared toward healthy athletes with adequate strength-training backgrounds and good motor skills. Thus, the sessions are intense and focus on powerful, speed-strength movements. Accordingly, sessions might last 15 to 30 minutes, but it is important to realize that for healthy athletes, plyometric training sessions are often periodized and performed with strength training sessions—plyometrics programs are often not standalone exercise sessions. For the athlete undergoing rehabilitation, this can still be a useful duration for a plyometric session. However, the duration could be lengthened to accommodate the need for lower-intensity exercise and longer recovery periods. Duration is a programming variable that is highly specific to the status of the patient and the goals established during the rehabilitation process.

Exercise Volume and Recovery

Volume

The volume of plyometric drills is a key component in that it is inherently related to the intensity and stress to which bones, articular cartilage, ligaments, muscles, and tendons are exposed. This is an especially important factor for avoidance of overuse injury in a patient who has progressed well in rehabilitation. Specifically, this patient has presumably reached all the goals for range of motion, strength, and flexibility in the athletic training room or clinic and has begun to tolerate plyometric drills at some level. Although the patient may be prepared to tolerate both

Table 26-2 Recommended Volumes and Intensity for Each Plyometric Training Session Based on Patient Status and Plyometric Experience

Patient/ Athlete	Number of Contacts	Intensity	Suggestions
Patient in an orthopedic/ sports medicine clinic	20-60	Low	Increase the number of contacts before increasing intensity; increases of 10% to 20%
Beginner	80-100	Low → medium	Primarily low, increase to medium during the midportion of the workout when not fatigued
Intermediate	100-120	Low → medium → high	Attempt high when not fatigued
Advanced	120-140	Low → medium → high	Primarily medium and high

low- and medium-intensity plyometric drills, the ability to tolerate the repetitive stress from volume may not be evident until an overuse injury, such as patellar tendinitis, has developed.

Volume in plyometrics is typically expressed as the number of foot contacts or throws of the medicine ball; the total distance jumped might also represent volume. Volume is also an expression of the amount of work performed. The analogue of volume in weight training is the product of the number of repetitions times the number of sets performed; repetitions and sets are appropriate terminology for most upper body plyometric exercises. Foot contacts are defined as the number of times that a foot, or both feet together, make contact with the surface during each workout session.

Again, it is important to consider whether the patient has regained endurance and glycolytic-oxidative capacity, in addition to musculoskeletal integrity, during the rehabilitation. The metabolic demands of plyometric training have been established in at least one study.[79] As always, the status of the patient dictates how much volume (and intensity, duration, and recovery) is appropriate. Table 26-2 provides general recommendations for volume and intensity in a plyometric training session.[4,7,8,84]

Recovery

Because plyometric drills tax the musculoskeletal system in a novel way during rehabilitation and might involve maximal effort on the part of the patient, recovery is extremely important. Recovery can include both rest between repetitions, sets, or drills within a given exercise session and the amount of rest that a patient needs between actual sessions (in days). As mentioned previously, recovery between drills during the session is an important factor in dictating the metabolic intensity of a workout.

There is a threshold of anaerobic or glycolytic endurance required for an athlete to tolerate a full plyometric training session. Generally speaking, the more intense a workout is, the more rest the athlete needs between sets, exercises, or drills during a particular training session. As the athlete gets fatigued during the session, the plyometric drills will be perceived to be more intense or difficult. Fatigue also increases the risk for injury. It is very important that recovery periods during the session be appropriate for the conditioning and skill level of the athlete, as well as for the prescribed volume/intensity of the program. One of the primary reasons for this is that plyometric drills are designed for developing functional speed-strength, not for improving overall conditioning. Moreover, as mentioned previously, type II fibers are more easily fatigued despite their force-generating capacity for plyometrics. Nonetheless, it is important to match the level of conditioning accompanying these drills to the specific metabolic demands of the sport. For example, a hurdler must be anaerobically conditioned enough to complete hurdles over a 10- to 30-second interval. A basketball player must be conditioned well enough to jump repetitively, as well as to run, cut, pivot, and leap intermittently, over the course of several minutes at a time. Depending on the height of the box, platform, or hurdle, high-intensity drills such as in-depth jumps and box jumps might require as much as 5 to 10 seconds of recovery between repetitions and 2 to 3 minutes between sets. In addition, the work-to-rest ratio should be dictated by the goals of the drill and the volume and intensity being used.[4]

As mentioned previously, muscle groups and joint complexes should not be subjected to plyometric drills on consecutive days. Two to 4 days between plyometric workouts is a general guideline, but this is mostly dictated by the intensity and status of the patient.[4,8] It is assumed that the athlete is performing strengthening and conditioning workouts on other days. An athlete may be able to perform some strength and endurance training on the same day as the plyometric workout, but use of body parts should be alternated. For example, one might perform upper body strength training on the same day that lower body plyometric exercises are performed. Alternatively, one might do a light-intensity endurance workout as part of the warm-up or cool-down on a plyometric training day.

According to Chu and Cordier, the work-to-rest ratio should be 1:5 to 1:10 to be certain that the intensity and proper execution of the movement are preserved.[8] Thus, a 10-second repetition of jumps should be followed by 50 to 100 seconds of rest before the next repetition is begun. If the set is composed of 10 repetitions, this would yield about 100 seconds of actual work for the set, and 500 to 1000 seconds of rest would need to be included in the set. Stone and Bryant, as cited by Chu and Cordier, suggested that about 1 to 5 minutes of rest is needed between plyometric exercises, depending on the intensity and volume of the workout.[8] Metabolically, high-intensity plyometrics uses the phosphagen and anaerobic energy systems, depending on the duration of a given drill. Recovery periods that are too short for adequate recovery limit athletes' ability to develop their phosphagen and anaerobic metabolic systems.

In contrast, as stated earlier, a basic level of endurance is needed to perform plyometric exercises and to perform in a given sport or activity. In the early stages of rehabilitation it is often necessary to incorporate an endurance component within the plyometric training program. In this case, the rest period needs to be shorter because the activity must also tax the aerobic or oxidative metabolic processes of the muscle. The clinician can monitor aerobic intensity via the training heart rate. It is well documented that training at 60% of the maximum heart rate is a minimum level of intensity to generate aerobic improvement.[78] In practical terms, this would indicate the need for a work-to-rest ratio of perhaps 1:1 or 1:2 to stress the oxidative and fast glycolytic energy systems.

In summary, if it has been determined that the patient is capable of tolerating maximal power exercise, longer rest periods can be implemented. To improve anaerobic power, more rest is needed. During the earlier stages of rehabilitation, it is probably more appropriate to use low- to medium-intensity plyometrics with longer intervals of recovery. Despite the fact that plyometrics has traditionally been reserved for healthy athletes attempting to maximize power and speed-strength, there is a place in the clinical setting for low-level plyometrics that stresses both the oxidative and glycolytic systems as a precursor to more aggressive plyometrics as the patient's condition improves. Indeed, low-intensity plyometrics can be focused on improving the patient's eccentric strength, coordination, and agility; promoting normal myotatic reflexes; and restoring functional ability.[8]

Muscle Fatigue, Muscle Damage, and Plyometrics

Plyometrics incorporates a significant amount of eccentric muscle activity, and unaccustomed eccentric anaerobic exercise has been associated with an immediate decrease in tension-generating capacity, a shift in the optimum muscle length, and changes in excitation-contraction coupling.[85] Eccentric resistance exercise has also been associated with increased delayed-onset muscle soreness, muscle tenderness, and weakness in healthy individuals.[43]

Exercise-induced muscle damage and injury have been studied by many investigators.[42] Kyrolainen et al investigated muscle damage after strenuous SSC exercise in power and endurance groups of athletes who performed 400 jumps and found elevated serum levels of creatine kinase, myoglobin, and carbonic anhydrase.[74] Levels of these blood proteins are often measured as an indication of skeletal muscle damage. Even in these athletic groups, the authors observed differences in physiologic responses between endurance and power athletes that they attributed to differences in muscle fiber type distribution, differences in the recruitment order of motor units, or differences in response to power-type strength exercises. Again, the importance of closely monitoring the volume, intensity, duration, and recovery time of plyometric training programs cannot be overemphasized.

Progression of Plyometric Exercise Training

Patients begin with low-intensity lower extremity drills and progress to medium- and high-intensity exercises only when they have regained enough strength, range of motion, and joint integrity and have mastered the basic plyometric movements. Chu and Cordier recommended that patients spend 12 to 18 weeks performing low- and medium-intensity plyometric drills.[8] Two-legged drills are a good starting point for lower extremity plyometrics, with progression to single-leg jumps and hops. A progression of lower extremity exercises is presented in Figures 26-1 to 26-12.

For the upper extremity, two-arm throws with a light ball are a good starting point. Cordaso et al used EMG recordings to determine muscle activity during the two-arm plyometric ball throw in 10 healthy males.[86] In the cocking phase, the upper trapezius, pectoralis major, and anterior deltoid muscles showed high activity (>40% to 60% maximum manual test), and the rotator cuff muscles had moderate activity (>20% to 40%). In the acceleration phase, five of the muscles demonstrated high levels of activity (>40% to 60%), and the upper trapezius and lower subscapularis muscles had very high levels of activity (>60%). Analysis of the deceleration phase revealed high activity in the upper trapezius muscle and moderate activity in all other muscles except the pectoralis major. The authors concluded that their findings support the use of medicine ball training as a bridge between static resistive training and dynamic throwing in the rehabilitation process. Fortun et al observed increases in both internal rotation strength and power following an 8-week plyometric program.[87] It should be acknowledged that rehabilitation specialists often use open chain plyometric exercises with a medicine ball and rebounder. Closed chain plyometric exercises are an additional option when working on shoulder stabilization exercises. Although "clap" push-ups might be a high-intensity drill, clinicians should consider bilateral upper extremity hops and jumps in place on an appropriate, padded surface.

In most cases, the athlete progresses from two-arm throws to one-arm throws. A progression of upper extremity exercises is shown in Figures 26-13 to 26-20 (see pp. 590-592).

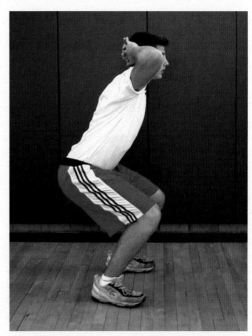

FIGURE 26-1 Squat jump (low intensity). With the feet shoulder width apart, the athlete begins by squatting down to approximately 90° of knee flexion while simultaneously maintaining lumbar lordosis and the weight equally distributed on the heels and forefeet; the hands should be behind the head with the fingers interlocked. With no arm movement, the athlete performs a maximal vertical jump and, on landing, immediately repeats the squat and jumps again. One set of 5 to 10 repetitions is performed. The amortization phase is slightly longer for this exercise to absorb the landing force until skill and strength improve.

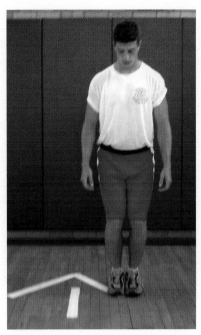

FIGURE 26-2 Ankle bounces (low intensity). With the feet 6 to 10 inches apart, the athlete jumps in the shape of a V, then laterally, and then forward/backward. Ten jumps in each direction should be performed for a total of 30 repetitions in 60 seconds; reduce the time allotted to increase agility and speed.

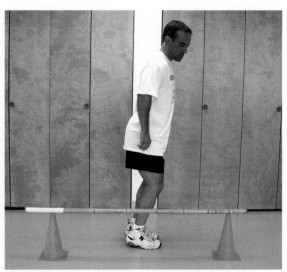

FIGURE 26-4 Lateral hurdle hops (low to medium intensity). Using a short cone or low 6- to 8-inch hurdle and keeping the feet together, the athlete jumps laterally over the hurdle as quickly as possible and repeats in the opposite direction. Most of the work should come from ankle action, but natural flexion of the knees and hips should be used to clear the hurdle. Three sets of 10 to 15 repetitions are performed.

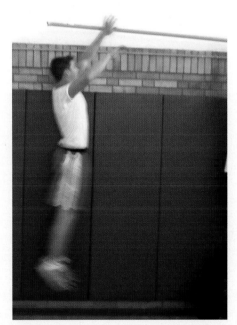

FIGURE 26-3 Standing jump and reach (low to medium intensity). Standing close to a target on the wall or near an object suspended overhead and the feet shoulder width apart, the athlete performs a half-squat using double-arm action (extension → flexion) and jumps to maximal height while reaching with one hand for the target each time. On landing, the athlete repeats the slight squat and jumps without taking any steps before jumping. The amortization time is slightly longer for beginners; progress to reducing amortization time. Three sets of 5 to 10 repetitions are performed.

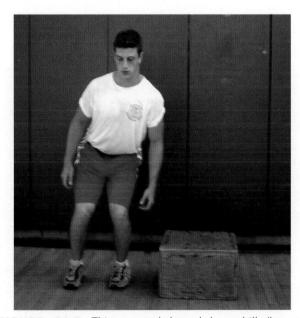

FIGURE 26-5 Thirty-second lateral box drill (low to medium intensity). Standing next to a 4- to 8-inch-high box or step with the feet shoulder width apart, the athlete jumps laterally with both feet onto the box, then off to the ground on the opposite side, and continues without stopping for 15 to 30 seconds. The ankles, knees, and hips should be used to absorb the force of landings. Progress to reducing amortization time or increasing the height of the step/box to increase intensity.

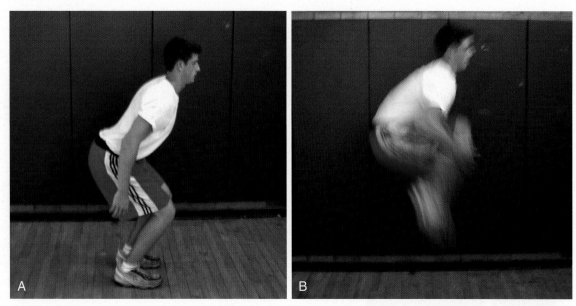

FIGURE 26-6 A and **B,** Double-leg tuck jump (medium intensity). Standing with the feet shoulder width apart, the athlete performs a half-squat with double-arm action, then immediately explodes vertically while pulling both knees to the chest and grasping the knees with both hands, and quickly releases them as descent begins. Spending minimal time on the ground, the athlete repeats the sequence. One set of 10 repetitions is performed.

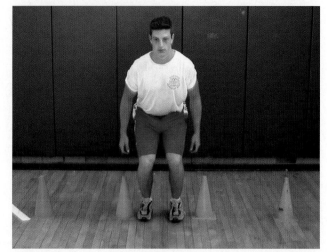

FIGURE 26-7 Lateral cone hops (medium intensity). Three to five cones or other obstacles are placed in a straight line about 3 feet apart, depending on the ability and height of the athlete. Standing with the feet shoulder width apart at the end of the row of cones, the athlete jumps laterally down the row of cones and lands on both feet. At the end of the row the athlete changes directions and returns, with minimal time spent on the ground. Three sets of 5 to 10 repetitions are performed (1 repetition = 1 lap, return to start position).

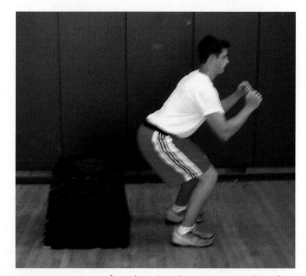

FIGURE 26-8 Jump from box (medium intensity). Standing on top of a 6- to 18-inch-high box with the feet shoulder width apart, the athlete squats slightly and jumps slightly from the box onto the floor while concentrating on absorbing the landing force and "sticking" the landing with no loss of balance or sway. A vertical jump from the box should *not* be performed; the jump direction is more horizontal than vertical. One set of 10 repetitions is performed.

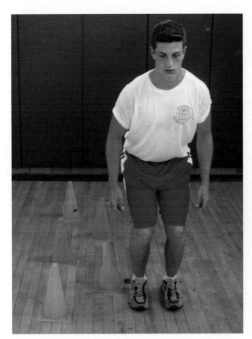

FIGURE 26-9 Double-leg zigzag cone hops (medium to high intensity). Five to 10 cones or similar obstacles are placed in a zigzag pattern about 20 to 30 inches apart. The athlete hops diagonally over each cone with minimal time spent on the ground between each cone while changing direction. The athlete should get as much vertical leap as possible and attempt to "hang" in the air to clear each cone with the shoulders maintained perpendicular to an imaginary straight line between the cones. One set of 5 to 10 repetitions is performed (1 repetition equals one trip down the row of cones).

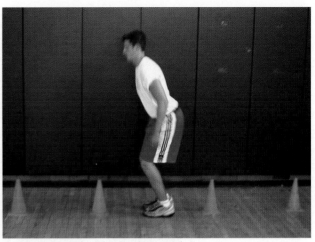

FIGURE 26-10 Hurdle jumps (medium to high intensity). Three to five hurdles are placed in a row. With the feet shoulder width apart, the athlete begins with a half-squat with double-arm action and leaps over hurdles consecutively while bringing the knees high and spending minimal time on the ground with each jump. Five to 10 repetitions are performed (1 repetition equals one trip down the row of hurdles).

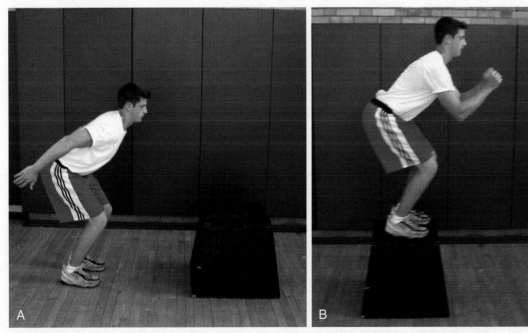

FIGURE 26-11 A and **B,** Box jumps (high intensity). Standing on the ground with the feet shoulder width apart about 2 feet in front of a box, the athlete performs a slight squat with double-arm action and jumps explosively forward and vertically onto the box. After a brief landing on the top of the box, the athlete jumps vertically and horizontally onto the ground. If multiple boxes are available, the athlete immediately jumps to the next box of equal height; if only one box is used, the athlete turns around and repeats. Two sets of 5 to 10 repetitions are performed.

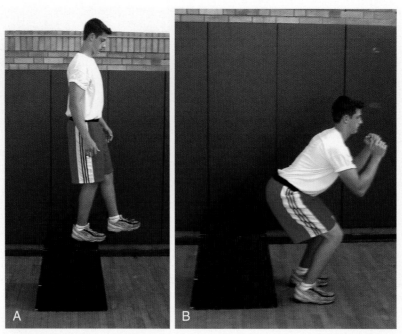

FIGURE 26-12 A and **B,** In-depth jumps (high intensity). The athlete starts by standing at the edge of the top of the box with the feet shoulder width apart, then steps (*not* jumps) off the box and lands on the balls of the feet to absorb the landing, but minimizes time on the ground and immediately jumps vertically or horizontally explosively using double-arm action. One set of 5 to 10 repetitions is performed.

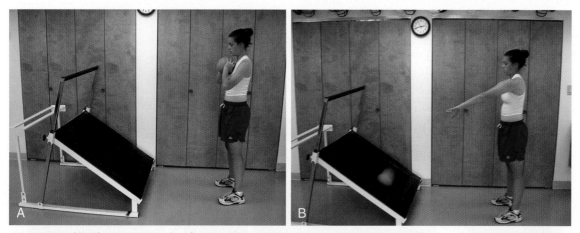

FIGURE 26-13 A and **B,** Chest pass. Standing facing a PlyoBack, the athlete uses both hands to hold a 3-lb medicine ball against the chest and pushes the ball away from the chest into the PlyoBack, with the ball allowed to return to the starting position as the athlete catches it.

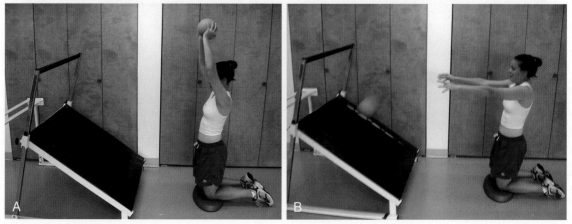

FIGURE 26-14 A and **B,** Two-hand overhead soccer throw. Standing or kneeling facing a PlyoBack, the athlete holds a 3- to 5-lb medicine ball in both hands, raises the ball overhead, and then throws it into the PlyoBack. The athlete catches the ball overhead as it rebounds.

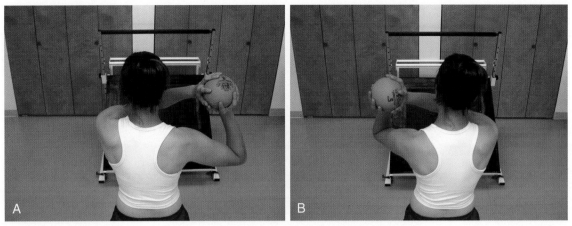

FIGURE 26-15 A and **B,** Two-handed side-to-side throw. Standing facing a PlyoBack, the athlete holds a 3- to 5-lb medicine ball with both hands positioned over one shoulder, throws the ball into the PlyoBack, then catches it with both hands over the opposite shoulder, and continues by alternating sides. This exercise can also be used to train rotation of the hips and trunk by allowing the body to rotate slightly as the ball is caught.

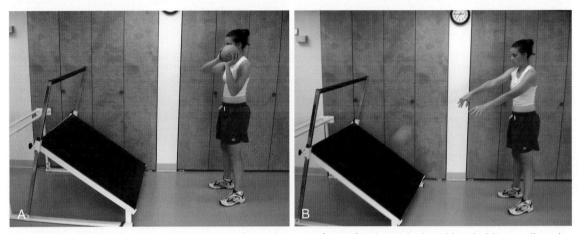

FIGURE 26-16 A and **B,** Two-handed side throw. Standing sideways in front of a PlyoBack, the athlete holds a small medicine ball in both hands, brings the ball over one shoulder, then throws it in a sidearm fashion into the PlyoBack, and catches the ball while allowing the body to turn slightly.

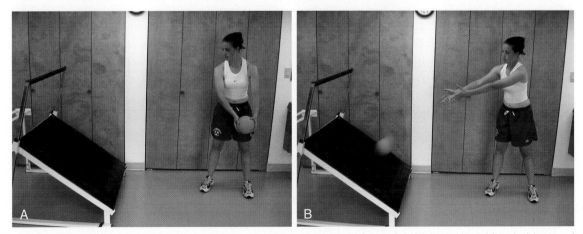

FIGURE 26-17 A and **B,** Two-handed underhand throw. Standing sideways in front of a PlyoBack, the athlete holds a medicine ball with both hands in front below waist level, brings the ball over to one side, throws it in an underhand fashion against the PlyoBack, catches the ball, and then throws it again.

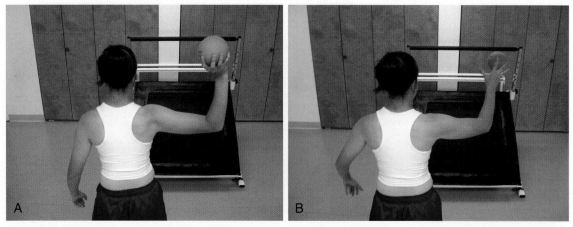

FIGURE 26-18 **A** and **B,** Baseball toss at 90/90. Standing facing a PlyoBack with the arm at a 90° angle away from the body and the elbow bent to 90° (cocking position), the athlete holds a 2-lb medicine ball, forcefully throws the ball into the PlyoBack, and then catches it as it rebounds while maintaining the same position of the arm and elbow. This exercise can also be used to train the legs and trunk to accelerate the arm by stepping out as the ball is thrown.

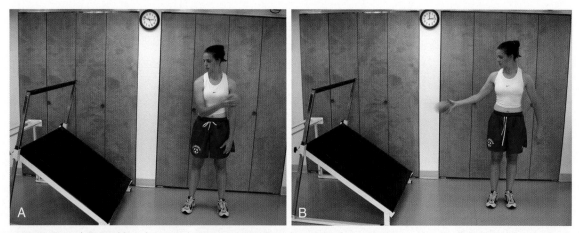

FIGURE 26-19 **A** and **B,** Backhand external rotation at 0°. Standing sideways with the involved side toward the PlyoBack, holding a 1- to 3-lb medicine ball in the involved hand, and keeping the upper part of the arm against the body with the elbow bent to 90°, the athlete rotates the arm toward the chest, forcefully rotates out, throws the ball into the PlyoBack, and tries to catch the ball as it rebounds with the palm toward the body and the upper part of the arm close to the side.

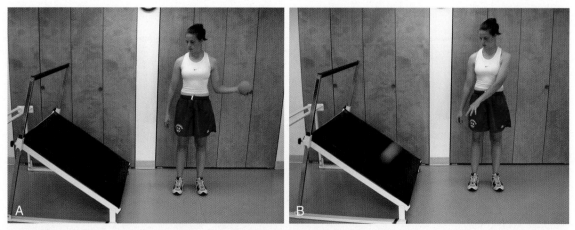

FIGURE 26-20 **A** and **B,** Backhand internal rotation at 0°. Standing sideways with the uninvolved side nearest the PlyoBack, holding a 1- to 3-lb medicine ball in the involved hand, and keeping the upper part of the arm on the involved side close to the body with the elbow bent at 90°, the athlete allows the arm to rotate out, forcefully throws the ball into the PlyoBack, and catches the ball while maintaining the upper part of the arm against the body.

CONCLUSION

Applied Anatomy/Physiology and Biomechanics of Plyometrics

- Plyometrics is based on the theory of the SSC, whereby active lengthening (eccentric contraction) of the agonist muscle produces energy that is stored in the musculotendinous unit to subsequently be used in a more powerful and efficient concentric contraction. This eccentric-concentric coupling forms the basis of the SSC.
- Three neuromuscular anatomic/physiologic areas are important in understanding the biomechanics of plyometrics: (1) the serial elastic and histologic components of muscles and tendons (i.e., sarcomeres, fiber types, sliding filaments, and metabolic properties), (2) proprioception mediated through muscle spindles and GTOs and their contribution to the stretch reflex, and (3) gross muscle-tendon complex architecture.
- The three phases of the SSC and plyometric exercise are the eccentric phase, amortization phase, and concentric phase. The eccentric phase consists of loading of the muscle spindle during the eccentric contraction and storage of elastic energy. The amortization phase is the transition from eccentric to concentric muscle activity; this phase should be as short as possible to minimize the loss of elastic energy as heat in the muscle. The explosive concentric contraction is the final phase.

Clinical Considerations for Plyometrics

- Patients must be thoroughly evaluated before they participate in a rehabilitation program with plyometrics, and goals established at the beginning of treatment should be considered. Generally, the patient must have no joint effusion or inflammation, normal range of motion, normal joint alignment and mobility, soft tissue integrity and flexibility, adequate strength both eccentrically and concentrically, normal reflexes, normal coordination, and no pain during exercise.
- Strength and conditioning are of the utmost importance for safe and effective plyometric training. Muscle performance tests via exercise, as well as functional tests of strength, should be administered before the clinician initiates plyometrics.
- Adequate warm-up and a variety of stretching exercises are warranted before plyometric training, including a full-body warm-up for 5 to 10 minutes followed by dynamic stretching and movements that mimic the drills to be performed. Controlled ballistic stretching and proprioceptive neuromuscular facilitation stretching are also useful adjuncts. Static stretching has been shown to reduce power output, so static stretching should be used as indicated by specific clinical need.

Programming and Implementation

- When a plyometric training program is initiated, a shock-absorbing surface and sturdy cross-training shoes are critical for safe performance of lower extremity drills. Equipment is generally simple and can include rubber-padded boxes or platforms, hurdles, cones, medicine balls, and physioballs.

- The frequency, intensity, volume, and duration components of exercise prescription are extremely important. By definition, plyometrics requires maximal effort, so manipulating these components for effective and safe training sessions is important to reduce the risk for overuse injury and overtraining. Volume is generally reflected as the total number of foot contacts during a given session. Intensity is mostly related to two-feet versus one-foot contacts, vertical and horizontal distances jumped, speed, height of jumps, body weight, and any added resistance applied. Frequency is simply the number of training sessions per week, and duration is the length of the workout session.
- For lower extremity plyometric exercises, two-feet contacts are generally less intense than one-foot contacts. Plyometric exercises are typically classified into low-, medium- and high-intensity categories. The individual exercises include jumps, hops, and bounds for the lower extremity. Upper extremity plyometric exercises often use a medicine ball and include weight-bearing push-up–type exercises.
- Recovery is a critical element of plyometric programming. As a general rule of thumb, plyometric workouts should be conducted only a maximum of two or three times per week. Track and field sports are traditionally more likely to use plyometric sessions more than twice per week. Major muscle groups should never be targeted in plyometric workouts on successive days. Although strength and endurance training can be performed concurrently with plyometrics in a comprehensive rehabilitation program, it is important to mix and match training sessions to prevent overuse and other injuries. For example, performing upper body strength training on the same day as lower extremity plyometrics would be a possible option.
- Overall, high-intensity plyometrics will rarely be used in athletic training rooms and clinics during rehabilitation. Rather, low- and medium-intensity drills will most likely be used. Patients in outpatient clinics will mostly be limited to low-intensity drills and roughly 20 to 60 contacts per workout to begin the program while working up to a volume of 80 to 100 contacts per workout.
- The clinician is encouraged to use creativity in customizing plyometric programming to achieve the best functional outcomes for patients.

REFERENCES

1. Adams, K., O'Shea, J.P., O'Shea, K.L., and Climstein, M. (1992): The effect of 6 weeks of squat, plyometric and squat-plyometric training on power production. J. Appl. Sport Sci. Res., 6:36–41.
2. Kraemer, W.J., and Newton, R.U. (2000): Training for muscular power. Phys. Med. Rehabil. Clin. North Am., 11:341–368.
3. Bobbert, M.F., Gerritsen, K.G., Litjens, M.C., and Van Soest, A.J. (1996): Why is countermovement jump height greater than squat jump height? Med. Sci. Sports Exerc., 28:1402–1412.
4. Potach, D.H., and Chu, D.A. (2008): Plyometric training. In Baechle, T.R., and Earle R.W., (eds.): Essentials of Strength and Conditioning, 3rd ed. Champaign, IL, Human Kinetics, pp. 414–456.
5. Saez-Saez de Villarreal, E., Elefthrerios, K., Kraemer, W.J., and Izquierdo, M. (2009): Determining variables of plyometric training for improving vertical jump height performance: A meta-analysis. J. Strength Cond. Res., 23:495–506.
6. Heiderscheit, B.C., McLean, K.P., and Davies, G.J. (1996): The effects of isokinetic vs. plyometric training on the shoulder internal rotators. J. Orthop. Sports Phys. Ther., 23:125–133.
7. Chu, D.A. (1992): Understanding plyometrics. In Chu, D.A. (ed.): Jumping into Plyometrics. Champaign, IL: Leisure Press, pp. 1–4.
8. Chu, D.A., and Cordier, D.J. (1998): Plyometrics—Specific applications in orthopedics. In: Orthopaedic Physical Therapy Home Study Course 98-A, Strength and Conditioning Applications in Orthopaedics. Orthopaedic Section, APTA, Inc., LaCrosse, WI.

9. Wilk, K.E., Voight, M.L., Keirns, M.A., et al. (1993): Stretch shortening drills for the upper extremities: Theory and clinical application. J. Orthop. Sports Phys. Ther., 17:305–317.

10. Davies, G.J., and Dickoff-Hoffman, S. (1993): Neuromuscular testing and rehabilitation of the shoulder complex. J. Orthop. Sports Phys. Ther., 18:449–458.

11. Hewett, T.E., Stroupe, A.L., Naunce, T.A., and Noyes, F.R. (1996): Plyometric training in female athletes. Decreased impact forces and increased hamstring torques. Am. J. Sports Med., 24:765–773.

12. Cavagna, G.A. (1977): Storage and utilization of elastic energy in skeletal muscle. Exerc. Sports Sci. Rev., 5:89–129.

13. Bosco, C., Tihanyi, J., Komi, P.V., et al. (1982): Store and recoil of elastic energy in slow and fast types of human skeletal muscles. Acta Physiol. Scand., 116:343–349.

14. Svantesson, U., Grimby, G., and Thomee, R. (1994): Potentiation of concentric plantar flexion torque following eccentric and isometric muscle actions. Acta Physiol. Scand., 152:287–293.

15. Helgeson, K., and Gajdosik, R. (1993): The stretch-shortening cycle of the quadriceps femoris muscle group measured by isokinetic dynamometry. J. Orthop. Sports Phys. Ther., 17:17–23.

16. Walshe, A.D., Wilson, G.J., and Ettema, G.J.C. (1998): Stretch-shorten cycle compared with isometric preload: Contributions to enhanced muscular performance. J. Appl. Physiol., 84:97–106.

17. Wilson, G.J., Murphy, A.J., and Pryor, J.F. (1994): Musculotendinous stiffness: Its relationship to eccentric, isometric, and concentric performance. J. Appl. Physiol., 76:2714–2719.

18. Brownstein, B., and Bronner, S. (1997): Functional Movement. New York: Churchill Livingstone.

19. Komi, P.V. (2000): Stretch-shortening cycle: A powerful model to study normal and fatigued muscle. J. Biomech., 33:1197–1206.

20. Kubo, K., Kanehisa, H., Takeshita, D., et al. (2000): In vivo dynamics of human medial gastrocnemius muscle-tendon complex during stretch-shortening cycle exercise. Acta Physiol. Scand., 170:127–135.

21. McCall, G.E., Byrnes, W.C., Dickinson, B.A., et al. (1996): Muscle fiber hypertrophy, hyperplasia and capillary density in college men after resistance training. J. Appl. Physiol., 81:2004–2012.

22. Narici, M.V., Roi, G.S., Landoni, L., et al. (1989): Changes in force, cross-sectional area and neural activation during strength training and detraining of the human quadriceps. Eur. J. Appl. Physiol., 59:310–319.

23. Staron, R.S., Hikida, R.S., Hagerman, F.C., et al. (1984): Human skeletal muscle fiber type adaptability to various workloads. J. Histochem. Cytochem., 32:146–152.

24. Young, P.A., and Young, P.H. (1997): Basic Clinical Neuroanatomy. Philadelphia, Williams & Wilkins.

25. Kandel, E.R., Schwartz, J.H., and Jessel, T.M. (1995): Essentials of Neural Science and Behavior. Stamford, CT: Appleton & Lange.

26. Benn, C., Forman, K., Mathewson, D., et al. (1998): The effects of serial stretch loading on stretch work and stretch-shorten cycle performance in the knee musculature. J. Orthop. Sports Phys. Ther., 27:412–422.

27. Goslow, G.E., Reinking, R.M., and Stuart, D.G. (1973): The cat step cycle: Hind limb joint angles and muscle lengths during unrestrained locomotion. J. Morphol., 141:1–42.

28. Hewett, T.E., Lindenfeld, T.N., Riccobene, J.V., and Noyes, F.R. (1999): The effect of neuromuscular training on the incidence of knee injury in female athletes. A prospective study. Am. J. Sports Med., 27:699–706.

29. Myer, G.D., Ford, K.R., McLean, S.G., and Hewett, T.E. (2006): The effects of plyometric versus dynamic stabilization and balance training on lower extremity biomechanics. Am. J. Sports Med., 34:445–455.

30. Risberg, M.A., and Holm, I. (2009): The long-term effect of 2 postoperative rehabilitation programs after anterior cruciate ligament reconstruction: A randomized controlled clinical trial with 2 years of follow-up. Am. J. Sports Med., 37:1958–1966.

31. Hewett, T.E., Ford, K.R., and Myer, G.D. (2006): Anterior cruciate ligament injuries in female athletes. Part 2, A met-analysis of neuromuscular interventions aimed at injury prevention. Am. J. Sports Med., 34:490–498.

32. Weiss, L.W., Fry, C., and Relyea, G.E. (2002): Explosive strength deficit as a predictor of vertical jumping performance. J. Strength Cond. Res., 16:83–86.

33. Huston, L.J., and Wojtys, E.M. (1996): Neuromuscular performance characteristics in elite female athletes. Am. J. Sports Med., 24:427–436.

34. Wojtys, E.M., Wylie, B.B., and Huston, L.J. (1996): The effects of muscle fatigue on neuromuscular function and anterior tibial translation in healthy knees. Am. J. Sports Med., 24:615–621.

35. Hewett, T.E., Stroupe, A.L., Nance, T.A., et al. (1996): Plyometric training in female athletes. Decreased impact forces and increased hamstring torques. Am. J. Sports Med., 24:765–773.

36. Ebben, W.P., VanderZanden, T., Wurm, B.J., and Petushek, E.J. (2010): Evaluating plyometric exercises using time to stabilization. J. Strength Cond. Res., 24:300–306.

37. Brown, C., Ross, S., Mynak, R., and Guskiewicz, K. (2004): Assessing functional ankle stability with joint position sense, time to stabilization and electromyography. J. Sport Rehabil., 13:122–134.

38. Markovic, G. (2007): Does plyometric training improve vertical jump height? A meta-analytical review. Br. J. Sports Med., 41:349–355.

39. Borkowski, J. (1990): Prevention of preseason muscle soreness: Plyometric exercise. Athl. Train., 25:122.

40. Gollhofer, A., Komi, P.V., Fujitsuka, N., et al. (1987): Fatigue during stretch-shortening cycle exercises. II. Changes in neuromuscular activation patterns of human skeletal muscle. Int. J. Sports Med., 8:38–47.

41. Nicol, C., Komi, P.V., Horita, T., et al. (1996): Reduced stretch reflex sensitivity after exhaustive stretch-shortening cycle (SSC) exercise. Eur. J. Appl. Physiol., 72:401–409.

42. Avela, J., Santos, P.M., and Komi, P.V. (1996): Effects of differently induced stretch loads on neuromuscular control in drop jump exercise. Eur. J. Appl. Physiol., 72:553–562.

43. Butterfield, T.A. (2010): Eccentric exercise in vivo: Strain-induced muscle damage and adaptation in a stable system. Exerc. Sport Sci. Rev., 38:51–60.

44. Kraemer, W.J., Ratamess, N.A., Volek, J.S., et al. (2000): The effect of the Meridian shoe on vertical jump and sprint performance following short-term combined plyometric/sprint and resistance training. J. Strength Cond. Res., 14:228–238.

45. Tofas, T., Jamurtas, A.Z., Fatouros, I.G., et al. (2008): The effects of plyometric exercise on muscle performance, muscle damage and collagen breakdown. J. Strength Cond. Res., 22:490–496.

46. Voight, M., and Tippett, S. (1994): Plyometric exercise in rehabilitation. In Prentice, W. E. (ed.): Rehabilitation Techniques in Sports Medicine, 2nd ed. St. Louis, Mosby, pp. 88–97.

47. Voight, M.L., and Draovitch, P. (1991): Plyometrics. In Albert, M. (ed.): Eccentric Muscle Training in Sports and Orthopaedics. New York, Churchill Livingstone, p. 45.

48. Byrne, P.J., Moran, K., Rankin, P., and Kinsella, S. (2010): A comparison of methods used to identify 'optimal' drop height for early phase adaptations in depth jump training. J. Strength Cond. Res., 24:2050–2055.

49. Enoka, R.M. (1996): Eccentric contractions require unique activation strategies by the nervous system. J. Appl. Physiol., 81:2339–2346.

50. Nardone, A., Romano, C., and Schieppetti, M. (1989): Selective recruitment of high-threshold human motor units during voluntary isotonic lengthening of active muscles. J. Physiol. (Lond.), 409:451–471.

51. Sale, D.G. (1988): Neural adaptation to resistance training. Med. Sci. Sports Exerc., 20:S135–S145.

52. McBride, J.M., Triplett-McBride, T., Davie, A., et al. (2002): The effect of heavy-vs. light-load jump squats on the development of strength, power and speed. J. Strength Cond. Res, 16:75–82.

53. Strojnik, V., and Komi, P.V. (2000): Fatigue after submaximal intensive stretch-shortening cycle exercise. Med. Sci. Sports Exerc., 32:1314–1319.

54. Ugarkovic, D., Matavulj, D., Kukolj, M., and Jaric, S. (2002): Standard anthropometric, body composition, and strength variables as predictors of jumping performance in elite junior athletes. J. Strength Cond. Res., 16:227–230.

55. Potdevin, F.J., Alberty, M.E., Chevutschi, A., et al. (2011): Effects of a 6-week plyometric training program on performances in pubescent swimmers. J. Strength Cond. Res., 25:80–86.

56. Rubley, M.D., Haase, A.C., Holcomb, W.R., et al. (2011): The effect of plyometric training on power and kicking distance in female adolescent soccer players. J. Strength Cond. Res., 25:129–134.

57. King, J.A., and Cipriani, D.J. (2010): Comparing preseason frontal and sagittal plane plyometric programs on vertical jump height in high school basketball players. J. Strength Cond. Res., 24:2109–2114.

58. Thomas, K., French, D., and Hayes, P.R. (2009): The effect of two plyometric training techniques on muscular power and agility in youth soccer players. J. Strength Cond. Res., 23:332–335.

59. Heinonen, A., Oja, P., Kannus, P., et al. (1995): BMD of female athletes representing sports with different loading characteristics of the skeleton. Bone, 17:197–203.

60. Lanyon, L.E. (1987): Functional strain in bone tissue as the objective and controlling stimulus for adaptive bone remodeling. J. Biomech., 20:1083–1095.

61. Grimston, S.K., Willows, N.D., and Hanley, D.A. (1993): Mechanical loading regime and its relationship to BMD in children. Med. Sci. Sports Exerc., 25:1203–1210.

62. Witzke, K.A., and Snow, C.M. (2000): Effects of plyometric jump training on bone mass in adolescent girls. Med. Sci. Sports Exerc., 32:1051–1057.

63. Aura, O., and Komi, P.V. (1986): The mechanical efficiency of locomotion in men and women with special emphasis on stretch-shortening cycle exercises. Eur. J. Appl. Physiol., 55:37–43.

64. Miyaguchi, K., and Demura, S. (2009): Gender differences in ability using the stretch-shortening cycle in the upper extremities. J. Strength Cond. Res., 23:231–236.

65. Thompson, L.V. (1994): Effects of age and training on skeletal muscle physiology and performance. Phys. Ther., 74:71–81.

66. Cuoco, A., Callahan, D.M., Sayers, S., et al. (2004): Impact of muscle power and force on gait speed in disabled older men and women. J. Gerontol. A Biol. Sci. Med. Sci., 59:1200–1206.

67. Jeffreys, I. (2008): Warm-up and stretching. In Baechle, T.R., and Earle R.W. (eds.): Essentials of Strength and Conditioning, 3rd ed. Champaign, IL, Human Kinetics, pp. 296–297.

68. Beckett, J.R., Schneiker, K.T., Wallman, K.E., et al. (2009): Effects of static stretching on repeated sprint and change of direction performance. Med. Sci. Sports Exerc., 41:444–450.

69. Thacker, S.B., Gilchrist, J., Stroup, D.F., Kinsey, C.D., Jr. (2004): The impact of stretching on sports injury risk: A systemic review of the literature. Med. Sci. Sports. Exerc., 36:371–378.

70. Taber's Cyclopedic Medical Dictionary (1993): 17th ed. Philadelphia, Davis.

71. Melvill-Jones, G., and Watt, D. (1971): Observation on control of jumping and hopping movements in man. J. Physiol., 219:709–727.

72. Avela, J., and Komi, P.V. (1998): Interaction between muscle stiffness and stretch reflex sensitivity after long-term stretch-shortening cycle exercise. Muscle Nerve, 21:1224–1227.

73. Komi, P.V., Gollhofer, A., Schmidtbleicher, D., et al. (1987): Interaction between man and shoe in running: Considerations for a more comprehensive measurement approach. Int. J. Sports Med., 8:196–202.

74. Kyrolainen, H., Takala, T.E.S., and Komi, P.V. (1998): Muscle damage induced by stretch-shortening cycle exercise. Med. Sci. Sports Exerc., 30:415–420.

75. Ball, N.B., Stock, C.G., and Scurr, J.C. (2010): Bilateral contact ground reaction forces and contact times during drop jumping. J. Strength Cond. Res., 24:2762–2769.

76. Besier, T.F., Lloyd, D.G., Cochrane, J.L., et al. (2001): External loading of the knee joint during running and cutting maneuvers. Med. Sci. Sports Exerc., 33:1168–1175.

77. McCann, M.R., and Flanagan, S.P. (2010): The effects of exercise selection and rest interval on postactivation potentiation of vertical jump performance. J. Strength Cond. Res., 24:1285–1291.

78. American College of Sports Medicine (2000): ACSM's Guidelines for Exercise Testing and Prescription, 6th ed. Philadelphia, Lippincott Williams & Wilkins. p. 141.

79. Brown, G.A., Ray, M.W., Abbey, B.M., et al. (2010): Oxygen consumption, heart rate, and blood lactate responses to an acute bout of plyometric depth jumps in college-aged men and women. J. Strength Cond. Res., 24:2475–2482.

80. Stemm, J.D., and Jacobson, B.H. (2007): Comparison of land and aquatic-based plyometric training on vertical jump performance. J. Strength Cond. Res., 21:568–571.

81. Martel, G.F., Harmer, M.L., Logan, J.M., and Parker, C.B. (2005): Aquatic plyometric training increases vertical jump in female volleyball players. Med. Sci. Sports Exerc., 37:1814–1819.

82. Allerheilegen, W.B. (1994): Speed development and plyometric training. In Baechle, T.R. (ed.): Essentials of Strength and Conditioning, 2nd ed. Champaign, IL, Human Kinetics, pp. 314–344.

83. Caffrey, E., Docherty, C.L., Schrader, J., and Klossner, J. (2009): The ability of 4 single-limb hopping tests to detect functional performance deficits in individuals with functional ankle instability. J. Orthop. Sports Phys. Ther., 39:799–806.

84. Bompa, T.O., and Haff, G.G. (2009): Periodization: Theory and Methodology of Training, 5th ed. Champaign, IL: Human Kinetics.

85. Morgan, D.L., and Allen, D.G. (1999): Early events in stretch-induced muscle damage. J. Appl. Physiol., 87:2007–2015.

86. Cordaso, F.A., Wolfe, I.N., Wooten, M.E., and Bigliani, L.U. (1996): An electromyographic analysis of the shoulder during a medicine ball rehabilitation program. Am. J. Sports Med., 34:386–392.

87. Fortun, C.M., Davies, G.J., and Kernozck, T.W. (1998): The effects of plyometric training on the shoulder internal rotators. Phys. Ther., 78(51):S87.

Index